T0075846

DiPiro's
Pharmacotherapy Handbook

Twelfth Edition

DiPiro's
Pharmacotherapy Handbook

Twelfth Edition

Terry L. Schwinghammer, PharmD, FCCP, FASHP, FAPhA
Professor Emeritus, Department of Clinical Pharmacy
School of Pharmacy
West Virginia University
Morgantown, West Virginia

Joseph T. DiPiro, PharmD, FCCP, FAAAS
Professor of Pharmacy and Associate Vice President for Health Sciences
Virginia Commonwealth University
Richmond, Virginia

Vicki L. Ellingrod, PharmD, FCCP, FACNP
Dean and John Gideon Searle Professor of Pharmacy, College of Pharmacy
Professor of Psychiatry, Medical School
Adjunct Professor of Psychology, College of Literature, Science, and the Arts
University of Michigan
Ann Arbor, Michigan

Cecily V. DiPiro, PharmD
Consultant Pharmacist
Midlothian, Virginia

New York   Chicago   San Francisco   Athens   London   Madrid   Mexico City
Milan   New Delhi   Singapore   Sydney   Toronto

1 2 3 4 5 6 7 8 9   LCR   28 27 26 25 24 23

ISBN 978-1-264-27791-9
MHID 1-264-27791-1

This book was set in Minion Pro by MPS Limited.
The editors were Michael Weitz and Peter J. Boyle.
The production supervisor was Catherine H. Saggese.
Project management was provided by Poonam Bisht, MPS Limited.

Library of Congress Control Number: 2023937871

Contents

Contents

SECTION 6: GYNECOLOGIC AND OBSTETRIC DISORDERS

Edited by Vicki L. Ellingrod

SECTION 7: HEMATOLOGIC DISORDERS

Edited by Cecily V. DiPiro

SECTION 8: INFECTIOUS DISEASES

Edited by Joseph T. DiPiro

SECTION 9: NEUROLOGIC DISORDERS

Edited by Vicki L. Ellingrod

SECTION 10: NUTRITION SUPPORT

Edited by Cecily V. DiPiro

SECTION 11: ONCOLOGIC DISORDERS

Edited by Cecily V. DiPiro

SECTION 12: OPHTHALMIC DISORDERS

Edited by Cecily V. DiPiro

SECTION 13: PSYCHIATRIC DISORDERS

Edited by Vicki L. Ellingrod

SECTION 14: RENAL DISORDERS

Edited by Cecily V. DiPiro

SECTION 15: RESPIRATORY DISORDERS

Edited by Terry L. Schwinghammer

Contents

SECTION 16: UROLOGIC DISORDERS

Edited by Cecily V. DiPiro

APPENDICES

Edited by Terry L. Schwinghammer

The 12th edition of this companion to *DiPiro's Pharmacotherapy: A Pathophysiologic Approach* is designed to provide practitioners and students with critical information to guide medication decision-making in collaborative, interprofessional healthcare settings. To ensure brevity, clarity, and portability, a bulleted format provides essential textual information along with key tables, figures, and treatment algorithms.

Corresponding to the major sections in *DiPiro's Pharmacotherapy* textbook, medical conditions are alphabetized within the following sections: Bone and Joint Disorders; Cardiovascular Disorders; Dermatologic Disorders; Endocrinologic Disorders; Gastrointestinal Disorders; Gynecologic and Obstetric Disorders; Hematologic Disorders; Infectious Diseases; Neurologic Disorders; Nutrition Support; Oncologic Disorders; Ophthalmic Disorders; Psychiatric Disorders; Renal Disorders; Respiratory Disorders; and Urologic Disorders. The *Handbook* includes nine tabular appendices involving: (1) pediatric pharmacotherapy, nutrition, and neonatal critical care; (2) geriatric assessment and pharmacotherapy; (3) critical care patient assessment and pharmacotherapy; (4) drug allergy; (5) drug-induced hematologic disorders; (6) drug-induced liver disease; (7) drug-induced pulmonary disease; (8) drug-induced kidney disease; and (9) drug-induced ophthalmic disorders. This edition also includes new chapters on coronavirus disease and multiple sclerosis.

Each chapter is organized in a consistent format:

• Disease state definition
• Pathophysiology
• Clinical presentation
• Diagnosis
• Treatment
• Evaluation of therapeutic outcomes

The Treatment section may include goals of treatment, general approach to treatment, nonpharmacologic therapy, drug selection guidelines, dosing recommendations, adverse effects, pharmacokinetic considerations, and important drug–drug interactions. For more in-depth information, the reader is encouraged to refer to the corresponding chapter in the primary textbook, *DiPiro's Pharmacotherapy: A Pathophysiologic Approach,* 12th edition. These chapters also provide guidance on application of the Pharmacists' Patient Care Process for specific conditions.

It is our hope that students and practitioners find this book to be helpful on their daily journey to provide the highest quality individualized, patient-centered care. We invite your comments on how we may improve subsequent editions of this work; you may write to pharmacotherapy@mcgraw-hill.com. Please indicate the author and title of this handbook in the subject line of your e-mail.

Terry L. Schwinghammer
Joseph T. DiPiro
Vicki L. Ellingrod
Cecily V. DiPiro

The Patient Care Process

Health professionals who provide direct patient care are often called *practitioners*. Health professionals *practice* when they use their unique knowledge and skills to serve patients. A healthcare practice is not a physical location or simply a list of activities; rather, a professional practice requires three essential elements: (1) a philosophy of practice, (2) a process of care, and (3) a practice management system.

A *practice philosophy* is the moral purpose and commonly held set of values that guides the profession. It is the critical foundation on which the practices of pharmacy, medicine, nursing, and dentistry are built. Although the concept of pharmaceutical care is not formally included in the code of ethics for the pharmacy profession or the oath of a pharmacist, pharmacists understand that they have a unique responsibility for addressing the drug-related needs of patients and should be held accountable for preventing, identifying, and resolving drug therapy problems.

The *patient care process* is a fundamental series of actions that guide the activities of health professionals. In 2014, the Joint Commission for Pharmacy Practitioners (JCPP)—representing 11 national pharmacy organizations—endorsed a framework for providing clinically oriented patient care services called the Pharmacists' Patient Care Process. This process includes five essential steps: (1) collecting subjective and objective information about the patient; (2) assessing the collected data to identify problems, determine the adequacy of current treatments, and set priorities; (3) creating an individualized care plan that is evidence-based and cost-effective; (4) implementing the care plan; and (5) monitoring the patient over time during follow-up encounters to evaluate the effectiveness of the plan and modify it as needed (Fig. 1). In addition to the five fundamental steps, a patient-centered approach to decision making is essential.

A *practice management system* is necessary to support the efficient and effective delivery of services, including physical, financial, and human resources with policies and procedures to carry out the work of patient care.

This chapter provides a brief summary of the patient care process applied to drug therapy management and the practice management issues influencing adoption and application of this process by pharmacists.

IMPORTANCE OF A STANDARD CARE PROCESS

The stimulus for developing the patient care process for pharmacy was the wide variation in pharmacists' practices as they provided direct patient care often using the same terminology to describe diverse services or, conversely, using different terminology to describe the same service. Without a consistent patient care process, it has been challenging for the pharmacy profession to communicate the pharmacist's role to external groups and establish the distinct value pharmacists bring to an interprofessional care team. Moreover, the patient must know and understand what is to be delivered to determine how best to receive the care provided. Likewise, other members of the healthcare team must determine how best to integrate the pharmacist's work into their efforts caring for the patient. A process of care must be built on a set of fundamental steps that can address the wide range of complexity that exists among patients. The process needs to be adaptable to varied settings, diverse populations, and different acuity levels.

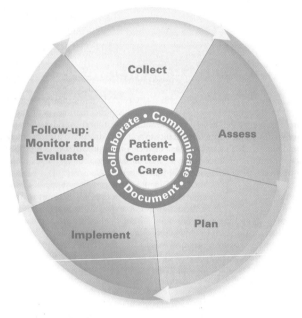

FIGURE 1. The pharmacists' patient care process. *Joint Commission of Pharmacy Practitioners. Pharmacists' Patient Care Process. May 29, 2014.* Available at: https://jcpp.net/.

THE PATIENT CARE PROCESS TO OPTIMIZE PHARMACOTHERAPY

The application or focus of a profession-specific process of care depends upon the profession's knowledge and expertise. For pharmacy, the patient care process is focused on patient's medication-related needs and experience with medication therapy. Each health profession then addresses patient's needs by assessing patient-specific information in a unique manner. For pharmacists providing comprehensive medication management (CMM), the assessment step involves a systematic examination of the *indication, effectiveness, safety,* and *adherence* for each of the patient's medications. This is a unique way of approaching a patient's health needs; no other discipline applies a systematic assessment process to medications and the medication experience in this manner.

The pharmacists' patient care process is standardized and is not specific to a care setting—it can be applied wherever CMM is performed. However, the type of information collected, its sources, and the duration of time to complete the process may vary depending on the practice setting and acuity of care. The subsequent sections in this chapter briefly describe the steps in the patient care process for pharmacists.

COLLECT PATIENT-SPECIFIC INFORMATION

Collect relevant subjective and objective information about the patient and analyze the data to understand the medical/medication history and clinical status of the patient. Information from the health record may include patient demographics, active medical problem list, admission and discharge notes, office visit notes, laboratory values, diagnostic tests, and medication lists. Conduct a comprehensive medication review with the patient that also includes alcohol, tobacco and caffeine use; immunization status; allergies; and adverse drug effects. Review social determinants of health relevant to medication use (eg, can the patient afford his/her medications, education level, housing arrangements, and means of transportation). Obtain and reconcile a complete medication list that includes all prescription and nonprescription medications as well as complementary and alternative medicine the patient is taking (ie, name, indication, strength and formulation, dose, frequency, duration, and response to medication). Review the indication, effectiveness, and safety of each medication with the patient. Gather past medication history, if pertinent. Collect information about the patient's medication experience (eg, beliefs, expectations, and cultural considerations related to medications). Ask about the patient's ability to access medications, manage medications at home, adhere to the therapy, and use medications appropriately. Gather additional important information (eg, physical assessment findings, review of systems, home-monitored blood glucose, blood pressure readings).

ASSESS INFORMATION AND FORMULATE A MEDICATION THERAPY PROBLEM LIST

Analyze the information collected to formulate a problem list consisting of the patient's active medical problems and medication therapy problems in order to prioritize medication therapy recommendations that achieve the patient's health goals. Assess the *indication* of each medication the patient is taking, including the presence of an appropriate indication; consider also whether the patient has an untreated medical condition that requires therapy. Assess the *effectiveness* of each medication, including progress toward achieving therapeutic goals; optimal selection of drug product, dose, and duration of therapy; and need for additional laboratory data to monitor medication response. Assess the *safety* of each medication by identifying adverse events; excessive doses; availability of safer alternatives; pertinent drug-disease, drug-drug, or drug-food interactions; and need for additional laboratory data to monitor medication safety. Assess *adherence* and the patient's ability to take each medication (eg, administration, access, affordability). Ensure that medication administration times are appropriate and convenient for the patient. From all of this information, formulate and prioritize a medication therapy problem list, classifying the patient's medication therapy problems based on indication, effectiveness, safety, and adherence (Table 1).

TABLE 1	Medication Therapy Problem Categories Framework
Medication-Related Needs	**Medication Therapy Problem Category**
Indication	Unnecessary medication therapy
	Needs additional medication therapy
Effectiveness	Ineffective medication
	Dosage too low
	Needs additional monitoring
Safety	Adverse medication event
	Dosage too high
	Needs additional monitoring
Adherence	Adherence
	Cost

Data from Pharmacy Quality Alliance. PQA Medication Therapy Problem Categories Framework. August 2017. Available at: https://www.pqaalliance.org/assets/Measures/PQA%20MTP%20 Categories%20Framework.pdf.

DEVELOP THE CARE PLAN

Working in collaboration with other healthcare professionals and the patient or caregiver, develop an individualized, patient-centered care plan that is evidence based and affordable for the patient. Design the plan to manage the patient's active medical conditions and resolve the identified medication therapy problems. Coordinate care with the primary care provider and other healthcare team members to reach consensus on the proposed care plan, when needed. Identify the monitoring parameters necessary to assess effectiveness, safety, and adherence, including frequency of follow-up monitoring. Design personalized education and interventions for the patient, and reconcile all medication lists (eg, from the medical record, patient, pharmacy) to arrive at an accurate and updated medication list. Determine who will implement components of the care plan (ie, patient, clinical pharmacist, other providers). Determine the appropriate time frame and mode for patient follow-up (eg, in person, by phone, electronically).

IMPLEMENT THE CARE PLAN

Implement the care plan in collaboration with other healthcare professionals and the patient or caregiver. Discuss the care plan with the patient, educate the patient about the medications and goals of therapy, make sure the patient understands and agrees with the plan, and implement recommendations that are within your scope of practice. For recommendations that cannot be independently implemented, communicate the care plan to the rest of the team, indicating where input is required by other team members. Document the encounter in the health record (eg, assessment, medication therapy care plan, rationale, monitoring, and follow-up). Arrange patient follow-up based on the determined time frame and communicate follow-up instructions with the patient.

FOLLOW-UP WITH THE PATIENT

Provide targeted follow-up and monitoring (whether in person, electronically, or via phone) to optimize the care plan and identify and resolve medication therapy problems. Modify the plan when needed in collaboration with other team members and the patient or caregiver to achieve patient and clinical goals of therapy. Plan for a CMM follow-up visit at least annually, and repeat all steps of the patient care process at that time to ensure continuity of care and ongoing medication optimization. Refer the patient back to the provider (and document accordingly) if it is determined that the patient no longer needs CMM services.

PRACTICE MANAGEMENT ISSUES

A practice management system is essential to the care process and includes the metrics to ensure patient health outcomes are being achieved; efficient workflow; communication and documentation using the power of information technology (IT); and data that accurately reflect the attribution and value the practitioner brings to patient care.

QUALITY METRICS

The patient care process sets a standard of achievable performance by defining the parameters of the process that can be measured. With the movement toward outcome-based healthcare models and value-based payment systems, it is critical to objectively measure the impact a patient care service has on a patient's health and well-being. For the process to be measurable, each element must be clearly defined and performed in a similar manner during each patient encounter. The lack of clarity and consistency has hindered collection of robust evidence to support the value of pharmacists' patient care services. The standard patient care process gives pharmacists an opportunity to show value on a large scale because the services are comparable and clearly understood across practice settings.

WORKFLOW, DOCUMENTATION, AND INFORMATION SYSTEMS

Healthcare systems are rapidly embracing the power of technology to analyze information and gain important insights about the health outcomes being achieved. The uniform patient care process sets a standard for the practice workflow that allows IT systems to capture and extract data for analysis and sharing. The ability to capture clinical data is currently available through a number of coding systems, such as the International Classification of Diseases 10th edition (ICD-10) and the Systematized Nomenclature of Medicine—Clinical Terms (SNOMED-CT). Practitioners need to understand how coding systems operate behind the scenes when performing and documenting their clinical activities. This will enable practitioners to assist information technologists to effectively design systems to accurately document the elements of the process that can produce the data on medication-related outcomes.

DOCUMENTATION, ATTRIBUTION, AND PAYMENT

Payment to healthcare providers for patient care services in the United States has traditionally been based on the documentation and reporting of standard processes of care. Rules and guidance from Medicare and the Centers for Medicare and Medicaid Services (CMS) are considered the billing and payment standard for healthcare providers both for governmental and commercial payers. Reporting the complexity of care provided is built on top of the documentation requirements; complexity is determined by the number of required elements in each documentation domain. A billing code is then assigned to the patient encounter that equates to a payment commensurate with the level of care provided. This process is the basis for the current fee-for-service payment structure, and it is likely that this general format will remain in any future payment model. The traditional SOAP (Subjective, Objective, Assessment, Plan) note format is often used by pharmacists when documenting patient care and is particularly appropriate when providing services incident to an eligible Medicare Part B provider. However, some elements of the SOAP note that are required when using certain billing codes are not routinely performed by pharmacists (eg, comprehensive physical examination). The pharmacists' patient care process establishes a standard framework that reflects the pharmacist's work. Using a standard care process accompanied with a standard documentation framework will result in efficiencies of practice, enable appropriate and accurate billing, and facilitate the attribution of care to desired patient outcomes needed in value-based payment models.

See Chapter 1, The Patient Care Process, authored by Stuart T. Haines, Mary Ann Kliethermes, and Todd D. Sorensen for a more detailed discussion of this topic.

CHAPTER 1

Gout and Hyperuricemia

- *Gout* involves an inflammatory response to precipitation of monosodium urate (MSU) crystals in both articular and nonarticular tissues.

ACUTE GOUTY ARTHRITIS

PATHOPHYSIOLOGY

- The underlying metabolic disorder is elevated serum uric acid (hyperuricemia), which is defined as a serum that is supersaturated with monosodium urate and begins to exceed the limit of solubility (>6.8 mg/dL [404 μmol/L]).
- Uric acid is the end product of purine degradation. An increased urate pool in individuals with gout may result from overproduction or underexcretion.
- Purines originate from dietary purine, conversion of tissue nucleic acid to purine nucleotides, and de novo synthesis of purine bases.
- Overproduction of uric acid may result from abnormalities in enzyme systems that regulate purine metabolism (eg, increased activity of phosphoribosyl pyrophosphate [PRPP] synthetase or deficiency of hypoxanthine-guanine phosphoribosyl transferase [HGPRT]).
- Uric acid may also be overproduced because of increased breakdown of tissue nucleic acids, as with myeloproliferative and lymphoproliferative disorders. Cytotoxic drugs can result in overproduction of uric acid due to lysis and the breakdown of cellular matter.
- Dietary purines are insignificant in generating hyperuricemia without some derangement in purine metabolism or elimination.
- Two-thirds of uric acid produced daily is excreted in urine. The remainder is eliminated through gastrointestinal (GI) tract after degradation by colonic bacteria. Decline in urinary excretion to a concentration below the rate of production leads to hyperuricemia and an increased pool of sodium urate.
- Drugs that decrease renal uric acid clearance include diuretics, nicotinic acid, salicylates (<2 g/day), ethanol, pyrazinamide, levodopa, ethambutol, cyclosporine, and cytotoxic drugs.
- Deposition of urate crystals in synovial fluid results in inflammation, vasodilation, increased vascular permeability, complement activation, and chemotactic activity for polymorphonuclear leukocytes. Phagocytosis of urate crystals by leukocytes results in rapid lysis of cells and discharge of proteolytic enzymes into cytoplasm. The ensuing inflammatory reaction causes intense joint pain, erythema, warmth, and swelling.
- Uric acid nephrolithiasis occurs in ~10% of patients with gout. Predisposing factors include excessive urinary excretion of uric acid, acidic urine (pH <6), and highly concentrated urine.
- In acute uric acid nephropathy, acute kidney injury occurs because of blockage of urine flow from massive precipitation of uric acid crystals in collecting ducts and ureters. Chronic urate nephropathy is caused by long-term deposition of urate crystals in the renal parenchyma.
- Tophi (urate deposits) are uncommon and are a late complication of hyperuricemia. The most common sites are the base of the fingers, olecranon bursae, ulnar aspect of forearm, Achilles tendon, knees, wrists, and hands.

CLINICAL PRESENTATION

- Acute gout attacks are characterized by rapid onset of excruciating pain, swelling, and inflammation. The attack is typically monoarticular, most often affecting the first metatarsophalangeal joint (podagra), and then, in order of frequency, the insteps, ankles, heels, knees, wrists, fingers, and elbows. Attacks commonly begin at night, with the patient awakening with excruciating pain. Affected joints are erythematous, warm, and swollen. Fever and leukocytosis are common. Untreated attacks last from 3 to 14 days before spontaneous recovery.
- Acute attacks may occur without provocation or be precipitated by stress, trauma, alcohol ingestion, infection, surgery, rapid lowering of serum uric acid by uric acid-lowering agents, and ingestion of drugs known to elevate serum uric acid concentrations.

DIAGNOSIS

- Definitive diagnosis requires aspiration of synovial fluid from the affected joint and identification of intracellular crystals of MSU monohydrate in synovial fluid leukocytes.
- When joint aspiration is not feasible, a presumptive diagnosis is based on presence of characteristic signs and symptoms as well as the response to treatment.

TREATMENT

- <u>Goals of Treatment</u>: Terminate the acute attack, prevent recurrent attacks, and prevent complications associated with chronic deposition of urate crystals in tissues.

NONPHARMACOLOGIC THERAPY

- Local ice application is the most effective adjunctive treatment.
- Dietary supplements (eg, flaxseed, cherry, celery root) are not recommended.

PHARMACOLOGIC THERAPY (FIG. 1-1)

- Most patients are treated successfully with nonsteroidal anti-inflammatory drugs (NSAIDs), corticosteroids, or colchicine. Treatment should begin as soon as possible after the onset of an attack.

NSAIDS

- NSAIDs have excellent efficacy and minimal toxicity with short-term use. Indomethacin, naproxen, and sulindac have Food and Drug Administration (FDA) approval for gout, but others are likely to be effective (Table 1-1).
- Start therapy within 24 hours of attack onset and continue until complete resolution (usually 5–8 days). Tapering may be considered after resolution, especially if comorbidities such as impaired hepatic or kidney function make prolonged therapy undesirable.
- The most common adverse effects involve the GI tract (gastritis, bleeding, and perforation), kidneys (renal papillary necrosis, reduced glomerular filtration rate), cardiovascular system (increased blood pressure, sodium and fluid retention), and central nervous system (impaired cognitive function, headache, and dizziness).
- Selective cyclooxygenase-2 inhibitors (eg, celecoxib) may be an option for patients unable to take nonselective NSAIDs, but cardiovascular risk must be considered.

Corticosteroids

- Corticosteroid efficacy is equivalent to NSAIDs; they can be used systemically or by intra-articular (IA) injection. With systemic therapy, a hypothetical risk exists for a rebound attack upon steroid withdrawal; therefore, gradual tapering is often employed.

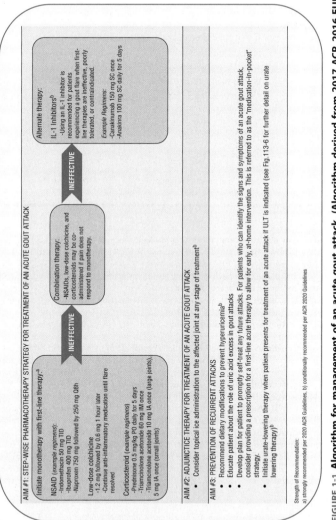

AIM #1: STEP-WISE PHARMACOTHERAPY STRATEGY FOR TREATMENT OF AN ACUTE GOUT ATTACK

Initiate monotherapy with first-line therapy[-a]

NSAID (*example regimens*):
-Indomethacin 50 mg TID
-Ibuprofen 400 mg TID
-Naproxen 750 mg followed by 250 mg Q8h

Low-dose colchicine
-1.2 mg followed by 0.6 mg 1 hour later
-Continue anti-inflammatory medication until flare resolved

Corticosteroid (*example regimens*)
-Prednisone 0.5 mg/kg PO daily for 5 days
-Triamcinolone acetonide 60 mg IM once
-Triamcinolone acetonide 10 mg IA once (large joints), 5 mg IA once (small joints)

INEFFECTIVE

Combination therapy:
-NSAIDs, low-dose colchicine, and corticosteroids may be co-administered if pain does not respond to monotherapy.

INEFFECTIVE

Alternate therapy:

IL-1 inhibitors[b]
-Using an IL-1 inhibitor is recommended for patients experiencing a gout flare when first-line therapies are ineffective, poorly tolerated, or contraindicated.

Example Regimens:
-Canakinumab 150 mg SC once
-Anakinra 100 mg SC daily for 5 days

AIM #2: ADJUNCTICE THERAPY FOR TREATMENT OF AN ACUTE GOUT ATTACK
- Consider topical ice administration to the affected joint at any stage of treatment[b]

AIM #3: PREVENTION OF RECURRENT ATTACKS
- Recommend dietary modifications to prevent hyperuricemia[b]
- Educate patient about the role of uric acid excess in gout attacks
- Develop plan for patient to promptly self-treat any future attacks. For patients who can identify the signs and symptoms of an acute gout attack, consider providing a prescription for a first-line acute therapy to allow for early, at-home intervention. This is referred to as the "medication-in-pocket" strategy.
- Initiate urate-lowering therapy when patient presents for treatment of an acute attack if ULT is indicated (see Fig.113-6 for further detail on urate lowering therapy)[b]

Strength of Recommendation:
a) strongly recommended per 2020 ACR Guidelines, b) conditionally recommended per ACR 2020 Guidelines

FIGURE 1-1 Algorithm for management of an acute gout attack. (Algorithm derived from 2017 ACP, 2016 EULAR, and 2012 ACR gout guidelines.)

TABLE 1-1	Dosage Regimens of Oral Nonsteroidal Anti-inflammatory Drugs for Treatment of Acute Gout	
Generic Name	**Initial Dose**	**Usual Range**
Etodolac	300 mg twice daily	300–500 mg twice daily
Fenoprofen	400 mg three times daily	400–600 mg three to four times daily
Ibuprofen	400 mg three times daily	400–800 mg three to four times daily
Indomethacin	50 mg three times daily	50 mg three times daily initially until pain is tolerable then rapidly reduce to complete cessation
Ketoprofen	75 mg three times daily or 50 mg four times daily	50–75 mg three to four times daily
Naproxen	750 mg followed by 250 mg every 8 hours until the attack has subsided	—
Piroxicam	20 mg once daily or 10 mg twice daily	—
Sulindac	200 mg twice daily	150–200 mg twice daily for 7–10 days
Meloxicam	5 mg once daily	7.5–15 mg once daily
Celecoxib	800 mg followed by 400 mg on day one, then 400 mg twice daily for 1 week	—

- **Prednisone** or **prednisolone** oral dosing strategies include (1) 0.5 mg/kg daily for 5–10 days followed by abrupt discontinuation, or (2) 0.5 mg/kg daily for 2–5 days followed by tapering for 7–10 days.
- **Methylprednisolone dose pack** is a 6-day regimen starting with 24 mg on day 1 and decreasing by 4 mg each day that may be considered.
- **Triamcinolone acetonide** 20–40 mg given by IA injection may be used if gout is limited to one or two joints; give 10–40 mg IA (large joints) or 5–20 mg IA (small joints). IA corticosteroids should be used with an oral NSAID, colchicine, or corticosteroid therapy.
- **Methylprednisolone** (a long-acting corticosteroid) given by a single intramuscular (IM) injection followed by a short course of oral corticosteroid therapy is another reasonable approach. Alternatively, IM corticosteroid monotherapy may be considered in patients with multiple affected joints who cannot take oral therapy.
- Short-term corticosteroid use is generally well tolerated. Use with caution in patients with diabetes, GI problems, bleeding disorders, cardiovascular disease, and psychiatric disorders. Avoid long-term use because of risk for osteoporosis, hypothalamic–pituitary–adrenal axis suppression, cataracts, and muscle deconditioning.
- **Adrenocorticotropic hormone (ACTH) gel:** 25–40 USP units subcutaneously and repeated as clinically indicated has been recommended in the past. Efficacy may be similar to systemic steroids, but other first-line agents are preferred over ACTH due to cost considerations.

Colchicine

- **Colchicine** is highly effective in relieving acute gout attacks; when it is started within the first 24 hours of onset, about two-thirds of patients respond within hours.
- Colchicine causes dose-dependent GI adverse effects (nausea, vomiting, and diarrhea). Non-GI effects include neutropenia and axonal neuromyopathy, which may be worsened in patients taking other myopathic drugs (eg, statins) or with impaired kidney function. Use colchicine with caution in patients taking P-glycoprotein or

strong CYP450 3A4 inhibitors (eg, clarithromycin) due to increased plasma colchicine levels and potential toxicity; colchicine dose reductions may be required. Also, use colchicine with caution in patients with impaired kidney or hepatic function.

- **Colcrys** is an FDA-approved colchicine product available in 0.6-mg oral tablets. The recommended dose is 1.2 mg (two tablets) initially, followed by 0.6 mg (one tablet) 1 hour later. Although not an FDA-approved regimen, the American College of Rheumatology (ACR) gout treatment guidelines suggest that colchicine 0.6 mg once or twice daily can be started 12 hours after the initial 1.2-mg dose and continued until the attack resolves. Colchicine is also available generically.

HYPERURICEMIA IN GOUT

- Recurrent gout attacks can be prevented by maintaining low uric acid levels, but nonadherence with nonpharmacologic and pharmacologic therapies is common.

NONPHARMACOLOGIC THERAPY

- Patient education should address the recurrent nature of gout and the objective of each lifestyle/dietary modification and medication.
- Promote weight loss through caloric restriction and exercise in all patients to enhance renal urate excretion.
- Alcohol restriction is important because increased consumption has been associated with an increased risk of gout attacks.
- Dietary recommendations include limiting consumption of high-fructose corn syrup and purine-rich foods (organ meats and some seafood), which have been linked to uric acid elevation. The DASH diet (Dietary Approaches to Stop Hypertension) may lower serum uric acid by ~1.0 mg/dL in hyperuricemic patients who are adherent.
- Evaluate the medication list for potentially unnecessary drugs that may elevate uric acid levels. When clinically appropriate, medications that increase serum uric acid (eg, hydrochlorothiazide) may be switched to equally effective medications without this effect. Low-dose aspirin for cardiovascular prevention should be continued despite its uric acid-elevating properties.

PHARMACOLOGIC THERAPY (FIG. 1-2)

- After the first attack of acute gout, prophylactic pharmacotherapy is recommended if patients have two or more attacks per year, even if serum uric acid is normal or only minimally elevated. Other indications include presence of tophi and radiographic evidence of damage attributable to gout.
- Urate-lowering therapy can be started during an acute attack if anti-inflammatory prophylaxis has been initiated.
- Apply a stepwise approach to hyperuricemia (Fig. 1-2). Xanthine oxidase inhibitors are recommended first-line therapy, with uricosurics reserved for patients with a contraindication or intolerance to xanthine oxidase inhibitors. In refractory cases, combination therapy with a xanthine oxidase inhibitor plus a drug with uricosuric properties (probenecid, losartan, or fenofibrate) is suggested. Pegloticase may be used in severe cases in which the patient cannot tolerate or is not responding to other therapies.
- The ACR guideline goal of urate-lowering therapy is to achieve and maintain serum uric acid <6 mg/dL (357 μmol/L). Urate lowering should be prescribed for long-term use.

Xanthine Oxidase Inhibitors

- Xanthine oxidase inhibitors reduce uric acid by impairing conversion of hypoxanthine to xanthine and xanthine to uric acid. Because they are effective in both overproducers and underexcretors of uric acid, they are the most widely prescribed agents for long-term prevention of recurrent gout attacks.
- **Allopurinol** lowers uric acid levels in a dose-dependent manner. ACR guidelines recommend a starting dose no greater than 100 mg daily in patients with normal

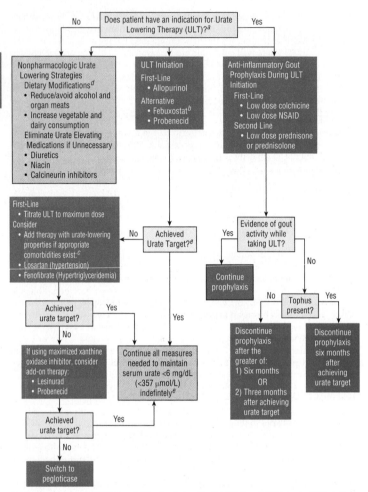

a) Indications for urate-lowering therapy include: 1) presence of tophus 2) ≥ 2 gout attacks per year 3) kidney disease 4) past urolithiasis. EULAR, but not ACR or ACP Guidelines, also recognize the following indications for ULT: 1) first diagnosis of gout at age < 40 years 2) uric acid > 8.0 mg/dL 3) high-risk comorbidities (hypertension, ischemic heart disease, hear failure)

b) Recognized as first line by ACR Guidelines but cardiovascular safety concerns have been reported since guideline publication

c) EULAR Guidelines also recognize calcium channel blockers and statins as add-on therapy for uric acid lowering when indicated for treatment of comorbidities

d) The effectiveness of dietary intervention in improving clinical outcomes is noted as an area of inconclusive evidence by 2017 ACP guidelines

e) Targeting and maintaining a specific urate level is noted as an area of inconclusive evidence by 2017 ACP guidelines

NSAID, nonsteroidal anti-inflammatory drug; ULT, urate-lowering therapy; XOI, xanthine oxidase inhibitor. (Algorithm derived from 2017 ACP, 2016 EULAR, and 2012 ACR gout guidelines.)

FIGURE 1-2 Algorithm for management of hyperuricemia in gout.

kidney function and no more than 50 mg/day in patients with chronic kidney disease (stage 4 or worse) to avoid allopurinol hypersensitivity syndrome and prevent acute gout attacks common during initiation of urate-lowering therapy. The dose should be titrated gradually based on serial serum uric acid measurements up to a maximum of 800 mg/day until the serum urate target is achieved.

- Mild adverse effects of allopurinol include skin rash, leukopenia, GI problems, headache, and urticaria. A more severe adverse reaction known as allopurinol hypersensitivity syndrome, which includes severe rash (toxic epidermal necrolysis, erythema multiforme, or exfoliative dermatitis), hepatitis, interstitial nephritis, and eosinophilia, occurs rarely but is associated with a 20%–25% mortality rate.

- **Febuxostat** (Uloric) also lowers serum uric acid in a dose-dependent manner. The recommended starting dose is 40 mg once daily, titrating to the maximum FDA-approved dose of 80 mg daily. Adverse events include nausea, arthralgias, and minor hepatic transaminase elevations. Clinical trial evidence demonstrated an increase in all-cause and cardiovascular mortality compared to allopurinol, resulting in a warning in the FDA-approved labeling that febuxostat should be reserved for patients unable to take allopurinol. Due to rapid mobilization of urate deposits during initiation, give concomitant therapy with colchicine or an NSAID for at least the first 8 weeks of therapy to prevent acute gout flares.

Uricosurics

- Uricosuric drugs increase renal clearance of uric acid by inhibiting the postsecretory renal proximal tubular reabsorption of uric acid. Patients with a history of urolithiasis should not receive uricosurics. Start uricosuric therapy at a low dose to avoid marked uricosuria and possible stone formation. Maintaining adequate urine flow and urine alkalinization during the first several days of therapy may also decrease the likelihood of uric acid stone formation. Uricosuric treatment is not generally recommended in patients with moderate to severe CKD.

- **Probenecid:** The initial dose is 250 mg twice daily for 1–2 weeks, then 500 mg twice daily for 2 weeks. Increase the daily dose thereafter by 500-mg increments every 1–2 weeks until satisfactory control is achieved or a maximum dose of 2 g/day is reached. Major side effects include GI irritation, rash and hypersensitivity, precipitation of acute gouty arthritis, and urolithiasis. Maintaining adequate fluid intake is important to reduce the risk of uric acid stone formation.

- **Lesinurad** (Zurampic) inhibits urate transporter 1 in proximal renal tubules, thereby increasing uric acid excretion. It is approved as combination therapy with a xanthine oxidase inhibitor for treatment of hyperuricemia associated with gout in patients who have not achieved target serum uric acid concentrations with xanthine oxidase inhibitor monotherapy. The approved lesinurad dose is 200 mg once daily in the morning with food and water in combination with a xanthine oxidase inhibitor. Adverse effects include urticaria and elevated levels of serum creatinine, lipase, and creatine kinase. It carries a black box warning highlighting an increased risk of acute renal failure when used in the absence of xanthine oxidase inhibitor therapy. Lesinurad retains FDA approval in the United States but is not currently being marketed.

Pegloticase

- **Pegloticase** (Krystexxa) is a pegylated recombinant uricase that reduces serum uric acid by converting uric acid to allantoin, which is water soluble. Pegloticase is indicated for antihyperuricemic therapy in adults refractory to conventional therapy.

- The dose is 8 mg by IV infusion over at least 2 hours every 2 weeks. Because of potential infusion-related allergic reactions, patients must be pretreated with antihistamines and corticosteroids. Pegloticase is substantially more expensive than first-line urate-lowering therapies.

- The ideal duration of pegloticase therapy is unknown. Patients may develop pegloticase antibodies that result in loss of efficacy after several months.

- Because of its limitations, reserve pegloticase for patients with refractory gout who are unable to take or have failed all other urate-lowering therapies.

Miscellaneous Urate-Lowering Agents

- **Fenofibrate** increases clearance of hypoxanthine and xanthine, leading to a sustained reduction in serum urate concentrations of 20%–30%. However, ACR guidelines recommend against changing cholesterol-lowering agents to fenofibrate because it is not a preferred therapy in current lipid guidelines.
- **Losartan** inhibits renal tubular reabsorption of uric acid and increases urinary excretion, properties that are not shared with other angiotensin II receptor blockers. It also alkalinizes the urine, which helps reduce the risk of stone formation. ACR guidelines recommend choosing losartan preferentially as antihypertensive therapy in patients with gout when feasible.

ANTI-INFLAMMATORY PROPHYLAXIS DURING INITIATION OF URATE-LOWERING THERAPY

- Initiation of urate-lowering therapy can precipitate an acute gout attack due to remodeling of urate crystal deposits in joints after rapid lowering of urate concentrations. Prophylactic anti-inflammatory therapy is recommended to prevent such gout attacks.
- The ACR guidelines strongly recommend low-dose oral colchicine (0.6 mg twice daily), low-dose NSAIDs (eg, naproxen 250 mg twice daily), or prednisone 10 mg daily during the first 3 to 6 months of urate-lowering therapy initiation, and longer as needed if gout flares persist. For patients on long-term NSAID prophylaxis, a proton pump inhibitor or other acid-suppressing therapy is indicated to protect from NSAID-induced gastric problems.

EVALUATION OF THERAPEUTIC OUTCOMES

- Check the serum uric acid level in patients suspected of having an acute gout attack, particularly if it is not the first attack, and a decision is to be made about starting prophylaxis. However, acute gout can occur with normal serum uric acid concentrations.
- Monitor patients with acute gout for symptomatic relief of joint pain as well as potential adverse effects and drug interactions related to drug therapy. Acute pain of an initial gout attack should begin to ease within about 8 hours of treatment initiation. Complete resolution of pain, erythema, and inflammation usually occurs within 48–72 hours.
- For patients receiving urate-lowering therapy, obtain baseline assessment of kidney function, hepatic enzymes, complete blood count, and electrolytes. Recheck the tests every 6–12 months in patients receiving long-term treatment.
- During titration of urate-lowering therapy, serial serum uric acid measurements should be obtained; after the urate target is achieved, monitor serum uric acid periodically (every 6–12 months).
- Because of the high rates of comorbidities associated with gout (diabetes, chronic kidney disease, hypertension, obesity, coronary heart disease, heart failure, and stroke), elevated serum uric acid concentrations or gout should prompt evaluation for these related comorbidities and implementation of appropriate risk reduction measures. Clinicians should also look for possible correctable causes of hyperuricemia (eg, medications, obesity, malignancy, and alcohol abuse).

See Chapter 113, Gout and Hyperuricemia, authored by Michelle A. Fravel and Michael E. Ernst, for a more detailed discussion of this topic.

CHAPTER 2

Osteoarthritis

- *Osteoarthritis* (OA) is a common, progressive disorder affecting primarily weight-bearing diarthrodial joints, characterized by progressive destruction of articular cartilage, osteophyte formation, pain, limitation of motion, deformity, and disability.

PATHOPHYSIOLOGY

- *Primary* (*idiopathic*) *OA*, the more common type, has no known cause.
- *Secondary OA* is associated with a known cause such as inflammation, trauma, metabolic or endocrine disorders, and congenital factors.
- OA usually begins with damage to articular cartilage through injury, excessive joint loading from obesity or other reasons, or joint instability. Damage to cartilage increases activity of chondrocytes in attempt to repair damage, leading to increased synthesis of matrix constituents with cartilage swelling. Normal balance between cartilage breakdown and resynthesis is lost, with increasing destruction and cartilage loss.
- Subchondral bone adjacent to articular cartilage undergoes pathologic changes and releases vasoactive peptides and matrix metalloproteinases. Neovascularization and increased permeability of adjacent cartilage occur, which contribute to cartilage loss and chondrocyte apoptosis.
- Cartilage loss causes joint space narrowing and painful, deformed joints. The remaining cartilage softens and develops fibrillations, followed by further cartilage loss and exposure of underlying bone. New bone formations (osteophytes) at joint margins distant from cartilage destruction are thought to help stabilize affected joints.
- Inflammatory changes can occur in the joint capsule and synovium. Crystals or cartilage shards in synovial fluid may contribute to inflammation. Interleukin-1, prostaglandin E_2, tumor necrosis factor-α, and nitric oxide in synovial fluid may also play a role. Inflammatory changes result in synovial effusions and thickening.
- Pain may result from distention of the synovial capsule by increased joint fluid; microfracture; periosteal irritation; or damage to ligaments, synovium, or the meniscus.

CLINICAL PRESENTATION

- Risk factors include increasing age, obesity, sex, certain occupations and sports activities, history of joint injury or surgery, and genetic predisposition.
- The predominant symptom is deep, aching pain in affected joints. Pain accompanies joint activity and decreases with rest.
- Joints most commonly affected are the distal interphalangeal (DIP) and proximal interphalangeal (PIP) joints of the hand, first carpometacarpal joint, knees, hips, cervical and lumbar spine, and first metatarsophalangeal (MTP) joint of the toe.
- Limitation of motion, stiffness, crepitus, and deformities may occur. Patients with lower extremity involvement may report weakness or instability.
- Upon arising, joint stiffness typically lasts less than 30 minutes and resolves with motion.
- Presence of warm, red, and tender joints suggests inflammatory synovitis.
- Physical examination of affected joints reveals tenderness, crepitus, and possibly enlargement. Heberden and Bouchard nodes are bony enlargements (osteophytes) of the DIP and PIP joints, respectively.

DIAGNOSIS

- Diagnosis is made through patient history, physician examination, radiologic findings, and laboratory testing.
- American College of Rheumatology criteria for classification of OA of the hips, knees, and hands include presence of pain, bony changes on examination, normal erythrocyte sedimentation rate (ESR), and radiographs showing osteophytes or joint space narrowing.
- For hip OA, patients must have hip pain and two of the following: (1) ESR <20 mm/h (5.6 µm/sec), (2) radiographic femoral or acetabular osteophytes, and/or (3) radiographic joint space narrowing.
- For knee OA, patients must have knee pain and radiographic osteophytes in addition to one or more of the following: (1) age >50 years, (2) morning stiffness lasting ≤30 minutes, (3) crepitus on motion, (4) bony enlargement, (5) bony tenderness, and/or (6) palpable joint warmth.
- ESR may be slightly elevated if inflammation is present. Rheumatoid factor is negative. Analysis of synovial fluid reveals high viscosity and mild leukocytosis (<2000 white blood cells/mm^3 [2 × 10^9/L]) with predominantly mononuclear cells.

TREATMENT

- Goals of Treatment: (1) Educate the patient, family members, and caregivers; (2) relieve pain and stiffness; (3) maintain or improve joint mobility; (4) limit functional impairment; and (5) maintain or improve quality of life.

NONPHARMACOLOGIC THERAPY

- Educate the patient about the disease process and extent, prognosis, and treatment options. Promote dietary counseling, exercise, and a weight loss program for overweight patients.
- Physical therapy—with heat or cold treatments and an exercise program—helps maintain range of motion and reduce pain and need for analgesics.
- Assistive and orthotic devices (canes, walkers, braces, heel cups, and insoles) can be used during exercise or daily activities.
- Surgical procedures (eg, osteotomy, arthroplasty, joint fusion) are indicated for functional disability and/or severe pain unresponsive to conservative therapy.

PHARMACOLOGIC THERAPY (TABLE 2-1)

General Approach

- Drug therapy is targeted at relief of pain. A conservative approach is warranted because OA often occurs in older individuals with other medical conditions.
- Apply an individualized approach (Figs. 2-1 and 2-2). Continue appropriate nondrug therapies when initiating drug therapy.

Knee and Hip OA

- **Acetaminophen** is a preferred first-line treatment; it may be less effective than oral nonsteroidal anti-inflammatory drugs (NSAIDs) but has a lower risk of serious gastrointestinal (GI) and cardiovascular (CV) events. Acetaminophen is usually well tolerated, but potentially fatal hepatotoxicity with overdose is well documented. It should be avoided in chronic alcohol users or patients with liver disease.
- **Nonselective NSAIDs** or **cyclooxygenase-2 (COX-2) selective inhibitors** (eg, **celecoxib**) are recommended if a patient fails acetaminophen. Nonselective NSAIDs may cause minor GI complaints such as nausea, dyspepsia, anorexia, abdominal pain, and diarrhea. They may cause gastric and duodenal ulcers and bleeding through direct (topical) or indirect (systemic) mechanisms. Risk factors for NSAID-associated ulcers and ulcer complications (perforation, gastric outlet obstruction, and GI bleeding) include longer duration of NSAID use, higher dosage, age older than 60 years,

TABLE 2-1	Medications for the Treatment of Osteoarthritis	
Drug	**Starting Dose**	**Usual Range**
Oral analgesics		
Acetaminophen	325–500 mg three times a day	325–650 mg every 4–6 hours or 1 g three to four times/day
Tramadol	25 mg in the morning	Titrate dose in 25-mg increments to reach a maintenance dose of 50–100 mg three times a day
Tramadol ER	100 mg daily	Titrate to 200–300 mg daily
Hydrocodone/ acetaminophen	5 mg/325 mg three times daily	2.5–10 mg/325–650 mg three to five times daily
Oxycodone/acetaminophen	5 mg/325 mg three times daily	2.5–10 mg/325–650 mg three to five times daily
Topical analgesics		
Capsaicin 0.025%–0.15%		Apply to the affected joint three to four times per day
Diclofenac 1% gel		Apply 2 or 4 g per site as prescribed, four times daily
Diclofenac 1.3% patch		Apply one patch twice daily to the site to be treated, as directed
Diclofenac 2% solution		Apply 40 mg (two pump actuations) twice daily drops to the affected knee, applying and rubbing in 10 drops at a time. Repeat for a total of four times daily.
Intra-articular corticosteroids		
Triamcinolone	5–15 mg per joint	10–40 mg per large joint (knee, hip, shoulder)
Methylprednisolone acetate	10–20 mg per joint	20–80 mg per large joint (knee, hip, shoulder)
NSAIDs		
Aspirin (plain, buffered, or enteric-coated)	325 mg three times a day	325–650 mg four times a day
Celecoxib	100 mg daily	100 mg twice daily or 200 mg daily
Diclofenac IR	50 mg twice a day	50–75 mg twice a day
Diclofenac XR	100 mg daily	100–200 mg daily
Diflunisal	250 mg twice a day	500–750 mg twice a day
Etodolac	300 mg twice a day	400–500 mg twice a day
Fenoprofen	400 mg three times a day	400–600 mg three to four times a day
Flurbiprofen	100 mg twice a day	200–300 mg/day in two to four divided doses

(Continued)

TABLE 2-1	Medications for the Treatment of Osteoarthritis *(Continued)*	
Drug	**Starting Dose**	**Usual Range**
Ibuprofen	200 mg three times a day	1200–3200 mg/day in three to four divided doses
Indomethacin	25 mg twice a day	Titrate dose by 25–50 mg/day until pain is controlled or maximum dose of 50 mg three times a day
Indomethacin SR	75 mg SR once daily	Can titrate to 75 mg SR twice daily if needed
Ketoprofen	50 mg three times a day	50–75 mg three to four times a day
Meclofenamate	50 mg three times a day	50–100 mg three to four times a day
Mefenamic acid	250 mg three times a day	250 mg four times a day
Meloxicam	7.5 mg daily	15 mg daily
Nabumetone	500 mg daily	500–1000 mg one to two times a day
Naproxen	250 mg twice a day	500 mg twice a day
Naproxen sodium	220 mg twice a day	220–550 mg twice a day
Naproxen sodium CR	750–1000 mg once daily	500–1500 mg once daily
Oxaprozin	600 mg daily	600–1200 mg daily
Piroxicam	10 mg daily	20 mg daily
Salsalate	500 mg twice a day	500–1000 mg two to three times a day

CR, controlled-release; ER, extended-release; IR, immediate-release; SR, sustained-release; XR, extended-release.

past history of peptic ulcer disease of any cause, history of alcohol use, and concomitant use of glucocorticoids or anticoagulants. Options for reducing the GI risk of nonselective NSAIDs include using (1) the lowest dose possible and only when needed, (2) misoprostol four times daily with the NSAID, and (3) a PPI or full-dose H_2-receptor antagonist daily with the NSAID.

- COX-2 inhibitors pose less risk for adverse GI events than nonselective NSAIDs, but this advantage is substantially reduced for patients taking aspirin. Both nonselective and selective NSAIDs are associated with an increased risk for CV events (hypertension, stroke, myocardial infarction, and death).
- NSAIDs may also cause kidney diseases, hepatitis, hypersensitivity reactions, rash, and CNS complaints of drowsiness, dizziness, headaches, depression, confusion, and tinnitus. NSAIDs inhibit COX-1–dependent thromboxane production in platelets, thereby increasing bleeding risk. Unlike aspirin, celecoxib and nonspecific NSAIDs inhibit thromboxane formation reversibly, with normalization of platelet function 1–3 days after drug discontinuation. Avoid NSAIDs in late pregnancy because of risk of premature closure of the ductus arteriosus. The most potentially serious drug interactions include use of NSAIDs with lithium, warfarin, oral hypoglycemics, methotrexate, antihypertensives, angiotensin-converting enzyme inhibitors, β-blockers, and diuretics.
- **Topical NSAIDs** are recommended for knee OA if acetaminophen fails, and they are preferred to oral NSAIDs in patients older than 75 years. Topical NSAIDs provide similar pain relief with fewer adverse GI events than oral NSAIDs but may be

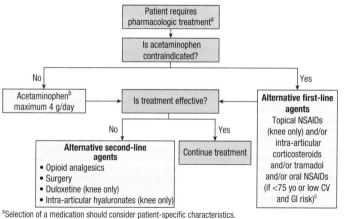

aSelection of a medication should consider patient-specific characteristics.
bThe patient must be counseled regarding all acetaminophen-containing products.
cWhen used for chronic management of OA, consider addition of a proton-pump inhibitor.

FIGURE 2-1 Treatment recommendations for hip and knee osteoarthritis.

associated with adverse events at the application site (eg, dry skin, pruritus, and rash). Patients using topical products should avoid oral NSAIDs to minimize the potential for additive side effects. Use of topical NSAIDs has not been linked with increased risk of CV events.

- **Intra-articular (IA) corticosteroid injections** are recommended for both hip and knee OA when analgesia with acetaminophen or NSAIDs is suboptimal. They can provide excellent pain relief, particularly when joint effusion is present. Local anesthetics such as lidocaine or bupivacaine are commonly combined with corticosteroids to provide rapid pain relief. Injections may also be given with concomitant oral analgesics for additional pain control. After aseptic aspiration of the effusion and corticosteroid injection, initial pain relief may occur within 24–72 hours, with peak relief occurring after 7–10 days and lasting for 4–8 weeks. Local adverse effects can include infection, osteonecrosis, tendon rupture, and skin atrophy at the injection site. Do not administer injections more frequently than once every 3 months to minimize systemic adverse effects. Systemic corticosteroid therapy is not recommended in OA, given the lack of proven benefits and well-known adverse effects with long-term use.

- **Tramadol** is recommended for hip and knee OA in patients who have failed scheduled full-dose acetaminophen and topical NSAIDs, who are not appropriate candidates for oral NSAIDs, and who are not able to receive IA corticosteroids. Tramadol can be added to partially effective acetaminophen or oral NSAID therapy. Tramadol is associated with opioid-like adverse effects such as nausea, vomiting, dizziness, constipation, headache, and somnolence. However, tramadol is not associated with life-threatening GI bleeding, CV events, or renal failure. The most serious adverse event is seizures. Tramadol is classified as a Schedule IV controlled substance due to its potential for dependence, addiction, and diversion. There is increased risk of serotonin syndrome when tramadol is used with other serotonergic medications, including duloxetine.

- **Opioids** should be considered in patients not responding adequately to nonpharmacologic and first-line pharmacologic therapies. Patients who are at high surgical risk and cannot undergo joint arthroplasty are also candidates for opioid therapy. Use opioid analgesics in the lowest effective dose and the smallest quantity needed. Avoid combinations of opioids and sedating medications whenever possible. Inform patients on how to use, store, and dispose of opioid medications. Sustained-release

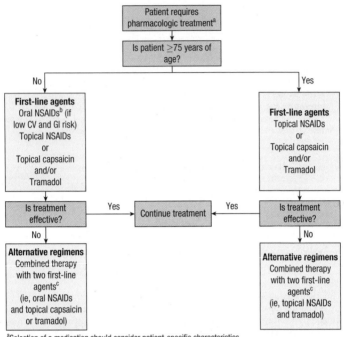


```
┌─────────────────────┐
│  Patient requires   │
│ pharmacologic treatmentᵃ│
└─────────────────────┘
         │
┌─────────────────────┐
│ Is patient ≥75 years of │
│        age?         │
└─────────────────────┘
```

No / Yes

First-line agents
Oral NSAIDsᵇ (if low CV and GI risk)
Topical NSAIDs
or
Topical capsaicin
and/or
Tramadol

First-line agents
Topical NSAIDs
or
Topical capsaicin
and/or
Tramadol

Is treatment effective? — Yes → Continue treatment ← Yes — Is treatment effective?

No / No

Alternative regimens
Combined therapy with two first-line agentsᶜ
(ie, oral NSAIDs and topical capsaicin or tramadol)

Alternative regimens
Combined therapy with two first-line agentsᶜ
(ie, topical NSAIDs and tramadol)

ᵃSelection of a medication should consider patient-specific characteristics.
ᵇWhen used for chronic management of OA, consider addition of a proton-pump inhibitor.
ᶜShould not combine topical NSAIDs and oral NSAIDs.

FIGURE 2-2 Treatment recommendations for hand osteoarthritis.

compounds usually offer better pain control throughout the day. Common adverse effects include nausea, somnolence, constipation, dry mouth, and dizziness. Opioid dependence, addiction, tolerance, hyperalgesia, and issues surrounding drug diversion may be associated with long-term treatment. Assess opioid use at least every 3 months, evaluating patient progress toward functional treatment goals, risks of harm, and adverse effects.

- **Duloxetine** can be used as adjunctive treatment of knee (not hip) OA in patients with partial response to first-line analgesics (acetaminophen, oral NSAIDs). It may be a preferred second-line medication in patients with both neuropathic and musculoskeletal OA pain. Pain reduction occurs after about 4 weeks of therapy. Duloxetine may cause nausea, dry mouth, constipation, anorexia, fatigue, somnolence, and dizziness. Serious rare events include Stevens-Johnson syndrome and liver failure. Concomitant use with other medications that increase serotonin concentration (including tramadol) increases risk of serotonin syndrome.

- **IA hyaluronic acid** (sodium hyaluronate) is not routinely recommended because injections have shown limited benefit for knee OA and have not been shown to benefit hip OA. Injections are usually well tolerated, but acute joint swelling, effusion, stiffness, and local skin reactions (eg, rash, ecchymoses, or pruritus) have been reported. IA preparations and regimens for OA knee pain include:
  - ✓ **Cross-linked hyaluronate 30 mg/3 mL** (Gel-One) single injection
  - ✓ **Hyaluronan 30 mg/2 mL** (Orthovisc) once weekly for three injections
  - ✓ **Hyaluronan 88 mg/4 mL** (Monovisc) single injection

✓ **Hylan G-F 20 16 mg/2 mL** (Synvisc) once weekly for three injections
✓ **Hylan G-F 20 48 mg/6 mL** (Synvisc-One) single injection
✓ **Sodium hyaluronate 20 mg/2 mL** (Hyalgan) once weekly for five injections
✓ **Sodium hyaluronate 20 mg/2 mL** (Euflexxa) once weekly for three injections
✓ **Sodium hyaluronate 25 mg/2.5 mL** (Supartz FX) once weekly for five injections
✓ **Sodium hyaluronate 25 mg/3 mL** (GenVisc 850) once weekly for five injections

• **Glucosamine and/or chondroitin** and **topical rubefacients** (eg, **methyl salicylate, trolamine salicylate**) lack uniform improvement in pain control or functional status for hip and knee pain and are not preferred treatment options. Glucosamine adverse effects are mild and include flatulence, bloating, and abdominal cramps. The most common adverse effect of chondroitin is nausea.

Hand OA

• **Topical NSAIDs** are a first-line option for hand OA. Topical diclofenac has efficacy similar to oral NSAIDs with fewer adverse GI events, albeit with some local application site events. Efficacy with topical NSAIDs typically occurs within 1–2 weeks.
• **Oral NSAIDs** are an alternative first-line treatment for patients who cannot tolerate the local skin reactions or who received inadequate relief from topical NSAIDs.
• **Capsaicin cream** is an alternative first-line treatment; small clinical trials have demonstrated about 50% reduction in pain scores. It is a reasonable option for patients unable to take oral NSAIDs. Capsaicin must be used regularly to be effective, and it may require up to 2 weeks to take effect. Adverse effects are primarily local and include burning, stinging, and/or erythema that usually subsides with repeated application. Warn patients not to get cream in their eyes or mouth and to wash hands after application. Application of the cream, gel, solution, or lotion is recommended four times daily.
• **Tramadol** is an alternative first-line treatment and is a reasonable option for patients who do not respond to topical therapy and are not candidates for oral NSAIDs because of high GI, CV, or renal risks. Tramadol may also be used in combination with partially effective acetaminophen, topical therapy, or oral NSAIDs.

EVALUATION OF THERAPEUTIC OUTCOMES

• To monitor efficacy, assess baseline pain with a visual analog scale, and assess range of motion for affected joints with flexion, extension, abduction, or adduction.
• Depending on the joint(s) affected, measurement of grip strength and 50-ft walking time can help assess hand and hip/knee OA, respectively.
• Baseline radiographs can document extent of joint involvement and follow disease progression with therapy.
• Other measures include the clinician's global assessment based on patient's history of activities and limitations caused by OA, the Western Ontario and McMaster Universities Arthrosis Index, Stanford Health Assessment Questionnaire, and documentation of analgesic or NSAID use.
• Ask patients about adverse effects of medications. Monitor for signs of drug-related effects, such as skin rash, headaches, drowsiness, weight gain, or hypertension from NSAIDs.
• Obtain baseline serum creatinine, hematology profile, and serum transaminases with repeat levels at 6- to 12-month intervals to identify specific toxicities to the kidney, liver, GI tract, or bone marrow.

_____

See Chapter 110, Osteoarthritis, authored by Lucinda M. Buys and Sara A. Wiedenfeld, for a more detailed discussion of this topic.

Osteoporosis

- *Osteoporosis* is a bone disorder characterized by low bone density, impaired bone architecture, and compromised bone strength predisposing to fracture.

PATHOPHYSIOLOGY

- Bone loss occurs when resorption exceeds formation, usually from a high bone turnover when the number or depth of bone resorption sites greatly exceeds the ability of osteoblasts to form new bone. Accelerated bone turnover can increase the amount of immature bone that is not adequately mineralized.
- Men and women begin to lose bone mass starting in the third or fourth decade because of reduced bone formation. Estrogen deficiency during menopause increases osteoclast activity, increasing bone resorption more than formation. Men are at a lower risk for developing osteoporosis and osteoporotic fractures because of larger bone size, greater peak bone mass, increase in bone width with aging, fewer falls, and shorter life expectancy. Male osteoporosis results from aging or secondary causes.
- Age-related osteoporosis results from hormone, calcium, and vitamin D deficiencies; decreased production or function of cytokines; decreased body water; less exercise; and other factors that result in accelerated bone turnover and reduced osteoblast formation.
- Drug-induced osteoporosis may result from systemic corticosteroids, excessive thyroid hormone replacement, antiepileptic drugs (eg, phenytoin, phenobarbital), depot medroxyprogesterone acetate, and other agents.

CLINICAL PRESENTATION

- Many patients are unaware that they have osteoporosis and only present after fracture. Fractures can occur after bending, lifting, or falling or independent of any activity.
- The most common fractures involve vertebrae, proximal femur, and distal radius (wrist or Colles fracture). Vertebral fractures may be asymptomatic or present with moderate to severe back pain that radiates down a leg. The pain usually subsides after 2–4 weeks, but residual back pain may persist. Multiple vertebral fractures decrease height and sometimes curve the spine (kyphosis or lordosis).
- Patients with a nonvertebral fracture frequently present with severe pain, swelling, and reduced function and mobility at the fracture site.

DIAGNOSIS

- The World Health Organization (WHO) Fracture Risk Assessment Tool (FRAX tool) uses the following risk factors to predict the percent probability of fracture in the next 10 years: age, race/ethnicity, sex, previous fragility fracture, parent history of hip fracture, body mass index, glucocorticoid use, current smoking, alcohol (≥ 3 drinks per day), rheumatoid arthritis, and select secondary causes with femoral neck or total hip bone mineral density (BMD) data optional.
- The Garvan calculator uses four risk factors (age, sex, low-trauma fracture, and falls) with the option to also use BMD. It calculates 5- and 10-year risk estimates of any osteoporotic/fragility fracture and hip fracture. This tool corrects some disadvantages of FRAX because it includes falls and the number of previous fractures, but it does not use as many other risk factors.
- Physical examination findings may include bone pain, postural changes (ie, kyphosis), and loss of height (>1.5 in [3.8 cm]).

- Laboratory testing: complete blood count, serum creatinine, calcium, phosphorus, electrolytes, alkaline phosphatase, albumin, thyroid-stimulating hormone, total testosterone (for men), 25-hydroxyvitamin D, and 24-hour urine concentrations of calcium and phosphorus.
- Measurement of central (hip and spine) BMD with dual-energy x-ray absorptiometry (DXA) is preferred for making therapeutic decisions. Measurement at peripheral sites (forearm, heel, and finger) with DXA or quantitative ultrasonography is used only for screening and for determining the need for further testing.
- A T-score compares the patient's BMD to the mean BMD of a healthy, young (20- to 29-year-old), sex-matched, White reference population. The T-score is the number of standard deviations from the mean of the reference population.
- Diagnosis of osteoporosis is based on low-trauma fracture or femoral neck, total hip, and/or spine DXA using WHO T-score thresholds. Normal bone mass has a T-score above −1, low bone mass (osteopenia) has a T-score between −1 and −2.4, and osteoporosis has a T-score at or below −2.5.

TREATMENT

- <u>Goals of Treatment</u>: The primary goal of osteoporosis care is prevention. Optimizing peak bone mass when young reduces the future incidence of osteoporosis. After low bone mass or osteoporosis develops, the objective is to stabilize or improve bone mass and strength and prevent fractures. Goals in patients with osteoporotic fractures include reducing pain and deformity, improving function, reducing falls and fractures, and improving quality of life.
- Figure 3-1 provides an osteoporosis management algorithm for postmenopausal women and men aged 50 and older.

NONPHARMACOLOGIC THERAPY

- All individuals should have a balanced diet with adequate intake of **calcium** and **vitamin D** (Table 3-1). Achieving daily calcium requirements from calcium-containing foods is preferred.
  - ✓ Consumers can calculate the amount of calcium in a food serving by adding a zero to the percentage of the daily value on food labels. One serving of milk (8 oz or 240 mL) has 30% of the daily value of calcium; this converts to 300 mg of calcium per serving.
  - ✓ To calculate the amount of vitamin D in a food serving, multiply the percent daily value of vitamin D listed on the food label by 4. For example, 20% vitamin D = 80 units.
- Protein is required for bone formation; the recommended dietary allowance (RDA) is 0.8 g/kg body weight per day for adults, increasing to 1–1.2 g/kg body weight in older adults.
- Alcohol consumption should not exceed 1–2 drinks per day for women and 2–3 drinks per day for men.
- Ideally, caffeine intake should be limited to two or fewer servings per day.
- Smoking cessation helps optimize peak bone mass, minimize bone loss, and ultimately reduce fracture risk.
- Weight-bearing aerobic and strengthening exercises can decrease the risk of falls and fractures by improving muscle strength, coordination, balance, and mobility.
- Fall prevention programs that are multifactorial can decrease falls, fractures, other injuries, and nursing home and hospital admissions.
- Vertebroplasty and kyphoplasty involve injection of cement into fractured vertebra(e) for patients with debilitating pain from compression fractures. Although intended to stabilize damaged vertebrae, reduce pain, and decrease opioid intake, research demonstrated only short-term benefit with no major pain relief and the potential for post-procedure complications.

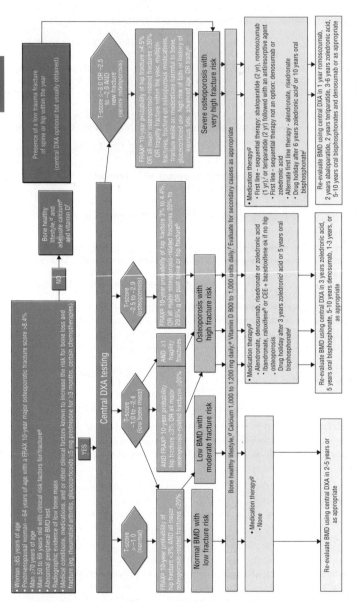

[a]Major clinical risk factors for fracture: advanced age, current smoker, low body weight or body mass index, personal history of fracture as an adult (after age 50 years), history of osteoporosis/low trauma fracture in a first-degree relative, excessive alcohol intake.
[b]Some providers use age adjusted FRAX thresholds versus set thresholds for all age groups.
[c]Fragility fracture is high risk for ES guidelines, and very high risk for AACE/ACE guideline.
[d]Bone-healthy lifestyle includes well-balanced diet with adequate calcium, vitamin D, and protein intakes; smoking cessation; limited alcohol intake; weight-bearing/resistance exercises; and fall prevention.

(Continued)

eDietary calcium preferred. If diet is inadequate, supplement as necessary.
fHigher vitamin D doses might be needed to achieve 25-hydroxyvitamin D concentrations >30 ng/mL.
gSome increased BMD effects will be seen for women using menopausal hormonal therapy and for men using testosterone for hypogonadism. For women and men on hormonal therapy and at high risk or very high risk for osteoporotic fractures, an osteoporosis medication will also be prescribed, creating a case for combination therapy.
hRaloxifene option for postmenopausal women <60 years old with low hip fracture, stroke, and venous thromboembolic risk and high breast cancer risk.
iRestart therapy when BMD goes below T-score ≤−2.5 or a fracture; alternative is to use raloxifene or denosumab, or in some cases a bone formation medication during the drug holiday.
jDo not use romosozumab in patients with at high risk for or past myocardial infarction and/or stroke.

BMD, bone mineral density; DXA, dual-energy x-ray absorptiometry; FRAX, World Health Organization Fracture Risk Assessment Tool.

FIGURE 3-1. Algorithm for the management of osteoporosis in postmenopausal women and men aged 50 and older.

PHARMACOLOGIC THERAPY

GENERAL APPROACH

- Alendronate, risedronate, zoledronic acid, and denosumab reduce both hip and vertebral fracture risks.
- Abaloparatide, calcitonin, ibandronate, raloxifene, romosozumab, and teriparatide reduce vertebral but not hip fracture risks.
- Calcitonin is the last-line therapy.
- Estrogen and testosterone are not used for osteoporosis treatment, but can have a positive bone effect when prescribed for other conditions.

TABLE 3-1	Calcium and Vitamin D RDAs and Tolerable Upper Intake Levels			
Group and Ages	**Elemental Calcium RDA (mg)**	**Calcium Tolerable Upper Intake Level (mg)**	**Vitamin D RDA (Units)[a]**	**Vitamin D Tolerable Upper Intake Level (Units)**
Infants				
Birth–6 months	200[b]	1000	400[b]	1000
7–12 months	260[b]	1500	400[b]	1500
Children				
1–3 years	700	2500	600	2500
4–8 years	1000	2500	600	3000
9–18 years	1300	3000	600	4000
Adults				
19–50 years	1000	2500	600[b,c]	4000
51–70 years (men)	1000	2000	600[b,c]	4000
51–70 years (women)	1200	2000	600[b,c]	4000
>70 years	1200	2000	800[b,c]	4000

RDA, recommended dietary allowance.
aSome guidelines recommend intake to achieve a 25-hydroxyvitamin D concentration >30 ng/mL (mcg/L; 75 nmol/L), which is higher than the Institute of Medicine goal of >20 ng/mL (mcg/L; 50 nmol/L).
bAdequate intake (evidence insufficient to determine an RDA).
cGuidelines recommend 800–1000 units or 1000–2000 units for adults with osteoporosis.

ANTIRESORPTIVE THERAPY

Calcium Supplementation

- Calcium generally maintains or increases BMD slightly, but its effects are less than those of other therapies. There are insufficient data to support using calcium and vitamin D supplementation to reduce fracture incidence. Because the fraction of calcium absorbed decreases with increasing dose, maximum single doses of 600 mg or less of elemental calcium are recommended.
- **Calcium carbonate** is the salt of choice because it contains the highest concentration of elemental calcium (40%) and is typically least expensive. It should be ingested with meals to enhance absorption in an acidic environment.
- **Calcium citrate** (21% calcium) has acid-independent absorption and need not be taken with meals. It may have fewer GI side effects than calcium carbonate.
- **Tricalcium phosphate** contains 38% calcium, but calcium-phosphate complexes could limit overall calcium absorption. It may be useful in patients with hypophosphatemia that cannot be resolved with increased dietary intake.
- Constipation is the most common calcium-related adverse reaction; treat with increased water intake, dietary fiber (given separately from calcium), and exercise. Calcium carbonate can sometimes cause flatulence or upset stomach. Calcium causes kidney stones rarely.
- Calcium can decrease the oral absorption of some drugs including iron, tetracyclines, quinolones, bisphosphonates, and thyroid supplements.

Vitamin D Supplementation

- **Vitamin D** supplementation using 700–800 units per day significantly reduces the incidence of both hip and nonvertebral fractures with small increases in BMD.
- Supplementation is usually provided with daily nonprescription cholecalciferol (vitamin D_3) products. Higher-dose prescription of ergocalciferol (vitamin D_2) regimens given weekly, monthly, or quarterly may be used for replacement and maintenance therapy. The RDAs in Table 3-1 should be achieved through food and supplementation.
- Current guidelines recommend treating patients with osteoporosis to a 25-hydroxyvitamin D concentration of at least 20 ng/mL (mcg/L; 50 nmol/L) or 30–50 ng/mL.
- Because the half-life of vitamin D is about 1 month, recheck the vitamin D concentration after about 3 months of therapy.
- Medications that can induce vitamin D metabolism include rifampin, phenytoin, barbiturates, valproic acid, and carbamazepine. Vitamin D absorption can be decreased by cholestyramine, colestipol, orlistat, and mineral oil. Vitamin D can enhance the absorption of aluminum; therefore, aluminum-containing products should be avoided to prevent aluminum toxicity.

Bisphosphonates

- Bisphosphonates (Table 3-2) mimic pyrophosphate, an endogenous bone resorption inhibitor. Therapy leads to decreased osteoclast maturation, number, recruitment, bone adhesion, and life span. Incorporation into bone gives bisphosphonates long biologic half-lives of up to 10 years.
- Bisphosphonates consistently increase BMD and reduce fracture risk, with differences in sites of fracture reduction among agents. Ibandronate is not a first-line therapy because of the lack of hip fracture reduction data.
- BMD increases are dose-dependent and greatest in the first 12 months of therapy. After discontinuation, the increased BMD is sustained for a prolonged period that varies per bisphosphonate.
- **Alendronate, risedronate,** and **IV zoledronic acid** are Food and Drug Administration (FDA) drugs indicated for postmenopausal, male, and glucocorticoid-induced osteoporosis. **IV and oral ibandronate** are indicated only for postmenopausal osteoporosis. Weekly alendronate, weekly and monthly risedronate, and monthly oral and quarterly IV ibandronate therapy produce equivalent BMD changes to their respective daily regimens.

TABLE 3-2 Medications Used to Prevent and Treat Osteoporosis

Drug	Brand Name	Dose	Comments
Antiresorptive Medications—Nutritional Supplements			
Calcium	Various	Adequate daily intake: IOM: 200–1200 mg/day, varies per age); supplement dose is difference between required adequate intake and dietary intake Immediate-release doses should be <500–600 mg	Recommend food first to achieve goal intake. Available in different salts including carbonate and citrate, absorption of other salts not fully quantified. Different formulations including chewable, liquid, gummy, softgel, drink, and wafer; different combination products. Review package to determine number of units to create a serving size and desired amount of elemental calcium. Give calcium carbonate with meals to improve absorption.
Vitamin D D₃ (cholecalciferol) D₂ (ergocalciferol)	Over the counter Tablets, 400, 1000, and 2000 units Capsule, 400, 1000, 2000, 5000, and 10,000 units Gummies, 300, 500, 1000 units Drops 300, 400, 1000, and 2000 units/mL or drop Solution, 400 and 5000 units/mL Spray 1000 and 5000 units/spray Creams and lotions 500 and 1000 units per ¼ teaspoonful Prescription Capsule, 50,000 units Solution, 8000 units/mL	Adequate daily intake: IOM: 400–800 units/day to achieve adequate intake; NOF: 800–1000 units orally daily; if low 25-hydroxyvitamin D concentrations, malabsorption, or altered metabolism higher doses (>2000 units daily) might be required. Vitamin D deficiency: 50,000 units orally once to twice weekly for 8–12 weeks; repeat as needed until therapeutic concentrations.	Vegetarians and vegans need to read label to determine if it is a plant-based product. Slight advantage of D₃ over D₂ for increasing serum 25-hydroxyvitamin D concentrations. For drops, make sure measurement is correct for desired dose. Ability of sprays, lotions, and creams to resolve deficiencies or maintain adequate intakes is unknown.

(Continued)

TABLE 3-2	Medications Used to Prevent and Treat Osteoporosis (*Continued*)	
Drug	**Brand Name**	**Dose**	**Comments**

Antiresorptive Prescription Medications

Bisphosphonates

Drug	Brand Name	Dose	Comments
Alendronate	Fosamax Fosamax Plus D Binosto (effervescent tab)	Treatment: 10 mg orally daily or 70 mg orally weekly Prevention: 5 mg orally daily or 35 mg orally weekly	Generic available for weekly tablet product. 70 mg dose is available as a tablet, effervescent tablet, oral liquid, or combination tablet with 2800 or 5600 units of vitamin D_3. Administered in the morning on an empty stomach with 6–8 ounces of plain water. Do not eat and remain upright for at least 30 minutes following administration. Do not coadminister with any other medication or supplements, including calcium and vitamin D.
Ibandronate	Boniva	Treatment: 150 mg orally monthly, 3 mg IV quarterly Prevention: 150 mg orally monthly	Generic available for oral product. Administration instructions are the same as for alendronate, except must delay eating and remain upright for at least 60 minutes.
Risedronate	Actonel Atelvia (delayed-release)	Treatment and prevention: 5 mg orally daily, 35 mg orally weekly, 150 mg orally monthly	Generic available for immediate-release product. 35 mg dose is also available as a delayed-release product. Administration instructions are the same as for alendronate, except delayed-release product is taken immediately following breakfast.

Zoledronic acid	Reclast	Treatment: 5 mg IV infusion yearly Prevention: 5 mg IV infusion every 2 years	Can premedicate with acetaminophen to decrease infusion reactions. Contraindicated if CrCl <35 mL/min Also marketed under the brand name Zometa (4 mg) for treatment of hypercalcemia and prevention of skeletal-related events from bone metastases from solid tumors with different dosing.
RANK Ligand Inhibitor			
Denosumab	Prolia	Treatment: 60 mg SC every 6 months	Administered by a healthcare practitioner. Correct hypocalcemia before administration. Also marketed under the brand name Xgeva (70 mg/ mL) for treatment of hypercalcemia and prevention of skeletal-related events from bone metastases from solid tumors with different dosing.
Estrogen Agonist/Antagonist and Tissue Selective Estrogen Complex			
Raloxifene	Evista	60 mg orally daily	Generic available.
Bazedoxifene with CEE	Duavee	20 mg plus 0.45 mg CEE orally daily	For postmenopausal women with a uterus; no progestogen needed. Bazedoxifene monotherapy available in some countries.
Calcitonin (salmon)	Fortical	200 units (1 spray) intranasally daily, alternating nares every other day	Generic available. Also available as an SC injection. Refrigerate nasal spray until opened for daily use, then room temperature. Prime with first use.

(Continued)

TABLE 3-2	Medications Used to Prevent and Treat Osteoporosis (*Continued*)		
Drug	**Brand Name**	**Dose**	**Comments**
Formation Medications			
Recombinant human parathyroid hormone (PTH 1–34 units)			
Teriparatide	Forteo	20 mcg SC daily for up to 2 years	First dose sitting or lying. Refrigerate before and after each use. Use new needle with each dose. Inject thigh or stomach. Discard after 28 days or if cloudy.
Human parathyroid hormone–related peptide (PTHrP[1–34]) analog			
Abaloparatide	Tymlos	80 mcg SC daily for up to 2 years	First dose sitting or lying. Refrigerate before use; then, keep at room temperature. Use new needle with each dose. Inject in abdomen. Discard after 30 days.
Formation and Antiresorptive Medication			
Sclerostin inhibitor			
Romosozumab	Evenity	210 mg SC monthly for 1 year; administered as two single-use 105-mg/1.17-mL prefilled syringes	Correct hypocalcemia before administration. Refrigerate. Leave at room temperature for at least 30 minutes before use. Inject in abdomen, thigh, or upper arm; preferably each injection at a different site.

CEE, conjugated equine estrogens; IOM, Institute of Medicine; IV, intravenously; NOF, National Osteoporosis Foundation; NSAID, nonsteroidal anti-inflammatory drug; SC, subcutaneously.

- Oral bisphosphonates must be administered correctly to optimize clinical benefit and minimize adverse GI effects. Each oral tablet should be taken in the morning with at least 6 oz (180 mL) of plain water (not coffee, juice, mineral water, or milk) and at least 30 minutes (60 minutes for oral ibandronate) before consuming any food, supplements, or medications. An exception is delayed-release risedronate, which is administered immediately after breakfast with at least 4 oz (120 mL) of plain water. The patient should remain upright (sitting or standing) for at least 30 minutes after alendronate and risedronate and 1 hour after ibandronate to prevent esophageal irritation and ulceration.
- If a patient misses a weekly dose, it can be taken the next day. If more than 1 day has elapsed, that dose is skipped. If a patient misses a monthly dose, it can be taken up to 7 days before the next scheduled dose.
- The most common bisphosphonate adverse effects include nausea, abdominal pain, and dyspepsia. Esophageal, gastric, or duodenal irritation, perforation, ulceration, or bleeding may occur. The most common adverse effects of IV bisphosphonates include fever, flu-like symptoms, and local injection-site reactions.
- Rare adverse effects include osteonecrosis of the jaw (ONJ) and subtrochanteric femoral (atypical) fractures. ONJ occurs more commonly in patients with cancer receiving higher-dose IV bisphosphonate therapy.
- The optimal duration of bisphosphonate therapy is unknown. Some experts recommend considering a bisphosphonate holiday (defined as disruption of therapy during which medication effects exist with a plan for medication reinstitution) in postmenopausal women after 5 years of oral bisphosphonates or 3 years of IV bisphosphonates if there is no significant fracture history, hip BMD T-score is above -2.5, and fracture risk is not high. In women with very high fracture risk, continuing oral bisphosphonates for 10 years or IV bisphosphonates for 6 years should be considered. Patients should be monitored during the drug holiday and restarting therapy considered if fractures occur or if there are significant BMD losses.

Denosumab

- **Denosumab** (Prolia) is a RANK ligand inhibitor that inhibits osteoclast formation and increases osteoclast apoptosis. It is FDA-approved for treatment of osteoporosis in postmenopausal women and men at high risk for fracture, for glucocorticoid-induced osteoporosis, to increase bone mass in men receiving androgen-deprivation therapy for nonmetastatic prostate cancer, and in women receiving adjuvant aromatase inhibitor therapy for breast cancer who are at high risk for fracture.
- Over 3 years, denosumab significantly decreased vertebral fractures, nonvertebral fractures, and hip fractures in postmenopausal women with low bone density. Continued increases in BMD occur with long-term treatment over 10 years.
- Denosumab is administered as a 60-mg subcutaneous (SC) injection in the upper arm, upper thigh, or abdomen once every 6 months.
- Adverse reactions not associated with the injection site include back pain, arthralgia, and infection. ONJ and atypical femoral shaft fracture occur rarely. Denosumab is contraindicated in patients with hypocalcemia until the condition is corrected.
- After 5–10 years of therapy, patients should be reevaluated for medication continuation, discontinuation, or switching to a different medication.

Mixed Estrogen Agonists/Antagonists and Tissue-Selective Estrogen Complexes

- **Raloxifene** (Evista) is an estrogen agonist/antagonist that is an estrogen agonist on bone receptors but an antagonist at breast receptors, with minimal effects on the uterus. It is approved for prevention and treatment of postmenopausal osteoporosis and for reducing the risk of invasive breast cancer in postmenopausal women with and without osteoporosis.
- **Bazedoxifene** is an estrogen agonist/antagonist that is an agonist at bone and antagonist at the uterus and breast; however, reduction in breast cancer risk has not yet been demonstrated. The proprietary product Duavee is combined with **conjugated**

equine estrogens (CEE), making it a tissue-selective estrogen complex. It is approved for prevention of postmenopausal osteoporosis and vasomotor menstrual symptoms.

- Raloxifene and bazedoxifene decrease vertebral but not hip fractures. The drugs increase spine and hip BMD, but to a lesser extent than bisphosphonates. However, the benefit is lost after discontinuation, and bone loss returns to age- or disease-related rates.
- Hot flushes are common with raloxifene but decreases with bazedoxifene/CEE. Raloxifene rarely causes endometrial thickening and bleeding; bazedoxifene decreases these events making progestogen therapy unnecessary when combined with CEE. Leg cramps and muscle spasms are common with these agents. Thromboembolic events are uncommon (<1.5%) but can be fatal. Bazedoxifene/CEE has all of the contraindications and precautions for estrogens as a class.

Calcitonin

- **Calcitonin** is FDA-approved for osteoporosis treatment for women at least 5 years past menopause. Intranasal calcitonin therapy (200 units daily) decreases only vertebral fractures. Once discontinued, the benefits are lost over the next 1–2 years. Calcitonin is considered as a last-line therapy because there are more effective treatment options.
- Intranasal calcitonin may provide some pain relief in patients with acute vertebral fractures, but such use should be short term (4 weeks) and not in place of other more appropriate analgesic or osteoporosis therapy.

Hormone Therapies

- **Estrogen** therapy is FDA-approved for prevention of postmenopausal osteoporosis but not for treatment. It can be considered for women going through early menopause when protection against bone loss is needed in addition to reduction of vasomotor symptoms. Other therapies are reserved for treatment closer to the average age of menopause.
- Estrogen with or without a progestogen significantly decreases fracture risk and bone loss in women. Oral and transdermal estrogens at equivalent doses and continuous or cyclic regimens have similar BMD effects. The effect on BMD is dose-dependent, with some benefits seen with lower estrogen doses. When estrogen therapy is discontinued, bone loss accelerates and fracture protection is lost.
- Testosterone is used to treat hypogonadism in men, but an osteoporosis medication should be added when risk for osteoporotic fracture is high. No fracture data are available, but some data support BMD improvements with testosterone use.

FORMATION MEDICATIONS

Parathyroid Hormone Analogs

- **Abaloparatide** (Tymlos) is an analog of parathyroid hormone–related peptide (PTHrP), and **teriparatide** (Forteo) is an analog of parathyroid hormone (PTH). These agents are indicated for the treatment of postmenopausal women with osteoporosis at high risk for fracture, defined as multiple risk factors for fracture, history of osteoporotic fracture, or failure or intolerance to other therapies. Teriparatide is also FDA-approved for osteoporosis in men who are at high risk for fracture, men intolerant to other osteoporosis medications, and patients with glucocorticoid-induced osteoporosis.
- Teriparatide increases bone formation with a minor increase in bone resorption for a net anabolic effect when administered intermittently (ie, subcutaneously once daily). Abaloparatide has a greater anabolic effect with less activation of bone resorption and remodeling than teriparatide. Both medications improve bone mass.
- Two years of teriparatide or abaloparatide reduces vertebral and nonvertebral fracture risk in postmenopausal women. Observational teriparatide data suggest a similar fracture benefit in men, whereas no data are available regarding abaloparatide use in men. Discontinuation of PTH analog therapy results in decreased BMD, which can be alleviated with subsequent antiresorptive therapy.

- Transient hypercalcemia can occur and is less common with abaloparatide than teriparatide (3.4% vs 6.4%, respectively). Because of an increased incidence of osteosarcoma in rats, both medications contain a box warning against use in patients at increased risk for osteosarcoma; this adverse effect has not occurred in people. PTH analogs should not be used in patients with hypercalcemia, metabolic bone diseases other than osteoporosis, metastatic or skeletal cancers, previous radiation therapy, or premenopausal women of childbearing potential.

FORMATION AND ANTIRESORPTIVE MEDICATION

Romosozumab

- **Romosozumab** (Evenity) is a humanized monoclonal antibody that binds to sclerostin to prevent inhibition of bone formation and decrease bone resorption, an activity that differentiates this medication from other anabolic therapies. It is FDA-approved for postmenopausal women at high risk for fracture, defined as multiple risk factors for fracture, a history of osteoporotic fracture, or failure or intolerance to other therapies.
- After 1 year of therapy in postmenopausal women, vertebral fractures decreased by 73%, with a nonsignificant decrease in nonvertebral fractures of 25%; lumbar spine and hip BMD statistically increase after 1 year of treatment. To prevent BMD loss after discontinuation, 1 year of denosumab or alendronate after romosozumab resulted in BMD continuing to increase at both sites.
- The most common adverse effects are headache and arthralgia; hypercalcemia occurs in <1% of patients. Mild injection site irritation occurs in 6%–8% of patients. Romosozumab antibodies may occur in 10%–20% of patients but are generally not neutralizing and do not reduce efficacy. Serious cardiovascular events have been reported, and the labeling contains a boxed warning of an increased risk of myocardial infarction (MI), stroke, and cardiovascular death. Romosozumab should not be used within 1 year of an MI or stroke, and benefit–risk evaluation should be conducted in patients with or at risk for these conditions. Rare cases of ONJ and atypical femoral fractures have been reported.
- Therapy should be limited to 12 monthly doses. If osteoporosis therapy remains warranted, continued therapy with an antiresorptive agent should be considered.

SEQUENTIAL AND COMBINATION THERAPY

- In sequential therapy, an anabolic agent is given first to increase bone remodeling units and bone mass, followed by an antiresorptive agent to continue with bone formation. This regimen is generally reserved for patients with severe osteoporosis because of the cost of anabolic agents.
  - ✓ Starting with an antiresorptive first and then switching to teriparatide results in lower BMD compared to starting with the bone formation medication first. Thus, starting teriparatide after antiresorption therapy is not recommended. However, this therapy may be useful for patients who have fractured or continue to lose bone mass while on antiresorptive therapy.
  - ✓ Small increases in BMD can occur after switching from an oral bisphosphonate to denosumab. This sequential therapy can be used during a bisphosphonate drug holiday or for bisphosphonate treatment failures (ie, no BMD changes or fracture).
- Combination therapy is rarely used because of no documented fracture benefit, increased cost, concern for dual suppression of bone turnover, and potential for more adverse effects. When raloxifene is used for breast cancer prevention, another antiresorptive agent is sometimes prescribed, especially if hip fracture risk is high.

GLUCOCORTICOID-INDUCED OSTEOPOROSIS

- Glucocorticoids decrease bone formation through decreased proliferation and differentiation as well as enhanced apoptosis of osteoblasts. They also increase the number of osteoclasts, increase bone resorption, decrease calcium absorption, and increase renal calcium excretion.

- All glucocorticoid doses and formulations have been associated with increased bone loss and fractures; however, risk is much greater with oral prednisone doses ≥5 mg daily (or equivalent) and oral therapy compared to inhaler or intranasal therapy.
- Bone losses are rapid, with up to 12%–15% loss over the first year; the greatest decrease occurs in the first 6 months of therapy. Bone loss is about 2%–3% per year after the first year.
- Perform an initial BMD assessment prior to or within 6 months of glucocorticoid initiation for adults ≥40 years of age and for adults <40 years of age with a history of fragility fracture or other risk factors. Repeat BMD testing is recommended every 2–3 years during osteoporosis therapy for those taking very high glucocorticoid doses (≥30 mg prednisone per day or a cumulative dose >5 g in the past year), a fracture 18 months or more after starting osteoporosis therapy, medication adherence or absorption concerns, or other risk factors for osteoporosis.
- All patients starting or receiving systemic glucocorticoid therapy (any dose or duration) should practice a bone-healthy lifestyle and ingest 1000–1200 mg elemental calcium and 600–800 units of vitamin D daily to achieve therapeutic 25-hydroxyvitamin D concentrations. Use the lowest possible corticosteroid dose and duration.
- Treatment guidelines divide recommendations for prescription medication use by fracture risk and age. Alendronate, risedronate, zoledronic acid, denosumab, and teriparatide are FDA-approved for glucocorticoid-induced osteoporosis.
- Standard osteoporosis therapy doses are used. Oral bisphosphonates are recommended first-line, although IV bisphosphonates can be used in nonadherent patients or those unable to take the oral preparations. Teriparatide is recommended for patients who cannot use bisphosphonate, and denosumab is recommended if neither bisphosphonate nor teriparatide can be used. Denosumab is not recommended as first-line therapy due to limited safety data in this population. Raloxifene does not have an FDA indication for this use, but there are clinical data documenting improved BMD at the lumbar spine in patients taking glucocorticoids.

EVALUATION OF THERAPEUTIC OUTCOMES

- Assess medication adherence and tolerability at each visit.
- Ask patients about possible fracture symptoms (eg, bone pain, disability) at each visit. Assessment of fracture, back pain, and height loss can help identify worsening osteoporosis.
- Obtain a central DXA BMD measurement after 1–2 years or 3–5 years after initiating a medication therapy to monitor response. Repeat a central DXA every 2 years until BMD is stable, at which time the reassessment interval can be lengthened. More frequent monitoring may be warranted in patients with conditions associated with high rates of bone loss (eg, glucocorticoid use).

See Chapter 112, Osteoporosis, authored by Mary Beth O'Connell, Jill S. Borchert, Erin M. Slazak, and Joseph P. Fava for a more detailed discussion of this topic.

Rheumatoid Arthritis

- *Rheumatoid arthritis* (RA) is a chronic, progressive autoimmune condition that primarily affects joints and the synovium but can also have systemic manifestations.

PATHOPHYSIOLOGY

- RA results from a combination of genetic susceptibility, nongenetic factors, and a triggering event. An unknown infectious process is thought to be the primary trigger.
- Antigen-presenting cells process and present antigens to T cells; activated T cells stimulate B cells to produce autoantibodies that form large complexes that deposit throughout the body. Antibodies to immunoglobulin G (IgG) are known as rheumatoid factor (RF) and have a strong correlation to the pathogenesis and poor prognosis of RA. B cells also produce proinflammatory cytokines, including tumor necrosis factor (TNF) and the interleukin (IL) system, which induce expression of adhesion molecules on the endothelium, further enhancing T-cell proliferation and differentiation, encouraging cell migration, and regulating matrix modeling.
- Overexpression of tumor suppressor gene p53 prevents normal DNA repair and interferes with appropriate cell apoptosis and increased anti-citrullinated protein antibodies (ACPA). ACPA positivity is associated with a worse prognosis in patients with RA.
- Migration of lymphocytes, macrophages, and mononuclear cells into the synovium and synovial cavity increases synovial mass, causing hypertrophy and angiogenesis. Angiogenesis is driven by IL-8, prostaglandins, vascular endothelial growth factor, and macrophage angiogenic factor. As the vessels develop, cytokines stimulate further migration of cells into the synovium, causing inflammation. The inflamed, fibrotic synovium (*pannus*) invades cartilage and bone around it, promoting further destruction and dysregulation.
- Cytokines within cartilage cause generation of reactive nitrogen and oxygen species and increase chondrocyte catabolism, inhibit chondrocyte anabolism, and increase extracellular matrix destruction. Proinflammatory cytokines travel to bone, provide the source for receptor activator of NFkB ligand (RANKL), and enhance osteoclast activity, leading to bone matrix destruction.
- Chronic inflammation in vascular endothelial and visceral, cutaneous, and pleural tissues leads to complications including vasculitis, fibrosis, anemia, and renal amyloidosis.

CLINICAL PRESENTATION

- Nonspecific prodromal symptoms developing over weeks to months include fatigue, weakness, low-grade fever, anorexia, and joint pain. Stiffness and myalgias may precede development of synovitis.
- Joint involvement tends to be symmetric and affects small joints of the hands, feet, wrists, and ankles; elbows, knees, shoulders, hips, cervical spine, and temporomandibular joints may also be affected.
- Joint stiffness is typically worse in the morning, usually exceeds 30 minutes, and may persist all day.
- On examination, joint swelling may be visible or apparent only by palpation. Tissue is soft, spongy, warm, and may be erythematous. If left untreated, long-term joint inflammation may lead to bony erosions and subluxations of wrists, metacarpophalangeal joints, and proximal interphalangeal joints (swan neck deformity, boutonnière deformity, and ulnar deviation).
- Extra-articular involvement may include rheumatoid nodules, interstitial lung disease, pleural effusions, vasculitis, ocular manifestations, pericarditis, cardiac conduction abnormalities, bone marrow suppression, and lymphadenopathy.

- RF is detected in 70%–80% of patients; higher titers generally reflect a more severe disease course. ACPA antibodies are more specific for RA and may be detectable very early in the disease; they generally predict a more aggressive disease course. Antinuclear antibodies are detected in 25% of patients with RA. Elevated erythrocyte sedimentation rate (ESR) and C-reactive protein (CRP) indicate the presence of a nonspecific inflammatory process. Normocytic anemia, thrombocytosis or thrombocytopenia, and leukopenia may also be present. Analysis of aspirated synovial fluid typically demonstrates a high white blood cell count without crystals or infection.
- Early radiologic findings include soft tissue swelling and periarticular osteoporosis. With disease progression, joint space narrowing, bony erosions, and joint subluxations and deviations may occur.

DIAGNOSIS

- The American College of Rheumatology (ACR) and the European League Against Rheumatism revised criteria for the diagnosis of RA in 2010. These criteria are intended for patients early in their disease to allow for earlier treatment targeted toward preventing structural joint damage. Patients with synovitis of at least one joint and no other explanation for the finding are candidates for assessment. The criteria use a scoring system with a combined score of 6 or more out of 10 indicating that the patient has definite RA.

TREATMENT

- Goals of Treatment: The ultimate goal is to induce complete remission or low disease activity (referred to as "treat to target"). Additional goals are to reduce inflammation and symptoms, maintain ability to function in daily activities, slow destructive joint changes, and delay disability.

NONPHARMACOLOGIC THERAPY

- Patient education about the disease and medications (eg, potential adverse effects, self-administration of injectable agents) is important.
- Physical therapy can reduce pain and inflammation while preserving joint function. Exercise and physical activity (including aerobic activity and muscle-strengthening exercises) can improve disease outcomes.
- Assistive devices and orthoses such as braces and supports are useful to improve pain and function. Occupational therapy can provide benefits such as appropriate footwear and splinting.
- Weight loss can help decrease stress on joints.
- Surgical options (eg, joint replacements) are reserved for patients with more severe disease with significant cartilage loss.

PHARMACOLOGIC THERAPY

General Approach

- Therapies to treat RA and slow disease progression include conventional and biologic disease-modifying antirheumatic drugs (DMARDs) and the small-molecule oral Janus-kinase (JAK) inhibitors.
  - ✓ Conventional DMARDs include **methotrexate, leflunomide, sulfasalazine,** and **hydroxychloroquine**.
  - ✓ Biologic DMARDs include TNF inhibitors (**adalimumab, certolizumab, etanercept, golimumab,** and **infliximab**) and non-TNF biologics (**abatacept, sarilumab, tocilizumab, rituximab,** and **anakinra**).
  - ✓ JAK inhibitors include **baricitinib, tofacitinib,** and **upadacitinib**.
- Current RA treatment guidelines recommend initiating conventional DMARDs irrespective of disease activity in treatment-naive patients once a diagnosis is established (**Fig. 4-1**).

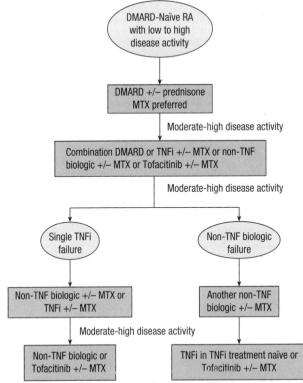

DMARD, disease-modifying antirheumatic drug; MTX, methotrexate; TNFi, tumor necrosis factor inhibitor.

FIGURE 4-1. Algorithm for treatment of rheumatoid arthritis (RA) in early (<6 months) or established (≥6 months) RA with low to high disease activity.

- The preferred conventional DMARD is methotrexate unless a contraindication exists. However, the choice of therapy may depend on the level of disease activity, comorbid conditions, patient preference, and insurance coverage.
- For patients with early RA (<6 months duration) and low disease activity, DMARD monotherapy is recommended. Double or triple DMARD therapy is recommended for moderate or high disease activity. A biologic agent can be used as monotherapy or with conventional DMARD(s) in patients with moderate or high disease activity. A JAK inhibitor is an alternate option if disease activity remains moderate or high with combination conventional DMARDs.
- If disease activity remains moderate or high despite conventional DMARDs or biologics, a low-dose glucocorticoid (prednisone ≤10 mg/day or equivalent) can be added for the shortest duration necessary. If patients achieve remission, DMARDs and biologic agents can be tapered, but patients should remain on DMARD therapy at some dosage level.
- For patients with established RA (duration ≥6 months), DMARD monotherapy is recommended despite disease activity in DMARD-naive patients. Combination conventional DMARDs, a biologic DMARD, or a JAK inhibitor can be used if disease activity remains moderate or high after an adequate trial with DMARD monotherapy. In patients taking TNF inhibitor monotherapy with moderate or high disease activity,

one or two conventional DMARDs can be added to the TNF inhibitor. A non-TNF biologic can be used in place of a TNF inhibitor if disease activity remains moderate or high on a TNF inhibitor and is recommended over a JAK inhibitor. Therapy can be switched to another non-TNF biologic if the first non-TNF agent cannot adequately control disease activity. A non-TNF biologic can also be started if separate courses of two different TNF inhibitors have not adequately controlled disease activity. A JAK inhibitor can be initiated if disease activity persists despite multiple TNF inhibitors in patients for whom non-TNF biologics are not an option. Dual biologic therapy should be avoided due to the risk of infection associated with immunosuppression. A glucocorticoid can be added if disease flares occur or disease activity is inadequately controlled despite DMARD, TNF inhibitor, or non-TNF biologic therapy.

- Because DMARDs can take weeks to months to take effect, nonsteroidal anti-inflammatory drugs (NSAIDs), glucocorticoids, and other analgesics (eg, acetaminophen) can be used to provide more rapid symptomatic relief ("bridge therapy"). NSAIDs do not slow disease progression, and glucocorticoids can have serious side effects, making both drug classes less desirable for long-term use.

- See Tables 4-1 and 4-2 for usual dosages and monitoring parameters for NSAIDs, glucocorticoids, and conventional and biologic DMARDs.

Conventional DMARDs

- **Methotrexate** inhibits dihydrofolate reductase, thereby inhibiting DNA synthesis and repair and cellular replication. Injectable (subcutaneous [SC], intramuscular [IM]) methotrexate has higher bioavailability than oral methotrexate and thus provides superior clinical efficacy; it is typically better tolerated with less potential to cause gastrointestinal (GI) side effects as well. Oral methotrexate doses >15 mg weekly may not have significant added clinical benefit; changing to SC methotrexate may increase bioavailability and clinical benefit in this situation. Clinical benefit can be seen 3–6 weeks after starting therapy. Methotrexate has numerous adverse effects (Table 4-2); concomitant folic acid 1–5 mg/day may reduce some adverse effects without loss of efficacy. Methotrexate is teratogenic, and patients should use contraception and discontinue the drug if conception is planned. Methotrexate is contra-indicated in pregnant and nursing women, chronic liver disease, immunodeficiency, and preexisting hematologic disorders (eg, leukopenia, thrombocytopenia). Methotrexate excretion is reduced in renal impairment and may require dose reduction or discontinuation in some cases.

- **Leflunomide** inhibits pyrimidine synthesis, which reduces lymphocyte proliferation and modulation of inflammation. It can be used as monotherapy or in combination with other DMARDs. Efficacy for RA is similar to that of methotrexate. A loading dose of 100 mg/day for 3 days may achieve steady state more rapidly but may increase the risk for toxicities. The usual maintenance dose of 20 mg/day may be lowered to 10 mg/day in cases of GI intolerance, alopecia, or other dose-related toxicity. Adverse effects are listed in Table 4-2. Leflunomide is teratogenic and should not be used in pregnant or nursing mothers or in patients with severe hepatic impairment.

- **Sulfasalazine** can be used as monotherapy or in combination with other DMARDs. Clinical benefit usually occurs in 4 weeks, but some patients may require 12 weeks. Sulfasalazine use is limited by GI adverse effects (Table 4-2). Sulfasalazine crosses the placenta and is present in breast milk but can be used in pregnant and nursing mothers with caution.

- **Hydroxychloroquine** is typically used in combination with other DMARDs, but it can be used as monotherapy in mild cases. Clinical benefit is delayed and may take several weeks. Its main advantage is that it does not require frequent, routine laboratory monitoring because it is not generally associated with infection risk or hepatic, renal, or blood cell abnormalities. GI side effects can sometimes be mitigated by taking the medication with food or splitting the dose into two doses. Hydroxychloroquine can be continued during pregnancy because no studies have shown an increased risk of birth defects or ocular toxicities. Hydroxychloroquine is excreted into breast milk, and caution should be used in nursing mothers. Periodic

TABLE 4-1 Usual Doses for Disease-Modifying Antirheumatic Drugs

Drugs	Brand Names	Routes of Administration	Starting Dose	Usual Ranges or Maintenance Dose	Comments
Conventional DMARDs					
Methotrexate	Rasuvo Trexall Otrexup (SC)	Oral, SC, IM	Oral: 7.5 mg once weekly or 2.5 mg every 12 hours for 3 doses once weekly SC/IM: 7.5 mg once weekly	7.5–20 mg every week	May be given with folic acid 1–5 mg/day to reduce adverse effects
Leflunomide	Arava	Oral	Loading dose: 100 mg daily for 3 days, then 20 mg daily or 10–20 mg daily without loading dose	10–20 mg daily	Not recommended in liver disease (ALT >3 times ULN)
Hydroxychloroquine	Plaquenil	Oral	200 mg twice daily or 400 mg daily	200 mg twice daily or 400 mg daily	Take with food or milk; use with caution in renal or hepatic impairment
Sulfasalazine	Azulfidine	Oral	500 mg once or twice daily	1000 mg twice daily (maximum 3000 mg/day if inadequate response after 12 weeks of 2000 mg/day)	Not recommended in renal or hepatic impairment
Tumor Necrosis Factor (TNF) Inhibitors					
Adalimumab	Humira	SC	40 mg every 2 weeks	40 mg every 2 weeks (may increase to 40 mg once weekly if not taking methotrexate)	

(Continued)

TABLE 4-1 Usual Doses for Disease-Modifying Antirheumatic Drugs (*Continued*)

Drugs	Brand Names	Routes of Administration	Starting Dose	Usual Ranges or Maintenance Dose	Comments
Certolizumab	Cimzia	SC	400 mg at 0, 2, 4 weeks	200 mg every other week or 400 mg every 4 weeks	
Etanercept	Enbrel	SC	50 mg once weekly or 25 mg twice weekly	Same as starting dose	
Golimumab	Simponi	SC	50 mg once monthly	Same as starting dose	
Infliximab	Remicade	IV	3 mg/kg at 0, 2, 6 weeks, and then every 8 weeks	3–10 mg/kg every 4–8 weeks	Give with methotrexate; pretreat with methylprednisolone, acetaminophen, and antihistamine
Costimulation Modulator					
Abatacept	Orencia	IV, SC	IV: <60 kg: 500 mg, 60–100 kg: 750 mg, >100 kg: 1000 mg at 0, 2, and 4 weeks or initial IV dose followed by 125 mg SC within 24 hours SC: 125 mg weekly	IV: dose based on weight every 4 weeks SC: 125 mg weekly	

IL-6 Receptor Antagonists

Drug	Brand	Route	Starting dose	Maintenance dose	Notes
Sarilumab	Kevzara	SC	200 mg every 2 weeks	Same as starting dose	
Tocilizumab	Actemra	IV, SC	IV: 4 mg/kg every 4 weeks, SC: <100 kg: 162 mg every other week, >100 kg: 162 mg weekly	IV: 4–8 mg/kg every 4 weeks (maximum 800 mg per infusion) SC: <100 kg: 162 mg every other week, followed by an increase to weekly injections if needed; >100 kg: 162 mg weekly	Can increase metabolism of CYP3A4 substrates

Janus Kinase (JAK) Inhibitors

Drug	Brand	Route	Starting dose	Maintenance dose	Notes
Baricitinib	Olumiant	Oral IR	2 mg once daily	Same as starting dose	1 mg once daily in patients taking strong OAT3 inhibitors (eg, probenecid)
Tofacitinib	Xeljanz	Oral	IR: 5 mg twice daily ER: 11 mg daily	Same as starting dose	5 mg once daily in moderate-to-severe renal insufficiency, moderate hepatic impairment, or concomitant CYP3A4 or CYP2C19 inhibitors
Upadacitinib	Rinvoq	Oral ER	15 mg once daily	Same as starting dose	Use with caution with strong CYP3A4 inhibitors; coadministration with strong CYP3A4 inducers is not recommended

(Continued)

TABLE 4-1 Usual Doses for Disease-Modifying Antirheumatic Drugs (*Continued*)

Drugs	Brand Names	Routes of Administration	Starting Dose	Usual Ranges or Maintenance Dose	Comments
Anti-CD20 Monoclonal Antibody					
Rituximab	Rituxan	IV	1000 mg in 2 doses given 2 weeks apart	Initial dose may be repeated every 16–24 weeks based on response	Pretreat with methylprednisolone, acetaminophen, and antihistamine
IL-1 Receptor Antagonist					
Anakinra	Kineret	SC	100 mg once daily	Same as starting dose	

ALT, alanine transaminase; CYP, cytochrome P; ER, extended release; IM, intramuscular; IR, immediate release; IV, intravenous; OAT3, organic anion transporter 3; SC, subcutaneous; ULN, upper limit of normal.

ophthalmologic examinations are necessary for early detection of irreversible retinal toxicity (Table 4-2).

Biologic DMARDs

- Biologic agents are genetically engineered proteins that decrease inflammation by various mechanisms. They are categorized as either TNF inhibitors or non-TNF biologics. They may be effective when conventional DMARDs fail to achieve adequate disease control but are considerably more expensive.
- Biologic DMARDs are associated with an increased risk of infection due to immunosuppressive effects. A tuberculin skin test or interferon gamma release assay blood test should be obtained before starting a biologic to detect and treat latent or active tuberculosis. Patients should also be screened for hepatitis B before starting biologic therapy because of the risk for reactivation.
- Biologics can be used in combination with conventional DMARDs, but multiple biologics should not be used concomitantly due to additive immunosuppressive effects. In general, if patients are switched from one biologic to another, the new agent should be initiated when the patient is due for a dose of the previous biologic. Because of immunosuppressive effects, patients taking biologics should notify their providers if they are being treated for an infection or plan to undergo major surgery. Treatment may need to be held until appropriate postsurgical healing and/or resolution of infection can be confirmed. Live vaccines should not be given to patients taking biologic agents.
- *Biosimilars* are biologic products that have been verified to have no clinically meaningful differences compared to an FDA-approved reference biologic product. These agents can increase access to RA treatment because their costs are lower than the originator products. However, concerns that limit their use include lack of regulatory guidelines about switching from the original biologic product to the biosimilar and uncertainty about extrapolation of indications for biosimilars from the original biologic product.

TNF-α Inhibitors

- TNF inhibitors block the proinflammatory cytokine TNF-α. It may take several weeks for clinical benefit to be noted and up to 3 months to achieve full clinical benefit. These agents are typically used when disease activity remains moderate or high despite conventional DMARD therapy. TNF inhibitors are more expensive than conventional DMARDs.
- Selection of a particular TNF inhibitor depends on cost and patient preference for route and frequency of administration. They should not be used in patients with moderate-to-severe heart failure (New York Heart Association [NYHA] class III/IV) because new-onset and worsening heart failure have been reported. These agents increase the risk of serious infection and malignancies (eg, lymphoma, skin cancers), and new-onset or exacerbation of demyelinating disorders such as multiple sclerosis has been observed.
- See Tables 4-1 and 4-2 for dosing and monitoring information.
  - ✓ **Adalimumab** (Humira) binds to TNF-α and blocks its interaction with the p55 and p75 cell surface TNF receptors. It is available as a prefilled syringe or pen for SC injection.
  - ✓ **Certolizumab** (Cimzia) is a pegylated humanized antibody Fab fragment of TNF-α monoclonal antibody. Because it lacks the Fc region, it does not induce complement activation, antibody-dependent cell-mediated cytotoxicity, or apoptosis. Pegylation allows for delayed elimination and extended half-life. It is available as a prefilled syringe for SC injection.
  - ✓ **Etanercept** (Enbrel) is a recombinant DNA-derived protein composed of TNF receptor linked to the Fc fragment of human IgG1. It is available as a prefilled syringe or pen for SC injection.
  - ✓ **Golimumab** (Simponi) is a human monoclonal antibody that binds to human TNF-α. It is available as a prefilled syringe or pen for SC injection. It is also available as an intravenous (IV) product.

TABLE 4-2	Clinical Monitoring of Drug Therapy in Rheumatoid Arthritis		
Drugs	**Adverse Drug Reactions**	**Initial Monitoring**	**Maintenance Monitoring**
NSAIDs	GI ulceration, bleeding, perforation; renal damage	SCr, CBC every 2–4 weeks after starting therapy	Same as initial plus stool guaiac every 6–12 months
Corticosteroids	Fluid retention, hyperglycemia, hypertension, behavioral and mood changes, increased appetite, weight gain, electrolyte imbalances, impaired healing, hirsutism, Cushing syndrome, HPA axis suppression, osteonecrosis of femoral and humeral heads, osteoporosis and fractures, myopathy, glaucoma, cataracts	Glucose, CBC periodically, BP every 3–6 months	Same as initial
Methotrexate	Infection, hepatic fibrosis, cirrhosis, interstitial pneumonitis, stomatitis, rash, GI perforation, diarrhea, thrombocytopenia, leukopenia	SCr, CBC with differential, AST, ALT, hepatitis B and C screening, tuberculosis screening	SCr, CBC with differential, AST, ALT, every 2–4 weeks for 3 months after starting or following a dose increase, then every 8–12 weeks during 3–6 months of therapy, and every 12 weeks after 6 months of therapy; signs of infection
Leflunomide	Hepatitis, diarrhea/nausea, alopecia, elevated BP	CBC with differential, SCr, ALT, AST, BP	CBC with differential, SCr, ALT, AST every 2–4 weeks for 3 months after starting or following a dose increase, then every 8–12 weeks during 3–6 months of therapy, and every 12 weeks after 6 months of therapy; BP periodically
Sulfasalazine	Rash, nausea, vomiting, diarrhea, photosensitivity, alopecia	CBC with differential, SCr, ALT, AST	CBC with differential, SCr, ALT, AST every 2–4 weeks for 3 months after starting or following a dose increase, then every 8–12 weeks during 3–6 months of therapy, and every 12 weeks after 6 months of therapy

Hydroxychloroquine	Retinal damage, rash, diarrhea	Ophthalmologic exam within 5 years of starting therapy	Ophthalmologic exam annually if risk factors for retinal damage present or annually beginning after 5 years of use if no risk factors
Etanercept, adalimumab, golimumab, certolizumab	Local injection-site reactions, infection, malignancy	Tuberculosis screening, hepatitis B screening, CBC with differential	Periodic skin examination, signs/symptoms of infection and malignancy, CBC with differential periodically
Infliximab	Immune reactions, infection, malignancy	Tuberculosis screening, hepatitis B screening, CBC with differential, LFTs	CBC with differential, LFTs, signs/symptoms of infection and malignancy
Abatacept	Immune reactions, infection, malignancy	Tuberculosis screening, hepatitis B screening	Signs/symptoms of infection and malignancy
Sarilumab	Local injection-site reactions, infection, malignancy	Tuberculosis screening, hepatitis B screening, CBC with differential, LFTs, lipid panel	CBC with differential and LFTs 4–8 weeks after starting and then every 3 months, FLP 4–8 weeks after starting and every 6 months during therapy, signs/symptoms of infection and malignancy
Tocilizumab	Local injection-site reactions, infection, malignancy, GI perforation, neutropenia, thrombocytopenia	Tuberculosis screening, hepatitis B screening, CBC with differential, AST, ALT, FLP	AST, ALT, CBC with differential every 4–8 weeks after starting then every 3 months; FLP after 4–8 weeks of starting then every 6 months; signs/symptoms of infection and malignancy
Baricitinib, tofacitinib, upadacitinib	Infection, malignancy, GI perforations, upper respiratory tract infections, neutropenia, lymphocytopenia, thrombosis	Tuberculosis screening, hepatitis B screening, CBC with differential, Hgb, LFTs, FLP, HR, and BP	CBC with differential and Hgb after 4–8 weeks and every 3 months, FLP after 4–8 weeks and periodically, LFTs periodically, periodic skin examinations, HR and BP, signs/symptoms of infection and malignancy

(Continued)

TABLE 4-2	Clinical Monitoring of Drug Therapy in Rheumatoid Arthritis (*Continued*)		
Drugs	**Adverse Drug Reactions**	**Initial Monitoring**	**Maintenance Monitoring**
Rituximab	Immune reactions, infection, malignancy	Tuberculosis screening, hepatitis B screening, CBC with differential	CBC with differential prior to each treatment course and at 2- to 4-month intervals, signs/symptoms of infection
Anakinra	Local injection site reactions, infection, malignancy	CBC with differential, tuberculosis screening, SCr, hepatitis B screening	CBC with differential every 3 months up to 1 year, SCr periodically, signs/symptoms of infection and malignancy

ALT, alanine transaminase; AST, aspartate transaminase; BP, blood pressure; CBC, complete blood count; FLP, fasting lipid panel; GI, gastrointestinal; Hgb, hemoglobin; HPA, hypothalamic–pituitary–adrenal; HR, heart rate; LFTs, liver function tests; NSAIDs, nonsteroidal anti-inflammatory drugs; SCr, serum creatinine.

✓ **Infliximab** (Remicade) is a chimeric monoclonal antibody that binds to human TNF-α. It is administered as an IV infusion. To prevent formation of an antibody response to this foreign protein, methotrexate must be given orally in doses used to treat RA for as long as the patient continues infliximab. Premedication with an antihistamine, acetaminophen, and/or a glucocorticoid can decrease development of infusion-related reactions. Patients on infliximab plus methotrexate have been shown to have a better clinical response than patients treated with methotrexate alone.

Costimulation Modulator

- **Abatacept** (Orencia) inhibits T-cell activation by binding to CD80 and CD86, which blocks the interaction between T cells CD28, thus inhibiting the activation of T cells. Abatacept is indicated for moderate-to-severe RA and can be used as monotherapy or in conjunction with conventional DMARDs. Abatacept is typically initiated if disease activity persists after conventional DMARD monotherapy and can be an alternative to TNF inhibitors with or without methotrexate. It can also be initiated in patients who have failed or have had an inadequate response to TNF inhibitors. Abatacept plus methotrexate has similar efficacy and incidence of adverse events as adalimumab plus methotrexate in biologic-naive patients who had an incomplete response to methotrexate. Abatacept is available in a prefilled syringe or auto-injector for SC injection and as an IV infusion.

IL-6 Receptor Antagonists

- **Sarilumab** (Kevzara) is indicated for treatment of patients with moderate-to-severe RA who have had an incomplete response or intolerance to one or more DMARDs. It can be used as monotherapy or with conventional DMARDs. It is available as pre-filled syringes for SC injection.
- **Tocilizumab** (Actemra) can be used for patients with moderate-to-severe RA who have had an incomplete response to one or more DMARDs. It can be used alone or in combination with conventional DMARDs. It is available as prefilled syringes for SC injection and as an IV infusion.

Anti-CD20 Monoclonal Antibody

- **Rituximab** (Rituxan) is a monoclonal antibody that binds the CD20 antigen on the surface of B cells. Binding of rituximab to B cells results in nearly complete depletion of peripheral B cells, with a gradual recovery over several months. Rituximab can be initiated in patients with moderate-to-severe RA who have had an incomplete response to one or more TNF inhibitors. Methotrexate should be given concurrently in the usual doses for RA to achieve optimal outcomes. An observational cohort study showed that patients who failed one TNF inhibitor had greater reductions in disease activity scores when treated with rituximab than with a second TNF inhibitor. Rituximab is given as two 1000-mg infusions separated by 2 weeks. Because recovery of B cells can take several months, rituximab can be given every 24 weeks. The decision to re-dose should be based on the return of RA symptoms. Methylprednisolone 100 mg IV is recommended 30 minutes before each infusion as well as acetaminophen and an antihistamine to reduce the incidence and severity of infusion reactions.

IL-1 Receptor Antagonist

- **Anakinra** (Kineret) is an IL-1 receptor antagonist; it is less effective than other biologics, is used infrequently, and is not included in the current ACR treatment recommendations. However, it can be used in patients with moderate-to-severe RA who have failed one or more DMARDs. Anakinra can be used alone or in combination with DMARDs other than TNF-α inhibitors.

Janus-Kinase Inhibitors

- **Baricitinib** (Olumiant), **tofacitinib** (Xeljanz), and **upadacitinib** (Rinvoq) are oral, small-molecule, nonbiologic JAK inhibitors. Baricitinib is FDA-approved for adults with moderately to severely active RA who have had an inadequate response to one or more TNF inhibitors; it may be used alone or in combination with methotrexate or other conventional DMARDs. Tofacitinib and upadacitinib have FDA approval for treatment of adults with moderately to severely active RA who have had an inadequate response or intolerance to methotrexate. These drugs may be used as monotherapy or in combination with methotrexate or other nonbiologic DMARDs. JAK inhibitors should not be given concomitantly with biologic agents.

- Labeling for all JAK inhibitors includes black-box warnings about serious infections, malignancies (including lymphoma), and thrombosis (eg, pulmonary embolism, deep vein thrombosis). Live vaccinations should not be given during treatment. Patients should be tested and treated for latent tuberculosis before starting therapy.

Nonsteroidal Anti-inflammatory Drugs

- NSAIDs inhibit prostaglandin synthesis, which is a small portion of the inflammatory cascade. They possess both analgesic and anti-inflammatory properties and reduce stiffness, but they do not slow disease progression or prevent bony erosions or joint deformity and should not be used as monotherapy for RA treatment. They have a more rapid onset of action than DMARDs and may be beneficial to "bridge" patients while DMARDs take effect. Common NSAID dosage regimens are shown in Table 4-3.

TABLE 4-3	Dosage Regimens for Nonsteroidal Anti-inflammatory Drugs		
	Recommended Total Daily Anti-inflammatory Dosage		
Drug	**Adult**	**Children**	**Dosing Schedule**
Aspirin	2.6–5.2 g	60–100 mg/kg	4 times daily
Celecoxib	200–400 mg	–	Once or twice daily
Diclofenac	150–200 mg	–	3 or 4 times daily; extended release: twice daily
Diflunisal	0.5–1.5 g	–	Twice daily
Etodolac	0.2–1.2 g (max. 20 mg/kg)	–	2–4 times daily
Fenoprofen	0.9–3 g	–	4 times daily
Flurbiprofen	200–300 mg	–	2–4 times daily
Ibuprofen	1.2–3.2 g	20–40 mg/kg	3 or 4 times daily
Indomethacin	50–200 mg	2–4 mg/kg (max. 200 mg)	2–4 times daily; extended release: once daily
Meclofenamate	200–400 mg	–	3–4 times daily
Meloxicam	7.5–15 mg	–	Once daily
Nabumetone	1–2 g	–	Once or twice daily
Naproxen	0.5–1 g	10 mg/kg	Twice daily; extended release: once daily
Naproxen sodium	0.55–1.1 g	–	Twice daily
Nonacetylated salicylates	1.2–4.8 g	–	2–6 times daily
Oxaprozin	0.6–1.8 g (max. 26 mg/kg)	–	1–3 times daily
Piroxicam	10–20 mg	–	Once daily
Sulindac	300–400 mg	–	Twice daily
Tolmetin	0.6–1.8 g	15–30 mg/kg	2–4 times daily

Glucocorticoids

- Glucocorticoids have anti-inflammatory and immunosuppressive properties; although they slow RA progression, glucocorticoids should not be used as monotherapy for RA due to the potential for serious, long-term adverse effects (Table 4-2). They should be used at the lowest effective dose for the shortest period of time. According to the ACR, short-term glucocorticoid therapy is defined as <3 months, and low-dose glucocorticoid is defined as prednisone ≤10 mg/day (or equivalent).
- Similar to NSAIDs, oral glucocorticoids (eg, **prednisone**, **methylprednisolone**) can be used to "bridge" patients while DMARDs take effect. They can also be used as adjuncts to DMARDs at the lowest dose possible in patients with refractory disease. High-dose, short-term bursts can be used as needed for acute flares of RA symptoms, followed by tapering to the lowest effective dose to control symptoms or until discontinued over several days.
- The IM route may be useful in nonadherent patients. Depot forms (**triamcinolone acetonide**, **triamcinolone hexacetonide**, and **methylprednisolone acetate**) provide 2–6 weeks of symptom control. Onset of effect may be delayed for several days. The depot effect provides a physiologic taper, avoiding hypothalamic–pituitary axis suppression.
- Intra-articular injections may be useful when only a few joints are involved. Injections should not be repeated more often than every 3 months because of the potential for accelerated loss of joint cartilage.

EVALUATION OF THERAPEUTIC OUTCOMES

- Assess disease activity at baseline and at each follow-up visit to evaluate therapeutic response. Clinical signs of improvement include reduction in joint pain, swelling, and tenderness; less morning stiffness; reduced fatigue; and improved ability to perform activities of daily living.
- Perform a physical examination at each visit to objectively evaluate the number of swollen and tender joints, joint mobility, and presence of deformity.
- Several assessment tools are available to measure RA disease activity, such as the Clinical Disease Activity Index (CDAI), Disease Activity Score (DAS28), Patient Activity Scale (PAS), Routine Assessment of Patient Index Data 3 (RAPID-3), and Simplified Disease Activity Index (SDAI).
- Laboratory monitoring of acute phase reactants such as CRP and ESR can be useful in assessing inflammation.
- Obtain plain radiographs of the hands, wrists, and forefeet at baseline and every 2 years in patients with low disease activity or in remission. Little to no evidence of RA disease progression should be evident if drug therapy is effective. Imaging may be needed more frequently in patients with moderate or high disease activity. Drug therapy should be modified if patients have radiographic changes suggestive of disease progression (eg, periarticular osteopenia, bone erosions, joint space narrowing).
- It is important to monitor and assess for clinical and laboratory adverse effects of the medications used to treat RA (Table 4-2).

See Chapter 111, Rheumatoid Arthritis, authored by Stephanie Gruber, Bianca Lezcano, and Susan Hylland, for a detailed discussion of this topic.

CHAPTER

5 | Acute Coronary Syndromes

- *Acute coronary syndrome* (ACS) involves acute myocardial ischemia resulting from an imbalance between myocardial oxygen demand and supply. Classification based on electrocardiographic (ECG) changes includes: (1) ST-segment-elevation myocardial infarction (STEMI) or (2) non–ST-segment-elevation ACS (NSTE-ACS), which includes non–ST-segment-elevation MI (NSTEMI) and unstable angina (UA).

PATHOPHYSIOLOGY

- Endothelial dysfunction, inflammation, and formation of fatty streaks contribute to development of atherosclerotic coronary artery plaques. Eventual plaque rupture and subsequent thrombus formation abruptly decreases myocardial blood flow and oxygen supply, leading to ischemia and, potentially, infarction.
- Atherosclerotic plaques that rupture typically have thin fibrous caps and tend to be nonobstructive, occluding <70% of the luminal diameter; thus, patients may not experience angina prior to plaque rupture due to adequate autoregulation that maintains blood flow and oxygen supply during increased myocardial oxygen demand. Increased catecholamine release during physical or emotional stress may enhance the likelihood of rupture of a thinning fibrous cap.
- Plaque rupture breaches the barrier between the necrotic plaque core and blood components; circulating platelets are attracted and adhere to the area of injury. Platelet adhesion occurs via platelet glycoprotein (GP) VI receptors binding to collagen within the damaged fibrotic cap, as well as platelet GP Ib-IX receptors and von Willebrand factor. Platelets are then activated by collagen, thrombin, thromboxane A_2, adenosine diphosphate (ADP), epinephrine, and serotonin. The binding of these activators to their specific receptors on the platelet surface (eg, $P2Y_{12}$ receptor for ADP, protease-activated receptor [PAR]-1 for thrombin) results in increased platelet surface area and release of further platelet activators from granules within platelets. Assembly of tenase and prothrombinase complexes within activated platelets produces most of the activated factor Xa and IIa (thrombin) in the coagulation cascade. A change in the conformation of the GP IIb/IIIa surface receptors of platelets cross-links platelets to each other through fibrinogen bridges, resulting in platelet aggregation and formation of a platelet plug in the area of plaque rupture.
- Activation of the clotting cascade forms a fibrin meshwork (thrombus) around the platelet plug that traps cellular components such as red blood cells and causes abrupt reduction in myocardial blood flow and oxygen supply. If ischemia is left untreated, myocyte necrosis and cell death may ensue.
- Subtypes of myocardial infarction (MI) are based on etiology: (1) rupture, fissure, or erosion of an atherosclerotic plaque (90% of cases); (2) reduced myocardial oxygen supply or increased demand in the absence of a coronary artery process; (3) MI resulting in death without the possibility of measuring biomarkers; (4) MI associated with percutaneous coronary intervention (PCI; Type 4a) or stent thrombosis (Type 4b); and (5) MI associated with coronary artery bypass graft (CABG) surgery.
- After MI, acute and chronic adaptations occur to prevent hemodynamic collapse but may also lead to ventricular remodeling and post-MI complications. Stimulation of the sympathetic nervous system (SNS) and renin–angiotensin–aldosterone system (RAAS) compensates for decreased cardiac output. However, chronic

hyperactivation of these systems can lead to ventricular hypertrophy and further impairment of contractility and cardiac output. The release of inflammatory mediators and collagen deposition contribute to myocardial fibrosis or scarring, which can lead to thinning of the left ventricular (LV) wall and eventual development of dilated cardiomyopathy.

- Complications of MI include ventricular arrhythmias, bradyarrhythmias, heart block, heart failure (HF), cardiogenic shock, LV free-wall or septal rupture, thromboembolism (including stroke secondary to LV thrombus embolization), aneurysm formation, and pericarditis. Many patients with ACS develop depression during the convalescent period.

CLINICAL PRESENTATION

- The patient is typically in acute distress and may present with or develop hypertensive crisis, acute HF, cardiogenic shock, or cardiac arrest.
- The classic symptom of ACS is abrupt-onset substernal chest pain or discomfort often described as a squeezing, heaviness, or tightness that persists for 10 minutes or longer. Symptoms may radiate to the arms and shoulders (especially on the left side), back, abdomen, or jaw. Nausea, vomiting, diaphoresis, or shortness of breath may also be present.
- Many patients have atypical symptoms without chest pain, such as epigastric pain, indigestion, pleuritic chest pain, and increasing exertional dyspnea. Older adults, women, and patients with diabetes mellitus (DM), impaired renal function, and dementia are more likely to present with atypical features.
- No physical examination findings are specific to ACS. Nonspecific findings include S_4 or paradoxical splitting of S_2 heart sounds on auscultation. Signs of acute decompensated HF include jugular venous distention, pulmonary edema, and an S_3 on auscultation. Patients may also present with arrhythmias, heart block, hypertension (HTN), hypotension, or shock.

DIAGNOSIS

- Obtain 12-lead ECG within 10 minutes of presentation. Changes suggestive of acute ischemia include ST-segment elevation (STE), ST-segment depression, and T-wave inversion. Presence of a new left bundle-branch block (LBBB) in patients with suspected ACS is strongly suggestive of acute MI. Some patients with ACS have no ECG changes, so appropriate evaluation and risk stratification must carefully assess medical history, presenting symptoms, and cardiac biomarkers.
- Cardiac troponin (either T or I) is measured at the time of presentation and repeated 3–6 hours later to detect myocardial injury; elevated blood levels (exceeding the 99th percentile of the upper reference limit) occur within 2–4 hours of myocyte injury or necrosis and may remain elevated as long as 2 weeks. Myocardial injury is considered acute if there is a dynamic rise and/or fall by 20% or more in serial troponin values. Elevated levels in a patient with ACS symptoms, ischemic changes on ECG, or other evidence of ischemia confirm the diagnosis of MI. Additional troponin levels should be obtained beyond 6 hours after symptom onset in patients with intermediate- to high-risk features of ACS but normal troponin levels during serial measurements.
- Elevated dynamic cardiac troponin levels with ST-segment elevation of at least 1 mm in two contiguous leads or new LBBB on the presenting ECG confirms the diagnosis of STEMI. In contrast, the diagnosis of NSTEMI is appropriate for patients with symptoms of ACS and elevated troponin levels without at least 1 mm ST-segment elevation on the ECG at presentation. Patients with symptoms consistent with ACS but in whom troponin is not elevated may have UA or an alternative diagnosis.

TREATMENT

- <u>Goals of Treatment</u>: Short-term goals include: (1) early restoration of blood flow to the affected artery to prevent infarct expansion (in the case of MI) or prevent complete occlusion and MI (in UA), (2) prevention of death and other complications, (3) prevention of coronary artery reocclusion, and (4) relief of ischemic chest discomfort. Long-term goals include control of cardiovascular (CV) risk factors, prevention of additional CV events, and improvement in quality of life.

GENERAL APPROACH TO TREATMENT OF ACS

- The clinical presentation, past medical history, ECG, and biomarkers are used to stratify patients as low, medium, or high risk and determine which patients may benefit from reperfusion therapy, an early invasive approach, or medical management. Treatment decisions are based on the initial and ongoing risk stratification (**Fig. 5-1**).
- Because STEMI has the highest short-term risk of death, these patients should be emergently referred for primary PCI; confirmation of elevated troponin should not delay treatment.
- General measures include hospital admission, oxygen administration if saturation is <90% (0.90), bed rest with continuous multilead ECG monitoring for arrhythmias and ischemia, frequent measurement of vital signs, ischemic pain relief, and prompt initiation of antithrombotic therapy.
- Assess kidney function (serum creatinine, creatinine clearance) to identify patients who may need dosing adjustments and those at high risk of morbidity and mortality.
- Measure serum potassium and magnesium levels, which may affect heart rhythm. Obtain complete blood cell count (CBC), fasting lipid panel, and coagulation tests (activated partial thromboplastin time [aPTT] or anti-Xa levels, INR) because most patients will receive antithrombotic therapy.

ACUTE SUPPORTIVE CARE FOR ACS

- **Aspirin** is recommended for all ACS patients without contraindications, regardless of the type of ACS or management strategy. The initial dose is 162–325 mg (nonenteric coated) given as soon as possible and chewed and swallowed to speed dissolution and onset of platelet inhibition (<30 minutes). After the initial dose, aspirin 81 mg daily is continued indefinitely. Contraindications to aspirin include hypersensitivity and major GI intolerance. In these cases, clopidogrel with a loading dose followed by a maintenance dose should be used as an alternative.
- **Nitroglycerin** (NTG) is indicated for relief of anginal symptoms, uncontrolled HTN, and acute HF. The sublingual (SL) dose is 0.3–0.4 mg every 5 minutes for up to 3 doses as needed for angina. Consider intravenous (IV) NTG for persistent angina despite SL NTG at an initial dose of 10 mcg/min titrated to symptom relief and desired blood pressure (BP). Continue IV NTG until symptoms have resolved, BP is controlled, and HF symptoms have subsided. Gradually taper the infusion upon discontinuation. Nitrate administration is contraindicated in patients who have recently taken oral phosphodiesterase-5 (PDE-5) inhibitors (eg, sildenafil).
- **Oxygen** administration (2–4 L/min) should be reserved for select patients, particularly those with oxygen saturation <90% (0.90), because data suggest that routine use may adversely affect patients with ACS by increasing coronary vascular resistance and reducing coronary blood flow.
- **Morphine** is an analgesic, anxiolytic, and venodilator that reduces oxygen demand, but its role in ACS is uncertain because some studies have shown adverse outcomes. Current guidelines recommend IV morphine for pain relief in patients with STEMI. Recommended doses are 4–8 mg IV × 1 (lower dose in elderly), then 2–8 mg IV every 5–15 minutes as needed. In NSTE-ACS, IV morphine use is recommended only in patients refractory to treatment with other anti-ischemic medications; doses between 1 and 5 mg every 5–30 minutes are recommended.
- **β-Blockers** should be administered to all patients without contraindications because they reduce angina and the risk of MI and arrhythmias, even though their mortality benefit in the reperfusion era is uncertain. Current guidelines recommend initiation of an oral β-blocker within the first 24 hours of ACS presentation and continuation for at least 3 years in patients with normal LV ejection fraction (LVEF). For ACS

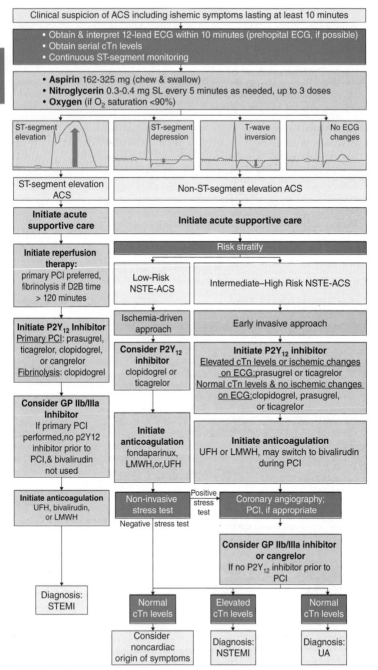

FIGURE 5-1. **Evaluation and initial management of patients with suspected ACS.**

patients with LV dysfunction (LVEF <40% [0.40]), β-blocker therapy is often life-long. Recommended doses include:

✓ **Carvedilol:** 6.25 mg orally twice daily; target dose is 25 mg twice daily as tolerated.

✓ **Metoprolol:** 25–50 mg orally every 6–12 hours for 2–3 days, then once daily (metoprolol succinate) or twice daily (metoprolol tartrate); target dose is 200 mg daily. The IV dose is 5 mg every 5 minutes as tolerated up to three doses, titrated to BP and heart rate (HR); the IV route should be reserved for STEMI patients with acute uncontrolled HTN or refractory symptoms.

- **Calcium channel blockers** (CCBs) have anti-ischemic effects but may not have beneficial effects on mortality, MI, or recurrent MI. Guidelines recommend nondihydropyridine CCBs (diltiazem, verapamil) for angina symptoms in patients with ACS who have a contraindication, have intolerance, or are refractory to β-blockers in the absence of LV dysfunction, risk factors for cardiogenic shock, and atrioventricular conduction defects. Long-acting CCBs are recommended for patients with ACS with known or suspected vasospasm. Recommended doses include:

✓ **Diltiazem:** 120–360 mg/day orally.

✓ **Verapamil:** 240–480 mg/day orally.

✓ **Amlodipine:** 5–10 mg orally once daily.

✓ **Nicardipine:** 60–120 mg/day orally.

✓ **Nifedipine extended-release** (ER): 30–120 mg orally once daily.

TREATMENT STRATEGIES IN STEMI

Primary PCI

- Mechanical reperfusion with PCI using intracoronary balloons, stents, or other devices within 90 minutes of first medical contact is the reperfusion treatment of choice. Patients presenting to hospitals unable to perform PCI should be transferred to a PCI-capable hospital to achieve reperfusion within 120 minutes of the first medical contact. Compared to reperfusion with fibrinolysis, primary PCI improves survival, establishes consistent revascularization to the infarct-related artery, reduces the risk of stroke and intracranial hemorrhage (ICH), and reduces reinfarction and recurrent ischemia.

Fibrinolysis

- Administer fibrinolysis to patients with STEMI when PCI cannot be performed within 120 minutes of first medical contact, provided no contraindications exist. Limit use of fibrinolytics between 12 and 24 hours after symptom onset to patients with clinical and/or ECG evidence of ongoing ischemia.
- Absolute contraindications to fibrinolytic therapy include any prior hemorrhagic stroke, ischemic stroke within 3 months, intracranial neoplasm or AV malformation, active internal bleeding, aortic dissection, considerable facial or closed head trauma in the past 3 months, intracranial or intraspinal surgery within 2 months, severe uncontrolled HTN, and for streptokinase, treatment within previous 6 months (if considering streptokinase again). Primary PCI is preferred in these situations.
- A fibrin-specific agent (alteplase, reteplase, or tenecteplase) is preferred over the non–fibrin-specific agent streptokinase because of greater reperfusion success and less systemic bleeding.
- Treat eligible patients within 30 minutes of hospital arrival with one of the following:
    ✓ **Alteplase:** 15-mg IV bolus over 1–2 minutes, then 0.75 mg/kg (maximum 50 mg) IV over 30 minutes, then 0.5 mg/kg (maximum 35 mg) IV over 60 minutes; maximum total dose 100 mg.
    ✓ **Reteplase:** 10 units IV over 2 minutes, followed 30 minutes later with another 10 units IV over 2 minutes.
    ✓ **Tenecteplase:** Single IV bolus given over 5 seconds based on patient weight: 30 mg if <60 kg; 35 mg if 60–69.9 kg; 40 mg if 70–79.9 kg; 45 mg if 80–89.9 kg; and 50 mg if ≥90 kg.

- Fibrinolytic therapy is associated with a slight but significant risk for stroke, largely attributed to ICH (0.9%–1.0% of patients). Predictors for ICH include advanced age, lower total body weight, female sex, preexisting cerebrovascular disease, and systolic and diastolic HTN at the time of presentation.

Antithrombotic Therapy

- Administer antithrombotic therapy with antiplatelet agents and parenteral anticoagulation concomitantly with both primary PCI and fibrinolysis to improve vessel patency and prevent reocclusion (see "Antithrombotic Therapy for ACS" section below).

TREATMENT STRATEGIES IN NSTE-ACS

Early Invasive Approach

- Patients presenting with NSTE-ACS typically have a partially occluded coronary artery with some residual perfusion; therefore, the need for and urgency to perform PCI is not as critical. With an early invasive approach, diagnostic angiography is typically performed within the first 24 hours with the intent to perform revascularization if appropriate. Guidelines recommend this strategy in patients with intermediate to high risk for death, MI, refractory angina, acute HF, cardiogenic shock, or arrhythmias.

Ischemia-Guided Approach (Medical Management)

- If an early invasive strategy using PCI is not considered appropriate, select low-risk patients may receive more conservative ischemia-guided medical management, where antiplatelet and anticoagulants are administered and PCI is not initially planned. Patients are evaluated for signs and symptoms of recurrent ischemia or hemodynamic instability (eg, with noninvasive stress testing) and taken for coronary angiography and possible PCI only if symptoms recur.

ANTITHROMBOTIC THERAPY FOR ACS

- Both antiplatelet and anticoagulant therapies are necessary in the acute treatment phase of ACS because platelets dominate the pathophysiologic processes in arterial thrombosis, and thrombin is involved in both platelet activation and coagulation. After hospital discharge, most patients are continued on long-term antiplatelet therapy only, although long-term anticoagulant therapy may benefit some high-risk individuals.

Antiplatelet Therapy

- **Aspirin:** A dose of 81 mg daily is continued indefinitely (after the initial 162–325 mg dose) in patients with either STEMI or NSTE-ACS, regardless of the management strategy employed. Patients undergoing PCI for STEMI or NSTE-ACS already receiving chronic aspirin 81 mg daily should be given an additional dose of 81–325 mg before the procedure.
- **$P2Y_{12}$ Inhibitors:** An oral agent (clopidogrel, prasugrel, ticagrelor) is typically given with aspirin as dual antiplatelet therapy (DAPT) to prevent stent thrombosis and thrombotic CV events. Cangrelor is an IV drug indicated as an adjunct to PCI to reduce periprocedural MI, repeat revascularization, and stent thrombosis in patients not receiving oral $P2Y_{12}$ inhibitors or planned GP IIb/IIIa inhibitors. Any of the four agents may be given with primary PCI, but only clopidogrel has been evaluated in large clinical trials in patients with STEMI receiving reperfusion with fibrinolysis. Recommended doses are as follows:
  - ✓ **Clopidogrel:** 600-mg oral loading dose before primary PCI for STEMI or NSTE-ACS. Give a 300-mg oral loading dose to patients receiving a fibrinolytic or who do not receive reperfusion therapy. Avoid a loading dose in patients age ≥75 years. The maintenance dose is 75 mg daily.
  - ✓ **Prasugrel:** 60-mg oral loading dose in patients undergoing PCI, followed by 10 mg orally once daily for patients weighing ≥60 kg; use 5 mg once daily for patients weighing <60 kg.

✓ **Ticagrelor:** 180-mg oral loading dose in patients undergoing PCI, followed by 90 mg orally twice daily.

✓ **Cangrelor:** 30 mcg/kg IV bolus prior to PCI followed by 4 mcg/kg/min infusion for duration of PCI or 2 hours, whichever is longer.

- Withhold clopidogrel and ticagrelor for at least 5 days and prasugrel for 7 days before elective surgery (eg, CABG surgery). Cangrelor can be continued until just a few hours before surgery because of its short duration of action.

Glycoprotein IIb/IIIa Inhibitors (GPIs)

- GPIs inhibit GP IIb/IIIa receptors on platelets, blocking the binding of fibrinogen to activated GP IIb/IIIa receptors, which is the final step in platelet aggregation.
- These agents must be given with unfractionated heparin (UFH) or a low-molecular-weight heparin (LMWH) that should be discontinued immediately after PCI to reduce the risk of major bleeding.
- The use of GPIs has been declining in recent years; patients likely to benefit most are those receiving PCI for NSTE-ACS with elevated troponin levels and patients with STEMI who have not been preloaded with a $P2Y_{12}$ inhibitor and are not being treated with bivalirudin. Recommended doses are as follows:
  ✓ **Abciximab:** 0.25 mg/kg IV bolus given 10–60 minutes before the start of PCI, followed by 0.125 mcg/kg/min (maximum 10 mcg/min) for 12 hours; alternatively, 0.25 mg/kg intracoronary bolus only.
  ✓ **Eptifibatide:** 180 mcg/kg IV bolus, repeated in 10 minutes, followed by IV infusion of 2 mcg/kg/min for 18–24 hours after PCI; reduce infusion dose by 50% if creatinine clearance (CrCl) is <50 mL/min (0.83 mL/sec).
  ✓ **Tirofiban:** 25 mcg/kg IV bolus, then 0.15 mcg/kg/min for up to 18–24 hours after PCI; reduce infusion dose by 50% if CrCl is ≤60 mL/min (1.0 mL/sec).
- GPIs are not beneficial and should not be used in patients with NSTE-ACS undergoing an ischemia-driven approach. GPIs should also be avoided in patients with STEMI receiving reperfusion with fibrinolytics because of significant increases in major bleeding and ICH.
- Besides bleeding, GPIs cause significant thrombocytopenia in about 0.5% of patients. Because GPIs are given with heparin, it is important to differentiate GPI-induced thrombocytopenia from heparin-induced thrombocytopenia (HIT).

Anticoagulants

- Although patients with ACS are typically on at least two antiplatelet agents for a year or more, a single anticoagulant is usually given for a short time (the initial few days of hospitalization).
- Current evidence in the acute management of ACS is with injectable anticoagulants. See Table 5-1 for anticoagulant indications and drug doses in ACS.
- **UFH** has been widely used in ACS management for several decades. Based on experience, UFH can be used across the spectrum of ACS and regardless of the management strategy. Because of significant interpatient variability in anticoagulant response, therapy must be monitored with the aPTT every 6 hours until two consecutive readings are within the institution's therapeutic range (1.5–2 times the control value), then every 24 hours for the duration of UFH therapy. The activated clotting time (ACT) is monitored during PCI because it can be measured at the bedside with rapid results. Platelet counts should also be monitored daily or every other day to detect HIT. If HIT is suspected, discontinue UFH and provide anticoagulation with an IV direct thrombin inhibitor.
- **LMWHs** provide a predicable anticoagulant dose response with no need for routine therapeutic monitoring. Anti-Xa level monitoring may be helpful in obese patients (>190 kg) and patients with severe renal insufficiency (eg, CrCl <30 mL/min [0.5 mL/sec]). The target peak anti-Xa level is 0.3–0.7 IU/mL (kIU/L) drawn 4 hours after the third dose. The utility of anti-Xa monitoring is limited because patients with ACS typically receive anticoagulant therapy for only a few days. Although the

TABLE 5-1 Anticoagulant Drug Use and Dosing for Treatment of Acute Coronary Syndrome

| | STEMI | | NSTE-ACS | |
Drug	Primary PCI	Fibrinolytic Perfusion	Early Invasive Strategy	Ischemia-Driven Strategy
Bivalirudin	0.75 mg/kg IV bolus, followed by 1.75 mg/kg/h IV infusion until completion of PCI CrCl <30 mL/min (0.5 mL/sec): reduce infusion to 1 mg/kg/h	No recommendation	0.10 mg/kg IV bolus, followed by 0.25 mg/kg/h IV infusion until completion of PCI	No recommendation
Enoxaparin	0.5 mg/kg one-time IV bolus	30 mg IV bolus, followed within 15 minutes by 1 mg/kg SC every 12 hours for up to 8 days or hospital discharge; cap first two SC doses at 100 mg CrCl <30 mL/min (0.5 mL/sec): 30 mg IV bolus, followed by 1 mg/kg SC every 24 hours; cap first dose at 100 mg Age ≥75 years: omit IV bolus and initiate 0.75 mg/kg SC every 12 hours; cap first two doses at 75 mg CrCl <30 mL/min (0.5 mL/sec) and age ≥75: omit IV bolus and initiate at 1 mg/kg every 24 hours	1 mg/kg SC every 12 hours until PCI; may give an initial 30 mg IV bolus Give 0.3 mg/kg IV bolus if PCI occurs before two SC doses have been given, or if the last dose was given 8 hours or more prior to PCI CrCl <30 mL/min (0.5 mL/s): 1 mg/kg SC every 24 hours	1 mg/kg SC every 12 hours for duration of hospitalization; may give an initial 30 mg IV bolus CrCl <30 mL/min (0.5 mL/sec): 1 mg/kg SC every 24 hours

Fondaparinux	No recommendation	2.5 mg IV first dose, followed by 2.5 mg SC daily for up to 8 days or hospital discharge	2.5 mg SC daily until PCI. At the time of PCI, if no GPI give 85 units/kg IV UFH[a] if with GPI give 60 units/kg IV UFH[a]	2.5 mg SC daily for up to 8 days or duration of hospitalization.
UFH	If no GPI, 70–100 units/kg IV bolus to achieve therapeutic ACT[a]. If taking GPI, 50–70 units/kg IV bolus to achieve therapeutic ACT[a]	60 units/kg (max. 4000 units) IV bolus, followed by 12 units/kg/h (max. initial infusion rate 1000 units/h)	60 units/kg (max. 4000 units) IV bolus, followed by 12 units/kg/h (max. initial infusion rate 1000 units/h)[a]	60 units/kg (max. 4000 units) IV bolus, followed by 12 units/kg/h (max. initial infusion rate 1000 units/h)

ACT, activated clotting time; CrCl, creatinine clearance; GPI, glycoprotein IIb/IIIa inhibitor; IV, intravenous; NSTE-ACS, non-ST-segment elevation acute coronary syndrome; PCI, percutaneous coronary intervention; SC, subcutaneous; STEMI, ST-segment elevation myocardial infarction; UFH, unfractionated heparin.

[a]Additional IV UFH boluses may be needed to maintain a therapeutic ACT.

incidence of HIT is lower with LMWHs (<2%) than with UFH (2%–5%), monitoring of platelet counts is still warranted. Due to 90% cross-reactivity between HIT antibodies from LMWH and UFH, LMWH is not a safe alternative in patients who develop HIT from UFH and vice versa.

✓ **Enoxaparin** is the most widely studied agent in ACS and is the only LMWH recommended in current guidelines. Data support its efficacy in patients with STEMI and NSTE-ACS, regardless of the perfusion or management strategy used. However, enoxaparin dosing varies across these different situations (Table 5-1). In patients with STEMI receiving reperfusion with fibrinolytics, enoxaparin significantly reduced death and MI compared to UFH. Based on clinical trial data, either UFH or enoxaparin is recommended in patients with NSTE-ACS.

- **Fondaparinux** provides a predicable anticoagulant dose response with no need for therapeutic monitoring (similar to LMWH). A clinical trial in NSTE-ACS patients receiving either an ischemia-driven or invasive management strategy demonstrated similar efficacy between fondaparinux and enoxaparin, with significantly less major bleeding in patients receiving fondaparinux. Although confounding factors may account for the bleeding difference, fondaparinux can be considered in patients undergoing an ischemia-driven approach who are at high risk of bleeding. Fondaparinux is not recommended in patients receiving primary PCI for STEMI because of clinical trial results demonstrating higher rates of catheter-related thrombosis compared to UFH. In patients with STEMI receiving fibrinolytics, fondaparinux had efficacy and safety similar to UFH. However, fondaparinux is rarely used in patients with STEMI based on the lack of superiority to UFH and the benefit shown with enoxaparin over UFH in this population.

- **Bivalirudin** is a direct thrombin inhibitor that is used only in patients with ACS who receive PCI and can be monitored with the ACT in the catheterization laboratory. Although current guidelines recommend bivalirudin use, UFH is often used instead because recent trials suggested that bivalirudin does not offer efficacy or safety benefits over UFH alone in the setting of primary PCI for STEMI. Bivalirudin has not been evaluated in patients with STEMI receiving reperfusion with fibrinolytics or in patients with NSTE-ACS undergoing an ischemia-driven approach.

SECONDARY PREVENTION OF ISCHEMIC EVENTS

- After a diagnosis of ACS, patients are considered to have atherosclerotic cardiovascular disease (ASCVD) and should be treated aggressively because they are at the highest risk of recurrent major adverse cardiovascular events (MACE).

- Aggressive risk factor modification strategies should be initiated and continued indefinitely (eg, increased physical activity, dietary modification, weight loss, BP modification, and smoking cessation).

- Pharmacotherapy, proven to decrease mortality, HF, reinfarction, stroke, and stent thrombosis, should be initiated prior to hospital discharge in all patients without contraindications. This includes anti-ischemic, antiplatelet, lipid-lowering, and antihypertensive therapies.

- Medication reconciliation at discharge should include assessment for the medication classes listed below as appropriate unless a contraindication exists; drug regimen examples within medication classes listed here are not intended to be exhaustive.

- **Aspirin:** Treat with aspirin 81 mg once daily indefinitely.

- **P2Y$_{12}$ inhibitor:** Because the ischemic risk following ACS is high, DAPT with aspirin plus a P2Y$_{12}$ receptor inhibitor is indicated for most patients for at least 12 months regardless of the management strategy employed. Continuation of DAPT beyond 12 months may be reasonable for patients at higher ischemic risk if they also have a low bleeding risk. For patients with STEMI treated with fibrinolysis, the minimum recommended duration of DAPT is 14 days.

  ✓ Clopidogrel: 75 mg once daily.
  ✓ Prasugrel: 10 mg once daily (5 mg daily if body weight <60 kg).
  ✓ Ticagrelor: 90 mg twice daily.

- **β-Blocker:**
  - ✓ Carvedilol: 6.25 mg twice daily; target dose (in patients with HF with reduced ejection fraction [HFrEF]) 25 mg twice daily as tolerated.
  - ✓ Metoprolol: 25–50 mg every 6–12 hours for 2–3 days, then once daily (metoprolol succinate) or twice daily (metoprolol tartrate); target dose (in patients with HFrEF) 200 mg daily.
  - ✓ Other β-blockers may be considered; in patients with HFrEF, use either metoprolol succinate, carvedilol, or bisoprolol; continue therapy for at least 3 years and indefinitely in patients with concomitant HFrEF.
- **Statin:** Initiate high-intensity statin therapy during the index hospitalization once the patient has been stabilized and continue treatment indefinitely. All patients should receive the highest dose of maximally tolerated statin:
  - ✓ Atorvastatin: 80 mg daily.
  - ✓ Rosuvastatin: 20–40 mg daily.
  Moderate-intensity statins or lower doses of high-intensity statins may be considered for ACS patients with a history of statin intolerance or those at high risk for statin-related adverse effects. Patients over age 75 may be prescribed a moderate-intensity statin as initial therapy. Reassess a lipid panel 4–6 weeks after initiation of therapy with the goal of a 50% reduction in LDL-C from baseline.
- **Nonstatin cholesterol-lowering medications:** For patients with very high-risk ASCVD (eg, post-ACS) and LDL-C >70 mg/dL (1.81 mmol/L) on maximally tolerated statin therapy.
  - ✓ Ezetimibe: 10 mg daily.
  - ✓ Simvastatin: 40 mg/ezetimibe 10 mg daily.
  - ✓ Alirocumab: 75 mg subcutaneous (SC) every 2 weeks or 300 mg SC every 4 weeks.
  - ✓ Evolocumab 140 mg SC every 2 weeks or 420 mg SC monthly.
- **Angiotensin-converting enzyme (ACE) inhibitor:** Early administration (within 48 hours of presentation) is associated with lower mortality within the first month of therapy with additional benefit observed during over longer treatment durations.
  - ✓ Lisinopril: 2.5–5 mg daily; target dose 10–40 mg daily.
  - ✓ Enalapril 2.5-5 mg twice daily; target dose 10-20 mg twice daily.
  - ✓ Captopril: 6.25–12.5 mg three times daily; target dose 25–50 mg three times daily.
  - ✓ Ramipril: 2.5 mg twice daily; target dose 5 mg twice daily.
  - ✓ Trandolapril: 0.5–1 mg daily; target dose 4 mg daily.
- **Angiotensin receptor blocker (ARB):** Patients intolerant to ACE inhibitors:
  - ✓ Valsartan: 20 mg twice daily; target dose 160 mg twice daily.
- **Aldosterone antagonist:** To reduce mortality, consider administration within the first 14 days after MI in patients treated with both an ACE inhibitor (or ARB) and β-blocker with LV dysfunction (LVEF ≤40% [0.40]) and either HF symptoms or DM.
  - ✓ Eplerenone: 25 mg daily; target dose 50 mg daily.
  - ✓ Spironolactone: 12.5–25 mg daily; target dose 25–50 mg daily.
- **Nitroglycerin:** All patients not taking PDE-5 inhibitors should be prescribed and instructed on appropriate use of short-acting NTG, either SL tablets (0.3–0.4 mg SL every 5 minutes, up to three doses) or lingual spray to relieve acute anginal symptoms on an as-needed basis.

EVALUATION OF THERAPEUTIC OUTCOMES

- Evaluation of short-term efficacy focuses on restoration or preservation of coronary blood flow, symptom relief, and prevention of MACE.
- Determine restoration of blood flow and relief of ischemia by resolution of ischemic ECG changes on presentation, which should occur soon after revascularization.
- Although troponin levels may remain elevated for several days, levels in patients with MI should peak within 12–24 hours and then decline steadily once ischemia is relieved.
- Monitor for development of ACS complications (eg, HF, arrhythmias) frequently.

- Prior to hospital discharge, perform echocardiogram or equivalent modality to identify patients with LV dysfunction (LVEF <40% [0.40]) who are at high risk of death and candidates for guideline-directed medical therapy and device therapy.
- Assure that evidence-based therapies shown to reduce the risk of MACE following ACS have been initiated.
- Long-term outcome evaluation is directed at maintaining functional capacity, quality of life, and continued focus on risk reduction.
- Monitor patients at every healthcare encounter for development of adverse effects from ACS pharmacotherapy (Table 5-2).

See Chapter 34, Acute Coronary Syndrome, authored by Robert J. DiDomenico, Paul P. Dobesh, and Shannon W. Finks, for a more detailed discussion of this topic.

TABLE 5-2	Adverse Drug Effect Monitoring for Acute Coronary Syndrome	
Drug	**Adverse Effects**	**Monitoring Parameters**
Fibrinolytics	Bleeding (ICH)	Clinical signs of bleeding[a]; baseline aPTT, INR; Hgb, Hct, platelet count at baseline then daily; mental status every 2 hours for signs of ICH
Aspirin	Dyspepsia, GI bleeding	Clinical signs of bleeding[a]; GI upset; Hgb, Hct, and platelet count at baseline and every 6 months
P2Y$_{12}$ inhibitors	Bleeding, rash	Clinical signs of bleeding[a]; evidence of rash; Hgb, Hct, platelet count at baseline and every 6 months
	Ticagrelor: dyspnea, ventricular pauses, bradycardia	Ticagrelor: dyspnea, HR, telemetry during hospitalization
Glycoprotein IIb/ IIIa inhibitors	Bleeding, thrombocytopenia (can be profound with abciximab)	Clinical signs of bleeding[a]; Hgb, Hct, and platelet count at baseline, 2 hours, then daily
		Eptifibatide and tirofiban: SCr at baseline then daily
Anticoagulants	Bleeding	Clinical signs of bleeding[a]; baseline aPTT, INR; Hgb, Hct, platelet count at baseline then daily
	UFH and LMWH: heparin-induced thrombocytopenia	UFH: aPTT every 6 hours until two consecutive aPTT values are at goal, then every 24 hours; monitor the ACT during PCI
		Enoxaparin, bivalirudin, and fondaparinux: SCr at baseline then daily
		Enoxaparin: may consider steady-state anti-Xa levels in select populations
β-Blockers	Hypotension, HF, bradycardia, cardiogenic shock, AV block, exacerbation of asthma or reactive airway disease	Continuous telemetry (while hospitalized); BP, HR, signs and symptoms of HF; monitor every 5 min before each IV bolus dose; monitor every shift while hospitalized then at each healthcare encounter after discharge
Nitroglycerin	Flushing, headache, hypotension, tachycardia	BP and HR; monitor every 5–15 min following dosage adjustment of IV NTG then every 1–2 hours; monitor every 5 min following administration of short-acting NTG
Morphine	Hypotension, respiratory depression, sedation, hypersensitivity	BP, HR, respiratory rate, sedation level 5 min after administration then every 1–2 hours for 4 hours after the last dose

(Continued)

TABLE 5-2	Adverse Drug Effect Monitoring for Acute Coronary Syndrome (Continued)	
Drug	**Adverse Effects**	**Monitoring Parameters**
Calcium channel blockers	Hypotension	BP and HR every shift while hospitalized, then at each healthcare encounter after discharge
	Verapamil and diltiazem: HF, cardiogenic shock, bradycardia, AV block	Verapamil and diltiazem: continuous telemetry (while hospitalized); signs and symptoms of HF every shift while hospitalized, then at each healthcare encounter after discharge
Statins	GI discomfort, arthralgia, myalgia, musculoskeletal pain, hepatotoxicity	Liver function tests at baseline (prior to discharge) and if signs or symptoms of hepatotoxicity develop; creatine kinase if severe myalgia or musculoskeletal symptoms occur; LDL-C at baseline, 4–12 weeks after initiation or dose adjustment, then every 3–12 months
Nonstatin therapies for cholesterol management	Ezetimibe and combination: GI discomfort, arthralgia, myalgia, musculoskeletal pain	Simvastatin/ezetimibe: liver function tests at baseline (prior to discharge) and if signs or symptoms of hepatotoxicity develop; creatinine kinase if severe myalgia or musculoskeletal symptoms occur; LDL-C at baseline, 4–12 weeks after initiation or dose adjustment, then every 3–12 months
	Alirocumab: injection site pain, hypersensitivity	Alirocumab: LDL-C at baseline and 4–8 weeks after initiation or dose adjustment; evaluation of injection site if injection site pain develops, signs and symptoms of hypersensitivity with each healthcare encounter
ACE inhibitors	Hypotension, hyperuricemia, hyperkalemia, worsening renal function, chronic cough, angioedema	BP every shift while hospitalized, 1–2 weeks after initiation or dose adjustment, then with each healthcare encounter; SCr and potassium at baseline, 1–2 weeks after initiation, then every 6–12 months; signs and symptoms of angioedema or cough with each healthcare encounter
ARBs	Hypotension, hyperuricemia, hyperkalemia, worsening renal function	BP every shift while hospitalized, 1–2 weeks after initiation or dose adjustment, then with each healthcare encounter; SCr and potassium at baseline, 1–2 weeks after initiation, then every 6–12 months
Aldosterone antagonist	Hyperkalemia, worsening renal function	BP every shift while hospitalized, 1–2 weeks after initiation or dose adjustment, then with each healthcare encounter; SCr and potassium at baseline, after initiation or dose adjustment at 3 days, 1 week, monthly for 3 months, then every 3 months

ACE, angiotensin-converting enzyme; ACT, activated clotting time; aPTT, activated partial thromboplastin time; ARB, angiotensin receptor blocker; AV, atrioventricular; BP, blood pressure; GI, gastrointestinal; Hct, hematocrit; HF, heart failure; Hgb, hemoglobin; HR, heart rate; ICH, intracranial hemorrhage; INR, international normalized ratio; IV, intravenous; LDL-C, low-density lipoprotein cholesterol; LMWH, low-molecular-weight heparin; NTG, nitroglycerin; PCI, percutaneous coronary intervention; SCr, serum creatinine; UFH, unfractionated heparin.
^aClinical signs of bleeding include bloody stools, melena, hematuria, hematemesis, bruising, and oozing from arterial or venous puncture sites.

Arrhythmias

- *Cardiac arrhythmia* involves a group of conditions in which the heartbeat is irregular, too slow, or too fast. *Supraventricular arrhythmias* occur above the ventricles, and *ventricular arrhythmias* occur within the ventricles.

PATHOPHYSIOLOGY

SUPRAVENTRICULAR ARRHYTHMIAS

Atrial Fibrillation and Atrial Flutter

- Atrial fibrillation (AF) has extremely rapid (400–600 atrial beats/min) and disorganized atrial activation. There is a loss of atrial contraction (atrial kick), and supraventricular impulses penetrate the atrioventricular (AV) conduction system to variable degrees, resulting in irregular ventricular activation and an irregularly irregular pulse. The AV node will not conduct most of the supraventricular impulses, causing the ventricular response to be considerably slower than the atrial rate.
- Atrial flutter has rapid (270–330 atrial beats/min) but regular atrial activation. Ventricular response usually has a regular pattern and a pulse of 300 beats/min. This arrhythmia is less common than AF but has similar precipitating factors, consequences, and drug therapy approach.
- AF may result from multiple atrial reentrant loops (or wavelets), triggered, or abnormal automaticity; whereas atrial flutter is caused by a single, dominant, reentrant substrate. Both abnormal rhythms usually occur in association with various forms of structural heart disease that causes atrial distension.

Paroxysmal Supraventricular Tachycardia

- Paroxysmal supraventricular tachycardia (PSVT) arising by reentrant mechanisms includes arrhythmias caused by AV nodal reentry (AVNRT), AV reentrant tachycardia (AVRT) due to an accessory pathway, sinoatrial (SA) nodal reentry, and intra-atrial reentry.

VENTRICULAR ARRHYTHMIAS

Premature Ventricular Complexes

- Premature ventricular complexes (PVCs) can occur in patients with or without structural heart disease (SHD). PVCs may be elicited by abnormal automaticity, triggered activity, or reentrant mechanisms. PVCs often occur in healthy individuals and have little, if any, prognostic significance in this situation. PVCs occur more frequently and in more complex forms in patients with SHD than in healthy individuals, and patients with some PVC forms (multifocal or couplets) are at higher risk of sudden cardiac death.

Ventricular Tachycardia

- Ventricular tachycardia (VT) is defined by three or more repetitive PVCs occurring at a rate of >100 beats/min. It is a wide QRS tachycardia that may result acutely from severe electrolyte abnormalities (hypokalemia, hypomagnesemia), hypoxia, drug toxicity (eg, digoxin), or (most commonly) in patients presenting with acute myocardial infarction (MI) or myocardial ischemia complicated by heart failure (HF). The chronic recurrent form is almost always associated with SHD (eg, idiopathic dilated cardiomyopathy or remote MI with left ventricular [LV] aneurysm).
- Sustained VT requires intervention to restore a stable rhythm or persists for a relatively long time (usually >30 seconds). Nonsustained VT self-terminates after a brief duration (usually <30 seconds). Incessant VT refers to VT occurring more

frequently than sinus rhythm, so that VT becomes the dominant rhythm. Monomorphic VT has a consistent QRS configuration, whereas polymorphic VT has varying QRS complexes. Torsades de pointes (TdP) is a polymorphic VT in which the QRS complexes appear to undulate around a central axis.

Ventricular Proarrhythmia

- Proarrhythmia is the development of a significant new arrhythmia, such as VT, ventricular fibrillation (VF), or TdP, or worsening of an existing arrhythmia. Proarrhythmia results from the same mechanisms that cause other arrhythmias or from an alteration in the underlying substrate due to an antiarrhythmic drug (AAD).
    ✓ Class Ic AADs can cause a rapid, sustained, monomorphic VT with a characteristic sinusoidal QRS pattern resulting from excessive sodium channel blockade and slowed conduction. The proarrhythmia risk continues as long as the AAD is continued. Predisposing factors include the presence of underlying ventricular arrhythmias, coronary artery disease (CAD), and LV dysfunction.
    ✓ TdP is a rapid form of polymorphic VT associated with evidence of delayed ventricular repolarization due to blockade of potassium conductance. TdP may be hereditary or acquired. Acquired forms are associated with many clinical conditions and drugs, especially class Ia and class III I_{Kr} blockers. Development of clinically significant QTc interval prolongation (ie, QTc interval >500 msec or an increase in QTc interval of >60–70 msec from baseline) after starting a drug is an indication to discontinue the agent or reduce its dose with careful monitoring.

Ventricular Fibrillation

- VF is electrical anarchy of the ventricle resulting in no cardiac output and cardiovascular (CV) collapse. Sudden cardiac death occurs most commonly in patients with CAD or LV dysfunction.

BRADYARRHYTHMIAS

- Sinus bradyarrhythmias (heart rate <60 beats/min) are common, especially in young, athletically active individuals, and are usually asymptomatic and do not require intervention. However, some patients have sinus node dysfunction (sick sinus syndrome) because of underlying SHD and the normal aging process, which attenuates SA nodal function. Sinus node dysfunction is usually representative of diffuse conduction disease, which may be accompanied by AV block and by paroxysmal tachycardias such as AF. Alternating bradyarrhythmias and tachyarrhythmias are referred to as the tachy–brady syndrome.
- AV block or conduction delay may occur in any area of the AV conduction system. AV block may be found in patients without underlying heart disease (eg, trained athletes) or during sleep when vagal tone is high. It may be transient when the underlying etiology is reversible (eg, myocarditis, myocardial ischemia, after CV surgery, or during drug therapy). β-Blockers, digoxin, or nondihydropyridine (non-DHP) calcium channel blockers (CCBs) may cause AV block, primarily in the AV nodal area. Class I AADs may exacerbate conduction delays below the level of the AV node. AV block may be irreversible if the cause is acute MI, rare degenerative diseases, primary myocardial disease, or congenital heart disease.

CLINICAL PRESENTATION

- Patients with AF or atrial flutter may complain of rapid heart rate, palpitations, chest pain, dyspnea, dizziness, and fatigue. Medical emergencies are severe HF (ie, pulmonary edema, hypotension) or AF occurring in the setting of acute MI. These arrhythmias are usually not directly life-threatening and do not generally cause hemodynamic collapse or syncope.
- PSVT caused by reentry can be transient, resulting in few, if any, symptoms. Patients may complain of intermittent episodes of rapid heart rate/palpitations that abruptly

start and stop, usually without provocation (but sometimes with exercise). Patients may also complain of chest pressure or a neck sensation. Life-threatening symptoms (syncope, hemodynamic collapse) are associated with an extremely rapid heart rate (eg, >200 beats/min) and AF associated with an accessory pathway.

- PVCs are non–life-threatening and usually asymptomatic. Patients occasionally complain of palpitations or uncomfortable heartbeats. Because the PVC occurs early and the ventricle contracts when incompletely filled, patients do not feel the PVC itself; rather, the sinus beat following the PVC and a compensatory pause is responsible for the symptoms.
- The symptoms of sustained VT (monomorphic VT or TdP) can range from nearly asymptomatic to pulseless hemodynamic collapse. Fast heart rates and underlying poor LV function result in more severe symptoms. Symptoms of nonsustained, self-terminating VT correlate with duration of episodes (eg, patients with 15-second episodes will be more symptomatic than those with 3-beat episodes).
- VF results in hemodynamic collapse, syncope, and cardiac arrest. Cardiac output and blood pressure are not recordable.
- Some patients who develop proarrhythmia may be asymptomatic, others may notice worsening symptoms, and some may die suddenly.
- Symptoms of bradyarrhythmias generally result from decreased cardiac output and may be associated with hypotension (eg, dizziness, syncope, fatigue, confusion). If LV dysfunction exists, patients may experience worsening HF symptoms. Except for recurrent syncope, symptoms associated with bradyarrhythmias are often subtle and nonspecific.

DIAGNOSIS

- On ECG, AF is an irregularly irregular rhythm with no discernible, consistent atrial activity (P waves). Ventricular rate is usually 90–170 beats/min and the pulse is irregular. Atrial flutter is usually a regular supraventricular rhythm with characteristic flutter waves reflecting more organized atrial activity; the ventricular rate is often in factors of 300 beats/min (eg, 150, 100, or 75 beats/min).
- The ECG in patients with PSVT commonly shows a rapid, narrow QRS tachycardia (regular in rhythm) that starts and stops abruptly. Atrial activity, although present, is difficult to ascertain on ECG because P waves are "buried" in the QRS complex or T wave.
- Proarrhythmia can be difficult to diagnose because of the variable nature of underlying arrhythmias.
- TdP is characterized by long QT intervals or prominent U waves on the ECG.
- First-degree AV block is 1:1 AV conduction with a prolonged PR interval. Second-degree AV block is divided into two forms: Mobitz I AV block (Wenckebach periodicity) is <1:1 AV conduction with progressively lengthening PR intervals until a ventricular complex is dropped; Mobitz II AV block is intermittently dropped ventricular beats in a random fashion without progressive PR lengthening. Third-degree AV block is complete heart block where AV conduction is totally absent (AV dissociation).

TREATMENT

- <u>Goals of Treatment</u>: The desired outcome depends on the underlying arrhythmia. For example, the goals of treating AF or atrial flutter are restoring sinus rhythm, preventing thromboembolic complications, and preventing further recurrences.

GENERAL APPROACH

- Use of AADs has declined because clinical trials showed increased mortality with their use due to proarrhythmic side effects and limited efficacy. AADs have been increasingly replaced by nonpharmacologic approaches such as ablation and the implantable cardioverter-defibrillator (ICD).

ANTIARRHYTHMIC DRUGS

- Drugs may depress the automatic properties of abnormal pacemaker cells by decreasing the slope of phase 4 depolarization and/or by elevating threshold potential. Drugs may alter conduction characteristics of the pathways of a reentrant loop.
- The Vaughan Williams classification system of AADs is frequently used for categorizing their electrophysiologic actions (Table 6-1).
  - ✓ Class Ia drugs are sodium channel blockers. Class Ia drugs slow conduction velocity, prolong refractoriness, and decrease the automatic properties of sodium-dependent (normal and diseased) conduction tissue. Class Ia drugs are effective for both supraventricular and ventricular arrhythmias, but they are infrequently used because of limited efficacy and significant toxicities.
  - ✓ Class Ib drugs probably act similarly to class Ia drugs, except that class Ib agents are considerably more effective in ventricular than supraventricular arrhythmias.
  - ✓ Class Ic drugs slow conduction velocity while leaving refractoriness relatively unaltered. Although effective for both ventricular and supraventricular arrhythmias, their use for ventricular arrhythmias has been limited by the risk of proarrhythmia.
  - ✓ Class II drugs include β-blockers; their antiarrhythmic effects result from anti-adrenergic actions. β-Blockers are most useful in tachycardias in which nodal tissues are abnormally automatic or are a portion of a reentrant loop. These agents are also helpful in slowing ventricular response in atrial tachycardias (eg, AF) by effects on the AV node.
  - ✓ Class III drugs prolong refractoriness in atrial and ventricular tissue and include very different drugs that share the common effect of delaying repolarization by blocking potassium channels. **Amiodarone** and **sotalol** are effective in most supraventricular and VTs. Amiodarone displays electrophysiologic characteristics

TABLE 6-1	Classification of AADs			
Class	**Drug**	**Conduction Velocity**[a]	**Refractory Period**	**Automaticity**	**Ion Block**
Ia	Quinidine	↓	↑	↓	Sodium (intermediate)
	Procainamide				
	Disopyramide				Potassium
Ib	Lidocaine	0/↓	↓	↓	Sodium (fast on–off)
	Mexiletine				
Ic	Flecainide	↓↓	0	↓	Sodium (slow on–off)
	Propafenone[b]				
II[c]	β-Blockers	↓	↑	↓	Calcium (indirect)
III	Amiodarone[d]	0	↑↑	0	Potassium
	Dofetilide				
	Dronedarone[d]				
	Sotalol[b]				
	Ibutilide				
IV[c]	Verapamil	↓	↑	↓	Calcium
	Diltiazem				

0, no change; ↑, increased; ↓, decreased.
[a]Variables for normal tissue models in ventricular tissue.
[b]Also has β-blocking actions.
[c]Variables for sinoatrial (SA) and atrioventricular (AV) nodal tissue only.
[d]Also has sodium, calcium, and β-blocking actions.

of all four Vaughan Williams classes. It is a sodium channel blocker with relatively fast on–off kinetics, has nonselective β-blocking actions, blocks potassium channels, and has slight calcium-blocking activity. Sotalol inhibits outward potassium movement during repolarization and also possesses nonselective β-blocking actions. **Dronedarone**, **ibutilide**, and **dofetilide** are indicated only for treatment of supraventricular arrhythmias.

✓ Class IV drugs include the non-DHP CCBs (**verapamil**, **diltiazem**), which inhibit calcium entry into cells, thereby slowing conduction, prolonging refractoriness, and decreasing SA and AV nodal automaticity. They are effective for automatic or reentrant tachycardias that arise from or use the SA or AV nodes.

- See Table 6-2 for recommended doses of oral AADs, Table 6-3 for usual IV antiarrhythmic doses, and Table 6-4 for common side effects.

ATRIAL FIBRILLATION OR ATRIAL FLUTTER

- The Atrial Fibrillation Better Care (ABC) approach to treating AF can be organized into several sequential goals: "A" Anticoagulation/Avoid stroke; "B" Better symptom management; and "C" Cardiovascular and Comorbidity optimization. This approach improves outcomes and reduces CV events and health-related costs (Fig. 6-1).

A—Anticoagulation/Avoid Stroke

- Traditionally, **warfarin** was used for stroke prevention in patients at moderate or high risk for stroke due to AF. If warfarin is used, the target INR range should be 2–3 and the time in therapeutic range (TTR) should ideally be >70%. Guidelines now recommend a direct oral anticoagulant (DOAC) over warfarin, including the direct thrombin inhibitor **dabigatran** and the factor Xa inhibitors **apixaban**, **edoxaban**, and **rivaroxaban**.
- Before selecting the most appropriate antithrombotic regimen, assess the patient's risk for stroke using the CHA_2DS_2VASc risk scoring system. If anticoagulation is indicated, evaluate the patient's risk for bleeding using the HAS-BLED score.

TABLE 6-2	Typical Maintenance Doses of Class I and Class III Oral AADs	
Drug	**Dose**	**Dose Adjusted**
Disopyramide	Immediate-release: 100–150 mg every 6 hours	HEP, REN
	Controlled-release: 200–300 mg every 12 hours	
Quinidine	200–300 mg sulfate every 6 hours	HEP
	324–648 gluconate every 8–12 hours	
Mexiletine	200–300 mg every 8 hours	HEP
Flecainide	50–200 mg every 12 hours	HEP, REN
Propafenone	150–300 mg every 8 hours	HEP
	225–425 mg every 12 hours (SR form)	
Amiodarone	400 mg 1–3 times daily until 10 g total, and then 100–400 mg daily[a]	None
Dofetilide	500 mcg every 12 hours	REN[b]
Dronedarone	400 mg twice daily (with meals)[c]	HEP
Sotalol	80–160 mg every 12 hours	HEP

HEP, hepatic disease; REN, renal impairment; SR, sustained release.
[a]Usual maintenance dose for atrial fibrillation is 200 mg/day (may further decrease dose to 100 mg/day with long-term use if patient clinically stable in order to decrease risk of toxicity); usual maintenance dose for ventricular arrhythmias is 300–400 mg/day.
[b]Dose should be based on creatinine clearance; should not be used when creatinine clearance <20 mL/min.
[c]Should not be used in severe hepatic impairment.

TABLE 6-3	Intravenous Antiarrhythmic Dosing	
Drug	**Clinical Situation**	**Dose**
Amiodarone	Pulseless VT/VF	300 mg IV/IO push (can give additional 150 mg IV/IO push if persistent VT/VF or if VT/VF recurs), followed by infusion of 1 mg/min for 6 hours, and then 0.5 mg/min × 18 hours
	Stable VT (with a pulse)	150 mg IV over 10 min, followed by infusion of 1 mg/min for 6 hours, and then 0.5 mg/min × 18 hours
	AF (termination)	150 mg IV over 10 min, followed by infusion of 1 mg/min for 6 hours, and then 0.5 mg/min × 18 hours
	AF (rate control)	300 mg IV over 1 hour, then 10–50 mg/h over 24 hours
Diltiazem	PSVT; AF (rate control)	0.25 mg/kg IV over 2 min (may repeat with 0.35 mg/kg IV over 2 min), followed by infusion of 5–15 mg/h
Ibutilide	AF (termination)	1 mg IV over 10 min (may repeat once if needed, 10 minutes after initial dose)
Lidocaine	Pulseless VT/VF	1–1.5 mg/kg IV/IO push (can give additional 0.5–0.75 mg/kg IV/IO push every 5–10 min if persistent VT/VF [maximum cumulative dose = 3 mg/kg]), followed by infusion of 1–4 mg/min (1–2 mg/min if liver disease or HF)
	Stable VT (with a pulse)	1–1.5 mg/kg IV push (can give additional 0.5–0.75 mg/kg IV push every 5–10 min if persistent VT [maximum cumulative dose = 3 mg/kg]), followed by infusion of 1–4 mg/min (1–2 mg/min if liver disease or HF)
Procainamide	AF (termination); stable VT (with a pulse)	15–18 mg/kg IV over 60 min, followed by infusion of 1–4 mg/min
Verapamil	PSVT; AF (rate control)	2.5–5 mg IV over 2 min (may repeat up to maximum cumulative dose of 20 mg); can follow with infusion of 2.5–10 mg/h

AF, atrial fibrillation; HF, heart failure; IO, intraosseous; IV, intravenous; PSVT, paroxysmal supraventricular tachycardia; VF, ventricular fibrillation; VT, ventricular tachycardia.

- After successful cardioversion, patients with AF and other risk factors for stroke should continue antithrombotic therapy because undetected episodes of paroxysmal AF may place them at risk for stroke.

B—Better Symptom Management

Ventricular Rate Control

- In patients with persistent AF, a rate control strategy (regulating only the ventricular rate while remaining remain in AF) has been compared with or rhythm control (restoring and maintaining normal sinus rhythm) in multiple clinical trials. Rhythm control does not offer any significant advantage over rate control, so the preferred strategy is driven primarily by the goal of improving the patient's quality of life.

TABLE 6-4	Adverse Drug Reactions of Class I and Class III AADs
Disopyramide	Anticholinergic symptoms (dry mouth, urinary retention, constipation, blurred vision), nausea, anorexia, HF, conduction disturbances, ventricular arrhythmias (eg, TdP)
Procainamide	Hypotension, worsening HF, conduction disturbances, ventricular arrhythmias (eg, TdP)
Quinidine	Cinchonism, diarrhea, abdominal cramps, nausea, vomiting, hypotension, worsening HF, conduction disturbances, ventricular arrhythmias (eg, TdP), fever
Lidocaine	Dizziness, sedation, slurred speech, blurred vision, paresthesia, muscle twitching, confusion, nausea, vomiting, seizures, psychosis, sinus arrest, conduction disturbances
Mexiletine	Dizziness, sedation, anxiety, confusion, paresthesia, tremor, ataxia, blurred vision, nausea, vomiting, anorexia, conduction disturbances, ventricular arrhythmias
Flecainide	Blurred vision, dizziness, dyspnea, headache, tremor, nausea, worsening HF, conduction disturbances, ventricular arrhythmias
Propafenone	Dizziness, fatigue, blurred vision, bronchospasm, headache, taste disturbances, nausea, vomiting, bradycardia or AV block, worsening HF, ventricular arrhythmias
Amiodarone	Tremor, ataxia, paresthesia, insomnia, corneal microdeposits, optic neuropathy/neuritis, nausea, vomiting, anorexia, constipation, TdP (<1%), bradycardia or AV block (IV and oral use), pulmonary fibrosis, liver function test abnormalities, hypothyroidism, hyperthyroidism, photosensitivity, blue-gray skin discoloration, hypotension (IV use), phlebitis (IV use)
Dofetilide	Headache, dizziness, TdP
Dronedarone	Nausea, vomiting, diarrhea, serum creatinine elevations, bradycardia, worsening HF, hepatotoxicity, pulmonary fibrosis, acute renal failure, TdP (<1%)
Ibutilide	Headache, TdP, bradycardia or AV block, hypotension
Sotalol	Dizziness, weakness, fatigue, nausea, vomiting, diarrhea, bradycardia or AV block, TdP, bronchospasm, worsening HF

AV, atrioventricular; HF, heart failure; IV, intravenous; TdP, torsades de pointes.

- For rate control, target a resting heart rate <110 beats/min for asymptomatic patients with preserved LV systolic function (left ventricular ejection fraction [LVEF] >40% [0.40]). For patients who are symptomatic or have LVEF ≤40% (0.40), consider targeting a resting heart rate <80 beats/min.
- In patients with preserved LV function, a β-blocker or nondihydropyridine (DHP) CCB (diltiazem or verapamil) is preferred over digoxin because of their relatively quick onset and maintained efficacy during exercise. Avoid CCBs in patients with HFrEF (LVEF ≤40% [0.40]) because of their negative inotropic effects; β-Blockers and digoxin are preferred in that situation.
- Amiodarone can be used if adequate rate control during rest and exercise cannot be achieved with β-blockers, non-DHP CCBs, and/or digoxin. However, amiodarone may stimulate the conversion of AF to sinus rhythm and place the patient at risk for a thromboembolic (TE) event.

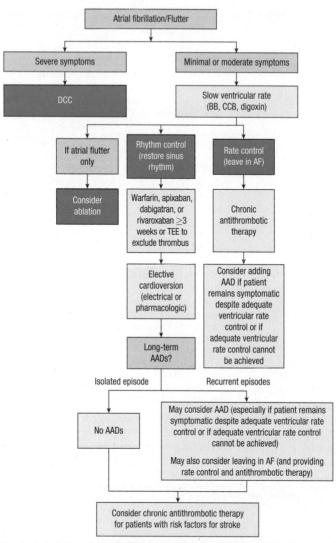

AAD, antiarrhythmic drug; AF, atrial fibrillation; AFl, atrial flutter; BB, β-blocker; CCB, calcium channel blocker (ie, verapamil or diltiazem); DCC, direct current cardioversion; TEE, transesophageal echocardiogram.

FIGURE 6-1 Algorithm for the treatment of AF and atrial flutter.

Rhythm Control

- Restoring sinus rhythm increases the risk for a TE event because return of effective atrial contraction may dislodge poorly adherent thrombi.
- Administering anticoagulant therapy prior to cardioversion prevents clot growth and the formation of new thrombi and allows existing thrombi to become organized and well adherent to the atrial wall.

- The risk of thrombus formation and a subsequent embolic event increases if the duration of the AF exceeds 48 hours. Patients undergoing elective electrical or pharmacologic cardioversion for AF lasting at least 48 hours or for an unknown duration should ideally receive anticoagulation with warfarin or a DOAC for at least 3 weeks before cardioversion. If 3 weeks of therapeutic oral anticoagulant therapy is not feasible, a screening transesophageal echocardiogram (TEE) can be performed prior to cardioversion to evaluate for the presence of thrombus in the heart chambers. If cardioversion is successful (ie, patient is now in SR), anticoagulation with warfarin (INR target range 2–3) or a DOAC should be continued for at least 4 weeks.
- Patients with AF less than 48 hours in duration do not require a prolonged period of anticoagulation prior to cardioversion because there has not been sufficient time to form atrial thrombi. However, an oral anticoagulant, LMWH or unfractionated heparin should be started as soon as possible.
- The two methods for restoring sinus rhythm are pharmacologic cardioversion and direct current cardioversion (DCCV). Disadvantages of pharmacologic cardioversion are the risk of significant side effects (eg, drug-induced TdP, drug–drug interactions) and lower efficacy of AADs compared with DCCV. DCC is quick and more often successful (80%–90% success rate), but it requires periprocedural sedation/anesthesia and has a small risk of serious complications, such as sinus arrest or ventricular arrhythmias. Clinicians may elect to use AADs first, and then resort to DCCV if these medications fail. Pharmacologic cardioversion is most effective when initiated within 7 days after the onset of AF. There is good evidence for cardioversion efficacy of class III pure Ik blockers (**ibutilide, dofetilide**), class Ic drugs (eg, **flecainide**, **propafenone**), and **amiodarone** (oral or IV).
- Single oral loading doses of propafenone (body weight >70 kg: 600 mg; <70 kg: 450 mg) and flecainide (body weight >70 kg: 300 mg; <70 kg: 200 mg) are effective for cardioversion of recent-onset AF. These regimens have been incorporated into the "pill in the pocket" approach, whereby outpatient, patient-controlled self-administration of a single oral dose of either flecainide or propafenone is used to terminate recent-onset AF in select patients without sinus or AV node dysfunction, bundle-branch block, or SHD. This method should only be considered for patients who have been successfully cardioverted with these medications on an inpatient basis.
- The following AADs are recommended for maintaining SR, depending on underlying SHD and other comorbidities: amiodarone, dofetilide, dronedarone, flecainide, propafenone, and sotalol. Amiodarone appears to be the most effective AAD to maintain SR, but because of potential toxicities it should only be used after considering its risks and when other agents have failed or are contraindicated.
- In patients with no SHD, **dofetilide**, **dronedarone**, **flecainide**, **propafenone**, or **sotalol** should be considered initially. **Amiodarone** is second-line if the patient fails or does not tolerate one of these drugs. In patients with HF, amiodarone or dofetilide are the AADs of first choice. In patients with CAD dofetilide, dronedarone, or sotalol can be used initially, with amiodarone as an alternative if the patient fails or does not tolerate one of the initial AADs. Flecainide and propafenone should be avoided in the presence of SHD because of the risk of proarrhythmia.

PAROXYSMAL SUPRAVENTRICULAR TACHYCARDIA

- Both pharmacologic and nonpharmacologic methods have been used to treat PSVT. Drugs can be divided into three broad categories: (1) those that directly or indirectly increase vagal tone to the AV node (eg, digoxin), (2) those that depress conduction through slow, calcium-dependent tissue (eg, adenosine, β-blockers, and non-DHP CCBs), and (3) those that depress conduction through fast, sodium-dependent tissue (eg, quinidine, procainamide, disopyramide, and flecainide). Drugs within these categories alter the electrophysiologic characteristics of the reentrant substrate so that PSVT cannot be sustained.

- Acute management for patients with AVNRT or orthodromic AVRT includes vagal maneuvers and/or adenosine. If these options are ineffective or unfeasible in a hemodynamically unstable patient, synchronized DCCV is the next step. If vagal techniques and adenosine are ineffective or unfeasible in a hemodynamically stable patient, the next step is administration of an IV β-blocker or non-DHP CCB. If AVNRT cannot be corrected with these measures, IV amiodarone can be used. For patients with AVRT, the next step is synchronized cardioversion.
- After an acute episode of AVNRT or AVRT is terminated, long-term prophylaxis is indicated if frequent episodes necessitate therapeutic intervention or if episodes are infrequent but severely symptomatic. AADs are no longer the treatment of choice to prevent recurrences of reentrant PSVT but may be necessary occasionally, particularly in patients with mild symptoms and infrequent recurrences. Drugs effective in preventing recurrences are the AV nodal blocking drugs (digoxin, β-blockers, non-DHP CCBs, and combinations of these agents) and the class Ic AADs (flecainide, propafenone). Sotalol, dofetilide, and amiodarone can be considered alternatives.
- Catheter ablation using radiofrequency current on the PSVT substrate is the preferred treatment strategy (over AADs) for patients with symptomatic PSVT. It is highly effective and curative, rarely results in complications, obviates need for chronic AAD therapy, and is cost effective.

PREMATURE VENTRICULAR COMPLEXES

- IPVCs carry little or no risk when the frequency is low in individuals without SHD; thus, medication therapy is unnecessary. In addition, AADs should not be used to suppress asymptomatic PVCs. In post-MI patients, β-blocker use is associated with a reduction in mortality and SCD, especially in the presence of LV dysfunction. β-Blockers and non-DHP CCBs can be used in patients without underlying SHD to suppress symptomatic PVCs.

VENTRICULAR TACHYCARDIA

Acute Ventricular Tachycardia

- Like other rapid tachycardias, the initial management of an acute episode of VT (with a pulse) requires a quick assessment of the patient's signs and symptoms. If VT is an isolated electrical event associated with a transient initiating factor (eg, acute myocardial ischemia or digitalis toxicity), there is no need for long-term antiarrhythmic therapy after precipitating factors are corrected.
- Patients presenting with an acute episode of sustained monomorphic VT and hemodynamically instability should have advanced cardiovascular life support (ACLS) initiated immediately, including DCCV to restore SR. In patients with stable monomorphic VT who have SHD, cardioversion should be implemented and IV procainamide, amiodarone, or sotalol can be considered. For patients without SHD, verapamil and β-blockers are first-line options.

Sustained Ventricular Tachycardia

- Once an acute episode of sustained VT has been successfully terminated by electrical or pharmacologic means and an acute MI has been ruled out, the possibility of recurrent episodes of VT should be considered. Patients who survive an acute episode of sustained VT are at extremely high risk for death, and the yield for finding an effective AAD via electrophysiologic testing is low.
- Numerous trials have established ICDs as superior to AADs not only for preventing SCD in patients who have been resuscitated from cardiac arrest or had sustained VT ("secondary prevention") but also for preventing an initial episode of SCD in certain high-risk patient populations ("primary prevention").

Ventricular Proarrhythmia

- The proarrhythmia caused by the class Ic AADs is often resistant to resuscitation with cardioversion or overdrive pacing. IV **lidocaine** (which competes for the sodium channel receptor) or **sodium bicarbonate** (which reverses the excessive sodium channel blockade) has been used successfully by some clinicians.

Torsades de Pointes

- For an acute episode of TdP, most patients require and respond to defibrillation. However, TdP tends to be paroxysmal and often recurs rapidly after defibrillation.
- IV **magnesium sulfate** is the drug of choice for preventing recurrences of TdP. If ineffective, institute strategies to increase heart rate and shorten ventricular repolarization (ie, temporary transvenous pacing at 105–120 beats/min or pharmacologic pacing with **isoproterenol**). Discontinue agents that prolong the QT interval and correct exacerbating factors (eg, hypokalemia and hypomagnesemia). Lidocaine is usually ineffective, and AADs that further prolong repolarization (eg, IV procainamide) are absolutely contraindicated.

Ventricular Fibrillation

- Patients with pulseless VT or VF should have ACLS initiated immediately, including defibrillation to restore SR.

BRADYARRHYTHMIAS

- Asymptomatic sinus bradyarrhythmias usually do not require treatment.
- Treatment of sinus node dysfunction involves eliminating symptomatic bradycardia and potentially managing alternating tachycardias such as AF. In general, permanent pacemaker implantation is the long-term therapy of choice. Drugs commonly used to treat supraventricular tachycardias should be used with caution, if at all, in the absence of a functioning pacemaker.
- Symptomatic carotid sinus hypersensitivity also should be treated with permanent pacemaker therapy. However, some patients still experience syncope or dizziness even after pacemaker implantation.
- Patients with vasovagal syncope should receive education targeting awareness and trigger avoidance (ie, prolonged standing or warm environments). First-line treatment includes counterpressure maneuvers (eg, laying on the ground, squatting), followed by increasing salt and fluid intake, when not contraindicated. The drug of choice is midodrine, an alpha-agonist that reduces the peripheral sympathetic neural outflow that causes venous pooling and vasodepression. β-Blockers are used to prevent episodes of vasovagal syncope in patients 42 years of age and older. Other drugs that have been used successfully include **fludrocortisone**, anticholinergics (**scopolamine patches** and **disopyramide**), α-adrenergic agonists (**midodrine**), adenosine analogues (**theophylline, dipyridamole**), and selective serotonin reuptake inhibitors (**sertraline, paroxetine**).

Atrioventricular Block

- If patients with second- or third-degree AV block develop signs or symptoms of poor perfusion (eg, altered mental status, chest pain, hypotension, shock) administer **atropine** (0.5 mg IV given every 3–5 minutes, up to 3 mg total dose). Transcutaneous pacing can be initiated in patients unresponsive to atropine. Infusions of **epinephrine** (2–10 mcg/min) or **dopamine** (2–10 mcg/kg/min) can also be used in the event of atropine failure. These agents usually do not help if the site of the AV block is below the AV node (Mobitz II or trifascicular AV block).
- Chronic symptomatic AV block warrants insertion of a permanent pacemaker. Patients without symptoms can sometimes be followed closely without the need for a pacemaker.

EVALUATION OF THERAPEUTIC OUTCOMES

• The most important monitoring parameters include: (1) mortality (total and sudden cardiac death), (2) arrhythmia recurrence (duration, frequency, and symptoms), (3) hemodynamic consequences (rate, blood pressure, and symptoms), and (4) treatment complications (adverse drug reactions or need for alternative or additional drugs, devices, or surgery).

See Chapter 40, Arrhythmias, authored by Jessica J. Tilton, Stephen T. Phillips, and Jerry L. Bauman, for a more detailed discussion of this topic.

Cardiac Arrest

- *Cardiac arrest* is defined as cessation of cardiac mechanical activity as confirmed by absence of signs of circulation (eg, detectable pulse, unresponsiveness, apnea).

PATHOPHYSIOLOGY

- Coronary artery disease is the most common finding in adults with cardiac arrest and causes ~75% of sudden cardiac deaths. In pediatric patients, cardiac arrest typically results from respiratory failure, asphyxiation, or progressive shock.
- Noncardiac causes include drowning, choking, asphyxia, electrocution, trauma, poisoning, severe asthma, pneumonia, drug overdose, and sudden infant death syndrome.
- Two different pathophysiologic conditions are associated with cardiac arrest:
  ✓ Primary: arterial blood is fully oxygenated at the time of arrest.
  ✓ Secondary: respiratory failure with lack of ventilation leads to severe hypoxemia, hypotension, and cardiac arrest.
- Cardiac arrest in adults usually results from arrhythmias. Historically, ventricular fibrillation (VF) and pulseless ventricular tachycardia (PVT) were most common, but data now indicate that nonshockable rhythms (ie, asystole, pulseless electrical activity [PEA]) are more prevalent. This change is of concern because survival rates to hospital discharge are higher after shockable rhythms like VF and PVT than after nonshockable rhythms like asystole and PEA.

CLINICAL PRESENTATION

- Cardiac arrest may be preceded by anxiety, shortness of breath, crushing chest pain, nausea, vomiting, and diaphoresis.
- Signs include apnea; hypotension; no detectable pulse; cyanosis; cold, clammy extremities; loss of consciousness; and syncope.

DIAGNOSIS

- Rapid diagnosis is vital to success and is made by observing clinical manifestations consistent with cardiac arrest.
- Electrocardiography (ECG) identifies the cardiac rhythm, which in turn determines drug therapy.
  ✓ VF is electrical anarchy of the ventricle resulting in no cardiac output and cardiovascular collapse.
  ✓ PEA is absence of a detectable pulse and presence of some type of electrical activity other than VF or PVT.
  ✓ Asystole occurs when there is no electrical activity in the heart, indicated by a flat line on the ECG.

TREATMENT

- Goals of Treatment: Resuscitation goals are to preserve life; restore health; relieve suffering; limit disability; and respect the individual's decisions, rights, and privacy. This can be accomplished via cardiopulmonary resuscitation (CPR) by return of spontaneous circulation (ROSC) with effective ventilation and perfusion quickly to minimize hypoxic damage to vital organs. After successful resuscitation, the primary outcome is survival to hospital discharge with good neurologic function.

GENERAL APPROACH

- The online American Heart Association (AHA) guidelines for CPR and emergency cardiovascular care (ECC) are updated continuously and emphasize timely implementation of the "chain of survival":
  ✓ For out-of-hospital arrests: (1) early recognition of cardiac arrest and activation of the emergency response system, (2) high-quality CPR, (3) rapid defibrillation, (4) advanced cardiac life support (ACLS), (5) post-arrest care, and (6) recovery.
  ✓ For in-hospital arrests: (1) early recognition and prevention of cardiac arrest, (2) activation of emergency response, (3) high-quality CPR, (4) prompt defibrillation, (5) post-arrest care, and (6) recovery.

Basic Life Support Given by Healthcare Providers

- The mnemonic for the CPR sequence is "CAB" (circulation, airway, breathing). Basic life support *given by healthcare providers trained in CPR* includes the following actions performed in this order:
  ✓ First, determine patient responsiveness. If unresponsive with no breathing or no normal breathing (ie, only gasping), activate the emergency medical response team and obtain an automated external defibrillator (AED).
  ✓ Check for a pulse, but if not definitely felt within 10 seconds, begin CPR with chest compressions and use the AED when available.
  ✓ Begin CPR with 30 chest compressions at a rate of 100–120/min and a compression depth of at least 2 in (5 cm) in adults and at least one-third of the anteroposterior chest diameter in infants and children (~1.5 in [4 cm] in infants and 2 in [5 cm] in children).
  ✓ Open the airway and deliver 2 rescue breaths, then repeat chest compressions. Follow each cycle of 30 chest compressions by 2 rescue breaths.
  ✓ Continue CPR until an AED is ready for use or ACLS providers take over care.
  ✓ If/when an AED is available, check rhythm to determine if defibrillation is advised. If so, deliver one shock with immediate resumption of chest compressions/rescue breaths for 2 minutes or until prompted by the AED to allow for another rhythm check.
  ✓ If the rhythm is not shockable, resume CPR immediately for 2 minutes or until prompted by the AED. Continue this cycle until ACLS providers take over or the victim starts to move.

Advanced Cardiac Life Support

- Once ACLS providers arrive, further definitive therapy is given following the ACLS algorithm shown in **Fig. 7-1**.
- A bag-mask device or an advanced airway (eg, endotracheal tube, supraglottic device) may be used to provide ventilation. One provider can deliver 1 breath every 6 seconds while a second provider performs continuous chest compressions.
- Central venous catheter access results in faster and higher peak drug concentrations than peripheral venous administration, but central line access is not needed in most resuscitation attempts. However, if a central line is already present, it is the access site of choice. If IV access (either central or peripheral) has not been established, insert a large peripheral venous catheter. If this is unsuccessful, insert an intraosseous (IO) device.
- If neither IV nor IO access can be established, **lidocaine**, **epinephrine**, **naloxone**, and **vasopressin** may be administered endotracheally. The endotracheal dose should generally be 2–2.5 times larger than the IV/IO dose. Dilute the medications in 5–10 mL of either sterile water (preferred) or normal saline.

TREATMENT OF VENTRICULAR FIBRILLATION AND PULSELESS VENTRICULAR TACHYCARDIA

Nonpharmacologic Therapy

- VF and PVT are shockable rhythms. CPR alone is not likely to terminate VF/PVT, and defibrillation is often necessary to restore cardiac rhythm.

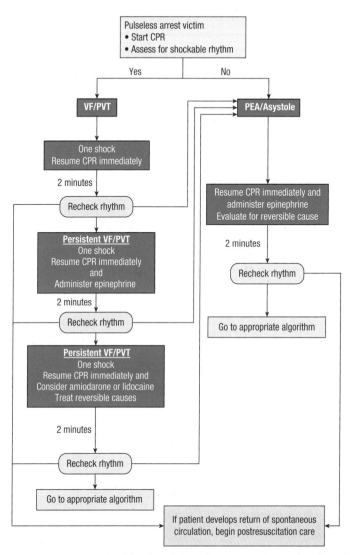

FIGURE 7-1. Treatment algorithm for adult cardiac arrest: Advanced cardiac life support (ACLS).

Pharmacologic Therapy

Epinephrine

- **Epinephrine** is the drug of first choice for treating VF, PVT, asystole, and PEA. It is an α- and β-receptor agonist, causing vasoconstriction and increased rate and forcefulness of heart contractions, thereby augmenting low coronary and cerebral perfusion pressures.

- The recommended adult dose of epinephrine is 1 mg administered by IV or IO injection every 3–5 minutes. Although higher doses have been studied, they are not recommended for routine use in cardiac arrest.

Vasopressin

- **Vasopressin** is a potent nonadrenergic vasoconstrictor that increases blood pressure (BP) and systemic vascular resistance. Despite some theoretical advantages, clinical outcomes are not superior to standard-dose epinephrine alone or to the combination of vasopressin and epinephrine.

Antiarrhythmics

- The purpose of antiarrhythmic drug therapy after unsuccessful defibrillation and vasopressor administration is to prevent development or recurrence of VF and PVT. However, clinical evidence demonstrating improved survival to hospital discharge is lacking.
- **Amiodarone** or **lidocaine** may be considered in adults with VF/PVT refractory to defibrillation and epinephrine.
- The amiodarone dose is 300 mg IV/IO followed by a second dose of 150 mg.
- The initial lidocaine dose is 1–1.5 mg/kg IV. Additional doses of 0.5–0.75 mg/kg can be administered at 5- to 10-minute intervals to a maximum total dose of 3 mg/kg if VF/PVT persists.

Magnesium

- Severe hypomagnesemia has been associated with VF/PVT, but routine administration of magnesium during cardiac arrest has not improved clinical outcomes. Two trials showed improved ROSC in cardiac arrests associated with torsades de pointes; therefore, limit magnesium administration to these patients. The dose is 1–2 g diluted in 10 mL of 5% dextrose in water administered IV/IO push over 15 minutes.

Thrombolytics

- Thrombolytic use during CPR has been investigated because most adult cardiac arrests are related to either myocardial infarction (MI) or pulmonary embolism (PE). However, a randomized trial of tenecteplase vs placebo showed no improvement in ROSC or survival to hospital discharge, and the incidence of intracranial hemorrhage was greater with the thrombolytic. Therefore, fibrinolytic therapy should not be used routinely in cardiac arrest but may be considered when PE is suspected.

TREATMENT OF PULSELESS ELECTRICAL ACTIVITY AND ASYSTOLE

Nonpharmacologic Therapy

- Successful treatment of PEA and asystole depends on diagnosis of the underlying cause. Potentially reversible causes include: (1) hypovolemia, (2) hypoxia, (3) acidosis, (4) hyper- or hypokalemia, (5) hypothermia, (6) hypoglycemia, (7) drug overdose, (8) cardiac tamponade, (9) tension pneumothorax, (10) coronary thrombosis, (11) pulmonary thrombosis, and (12) trauma.
- PEA and asystole are treated the same way. Both conditions require CPR, airway control, and IV access. Avoid defibrillation because the resulting parasympathetic discharge can reduce the chance of ROSC and decrease the likelihood of survival.

Pharmacologic Therapy

- **Epinephrine** (1 mg by IV or IO injection every 3–5 minutes) is the primary pharmacologic agent used and should be administered as soon as possible.

ACID–BASE MANAGEMENT

- Acidosis occurs during cardiac arrest because of decreased blood flow or inadequate ventilation. Chest compressions generate only about 25% of normal cardiac output, leading to inadequate organ perfusion, tissue hypoxia, and metabolic acidosis. Lack of ventilation causes CO_2 retention, leading to respiratory acidosis. Acidosis reduces myocardial contractility and lowers the fibrillation threshold.

- Routine use of sodium bicarbonate in cardiac arrest is not recommended because it has not been shown to improve ROSC or survival to hospital discharge, and it may have detrimental effects. It can be used in special circumstances (eg, hyperkalemia, tricyclic antidepressant overdose, salicylate toxicity).

POSTRESUSCITATIVE CARE

- ROSC from a cardiac arrest may be followed by a post-cardiac arrest syndrome characterized by hypoxic brain injury, myocardial dysfunction, systemic ischemia-reperfusion response, and the underlying persistent precipitating pathology.
- It is imperative to ensure adequate airway and oxygenation. After use of 100% oxygen during the resuscitation effort, titrate the oxygen fraction down as tolerated to maintain an oxyhemoglobin saturation of 92-98% (0.92-0.98). Overventilation can be avoided by using end-tidal (ET) CO_2 measurements.
- Evaluate for ECG changes consistent with acute MI immediately and perform revascularization if present.
- Because cerebral hypoperfusion may persist for several hours after resuscitation, augmenting BP to achieve a goal of mean arterial pressure (MAP) >80 mm Hg has been recommended.
- Therapeutic hypothermia or targeted temperature management (TTM) can protect against cerebral injury by suppressing chemical reactions that occur after restoration of blood flow. Although randomized controlled trials produced mixed results with respect to improved neurologic function and survival, guidelines recommend TTM between 32°C and 36°C for at least 24 hours. Prevent fever after the TTM period. Potential complications of TTM include coagulopathy, dysrhythmias, bradycardia, diuresis, electrolyte disorders, hyperglycemia, infection risks, and effects on drug distribution and clearance.

EVALUATION OF THERAPEUTIC OUTCOMES

- The optimal outcome following CPR is an awake, responsive, spontaneously breathing patient. Patients must remain neurologically intact with minimal morbidity after resuscitation if it is to be considered successful.
- In many cases, rhythm assessment via ECG and pulse checks are the only physiologic parameters available to guide therapy. However, palpating a pulse to determine efficacy of blood flow during CPR has not been shown to be useful.
- Invasive hemodynamic monitoring (eg, coronary perfusion pressure, central venous oxygenation) can provide useful information during CPR but is seldom available. Arterial diastolic pressure may be a reasonable surrogate for coronary perfusion pressure with a suggested goal of >25 mm Hg. An arterial central venous oxygen saturation <30% (0.30) indicates poor CPR quality.
- $ETCO_2$ monitoring is a useful method to assess cardiac output during CPR and has been associated with ROSC. Persistently low $ETCO_2$ values (<10 mm Hg [1.3 kPa]) during CPR in intubated patients suggest that ROSC is unlikely.
- In the postresuscitative phase, monitoring should be directed toward the components of the post-cardiac arrest syndrome. Identify and treat the precipitating cause of the arrest. Optimize hemodynamics with avoidance of hypotension (MAP <65 mm Hg or SBP <90 mm Hg). Monitor oxygenation closely and maintain arterial blood oxygen saturation >94% (0.94). Because seizures can occur after cardiac arrest, EEG monitoring is indicated. Avoid hyperthermia and maintain normoglycemia. A complete review of systems is recommended because the post-cardiac arrest syndrome can affect most organ systems.

- Many cardiac arrest survivors experience prolonged emotional, cognitive, physical, and neurologic symptoms. In the recovery phase, provide a multimodal plan at hospital discharge that includes instructions for treatment, rehabilitation, and surveillance. Define short- and long-term expectations clearly with appropriate action plans for each phase of the recovery.

See Chapter 41, Cardiac Arrest, authored by Jeffrey F. Barletta, for a more detailed discussion of this topic.

8 Dyslipidemia

- *Dyslipidemia* is defined as elevated total cholesterol (TC), low-density lipoprotein cholesterol (LDL-C), or triglycerides (TG); low high-density lipoprotein cholesterol (HDL-C); or a combination of these abnormalities.

PATHOPHYSIOLOGY

- Cholesterol, triglycerides, and phospholipids are transported in blood as complexes of lipids and proteins (lipoproteins). Lipid abnormalities increase the risk of coronary, cerebrovascular, and peripheral arterial disease, collectively known as atherosclerotic cardiovascular disease (ASCVD).
- Atherogenesis is a progressive process initiated by migration of LDL-C and remnant lipoprotein particles into vessel walls. These particles undergo oxidation and are taken up by macrophages, which induces endothelial cell dysfunction that reduces the ability of the endothelium to dilate the artery and causes a prothrombotic state. Unregulated uptake of cholesterol by macrophages leads to foam cell formation and the development of atherosclerotic plaques. Macrophages eventually produce and secrete matrix metalloproteinases, which degrade the collagen matrix of the plaques and cause them to be unstable.
- Repeated injury and repair within an atherosclerotic plaque eventually lead to a fibrous cap protecting the underlying core of lipids, collagen, calcium, and inflammatory cells. Maintenance of the fibrous plaque is critical to prevent plaque rupture and coronary thrombosis. Potential clinical outcomes include angina, myocardial infarction (MI), arrhythmias, stroke, peripheral arterial disease, abdominal aortic aneurysm, and sudden death.
- Primary dyslipidemias include genetic defects resulting in hypercholesterolemia, hypertriglyceridemia, combined hyperlipidemia, and disorders of HDL-C metabolism and an excess of lipoproteins. These disorders have an increased risk of premature ASCVD due to significant elevations in cholesterol levels. In homozygous and heterozygous familial hypercholesterolemia (FH), the primary defect is the inability to bind LDL-C to LDL-C receptors. This leads to lack of LDL-C degradation by cells and unregulated biosynthesis of cholesterol.
- Secondary or acquired dyslipidemias can accompany genetic disorders and may be associated with diet (excessive alcohol use, anorexia, weight gain, excessive intake of carbohydrates or saturated fat), medications (eg, progestins, thiazide diuretics, glucocorticoids, β-blockers, isotretinoin, protease inhibitors, cyclosporine, mirtazapine, sirolimus), and comorbid conditions (eg, nephrotic syndrome, renal failure, hypothyroidism, obesity, diabetes).

CLINICAL PRESENTATION AND DIAGNOSIS

- Most patients are asymptomatic for years before they develop ASCVD, which may produce symptoms including chest pain, palpitations, sweating, anxiety, shortness of breath, loss of consciousness, difficulty with speech or movement, or abdominal pain.
- Perform a thorough medical history in patients presenting with dyslipidemia, including individual characteristics (age, race, gender, pregnancy), history of high-risk comorbid conditions (eg, hypertension, diabetes, peripheral arterial disease, coronary heart disease [CHD], chronic kidney disease [CKD], carotid artery stenosis), family history (eg, early-onset CHD), current medication and prior lipid-lowering medication use, lifestyle assessment (smoking status, exercise, diet, alcohol use), and ischemic symptoms.

- Measure height, weight, body mass index (BMI), and blood pressure. Physical signs may include eruptive xanthomas, peripheral polyneuropathy, increased blood pressure, and abdominal obesity.
- Laboratory tests may show elevated TC, LDL-C, TG, apolipoprotein B, and high-sensitivity C-reactive protein (hsCRP); HDL-C may be low. Perform other baseline testing (eg, AST/ALT, TSH, glucose, serum creatinine, BUN, and urinalysis). Calculate 10-year ASCVD risk in primary prevention situations.
- Screening may be conducted for manifestations of vascular disease, including carotid ultrasound, coronary calcium score, ankle-brachial index, and heart catheterization.

TREATMENT

- Goals of Treatment: Prevent ASCVD-related morbidity and mortality, including revascularization procedures, MI, and ischemic stroke. Surrogate markers include achieving desired levels of TC, LDL-C, HDL-C, and TG (Table 8-1).

GENERAL APPROACH

- A comprehensive approach to treating dyslipidemia and modifiable ASCVD risk factors is required to reduce the risk of first and recurrent ASCVD events. Therapeutic lifestyle changes (TLC) are first-line therapy for any lipoprotein disorder, including reducing the percent of calories from saturated and trans fats, increased intake of soluble fiber, weight reduction if overweight or obese, increased physical activity, and avoiding or quitting tobacco use. Hypertensive patients should achieve optimal blood pressure control, and persons with diabetes mellitus should receive glucose-lowering therapies that reduce ASCVD risk.
- If TLC is insufficient, lipid-lowering agents should be chosen based on which lipid is at an undesirable level and the degree to which it is expected to increase the risk of ASCVD. The decision to initiate lipid-lowering therapy should be based on an individual's ASCVD risk and not merely plasma levels of atherogenic lipoproteins

TABLE 8-1	Classification of Total-, LDL-, HDL-Cholesterol, and Triglycerides in Adults
Total Cholesterol	
<200 mg/dL (5.17 mmol/L)	Desirable
200–239 mg/dL (5.17–6.20 mmol/L)	Borderline high
≥240 mg/dL (6.21 mmol/L)	High
Low-Density Lipoprotein Cholesterol	
<100 mg/dL (2.59 mmol/L)	Optimal
100–129 mg/dL (2.59–3.35 mmol/L)	Near or above optimal
130–159 mg/dL (3.36–4.13 mmol/L)	Borderline high
160–189 mg/dL (4.14–4.90 mmol/L)	High
≥190 mg/dL (4.91 mmol/L)	Very high
High-Density Lipoprotein Cholesterol	
<40 mg/dL (1.03 mmol/L)	Low (Men)
<50 mg/dL (1.3 mmol/L)	Low (Women)
Triglycerides	
<150 mg/dL (1.70 mmol/L)	Normal
150–199 mg/dL (1.70–2.25 mmol/L)	Borderline high
200–499 mg/dL (2.26–5.64 mmol/L)	High
≥500 mg/dL (5.65 mmol/L)	Very high

(eg, LDL-C) alone. Patients with established ASCVD are at highest risk and most likely to benefit from lipid-lowering therapy. Risk assessment in patients without established ASCVD requires careful consideration of risk factors, the risks of lipid-lowering therapy, and patient preference. For patients between 40 and 79 years of age and no history of ASCVD, the ASCVD Risk Estimator Plus (www.tools.acc.org/ascvd-risk-estimator-plus) should be used to facilitate a clinician–patient discussion regarding the benefits and risks of lipid-lowering therapy, especially in patients whose 10-year risk is ≥7.5%. An estimated lifetime risk for ASCVD can also be performed for patients between ages 20 and 39, but the results should only be used to justify the need for lifestyle changes and not initiation of lipid-lowering therapy.

- HMG-CoA reductase inhibitors (statins) are the drugs of choice for most patients with dyslipidemia based on demonstrated effectiveness in reducing first and recurrent cardiovascular (CV) events, CV mortality, and all-cause mortality. The 2018 American College of Cardiology/American Heart Association (ACC/AHA) Blood Cholesterol Guideline identified patient groups for whom clinical trial data demonstrate clear evidence that the benefits of statin therapy outweigh the potential risks.

- For primary ASCVD prevention (Fig. 8-1), patient groups with an untreated LDL-C ≥190 mg/dL (4.91 mmol/L) or type 1 or 2 diabetes (age 40–75 years) are eligible for statin therapy without estimating ASCVD risk using the Pooled Cohorts Equation. Given limited data in adults over age 75, a patient–clinician discussion regarding the benefits and risks of statin therapy is warranted. For all others, age is a primary consideration to determine the appropriate method of risk assessment and treatment recommendations.

- For secondary prevention (patients with established ASCVD; Fig. 8-2), high-intensity statin therapy is indicated. Moderate-intensity statin should only be considered in adults >75 years of age and those unable to tolerate high-intensity statins therapy. After high-intensity statin therapy is initiated, ezetimibe may be added if the LDL-C remains ≥70 mg/dL (1.81 mmol/L). In select, very high-risk patients, adding a PCSK9 inhibitor is reasonable if the LDL-C remains ≥70 mg/dL (1.81 mmol/L) after adding ezetimibe.

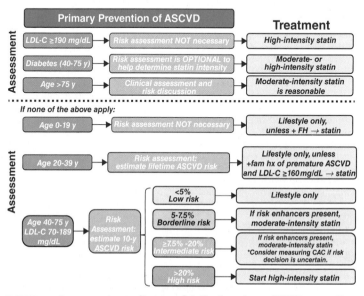

FIGURE 8-1. Assessment regarding use of statins for primary ASCVD prevention.

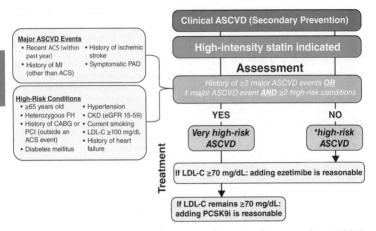

FIGURE 8-2. Assessment regarding use of statins for secondary ASCVD prevention.

- Nonstatin therapies (ezetimibe, bempedoic acid, PCSK9 inhibitors) may be added when adequate LDL-C lowering cannot be achieved with statins alone or in patients unable to tolerate the recommended dose of a statin.

NONPHARMACOLOGIC THERAPY

- Employ TLC in all patients, including those receiving lipid-lowering therapy. Lifestyle modification alone is inappropriate for patients with established ASCVD given the benefit of statins in these high-risk patients.
- Determine weight and BMI at each visit and discuss lifestyle changes to induce a 5%–10% weight loss in overweight or obese persons.
- Recommend moderate-to-vigorous intensity physical activity three to four times per week with each session lasting 40 minutes on average.
- Counsel all patients to stop smoking and avoid tobacco products altogether.
- Advise patients to reduce the percent of daily calories from saturated and trans fats by following a diet that emphasizes vegetables, fruits, whole grains, low-fat dairy, poultry, fish, legumes, and nuts while limiting intake of sweets, sugary beverages, and red meat. Adapt the dietary pattern to a patient's caloric requirements, cultural food preferences, and other medical conditions (eg, diabetes mellitus). It is important to involve all family members, especially if the patient is not the primary person preparing food.
- Increased intake of soluble fiber (oat bran, pectins, certain gums, and psyllium) can reduce total and LDL cholesterol but has little effect on HDL-C or TG. Total daily fiber intake should be about 25 g/day. Fiber products may also help manage constipation associated with bile acid sequestrants (BAS).
- Ingestion of modest to large amounts of oily, cold-water fish (eg, salmon, tuna) may provide CV benefits; however, there are concerns about environmental contaminants and long-term sustainability. Alternatively, fish oil supplementation provides a consistent daily intake of omega-3 polyunsaturated fatty acids (PUFA) such as eicosapentaenoic acid (EPA) and docosahexaenoic acid (DHA) (see "Pharmacologic Therapy" section below).
- Ingestion of 2–3 g daily of plant sterols and stanols isolated from vegetable oils reduces LDL-C by 5%–15%. They are usually available in butter-like spreads (eg, Benecol). Phytosterols should be administered 2–4 hours before or after BAS to avoid binding of phytosterols in the gut.

- Red yeast rice contains monacolin K, which is chemically identical to lovastatin. However, the amount of monacolin K in OTC products varies by over 120-fold, with some products containing negligible amounts and others likely having higher levels than described on the label, resulting in cases of rhabdomyolysis, liver toxicity, and renal failure. Red yeast rice is not a suitable alternative to statins, but if patients choose to take it, recommend that they purchase a reputable product and avoid concurrent use with prescription statins.

PHARMACOLOGIC THERAPY

- Evidence from controlled clinical trials demonstrates that reducing LDL-C lowers ASCVD event rates in the setting of primary and secondary prevention. Epidemiological studies suggest that every 38 mg/dL (0.98 mmol/L) reduction in LDL-C produces a 21% reduction in ASCVD event rates over 5 years. There is a dose-dependent, log-linear association between LDL-C and ASCVD risk, and evidence suggests that lower levels of LDL-C achieve greater risk reductions.
- Lipid-lowering drugs can be broadly divided into agents that primarily decrease atherogenic cholesterol-containing lipoprotein particles (eg, statins) and those that primarily decrease TG levels (eg, fibrates).

Statins

- Statins inhibit 3-hydroxy-3-methylglutaryl coenzyme A (HMG-CoA) reductase, interrupting conversion of HMG-CoA to mevalonate, the rate-limiting step in cholesterol biosynthesis. Reduced LDL synthesis and enhanced LDL catabolism mediated through LDL receptors appear to be the principal mechanisms for lipid-lowering effects.
- Statins significantly reduce LDL-C (20%–60%), modestly increase HDL-C (6%–12%), and decrease TG (10%–29%).
- Statins are first-line lipid-lowering therapy for dyslipidemia due to strong evidence from many controlled trials demonstrating significant reduction in the risk of first (primary prevention) and recurrent (secondary prevention) CV events.
- Statin selection is primarily based on the indicated intensity (Table 8-2). Products in order of decreasing LDL-C lowering potency include **rosuvastatin**, **atorvastatin**, **pitavastatin**, **simvastatin**, **lovastatin**, **pravastatin**, and **fluvastatin**.
- Statins are generally well tolerated. Statin-associated muscle symptoms (SAMS) are reported by 10%–25% of users and are often a reason for discontinuation. Myalgia is

TABLE 8-2	Intensity of Statin Therapy by Drug and Dose	
High-Intensity Therapy	**Moderate-Intensity Therapy**	**Low-Intensity Therapy**
Daily dose lowers LDL on average by ≥50%	Daily dose lowers LDL on average by 30% to <50%	Daily dose lowers LDL on average by <30%
Atorvastatin 40–80 mg	**Atorvastatin 10–20 mg**	Simvastatin 10 mg
Rosuvastatin 20–40 mg	**Rosuvastatin 5–20 mg**	**Pravastatin 10–20 mg**
	Simvastatin 20–40 mg[a]	**Lovastatin 20 mg**
	Pravastatin 40–80 mg	Fluvastatin 20–40 mg
	Lovastatin 40 mg	Pitavastatin 1 mg
	Fluvastatin XL 80 mg	
	Fluvastatin 40 mg BID	
	Pitavastatin 2–4 mg	

[a]Simvastatin is not recommended by the U.S. Food and Drug Administration (FDA) to be started at 80 mg/day due to increased risk of myopathy and rarely rhabdomyolysis.
Boldface type indicates medications that have cardiovascular outcome data from randomized controlled trials when given in the specified dose.

the most common SAMS and involves bilateral muscle achiness, weakness, or cramps affecting larger muscle groups (such as thighs and back). The most concerning SAMS is rhabdomyolysis, which is rapid breakdown of skeletal muscle resulting in creatine kinase (CK) elevations >10 times the upper limit of normal and potentially acute kidney injury. Rhabdomyolysis may be associated with dark ("tea-colored") urine, nausea, vomiting, confusion, coma, cardiac arrhythmias, electrolyte disturbances, and even death. Fortunately, rhabdomyolysis is quite rare (0.1% of statin-treated patients versus 0.04% of patients receiving placebo in controlled clinical trials). Risk factors for developing SAMS include advanced age, female gender, low BMI, frequent heavy exercisers, comorbidities (eg, kidney disease, hypothyroidism), and increased serum statin concentrations due to drug–drug interactions. Lower starting doses may be advisable for patients with multiple risk factors, with dose titration to the desired potency after the initial dose is tolerated.

- Statins (except pravastatin) are metabolized to some degree by CYP isoenzymes. Lovastatin, simvastatin, and atorvastatin have more significant drug–drug interactions because they are predominantly metabolized by CYP3A4, whereas fluvastatin, pitavastatin, and rosuvastatin are metabolized by other CYP isoenzymes (eg, CYP2C9, CYP2C8, CYP2C19). Concurrent medications that compete with or inhibit the same CYP isoenzyme (eg, verapamil) can increase serum statin concentrations and the risk for SAMS. Concurrent use of medications such as gemfibrozil that interfere with statin glucuronidation, which is responsible for statin clearance, also increase the risk of SAMS.

- A Statin Intolerance App (http://www.acc.org/statinintoleranceapp) can be used to determine the possibility of SAMS and provide guidance on managing patients with possible SAMS. Statin therapy should generally be discontinued in patients with intolerable symptoms. If symptoms resolve, start a different statin at a lower dose. Additionally, hydrophilic statins (eg, rosuvastatin) may be better tolerated than lipophilic statins (eg, simvastatin). If symptoms do not improve, investigate other potential causes of muscle pain (eg, hypothyroidism, severe vitamin D deficiency) before a statin rechallenge. Every-other-day dosing using statins with long half-lives (eg, atorvastatin, rosuvastatin) may also be considered. Nonstatin therapies may be considered in patients who fail multiple statins. Routine CK monitoring is not recommended, but testing in a patient with symptoms can be used to exclude rhabdomyolysis and help confirm myalgia.

- Mild elevations in serum transaminase levels (primarily alanine aminotransferase [ALT]) may occur, but routine monitoring of liver enzymes is not required. Obtain hepatic enzymes before starting statin therapy as a baseline value for comparison if enzymes are later found to be elevated. Statins may be initiated in patients with chronic liver disease, compensated cirrhosis, and nonalcoholic fatty liver disease but are contraindicated in decompensated cirrhosis or acute liver failure.

- Statin use is also associated with a small (<1%) increased risk of new-onset diabetes. Common attributes of statin users who develop new-onset diabetes include higher statin doses and presence of other risk factors for diabetes, including obesity, impaired fasting glucose, A1C >6% (0.06; 42 mmol/mol Hb), or metabolic syndrome.

- Statin products and usual adult starting doses are provided in Table 8-3.

Cholesterol Absorption Inhibitors

- **Ezetimibe** (Table 8-3) is a preferred adjunct therapy because it modestly reduces the risk of recurrent CV events when used in combination with statin therapy. Its primary effect is modest reduction in LDL-C (15%–24%) with higher reductions achievable in combination with statin therapy. Ezetimibe reduces LDL-C by inhibiting the NPC1L1 protein, an important transporter of cholesterol absorption in the small intestine and hepatocytes. Ezetimibe is generally well tolerated and is associated with mild gastrointestinal (GI) complaints (eg, diarrhea), myalgia, and ALT elevations when used with statins. Ezetimibe has no effects on the CYP450 enzyme system; however, concomitant use with cyclosporine can lead to increased exposure to both ezetimibe and cyclosporine.

TABLE 8-3 Select Drugs Used for Treatment of Dyslipidemia

Generic (Brand) Name	Dosage Forms	Recommended Adult Starting Dose	Maximum Total Daily Dose
Statins			
Rosuvastatin (Crestor)	5, 10, 20, 40 mg tablets	5 mg once daily	40 mg
Atorvastatin (Lipitor)	10, 20, 40, 80 mg tablets	10–20 mg once daily	80 mg
Pitavastatin (Livalo)	1, 2, 4 mg tablets	2 mg once daily	4 mg
Simvastatin (Zocor)	5, 10, 20, 40, 80 mg tablets	10–20 mg once daily	80 mg
Lovastatin (Mevacor)	20, 40 mg tablets	20 mg once daily with the evening meal	80 mg
Pravastatin (Pravachol)	20, 40, 80 mg tablets	40 mg once daily	80 mg
Fluvastatin (Lescol)	20, 40 mg capsules; 80 mg XL tablets	40–80 mg once daily	80 mg
Cholesterol Absorption Inhibitors			
Ezetimibe (Zetia)	10 mg tablets	10 mg once daily	10 mg
Colesevelam (Welchol)	625 mg tablets; 3.75 and 1.875 g oral suspension packets	6 tablets once daily or 3 tablets twice daily; suspension: 3.75 g packet once daily or one 1.875 g packet twice daily	3750 mg
Colestipol hydrochloride (Colestid)	1 g tablets; 5 g granule packets, bulk powder	Tablets: 2 g once or twice daily; granules: 5 g once or twice daily	16 g tablets; 30 g packets
Cholestyramine (Questran)	4 g packets, bulk powder	4 g once or twice daily	24 g
Proprotein Convertase Subtilisin/Kexin Type 9 (PCSK9) Inhibitors			
Alirocumab (Praluent)	75 mg, 150 mg SC injection	75 mg SC every 2 weeks	150 mg
Evolocumab (Repatha)	140 mg, 420 mg SC injection	140 mg SC every 2 weeks or 420 mg SC once monthly	420 mg

(Continued)

TABLE 8-3   Select Drugs Used for Treatment of Dyslipidemia *(Continued)*

Generic (Brand) Name	Dosage Forms	Recommended Adult Starting Dose	Maximum Total Daily Dose
Adenosine Triphosphate–Citrate Lyase (ACL) Inhibitor			
Bempedoic acid (Nexletol)	180 mg tablets	180 mg once daily with or without food	180 mg
Fibric Acid Derivatives (Fibrates)			
Gemfibrozil (Lopid)	600 mg capsules	600 mg twice daily	1200 mg
Fenofibrate (Tricor, others)	(product dependent)	(product dependent)	(product dependent)
Omega-3 Polyunsaturated Fatty Acids (PUFA)			
Omega-3-acid ethyl esters (Lovaza)	1 g capsules	4 capsules once daily or 2 capsules twice daily	4 g
Omega-3-carboxylic acids (Epanova)	1 g capsules	2 or 4 capsules once daily	4 g
Icosapent ethyl (Vascepa)	0.5, 1 g capsules	Four 0.5 g capsules or two 1 g capsules twice daily	2 g
Niacin			
Niacin (generic)	50, 100, 250, 500 mg tablets; others	250 mg once daily	6 g
Extended-release niacin (Niaspan)	500, 750, 1000 mg tablets	500 mg once daily	2 g
Mipomersen (Kynamro)	200 mg SC injection	200 mg SC once weekly	200 mg
Lomitapide (Juxtapid)	5, 10, 20 mg capsules	5 mg once daily	60 mg

Select Combination Products

Extended-release niacin + lovastatin tablets (Advicor)	Niacin/lovastatin 500 mg/20 mg, 750 mg/20 mg, 1000 mg/20 mg, 1000 mg/40 mg	500 mg/20 mg once daily at bedtime	1000 mg/40 mg
Ezetimibe + simvastatin tablets (Vytorin)	Ezetimibe/simvastatin 10 mg/10 mg, 10 mg/20 mg, 10 mg/40 mg, 10 mg/80 mg	10 mg/10 mg or 10 mg/20 mg once daily	10 mg/80 mg
Bempedoic acid + ezetimibe (Nexlizet)	Bempedoic acid/ezetimibe 180 mg/10 mg	180 mg/10 mg once daily with or without food	180 mg/10 mg

SC, subcutaneously.

- **Colesevelam**, **colestipol**, and **cholestyramine** are BAS that modestly reduce LDL-C (13%–20%) and reduce CV events when used as monotherapy (**Table 8-3**). They are generally combined with statins when desired LDL-C levels are not achieved with statins alone. BAS are considered first line during pregnancy because they are not systemically absorbed and pose no risk to the fetus.

  ✓ BAS bind bile acids in the intestinal lumen, interrupting enterohepatic circulation of bile acids, which decreases the bile acid pool size and stimulates hepatic synthesis of bile acids from cholesterol. Depletion of the hepatic cholesterol pool increases cholesterol biosynthesis and the number of LDL receptors on hepatocyte membranes, which enhances the rate of catabolism from plasma and lowers LDL levels. Increased hepatic cholesterol biosynthesis may be paralleled by increased hepatic VLDL production; consequently, BAS may aggravate hypertriglyceridemia and should be avoided in patients with TG levels >300 mg/dL (3.39 mmol/L).

  ✓ Cholestyramine powders that require mixing with water or juice to create a slurry for oral administration are associated with GI complaints of constipation, bloating, epigastric fullness, nausea, and flatulence. These effects can be minimized by increasing fluid intake, increasing dietary bulk, and using stool softeners. Tablet forms of colesevelam are generally better tolerated than resin powders. Other potential adverse effects include impaired absorption of fat-soluble vitamins A, D, E, and K; GI obstruction; and reduced bioavailability of other drugs such as warfarin, levothyroxine, and phenytoin. Drug–drug interactions may be avoided by taking other medications 1 hour before or 4 hours after the BAS.

  ✓ Given the better safety and tolerability profile of ezetimibe, BAS should be reserved for patients unable to tolerate ezetimibe who need additional LDL-C lowering despite maximally tolerated statin therapy.

Proprotein Convertase Subtilisin/Kexin Type 9 (PCSK9) Inhibitors

- **Alirocumab** and **evolocumab** are fully human monoclonal antibodies to PCSK9; inhibiting PCSK9 promotes intracellular degradation of hepatic LDL-C, prevents LDL receptor recycling to the cell surface, and reduces LDL-C clearance from the circulation. They reduce LDL-C by as much as 60% when added to statin therapy. Clinical trials have shown that these agents reduce recurrent CV events when added to statin therapy. The drugs are administered by subcutaneous injection either biweekly or once monthly.

- The most common adverse effect is injection site reactions, which can be minimized by allowing the injection to come to room temperature before use and icing the site before injecting. Some patients report flu-like symptoms after the injection. Patients who reach low LDL-C levels (<20 mg/dL [0.53 mmol/L]) do not appear to be at increased risk of adverse events. Nevertheless, the long-term effects of achieving low LDL-C levels remain unknown.

- Despite their favorable clinical benefits, alirocumab and evolocumab frequently require a prior authorization due to high cost. Although these agents should primarily be used in combination with maximally tolerated statins in high-risk patients unable to achieve desired LDL-C levels with a statin alone, both drugs are FDA-approved for use as monotherapy in patients with primary hyperlipidemia (such as heterozygous FH).

- **Inclisiran** (Leqvio) is a small interfering RNA (siRNA) molecule that reduces PCSK9 production by inhibiting messenger RNA. It has a sustained effect on LDL lowering and is given subcutaneously every 3–6 months. In Phase 3 clinical trials, inclisiran reduced LDL-C by an average of 50% when given as add-on therapy in patients treated with a high-intensity statin but had not achieved their LDL-C goal. Inclisiran is approved as an additional treatment to maximally tolerated statin therapy to further lower LDL-C in adults with HeFH or ASCVD. The most common adverse effects reported are transient and mild injection-site reactions. The effect of Inclisiran on cardiovascular event rates is currently being investigated.

Adenosine Triphosphate-Citrate Lyase Inhibitor

- **Bempedoic acid** (Nexletol) inhibits adenosine triphosphate-citrate lyase (ACL), a cytoplasmic enzyme that generates acetyl coenzyme A, which is needed for synthesis of fatty acids and cholesterol. ACL inhibitors prevent cholesterol production upstream from statins, and the two strategies can be used in combination. Oral bempedoic acid produces modest reductions in LDL-C (15%-20%) when combined with statin therapy or as monotherapy in patients unable to tolerate statins. Bempedoic acid plus ezetimibe resulted in a 36% reduction in LDL-C from baseline in a Phase 3 clinical trial. Bempedoic acid is generally well tolerated but may cause hyperuricemia and (rarely) tendon rupture. Until results of a long-term cardiovascular outcomes trial are published, bempedoic acid use should be limited to patients unable to achieve desired treatment goals on maximally tolerated statin plus ezetimibe who prefer a noninjectable therapeutic option.

Fibric Acid Derivatives (Fibrates)

- **Gemfibrozil** and **fenofibrate** are potent TG-lowering therapies (20%–50%) but may cause a modest reciprocal rise in LDL-C in patients with severely elevated TG levels. Plasma HDL concentrations may rise 10%–15% or more with fibrates. Gemfibrozil increases the activity of lipoprotein lipase (LPL) and reduces secretion of VLDL from the liver into the plasma. Fenofibrate increases LPL activity and reduces apoprotein C-III (an inhibitor of LPL) by activating peroxisome-proliferator-activated receptor α (PPARα), which regulates the expression of genes involved in the regulation of lipids and other metabolic processes.

- Fibrates have been shown to reduce CV events when used as monotherapy, but there is less evidence to support combination therapy with statins. Fibrates are primarily used in patients with TG levels >500 mg/dL (5.65 mmol/L) to reduce the risk of acute pancreatitis.

- Fibrates are generally well tolerated, but GI complaints and transient hepatic transaminase elevations have been reported. Both agents require dose adjustments for significant renal impairment, and fenofibrate has been reported to transiently worsen renal function.

- SAMS can occur when fibrates are used alone but are more common when used in combination with statins. Gemfibrozil and its glucuronide metabolite have potent effects on CYP450 enzymes (such as CYP3A4) and intestinal, hepatic, and renal transporters making it highly prone to significantly increase serum statin concentrations and the risk of SAMS. Consequently, current guidelines do not recommend gemfibrozil in patients receiving statin therapy; fenofibrate should be used instead.

- Fenofibrate and gemfibrozil may rarely enhance gallstone formation. Fibrates may potentiate the effects of warfarin; the international normalized ratio (INR) should be monitored closely with this combination.

Omega-3 Polyunsaturated Fatty Acids (PUFA)

- High doses of omega-3 PUFA (2–4 g/day of EPA/DHA) significantly reduce TG and VLDL cholesterol levels (20%–50%), but PUFA supplementation has either no effect on TC and LDL-C or may cause slight elevations. Omega-3 PUFA reduce TG levels by increasing hepatic oxidation of free fatty acids, increasing LDL hydrolysis by activating PPARα, and inhibiting apoprotein C-III.

- The omega-3 PUFA formulations approved by the FDA for treating TG levels ≥500 mg/dL (5.65 mmol/L) include **omega-3-acid ethyl esters of EPA/DHA** (Lovaza), **omega-3-carboxylic acids of EPA/DHA** (Epanova), and **ethyl ester of EPA only** (icosapent ethyl; Vascepa). Prescription omega-3 PUFA products contain approximately 1 g of EPA/DHA per capsule, whereas the EPA/DHA content of non–FDA-regulated OTC fish oil supplements is often <300 mg per capsule. Unless patient affordability is an issue, prescription omega-3 PUFA are preferred to minimize pill burden and ensure product quality.

- Randomized clinical trials of omega-3 PUFA have shown mixed results due to variability in study designs and products used. Low doses (<2 g/day) of omega-3 PUFA did not reduce the risk of ASCVD events. Low-dose omega-3 PUFA supplementation is not recommended for primary prevention, especially in patients with diabetes. In late 2019, icosapent ethyl received U.S. FDA approval for reducing the risk of CV events in adults with triglyceride levels ≥150 mg/dL and with established CV disease or diabetes plus at least two other CV risk factors and who are already taking maximally tolerated doses of statins.

- GI complaints (eg, abdominal pain, "fishy burps") are common with OTC omega-3 PUFA products but may be minimized by refrigerating the capsules. These products should be used with caution in patients with known sensitivities or allergies to fish or shellfish. Drug–drug interactions are minimal with omega-3 PUFA, although caution is advised when used concomitantly with antiplatelet agents or anticoagulants because omega-3 PUFA may prolong bleeding time.

Niacin

- **Niacin (nicotinic acid)** lowers TG levels (20%–50%) by inhibiting lipolysis with a decrease in free fatty acids in plasma and decreased hepatic esterification of TG. It also significantly raises HDL-C (5%–30%) by reducing its catabolism and decreasing hepatic removal. Niacin reduces hepatic synthesis of VLDL, leading to a modest dose-dependent decrease in LDL-C (5%–20%). Despite these favorable changes, niacin has not been shown to improve CV outcomes in patients already receiving statin therapy with relatively well-controlled lipids at baseline.

- Adverse events frequently limit niacin use. Cutaneous flushing and itching appear to be prostaglandin mediated and can be reduced by taking aspirin 325 mg shortly before niacin ingestion. Flushing seems to be related to rising plasma niacin concentrations and use of immediate-release formulations; taking the dose with meals and slowly titrating the dose upward may also minimize these effects. Concomitant alcohol and hot drinks may magnify flushing and pruritus with niacin and should be avoided at the time of ingestion.

- Niaspan, the only prescription form, is an extended-release product with pharmacokinetics intermediate between immediate- and sustained-release products that are sold as OTC dietary supplements. In controlled trials, Niaspan had fewer dermatologic reactions and a lower risk for hepatotoxicity.

- Niacin therapy may be associated with elevated hepatic enzymes, hyperuricemia, and hyperglycemia. It is contraindicated in patients with active liver disease and active peptic ulcer disease. Nicotinamide should not be used as an alternative to niacin because it does not effectively lower cholesterol or triglyceride levels.

Mipomersen

- **Mipomersen** is indicated as an adjunct to diet and lipid-lowering treatments to reduce LDL-C, TC, apolipoprotein B, and non-HDL-C in patients with homozygous FH. It is an oligonucleotide inhibitor of apolipoprotein B-100 synthesis. When given in combination with maximum tolerated doses of lipid-lowering therapy, mipomersen can produce an additional 25% reduction in LDL-C. Adverse reactions include injection site reactions, flu-like symptoms, nausea, headache, and elevations in serum transaminases. The labeling contains a black box warning for severe hepatotoxicity, and mipomersen is only available through a restricted Risk Evaluation and Mitigation Strategy (REMS) program.

Lomitapide

- **Lomitapide** has the same indication for FH as mipomersen. Lomitapide is a microsomal triglyceride transfer protein (MTP) inhibitor that reduces the amount of cholesterol that the liver and intestines assemble and secrete into the circulation. It may reduce LDL cholesterol by about 40% in patients on maximum tolerated lipid-lowering therapy and LDL apheresis. Like mipomersen, lomitapide contains a black box warning for severe hepatotoxicity and is only available through a restricted REMS program.

TREATMENT RECOMMENDATIONS

Familial Hypercholesterolemia

- Persons with FH have a very high lifetime risk of developing ASCVD. FH should be suspected in adults with untreated LDL-C levels ≥190 mg/dL (4.91 mmol/L) or non-HDL-C levels ≥220 mg/dL (5.69 mmol/L) who have a family history of high cholesterol or ASCVD in first-degree relatives.
- Intensive lifestyle and pharmacologic therapy are often necessary for adults with FH. Patients who have not had an ASCVD event should receive a high-intensity statin; those with an LDL-C ≥100 mg/dL (2.59 mmol/L) despite maximum tolerated statin should receive ezetimibe, bempedoic acid, and/or a PCSK9 inhibitor. For patients with a history of ASCVD, the LDL-C threshold to consider nonstatin therapies is ≥70 mg/dL (1.81 mmol/L).
- Mipomersen and lomitapide are indicated for patients with FH and reduce LDL-C levels by ~25% and ~40%, respectively, when added to maximum tolerated doses of lipid-lowering therapy.
- **Evinacumab-dgnb** (Evkeeza) is a humanized monoclonal antibody that inhibits angiopoietinlike 3 (ANGPTL3) protein and is approved to lower LDL-C in patients age 12 and older with homozygous FH. It is administered as an IV infusion every 4 weeks. Evinacumab reduces LDL-C by ~50% and also reduces TG by ~55%. Adverse effects include infusion-site reactions, flu-like illness, and rhinorrhea. It is unknown whether evinacumab reduces ASCVD events.
- Other treatment options for FH patients include LDL apheresis (a process that removes LDL from the blood) and liver transplantation.

Hypertriglyceridemia

- Elevated TG levels are strongly associated with increased ASCVD risk, but the direct role of TG in ASCVD development is debated.
- Advise all patients with elevated TG to implement lifestyle interventions that reduce TG levels, including 5%–10% reduction in body weight, reduced consumption of sugar and refined carbohydrates, increased physical activity, smoking cessation, and restricted alcohol intake.
- Identify and address secondary causes of hypertriglyceridemia (eg, uncontrolled diabetes and CKD, medications such as protease inhibitors and atypical antipsychotics).
- Statins are generally considered first-line therapy after optimizing lifestyle interventions and addressing secondary causes; they can reduce TG levels by up to 30% at higher doses and help achieve desired levels of LDL-C.
- Fibrates effectively lower TG levels but are not routinely used for borderline-high TG levels because there is no evidence that they reduce ASCVD risk. Omega-3 PUFA also significantly lower TG levels at higher doses (24 g/day) but only the icosapent ethyl (EPA only) prescription product is indicated for borderline-high TG levels and to reduce ASCVD risk.
- Fasting TG levels >500 mg/dL (5.65 mmol/L) are associated with pancreatitis and other complications. Dietary fat restriction is essential because it reduces synthesis and entry of additional chylomicrons into the circulation. Lipid-lowering therapies that primarily lower TG (fibrates and omega-3 PUFA) are recommended as first-line agents. Statins may be reasonable first-line options in patients with an ASCVD risk of ≥7.5%. Treatment success is defined as reducing TG below 500 mg/dL (5.65 mmol/L) and preventing pancreatitis.

Low HDL Cholesterol

- Low HDL-C is a strong independent risk predictor of ASCVD and is defined as <40 mg/dL (1.03 mmol/L) for men and <50 mg/dL (1.29 mmol/L) for women.

There is no specified goal for HDL-C raising, and the primary target in these patients remains lowering LDL-C.

- Lifestyle modifications (eg, smoking cessation, increasing physical activity) are the preferred treatment approach.
- Niacin can produce the greatest increase in HDL-C compared to other lipid-lowering therapies, but no randomized clinical trial data have shown reduction in ASCVD risk by increasing HDL-C.

Patients with Diabetes

- Diabetic dyslipidemia is often characterized by hypertriglyceridemia, low HDL-C, and modestly elevated but dense LDL-C forms that are highly atherogenic. Statins are the first-line therapy based on evidence from randomized clinical trials that statins reduce ASCVD events and mortality in persons with diabetes. However, the risk among patients with no history of ASCVD varies, so the 10-year ASCVD risk score is used to determine the appropriate statin intensity (Fig. 8-1). High-intensity statin therapy is preferred in patients with a history of ASCVD (secondary prevention) because these patients are at high risk of recurrent ASCVD events.
- The role of nonstatin therapies in patients with diabetes is complex. Both ezetimibe and evolocumab have shown improved outcomes when added to statin therapy. Although diabetes is associated with a mixed dyslipidemia, the combination of fenofibrate and a statin did not reduce the rate of CV events compared to simvastatin alone in patients with type 2 diabetes. Fenofibrate may offer potential benefit with TG levels >204 mg/dL (2.31 mmol/L) and HDL-C <34 mg/dL (0.88 mmol/L), but this has not been evaluated in a prospective clinical trial. Additionally, fenofibrate reduces the progression of diabetic retinopathy and the need for laser treatment. Colesevelam is FDA-approved to improve both glycemic and lipid control, but it can exacerbate hypertriglyceridemia, which is common in diabetes. Niacin modestly increases fasting plasma glucose (4%–5%) and A1C levels (~0.25%); consequently, niacin should not be routinely used in persons with diabetes.

EVALUATION OF THERAPEUTIC OUTCOMES

- For short-term evaluation, obtain a complete lipid panel 4–12 weeks after initiation or following a dose adjustment of lipid-lowering therapy to assess therapeutic response.
- For long-term evaluation, obtain a repeat lipid panel every 3–12 months to ensure adherence to lipid-lowering therapy and maintenance of desired levels of LDL-C.
  ✓ Although TC, HDL-C, and TG levels are directly measured, LDL-C is typically estimated using the Friedewald equation: LDL-C = TC - HDL-C - (TG/5) [or LDL-C = TC - HDL-C - (TG/2.2) when lipid levels are all expressed in mmol/L]. However, the equation does not provide an accurate estimate of VLDL-C and can underestimate LDL-C in patients with high TG or very low LDL-C. Useful alternatives in these patients include non-HDL-C (TC - HDL-C) and direct LDL-C measurements, which are more accurate than estimated LDL-C using the Friedewald equation.
  ✓ A nonfasting lipid panel is generally acceptable except in patients with hypertriglyceridemia, where a fasting lipid panel is preferred to minimize interference from chylomicrons.
- Routine safety monitoring of hepatic function and CK levels is not recommended in statin-treated patients, but these may be obtained if the patient has signs or symptoms suggestive of liver or muscle injury. Perform hepatic function tests in patients taking niacin at baseline, after each dosage increase, and every 6 months thereafter while taking a stable dose.
- Monitor A1C periodically in persons with diabetes receiving niacin and patients treated with statins who are at high risk for developing diabetes.

- In patients treated with lipid-lowering therapy for secondary prevention, symptoms such as angina or intermittent claudication may improve over months to years. Xanthomas or other external manifestations of dyslipidemia should regress with therapy.
- Evaluate modifiable risk factors such as hypertension, smoking, exercise, weight control, and glycemic control in persons with diabetes. Use of food diaries and recall surveys enable collection of information about diet in a systematic manner and may improve patient adherence to dietary recommendations.

See Chapter 32, Dyslipidemia, authored by Dave L. Dixon, Daniel M. Riche, and Michael S. Kelly for a more detailed discussion of this topic.

Heart Failure

9 CHAPTER

- *Heart failure* (HF) is a syndrome associated with signs and symptoms due to abnormalities in cardiac structure or function substantiated by the presence of increased natriuretic peptide plasma concentrations or objective evidence of pulmonary or systemic congestion of cardiogenic origin. HF may be caused by an abnormality that affects systolic function, diastolic function, or both. HF with reduced systolic function (ie, reduced left ventricular ejection fraction, LVEF) is referred to as HF with reduced ejection fraction (HFrEF). Diastolic dysfunction with normal LVEF is termed HF with preserved ejection fraction (HFpEF).

PATHOPHYSIOLOGY

- Causes of systolic dysfunction (decreased contractility) include reduced muscle mass (eg, myocardial infarction [MI]), dilated cardiomyopathies, and ventricular hypertrophy. Ventricular hypertrophy can be caused by pressure overload (eg, systemic or pulmonary hypertension and aortic or pulmonic valve stenosis) or volume overload (eg, valvular regurgitation, shunts, high-output states).
- Causes of diastolic dysfunction (restriction in ventricular filling) include increased ventricular stiffness, ventricular hypertrophy, infiltrative myocardial diseases, myocardial ischemia and MI, mitral or tricuspid valve stenosis, and pericardial disease (eg, pericarditis and pericardial tamponade).
- The leading causes of HF are coronary artery disease and hypertension.
- Regardless of the index event, decreased cardiac output (CO) results in activation of compensatory responses to maintain circulation: (1) tachycardia and increased contractility through sympathetic nervous system activation, (2) the Frank–Starling mechanism, whereby increased preload (through sodium and water retention) increases stroke volume, (3) vasoconstriction, and (4) ventricular hypertrophy and remodeling. Although these compensatory mechanisms initially maintain cardiac function, they are responsible for the symptoms of HF and contribute to disease progression.
- In the *neurohormonal model* of HF, an initiating event (eg, acute MI) leads to decreased CO; the HF state then becomes a systemic disease whose progression is mediated largely by neurohormones and autocrine/paracrine factors that drive myocyte injury, oxidative stress, inflammation, and extracellular matrix remodeling. These substances include angiotensin II, norepinephrine, aldosterone, natriuretic peptides, and arginine vasopressin (AVP).
- Chronic activation of the neurohormonal systems results in a cascade of events that affect the myocardium at the molecular and cellular levels. These events lead to changes in ventricular size (left ventricular hypertrophy), shape, structure, and function known as *ventricular remodeling*. The alterations in ventricular function result in further deterioration in cardiac systolic and diastolic functions that further promotes the remodeling process.
- Common precipitating factors that may cause a previously compensated HF patient to decompensate include myocardial ischemia and MI, pulmonary infections, nonadherence with diet or drug therapy, and inappropriate medication use. Drugs may precipitate or exacerbate HF through negative inotropic effects, direct cardiotoxicity, or increased sodium and water retention.

CLINICAL PRESENTATION

- Patient presentation may range from asymptomatic to cardiogenic shock.
- Primary symptoms are dyspnea (especially on exertion) and fatigue, which lead to exercise intolerance. Other pulmonary symptoms include orthopnea, paroxysmal nocturnal dyspnea (PND), tachypnea, and cough.

- Fluid overload can result in pulmonary congestion and peripheral edema.
- Nonspecific symptoms may include fatigue, nocturia, hemoptysis, abdominal pain, anorexia, nausea, bloating, ascites, poor appetite or early satiety, and weight gain or loss.
- Physical examination may reveal pulmonary crackles, S_3 gallop, cool extremities, Cheyne–Stokes respiration, tachycardia, narrow pulse pressure, cardiomegaly, symptoms of pulmonary edema (extreme breathlessness and anxiety, sometimes with coughing and pink, frothy sputum), peripheral edema, jugular venous distention (JVD), hepatojugular reflux (HJR), hepatomegaly, and mental status changes.

DIAGNOSIS

- Consider the diagnosis of HF in patients with characteristic signs and symptoms. A complete history and physical examination with appropriate laboratory testing are essential in evaluating patients with suspected HF.
- Laboratory tests for identifying disorders that may cause or worsen HF include complete blood cell count; serum electrolytes (including calcium and magnesium); renal, hepatic, thyroid function tests, and iron studies; urinalysis; lipid profile; and A1C. Hyponatremia (serum sodium <130 mEq/L [mmol/L]) may indicate worsening volume overload and/or disease progression and is associated with reduced survival. Serum creatinine may be increased due to hypoperfusion; preexisting renal dysfunction can contribute to volume overload. B-type natriuretic peptide (BNP) is typically >35 pg/mL (ng/L; 10 pmol/L) for ambulatory patients and >100 pg/mL (ng/L; 29 pmol/L) for patients hospitalized or with decompensated HF. NT-proBNP is usually >125 pg/mL (ng/L; 15 pmol/L) for ambulatory patients and >300 pg/mL (ng/L; 35 pmol/L) for patients hospitalized or with decompensated HF.
- Ventricular hypertrophy can be demonstrated on chest radiograph or electrocardiogram (ECG). Chest radiograph may also show pleural effusions or pulmonary edema.
- Echocardiogram can identify abnormalities of the pericardium, myocardium, or heart valves and quantify LVEF to determine if systolic or diastolic dysfunction is present.
- The New York Heart Association Functional Classification System is intended primarily to classify symptoms according to the physician's subjective evaluation. Functional class (FC)-I patients have no limitation of physical activity, FC-II patients have slight limitation, FC-III patients have marked limitation, and FC-IV patients are unable to carry on physical activity without discomfort.

TREATMENT OF CHRONIC HEART FAILURE

- <u>Goals of Treatment</u>: Improve quality of life, relieve or reduce symptoms, prevent or minimize hospitalizations, slow disease progression, and prolong survival.

GENERAL APPROACH

- The first step is to determine the classification of HF based on LVEF and symptoms based on NYHA functional class and any precipitating factors. Treatment of underlying disorders (eg, hyperthyroidism) may obviate the need for treating HF.
- An international group developed a staging system to emphasize that HF is a continuum and includes risk factor modification and preventive strategies.
- *Stage A (at risk for HF):* Patients with no HF signs or symptoms and no structural or biomarker evidence of HF but who are at risk for developing HF because of the presence of risk factors. Identify and modify risk factors to prevent development of structural heart disease and subsequent HF. Strategies include smoking cessation and control of hypertension, diabetes mellitus, and dyslipidemia. Angiotensin-converting enzyme (ACE) inhibitors or angiotensin receptor blockers (ARBs) are recommended for HF prevention in select patients with ASCVD or diabetes. Consider sodium-glucose cotransporter type 2 (SGLT2) inhibitors in patients with diabetes because they reduce the risks of adverse cardiovascular events and hospitalization for HF.

- *Stage B (pre-HF):* Patients with no current or prior HF signs or symptoms but with structural heart disease, abnormal cardiac function, or increased natriuretic peptide levels. Treatment is targeted at minimizing additional injury and preventing or slowing the remodeling process. In addition to treatment measures outlined for stage A, patients an LVEF (<40%) should receive an ACE inhibitor (or ARB) and a β-blocker, especially if there is a history of MI. Consider an aldosterone antagonist post-MI if LVEF is <40% (0.4) and an SGLT2 inhibitor in patients with DM to prevent HF development.
- *Stage C (HF):* Patients with structural heart disease and previous or current HF symptoms. Most patients with HFrEF in stage C should receive guideline-directed medical therapy (GDMT) proven to reduce morbidity and mortality. Consider hydralazine–isosorbide dinitrate (ISDN), loop diuretics, digoxin, ivabradine, and vericiguat in select patients (Fig. 9-1). Loop diuretics, ISDN, digoxin, and ivabradine are also used in select patients.
- *Stage D (advanced HF):* These patients have persistent HF symptoms despite maximally tolerated GDMT. In addition to standard treatments for Stages A to C, they should be considered for referral to HF management programs so specialized interventions, including mechanical circulatory support, continuous IV positive inotropic therapy, cardiac transplantation, or hospice care (when no additional treatments are appropriate).

NONPHARMACOLOGIC THERAPY OF CHRONIC HEART FAILURE

- Interventions include cardiac rehabilitation and restriction of fluid intake and dietary sodium intake (<2–3 g of sodium/day) with daily weight measurements.
- In patients with hyponatremia (serum sodium <130 mEq/L [mmol/L]) or persistent volume retention despite high diuretic doses and sodium restriction, limit daily fluid intake to 2 L/day from all sources.
- Revascularization or anti-ischemic therapy in patients with coronary disease may reduce HF symptoms.
- Drugs that can aggravate HF should be discontinued if possible.

PHARMACOLOGIC THERAPY OF CHRONIC HEART FAILURE

- In general, patients with stage C HFrEF should receive an ACE inhibitor, ARB, or ARNI along with an evidence-based β-blocker, plus an aldosterone antagonist in select patients (Fig. 9-1). Administer a diuretic if there is evidence of fluid retention. A hydralazine–nitrate combination, ivabradine, or digoxin may be considered in select patients. Dosing recommendations for GDMT used to treat patients with HFrEF and HFpEF are provided in Table 9-1.

Angiotensin-Converting Enzyme Inhibitors

- ACE inhibitors decrease angiotensin II and aldosterone, attenuating many of their deleterious effects that drive HF initiation and progression. ACE inhibitors also inhibit the breakdown of bradykinin, which increases vasodilation and also leads to cough. ACE inhibitors improve symptoms, slow disease progression, and decrease mortality in patients with HFrEF. Prior guidelines recommended that all patients with HFrEF, regardless of whether or not symptoms are present, should receive an ACE inhibitor to reduce morbidity and mortality, unless there are contraindications. However, recent evidence suggests that sacubitril/valsartan is preferred over ACE inhibitors (or ARBs) for HFrEF unless other circumstances (eg, affordability) are present in individual patients.
- Start therapy with low doses followed by gradual titration as tolerated to the target or maximally tolerated doses (Table 9-1). Dose titration is usually accomplished by doubling the dose every 2 weeks. Evaluate blood pressure (BP), renal function, and serum potassium at baseline and within 1–2 weeks after the start of therapy and after each dose increase. Although symptoms may improve within a few days of starting therapy, it may take weeks to months before the full benefits are apparent. Even if symptoms do not improve, continue long-term therapy to reduce mortality and hospitalizations.

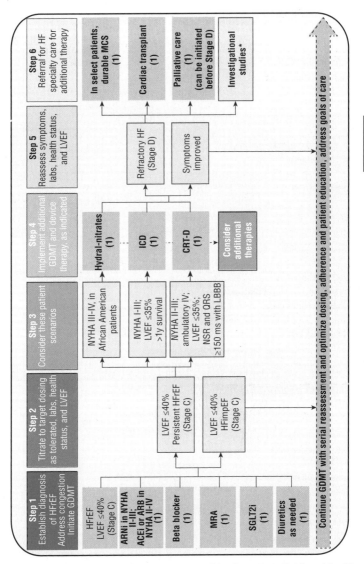

FIGURE 9-1. Treatment of HFrEF Stages C and D. (Data from Heidenreich PA, Bozkurt B, Aguilar D, et al. 2022 AHA/ACC/HFSA guideline for the management of heart failure: a report of the American College of Cardiology/American Heart Association Joint Committee on Clinical Practice Guidelines. *J Am Coll Cardiol* 2022;79:e263–e421.)

- The most common adverse effects include hypotension, renal dysfunction, and hyperkalemia. A dry, nonproductive cough (occurring in 15%–20% of patients) is the most common reason for discontinuation. Because cough is a bradykinin-mediated effect, replacement with sacubitril/valsartan or an ARB is reasonable; however,

TABLE 9-1	Guideline Recommended Drug Therapies and Doses for HFrEF and HFpEF	
Generic (Brand) Name	Initial Dose	Usual Range with Normal Renal Function
Loop Diuretics		
Furosemide (Lasix)	20–40 mg once or twice daily	20–160 mg once or twice daily
Bumetanide (Bumex)	0.5–1 mg once or twice daily	1–2 mg once or twice daily
Torsemide (Demadex)	10–20 mg once daily	10–80 mg once daily
ACE Inhibitors		
Captopril (Capoten)	6.25 mg three times daily	50 mg three times daily[a]
Enalapril (Vasotec)	2.5 mg twice daily	10–20 mg twice daily[a]
Lisinopril (Prinivil, Zestril)	2.5–5 mg once daily	20–40 mg once daily[a]
Quinapril (Accupril)	5 mg twice daily	20–40 mg twice daily
Ramipril (Altace)	1.25–2.5 mg once daily	10 mg once daily[a]
Fosinopril (Monopril)	5–10 mg once daily	40 mg once daily
Trandolapril (Mavik)	1 mg once daily	4 mg once daily[a]
Perindopril (Aceon)	2 mg once daily	8–16 mg once daily
Angiotensin Receptor Blockers		
Candesartan (Atacand)	4–8 mg once daily	32 mg once daily[a]
Valsartan (Diovan)	20–40 mg twice daily	160 mg twice daily[a]
Losartan (Cozaar)	25–50 mg once daily	150 mg once daily[a]
Angiotensin Receptor Blocker–Neprilysin Inhibitor		
Sacubitril/Valsartan (Entresto)	49/51 mg sacubitril–valsartan twice daily	97/103 mg sacubitril–valsartan twice daily[a]
β-Blockers		
Bisoprolol (Zebeta)	1.25 mg once daily	10 mg once daily[a]
Carvedilol (Coreg)	3.125 mg twice daily	25 mg twice daily[a]
Carvedilol phosphate (Coreg CR)	10 mg once daily	80 mg once daily
Metoprolol succinate CR/XL (Toprol-XL)	12.5–25 mg once daily	200 mg once daily[a]
Aldosterone Antagonists		
Spironolactone (Aldactone)	12.5–25 mg once daily	25–50 mg once daily[a]
Eplerenone (Inspra)	25 mg once daily	50 mg once daily[a]
SGLT2 Inhibitors		
Dapagliflozin (Farxiga)	10 mg daily	10 mg daily
Empagliflozin (Jardiance)	10 mg daily	10 mg daily
Other		
Hydralazine–Isosorbide Dinitrate (Bidil)	Hydralazine 37.5 mg three times daily	Hydralazine 75 mg three times daily[a]
	Isosorbide dinitrate 20 mg three times daily	Isosorbide dinitrate 40 mg three times daily[a]
Digoxin (Lanoxin)	0.125–0.25 mg once daily	0.125–0.25 mg once daily
Ivabradine (Corlanor)	5 mg twice daily	5–7.5 mg twice daily
Vericiguat (Verquvo)	2.5 mg once daily	10 mg once daily

ACEI, angiotensin-converting enzyme inhibitor; ARB, angiotensin receptor blocker.
[a]Regimens proven in large clinical trials to reduce mortality.

caution is required because crossreactivity has been reported. Angioedema occurs in approximately 1% of patients and is potentially life threatening; ACE inhibitors are contraindicated in patients with a history of angioedema. ACE inhibitors are contraindicated in pregnancy due to various congenital defects.

Angiotensin Receptor Blockers

- The ARBs block the angiotensin II receptor subtype AT_1, preventing the deleterious effects of angiotensin II on ventricular remodeling. Because they do not affect the ACE enzyme, ARBs do not affect bradykinin, which is linked to ACE inhibitor cough and angioedema.
- Although ARBs are a guideline-recommended alternative in patients who are unable to tolerate an ACE inhibitor due to cough or angioedema, sacubitril/valsartan is preferred for ACE inhibitor-associated cough. Although numerous ARBs are available, only **candesartan**, **valsartan**, and **losartan** are recommended in the guidelines because efficacy has been demonstrated in clinical trials. As with ACE inhibitors, initiate therapy with low doses and then titrate to target doses. Evaluate BP, renal function, and serum potassium within 1–2 weeks after starting therapy and after dosage increases, with these parameters used to guide subsequent dose changes.
- ARBs are not suitable alternatives in patients with hypotension, hyperkalemia, or renal insufficiency due to ACE inhibitors because they are just as likely to cause these adverse effects. Careful monitoring is required when an ARB is used with another inhibitor of the renin–angiotensin–aldosterone (RAAS) system (eg, ACE inhibitor or aldosterone antagonist) because this combination increases the risk of these adverse effects. Because ARBs do not affect bradykinin, they are not associated with cough and have a lower risk of angioedema than ACE inhibitors. Caution should be exercised when ARBs are used in patients with angioedema from ACE inhibitors because crossreactivity has been reported. Similar to ACE inhibitors, ARBs are contraindicated in pregnancy.

Angiotensin Receptor–Neprilysin Inhibitor

- **Valsartan/Sacubitril** is an ARNI approved to reduce the risk of cardiovascular death and hospitalization for HF in patients with NYHA class II–IV HF and reduced LVEF. Neprilysin is an enzyme that degrades bradykinin and other endogenous vasodilator and natriuretic peptides. By reducing neprilysin-mediated breakdown of these compounds, vasodilation, diuresis, and natriuresis are enhanced, and renin and aldosterone secretion is inhibited.
- In patients with HFrEF, ARNI is preferred over either ACE inhibitors or ARBs to improve survival, slow disease progression, reduce hospitalizations, and improve quality of life. Patients receiving ACE inhibitors or ARBs can be switched to ARNI or ARNI can be used as initial treatment in patients with newly detected HFrEF without previous exposure to ACE inhibitors or ARBs. Discontinue ACE inhibitors 36 hours prior to initiating the ARNI; no waiting period is needed in patients receiving an ARB. The initial starting dose for most HFrEF patients is 49/51 mg sacubitril/valsartan twice daily and titrated to the target dose of 97/103 mg sacubitril/valsartan twice daily after 2–4 weeks (see Table 9-1). Closely monitor BP, serum potassium, and renal function after the start of therapy and after each titration step.
- The most common adverse effects include hypotension, kidney dysfunction, and hyperkalemia. Angioedema is more common with sacubitril/valsartan than with enalapril (0.5% vs 0.2%, respectively). Sacubitril/valsartan is contraindicated in patients with a history of angioedema associated with an ACE inhibitor or ARB. It is also contraindicated in pregnancy and should not be used concurrently with ACE inhibitors or other ARBs.

β-Blockers

- β-Blockers antagonize the detrimental effects of the sympathetic nervous systems in HF and slow disease progression. β-Blockers reduce morbidity and mortality in patients with HFrEF.

- The ACC/AHA guidelines recommend use of β-blockers in all stable patients with HFrEF in the absence of contraindications or a clear history of β-blocker intolerance. Patients should receive a β-blocker even if symptoms are mild or well controlled with other GDMT. It is not essential that doses of other agents be optimized before a β-blocker is started because the addition of a β-blocker is likely to be of greater benefit than an increase in the dose of other medications.
- β-Blockers are also recommended for asymptomatic persons with a reduced LVEF (stage B) to decrease the risk of progression to HF.
- **Carvedilol**, **metoprolol succinate (CR/XL)**, and **bisoprolol** are the only β-blockers shown to reduce mortality in large HF trials. Because bisoprolol is not available in the necessary starting dose of 1.25 mg, the choice is typically limited to either carvedilol or metoprolol succinate. Target doses are those associated with reductions in mortality in placebo-controlled clinical trials (Table 9-1).
- Initiate β-blockers in stable patients who have no or minimal evidence of fluid overload. Because of their negative inotropic effects, start β-blockers in very low doses with slow upward dose titration to avoid symptomatic worsening or acute decompensation. Doses should be doubled no more often than every 2 weeks, as tolerated, until the target or maximally tolerated dose is reached.
- Inform patients that β-blocker therapy is expected to positively influence disease progression and survival even if there is little symptomatic improvement. In addition, dose titration is a long, gradual process; response to therapy may be delayed; and HF symptoms may actually worsen during the initiation period.
- Adverse effects include bradycardia or heart block, hypotension, fatigue, impaired glycemic control in diabetic patients, bronchospasm in patients with asthma, and worsening HF. Absolute contraindications include uncontrolled bronchospastic disease, symptomatic bradycardia, advanced heart block without a pacemaker, and acute decompensated HF. However, β-blockers may be tried with caution in patients with asymptomatic bradycardia, COPD, or well-controlled asthma.

Aldosterone Antagonists

- **Spironolactone** and **eplerenone** block mineralocorticoid receptors, the target for aldosterone. In the kidney, aldosterone antagonists inhibit sodium reabsorption and potassium excretion. However, diuretic effects with low doses are minimal, suggesting that their therapeutic benefits result from other actions. In the heart, aldosterone antagonists inhibit cardiac extracellular matrix and collagen deposition, thereby attenuating cardiac fibrosis and ventricular remodeling. Aldosterone antagonists also attenuate the systemic proinflammatory state, atherogenesis, and oxidative stress caused by aldosterone.
- Current guidelines recommend adding a low-dose aldosterone antagonist to standard therapy to improve symptoms, reduce the risk of HF hospitalization, and increase survival in select patients provided that serum potassium and renal function can be carefully monitored. Guidelines recommend adding an aldosterone antagonist to decrease the risk for hospitalization for HF in patients with HFpEF, especially if plasma natriuretic peptide levels are elevated.
- Start with low doses (spironolactone 12.5 mg/day or eplerenone 25 mg/day) especially in older persons and those with diabetes or a creatinine clearance <50 mL/min/1.73m^2 (0.48 mL/sec/m^2) (Table 9-1).
- Avoid aldosterone antagonists in patients with renal impairment, elevated serum potassium (>5 mEq/L [mmol/L]), or history of severe hyperkalemia. Spironolactone also interacts with androgen and progesterone receptors, which may lead to gynecomastia, impotence, and menstrual irregularities in some patients.

Sodium-Glucose Cotransporter Type 2 (SGLT2) Inhibitors

- SLGT2 inhibitors inhibit glucose and sodium reabsoprtion in the proximal kidney tubules, which leads to osmotic diuresis and natriuresis, reduction in arterial pressure and stiffness, and a shift to ketone-based myocardial metabolism.

- **Dapagliflozin** and **empagliflozin** reduce the risk of worsening HF and cardiovascular death in patients with HFrEF (with or without diabetes) and are FDA-approved for this use.
- Patients should be advised to weigh daily and contact their healthcare provider if their weight starts to decline and to avoid abrupt changes in position as orthostasis may occur in the setting of overdiuresis.

Diuretics

- Compensatory mechanisms in HF stimulate excessive sodium and water retention, often leading to systemic and pulmonary congestion. Consequently, diuretic therapy (in addition to sodium restriction) is recommended for all patients with clinical evidence of fluid retention. However, because they do not alter disease progression or prolong survival, diuretics are not required for patients without fluid retention.
- Thiazide diuretics (eg, **hydrochlorothiazide**) are relatively weak and are infrequently used alone in HF. However, thiazides or the thiazide-like diuretic **metolazone** can be used in combination with a loop diuretic to promote very effective diuresis. Thiazides may be preferred over loop diuretics in patients with only mild fluid retention and elevated BP because of their more persistent antihypertensive effects.
- Loop diuretics (**furosemide**, **bumetanide**, and **torsemide**) are usually necessary to restore and maintain euvolemia in HF. In addition to acting in the thick ascending limb of the loop of Henle, they induce a prostaglandin-mediated increase in renal blood flow that contributes to their natriuretic effect. Unlike thiazides, loop diuretics maintain their effectiveness in the presence of impaired renal function, although higher doses may be necessary.
- Adverse effects of diuretics include hypovolemia, hypotension, hyponatremia, hypokalemia, hypomagnesemia, hyperuricemia, and renal dysfunction.

Nitrates and Hydralazine

- **Isosorbide dinitrate (ISDN)** is a venodilator that reduces preload, whereas **hydralazine** is a direct arterial vasodilator that reduces systemic vascular resistance (SVR) and increases stroke volume and CO. The beneficial effects of combining a nitrate with hydralazine extend beyond their complementary hemodynamic actions and are likely related to attenuating the biochemical processes driving HF progression.
- Guidelines recommend adding hydralazine/ISDN to Black patients with HFrEF and persistent symptoms despite ARNI, β-blocker, aldosterone antagonist, and SGLT2 inhibitor therapy. The combination can also be useful in patients unable to tolerate either an ACE inhibitor or ARB because of renal insufficiency, hyperkalemia, or hypotension.
- Obstacles to successful therapy with the combination include the need for frequent dosing (ie, three times daily with the fixed-dose combination product), high frequency of adverse effects (eg, headache, dizziness, and GI distress), and increased cost for the fixed-dose combination product.
- In patients with HFpEF, nitrates reduce exercise capacity and do not improve quality of life or plasma NTproBNP concentrations. Adverse events, including worsening HF and presyncope/syncope, are more frequent with nitrate treatment. In the absence of another indication for nitrate therapy (eg, angina), nitrates provide no benefits to patients with HFpEF.

Ivabradine

- Ivabradine inhibits the I_f current in the sinoatrial node that is responsible for controlling HR, thereby slowing spontaneous depolarization of the sinus node and resulting in a dose-dependent slowing of the HR. It does not affect AV conduction, BP, or myocardial contractility. Elevated resting heart rate (HR) (>70–80 bpm) is an independent risk factor for adverse HFrEF outcomes, and β-blockers are frequently underdosed in clinical practice for a variety of reasons. Because of the clear benefits of β-blockers on mortality, clinicians should titrate to the maximum tolerated doses before considering use of ivabradine.

- Ivabradine is indicated to reduce the risk of hospitalization for worsening HF in patients with LVEF ≤35% who are in sinus rhythm with resting HR ≥70 bpm and are either on a maximally tolerated dose of a β-blocker or have a contraindication to β-blocker use.
- The usual starting dose is 5 mg twice daily with meals (Table 9-1). After 2 weeks of treatment, if the resting HR is between 50 and 60 bpm, the dose should be continued. If the HR is >60 bpm, the dose can be increased to the maximum of 7.5 mg twice daily. If at any point the HR is <50 bpm or the patient has symptomatic bradycardia, the dose should be reduced by 2.5 mg twice daily; if the patient is only receiving 2.5 mg twice daily, ivabradine should be discontinued.
- The most common adverse effects are bradycardia, atrial fibrillation, and visual disturbances.

Digoxin

- Although digoxin has positive inotropic effects, its benefits in HF are related to its neurohormonal effects. It attenuates the excessive sympathetic nervous system activation in HF and increases parasympathetic activity, thereby decreasing HR and enhancing diastolic filling. Observational studies of digoxin conducted in the context of contemporary HF therapy showed either neutral effects or reductions in hospitalizations and either neutral or detrimental effects of digoxin on mortality.
- Digoxin is not considered a first-line agent in HF, but a trial may be considered in conjunction with GDMT in patients with symptomatic HFrEF to improve symptoms and reduce hospitalizations. Digoxin may also be considered to help control ventricular rate in patients with HFrEF and supraventricular arrhythmias.
- The target serum digoxin concentration for most patients is 0.5–0.9 ng/mL (0.6–1.2 nmol/L). Most patients with normal renal function can achieve this level with a dose of 0.125 mg/day. Patients with decreased renal function, low body weight, advanced age, or interacting drugs (eg, amiodarone) should receive 0.125 mg every other day.

Vericiguat

- Vericiguat modulates endothelial dysfunction; it is a soluble guanylate cyclase activator (sGC) that enhances the effect of nitric oxide (NO) to increase cGMP activity and regulate contractility and diastolic function.
- In a clinical trial, patients with HFrEF receiving vericiguat demonstrated a significant, but modest, reduction in the primary endpoint of cardiovascular death or HF hospitalization. The drug was well tolerated overall, but there was an unexplained greater incidence of anemia in patients treated with vericiguat.
- Its place in therapy is unclear given the limited benefit, but it may lie in the lack of significant hemodynamic, renal, and electrolyte effects in high-risk patients who often do not tolerate GDMT. It is not indicated in HFpEF due to lack of benefit and safety data.

PHARMACOLOGIC THERAPY FOR HFpEF

- Treatment includes controlling HR and BP, alleviating causes of myocardial ischemia, reducing volume, and restoring and maintaining sinus rhythm in patients with atrial fibrillation. Many of the drugs are the same as those used to treat HFrEF, but the rationale and dosing may be different.
- ACE inhibitors, ARBs, and β-blockers have not demonstrated efficacy in the absence of other comorbid conditions such as HTN or myocardial infarction.
- The diuretic doses used to treat HFpEF are generally much lower than those used to treat HFrEF.
- Calcium channel blockers (eg, diltiazem, amlodipine, verapamil) may be useful when treating HTN.
- ARNIs and SGLT2 inhibitors are beneficial in select patients with HFpEF.

TREATMENT OF ACUTE DECOMPENSATED HEART FAILURE (ADHF)

GENERAL APPROACH

- *Acute decompensated heart failure* involves patients with new or worsening signs or symptoms (often resulting from volume overload and/or low CO) requiring medical intervention, such as emergency department visit or hospitalization.
- <u>Goals of Treatment</u>: The overall goals are to relieve symptoms, improve hemodynamic stability, and reduce short-term mortality so the patient can be discharged in a stable compensated state on oral drug therapy.
- Consider hospitalization based on clinical findings. Admission to an intensive care unit (ICU) may be required if the patient experiences hemodynamic instability requiring frequent monitoring of vital signs, invasive hemodynamic monitoring, or rapid titration of IV medications with close monitoring.
- Focus on the history and physical exam on potential etiologies of ADHF; presence of precipitating factors; onset, duration, and severity of symptoms; and a careful medication history.
- Symptoms of volume overload include dyspnea, orthopnea, PND, ascites, GI symptoms (poor appetite, nausea, early satiety), peripheral edema, and weight gain. Low output symptoms include altered mental status, fatigue, GI symptoms (similar to volume overload), and decreased urine output.
- Signs of volume overload include pulmonary crackles, elevated jugular venous pressure, HJR, S_3 gallop, and peripheral edema. Low output signs include tachycardia, hypotension (more commonly) or hypertension, narrow pulse pressure, cool extremities, pallor, and cachexia.
- Laboratory tests: B-type natriuretic peptide (BNP) <100 pg/mL (ng/L; 29 pmol/L) and N-terminal BNP <300 pg/mL (ng/L; 35 pmol/L) are negatively predictive for congestive ADHF; serum sodium concentration <130 mEq/L (mmol/L); elevated alkaline phosphatase; elevated gamma-glutamyl transferase.
- Ascertain hemodynamic status to guide initial therapy. Patients may be categorized into one of four hemodynamic subsets based on volume status (euvolemic or "dry" vs volume overloaded or "wet") and CO (adequate CO or "warm" vs hypoperfusion or "cold") (Fig. 9-2).
- In patients who require invasive hemodynamic monitoring, measure pulmonary capillary wedge pressure (PCWP) and cardiac Index.
- Assess medications being taken prior to admission and determine whether adjustment or discontinuation is required.
- If fluid retention is evident on physical exam, pursue aggressive diuresis, preferably with IV diuretics.
- In the absence of cardiogenic shock or symptomatic hypotension, strive to continue all GDMT for HF. β-blockers may be temporarily held or dose-reduced if recent changes are responsible for acute decompensation. Other GDMT (ACE inhibitors, ARBs, ARNI, and aldosterone antagonists) may also need to be temporarily withheld in the presence of renal dysfunction, with close monitoring of serum potassium. Most patients may continue to receive digoxin at doses targeting a trough serum concentration of 0.5–0.9 ng/mL (mcg/L; 0.6–1.2 nmol/L).

NONPHARMACOLOGIC THERAPY FOR ADHF

- Place all patients with congestive symptoms on sodium restriction (<2 g daily) and consider fluid restriction for refractory symptoms.
- Consider noninvasive ventilation for patients in respiratory distress due to acute pulmonary edema, particularly those at risk for intubation.
- Provide pharmacologic thromboprophylaxis with unfractionated heparin or low-molecular-weight heparin for most patients with limited mobility; consider mechanical thromboprophylaxis with intermittent pneumatic compression devices in patients at high risk for bleeding.

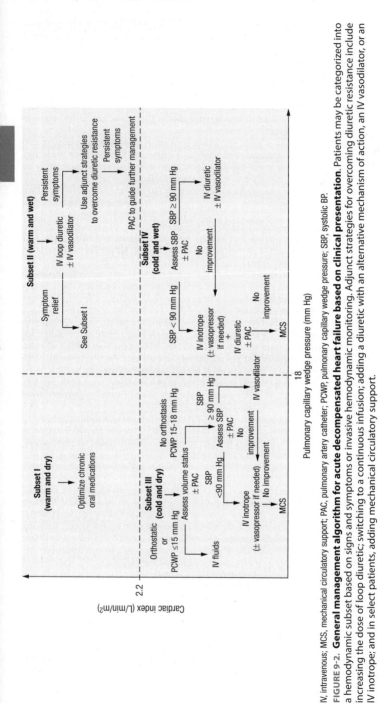

FIGURE 9-2. **General management algorithm for acute decompensated heart failure based on clinical presentation.** Patients may be categorized into a hemodynamic subset based on signs and symptoms or invasive hemodynamic monitoring. Adjunct strategies for overcoming diuretic resistance include increasing the dose of loop diuretic; switching to a continuous infusion; adding a diuretic with an alternative mechanism of action, an IV vasodilator, or an IV inotrope; and in select patients, adding mechanical circulatory support.

IV, intravenous; MCS, mechanical circulatory support; PAC, pulmonary artery catheter; PCWP, pulmonary capillary wedge pressure; SBP, systolic BP.

- Most nonpharmacologic therapies for ADHF are reserved for patients failing pharmacologic therapy. Ultrafiltration and wireless invasive hemodynamic monitoring (W-IHM) may be used to manage congestive symptoms. Temporary mechanical circulatory support (MCS) with an intra-aortic balloon pump (IABP), ventricular assist device (VAD), or extracorporeal membrane oxygenation (ECMO) may be considered for hemodynamic stabilization until the underlying etiology of cardiac dysfunction resolves or has been corrected ("bridge to recovery") or until evaluation for definitive therapy (eg, durable MCS or cardiac transplantation) can be completed ("bridge to decision"). IV vasodilators and inotropes may be used with temporary MCS to maximize hemodynamic and clinical benefits or facilitate device removal. Systemic anticoagulant therapy is generally required to prevent device thrombosis, regardless of the method selected.
- Durable MCS with temporary device implantation is used for patients awaiting heart transplantation who are unlikely to survive until a suitable donor is identified ("bridge to transplantation"). Permanent device implantation is used in patients ineligible for heart transplantation due to advanced age or comorbid conditions ("destination therapy").
- Cardiac transplantation is the best option for patients with irreversible advanced HF. New surgical strategies such as ventricular aneurysm resection and myocardial cell transplantation offer additional options for patients ineligible for VAD implantation or heart transplantation.

PHARMACOLOGIC THERAPY FOR ADHF

Loop Diuretics

- Current guidelines recommend IV loop diuretics (**furosemide**, **bumetanide**) as first-line therapy for ADHF patients with volume overload.
- Bolus administration reduces preload by functional venodilation within 5–15 minutes and later (>20 minutes) via sodium and water excretion, thereby improving pulmonary congestion. Although patients with HFrEF can tolerate significant reductions in preload without compromising stroke volume, excessive diuresis can decrease CO. Excessive reductions in venous return may also compromise CO in diastolic dysfunction, intravascular volume depletion, or patients in whom CO is significantly dependent on adequate filling pressure (ie, preload-dependent). Reflex increases in neurohormonal activation (ie, elevated renin, norepinephrine, and AVP) may result in arteriolar and coronary vasoconstriction, tachycardia, and increased myocardial oxygen consumption.
- Use low doses (equivalent to IV furosemide 20–40 mg) initially in ADHF patients who are naïve to loop diuretics. For patients taking loop diuretics prior to admission, a total daily dose of 1- to 2.5-times their home dose is recommended. Higher doses are associated with more rapid relief of congestive symptoms but may also increase the risk of transient worsening of renal function. Doses may be administered as either an IV bolus (ie, divided every 12 hours) or continuous IV infusion. Use diuretic therapy judiciously to obtain the desired improvement in congestive symptoms while avoiding a reduction in CO, symptomatic hypotension, or worsening renal function.
- Diuretic resistance may be improved by administering larger IV bolus doses, transitioning from IV bolus to continuous IV infusions, or adding a second diuretic with a different mechanism of action, such as a distal tubule blocker (eg, oral **metolazone**, oral **hydrochlorothiazide**, or IV **chlorothiazide**). Sequential nephron blockade with a loop and thiazide-type diuretic should generally be reserved for inpatients who can be monitored closely for development of severe electrolyte and intravascular volume depletion.

Vasopressin Antagonists

- Vasopressin receptor antagonists affect one or two AVP (antidiuretic hormone) receptors, V_{1A} or V_2. Stimulation of V_{1A} receptors (located in vascular smooth muscle cells and myocardium) results in vasoconstriction, myocyte hypertrophy, coronary vasoconstriction, and positive inotropic effects. V_2 receptors are located in renal tubules, where they regulate water reabsorption.

✓ **Tolvaptan** selectively binds to and inhibits the V_2 receptor. It is an oral agent indicated for hypervolemic and euvolemic hyponatremia in patients with syndrome of inappropriate antidiuretic hormone (SIADH), cirrhosis, or HF. Tolvaptan is typically initiated at 15 mg orally daily and then titrated to 30 or 60 mg daily as needed to resolve hyponatremia. It is a substrate of cytochrome P450-3A4 and is contraindicated with potent inhibitors of this enzyme. The most common side effects are dry mouth, thirst, urinary frequency, constipation, and hyperglycemia.

✓ **Conivaptan** nonselectively inhibits both the V_{1A} and V_2 receptors. It is an IV agent indicated for hypervolemic and euvolemic hyponatremia due to a variety of causes but is not indicated for patients with ADHF.

• Monitor patients closely to avoid an excessively rapid rise in serum sodium (>12 mEq/L [mmol/L] per 24 hours); fluid restrictions should be liberalized to reduce this risk.

Vasodilators

• Venodilators reduce preload by increasing venous capacitance, improving symptoms of pulmonary congestion in patients with high ventricular filling pressures. Arterial vasodilators counteract the peripheral vasoconstriction and impaired CO that can result from activation of the sympathetic nervous system, RAAS, and other neurohormonal mediators in HF. Arterial vasodilators reduce impedance, decreasing afterload and causing reflex improvement in LV performance and increased CO. Mixed vasodilators act on both arterial resistance and venous capacitance vessels, reducing congestive symptoms while increasing CO.

• IV vasodilators should be considered before positive inotropic therapy in patients with low CO and elevated SVR (or elevated BP in those without a pulmonary artery catheter). However, hypotension may preclude their use in patients with preexisting low BP or SVR.

• **IV nitroglycerin** is often preferred for preload reduction in ADHF, especially in patients with pulmonary congestion. It reduces preload and pulmonary capillary wedge pressure (PCWP) via functional venodilation and mild arterial vasodilation. In higher doses, nitroglycerin displays potent coronary vasodilating properties and beneficial effects on myocardial oxygen demand and supply, making it the vasodilator of choice for patients with severe HF and ischemic heart disease.

✓ Initiate nitroglycerin at 5–10 mcg/min (0.1 mcg/kg/min) and increase every 5–10 minutes as necessary and tolerated. Maintenance doses usually range from 35 to 200 mcg/min (0.5–3 mcg/kg/min). Hypotension and excessive decrease in PCWP are important dose-limiting side effects. Tolerance to the hemodynamic effects may develop over 12–72 hours of continuous administration.

• **Sodium nitroprusside** is a mixed arteriovenous vasodilator that increases cardiac index (CI) to a similar degree as dobutamine and milrinone despite having no direct inotropic activity. However, nitroprusside generally produces greater decreases in PCWP, SVR, and BP.

✓ Hypotension is an important dose-limiting adverse effect of nitroprusside, and its use should be primarily reserved for patients with elevated SVR. Close monitoring is required because even modest HR increases can have adverse consequences in patients with underlying ischemic heart disease or resting tachycardia.

✓ Nitroprusside is effective in the short-term management of severe HF in a variety of settings (eg, acute MI, valvular regurgitation, after coronary bypass surgery, and ADHF). It does not usually worsen, and may improve, the balance between myocardial oxygen demand and supply. However, an excessive decrease in systemic arterial pressure can decrease coronary perfusion and worsen ischemia.

✓ Nitroprusside has a rapid onset and a duration of action <10 minutes, necessitating continuous IV infusions. Initiate therapy with a low dose (0.1–0.2 mcg/kg/min) to avoid excessive hypotension, and increase by small increments (0.1–0.2 mcg/kg/min) every 5–10 minutes as tolerated. Usual effective doses range from 0.5 to 3 mcg/kg/min. Taper nitroprusside slowly when transitioning to oral medications to avoid the rebound phenomenon of reflex neurohormonal activation after abrupt withdrawal. Nitroprusside-induced cyanide and thiocyanate toxicity are unlikely when doses <3 mcg/kg/min are administered for less than 3 days, except in patients with significant renal impairment (ie, serum creatinine >3 mg/dL [265 μmol/L]).

Inotropes

- Prompt correction of low CO in patients with "cold" subsets (III and IV) is required to restore peripheral tissue perfusion and preserve end-organ function. Although IV inotropes can improve hypoperfusion by enhancing cardiac contractility, potential adverse outcomes limit their use to select patients with refractory ADHF. Inotropes should be considered only as a temporizing measure to maintain end-organ perfusion in patients with cardiogenic shock or severely depressed CO and low systolic BP (ie, ineligible for IV vasodilators) until definitive therapy can be initiated, as a "bridge" for patients with advanced HF who are eligible for MCS or cardiac transplantation, or for palliation of symptoms in patients with advanced HF who are ineligible for MCS or cardiac transplantation.

- Dobutamine and milrinone produce similar hemodynamic effects, but dobutamine usually causes more pronounced increases in HR, and milrinone is associated with greater relaxation in arterial smooth muscle.

- **Dobutamine** is a β_1- and β_2-receptor agonist with some α_1-agonist effects; its positive inotropic effects are due to effects on β_1-receptors. Stimulation of cardiac β_1-receptors does not generally produce a significant increase in HR. Modest peripheral β_2-receptor-mediated vasodilation tends to offset minor α_1-receptor-mediated vasoconstriction; the net vascular effect is usually vasodilation.

  ✓ CI is increased because of inotropic stimulation, arterial vasodilation, and a variable increase in HR. It causes relatively little change in mean arterial pressure (MAP) compared with the more consistent increases observed with dopamine. Dobutamine should be considered over milrinone when a significant decrease in MAP might further compromise hemodynamic function.

  ✓ Vasodilation usually reduces PCWP, making dobutamine particularly useful in the presence of low CI and an elevated LV filling pressure; however, these effects may be detrimental in the presence of reduced filling pressure.

  ✓ Initial doses of 2.5–5 mcg/kg/min may be increased progressively to 20 mcg/kg/min based on clinical and hemodynamic responses. The dose should be tapered rather than abruptly discontinued.

  ✓ Dobutamine's major adverse effects are tachycardia and ventricular arrhythmias. Potentially detrimental increases in oxygen consumption have also been observed.

- **Milrinone** inhibits phosphodiesterase III and produces positive inotropic and arterial and venous vasodilating effects (an inodilator). It has supplanted use of amrinone, which has a higher rate of thrombocytopenia.

  ✓ During IV administration, milrinone increases stroke volume and CO with minimal change in HR. However, the vasodilating effects may predominate, leading to decreased BP and a reflex tachycardia. Use milrinone cautiously in severely hypotensive HF patients because it does not increase, and may even decrease, arterial BP.

  ✓ Most patients are started on a continuous IV infusion of 0.1–0.3 mcg/kg/min, titrated to a maximum of 0.75 mcg/kg/min. A loading dose of 50 mcg/kg over 10 minutes can be given if rapid hemodynamic changes are required, but its use is uncommon due to an increased risk of hypotension.

  ✓ The most notable adverse events are arrhythmia, hypotension, and thrombocytopenia. Measure the platelet count before and during therapy.

- **Norepinephrine** and **dopamine** have combined inotropic and vasopressor activity. Although therapies that increase SVR are generally avoided in ADHF, they may be required in select patients where marked hypotension precludes use of traditional inotropes (eg, septic shock, refractory cardiogenic shock). These agents are sometimes combined with traditional inotropes so each drug can be adjusted independently to achieve the desired hemodynamic response, although little data exist to support that practice.

✓ Norepinephrine stimulates α_1- and β_1-adrenergic receptors. Stimulation of β_1-receptors in myocardial tissue increases HR, contractility, and therefore CO, but peripheral α_1-receptor-induced vasoconstriction is the predominant clinical hemodynamic effect. Lack of affinity for β_2-receptors may be responsible for the limited impact of norepinephrine on CO.

✓ Dopamine is an endogenous precursor of norepinephrine that stimulates α_1, β_1, β_2, and D_1 (vascular dopaminergic) receptors. Positive inotropic effects mediated primarily by β_1-receptors are prominent with doses of 2–5 mcg/kg/min. The CI is increased with minimal changes in SVR. At doses between 5 and 10 mcg/kg/min, chronotropic and α_1-mediated vasoconstriction become more prominent and MAP usually increases as a result of increases in both CI and SVR.

✓ Administration of low doses of dopamine (ie, 2–5 mcg/kg/min), does not consistently improve congestive symptoms or diuresis but increases the risk of tachyarrhythmias. Because of β-mediated effects at lower infusion rates, dopamine likely does not provide any advantages over a traditional inotrope in this setting.

EVALUATION OF THERAPEUTIC OUTCOMES

CHRONIC HEART FAILURE

- Ask patients about the presence and severity of symptoms and how symptoms affect daily activities.
- Evaluate efficacy of diuretic treatment by disappearance of the signs and symptoms of excess fluid retention. Focus the physical examination on body weight, extent of JVD, presence of HJR, and presence and severity of pulmonary congestion (crackles, dyspnea on exertion, orthopnea, and PND) and peripheral edema.
- Other outcomes are improvement in exercise tolerance and fatigue, decreased nocturia, and decreased HR.
- Monitor BP to ensure that symptomatic hypotension does not develop as a result of drug therapy.
- Body weight is a sensitive marker of fluid loss or retention, and patients should weigh themselves daily and report changes of 3–5 lb (1.4–2.3 kg) to their healthcare provider so adjustments can be made in diuretic doses.
- Symptoms may worsen initially on β-blocker therapy, and it may take weeks to months before patients notice symptomatic improvement.
- Routine monitoring of serum electrolytes (especially potassium and magnesium) and renal function (BUN, serum creatinine, eGFR) is mandatory in patients with HF.

ACUTE DECOMPENSATED HEART FAILURE

- Assess the efficacy of drug therapy with daily monitoring of weight, strict fluid intake and output measurements, and HF signs/symptoms. Monitor frequently for electrolyte depletion, symptomatic hypotension, and renal dysfunction. Assess vital signs frequently throughout the day.
- Patients should not be discharged until optimal volume status is achieved, they have been successfully transitioned from IV to oral diuretics, and IV inotropes and vasodilators have been discontinued for at least 24 hours.
- Optimize GDMT in hemodynamically stable patients without contraindications, including reinitiation of therapies withheld earlier in the admission. Low-dose β-blockers may be safely initiated at discharge without increasing the risk of readmission. Transitioning eligible patients to the ARNI sacubitril/valsartan may also be considered.

- Schedule a follow-up appointment at 7–10 days postdischarge and a nurse visit or phone call at 3 days for select patients. Also schedule pertinent follow-up labs (eg, potassium, serum creatinine, INR, serum digoxin concentration).
- All patients should be considered for referral to a formal disease management program.

See Chapter 36, Chronic Heart Failure, authored by Robert B. Parker and Jo Ellen Rodgers, and Chapter 37, Acute Decompensated Heart Failure, authored by Brent N. Reed, Stormi E. Gale, and Zachary L. Cox, for more detailed discussions of these topics.

Hypertension

- *Hypertension* is defined as persistently elevated arterial blood pressure (BP). See Table 10-1 for the classification of BP in adults.
- Isolated systolic hypertension is diastolic blood pressure (DBP) <80 mm Hg and systolic blood pressure (SBP) ≥130 mm Hg.
- Hypertensive crisis (BP >180/120 mm Hg) is categorized as hypertensive emergency (extreme BP elevation with acute or progressing end-organ damage) or hypertensive urgency (extreme BP elevation without acute or progressing end-organ injury).
- This chapter incorporates elements of the 2017 American College of Cardiology/American Heart Association (ACC/AHA) Guideline for the Prevention, Detection, Evaluation, and Management of High Blood Pressure in Adults, the most recent evidence-based U.S. guideline for hypertension management.

PATHOPHYSIOLOGY

- Hypertension may result from an unknown etiology (primary or essential hypertension) or from a specific cause (secondary hypertension). Secondary hypertension (<10% of cases) is usually caused by chronic kidney disease (CKD) or renovascular disease. Other conditions are Cushing syndrome, coarctation of the aorta, obstructive sleep apnea, hyperparathyroidism, pheochromocytoma, primary aldosteronism, and hyperthyroidism. Examples of drugs that may increase BP include corticosteroids, estrogens, nonsteroidal anti-inflammatory drugs (NSAIDs), amphetamines, cyclosporine, tacrolimus, erythropoietin, and venlafaxine.
- Factors contributing to development of primary hypertension include:
  - ✓ Humoral abnormalities involving the renin–angiotensin–aldosterone system (RAAS), natriuretic hormone, and hyperinsulinemia;
  - ✓ Disturbances in the central nervous system (CNS), autonomic nerve fibers, adrenergic receptors, or baroreceptors;
  - ✓ Abnormalities in renal or tissue autoregulatory processes for sodium excretion, plasma volume, and arteriolar constriction;
  - ✓ Deficiency in synthesis of vasodilating substances in vascular endothelium (prostacyclin, bradykinin, nitric oxide) or excess vasoconstricting substances (angiotensin II, endothelin I);
  - ✓ High sodium intake or lack of dietary calcium.
- Major causes of death include cerebrovascular events, cardiovascular (CV) events, and renal failure. Probability of premature death correlates with the severity of BP elevation.

TABLE 10-1	Classification of Blood Pressure in Adults		
Classification	**Systolic (mm Hg)**		**Diastolic (mm Hg)**
Normal	<120	and	<80
Elevated	120–129	or	<80
Stage 1 hypertension	130–139	or	80–89
Stage 2 hypertension	≥140	or	≥90

CLINICAL PRESENTATION

- Patients with uncomplicated primary hypertension are usually asymptomatic initially.
- Patients with secondary hypertension may have symptoms of the underlying disorder:
  - ✓ Pheochromocytoma—headaches, sweating, tachycardia, palpitations, orthostatic hypotension;
  - ✓ Primary aldosteronism—hypokalemic symptoms of muscle cramps and weakness;
  - ✓ Cushing syndrome—moon face, buffalo hump, hirsutism, weight gain, polyuria, edema, menstrual irregularities, acne, muscle weakness.

DIAGNOSIS

- Elevated BP may be the only sign of primary hypertension on physical examination. Diagnosis should be based on the average of two or more readings taken at each of two or more clinical encounters. Refer to Chapter 30, "Hypertension," in *DiPiro's Pharmacotherapy: A Pathophysiologic Approach*, 12 ed., for the correct procedure for BP measurement.
- Signs of end-organ damage occur primarily in the eyes, brain, heart, kidneys, and peripheral vasculature.
- Funduscopic examination may reveal arteriolar narrowing, focal arteriolar constriction, arteriovenous nicking, retinal hemorrhages and exudates, and disk edema. Presence of papilledema usually indicates a hypertensive emergency requiring rapid treatment.
- Cardiopulmonary examination may reveal abnormal heart rate or rhythm, left ventricular (LV) hypertrophy, coronary artery disease, or heart failure (HF).
- Peripheral vascular examination may reveal aortic or abdominal bruits, distended veins, diminished or absent peripheral pulses, or lower extremity edema.
- Patients with renal artery stenosis may have an abdominal systolic-diastolic bruit.
- Baseline hypokalemia may suggest mineralocorticoid-induced hypertension. Protein, blood cells, and casts in the urine may indicate renovascular disease.
- *Laboratory tests*: Blood urea nitrogen (BUN), serum creatinine with estimated glomerular filtration rate (eGFR, using the CKD-EPI creatinine equation), fasting lipid panel, fasting blood glucose, serum electrolytes (sodium, potassium, calcium), uric acid, hemoglobin and hematocrit, and spot urine albumin-to-creatinine ratio. A 12-lead electrocardiogram (ECG) should also be obtained.
- *Laboratory tests to diagnose secondary hypertension*: Baseline hypokalemia may suggest mineralocorticoid-induced hypertension. Protein, red blood cells, and casts in the urine may indicate renovascular disease. Obtain plasma norepinephrine and urinary metanephrine levels for pheochromocytoma; plasma and urinary aldosterone concentrations for primary aldosteronism; and plasma renin activity, captopril stimulation test, renal vein renin, and renal artery angiography for renovascular disease.

TREATMENT

- Goals of Treatment: The overall goal is to reduce morbidity and mortality from CV events. The 2017 ACC/AHA guideline recommends a goal BP of <130/80 mm Hg for most patients, including those with clinical arteriosclerotic cardiovascular disease (ASCVD), diabetes, or CKD. For older ambulatory, community-dwelling patients, the goal is SBP <130 mm Hg. For institutionalized older patients and those with a high disease burden or limited life expectancy, consider a relaxed SBP goal of <150 mm Hg (or <140 mm Hg if tolerated).

NONPHARMACOLOGIC THERAPY

- Implement lifestyle modifications in all patients with elevated BP or stage 1 or 2 hypertension. These measures alone are appropriate initial treatment for patients with elevated BP or stage 1 hypertension who are at low risk of ASCVD (ie, primary prevention with a 10-year ASCVD risk <10%). Start drug therapy for these patients when BP is ≥140/90 mm Hg. For patients with stage 1 or 2 hypertension who already have ASCVD (secondary prevention) or an elevated 10-year ASCVD risk ≥10%, the threshold for starting drug therapy is ≥130/80 mm Hg with a goal BP of <130/80 mm Hg.
- Lifestyle modifications shown to lower BP include (1) weight loss if overweight or obese, (2) the Dietary Approaches to Stop Hypertension (DASH) eating plan, (3) reduced salt intake, ideally to 1.5 g/day sodium (3.8 g/day sodium chloride), (4) physical activity (90–150 min/week of aerobic or dynamic resistance training), and (5) moderation of alcohol intake (≤2 drinks/day in men and ≤1 drink/day in women). Although smoking cessation does not control BP, it reduces CV disease risk and should be encouraged.

PHARMACOLOGIC THERAPY

General Approach to Treatment

- Initial drug selection depends on the degree of BP elevation and presence of compelling indications for certain drugs.
- Use a single first-line drug as initial therapy in most patients with newly diagnosed stage 1 hypertension. Start combination drug therapy (preferably with two first-line drugs) as the initial regimen in patients with newly diagnosed stage 2 hypertension (Fig. 10-1).
- The four first-line options are **angiotensin-converting enzyme inhibitors (ACEi)**, **angiotensin II receptor blockers (ARBs)**, **calcium channel blockers (CCBs)**, and **thiazide diuretics**.
- **β-Blockers** should be reserved to treat a specific compelling indication or in combination with a first-line antihypertensive agent for patients without a compelling indication.
- Other antihypertensive drug classes (α_1-blocker, **mineralocorticoid receptor antagonist [MRA]**, **central α_2-agonist**, adrenergic inhibitor, and **direct arterial vasodilator**) may be used for select patients after implementing first-line agents. They are generally reserved for resistant hypertension or as add-on therapy with multiple other first-line agents. However, they either lack convincing evidence showing reduced morbidity and mortality in hypertension or have a high incidence of adverse effects that hinders tolerability.

COMPELLING INDICATIONS

- Compelling indications are specific comorbid conditions for which clinical trial data support using specific antihypertensive drug classes to treat both hypertension and the compelling indication (Fig. 10-2). Selection of drug therapy should follow an evidence-based order.

Heart Failure with Reduced Ejection Fraction (HFrEF)

- Guideline-directed medical therapy consists of an ACE inhibitor or ARB (although ARB with a neprilysin inhibitor [also called angiotensin receptor neprilysin inhibitor; ARNI] is preferred ahead of an ACEi or ARB alone), an evidence-based β-blocker (ie, bisoprolol, carvedilol, metoprolol succinate) titrated to the maximum dose, and then possibly an MRA.
- Start an ACE inhibitor or ARB in low doses to avoid orthostatic hypotension because of the high renin state in HF.
- Diuretics reduce edema, and loop diuretics are often needed, especially in patients with advanced HF and/or CKD.

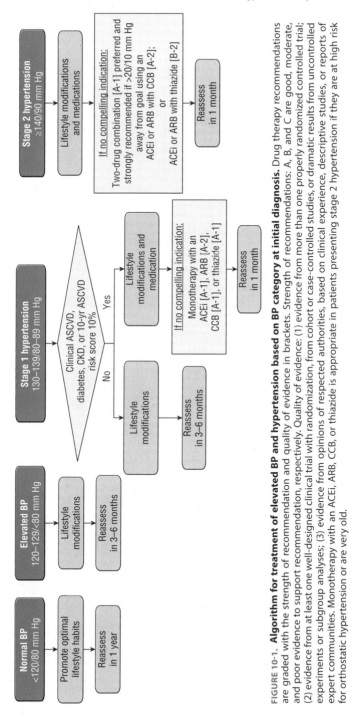

FIGURE 10-1. Algorithm for treatment of elevated BP and hypertension based on BP category at initial diagnosis. Drug therapy recommendations are graded with the strength of recommendation and quality of evidence in brackets. Strength of recommendations: A, B, and C are good, moderate, and poor evidence to support recommendation, respectively. Quality of evidence: (1) evidence from more than one properly randomized controlled trial; (2) evidence from at least one well-designed clinical trial with randomization, from cohort or case-controlled studies, or dramatic results from uncontrolled experiments or subgroup analyses; (3) evidence from opinions of respected authorities, based on clinical experience, descriptive studies, or reports of expert communities. Monotherapy with an ACEi, ARB, CCB, or thiazide is appropriate in patients presenting stage 2 hypertension if they are at high risk for orthostatic hypertension or are very old.

117

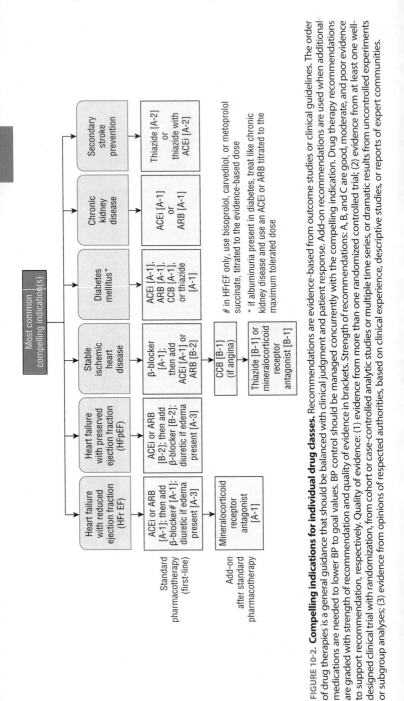

FIGURE 10-2. Compelling indications for individual drug classes. Recommendations are evidence-based from outcome studies or clinical guidelines. The order of drug therapies is a general guidance that should be balanced with clinical judgment and patient response. Add-on recommendations are used when additional medications are needed to lower BP to goal values. BP control should be managed concurrently with the compelling indication. Drug therapy recommendations are graded with strength of recommendation and quality of evidence in brackets. Strength of recommendations: A, B, and C are good, moderate, and poor evidence to support recommendation, respectively. Quality of evidence: (1) evidence from more than one randomized controlled trial; (2) evidence from at least one well-designed clinical trial with randomization, from cohort or case-controlled analytic studies or multiple time series, or dramatic results from uncontrolled experiments or subgroup analyses; (3) evidence from opinions of respected authorities, based on clinical experience, descriptive studies, or reports of expert communities.

- β-Blockers modify disease in HFrEF and are part of standard treatment; adding a β-blocker to a diuretic with an ACE inhibitor or ARB (or ARNI) reduces CV morbidity and mortality. Because of the risk of exacerbating HF, β-blockers must be started in low doses and titrated slowly to high doses based on tolerability. **Bisoprolol**, **carvedilol**, and **metoprolol succinate** are the only β-blockers proven to be beneficial in HFrEF.
- After implementing a standard regimen, other agents may be added to further reduce CV morbidity and mortality, and reduce BP if needed, such as an MRA (**spironolactone** or **eplerenone**).

Heart Failure with Preserved Ejection Fraction (HFpEF)

- Unlike interventions in HFrEF that decrease morbidity and mortality, trials using the same medications in HFpEF have not shown similar benefits. Therefore, treatment should be targeted at signs and symptoms (eg, dyspnea, fatigue, edema), appropriate management of underlying coronary artery disease, and attainment of goal BP to prevent HF progression.
- Patients should use a β-blocker or an ACE inhibitor (or ARB) to treat hypertension, and they should receive a diuretic if signs and symptoms of edema are present.

Stable Ischemic Heart Disease (SIHD)

- β-Blockers (without ISA) are first-line therapy in SIHD; they reduce BP and improve angina symptoms by decreasing myocardial oxygen consumption and demand. β-Blockers should be used to treat hypertension in patients with SIHD. An ACE inhibitor or ARB has been shown to reduce CV events as an add-on to a β-blocker.
- A long-acting nondihydropyridine CCB is an alternative to a β-blocker in SIHD, but β-blockers are the therapy of choice.
- A dihydropyridine CCB may be considered as add-on therapy in SIHD patients who have ongoing ischemic symptoms, but cardiac stimulation makes these agents less desirable.
- For acute coronary syndromes, first-line therapy includes a β-blocker and ACE inhibitor (or ARB); the combination lowers BP, controls acute ischemia, and reduces CV risk.

Diabetes Mellitus

- All four first-line antihypertensive classes (ACE inhibitors, ARBs, CCBs, thiazides) reduce CV events in patients with diabetes, with no evidence of difference in all-cause mortality, CV mortality, HF, or stroke. The risk of kidney disease progression is low in the absence of albuminuria (urine albumin-to-creatinine ratio ≥30 mg/g [3.4 mg/mmol creatinine]). Therefore, any first-line agent can be used to control hypertension in patients with diabetes in the absence of albuminuria. Regardless of the initial agent selected, most patients require combination therapy, which typically includes an ACE inhibitor (or ARB) with a CCB or thiazide.
- After first-line agents, a β-blocker is a useful add-on therapy for BP control in patients with diabetes. However, they may mask symptoms of hypoglycemia (tremor, tachycardia, and palpitations but not sweating) in tightly controlled patients, delay recovery from hypoglycemia, and elevate BP due to vasoconstriction caused by unopposed β-receptor stimulation during the hypoglycemic recovery phase. Despite these potential concerns, β-blockers can be used safely in patients with diabetes.

Chronic Kidney Disease

- In addition to lowering BP, ACE inhibitors and ARBs reduce intraglomerular pressure, which may further slow CKD progression.

- Start with low doses and evaluate the serum creatinine soon after starting therapy to minimize the risk of rapid and profound BP drops that could precipitate acute kidney injury (AKI).

Secondary Stroke Prevention

- A thiazide diuretic, either alone or combined with an ACE inhibitor, is recommended for patients with history of stroke or transient ischemic attack. Implement antihypertensive drug therapy only after patients have stabilized after an acute cerebrovascular event.
- The threshold for starting antihypertensive drug therapy in patients with a history of stroke is when BP is >140/90 mm Hg. Once therapy is initiated, patients should be treated to a goal of <130/80 mm Hg.

FIRST-LINE ANTIHYPERTENSIVE AGENTS (TABLE 10-2)

Angiotensin-Converting Enzyme Inhibitors

- ACE inhibitors block conversion of angiotensin I to angiotensin II, a potent vasoconstrictor and stimulator of aldosterone secretion. ACE inhibitors also block degradation of bradykinin and stimulate synthesis of other vasodilating substances (prostaglandin E_2 and prostacyclin).
- Starting doses should be low with slow dose titration. Acute hypotension may occur at the onset of therapy, especially in patients who are sodium or volume depleted, in HF exacerbation, very elderly, or on concurrent vasodilators or diuretics. Starting doses in such patients should be half the normal dose followed by slow dose titration.
- ACE inhibitors decrease aldosterone and can increase serum potassium concentrations. Hyperkalemia occurs primarily in patients with CKD or those also taking potassium supplements, potassium-sparing diuretics, MRAs, ARBs, or direct renin inhibitors.
- AKI is an uncommon but serious side effect; preexisting kidney disease increases risk. Bilateral renal artery stenosis or unilateral stenosis of a solitary functioning kidney renders patients dependent on the vasoconstrictive effect of angiotensin II on efferent arterioles, making them particularly susceptible to AKI.
- GFR decreases somewhat when ACE inhibitors are started because of inhibition of angiotensin II vasoconstriction on efferent arterioles. Serum creatinine concentrations often increase, but modest elevations (eg, absolute increases <1 mg/dL [88 μmol/L]) do not warrant treatment changes. Discontinue therapy or reduce dose if larger increases occur.
- Angioedema occurs in <1% of patients. Drug withdrawal is necessary, and some patients may require drug treatment and/or emergent intubation to support respiration. An ARB can generally be used in patients with a history of ACE inhibitor-induced angioedema, with careful monitoring.
- A persistent dry cough occurs in up to 20% of patients and is thought to be due to inhibition of bradykinin breakdown.
- ACE inhibitors (as well as ARBs and direct renin inhibitors) are contraindicated in pregnancy.

Angiotensin II Receptor Blockers

- Angiotensin II is generated by the renin–angiotensin pathway (which involves ACE) and an alternative pathway that uses other enzymes such as chymases. ACE inhibitors block only the renin–angiotensin pathway, whereas ARBs inhibit angiotensin II generated by either pathway. The ARBs directly block the angiotensin II type 1 receptor that mediates the effects of angiotensin II.
- Unlike ACE inhibitors, ARBs do not block bradykinin breakdown. Although this accounts for the lack of cough as a side effect, some of the antihypertensive effect of ACE inhibitors may be due to bradykinin.

TABLE 10-2 Most Common First-Line and Other Antihypertensive Agents

Class	Subclass	Medication (Brand Name)	Usual Dose Range (mg/ day)	Daily Frequency
ACEi		Benazepril (Lotensin)	10–40	1 or 2
		Captopril (Capoten)	12.5–150	2 or 3
		Enalapril (Vasotec)	5–40	1 or 2
		Fosinopril (Monopril)	10–40	1
		Lisinopril (Prinivil, Zestril)	10–40	1
		Moexipril (Univasc)	7.5–30	1 or 2
		Perindopril (Aceon)	4–16	1
		Quinapril (Accupril)	10–80	1 or 2
		Ramipril (Altace)	2.5–10	1 or 2
		Trandolapril (Mavik)	1–4	1
ARB		Azilsartan (Edarbi)	40–80	1
		Candesartan (Atacand)	8–32	1 or 2
		Eprosartan (Teveten)	600–800	1 or 2
		Irbesartan (Avapro)	150–300	1
		Losartan (Cozaar)	50–100	1 or 2
		Telmisartan (Micardis)	20–40	1
		Olmesartan (Benicar)	20–80	1
		Valsartan (Diovan)	80–320	1
Calcium channel blocker	Dihydropyridine	Amlodipine (Norvasc)	2.5–10	1
		Felodipine (Plendil)	5–20	1
		Nifedipine long-acting (Afeditab CR Adalat CC, Nifediac CC, Nifedical XL, Procardia XL)	30–90	1
		Nisoldipine (Sular)	10–40	1
	Nondihydropyridine	Diltiazem sustained release (Cardizem CD, Cartia XT, Dilacor XR, Diltia XT, Tiazac, Taztia XT)	120–480	1
		Diltiazem extended release (Cardizem LA, Matzim LA)	180–480	1 (morning or evening)
		Verapamil sustained release (Calan SR, Isoptin SR, Verelan)	180–420	1 or 2
		Verapamil chronotherapeutic oral drug absorption system (Verelan PM)	100–400	1 (in the evening)

(Continued)

TABLE 10-2 Most Common First-Line and Other Antihypertensive Agents (*Continued*)

Class	Subclass	Medication (Brand Name)	Usual Dose Range (mg/day)	Daily Frequency
Diuretic	Thiazide	Chlorthalidone (Thalitone)	12.5–25	1
		Hydrochlorothiazide (Microzide)	12.5–50	1
		Indapamide (Lozol)	1.25–2.5	1
		Metolazone (Zaroxolyn)	2.5–10	1
	Loop	Bumetanide (Bumex)	0.5–4	2
		Furosemide (Lasix)	20–80	2
		Torsemide (Demadex)	5–10	1
	Potassium sparing	Amiloride (Midamor)	5–10	1 or 2
		Amiloride/ Hydrochlorothiazide (Moduretic)	5–50	1
		Triamterene (Dyrenium)	50–100	1 or 2
		Triamterene/ Hydrochlorothiazide (Dyazide, Maxide)	37.5–75/25–50	1
	Mineralocorticoid receptor antagonist	Eplerenone (Inspra)	50–100	1 or 2
		Spironolactone (Aldactone, CaroSpir)	25–50	1 or 2
β-Blocker	Cardioselective	Atenolol (Tenormin)	25–100	1 or 2
		Betaxolol (Kerlone)	5–20	1
		Bisoprolol (Zebeta)	2.5–10	1
		Metoprolol tartrate (Lopressor)	100–200	2
		Metoprolol succinate extended release (Toprol XL)	50–200	1
		Nebivolol (Bystolic)	5–20	1
	Nonselective	Nadolol (Corgard)	40–120	1
		Propranolol (Inderal)	160–480	2
		Propranolol long acting (Inderal LA, Inderal XL, InnoPran XL)	80–320	1
		Timolol (Blocadren)	10–40	1
	Mixed α- and β-blockers	Carvedilol (Coreg)	12.5–50	2
		Carvedilol phosphate (Coreg CR)	20–80	1
		Labetalol (Normodyne, Trandate)	200–800	2

- The combination of an ACE inhibitor and ARB has no additional CV event lowering but is associated with a higher risk of side effects (renal dysfunction, hypotension) and should be avoided.
- All ARBs have similar antihypertensive efficacy and fairly flat dose-response curves. Addition of a CCB or thiazide diuretic significantly increases antihypertensive efficacy.
- ARBs have a low incidence of side effects. Like ACE inhibitors, they may cause renal insufficiency, hyperkalemia, and orthostatic hypotension. ARBs are contraindicated in pregnancy and should not be used with an ACEi or direct renin inhibitor.

Calcium Channel Blockers

- Dihydropyridine and nondihydropyridine CCBs are first-line antihypertensive therapies and are also used in addition to or instead of other first-line agents for the compelling indication of ischemic heart disease.
- CCBs cause relaxation of cardiac and smooth muscle by blocking voltage-sensitive calcium channels, thereby reducing entry of extracellular calcium into cells. This leads to vasodilation and a corresponding reduction in BP. Dihydropyridine CCBs may cause reflex sympathetic activation, and all agents (except **amlodipine** and **felodipine**) may have negative inotropic effects.
- **Verapamil** decreases heart rate, slows atrioventricular (AV) nodal conduction, and produces a negative inotropic effect that may precipitate HF in patients with borderline cardiac reserve. **Diltiazem** decreases AV conduction and heart rate to a lesser extent than verapamil.
- Diltiazem and verapamil can cause cardiac conduction abnormalities such as bradycardia, AV block, and HF. Both can cause peripheral edema and hypotension. Verapamil causes constipation in about 7% of patients.
- Dihydropyridines cause a baroreceptor-mediated reflex increase in heart rate because of potent peripheral vasodilating effects. Dihydropyridines do not decrease AV node conduction and are not effective for treating supraventricular tachyarrhythmias.
- Short-acting nifedipine may rarely increase frequency, intensity, and duration of angina in association with acute hypotension. This effect may be obviated by using sustained-release formulations of nifedipine or other dihydropyridines. Other side effects of dihydropyridines are dizziness, flushing, headache, gingival hyperplasia, and peripheral edema.

Diuretics

- Thiazides are the preferred type of diuretic and are a first-line option for most patients with hypertension. **Chlorthalidone** (thiazide-like) is preferred over **hydrochlorothiazide**, especially in resistant hypertension, because it is more potent on a milligram-per-milligram basis.
- Loop diuretics are more potent for inducing diuresis but are not ideal antihypertensives unless edema treatment is also needed. Loop diuretics are sometimes required over thiazides in patients with severe CKD when eGFR is <30 mL/min/1.73 m², especially when edema is present.
- Potassium-sparing diuretics are weak antihypertensives when used alone and do not enhance antihypertensive effects when combined with a thiazide or loop diuretic. Their primary use is in combination with another diuretic to counteract potassium-wasting properties.
- MRAs (**spironolactone** and **eplerenone**) are also potassium-sparing diuretics that are usually used to treat resistant hypertension because elevated aldosterone concentrations are prevalent in this setting. They are also used as add-on agents in patients with HFrEF with or without concomitant hypertension.
- Acutely, diuretics lower BP by causing diuresis. The reduction in plasma volume and stroke volume associated with diuresis decreases cardiac output and BP. The initial drop in cardiac output causes a compensatory increase in peripheral vascular

resistance. With chronic therapy, extracellular fluid volume and plasma volume return to near pretreatment levels, and peripheral vascular resistance falls below baseline. Reduced peripheral vascular resistance is responsible for persistent hypotensive effects. Thiazides also mobilize sodium and water from arteriolar walls, which may contribute to decreased peripheral vascular resistance and lowered BP.

- Combining diuretics with other antihypertensive agents usually results in an additive hypotensive effect because of independent mechanisms of action. Furthermore, many nondiuretic antihypertensive agents induce sodium and water retention, which is counteracted by concurrent diuretic use.
- Side effects of thiazides include hypokalemia, hypomagnesemia, hypercalcemia, hyperuricemia, hyperglycemia, dyslipidemia, and sexual dysfunction. Loop diuretics have less effect on serum lipids and glucose, but hypokalemia is more pronounced, and hypocalcemia may occur.
- Hypokalemia and hypomagnesemia may cause muscle fatigue or cramps, and severe electrolyte abnormalities may result in serious cardiac arrhythmias. Low-dose therapy (eg, 25 mg hydrochlorothiazide or 12.5 mg chlorthalidone daily) causes less electrolyte disturbances than higher doses.
- Potassium-sparing diuretics may cause hyperkalemia, especially in patients with CKD or diabetes and in patients receiving concurrent treatment with an MRA, ACE inhibitor, ARB, direct renin inhibitor, or potassium supplement. Eplerenone has an increased risk for hyperkalemia and is contraindicated in patients with impaired renal function or type 2 diabetes with proteinuria. Spironolactone may cause gynecomastia in up to 10% of patients; this effect occurs rarely with eplerenone.

ALTERNATIVE ANTIHYPERTENSIVE AGENTS (TABLES 10-2 AND 10-3)

β-Blockers

- Evidence suggests that β-blockers may not reduce CV events as well as ACE inhibitors, ARBs, CCBs, or thiazides when used as the initial drug in patients who do not have a compelling indication for a β-blocker.
- β-Blockers are appropriate first-line agents when used to treat specific compelling indications (Fig. 10-2) or when an ACE inhibitor, ARB, CCB, or thiazide cannot be used. β-Blockers also have an important role as add-on therapy to first-line agents in patients with hypertension but no compelling indications.

TABLE 10-3	Alternative Antihypertensive Agents	
Class Drug (Brand Name)	**Usual Dose Range (mg/day)**	**Daily Frequency**
α₁-Blockers		
Doxazosin (Cardura)	1–8	1
Prazosin (Minipress)	2–20	2 or 3
Terazosin (Hytrin)	1–20	1 or 2
Direct renin inhibitor		
Aliskiren (Tekturna)	150–300	1
Central α₂-agonists		
Clonidine (Catapres)	0.1–0.8	2
Clonidine patch (Catapres-TTS)	0.1–0.3	1 weekly
Methyldopa (Aldomet)	250–1000	2
Direct arterial vasodilators		
Minoxidil (Loniten)	10–40	1 or 2
Hydralazine (Apresoline)	20–100	2–4

- Their hypotensive mechanism may involve decreased cardiac output through negative chronotropic and inotropic cardiac effects and inhibition of renin release from the kidney.
- **Atenolol, betaxolol, bisoprolol, metoprolol**, and **nebivolol** are cardioselective at low doses and bind more avidly to β_1-receptors than to β_2-receptors. As a result, they are less likely to provoke bronchospasm and vasoconstriction and are safer than nonselective β-blockers in patients with asthma or diabetes who have a compelling indication for a β-blocker. Cardioselectivity is a dose-dependent phenomenon, and the effect is lost at higher doses.
- **Acebutolol, carteolol**, and **pindolol** possess intrinsic sympathomimetic activity (ISA) or partial β-receptor agonist activity. When sympathetic tone is low, as in resting states, β-receptors are partially stimulated, so resting heart rate, cardiac output, and peripheral blood flow are not reduced when receptors are blocked. Theoretically, these drugs may have advantages in select patients with HF or sinus bradycardia. Unfortunately, they do not reduce CV events as well as other β-blockers and may increase CV risk in patients with SIHD. Thus, agents with ISA are rarely needed and have no role in hypertension management.
- **Atenolol** and **nadolol** have relatively long half-lives and are excreted renally; the dosage may need to be reduced in patients with renal insufficiency. Even though the half-lives of other β-blockers are shorter, once-daily administration still may be effective.
- Cardiac side effects include bradycardia, AV conduction abnormalities, and acute HF. Blocking β_2-receptors in arteriolar smooth muscle may cause cold extremities and aggravate intermittent claudication or Raynaud phenomenon because of decreased peripheral blood flow. Increases in serum lipids and glucose appear to be transient and of little clinical significance.
- Abrupt cessation of β-blocker therapy can produce cardiac ischemia (angina, chest pain), a CV event, or even death in patients with coronary artery disease. In patients without heart disease, abrupt discontinuation of β-blockers may be associated with tachycardia, sweating, and generalized malaise in addition to increased BP. For these reasons, the dose should always be tapered gradually over 1–2 weeks before discontinuation.

α_1-Receptor Blockers

- **Prazosin, terazosin**, and **doxazosin** are selective α_1-receptor blockers that inhibit catecholamine uptake in smooth muscle cells of peripheral vasculature, resulting in vasodilation and BP lowering.
- A first-dose phenomenon characterized by orthostatic hypotension accompanied by transient dizziness or faintness, palpitations, and even syncope may occur within 1–3 hours of the first dose or after later dosage increases. The patient should take the first dose (and subsequent first increased doses) at bedtime. Occasionally, orthostatic hypotension and dizziness persist with chronic administration.
- Sodium and water retention can occur; these agents are most effective when given with a thiazide to maintain antihypertensive efficacy and minimize edema.
- These agents block postsynaptic α_1-adrenergic receptors on the prostate capsule, causing relaxation and decreased resistance to urinary outflow. Although they can provide symptomatic benefit in men with benign prostatic hyperplasia, they should be used to lower BP only in combination with first-line antihypertensive agents.

Direct Renin Inhibitor

- **Aliskiren** blocks the RAAS at its point of activation, resulting in reduced plasma renin activity and BP. It should not be used with an ACE inhibitor or an ARB because of a higher risk of adverse effects without providing any additional reduction in CV events. Its role in the management of hypertension is limited.
- Many of the cautions and adverse effects seen with ACE inhibitors and ARBs apply to aliskiren. It is contraindicated in pregnancy due to known teratogenic effects.

Central α_2-Agonists

- **Clonidine, guanfacine**, and **methyldopa** lower BP primarily by stimulating α_2-adrenergic receptors in the brain, which reduces sympathetic outflow from the vasomotor center and increases vagal tone. Stimulation of presynaptic α_2-receptors peripherally may contribute to reduced sympathetic tone. Consequently, there may be decreases in heart rate, cardiac output, total peripheral resistance, plasma renin activity, and baroreceptor reflexes.
- Clonidine is usually reserved for resistant hypertension, and methyldopa is primarily used for pregnancy-induced hypertension.
- Chronic use results in sodium and fluid retention. Other side effects include depression, orthostatic hypotension, dizziness, and anticholinergic effects (eg, dry mouth, sedation).
- Abrupt cessation may lead to rebound hypertension, perhaps from a compensatory increase in norepinephrine release that follows discontinuation of presynaptic α-receptor stimulation. The transdermal form should be used instead of tablets when clonidine therapy is needed.
- Methyldopa rarely causes hepatitis or hemolytic anemia. Discontinue therapy if persistent increases in liver function tests occur, because this may herald onset of fulminant, life-threatening hepatitis. Coombs-positive hemolytic anemia occurs rarely, and 20% of patients exhibit a positive direct Coombs test without anemia. For these reasons, methyldopa has limited usefulness except in pregnancy.

Direct Arterial Vasodilators

- **Hydralazine** and **minoxidil** directly relax arteriolar smooth muscle, resulting in vasodilation and BP lowering. Compensatory activation of baroreceptor reflexes increases sympathetic outflow, thereby increasing heart rate, cardiac output, and renin release. Consequently, hypotensive effectiveness of direct vasodilators diminishes over time unless the patient is also taking a diuretic and a β-blocker. The diuretic minimizes the side effect of sodium and water retention. Direct vasodilators can precipitate angina in patients with underlying SIHD unless the baroreceptor reflex mechanism is blocked with a β-blocker. Nondihydropyridine CCBs can be used as an alternative to β-blockers in patients with contraindications to β-blockers.
- Hydralazine may cause a dose-related, reversible lupus-like syndrome, which is more common in slow acetylators. Lupus-like reactions can usually be avoided by limiting the maximum total daily dose to 200 mg. Because of side effects, hydralazine has limited usefulness for chronic hypertension management.
- Minoxidil is a more potent vasodilator than hydralazine, and compensatory increases in heart rate, cardiac output, renin release, and sodium retention are more dramatic. Due to significant water retention, a loop diuretic is often more effective than a thiazide. Reversible hypertrichosis on the face, arms, back, and chest may be troublesome. Minoxidil is reserved for resistant hypertension and for patients requiring hydralazine who experience drug-induced lupus.

SPECIAL POPULATIONS

Older Persons

- Older patients may present with either isolated systolic hypertension or elevation in both SBP and DBP. CV morbidity and mortality are more directly correlated to SBP than to DBP in patients aged 50 and older.
- First-line antihypertensives provide significant benefits and can be used safely in older patients, but smaller-than-usual initial doses must be used.
- Although the most appropriate BP goal for older patients has been debated, the totality of evidence indicates that older ambulatory patients should be treated to an SBP goal of <130 mm Hg, with careful monitoring. In patients with multiple comorbidities, a relaxed SBP goal of <150 mm Hg (or <140 mm Hg if tolerated) may be considered.

Children and Adolescents

- In children, hypertension is defined as SBP or DBP that is >95th percentile for sex, age, and height on at least three occasions. For adolescents, BP values between the 90th and 95th percentile, or >120/80 mm Hg, is considered elevated BP.
- Because secondary hypertension is more common in children and adolescents than in adults, an appropriate workup is required if elevated BP is identified.
- Nonpharmacologic treatment (eg, weight loss if overweight or obese, healthy diet, physical activity) is the cornerstone of therapy for primary hypertension.
- The goal is to reduce the BP to <90th percentile for sex, age, and height and <130/80 mm Hg in adolescents age 13 years and older.
- ACE inhibitors, ARBs, β-blockers, CCBs, and thiazide diuretics are all acceptable drug therapy choices.
- ACE inhibitors, ARBs, and direct renin inhibitors are contraindicated in sexually active girls because of potential teratogenic effects.

Pregnancy

- *Preeclampsia* is defined as hypertension (elevated BP ≥140/90 mm Hg on more than two occasions at least 4 hours apart after 20 weeks' gestation or ≥160/110 mm Hg confirmed within a short interval) and either proteinuria or new-onset hypertension with the onset of thrombocytopenia, impaired liver function, new-onset renal insufficiency, pulmonary edema, or new-onset cerebral or visual disturbances. It can lead to life-threatening complications for both mother and fetus.
- *Eclampsia* is the onset of convulsions in preeclampsia and is a medical emergency.
- Definitive treatment of preeclampsia is delivery, and labor induction is indicated if eclampsia is imminent or present. Otherwise, management consists of restricting activity, bed rest, and close monitoring. Salt restriction or other measures that contract blood volume should be avoided. Antihypertensives are used before induction of labor if DBP is >105 mm Hg, with a target DBP of 95–105 mm Hg. Intravenous (IV) hydralazine is most commonly used; IV labetalol is also effective.
- *Chronic hypertension* is hypertension that predates pregnancy. Labetalol, long-acting nifedipine, or methyldopa is recommended as first-line therapy due to favorable safety profiles. Other β-blockers (except atenolol) and CCBs are also reasonable alternatives. ACE inhibitors, ARBs, and the direct renin inhibitor aliskiren are known teratogens and contraindicated in pregnancy.

Black Patients

- Hypertension is more common and more difficult to control in Black patients than in those of other races; treatment usually requires two or more antihypertensives to reach a BP goal of <130/80 mm Hg.
- CCBs and thiazides are most effective in Black patients and should be first-line in the absence of a compelling indication. Antihypertensive response is significantly increased when either class is combined with a β-blocker, ACE inhibitor, or ARB, perhaps due to the low-renin pattern of hypertension in Black patients.
- Medications recommended for specific compelling indications should be used, even if the antihypertensive effect may not be as great as with another drug class (eg, use a β-blocker first-line for hypertension in Black patients with SIHD).

Pulmonary Disease and Peripheral Arterial Disease

- Although β-blockers (especially nonselective agents) have generally been avoided in hypertensive patients with asthma and COPD because of fear of inducing bronchospasm, cardioselective β-blockers can be used safely. Consequently, cardioselective agents should be used to treat a compelling indication (ie, SIHD or HF) in patients with reactive airway disease.

- Because PAD is a noncoronary form of ASCVD, patients with PAD are at increased risk of stroke and CV events. β-Blockers can theoretically be problematic because of possible decreased peripheral blood flow secondary to unopposed stimulation of α_1-receptors that results in vasoconstriction. However, available data indicate that β-blockers do not worsen claudication symptoms or cause functional impairment. Therefore, antihypertensive treatment for patients with PAD should follow the same general principles as patients without PAD.

HYPERTENSIVE URGENCIES AND EMERGENCIES

- *Hypertensive urgencies* are ideally managed conservatively by initiating, reinitiating, or intensifying oral antihypertensive medications and implementing nonpharmacologic interventions. Aggressive BP lowering with IV antihypertensives is not indicated in the absence of target organ damage. Acute administration of a short-acting oral drug (**captopril**, **clonidine**, or **labetalol**) followed by careful observation for several hours to ensure a gradual BP reduction is an option.
  - ✓ Captopril 25–50 mg orally may be given at 1- to 2-hour intervals. The onset of action is 15–30 minutes.
  - ✓ For treatment of hypertensive rebound after withdrawal of clonidine, 0.2 mg orally is given initially, followed by 0.2 mg hourly until the DBP falls below 110 mm Hg or a total of 0.7 mg has been administered; a single dose may be sufficient.
  - ✓ Labetalol 200–400 mg orally can be given, followed by additional doses every 2–3 hours.
- *Hypertensive emergencies* require immediate BP reduction with a parenteral agent to limit new or progressing end-organ damage. Admission to an intensive care unit is required to accommodate frequent monitoring and administration of antihypertensive therapy via continuous IV infusion. The rate of BP reduction depends on the presence of various compelling indications (see Chapter e31, "Acute Hypertensive Crisis," in *DiPiro's Pharmacotherapy: A Pathophysiologic Approach*, 12 ed.). Dosing guidelines and adverse effects of parenteral agents for treating hypertensive emergency are listed in Table 10-4.

EVALUATION OF THERAPEUTIC OUTCOMES

- Both clinic-based and self-measurement home BP monitoring are important for monitoring and managing hypertension. Encourage patients to obtain a home BP monitor, record the results, and bring them to follow-up clinic visits.
- Evaluate BP response in the clinic 4 weeks after initiating or making changes in therapy and compare the results to home BP readings. Once goal BP is obtained, monitor BP every 3–6 months, assuming no signs or symptoms of acute end-organ damage. Evaluate more frequently in patients with a history of poor control, nonadherence, progressive end-organ damage, or symptoms of adverse drug effects.
- Automated BP monitoring can be useful to establish effective 24-hour control and confirm white coat or masked uncontrolled hypertension.
- Monitor patients routinely for adverse drug events, which may require dosage reduction or substitution with an alternative antihypertensive agent. Perform laboratory monitoring 4 weeks after starting a new agent or dose increase, and then every 6–12 months in stable patients. For patients treated with an MRA (eplerenone or spironolactone), monitor potassium concentrations and kidney function within 3 days of initiation and again at 1 week to detect potential hyperkalemia.
- Monitor patients for signs and symptoms of hypertension-associated complications. Take a careful history for ischemic chest pain (or pressure), palpitations, dizziness, dyspnea, orthopnea, headache, sudden change in vision, one-sided weakness, slurred speech, and loss of balance.
- Monitor funduscopic changes on eye examination, LV hypertrophy on ECG, albuminuria, and changes in kidney function periodically.

TABLE 10-4 Parenteral Antihypertensive Agents for Hypertensive Emergency

Drug	Dose	Onset (Minutes)	Duration (Minutes)	Adverse Effects
Clevidipine	1–2 mg/h (32 mg/h max)	2–4	5–15	Headache, nausea, tachycardia, hypertriglyceridemia
Enalaprilat	1.25–5 mg IV every 6 hours	15–30	360–720	Precipitous fall in BP in high-renin states; variable response
Esmolol hydrochloride	250–500 mcg/kg/min IV bolus, then 50–100 mcg/kg/min IV infusion; may repeat bolus after 5 min or increase infusion to 300 mcg/min	1–2	10–20	Hypotension, nausea, asthma, first-degree heart block, heart failure
Fenoldopam mesylate	0.1–0.3 mcg/kg/min IV infusion	<5	30	Tachycardia, headache, nausea, flushing
Hydralazine hydrochloride	12–20 mg IV 10–50 mg IM	10–20 20–30	60–240 240–360	Tachycardia, flushing, headache, vomiting, aggravation of angina
Labetalol hydrochloride	20–80 mg IV bolus every 10 min; 0.5–2 mg/min IV infusion	5–10	180–360	Vomiting, scalp tingling, bronchoconstriction, dizziness, nausea, heart block, orthostatic hypotension
Nicardipine hydrochloride	5–15 mg/h IV	5–10	15–30; may exceed 240	Tachycardia, headache, flushing, local phlebitis
Nitroglycerin	5–200 mcg/min IV infusion	2–5	5–10	Headache, vomiting, methemoglobinemia, tolerance with prolonged use
Sodium nitroprusside	0.25–10 mcg/kg/min IV infusion (requires special delivery system)	Immediate	1–2	Nausea, vomiting, muscle twitching, sweating, thiocyanate and cyanide intoxication

BP, blood pressure; IM, intramuscular; IV, intravenous.

• Assess patient adherence with the regimen regularly. Ask patients about changes in their general health perception, physical functioning, and overall satisfaction with treatment.

See Chapter 30, Hypertension, authored by Eric J. MacLaughlin and Joseph J. Saseen; and Chapter e31, Acute Hypertensive Crisis, authored by Jeffrey J. Mucksavage, Danielle M. Tompkins, and Eric J. MacLaughlin, for a more detailed discussion of these topics.

CHAPTER 11

Ischemic Heart Disease

- *Ischemic heart disease* (IHD) is defined as lack of oxygen and decreased or no blood flow to the myocardium resulting from coronary artery narrowing or obstruction. It may present as acute coronary syndrome (ACS), which includes unstable angina and non–ST-segment elevation (NSTE) or ST-segment elevation (STE) myocardial infarction (MI), chronic stable exertional angina, ischemia without symptoms, microvascular angina, or ischemia due to coronary artery vasospasm (variant or Prinzmetal angina). The focus of this chapter is stable IHD.

PATHOPHYSIOLOGY

- Angina pectoris usually results from increased myocardial oxygen demand (MVO_2) in the setting of a fixed decrease in myocardial oxygen supply because of atherosclerotic plaque.
- Major determinants of MVO_2 are heart rate (HR), myocardial contractility, and intramyocardial wall tension during systole. A doubling in any of these individual parameters requires a 50% increase in coronary flow to maintain myocardial supply.
- Coronary atherosclerotic plaques typically develop in larger epicardial (R_1 or conductance) vessels, which normally offer little resistance to myocardial flow. As plaques grow and narrow the lumen, the affected vessel begins to provide considerable resistance to blood flow. Smaller endocardial (R_2 or resistance) vessels provide most resistance to flow in normal coronary arteries and can contract and dilate to maintain blood flow based on metabolic demands of the myocardium (referred to as autoregulation). As a result, coronary plaques that occupy less than 50%–70% of the vessel luminal diameter rarely produce ischemia or angina. However, smaller plaques have a lipid-rich core and thin fibrous cap and are more prone to rupture and cause acute thrombosis. When the luminal diameter of epicardial vessels is reduced by 70% or more, endocardial vessels are maximally dilated, much of the coronary flow reserve has been used to preserve resting coronary blood flow, and minimal physical exertion may result in a flow deficit with myocardial ischemia and often angina. When epicardial stenosis exceeds 90%, endocardial flow reserve is exhausted (referred to as critical stenosis).
- When coronary stenosis exceeds 70%, ischemic episodes lead to production of vascular endothelial growth factor and basic fibroblast growth factor which, combined with endogenous vasodilators (eg, nitrous oxide, prostacyclin), cause native collateral vessels to increase in diameter (arteriogenesis) to maintain perfusion. New collateral vessels can also develop (angiogenesis).
- Inflammation also plays a role in IHD; macrophages and T-lymphocytes produce cytokines, chemokines, and growth factors that activate endothelial cells, increase vasoreactivity, and cause proliferation of vascular smooth muscle cells. C-reactive protein may be elevated and correlates with adverse cardiovascular events.
- Some patients have plaque that causes a fixed decrease in supply but also have reduced myocardial oxygen supply transiently due to vasospasm at the site of the plaque. Vasospasm is typically caused by endothelial damage induced by the plaque. Patient symptoms depend on the extent of the fixed obstruction and the degree of dynamic change in coronary arterial tone. The pattern of ischemic symptoms can change due to a variable amount of vasospasm under certain conditions (referred to as *variable threshold angina*). Ischemic episodes may be more common in the morning hours (due to circadian release of vasoconstrictors) and be precipitated by cold exposure and emotional or mental stress.
- Patients with *variant (Prinzmetal) angina* usually do not have a coronary flow-obstructing plaque but instead have significant reduction in myocardial oxygen supply due to vasospasm in epicardial vessels.

CLINICAL PRESENTATION

- Patients typically complain of chest pain precipitated by exertion or activities of daily living that is described as squeezing, crushing, heaviness, or chest tightness. Symptoms may radiate to the arms, shoulders, back, abdomen, or jaw. Nausea, vomiting, diaphoresis, or shortness of breath may also be present. Chest pain generally lasts from 5 to 20 minutes and is usually relieved by rest or sublingual nitroglycerin (SL NTG).
- Some patients (especially women and older individuals) present with atypical chest pain, characterized by midepigastric discomfort, effort intolerance, dyspnea, and excessive fatigue. Patients with diabetes mellitus may have decreased pain sensation due to neuropathy.
- Patients with variant (Prinzmetal) angina are typically younger and may present with chest pain at rest, often early in the morning, and may have transient STE on the ECG.

DIAGNOSIS

- Obtain the medical history to identify the quality and severity of chest pain, precipitating factors, location, duration, pain radiation, and response to nitroglycerin or rest. Ischemic chest pain may resemble pain from noncardiac sources, and diagnosis of anginal pain may be difficult based on history alone.
- Assess nonmodifiable risk factors for coronary artery disease (CAD): age, sex, and family history of premature atherosclerotic disease in first-degree relatives (male onset before age 55 or female before age 65). Identify the presence of modifiable CAD risk factors: hypertension, diabetes mellitus, dyslipidemia, and cigarette smoking.
- Physical exam findings are usually nonspecific, but patients having an ischemic episode may present with tachycardia, diaphoresis, shortness of breath, nausea, vomiting, and lightheadedness. Other findings related to CAD risk factors may include increased blood pressure (BP) and a fourth heart sound reflecting longstanding hypertension. Other positive findings may include pulmonary crackles, displaced point of maximal impulse, and a third heart sound in patients with heart failure with reduced ejection fraction (HFrEF).
- Markers of inflammation, such as high-sensitivity C-reactive protein (hs-CRP), may be elevated.
- Cardiac troponin concentrations are not typically elevated in stable IHD.
- Resting ECG is normal in at least half of patients with angina who are not experiencing acute ischemia. About 50% of patients develop ischemic ST-T wave changes during an episode of angina, which can be observed on the ECG during an exercise stress test. Patients who cannot endure stress testing can have the myocardium stressed pharmacologically with adenosine, regadenoson, dipyridamole, or dobutamine.
- Coronary angiography is the most accurate test for confirming CAD but is invasive and requires arterial access. Myocardial perfusion imaging, cardiac magnetic resonance, coronary artery calcium scoring, and CT angiography can also be used to detect CAD.

TREATMENT

- <u>Goals of Treatment</u>: A primary goal of therapy is complete (or nearly complete) elimination of anginal chest pain and return to normal activities. Long-term goals are to slow progression of atherosclerosis and prevent complications such as MI, heart failure, stroke, and death.

NONPHARMACOLOGIC THERAPY

- Risk factor modification is the primary nondrug approach for primary and secondary prevention of CAD events. Lifestyle modifications include daily physical activity, weight management, dietary therapy (reduced intake of saturated fats, trans-fatty acids, and cholesterol), smoking cessation, psychological interventions (eg, screening

and treatment for depression if appropriate), limitation of alcohol intake, and avoiding exposure to air pollution.
- Surgical revascularization options for select patients include coronary artery bypass grafting (CABG) or percutaneous coronary intervention (PCI) with or without stent placement.

PHARMACOLOGIC THERAPY

- Guideline-directed medical therapy (GDMT) reduces the rates of death and MI similar to revascularization therapy. See Fig. 11-1 for a treatment algorithm based

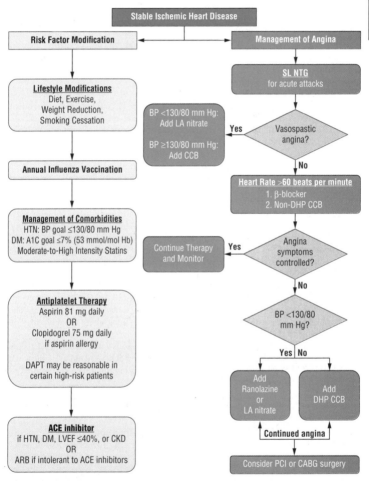

ACE, angiotensin-converting enzyme; ARB, angiotensin receptor blocker; BP, blood pressure; CABG, coronary artery bypass graft; CCB, calcium channel blocker; CKD, chronic kidney disease; DAPT, dual antiplatelet therapy; DHP, dihydropyridine; DM, diabetes mellitus; Hb, hemoglobin; HTN, hypertension; LA, long-acting; LVEF, left ventricular ejection fraction; PCI, percutaneous coronary intervention; SL NTG, sublingual nitroglycerin.

FIGURE 11-1. Algorithm for treatment of stable ischemic heart disease (guideline-directed medical therapy).

on the American College of Cardiology/American Heart Association (ACC/AHA) guidelines.

- Approaches to risk factor modification include the following recommendations:
  ✓ Dyslipidemia: Use moderate- or high-dose statin therapy in the absence of contraindications or adverse effects, in addition to lifestyle changes. Addition of ezetimibe, a PCSK9 inhibitor, or bile acid sequestrant may be considered for patients who do not tolerate statins or do not attain a 50% decrease in LDL cholesterol (or LDL remains above 70–100 mg/dL).
  ✓ Blood pressure: If BP is ≥130/80 mm Hg, institute drug therapy in addition to or after a trial of lifestyle modifications.
  ✓ Diabetes mellitus: Pharmacotherapy to achieve a target A1C of ≤7% (53 mmol/mol Hb) is reasonable for select patients (eg, short duration of diabetes and long life expectancy). An A1C goal of <8% is reasonable for other patients, such as those with micro- or macrovascular complications or coexisting medical conditions.
  ✓ Annual influenza vaccinations are recommended.

Antithrombotic Therapy

- Aspirin irreversibly blocks cyclooxygenase-1 (COX-1) activity and subsequent thromboxane A_2 production, leading to reduced platelet activation and aggregation. A small percentage of patients are nonresponsive to aspirin's antiplatelet effects. Nonsteroidal anti-inflammatory drugs (NSAIDs) may interfere with aspirin's antiplatelet effect when coadministered by competing for the site of action in the COX-1 enzyme. The ACC/AHA guidelines contain the following recommendations for stable IHD:
  ✓ **Aspirin:** 75–162 mg daily should be continued indefinitely in the absence of contraindications.
  ✓ **Clopidogrel:** 75 mg daily is a suitable alternative for patients unable to take aspirin due to allergy or intolerance. Patient responsiveness to clopidogrel is highly variable, with estimates of nonresponsiveness ranging from 5% to 44% of patients. The most common cause of nonresponsiveness is nonadherence, but genetic polymorphisms to CYP2C19 may contribute in some patients. There may also be drug interactions with CYP2C19, such as proton pump inhibitors, that may alter clopidogrel's effectiveness.
  ✓ **Dual antiplatelet therapy (DAPT)** with aspirin plus a $P2Y_{12}$ inhibitor (clopidogrel, prasugrel, ticagrelor) is beneficial after PCI with coronary stent placement and after treatment for ACS. Its benefits in other situations are less clear. The combination of aspirin (75–162 mg daily) and clopidogrel 75 mg daily may be reasonable in certain high-risk patients.
  ✓ **Rivaroxaban**, a direct factor Xa inhibitor, has demonstrated benefit in patients with CAD when added to aspirin therapy. Supporting data were not available when the ACC/AHA guidelines were published, but the combination is recommended by the American Diabetes Association.

Angiotensin-Converting Enzyme (ACE) Inhibitors and Angiotensin Receptor Blockers (ARBs)

- In the setting of IHD, ACE inhibitors stabilize coronary plaque, restore or improve endothelial function, inhibit vascular smooth muscle cell growth, decrease macrophage migration, and possibly prevent oxidative stress. However, ACE inhibitors have not been shown to improve symptomatic ischemia or reduce chest pain episodes. Clinical trials of the role of ACE inhibitors or ARBs in reducing cardiovascular events (eg, cardiovascular death, MI, stroke) in high-risk patients have produced conflicting results. The ACC/AHA guidelines for stable IHD recommend the following strategies:
  ✓ Use ACE inhibitors in patients who also have hypertension, diabetes, HFrEF, or chronic kidney disease, unless contraindicated.

✓ ARBs are recommended for the same populations if patients are intolerant to ACE inhibitors.
✓ Combination ACE inhibitor/ARB therapy should be avoided due to the lack of additional benefit and a higher risk of adverse events (eg, hypotension, syncope, renal dysfunction).
✓ Table 11-1 provides the usual dosage ranges for ACE inhibitors and ARBs in stable IHD.

TABLE 11-1	Drugs and Regimens for Stable Ischemic Heart Disease
Drug Class and Generic Names	**Usual Dosage Range[a]**
Angiotensin-Converting Enzyme Inhibitors	
Captopril	6.25–50 mg three times daily
Enalapril	2.5–40 mg daily in one to two divided doses
Fosinopril	10–80 mg daily in one to two divided doses
Lisinopril	2.5–40 mg once daily
Perindopril	4–8 mg once daily
Quinapril	5–20 mg twice daily
Ramipril	2.5–10 mg daily in one to two divided doses
Trandolapril	1–4 mg once daily
Angiotensin Receptor Blockers	
Candesartan	4–32 mg once daily
Valsartan	80–320 mg daily in one to two divided doses
Telmisartan	20–80 mg once daily
β-Adrenergic Blockers	
Atenolol[b]	25–200 mg once daily
Betaxolol[b]	5–20 mg once daily
Bisoprolol[b]	2.5–10 mg once daily
Carvedilol[c]	3.125–25 mg twice daily
Carvedilol phosphate[c]	10–80 mg once daily
Labetalol[c]	100–400 mg twice daily
Metoprolol[b]	50–200 mg twice daily (once daily for extended release)
Nadolol[d]	40–120 mg once daily
Nebivolol	5–10 mg once daily
Propranolol[d]	20–120 mg twice daily (60–240 mg once daily for long-acting formulation)
Timolol[d]	10–20 mg twice daily
Calcium Channel Blockers: Nondihydropyridine Type	
Diltiazem, extended release	120–360 mg once daily
Verapamil, extended release	180–480 mg once daily

(Continued)

TABLE 11-1 Drugs and Regimens for Stable Ischemic Heart Disease (*Continued*)

Drug Class and Generic Names	Usual Dosage Range[a]
Calcium Channel Blockers: Dihydropyridine Type	
Amlodipine	5–10 mg once daily
Felodipine	5–10 mg once daily
Nifedipine, extended release	30–90 mg once daily
Nicardipine	20–40 mg three times daily
Nitrates	
Nitroglycerin extended-release capsules	2.5 mg three times daily initially, with up-titration according to symptoms and tolerance; allow a 10- to 12-hour nitrate-free interval
Isosorbide dinitrate tablets	5–20 mg two to three times daily, with a daily nitrate-free interval of at least 14 hours (eg, dose at 7 AM, noon, and 5 PM)
Isosorbide dinitrate slow-release capsules	40 mg one to two times daily, with a daily nitrate-free interval of at least 18 hours (eg, dose at 8 AM and 2 PM)
Isosorbide mononitrate tablets	5–20 mg two times daily initially, with up-titration according to symptoms and tolerance; doses should be taken 7 hours apart (eg, 8 AM and 3 PM)
Isosorbide mononitrate extended-release tablets	30–120 mg once daily
Nitroglycerin transdermal extended-release film	0.2–0.8 mg/h, on for 12–14 hours, off for 10–12 hours

[a]Consult official prescribing information. In patients with renal and hepatic dysfunction, adjust initial and maintenance doses for all agents as appropriate based on FDA-approved labeling.
[b]Relatively β_1-selective (selectively is lost at higher doses).
[c]Blocks α_1, β_1, and β_2 receptors.
[d]Nonselective (blocks both β_1 and β_2 receptors).
Data from Landup D, Havrda D. Stable ischemic heart disease. In: Chisholm-Burns MA, et al., eds. Pharmacotherapy Principles & Practice. 6th ed. New York: McGraw-Hill Education; 2022.

β-Adrenergic Blockers

- β-Blockers competitively inhibit the effects of neuronally released and circulating catecholamines on β-adrenoceptors. Blockade of β_1-receptors in the heart and kidney reduces HR, contractility, and BP, thereby decreasing MVO_2.
- β-Blockers are recommended over calcium channel blockers (CCBs) for initial control of angina episodes in patients with stable IHD. The target is to lower the resting HR to 50–60 beats/min and the exercise HR to <100 beats/min. For patients (eg, older adults) who cannot tolerate these ranges, the target HR should be as low as can be tolerated above 50 beats/min. β-Blockers may be combined with CCBs or long-acting nitrates when initial treatment with β-blockers alone is unsuccessful.
- Only the β-blockers **carvedilol**, **metoprolol succinate**, and **bisoprolol** should be used in patients with HFrEF, starting with low doses and titrating upward slowly.
- Selection of a particular agent depends on the presence of comorbid states, preferred dosing frequency, and cost. β_1-Selective agents are preferred in patients with chronic obstructive pulmonary disease, peripheral arterial disease (PAD), diabetes, dyslipidemia, and sexual dysfunction. Drugs with combined α_1- and β-blockade are effective for IHD, but agents with intrinsic sympathomimetic activity provide little

to no reduction in resting HR and are not preferred except perhaps in patients with PAD or dyslipidemia.

- Common adverse effects include bradycardia, hypotension, heart block, impaired glucose metabolism, altered serum lipids (transiently increased triglycerides, decreased HDL-C, and no change in LDL-C), fatigue, depression, insomnia, and malaise. β-Blockers are contraindicated in patients with preexisting bradycardia, hypotension, second- or third-degree atrioventricular (AV) block, uncontrolled asthma, severe PAD, hypotension, HFrEF with unstable fluid status, and diabetes associated with frequent episodes of hypoglycemia.
- If β-blocker therapy must be discontinued, doses should be tapered over 2–3 weeks to prevent abrupt withdrawal, which can significantly increase in MVO_2 and induce ischemia and even MI because of up-regulation of β-receptors in the myocardium.
- See Table 11-1 for the usual dosage ranges of β-blockers in stable IHD.

Calcium Channel Blockers

- CCBs modulate calcium entry into the myocardium, vascular smooth muscle, and other tissues, which reduces the cytosolic concentration of calcium responsible for activation of the actin–myosin complex and contraction of vascular smooth muscle and myocardium. All CCBs reduce MVO_2 by reducing wall tension via lowering arterial BP and (to a minor extent) depressing contractility. CCBs also provide some increase in supply by inducing coronary vasodilation and preventing vasospasm.
- CCBs or long-acting nitrates should be prescribed for relief of symptoms when β-blockers are contraindicated or cause unacceptable side effects.
- Dihydropyridine CCBs (eg, **nifedipine**, **amlodipine**, **isradipine**, and **felodipine**) primarily affect vascular smooth muscle with little effect on the myocardium. These drugs produce minimal reduction in contractility and either no change or increased HR due to reflex tachycardia from direct arterial dilation. Nifedipine produces more impairment of LV function than amlodipine and felodipine. Short-acting agents should not be used because of their greater propensity to cause reflex tachycardia. Other side effects of these CCBs include hypotension, headache, gingival hyperplasia, and peripheral edema. Although most CCBs are contraindicated in patients with HFrEF, amlodipine and felodipine are considered safe options in these patients.
- Nondihydropyridine CCBs (**verapamil** and **diltiazem**) mostly affect the myocardium with minimal effects on vascular smooth muscle; they reduce HR, contractility, and MVO_2. Initial therapy for relief of symptoms with a long-acting nondihydropyridine CCB instead of a β-blocker is a reasonable approach. Common side effects of these CCBs include bradycardia, hypotension, AV block, and symptoms of LV depression. These agents should be avoided in patients with concomitant HFrEF due to negative inotropic effects. Verapamil may cause constipation in ~8% of patients. Verapamil and diltiazem inhibit clearance of drugs that utilize the cytochrome P450 3A4 isoenzyme such as carbamazepine, cyclosporine, lovastatin, simvastatin, and benzodiazepines. Verapamil, and to a lesser extent diltiazem, also inhibit P-glycoprotein–mediated drug transport, which can increase concentrations of digoxin and cyclosporine. Verapamil also decreases digoxin clearance. Agents that induce the 3A4 isoenzyme can reduce the effectiveness of all CCBs.
- See Table 11-1 for the usual dosage ranges of CCBs in stable IHD.

Nitrates

- Nitrates increase concentrations of cyclic guanosine monophosphate in vascular endothelium, leading to reduced cytoplasmic calcium and vasodilation. Most vasodilation occurs on the venous side, leading to reduced preload, myocardial wall tension, and MVO_2. Arterial vasodilation increases as doses are escalated, which can produce reflex tachycardia that can negate some of the antianginal benefits. This effect can be mitigated with concomitant β-blocker therapy. Nitrates also produce vasodilation of stenotic epicardial vessels and intracoronary collateral vessels, increasing oxygen supply to the ischemic myocardium.

- All patients should have access to SL NTG 0.3 or 0.4 mg tablets or spray to treat acute angina episodes. Relief typically occurs within 5 minutes of administration.
- SL nitrates can also be used to prevent acute episodes if given 2–5 minutes before activities known to produce angina; protection can last for up to 30 minutes with SL NTG and up to 1 hour with SL isosorbide dinitrate (ISDN).
- Long-acting nitrates (or CCBs) should be prescribed for relief of symptoms when β-blockers are contraindicated or cause unacceptable side effects. Various nitrate formulations are available for acute and chronic use (Table 11-1).
- Transdermal patches and isosorbide mononitrate (ISMN) are most commonly prescribed for long-term prevention of angina episodes. ISDN is also effective, but the three-times daily regimen requires dosing every 4–5 hours during the day to provide a nitrate-free interval. Chronic nitrate use should incorporate a 10- to 14-hour nitrate-free interval each day to reduce nitrate tolerance. Because this approach places the patient at risk for angina episodes, the nitrate-free interval is usually provided during the nighttime hours when the patient has a reduced MVO_2 while sleeping. The extended-release ISMN products that are dosed twice daily should be given 7 hours apart (eg, 7:00 AM and 2:00 PM). An extended-release, once-daily ISMN product is available that provides 12 hours of nitrate exposure followed by a 12-hour nitrate-free interval. Transdermal NTG patches are typically prescribed as "on in the AM and off in the PM" but patients should be given specific application and removal times (eg, apply at 8:00 AM and remove at 8:00 PM).
- Nitrates should not be used routinely as monotherapy for stable IHD because of the lack of angina coverage during the nitrate-free interval, lack of protection against circadian rhythm (nocturnal) ischemic events, and potential for reflex tachycardia. Concomitant β-blocker or diltiazem therapy can prevent rebound ischemia during the nitrate-free interval.
- Common nitrate adverse reactions include headache, flushing, nausea, postural hypotension, and syncope. Headache can be treated with acetaminophen and usually resolves after about 2 weeks of continued therapy. Transdermal NTG may cause skin erythema and inflammation. Initiating therapy with smaller doses and/or rotating the application site can minimize transdermal nitroglycerin side effects.

Ranolazine

- Ranolazine reduces ischemic episodes by selective inhibition of late sodium current (I_{Na}), which reduces intracellular sodium concentration and improves myocardial function and perfusion. It does not impact HR, BP, the inotropic state, or increase coronary blood flow.
- Ranolazine is effective as monotherapy for relief of angina symptoms but should only be used if patients cannot tolerate traditional agents due to hemodynamic or other adverse effects. Because it does not substantially affect HR and BP, it is recommended as add-on therapy to traditional antianginal agents for patients who achieve goal HR and BP and still have exertional angina symptoms, patients who cannot achieve these hemodynamic goals due to adverse effects, and patients who reach maximum doses of traditional agents but still have angina symptoms.
- The initial ranolazine dose is 500 mg twice daily, increased to 1000 mg twice daily within the next 1–2 weeks if tolerated. It can be combined with a β-blocker when initial treatment with β-blockers alone is unsuccessful.
- Adverse effects include constipation, nausea, dizziness, and headache. Ranolazine can prolong the QTc interval and should be used with caution in patients receiving concomitant QTc-prolonging agents.
- Potent inhibitors of CYP3A4 and P-glycoprotein (ketoconazole, itraconazole, protease inhibitors, clarithromycin, and nefazodone) or potent inducers of CYP3A4 and P-glycoprotein (phenytoin, phenobarbital, carbamazepine, rifampin, rifabutin, rifapentine, St. John's wort) are contraindicated with ranolazine due to significant increases and decreases in ranolazine drug concentrations, respectively. Moderate

CYP3A4 inhibitors (eg, diltiazem, verapamil, erythromycin, and fluconazole) can be used with ranolazine, but the maximum dose should not exceed 500 mg twice daily.

TREATMENT OF VARIABLE THRESHOLD ANGINA AND PRINZMETAL ANGINA

- Patients with variable threshold angina require pharmacotherapy for vasospasm. Most patients respond well to SL NTG for acute attacks.
- Both CCBs and nitrates are effective for chronic therapy. CCBs may be preferred because they are dosed less frequently. Nifedipine, verapamil, and diltiazem are equally effective as single agents for initial management of coronary vasospasm; dose titration is important to maximize the response. Patients unresponsive to CCBs alone may have nitrates added.
- β-Blockers are not useful for vasospasm because they may induce coronary vasoconstriction and prolong ischemia.

EVALUATION OF THERAPEUTIC OUTCOMES

- Assess for symptom improvement by number of angina episodes, weekly SL NTG use, and increased exercise capacity or duration of exertion needed to induce angina.
- Use statins for dyslipidemia, strive to achieve BP and A1C goals, and implement the lifestyle modifications of dietary modification, smoking cessation, weight loss, and regular exercise.
- Once patients have been optimized on medical therapy, symptoms should improve over 2–4 weeks and remain stable until the disease progresses. Patients may require evaluation every 1–2 months until target endpoints are achieved; follow-up every 6–12 months thereafter is appropriate.
- The Seattle Angina Questionnaire, Specific Activity Scale, and Canadian Cardiovascular Society classification system can be used to improve reproducibility of symptom assessment.
- If the patient is doing well, no other assessment may be necessary. Although follow-up exercise tolerance testing with or without cardiac imaging can be performed to objectively assess control of ischemic episodes, this is rarely done if patients are doing well because of the expense involved.
- Monitor for adverse drug effects such as headache and dizziness with nitrates; fatigue and lassitude with β-blockers; and peripheral edema, constipation, and dizziness with CCBs.

See Chapter 33, Stable Ischemic Heart Disease, authored by Paul P. Dobesh, Robert J. DiDomenico, and Kelly C. Rogers, for a more detailed discussion of this topic.

Shock Syndromes

- *Shock* involves a group of syndromes that cause acute, generalized circulatory failure associated with inadequate tissue and organ perfusion. Shock is characterized by systolic blood pressure (SBP) <90 mm Hg (or reduction of at least 40 mm Hg from baseline) or mean arterial blood pressure (MAP) <70 mm Hg with tachycardia and organ perfusion abnormalities.
- Classes of shock based on etiologic mechanisms include (1) hypovolemic, (2) cardiogenic, (3) obstructive, and (4) vasodilatory/distributive. Patients may have components of more than one shock syndrome upon presentation.

PATHOPHYSIOLOGY

- Circulatory shock develops when the cardiovascular system is unable to deliver an adequate oxygen supply to meet tissue demands, resulting in cellular dysfunction, a shift in cellular metabolism to anaerobic pathways, and elevated blood lactate concentrations.
- *Hypovolemic shock* is caused by inadequate venous return because of internal or external loss of intravascular fluids (eg, trauma, surgery, hemorrhage), resulting in insufficient cardiac preload and decreased stroke volume.
- *Cardiogenic shock* results from loss of pump function because of decreased cardiac contractility (eg, acute myocardial infarction [AMI]), acute valvular abnormality, or arrhythmia (eg, ventricular tachycardia).
- *Obstructive shock* results from extracardiac obstruction to blood flow into or out of the heart, such as tension pneumothorax, cardiac tamponade, or pulmonary embolism.
- *Vasodilatory/distributive shock* is characterized by loss of vascular tone; this involves tissue hypoperfusion due to decreased systemic vascular resistance (or hypoperfusion despite normal or elevated cardiac output). Distributive shock is a subset of vasodilatory shock characterized by maldistribution of blood flow in organ microcirculation. Most cases of vasodilatory shock result in distributive shock. Almost all cases of septic shock result in vasodilatory/distributive shock.
- The body responds to an abrupt decrease in tissue perfusion with subsequent restoration of perfusion, leading to a systemic inflammatory response syndrome (SIRS) with release of numerous mediators that interact to cause further injury. This "ischemia-reperfusion injury" results in edematous obstruction of capillaries, oxygen free-radical damage of cell membranes, activation of cellular (eg, white blood cells, platelets) and humoral (eg, procoagulants, anticoagulants, complement, kinins) components, release of other inflammatory mediators, and formation of microthrombi.
- As part of the stress response, anti-inflammatory pathways are also activated to counterbalance the proinflammatory effects on tissues. Vagal nerve-mediated release of acetylcholine leads to suppression of proinflammatory cytokines by macrophages. The renin–angiotensin–aldosterone and hypothalamic–pituitary–adrenocortical systems are activated, with release of angiotensin II, vasopressin, and cortisol to maintain blood pressure (BP) via vasoconstriction and renal sodium and water retention. Cortisol and catecholamine release from the adrenal glands also inhibits proinflammatory cytokine production.

CLINICAL PRESENTATION

- Patients may report dizziness, lightheadedness, confusion, and low urine production.
- Symptoms related to the underlying shock etiology will be present (eg, cough, fever, malaise with pneumonia; chest pain with AMI).

- Vital signs may reveal tachycardia (eg, >120 bpm), tachypnea (eg, >30 breaths/min), hypotension (eg, SBP <90 mm Hg), and low or normal body temperature (eg, 36°C–37°C [96.8°F–98.6°F]) in the absence of infection. Temperature may be elevated if infection is present (eg, >38.3°C [101°F]).
- Physical exam findings of tissue hypoperfusion may include neurologic (eg, confusion, obtundation), cutaneous (eg, warm skin with vasodilation and cool, clammy skin with vasoconstriction), and renal (eg, low urine production) system abnormalities. Capillary refill is usually impaired.
- Laboratory test abnormalities may include elevated blood lactate concentration (>2 mmol/L), increased blood urea nitrogen (BUN) and serum creatinine and decreased urine output (<0.5 to 1 mL/kg/h) with renal dysfunction, elevated transaminase levels with hepatic dysfunction, decreased hemoglobin/hematocrit with hemorrhage, and elevated cardiac troponin concentration with AMI. In septic shock, the white blood cell (WBC) count is usually >12,000 cells/mm^3 (12×10^9/L), and thrombocytopenia may occur. In hemorrhagic and septic shock, the prothrombin time (PT) and international normalized ratio (INR) may increase over time.

DIAGNOSIS AND MONITORING

- Rapid assessment by cardiac echocardiography is indicated when the shock etiology is unclear. Transthoracic echocardiograms can lead to rapid (within 5 minutes) diagnosis of the shock type.
- Initial monitoring in suspected circulatory shock should include vital signs, blood lactate concentration, urine production, and physical examination, including mental status.
- Advanced hemodynamic monitoring (eg, central venous catheterization) may be needed to measure central venous pressure (CVP), obtain venous samples for laboratory testing (including central venous oxygen saturation or $ScvO_2$), and administer drugs (including vasopressors) or fluids directly into the central circulation.
- Tissue metabolic requirements are met by both adequate MAP and adequate oxygen delivery (Do_2). MAP is the driving pressure for peripheral blood flow and end-organ perfusion and is a surrogate estimate of tissue blood flow. Because the components of BP are cardiac output (CO) and systemic vascular resistance (SVR) and CO is a determinant of Do_2, BP is integrally related to Do_2. However, compensatory mechanisms such as vasoconstriction may preserve BP while tissue perfusion is inadequate. Therefore, while low BP is commonly present in patients with shock, it is not required to define shock.
- Inadequate Do_2 leads to organ damage in critical illness. In normal individuals, oxygen consumption (Vo_2) depends on Do_2 up to a certain critical level (Vo_2 flow dependency). At this point, tissue oxygen requirements are satisfied and further increases in Do_2 will not alter Vo_2 (Vo_2 flow independency). The point that Vo_2 becomes dependent on Do_2 represents a pathologic transition from aerobic to anaerobic cellular metabolism and lactate production. However, studies in critically ill patients show a continuous, pathologic dependence relationship of Vo_2 with Do_2. The parameters are calculated as follows:

$$Do_2 = CO \times Cao_2 \text{ and } Vo_2 = CO \times (Cao_2 - Cvo_2)$$

where CO = cardiac output, Cao_2 = arterial oxygen content determined by hemoglobin concentration and arterial oxygen saturation (Sao_2), and Cvo_2 = mixed venous oxygen content determined by hemoglobin concentration and venous oxygen saturation (Svo_2).

- Venous oximetry (ie, venous oxygen saturations) reflects the adequacy of tissue oxygenation. Svo_2 and central venous oxygen saturation ($Scvo_2$) are the oxyhemoglobin saturation of venous blood obtained from the pulmonary artery and a central vein in the thorax, respectively, and are expressed as a percentage. When tissue oxygen demand exceeds supply, the oxygen extraction ratio (O_2ER) increases and values of

Svo_2 and $Scvo_2$ are low. When hemoglobin, Sao_2, and Vo_2 are stable, Svo_2 or $Scvo_2$ values reflect CO. Thus, venous oximetry may be used as a surrogate for CO and can be useful in shock state differentiation.

- Generally, Svo_2 values >70% (0.70) are considered adequate and normal. However, Svo_2 values <50% (0.50) are low and may approach the critical O_2ER where anaerobic metabolism occurs and lactate concentrations increase. High Svo_2 (>80% [0.80]) can represent a high CO but may also be a poor prognostic sign indicating adequate Do_2 but poor capacity of tissues to extract oxygen.

TREATMENT

- Goals of Treatment: The desired outcome is to reduce morbidity and mortality by preventing organ damage and, to the extent possible, halt or reverse existing organ dysfunction. Treatment of circulatory shock can be divided into four phases, each with different (but sometimes overlapping) treatment goals and strategies: (1) *Salvage*, with goals of obtaining a minimum perfusion pressure and CO to ensure survival and treating the underlying shock etiology (eg, hemostasis, antimicrobials, coronary revascularization); (2) *optimization*, ensuring adequate organ perfusion and Do_2; (3) *stabilization*, to prevent further end-organ dysfunction; and (4) *de-escalation*, which targets patient recovery with goals of weaning (or stopping) vasoactive medications and fluids. This chapter focuses on salvage and optimization, but recognizing the phase of a patient's circulatory shock is necessary to establish treatment goals and therapeutic approaches.

GENERAL APPROACH

- Figure 12-1 presents an algorithm for managing patients with shock using a stepwise approach to optimize MAP, first with crystalloid fluid resuscitation followed by the vasopressor norepinephrine if appropriate.
- Hospitalization is indicated for patients with circulatory insufficiency that does not respond readily to fluid resuscitation.
- Venous access is generally obtained during the initial examination process. Large-bore peripheral IV lines are preferred over central lines for initial fluid resuscitation, but vasopressors should preferentially be administered via a central venous catheter.
- The stabilization phase should include general supportive care measures such as assessment and management of pain, anxiety/agitation, delirium, immobility, sleep disturbances, nutrition, glycemic control, and thromboembolism prophylaxis.
- A goal MAP >65 mm Hg is often targeted to maintain adequate perfusion to critical organs.
- Consider patient-specific characteristics when establishing a BP goal and determining an adequate perfusion response to resuscitation.
- If MAP or SBP remains below goal, then initiate vasopressors to ensure tissue perfusion.
- Determine adequacy of Do_2 by assessing markers of end-organ perfusion (eg, urine production), lactate concentrations, and capillary refill time. Obtain serial lactate concentrations in the early treatment phases because lactate clearance and normalization correspond with improved global tissue perfusion.
- After the salvage treatment phase, give fluids only to patients with ineffective tissue perfusion who are predicted or known to be fluid responsive. The benefits of continued fluid administration (improved CO and tissue perfusion) must be balanced against the risks of fluid overload (eg, pulmonary edema).

NONPHARMACOLOGIC THERAPY

- Give all patients the basic life support measures of a secure airway with appropriate oxygenation.
- For hypovolemic shock, additional measures may include surgery, control of blood loss, blood component transfusion, and prevention of heat loss with hypothermia or cooling measures with heat exposure (eg, heat stroke).

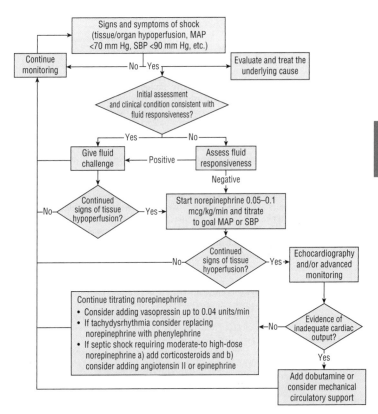

FIGURE 12-1. Algorithm for the management of patients with shock.

- For patients with thermal injuries, cover wound sites with cool, moist sterile dressings until more definitive care can be provided.
- Patients with cardiogenic shock secondary to AMI should undergo emergent coronary revascularization and be considered for CO augmentation via mechanical device (eg, temporary percutaneous circulatory support).
- Measures for obstructive shock may include pericardiocentesis or surgical evacuation of fluid for cardiac tamponade, needle decompression and/or chest tube thoracostomy for tension pneumothorax, and surgical or catheter thrombectomy for pulmonary embolism.
- Patients with vasodilatory/distributive shock secondary to septic shock should have infectious source control with consideration given to fever control via external cooling.

PHARMACOLOGIC THERAPY

Intravenous Fluids and Blood Products

- The goal of administering IV fluids is to increase venous return in order to increase stroke volume, cardiac output, Do_2, and BP. Blood products may also be administered to replace cellular and plasma losses with the added benefit of increasing venous return.

Crystalloids

- Isotonic (or near isotonic) crystalloid solutions (eg, **lactated Ringer's** and **0.9% sodium chloride** [normal saline]) are the initial fluid of choice for resuscitation, and large volumes should be administered (except for patients with cardiogenic shock). Balanced salt solutions (eg, lactated Ringer's) and **multiple electrolytes injection** (eg, Plasma-Lyte A) and normal saline have similar efficacy in expanding plasma volume, but balanced salt solutions may be safer. Excess chloride administration with normal saline may be more likely to lead to hyperchloremic metabolic acidosis and possibly acute kidney injury (AKI). However, balanced salt solutions should be used with extreme caution in brain-injured patients because they may exacerbate cerebral edema. If there are signs of tissue hypoperfusion and the clinical syndrome is consistent with a shock state that is fluid responsive (eg, hypovolemic), administer an initial fluid challenge of at least 500 mL of crystalloid.
- **3% sodium chloride** (hypertonic saline) causes redistribution of fluid from the intracellular space, resulting in rapid expansion of the intravascular compartment; however, its use is not associated with improved outcomes when used for initial fluid resuscitation in shock. In addition, potential dosing and administration errors can lead to adverse events, and dramatic fluid shifts may be associated with hypernatremia, metabolic acidosis from hyperchloremia, and peripheral vein damage due to high osmolality (1026 mOsm/L).

Colloids

- **Albumin (5% or 25%), hydroxyethyl starch**, and **dextran** are large molecular weight solutions that have a prolonged intravascular retention time compared to crystalloid solutions; colloids remain in the intravascular space for hours or days, depending on the size of the colloid molecules and capillary permeability. However, colloids are expensive and have been associated with fluid overload, renal dysfunction, and bleeding. When compared with alternative resuscitation solutions, hydroxyethyl starch was associated with increased mortality, AKI, and need for renal replacement therapy. Consequently, the US product labeling was changed to state that starch products are contraindicated in critically ill patients; therefore, they should not be used for fluid resuscitation.

Blood products

- Some patients require blood products (**packed red blood cells, fresh frozen plasma, platelets,** or **cryoprecipitate**) to ensure maintenance of O_2-carrying capacity, as well as clotting factors and platelets for blood hemostasis. Blood products may be associated with circulatory overload, transfusion-related reactions, virus transmission (rarely), hypocalcemia from added citrate, increased blood viscosity from supranormal hematocrit elevations, and hypothermia from failure to appropriately warm solutions before administration.

Fluid Resuscitation in Distributive (Septic) Shock

- The initial fluid challenge volume is unclear; the Surviving Sepsis Campaign guidelines suggest 30 mL/kg crystalloids given within the first 3 hours of shock recognition, but supporting evidence for this specific volume is of low quality. Several approaches exist for fluid resuscitation during the first 6 hours: (1) liberal fluid administration (50–75 mL/kg) while reserving vasopressors; and (2) relatively restrictive initial fluid administration (≤30 mL/kg) with earlier vasopressor use to maintain tissue perfusion. More than 30 mL/kg of crystalloid fluids may be needed to obtain goal MAP, reverse global hypoperfusion (lactate clearance, $SCVo_2$ ≥70% [0.70]), or achieve clinical indication of regional organ-specific perfusion (eg, urine production). An isolated bolus (eg, 250–500 mL) in an adult patient is unlikely to cause a substantial change in BP or acid–base balance. Therefore, multiple fluid boluses are often needed to achieve hemodynamic stability. However, excessive fluid administration has been associated with higher mortality, and overly aggressive fluid administration should be avoided, especially in patients with heart failure or impending pulmonary edema.

Because intravenous medication diluents can contribute significantly to total fluid volume, the total fluid administration should be accounted for, and dynamic fluid response with clinical assessment should occur frequently after each fluid challenge.

Fluid Resuscitation in Hypovolemic (Hemorrhagic/Traumatic) Shock

- Immediate treatment of hemorrhagic shock with plasma expanders (crystalloids or colloids) seems logical, but no large, well-controlled clinical trials have supported this practice. To the contrary, fluid resuscitation beyond minimal levels (ie, MAP ≥60 mm Hg) is harmful in patients with abdominal trauma due to hemodilution and clot destabilization.
- Instead of immediate plasma expansion in all preoperative patients with circulatory insufficiency caused by hemorrhage, the initial priority should be surgical control of the bleeding source; until this is possible, fluids should be given in small aliquots to yield a palpable pulse and to maintain MAP values no more than 60 mm Hg and SBP no more than 90 mm Hg.
- Isotonic crystalloids are the fluid of choice because they are equal in efficacy to hypertonic sodium chloride solutions with a lower risk of adverse effects. Balanced salt solutions may be used as an alternative to normal saline but should be avoided in patients with severe traumatic brain injury because it may worsen cerebral edema. Hypotonic solutions should be avoided in this population given their relatively poor intravascular expansion and association with poor outcomes in animal models of closed head injury.
- Once hemostasis has been achieved in a patient with hemorrhage, a relatively restrictive transfusion strategy (ie, transfusion if hemoglobin ≤7 g/dL [70 g/L; 4.34 mmol/L]) is indicated unless a patient has active cardiac ischemia. Additional blood product administration should be guided by laboratory parameters (eg, PT/INR, platelets) or viscoelastic testing (eg, thromboelastography). Reversal of antithrombotic therapy (eg, prothrombin complex concentrates for warfarin) may also be used for severe bleeding.

Vasopressors and Inotropes

- Vasopressors and inotropes are required when volume resuscitation is not indicated or fails to maintain adequate BP (MAP ≥65 mm Hg) and organs and tissues remain hypoperfused. Vasopressors may also be needed temporarily to treat life-threatening hypotension when tissue perfusion is inadequate despite ongoing aggressive fluid resuscitation. Inotropes are frequently used to optimize Do_2 in septic shock and cardiac function in cardiogenic shock.
- Table 12-1 lists the usual dosage range, receptor selectivity, and potential adverse effects of vasopressors and inotropes used in shock.
- Norepinephrine has combined strong α_1-agonist activity and less potent β_1-agonist effects while maintaining weak vasodilatory effects of β_2-receptor stimulation. It produces vasoconstriction primarily via its more prominent α-effects on all vascular beds, thus increasing SVR; it also produces a small (10%–15%) increase in stroke volume. Norepinephrine is the vasopressor of choice in patients in most shock states because (1) it may decrease mortality in septic shock; (2) it reverses inappropriate vasodilation and low global oxygen extraction; (3) it attenuates myocardial depression at unchanged or increased CO and increased coronary blood flow; (4) it improves renal perfusion pressure and renal filtration; (5) it enhances splanchnic perfusion; and (6) it is less likely than many other vasopressors to cause tachydysrhythmias. Norepinephrine 0.05–2 mcg/kg/min improves hemodynamic parameters to "normal" values in most patients with shock. As with other vasopressors, norepinephrine dosages exceeding those recommended by most references are frequently needed in critically ill patients with shock to achieve predetermined goals. A significant increase in MAP is caused by an increase in SVR. Heart rate generally decreases because of reflex bradycardia from increased SVR. Increasing doses to maintain higher MAPs may increase heart rate, cardiac index, Do_2, and cutaneous blood flow, but these results are inconsistent. Norepinephrine may be associated with

TABLE 12-1	Receptor Pharmacology and Adverse Events of Selected Vasopressor and Inotropic Agents Used in Shock[a]						
Agent (Adverse Events)	α_1	α_2	β_1	β_2	D	V_1	V_2
Angiotensin II (5000–10,000 ng/mL NS)	Tachycardia, thrombosis, peripheral ischemia, lactic acidosis, bronchospasm, infection						
1.25–80 ng/kg/min	0	0	0	0	0	0	0
Dobutamine (500–4000 mcg/mL D_5W or NS)	Tachycardia, dysrhythmias, hypotension						
2–10 mcg/kg/min	+	0	++++	++	0	0	0
>10–20 mcg/kg/min	++	0	++++	+++	0	0	0
Dopamine (800–3200 mcg/mL D_5W or NS)	Tachycardia, dysrhythmias, decreased PaO_2, mesenteric hypoperfusion, gastrointestinal motility inhibition, T-cell inhibition						
1–3 mcg/kg/min	0	0	+	0	++++	0	0
3–10 mcg/kg/min	0/+	0	++++	+	++++	0	0
>10–20 mcg/kg/min	+++	0	++++	+	0	0	0
Epinephrine (8–16 mcg/mL D_5W or NS)	Tachycardia, dysrhythmias, decreased PaO_2, mesenteric hypoperfusion, increased lactate, hyperglycemia, immunomodulation						
0.01–0.05 mcg/kg/min	++	++	++++	+++	0	0	0
0.05–3 mcg/kg/min	++++	++++	+++	+	0	0	0
Norepinephrine (16–64 mcg/mL D_5W)	Mixed effects on myocardial performance and mesenteric perfusion, peripheral ischemia						
0.02–3 mcg/kg/min	+++	+++	+++	+/++	0	0	0
Phenylephrine (100–400 g/mL D_5W or NS)	Mixed effects on myocardial performance, peripheral ischemia						
0.5–9 mcg/kg/min	+++	+	+	0	0	0	0
Vasopressin (0.2–1 units/mL D_5W or NS)	Mixed effects on myocardial performance, mesenteric hypoperfusion, peripheral ischemia, hyponatremia, thrombocytopenia, hyperbilirubinemia						
0.01–0.1 units/min	0	0	0	0	0	+++	+++

AT, angiotensin; D, dopamine; D_5W, dextrose 5% in water; NS, normal saline; PaO_2, partial pressure of arterial oxygen; V, vasopressin.

[a]Activity ranges from no activity (0) to maximal (++++) activity. Angiotensin II has ++++ activity at AT-1 and AT-2 receptors but no activity at other receptors.

tachydysrhythmias, which is more common with higher doses. Norepinephrine is not commercially available as a premixed ready-to-use solution, so its use requires preparation time.

- **Epinephrine** has combined α- and β-agonist effects. At low doses (0.01–0.05 mcg/kg/min) β-adrenergic effects predominate with an increase in stroke volume and CO. For this reason, low doses may be used as an inotrope after cardiac surgery. When higher dosages are used, α-adrenergic effects are predominant and SVR and MAP are increased. Epinephrine is an acceptable choice for hemodynamic support of patients with shock because of its combined vasoconstrictor and inotropic effects. It is as effective as norepinephrine for MAP response in vasodilatory/distributive shock. Epinephrine doses of 0.04–1 mcg/kg/min alone increase hemodynamic and oxygen-transport variables to "supranormal" values in shock patients without coronary artery disease. Large doses (0.5–3 mcg/kg/min) are often required, particularly for patients with septic shock. Smaller doses (0.1–0.5 mcg/kg/min) are effective when epinephrine is added to other vasopressors and inotropes. In addition, younger patients appear to respond better to epinephrine, possibly due to greater β-adrenergic reactivity. Despite rapid improvement of hemodynamic variables and Do_2, it can have deleterious effects on renal hemodynamics and oxygen utilization. Like norepinephrine, epinephrine is not commercially available as a premixed ready-to-use solution.
- **Phenylephrine** is a pure α_1-agonist and increases BP primarily through vasoconstriction. It improves MAP by increasing SVR and stroke index through enhanced venous return to the heart. Given the presence of cardiac α_1-receptors, phenylephrine may also increase contractility and CO. Tachydysrhythmias are infrequent, particularly when phenylephrine is used as a single agent or at higher doses because it exerts little activity on β_1-adrenergic receptors. Phenylephrine may be a useful alternative in patients who cannot tolerate tachycardia or tachydysrhythmias from norepinephrine or epinephrine. As with other vasopressors, the doses required to achieve therapeutic goals are significantly higher than those traditionally recommended. Phenylephrine 0.5–9 mcg/kg/min, used alone or in combination with dobutamine or low dopamine doses, improves BP and myocardial performance in fluid-resuscitated patients with vasodilatory/distributive shock. In septic shock, phenylephrine does not significantly impair the cardiac index, pulmonary artery occlusion pressure (PAOP), or peripheral perfusion. Like norepinephrine and epinephrine, phenylephrine is not commercially available as a premixed ready-to-use solution.
- **Dopamine** has been described as having dose-related receptor activity at D_1-, D_2-, β_1-, and α_1-receptors, but this dose-response relationship has not been confirmed in critically ill patients. In patients with shock, a significant overlap of hemodynamic effects occurs, even at doses as low as 3 mcg/kg/min. Low-dose dopamine does not enhance renal function or survival in critically ill patients. Dopamine is a natural precursor to norepinephrine and epinephrine but is generally not as effective for achieving goal MAP in patients with shock. Doses of 5–10 mcg/kg/min increase CO by improving contractility and heart rate, primarily from β_1 effects. At higher doses (>10 mcg/kg/min), it increases MAP as a result of both increased CO and SVR due to its combined β_1 and α_1 effects. The clinical utility of dopamine as a vasopressor in shock is limited because large doses are frequently necessary to maintain CO and MAP. At doses >20 mcg/kg/min, further improvement in cardiac performance and regional hemodynamics is limited. In addition, its clinical use is often hampered by tachycardia and tachydysrhythmias, which may lead to myocardial ischemia. For these reasons, dopamine is no longer considered a first-line therapy for shock. Dopamine is commercially available as premixed ready-to-use solution of various concentrations.
- **Dobutamine** is primarily a selective β_1-agonist with mild β_2- and vascular α_1-activity, resulting in strong positive inotropic activity without concomitant vasoconstriction. Compared to dopamine, dobutamine produces a larger increase in CO and is less arrhythmogenic. β_2-induced vasodilation and increased myocardial contractility with subsequent reflex reduction in sympathetic tone lead to decreased SVR. Optimal uses of dobutamine in shock are for patients with low CO and high filling pressures

(eg, left ventricular dysfunction on echocardiography) or ongoing signs of global or regional hypoperfusion despite adequate resuscitation; however, vasopressors may be needed to counteract arterial vasodilation. Dobutamine is an inotrope with vasodilatory properties (an "inodilator"). It is used for treatment of septic and cardiogenic shock to increase CO, typically by 25%–50%. Dobutamine increases stroke volume, left ventricular stroke work index, and thus cardiac index and Do_2 without increasing PAOP. Because dobutamine increases myocardial oxygen demand, it should be used cautiously in patients with cardiogenic shock. The combination of dobutamine and norepinephrine results in a lower increase in heart rate than use of epinephrine alone. Dobutamine is commercially available as a premixed ready-to-use solution.

- **Vasopressin** causes rapid and sustained vasoconstriction that increases SVR and BP, which allows for reductions in the dosage requirements of catecholamines and adrenergic agents in vasodilatory/distributive shock. These effects occur with doses up to 0.04 units/min. Doses >0.04 units/min may be associated with negative changes in CO and mesenteric mucosal perfusion. Cardiac ischemia occurs rarely with low doses; use of higher doses in septic shock patients with cardiac dysfunction warrants extreme caution. Vasopressin decreases heart rate after initiation because of reflex bradycardia from increased SVR. Unlike adrenergic agonists, the vasoconstrictive effects are preserved during hypoxemia and severe acidemia, and pulmonary arterial pressures do not increase. After treatment initiation, organ-specific vasodilation may preserve cardiac and renal function. Whereas V_2 stimulation promotes water retention from the distal kidney tubules and collecting ducts, V_1-receptors constrict efferent arterioles and dilate afferent arterioles to increase glomerular perfusion pressure and filtration rate, enhancing urine production. Vasopressin is not available as a premixed ready-to-use solution.
- **Angiotensin II** increases SVR and may be used for vasodilatory/distributive shock. BP rapidly increases after initiation in patients with low SVR. The starting dose is 10–20 ng/kg/min with rapid titration (as quickly as every 5 minutes) to MAP goal. In the first 3 hours of treatment, the dose may be increased up to 80 ng/kg/min; thereafter, the dose should not exceed 40 ng/kg/min. The effects of angiotensin II on myocardial performance, oxygen transport parameters, and regional organ perfusion are unclear. However, it may have a deleterious effect on regional tissue perfusion because its risk of lactic acidosis and delirium is higher. Angiotensin II has only been evaluated in patients without depressed CO so it should be used with extreme caution in patients with impaired left ventricular systolic function. Angiotensin II also increases glomerular perfusion pressure and filtration, but its effects on kidney function are unclear. Heart rate increases significantly after initiation, so it should be used cautiously in vulnerable patients (eg, older patients with coronary artery disease). Because it increases the risk of thromboembolic events, concurrent thromboembolism prophylaxis should be employed. Patients receiving angiotensin II have a higher risk for secondary infection. It has been associated with bronchospasm and should be avoided in patients with asthma or current bronchospasm.

Use of Vasopressors and Inotropes in Distributive (Septic) Shock

- Norepinephrine should be started when a MAP ≥65 mm Hg and/or adequate tissue perfusion are not achieved with fluid resuscitation. Infusions are initiated at 0.05–0.1 mcg/kg/min and rapidly titrated to preset BP goals (usually MAP ≥65 mm Hg) and/or improvement in global and regional peripheral perfusion (eg, decrease blood lactate or restore urine production).
- Epinephrine is considered adjunctive therapy to norepinephrine because it is associated with tachydysrhythmias, lactate elevation, and variable pH values.
- Phenylephrine improves myocardial performance in hyperdynamic, normotensive patients with sepsis but worsens myocardial performance in patients with cardiogenic shock because of decreased CO and increased SVR. Therefore, phenylephrine use warrants caution, and it should not be used as an initial vasopressor in shock patients with impaired myocardial performance.

- Dopamine is no longer recommended as a first-line vasopressor because of the limitations described previously.
- Current guidelines recommend a trial of dobutamine for patients with septic shock in the presence of myocardial dysfunction. However, administration of dobutamine purely to achieve a normal CO, Do_2, or $SCVo_2$ in the absence of other signs of tissue hypoperfusion (eg, low urine production) is not recommended. Dobutamine should be started at doses ranging from 2.5 to 5 mcg/kg/min up to a maximum of 20 mcg/kg/min. Doses >20 mcg/kg/min are limited by tachycardia, myocardial ischemia, hypertension, and tachydysrhythmias. Like other inotropes, dobutamine is usually given until improvement in myocardial function with resolution of the underlying etiology or dose-limiting adverse reactions are observed.
- Additional vasoactive agents (eg, vasopressin, angiotensin II, corticosteroids) may be added to improve MAP or decrease catecholamine requirements. However, specific catecholamine dosage thresholds indicating the initiation of these adjunctive agents are unclear. Adjunctive use of vasopressin to prevent dose escalation of adrenergic agents, decrease norepinephrine dosage, or increase MAP should be considered in patients with vasodilatory/distributive shock. Doses are generally fixed at 0.03–0.04 units/min, with higher doses reserved for salvage therapy. Increased arterial pressure should be evident within the first hour of vasopressin therapy, at which time the dose(s) of adrenergic agent(s) should be reduced while maintaining goal MAP.
- The role of angiotensin II is unclear, but it is most frequently used as adjunctive therapy to norepinephrine and vasopressin.
- Corticosteroid therapy in septic shock improves hemodynamic variables and allows lower catecholamine vasopressor dosages with minimal adverse effects on patient safety. Corticosteroids should be considered when fluids and vasopressors are unable to restore hemodynamic stability, or when weaning of vasopressor therapy proves futile. They should also be started in cases of shock when adrenal insufficiency is suspected (eg, patients receiving long-term corticosteroid therapy for other indications prior to the onset of shock); however, assessment of adrenal function to guide therapy is not recommended. Adverse events are few because corticosteroids are administered for a short period, usually 7 days. Studies suggest that short-term, low-dose corticosteroids do not increase rates of gastrointestinal bleeding and superinfections but do increase the risk for hypernatremia, hyperglycemia, and perhaps neuromuscular weakness. Acutely elevated serum BUN and WBC count may also occur.

Use of Vasopressors and Inotropes in Hypovolemic (Hemorrhagic/Traumatic) Shock

- In contrast to other forms of shock, medications are a distant alternative to fluid resuscitation, which is the primary therapy for hypovolemic shock. In hypovolemic shock, peripheral resistance is high due to compensatory mechanisms aimed at maintaining tissue perfusion. Early or overzealous use of vasopressors in lieu of fluids may exacerbate this resistance to the point that flow is stopped.
- Vasopressors are only used as a temporizing measure or as a last resort when all other measures to maintain perfusion have been exhausted. Few studies have compared the various agents, but norepinephrine is considered the first-line vasopressor of choice.

EVALUATION OF THERAPEUTIC OUTCOMES

- The initial goals of therapy are to restore effective tissue and organ perfusion. Place priority on the ABCs of life support (ie, airway, breathing, and circulation), assessing vital signs and mental status, and determining tissue perfusion (eg, urine production after catheterization).
- Evaluate the underlying cause of tissue hypoperfusion to identify the correct treatment approach.
- For patients with sepsis, measure blood lactate concentration (and remeasure if initial lactate is >2 mmol/L), begin rapid administration of 30 mL/kg of crystalloid for

hypotension, and obtain MAP ≥65 mm Hg with vasopressors if patient is hypotensive during or after fluid resuscitation, all started within 1 hour of recognition. Usual care must include rapid (ie, within 1 hour of recognition) antibiotic administration and aggressive fluid resuscitation.

- Goals of initial fluid resuscitation should include crystalloids if the patient is fluid responsive, vasopressors to achieve MAP at least 65 mm Hg (or SBP 80–90 mm Hg in trauma patients), and frequent clinical assessments to meet perfusion goals (eg, additional fluid challenge or inotropic therapy to achieve lactate clearance ≥20%, capillary refill time <3 seconds, $SCvo_2$ ≥70% (0.70), or urine production ≥0.5 mL/kg/h).

- Initiate vasopressors/inotropes if tissue perfusion is not responding to fluid challenges. Titration and monitoring should be guided by the "best clinical response," lactate clearance, and capillary refill time. Although doses required for efficacy may be much higher than recommended by most references, use the lowest effective dosage while minimizing evidence of global hypoperfusion (lactate, $SCvo_2$, capillary refill time) and regional hypoperfusion such as myocardial (eg, tachydysrhythmias, electrocardiographic changes, troponin elevations), renal (decreased glomerular filtration rate and/or urine production), splanchnic/gastric (bowel ischemia, elevated transaminases), pulmonary (worsening Pao_2), or peripheral (cold extremities) ischemia. Continue vasopressors/inotropes until myocardial depression and/or BP improve, usually measured in hours to days.

- Monitor patients frequently for their response to therapy. If perfusion is not restored with the initial treatment approach, perform echocardiography with additional treatment options implemented based on the findings.

- Consider hemodynamic monitoring with a pulmonary artery (Swan-Ganz) catheter in complex patients (eg, mixed shock states) or when the validity of measurements from other monitoring devices is in question. The catheter provides multiple cardiovascular parameters, including CVP, pulmonary artery pressure, PAOP (wedge pressure), CO, SVR, and SVo_2. However, the pulmonary artery catheter should not be used routinely for patients with shock because it is more invasive (leading to a higher risk of complications) than a central venous catheter and is not associated with improved clinical outcomes.

- Laboratory tests for monitoring of shock include serum electrolytes, BUN, serum creatinine, and complete blood count to identify possible infection (WBC count), oxygen-carrying capacity of the blood (hemoglobin, hematocrit), and ongoing bleeding (hemoglobin, hematocrit, platelet count). Hepatic transaminases may be acutely elevated when blood flow to the liver is reduced because of sustained hypotension ("shock liver"), although the concentrations should decrease over time with recovery.

- In bleeding patients, monitor coagulation function via PT/INR, platelets, and perhaps viscoelastic tests (eg, thromboelastography) with initiation of appropriate support measures as indicated.

- Observe for an increased blood lactate concentration and arterial base deficit or a decreasing bicarbonate concentration, which indicates inadequate perfusion leading to anaerobic metabolism.

- In patients responding to initial therapy, the goal is to discontinue vasopressors and inotropes as soon as the patient is hemodynamically stable. However, taper vasopressor/inotrope therapy slowly, and monitor the patient carefully to avoid worsening hemodynamics. Reevaluate fluid responsiveness frequently so the patient can be weaned from the vasopressor as soon as possible. Titrate doses downward approximately every 10 minutes to determine if the patient can tolerate gradual withdrawal and eventual discontinuation. Shock requiring vasopressor and/or inotropic support usually resolves within several days to 1 week.

See Chapter e42, Shock Syndromes, authored by Seth R. Bauer, Robert MacLaren, and Brian L. Erstad, for a more detailed discussion of this topic.

CHAPTER 13

Stroke

- *Stroke* involves the abrupt onset of focal neurologic dysfunction that lasts at least 24 hours and is caused by cerebral, spinal, or retinal infarction. Stroke can be either ischemic or hemorrhagic. Transient ischemic attacks (TIAs) are focal ischemic neurologic deficits lasting <24 hours and usually <30 minutes.

PATHOPHYSIOLOGY

ISCHEMIC STROKE

- Ischemic stroke (87% of all strokes) results from occlusion of a cerebral artery, causing reduced cerebral blood flow and neuronal ischemia. Ischemic strokes are due either to local thrombus formation or emboli from a distant site. Atherosclerosis of large intracranial or extracranial arteries or small artery disease can result in ischemic stroke. Emboli can arise from the heart in patients with atrial fibrillation, valvular heart disease, or other prothrombotic heart problems and cause about 25% of ischemic strokes. The stroke cause is undetermined in some cases.
- Decreased cerebral blood flow can lead to infarction of cerebral tissue with a surrounding area that is ischemic but may maintain membrane integrity (the ischemic penumbra). This penumbra is an area of brain tissue that is potentially salvageable with urgent pharmacologic and endovascular treatment interventions.
- Insufficient oxygen supply in ischemic tissue leads to adenosine triphosphate (ATP) depletion and anaerobic metabolism. This results in accumulation of intracellular lactate, sodium, and water, which may cause cytotoxic edema and eventual cell lysis. An influx of intracellular calcium activates lipases and proteases that degrade proteins and release free fatty acid release from cellular membranes. Release of excitatory amino acids (eg, glutamate, aspartate) in ischemic tissue perpetuates neuronal damage and produces damaging prostaglandins, leukotrienes, and reactive oxygen species. These processes occur within 2–3 hours from the onset of ischemia and ultimately lead to cellular apoptosis and necrosis.
- The most common modifiable risk factors for ischemic stroke include hypertension, cigarette smoking, diabetes, atrial fibrillation, and dyslipidemia.

HEMORRHAGIC STROKE

- Hemorrhagic strokes (13% of strokes) include subarachnoid hemorrhage (SAH) and intracerebral hemorrhage (ICH). SAH may result from trauma or rupture of an intracranial aneurysm or arteriovenous malformation (AVM). ICH occurs when bleeding in the brain parenchyma results in hematoma formation.
- Intracranial hematoma causes mechanical compression of brain parenchyma. Early hematoma expansion often occurs within 3 hours of hemorrhage onset, contributing to worsened functional outcome and increased mortality.
- Secondary mechanisms of injury are mediated by the subsequent inflammatory response, cerebral edema, and damage from blood product degradation.

CLINICAL PRESENTATION

- Patients may be unable to provide a reliable history because of cognitive or language deficits. Family members or other witnesses may need to provide this information.
- Symptoms include unilateral weakness, inability to speak, loss of vision, vertigo, or falling. Ischemic stroke is not usually painful, but some patients complain of headache. Pain and headache are more common and severe in hemorrhagic stroke.
- Neurologic deficits on physical examination depend on the brain area involved. Hemi- or monoparesis and hemisensory deficits are common. Patients with posterior circulation involvement may have vertigo and diplopia. Anterior circulation strokes

commonly result in aphasia. Patients may experience dysarthria, visual field defects, and altered levels of consciousness.

DIAGNOSIS

- Blood glucose, platelet count, and coagulation parameters (eg, prothrombin time, aPTT) are used to determine treatment eligibility.
- Tests for hypercoagulable states (protein C and S deficiency, antiphospholipid antibody) should be done only when the etiology cannot be determined based on presence of well-known risk factors.
- Computed tomography (CT) and magnetic resonance imaging (MRI) head scans can reveal areas of hemorrhage and infarction.
- Vascular imaging with computed tomography angiography (CTA) is recommended in patients with endovascular treatment indications.
- Carotid Doppler (CD), electrocardiogram (ECG), transthoracic echocardiogram (TTE), and transcranial Doppler (TCD) studies can each provide valuable diagnostic information.

TREATMENT

- <u>Goals of Treatment</u>: The goals are to (1) minimize ongoing neurologic injury acutely to reduce mortality and long-term disability; (2) prevent complications secondary to immobility and neurologic dysfunction; and (3) prevent stroke recurrence.

GENERAL APPROACH

- In patients with presumed acute stroke, perform a CT scan urgently to identify the type of injury (eg, ischemic or hemorrhagic) if respiratory and cardiac indices are stable.
- Evaluate ischemic stroke patients presenting within hours of symptom onset for pharmacologic and mechanical reperfusion therapy.
- Patients with TIA require urgent assessment and intervention to reduce the risk of stroke, which is highest in the first few days after TIA.
- In patients with an ischemic stroke and blood pressure (BP) <220/120 mm Hg without comorbid conditions requiring acute antihypertensive treatment, acute BP lowering in the first 48–72 hours does not improve survival. *Permissive hypertension* (BP up to 220/120 mm Hg) is often allowed. In patients with intracranial hemorrhage and elevated systolic blood pressure (SBP) (150–220 mm Hg), acute SBP lowering to <140 mm Hg is safe and may improve functional outcomes.
- Assess patients with hemorrhagic stroke to determine whether they are candidates for surgical intervention.
- After the acute phase (the first week after the event), focus on preventing worsening of stroke, minimizing complications, and instituting secondary prevention strategies.

NONPHARMACOLOGIC THERAPY

Ischemic Stroke

- Endovascular intervention and thrombectomy to reperfuse ischemic brain tissue is recommended by the American Heart Association (AHA) and American Stroke Association (ASA). Thrombectomy is strongly recommended for patients with anterior circulation occlusion in the internal carotid artery (ICA) or the M1 segment of the middle cerebral artery (MCA) who are within 6 hours of symptom onset and may be considered in select patients within 6–24 hours of symptom onset. The benefit of mechanical thrombectomy is less clear in posterior circulation occlusions and should be considered on a case-by-case basis.
- Decompressive hemicraniectomy is a surgical procedure to reduce intracranial pressure (typically due to cerebral edema) and can reduce mortality and improve functional outcome in select patients.

- For all ischemic stroke patients, coordinated care with a multidisciplinary approach to assessment and early rehabilitation reduces overall disability due to stroke.
- In secondary prevention, carotid endarterectomy of an ulcerated or stenotic carotid artery is effective in reducing stroke incidence and recurrence in appropriate patients if performed in centers where operative morbidity and mortality are low. Carotid stenting is a less invasive alternative and can reduce recurrent stroke risk when combined with aspirin and clopidogrel therapy.
- Other secondary stroke prevention approaches include diet modification, exercise, smoking cessation, avoidance of environmental tobacco smoke, moderation of alcohol consumption, and avoidance of stimulants such as amphetamines and cocaine.

Hemorrhagic Stroke

- In SAH from ruptured intracranial aneurysm or AVM, early intervention with either surgical clipping or endovascular coiling of the vascular abnormality reduces mortality from rebleeding.
- Early surgical intervention and hematoma removal is recommended for patients with cerebellar hemorrhage and neurologic deterioration, brainstem compression, or hydrocephalus from ventricular obstruction. The usefulness of surgical hematoma evacuation is not well-established for patients with cerebral hemorrhage.
- Ventricular drainage with an extraventricular drain (EVD) is reasonable in patients with hydrocephalus causing decreased consciousness.

Temperature Management

- Fever worsens outcomes in patients with both hemorrhagic and ischemic stroke. Identification of the source and pharmacologic and/or nonpharmacologic management is recommended to maintain normothermia range. Because of limited supporting data, induced hypothermia should be done only in the setting of controlled clinical trials.

PHARMACOLOGIC THERAPY OF ISCHEMIC STROKE

- Table 13-1 provides evidence-based recommendations for pharmacotherapy of ischemic stroke.
- **Alteplase** initiated within 4.5 hours of symptom onset improves functional ability after ischemic stroke. Adherence to a guideline-recommended protocol is essential to achieve positive outcomes: (1) activate the stroke team; (2) obtain CT scan to rule out hemorrhage; (3) treat as early as possible within 4.5 hours of symptom onset; (4) meet all inclusion criteria with no contraindications (Table 13-2); (5) administer alteplase 0.9 mg/kg IV total dose (maximum 90 mg), with 10% infused as an initial bolus over 1 minute and the remainder given over 1 hour; (6) avoid anticoagulant and antiplatelet therapy for 24 hours after alteplase; and (7) monitor the patient closely for elevated blood pressure (BP), neurologic status, and hemorrhage.
- **Aspirin** 160–325 mg/day started within 24–48 hours of symptom onset (and 24 hours after alteplase completion) reduces long-term death and disability. An alternate antiplatelet agent may be considered for patients with aspirin allergy or other contraindications.
- For patients with elevated BP who are eligible for alteplase, treatment to a goal BP <185/110 mm Hg is recommended before thrombolytic administration. While data are limited, it is also reasonable to maintain BP <185/110 mm Hg for patients undergoing mechanical thrombectomy. For patients not requiring IV thrombolysis or endovascular intervention, *permissive hypertension*, allowing BP to rise as high as 220/120 mm Hg for the first 48–72 hours is often used because early BP reduction does not prevent death or dependency. For patients with comorbid conditions requiring BP lowering, a reduction of 15% is reasonable. If BP is treated, short-acting and easily titrated IV agents are preferred:
  ✓ **Labetalol:** 10–20 mg IV over 1–2 minutes; may repeat
  ✓ **Nicardipine:** 5 mg/h IV; titrate up by 2.5 mg/h every 5–15 minutes; maximum 15 mg/h

TABLE 13-1	Recommendations for Pharmacotherapy of Ischemic Stroke	
	Recommendation	**Evidence[a]**
Acute treatment	Alteplase 0.9 mg/kg IV (maximum 90 mg), 10% as a bolus with remainder given over 1 hour in select patients within 3 hours of onset	IA
	Alteplase in dose above given between 3 and 4.5 hours of onset	IB-R
	Tenecteplase 0.25 mg/kg IV bolus (maximum 25 mg) may be a reasonable alternative for patients eligible to undergo mechanical thrombectomy	IIbB-R
	Aspirin 160–325 mg daily started within 48 hours of onset	IA
Secondary prevention		
Noncardioembolic	Antiplatelet therapy	
	Aspirin 50–325 mg daily	IA
	Aspirin 25 mg + extended-release dipyridamole 200 mg twice daily	IA
	Clopidogrel 75 mg daily	IA
Cardioembolic (especially atrial fibrillation)	Anticoagulant therapy	
	Vitamin K antagonist (warfarin; target INR = 2–3)	IA
	Apixaban 5 mg twice daily	IA
	Dabigatran 150 mg twice daily	IA
	Edoxaban 60 mg daily	IA
	Rivaroxaban 20 mg daily	IA
LDL cholesterol >100 mg/dL (2.59 mmol/L) with no known CHD and no major cardiac sources of embolism	Atorvastatin 80 mg daily	IA
Patients with atherosclerotic disease	Statins and ezetimibe, if needed; goal LDL cholesterol <70 mg/dL (1.81 mmol/L)	IA
BP >130/80 mm Hg	BP reduction; goal <130/80 mm Hg	IB-R

[a]Classes: I, evidence or general agreement about usefulness and effectiveness; II, conflicting evidence about usefulness; IIa, weight of evidence in favor of the treatment; IIb, usefulness less well-established; III, not useful and maybe harmful. Levels of evidence: A, multiple randomized clinical trials; B, a single randomized trial or nonrandomized studies; C, expert opinion or case studies; B-R, moderate-quality evidence from one or more randomized controlled trials or meta-analyses of moderate-quality randomized controlled trials.
CHD, coronary heart disease;
INR, international normalized ratio; IV, intravenous.

✓ **Clevidipine:** 1–2 mg/h IV; titrate by doubling the dose every 2–5 minutes; maximum 21 mg/h

✓ Other potential agents: **hydralazine**, **enalaprilat**, **nitroprusside** IV infusion, labetalol IV infusion

TABLE 13-2 Inclusion Criteria and Contraindications to Alteplase Use in Acute Ischemic Stroke

Inclusion criteria
- Age 18 years or older
- Clinical diagnosis of ischemic stroke with neurologic deficit
- Time of symptom onset well-established to be <4.5 hours before treatment would begin

Contraindications
- History of intracerebral hemorrhage
- History of ischemic stroke within prior 3 months
- Symptoms/imaging consistent with SAH or acute intracerebral hemorrhage
- Current use of direct thrombin inhibitors or direct factor Xa inhibitors in prior 48 hours
- Use of treatment-dose low-molecular-weight heparin in prior 24 hours
- Infective endocarditis
- Intra-axial, intracranial neoplasm
- Aortic arch dissection
- Active internal bleeding or coagulopathy (platelets <100,000/mm³ [100 × 10⁹/L], INR>1.7, aPTT >40 sec, PT >15 sec)
- Severe head trauma in prior 3 months
- Gastrointestinal malignancy or bleeding within prior 21 days

Warnings/Use Clinical Judgment
- Unruptured/unsecured AVM or aneurysm >10 mm
- Major surgery or nonhead trauma
- History of bleeding diathesis
- Extensive regions of clear hypoattenuation on initial CT scan

aPTT, activated partial thromboplastin time; AVM, arteriovenous malformation; CT, computed tomography; INR, international normalized ratio; PT, prothrombin time; SAH, subarachnoid hemorrhage.

- Therapeutic anticoagulation (eg, unfractionated heparin or low-molecular-weight heparin) is not routinely recommended in the early phase of acute ischemic stroke treatment. Anticoagulation for nonstroke indications (eg, prophylaxis of venous thromboembolism) should be weighed against the risk of intracranial hemorrhagic conversion.

- Secondary prevention of ischemic stroke:

  ✓ All patients who have had an acute ischemic stroke or TIA should receive long-term antithrombotic therapy for secondary prevention. Antiplatelet therapy should be used in noncardioembolic stroke. Aspirin, extended-release dipyridamole plus aspirin, clopidogrel, and ticagrelor are all recommended. In patients with atrial fibrillation, oral anticoagulation with apixaban, dabigatran, edoxaban, rivaroxaban, or warfarin is recommended (Table 13-1).

  ✓ Adults with previously treated hypertension who experience a stroke or TIA should be restarted on antihypertensive treatment after the first few days of the index event to reduce the risk of recurrent stroke and other vascular events. Treatment with a **thiazide diuretic**, **angiotensin-converting enzyme (ACE) inhibitor**, or **angiotensin II receptor blocker** is useful. Adults not previously treated for hypertension who experience a stroke or TIA and have an average BP ≥130/80 mm Hg should be prescribed antihypertensive treatment several days after the index event. For adults who experienced a stroke or TIA, a BP goal of <130/80 mm Hg is recommended.

  ✓ Patients without known heart disease but who have LDL cholesterol >100 mg/dL (2.59 mmol/L) should be given **atorvastatin** 80 mg daily to reduce the risk of stroke recurrence. Patients who have atherosclerotic cardiovascular disease (ASCVD) should be given a high-intensity statin (and **ezetimibe** if necessary) to reach a goal of LDL cholesterol <70 mg/dL (1.81 mmol/L). A **proprotein convertase subtilisin/kexin type 9 (PCSK9) inhibitor** may be considered in very high-risk patients who are taking maximally tolerated statins and ezetimibe with LDL cholesterol ≥70 mg/dL (1.81 mmol/L).

✓ **Icosapent ethyl** is recommended for patients with hypertriglyceridemia provided they have A1C <10% (86 mmol/mol) and no history of pancreatitis, atrial fibrillation, or severe heart failure.

PHARMACOLOGIC THERAPY OF HEMORRHAGIC STROKE

- The usefulness of pharmacotherapy is limited in spontaneous ICH.
- Because hypertension in hemorrhagic stroke increases the risk of hematoma expansion, it is reasonable for patients with a SBP >220 mm Hg to receive aggressive BP lowering with continuous IV infusion medications. Acute lowering of SBP to a goal of 140 mm Hg is safe and may improve functional outcomes. For patients with SAH due to aneurysm rupture, BP control to at least a SBP <160 mm Hg is reasonable in the period from symptom onset to aneurysm obliteration.
- When intracranial hemorrhage occurs in a patient on anticoagulants, use of reversal agents to correct the medication-induced coagulopathy should be considered (Table 13-3).

TABLE 13-3	Select Anticoagulant Reversal	
Drug	**First-Line Reversal Recommendation**	**Alternate Treatment**
Warfarin	Vitamin K 10 mg IV × 1 -and- 4PCC INR 2 to <4: 25 units/kg, max 2500 units INR 4–6: 35 units/kg, max 3500 units INR >6: 50 units/kg, max 5000 units	Vitamin K 10 mg IV × 1 -and- FFP 10–15 mL/kg
Dabigatran	Idarucizumab 5 g IV × 1	Hemodialysis 4PCC 50 units/kg
Rivaroxaban ≤10 mg	Andexanet alfa 400 mg IV bolus at rate of 30 mg/min, followed by 4 mg/min IV infusion up to 120 min	4PCC 50 units/kg
Rivaroxaban >10 mg or unknown dose	If <8 hours since last dose or unknown time, andexanet alfa 800 mg IV bolus at rate of 30 mg/min, followed by 8 mg/min IV infusion up to 120 min If ≥8 hours since last dose, andexanet alfa 400 mg IV bolus at rate of 30 mg/min, followed by 4 mg/min IV infusion up to 120 min	4PCC 50 units/kg
Apixaban ≤5 mg	Andexanet alfa 400 mg IV bolus at rate of 30 mg/min, followed by 4 mg/min IV infusion up to 120 min	4PCC 50 units/kg
Apixaban >5 mg or unknown dose	If <8 hours since last dose or unknown time, andexanet alfa 800 mg IV bolus at rate of 30 mg/min, followed by 8 mg/min IV infusion up to 120 min If ≥8 hours since last dose, andexanet alfa 400 mg IV bolus at rate of 30 mg/min, followed by 4 mg/min IV infusion up to 120 min	4PCC 50 units/kg
Edoxaban	Andexanet alfa not studied	4PCC 50 units/kg

FFP, fresh frozen plasma; IV, intravenous; 4PCC, 4-factor prothrombin complex concentrate; INR, international normalized ratio.

EVALUATION OF THERAPEUTIC OUTCOMES

- Monitor patients with acute stroke intensely for development of neurologic worsening (recurrence or extension of stroke), complications (venous thromboembolism, infection), and adverse treatment effects.
- The most common reasons for clinical deterioration in stroke patients include: (1) extension of the original lesion in the brain; (2) development of cerebral edema and elevated intracranial pressure; (3) hypertensive emergency; (4) infection (eg, urinary and respiratory tract); (5) venous thromboembolism; (6) electrolyte abnormalities and rhythm disturbances; and (7) recurrent stroke.
- For patients receiving alteplase therapy, monitor for bleeding with neurologic examination and BP every 15 minutes for 1 hour, then every half-hour for 6 hours, then every hour for 17 hours, then once every shift thereafter.
- For aspirin, clopidogrel, extended-release dipyridamole plus aspirin, warfarin, and other oral anticoagulants, monitor for bleeding daily.
- For patients receiving warfarin, check the PT/INR and hemoglobin/hematocrit daily.

See Chapter 39, Stroke, authored by Melody Ryan and Melisa Nestor, for a more detailed discussion of this topic.

Venous Thromboembolism

- *Venous thromboembolism* (VTE) results from clot formation in the venous circulation and is manifested as deep vein thrombosis (DVT) and pulmonary embolism (PE).

PATHOPHYSIOLOGY

- Risk factors for VTE include increasing age, history of VTE, and aspects related to Virchow's triad: (1) blood stasis (eg, immobility and obesity); (2) vascular injury (eg, surgery, trauma, venous catheters); and (3) hypercoagulability (eg, malignancy, coagulation factor abnormalities, antiphospholipid antibodies, certain drugs).
- The most common inherited hypercoagulability disorder is activated protein C (aPC) resistance (Caucasian prevalence 2%–7%), which increases the risk of VTE three-fold. Most aPC resistance results from a factor V gene mutation (known as factor V Leiden) that renders it resistant to degradation by aPC.
- The prothrombin G20210A mutation is the second most frequent inherited hypercoagulability disorder (Caucasian prevalence 2%–4%) and imparts a threefold increased risk of VTE. The mutation increases circulating prothrombin, enhancing thrombin generation.
- Inherited deficiencies of protein C, protein S, and antithrombin occur in <1% of the population and may increase the lifetime VTE risk by as much as sevenfold.
- Normal hemostasis maintains circulatory system integrity after blood vessel damage. Disruption of the endothelial cell lining with injury results in platelet activation and tissue-factor–mediated clotting factor cascade initiation, culminating in thrombin formation and ultimately a fibrin clot. In contrast to physiologic hemostasis, pathologic VTE often occurs without gross vessel wall damage and may be triggered by tissue factor (TF) brought to the growing thrombus by circulating microparticles. Clots causing VTE impair blood flow and often cause complete vessel occlusion.
- Exposure of blood to damaged vessel endothelium causes platelets to become activated after binding to adhesion proteins (eg, von Willebrand factor, collagen). Activated platelets recruit additional platelets, causing growth of the platelet thrombus. Activated platelets change shape and release components that sustain further thrombus formation at the site. Activated platelets express the adhesion molecule P-selectin, which facilitates capture of TF-bearing microparticles, resulting in fibrin clot formation via the coagulation cascade.
- The conceptual coagulation cascade model involves reactions that occur on cell surfaces in three overlapping phases (**Fig. 14-1**):
  ✓ *Initiation*: A TF/VIIa complex (known as extrinsic tenase or X-ase) on cells bearing TF that have been exposed after vessel injury or captured via P-selectin activates limited amounts of factors IX and X. Factor Xa then associates with factor Va to form the prothrombinase complex, which cleaves prothrombin (factor II) to generate a small amount of thrombin (factor IIa), which activates factors V, VIII, and XI on platelet surfaces. Factor IXa moves to the surface of activated platelets in the growing platelet thrombus. Tissue factor pathway inhibitor (TFPI) regulates TF/VIIa-induced coagulation, rapidly terminating the initiation phase.
  ✓ *Amplification:* Thrombin produced during the initiation phase activates factors V and VIII, which bind to platelet surfaces and support the large-scale thrombin generation occurring during the propagation phase. Platelet-bound factor XI is also activated by thrombin during amplification.
  ✓ *Propagation:* A burst of thrombin generation occurs as factor VIIIa/IXa complex (known as intrinsic tenase) promotes factor Xa formation and prothrombinase complexes assemble on the surface of activated platelets, accelerating thrombin generation. Thrombin generation is further supported by factor XIa bound to platelet surfaces, which activates factor IX to form additional intrinsic tenase.

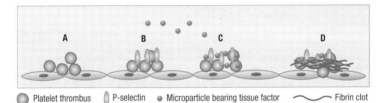

Platelet thrombus   P-selectin   Microparticle bearing tissue factor   Fibrin clot

FIGURE 14-1. Model of pathologic thrombus formation: (A) activated platelets adhere to vascular endothelium; (B) activated platelets express P-selectin; (C) pathologic microparticles express active tissue factor and are present at a high concentration in the circulation—these microparticles accumulate, perhaps by binding to activated platelets expressing P-selectin; and (D) tissue factor can lead to thrombin generation, and thrombin generation leads to platelet thrombus formation and fibrin generation.

- Thrombin then converts fibrinogen to fibrin monomers that precipitate and polymerize to form fibrin strands. Factor XIIIa (also activated by thrombin) covalently bonds these strands to form an extensive meshwork that encases the aggregating platelet thrombus and red cells to form a stabilized fibrin clot.
- Hemostasis is controlled by antithrombotic substances produced by intact endothelium adjacent to damaged tissue. Thrombomodulin modulates thrombin activity by converting protein C to its activated form (aPC), which joins with protein S to inactivate factors Va and VIIIa. This prevents coagulation reactions from spreading to uninjured vessel walls. In addition, circulating antithrombin inhibits thrombin and factor Xa. Heparan sulfate is secreted by endothelial cells and accelerates antithrombin activity. These self-regulatory mechanisms limit fibrin clot formation to the zone of vessel injury.
- The fibrinolytic system dissolves formed blood clots; inactive plasminogen is converted to plasmin by tissue plasminogen activator (tPA). Plasmin is an enzyme that degrades the fibrin mesh into soluble end products (known as fibrin degradation products including D-dimer).
- Most venous thrombi begin in the leg(s). Isolated calf vein thrombi seldom embolize; those involving the popliteal and larger veins above the knee are more likely to embolize and lodge in the pulmonary artery or one of its branches, occluding blood flow to the lung and impairing gas exchange. Without treatment, the affected lung area becomes necrotic and oxygen delivery to other vital organs may decrease, potentially resulting in fatal circulatory collapse.

CLINICAL PRESENTATION

- Some patients with DVT are asymptomatic. Symptoms may include unilateral leg swelling, pain, tenderness, erythema, and warmth. Physical signs may include a palpable cord and a positive Homan sign.
- Symptoms of PE may include cough, chest pain or tightness, shortness of breath, palpitations, hemoptysis, dizziness, or lightheadedness. Signs of PE include tachypnea, tachycardia, diaphoresis, cyanosis, hypotension, shock, and cardiovascular collapse.
- Postthrombotic syndrome may produce chronic lower extremity swelling, pain, tenderness, skin discoloration, and ulceration.

DIAGNOSIS

- Assessment should focus on identifying risk factors (see section Pathophysiology).
- Compression ultrasound (CUS) and computed tomography pulmonary angiography (CTPA) are used most often for initial evaluation of suspected VTE.

- Radiographic contrast studies (venography, pulmonary angiography) are the most accurate and reliable diagnostic methods but are expensive, invasive, and difficult to perform and evaluate. The ventilation-perfusion (V/Q) scan is an alternative PE diagnostic test.
- Serum concentration of D-dimer is nearly always elevated; values <500 ng/mL (mcg/L) combined with clinical probability scores are useful in ruling out VTE.
- Clinical assessment checklists (eg, Wells score) can be used to determine whether a patient is likely or unlikely to have DVT or PE.

TREATMENT

- Goals of Treatment: The initial goal is to prevent VTE in at-risk populations. Treatment of VTE is aimed at preventing thrombus extension and embolization, reducing recurrence risk, and preventing long-term complications (eg, postthrombotic syndrome, chronic thromboembolic pulmonary hypertension).

PREVENTION OF VTE

- Nonpharmacologic methods improve venous blood flow by mechanical means and include early ambulation, graduated compression stockings, intermittent pneumatic compression (IPC) devices, and inferior vena cava filters.
- Hospitalized and acutely ill medical patients at high VTE risk and low bleeding risk should receive pharmacologic prophylaxis with **low-dose unfractionated heparin** (**LDUH**), **low-molecular-weight heparin** (**LMWH**), **fondaparinux**, or **rivaroxaban** during hospitalization or until fully ambulatory. Routine pharmacologic prophylaxis is not warranted in low-risk medical patients.
- Most patients undergoing general, gynecologic, cardiac, and vascular surgery should receive pharmacologic prophylaxis with LMWH or lowdose UFH to prevent VTE. Patients unable to receive pharmacologic prophylaxis should use IPCs or compression stockings.
- Recommended VTE prophylaxis following joint replacement surgery may include **aspirin**, adjusted-dose **warfarin**, **LDUH**, **LMWH**, **fondaparinux**, **dabigatran**, **apixaban**, or **rivaroxaban** for at least 10 days postsurgery.
- VTE prophylaxis after surgery should be given throughout the period of increased VTE risk. Guidelines support extended VTE prophylaxis for up to 42 days after major surgery. Most clinical trials support use of prophylaxis for 15–42 days after total knee or hip replacement surgery.

GENERAL APPROACH TO TREATMENT OF VTE

- Anticoagulation is the primary treatment for VTE; DVT and PE are treated similarly (Fig. 14-2).
- After VTE is confirmed objectively, therapy with a rapid-acting anticoagulant should be instituted as soon as possible. Anticoagulants can be administered in the outpatient setting in most patients with DVT and in carefully selected hemodynamically stable patients with PE.
- Stable patients with DVT or PE who have normal vital signs, low bleeding risk, and no other uncontrolled comorbid conditions requiring hospitalization can be discharged early or treated entirely on an outpatient basis (if considered appropriate candidates). Hemodynamically unstable patients with PE should be admitted for initiation of anticoagulation therapy.
- Three months is the appropriate initial duration of anticoagulation therapy for the acute first episode of VTE for all patients. This duration is also recommended when the initial thrombotic event was associated with a major transient or reversible risk factor (eg, surgery, hospitalization).
- Continuing anticoagulation is required to prevent new VTE episodes not directly related to the preceding episode. Consider extended therapy beyond 3 months for patients with a first unprovoked (idiopathic) VTE when feasible because of a

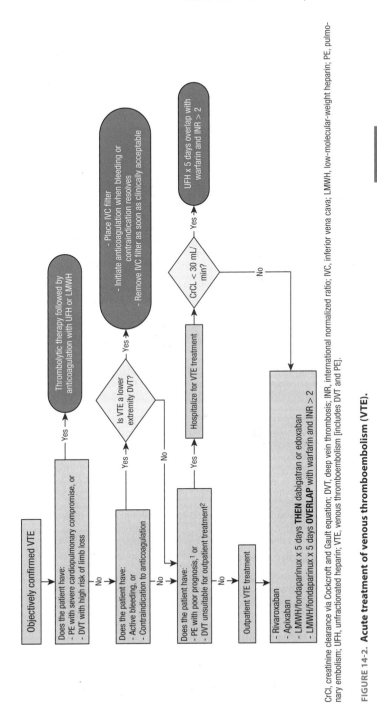

FIGURE 14-2. Acute treatment of venous thromboembolism (VTE).

CrCl, creatinine clearance via Cockcroft and Gault equation; DVT, deep vein thrombosis; INR, international normalized ratio; IVC, inferior vena cava; LMWH, low-molecular-weight heparin; PE, pulmonary embolism; UFH, unfractionated heparin; VTE, venous thromboembolism [includes DVT and PE].

relatively high recurrence rate. In patients with VTE and active cancer, extended therapy is rarely stopped because of a high recurrence risk.

NONPHARMACOLOGIC THERAPY

- Encourage patients to ambulate as much as symptoms permit.
- Ambulation in conjunction with graduated compression stockings results in a faster reduction in pain and swelling than strict bedrest with no increase in embolization rate.
- Inferior vena cava filters should only be used when anticoagulants are contraindicated due to active bleeding.
- Elimination of the obstructing thrombus via thrombolysis or thrombectomy may be warranted in life- or limb-threatening DVT.

PHARMACOLOGIC THERAPY

Direct Oral Anticoagulants (DOACs)

- **Rivaroxaban**, **apixaban**, and **edoxaban** are oral selective inhibitors of both free and clot-bound factor Xa and do not require antithrombin to exert their anticoagulant effect. **Dabigatran** is an oral selective, reversible, direct factor IIa (thrombin) inhibitor.
- See Table 14-1 for DOAC indications and dosing. Use DOACs with caution in patients with renal dysfunction.
- Single-drug oral therapy with rivaroxaban or apixaban produces similar rates of recurrent VTE compared to traditional therapy with warfarin overlapped with enoxaparin and perhaps less major bleeding. Both drugs are initiated with a higher dose and subsequently reduced to a maintenance dose. Neither drug requires routine anticoagulation monitoring, but the high acquisition cost may be a barrier for some patients.
- Edoxaban and dabigatran must be given only after at least 5 days of subcutaneous (SC) anticoagulation with UFH, LMWH, or fondaparinux. These regimens were noninferior to warfarin in patients with acute VTE for the outcome of recurrent VTE. Compared to warfarin, dabigatran caused similar major bleeding and edoxaban caused significantly less bleeding.
- Bleeding is the most common adverse effect with DOAC therapy. Patients experiencing significant bleeding should receive routine supportive care and discontinuation of anticoagulant therapy. **Idarucizumab** (Praxbind) 5 g IV rapidly reverses the dabigatran anticoagulant effect when needed during emergency situations (eg, life-threatening bleeding) and when there is need for urgent surgical intervention. **Recombinant coagulation factor Xa** (also known as **andexanet alfa**; Andexxa) can reverse life-threatening bleeding in patients taking rivaroxaban or apixaban. Adding aspirin to DOAC therapy nearly doubles bleeding rates and should be avoided in most patients with VTE. All DOACs are P-gp substrates and subject to changes in anticoagulant effect when coadministered with P-gp inhibitors or inducers. Rivaroxaban and apixaban are subject to interactions involving inhibitors or inducers of CYP 3A4.

Low-Molecular-Weight Heparin

- LMWH fragments produced by either chemical or enzymatic depolymerization of UFH are heterogeneous mixtures of sulfated glycosaminoglycans with approximately one-third of the mean UFH molecular weight. LMWH prevents thrombus propagation by accelerating the activity of antithrombin similar to UFH.
- LMWH given SC in fixed, weight-based doses is at least as effective as UFH given IV for VTE treatment. LMWH has largely replaced UFH for initial VTE treatment due to improved pharmacokinetic and pharmacodynamic profiles and ease of use. Advantages of LMWH over UFH include: (1) predictable anticoagulation dose response; (2) improved SC bioavailability; (3) dose-independent clearance; (4) longer biologic half-life; (5) lower incidence of thrombocytopenia; and (6) less need for routine laboratory monitoring.

TABLE 14-1 Approved Indications and Dosing for the Direct Oral Anticoagulants

Generic (Brand) Name	VTE Prophylaxis	Acute VTE Treatment	Reduction in Risk of Recurrent VTE in Patients at Continued Risk
Dabigatran (Pradaxa)	Hip replacement surgery: CrCl >30 mL/min: 110 mg the first day beginning 1–4 hours after surgery once hemostasis is achieved, then 220 mg once daily for 28–35 days CrCl ≤30 mL/min or on dialysis: Dosing recommendations cannot be provided	150 mg PO twice daily with or without food FOLLOWING at least 5 days of parenteral anticoagulant therapy	150 mg PO twice daily with or without food
Rivaroxaban (Xarelto)	Hip or knee replacement surgery: 10 mg PO once daily with or without food beginning 6–10 hours after surgery once hemostasis is achieved and continuing for 12 (knee) to 35 (hip) days	15 mg PO twice daily with food for days 1–21, then 20 mg PO once daily with food beginning on day 22	10 mg PO once daily with or without food
Apixaban (Eliquis)	Hip or knee replacement surgery: 2.5 mg PO twice daily with or without food beginning 12–24 hours after surgery and continuing for 12 (knee) or 35 (hip) days	10 mg PO twice daily with or without food on days 1–7, then 5 mg PO twice daily beginning on day 8	2.5 mg PO twice daily with or without food
Edoxaban (Savaysa)	Not approved for use	60 mg PO once daily with or without food FOLLOWING at least 5 days of parenteral anticoagulant therapy; 30 mg once daily with CrCl 15–50 mL/min (0.25–0.83 mL/sec) or body weight ≤60 kg or who use certain P-gp inhibitors	Not approved for use
Betrixaban (Bevyxxa)	Adults hospitalized for acute medical illness: Initial single dose of 160 mg PO with food, followed by 80 mg once daily with food for 35–42 days	Not approved for use	Not approved for use

PO, by mouth; CrCl, creatinine clearance; P-gp, P-glycoprotein; VTE, venous thromboembolism.

- Recommended doses (based on actual body weight) include:
  - ✓ **Enoxaparin** (Lovenox): For acute DVT treatment with or without PE, 1 mg/kg SC every 12 hours or 1.5 mg/kg every 24 hours;
  - ✓ **Dalteparin** (Fragmin): For acute DVT treatment, 200 units/kg SC once daily or 100 units/kg SC twice daily (not FDA approved in the United States for this indication). For VTE in patients with cancer, 200 units/kg SC every 24 hours for 30 days, followed by 150 units SC every 24 hours. The maximum total daily dose is 18,000 units.

- In patients without cancer, acute LMWH treatment is generally transitioned to long-term warfarin therapy after 5–10 days.
- Routine laboratory monitoring is unnecessary because LMWH anticoagulant response is predictable when given SC. Prior to initiating therapy, obtain a baseline complete blood cell count (CBC) with platelet count and serum creatinine. Check the CBC every 5–10 days during the first 2 weeks of LMWH therapy and every 2–4 weeks thereafter to monitor for occult bleeding. Measuring anti–factor Xa activity is the most widely used method to monitor LMWH; routine measurement is unnecessary in stable, uncomplicated patients. Monitoring may be considered in patients who have significant renal impairment, are morbidly obese, or are pregnant.
- As with other anticoagulants, bleeding is the most common adverse effect of LMWH therapy, but major bleeding may be less common than with UFH. If major bleeding occurs, IV **protamine sulfate** can be administered, but it cannot neutralize the anticoagulant effect completely. The recommended protamine sulfate dose is 1 mg per 1 mg of enoxaparin or 1 mg per 100 anti–factor Xa units of dalteparin administered in the previous 8 hours. A second dose of 0.5 mg per 1 mg or 100 anti–factor Xa units can be given if bleeding continues. Smaller protamine doses can be used if the LMWH dose was given in the previous 8–12 hours. Protamine sulfate is not recommended if the LMWH was given more than 12 hours earlier.
- Thrombocytopenia can occur with LMWHs, but the incidence of heparin-induced thrombocytopenia (HIT) is one-third that of UFH. The risk of osteoporosis appears to be lower with LMWH than with UFH.

Fondaparinux

- **Fondaparinux** (Arixtra) prevents thrombus generation and clot formation by indirectly inhibiting factor Xa activity through its interaction with antithrombin. Unlike UFH or LMWH, fondaparinux inhibits only factor Xa activity.
- Fondaparinux is a safe and effective alternative to LMWH for acute VTE treatment and is likewise followed by long-term warfarin therapy.
- Fondaparinux is dosed once daily via weight-based SC injection: 5 mg if <50 kg, 7.5 mg if 50–100 kg, and 10 mg if >100 kg.
- Patients receiving fondaparinux do not require routine coagulation testing. Determine baseline kidney function before starting therapy because fondaparinux is contraindicated if CrCl is <30 mL/min (0.5 mL/sec).
- Bleeding is the primary adverse effect associated with fondaparinux therapy. Measure CBC at baseline and periodically thereafter to detect occult bleeding. Monitor for signs and symptoms of bleeding daily. There is no specific antidote to reverse the antithrombotic activity of fondaparinux.

Unfractionated Heparin

- **Unfractionated heparin** binds to antithrombin, provoking a conformation change that makes it much more potent in inhibiting the activity of factors IXa, Xa, XIIa, and IIa. This prevents thrombus growth and propagation allowing endogenous thrombolytic systems to lyse the clot. Because some patients fail to achieve an adequate response, IV UFH has largely been replaced by LMWH, fondaparinux, and DOACs. UFH continues to have a role in patients with CrCl <30 mL/min (0.5 mL/sec) and unstable patients.

TABLE 14-2	Weight-Based[a] Dosing for Unfractionated Heparin Administered by Continuous IV Infusion	
Indication	**Initial Loading Dose**	**Initial Infusion Rate**
Deep venous thrombosis/ pulmonary embolism	80–100 units/kg	17–20 units/kg/h
	Maximum = 10,000 units	Maximum = 2300 units/h
Activated Partial Thromboplastin Time (seconds)	**Maintenance Infusion Rate**	
	Dose Adjustment	
<37 (or anti–factor Xa <0.20 unit/ mL [kU/L])	80 units/kg bolus, and then increase infusion by 4 units/kg/h	
37–47 (or anti–factor Xa 0.20–0.29 unit/mL [kU/L])	40 units/kg bolus, and then increase infusion by 2 units/kg/h	
48–71 (or anti–factor Xa 0.30–0.70 unit/mL [kU/L])	No change	
72–93 (or anti–factor Xa 0.71–1 unit/mL [kU/L])	Decrease infusion by 1–2 units/kg/h	
>93 (or anti–factor Xa >1 unit/ mL [kU/L])	Hold infusion for 1 hour, and then decrease by 3 units/kg/h	

[a]Use actual body weight for all calculations. Adjusted body weight may be used for obese patients (>130% of ideal body weight).

- When immediate and full anticoagulation is required, a weight-based IV loading dose followed by a continuous IV infusion is preferred (Table 14-2). Subcutaneous UFH (initial dose 333 units/kg followed by 250 units/kg every 12 hours) also provides adequate anticoagulation for treatment of acute VTE.
- The activated partial thromboplastin time (aPTT) is generally recommended for monitoring UFH, provided that institution-specific therapeutic ranges are defined. Measure aPTT prior to initiation of therapy and 6 hours after the start of therapy or a dose change. Adjust the UFH dose based on patient response and the institution-specific aPTT therapeutic range.
- Monitor patients closely for bleeding signs and symptoms during UFH therapy. If major bleeding occurs, discontinue UFH immediately, identify and treat the underlying bleeding source, and give **protamine sulfate** by slow IV infusion over 10 minutes (1 mg/100 units of UFH infused during the previous 4 hours; maximum 50 mg).
- HIT is a rare immunologic reaction requiring immediate intervention and that may be fatal. The most common complication of HIT is VTE; arterial thrombosis occurs less frequently. Thrombocytopenia is the most common clinical manifestation, but serologic confirmation of heparin antibodies is required to diagnose HIT. The use of a clinical prediction rule, such as the 4Ts score (Thrombocytopenia, Timing of platelet count fall or thrombosis, Thrombosis, oTher explanations for thrombocytopenia), can improve the predictive value of platelet count monitoring and heparin antibody testing. Discontinue all heparin if new thrombosis occurs in the setting of falling platelets in conjunction with a moderate or high 4Ts score. Alternative anticoagulation with a direct thrombin inhibitor should then be initiated.
- Using UFH doses of 20,000 units/day or more for longer than 6 months, especially during pregnancy, is associated with significant bone loss and may lead to osteoporosis.

Warfarin

- **Warfarin** inhibits enzymes responsible for cyclic interconversion of vitamin K in the liver. Reduced vitamin K is a cofactor required for carboxylation of the vitamin K–dependent coagulation factors II (prothrombin), VII, IX, and X and the endogenous anticoagulant proteins C and S. By inhibiting the reduced vitamin K supply needed for production of these proteins, warfarin therapy produces coagulation proteins with less activity. By suppressing clotting factor production, warfarin prevents initial thrombus formation and propagation. The time required to achieve its anticoagulant effect depends on the elimination of half-lives of the coagulation proteins (6 hours for factor VII and 72 hours for prothrombin). Full antithrombotic effect is not achieved for at least 6 days after warfarin therapy initiation.

- Because of its slow onset of effect, warfarin must be started concurrently with rapid-acting injectable anticoagulant therapy with an overlap of at least 5 days and until an international normalized ratio (INR) of 2 or greater has been achieved for at least 24 hours.
- Guidelines for initiating warfarin therapy are given in Fig. 14-3. The initial dose should be 5–10 mg for most patients. Lower starting doses may be acceptable in

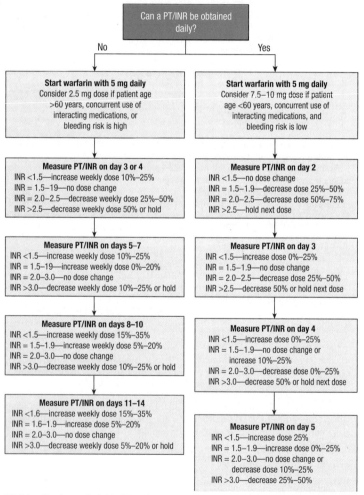

INR, international normalized ratio; PT, prothrombin time.

FIGURE 14-3. **Initiation of warfarin therapy.**

patients with advanced age, malnutrition, liver disease, or heart failure. Starting doses more than 10 mg should be avoided.

- Monitor warfarin therapy by the INR; the recommended target INR for VTE treatment is 2.5, with an acceptable range of 2–3. After an acute thromboembolic event, obtain a baseline INR and CBC prior to initiating warfarin and every 1–3 days until stabilized. Once the patient's dose response is established, obtain an INR every 7–14 days until it stabilizes, then ideally every 4–12 weeks thereafter.
- In general, maintenance dose changes should not be made more frequently than every 3 days. Adjust maintenance doses by calculating the weekly dose and reducing or increasing it by 5%–25%. The full effect of a dose change may not become evident for 5–7 days.
- Warfarin's primary adverse effect is bleeding that can range from mild to life-threatening. It does not cause bleeding per se, but it exacerbates bleeding from existing lesions and enables massive bleeding from ordinarily minor sources. The likelihood of bleeding rises with increasing INR values; therefore, maintaining the INR within the target range is important to reduce bleeding risk:
  - ✓ When the INR is >4.5 without evidence of bleeding, the INR can be lowered by withholding warfarin, adjusting the warfarin dose, and/or providing a small dose of vitamin K to shorten the time to return to normal INR. Although vitamin K can be given parenterally or orally, the oral route is preferred in the absence of serious bleeding.
  - ✓ If the INR is between 5 and 10 and no bleeding is present, routine vitamin K use is not recommended because it has not been shown to affect the risk of developing subsequent bleeding or thromboembolism compared to simply withholding warfarin alone.
  - ✓ For INR >10 without evidence of bleeding, oral vitamin K (**phytonadione** 2.5 mg) is suggested. Use vitamin K with caution in patients at high risk of recurrent thromboembolism because of the possibility of INR overcorrection.
- Patients with warfarin-associated major bleeding require supportive care. Rapid reversal of anticoagulation with a four-factor prothrombin complex concentrate and 5–10 mg of vitamin K given by slow IV injection are also recommended.
- Nonhemorrhagic adverse effects of warfarin include the rare "purple toe" syndrome and skin necrosis.
- Because of the large number of food–drug and drug–drug interactions with warfarin, close monitoring and additional INR determinations may be indicated when other medications are initiated or discontinued or a change in consumption of vitamin K–containing foods occurs.

Thrombolytics

- Thrombolytic agents are proteolytic enzymes that enhance conversion of plasminogen to plasmin, which subsequently degrades the fibrin matrix.
- Most patients with VTE do not require thrombolytic therapy. Treatment should be reserved for patients who present with extensive proximal (eg, ileofemoral) DVT within 14 days of symptom onset, have good functional status, and are at low risk of bleeding.
- Patients with massive PE and evidence of hemodynamic compromise (hypotension or shock) should receive thrombolytic therapy unless contraindicated by bleeding risk.
- The same duration and intensity of anticoagulation therapy is recommended as for DVT patients not receiving thrombolysis. Patients with DVT involving the iliac and common femoral veins are at highest risk for postthrombotic syndrome and may receive the greatest benefit from thrombus removal strategies.
- For patients with massive PE manifested by shock and cardiovascular collapse (~5% of patients with PE), thrombolytic therapy is considered necessary in addition to aggressive interventions such as volume expansion, vasopressor therapy, intubation, and mechanical ventilation. Administer thrombolytic therapy in these patients

without delay to reduce the risk of progression to multisystem organ failure and death. However, the risk of death from PE should outweigh the risk of serious bleeding associated with thrombolytic therapy.

- **Alteplase** (Activase) 100 mg by IV infusion over 2 hours is the most commonly used thrombolytic therapy for patients with PE.
- Before giving thrombolytic therapy for PE, IV UFH should be administered in full therapeutic doses. During thrombolytic therapy, IV UFH may be either continued or suspended; the most common practice in the United States is to suspend UFH.
- Measure the aPTT after completion of thrombolytic therapy. If the aPTT is <80 seconds, start UFH infusion and adjust to maintain the aPTT in the therapeutic range. If the posttreatment aPTT is >80 seconds, remeasure it every 2–4 hours and start UFH infusion when the aPTT is <80 seconds.

EVALUATION OF THERAPEUTIC OUTCOMES

- Monitor patients for resolution of symptoms, development of recurrent thrombosis, symptoms of postthrombotic syndrome, and adverse anticoagulant effects.
- Monitor hemoglobin, hematocrit, and blood pressure carefully to detect bleeding from anticoagulant therapy.
- Perform coagulation tests (aPTT, PT, INR) prior to initiating therapy to establish the patient's baseline values and guide later anticoagulation.
- Ask outpatients taking warfarin about medication adherence to prior dosing instructions, other medication use, changes in health status, and symptoms related to bleeding and thromboembolic complications. Any changes in concurrent medications should be carefully explored, and dietary intake of vitamin K–rich foods should be assessed.

See Chapter 38, Venous Thromboembolism, authored by Daniel M. Witt, Nathan P.
Clark, and Sara R. Vazquez, for a more detailed discussion of this topic.

15 Acne Vulgaris

- *Acne* is a chronic skin disease characterized by open or closed comedones and inflammatory lesions, including papules, pustules, and nodules (cysts).

PATHOPHYSIOLOGY

- Acne usually begins during prepuberty and progresses as androgen production and sebaceous gland activity increase with gonad development.
- Acne progresses through four stages: (1) increased sebum production by sebaceous glands, (2) *Cutibacterium acnes* (formerly *Propionibacterium acnes*) follicular colonization (and bacterial lipolysis of sebum triglycerides to free fatty acids), (3) release of inflammatory mediators, and (4) increased follicular keratinization.
- Circulating androgens cause sebaceous glands to increase their size and activity. There is increased keratinization of epidermal cells and development of an obstructed sebaceous follicle, called a *microcomedone*. Cells adhere to each other, forming a dense keratinous plug. Sebum, produced in increasing amounts, becomes trapped behind the keratin plug and solidifies, contributing to open or closed comedone formation.
- Pooling of sebum in the follicle facilitates proliferation of the anaerobic bacterium *C. acnes*, which generates a T-cell response resulting in inflammation. *C. acnes* produces a lipase that hydrolyzes sebum triglycerides into free fatty acids that may increase keratinization and lead to microcomedone formation.
- *Noninflammatory acne* lesions include closed comedones (whiteheads) and open comedones (blackheads). Closed comedones are the first visible lesion in acne; they are almost completely obstructed to drainage and tend to rupture. Open comedones are formed as the plug extends to the upper canal and dilates its opening.
- *Inflammatory acne* lesions include papules, pustules, and nodules. Pus formation occurs due to recruitment of neutrophils into the follicle during the inflammatory process and release of *C. acnes*–generated chemokines. *C. acnes* also produces enzymes that increase permeability of the follicular wall, causing it to rupture, thereby releasing keratin, lipids, and irritating free fatty acids into the dermis.

CLINICAL PRESENTATION

- Lesions usually occur on the face, back, neck, shoulders, and chest and may extend to the buttocks or extremities. One or more anatomic areas may be involved; once present, the pattern of involvement tends to remain constant. The skin, scalp, and hair are frequently oily.
- Lesions may take months to heal completely. Nodules and deep lesions may result in scarring. Resolution of inflammatory lesions may leave erythematous or pigmented macules (hyperpigmentation) that persist for months or longer, especially in dark-skinned individuals.

DIAGNOSIS

- Diagnosis is established by patient assessment, which includes observation of lesions and excluding other potential causes (eg, drug-induced acne). Several different systems are in use to grade acne severity.

TREATMENT

- <u>Goals of Treatment</u>: Reduce the number and severity of lesions, improve appearance, slow progression, limit duration and recurrence, prevent disfigurement from scarring and hyperpigmentation, and avoid psychologic suffering.

GENERAL APPROACH

- Acne is a chronic disease that warrants early and aggressive treatment (Fig. 15-1). Maintenance therapy is often needed for optimal outcomes. Patient adherence to lengthy treatment regimens is crucial to long-term control.
- Eliminating follicular occlusion will arrest the acne cascade. Nondrug and pharmacologic measures should be directed toward cleansing, reducing triggers, and combination therapy targeting all four pathogenic mechanisms.
- Combination therapy is often more effective than single therapy and may decrease side effects and minimize resistance or tolerance to individual treatments.
- Topical therapy is standard treatment for mild-to-moderate acne, whereas systemic therapy is required for moderate-to-severe acne.
- First-, second-, and third-line therapies should be selected and altered as appropriate for the severity and staging of the disease. Treatment is directed at control, not cure. Regimens should be tapered over time, adjusting to response.
- Combine the smallest number of agents at the lowest possible dosages to ensure efficacy, safety, avoidance of resistance, and patient adherence. Once control is achieved, simplify the regimen but continue with some suppressive therapy.

NONPHARMACOLOGIC THERAPY

- Encourage patients to avoid aggravating factors (eg, mechanical occlusion, cosmetics), maintain a balanced low-glycemic-load diet, and control stress.
- Patients should wash twice daily with a mild, nonfragranced opaque or glycerin soap or a soapless cleanser. Scrubbing should be minimized to prevent follicular rupture.
- Males using a safety razor for shaving should soften the beard with soap and warm water or shaving gel. Shaving should be done lightly and infrequently, using a sharp blade and being careful to avoid nicking lesions. Strokes should be in the direction of hair growth, shaving each area only once to minimize irritation.

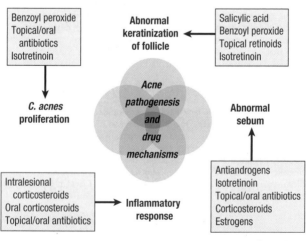

© Debra Sibbald

FIGURE 15-1. **Acne pathogenesis and drug mechanisms.**

- Comedone extraction results in immediate cosmetic improvement but has not been widely tested in clinical trials.
- Light therapies are believed to work by killing *C. acnes* and by damaging and shrinking sebaceous glands, reducing sebum output with few or temporary adverse effects. Light therapies may be used once or twice weekly over a course of 6–10 treatments, with each irradiation lasting 10–20 minutes. Home-use blue light therapy is now available.

PHARMACOLOGIC THERAPY

- *Comedonal noninflammatory acne*: Select topical agents that target the increased keratinization by producing exfoliation. Topical retinoids (especially adapalene) or a fixed combination with a retinoid (eg, adapalene plus benzoyl peroxide) are drugs of choice. Benzoyl peroxide, azelaic acid, or salicylic acid are second-line alternatives.
- *Mild-to-moderate papulopustular inflammatory acne*: It is important to reduce the population of *C. acnes* in follicles. Either the fixed-dose combination of adapalene plus benzoyl peroxide or benzoyl peroxide, topical retinoid, or azelaic acid are recommended as first-choice therapy. In moderate papulopustular inflammatory acne, the fixed-dose combination is preferred, with or without hormonal therapy and/or antibiotic, particularly if the trunk is involved. If there are limitations in use of first-choice agents, alternatives include blue light monotherapy, alternate combination therapy (such as a fixed-dose combination of erythromycin plus tretinoin), or oral zinc. In cases of widespread disease, combining an oral antibiotic with topical benzoyl peroxide with or without adapalene can be considered.
- *Moderately severe or severe papulopustular or moderate nodular acne*: An oral antibiotic plus the fixed-dose topical combination is preferred. Alternatively, oral isotretinoin or oral hormonal therapy can be added. If there are limitations to use of these agents, consider oral antiandrogens in combination with oral antibiotics or topical treatments.
- *Nodular or conglobate acne*: Monotherapy with oral isotretinoin is first choice. As alternatives, a retinoid fixed combination or oral antibiotic can be recommended. For females, oral isotretinoin plus antiandrogenic hormonal therapy is preferred. Alternatively, a fixed combination retinoid with oral antibiotics and/or an oral antiandrogen can be recommended.
- *Maintenance acne therapy*: A topical retinoid alone or a retinoid plus benzoyl peroxide fixed-dose combination is most commonly recommended. Topical azelaic acid is an alternative. Maintenance is usually begun after a 12-week induction period and continues for 3–4 months. A longer duration may be necessary to prevent relapse upon discontinuation. Long-term therapy with antibiotics is not recommended to minimize antibiotic resistance.

Exfoliants (Peeling Agents)

- Exfoliants induce continuous mild drying and peeling by irritation, damaging superficial skin layers and inciting inflammation. This stimulates mitosis, thickening the epidermis and increasing horny cells, scaling, and erythema. Decreased sweating results in a dry, less oily surface and may resolve pustular lesions.
- **Resorcinol** is less keratolytic than salicylic acid and, when used alone, is classified by the Food and Drug Administration (FDA) as category II (not generally recognized as safe and effective). The FDA considers resorcinol 2% and resorcinol monoacetate 3% to be safe and effective when used in combination with sulfur 3%–8%. Resorcinol is an irritant and sensitizer and should not be applied to large areas or on broken skin. It produces a reversible dark brown scale on some dark-skinned individuals.
- **Salicylic acid** is a comedolytic agent available over the counter in 0.5%–2% strengths; concentrations between 3% and 6% are keratolytic, softening the horny layer and producing shedding of scales. It has mild antibacterial activity against *C. acnes* and offers slight anti-inflammatory activity at concentrations up to 5%. Salicylic acid is recognized by the FDA as safe and effective, but it offers no advantages over benzoyl

peroxide or topical retinoids. Salicylic acid products are often used as first-line therapy for mild acne because of their availability without a prescription in alcohol–detergent impregnated pads, washes, bars, and semisolid vehicles. Both wash-off and leave-on preparations are well tolerated. Lower concentrations are sometimes combined with sulfur to produce an additive keratolytic effect. Concentrations of 5%–10% can also be used by prescription, beginning with a low concentration and increasing as tolerance develops to the irritation. Salicylic acid is often used when patients cannot tolerate topical retinoids because of skin irritation.

- **Sulfur** is keratolytic and has antibacterial activity. It can quickly resolve pustules and papules, mask lesions, and produce irritation that leads to skin peeling. Sulfur is used in the precipitated or colloidal form in concentrations of 2%–10%. Although it is often combined with salicylic acid or resorcinol to increase effect, use is limited by offensive odor and availability of more effective agents.

Topical Retinoids

- Retinoids reduce obstruction within the follicle and are useful for both comedonal and inflammatory acne. They reverse abnormal keratinocyte desquamation and are active keratolytics. They inhibit microcomedone formation, decreasing the number of mature comedones and inflammatory lesions.

- Topical retinoids are safe, effective, and economical for treating all but the most severe cases of acne. They should be the first step in moderate acne, alone or with antibiotics and benzoyl peroxide, reverting to retinoids alone for maintenance once adequate results are achieved. Combination products containing benzoyl peroxide or topical antimicrobials are available.

- Retinoids can produce extended periods of remission if accompanying irritation does not impede patient adherence. Side effects of dryness, peeling, erythema, and irritation can be mitigated by reduced frequency of application.

- Retinoids should be applied at night, a half-hour after cleansing, starting with every other night for 1–2 weeks to adjust to irritation. Doses can be increased only after 4–6 weeks of the lowest concentration and least irritating vehicle. Gels and creams are less irritating than solutions.

- **Tretinoin** (retinoic acid, vitamin A acid) is available in various strengths in creams, gels, and pumps. Tretinoin should not be used in pregnant women because of risk to the fetus.

- **Adapalene** (Differin) is as effective as and less irritating than other topical retinoids. Adapalene is available as 0.1% gel (nonprescription for once-daily application by patients age 12 years and older), cream, solution, lotion, and pads. A 0.3% gel is also available. It is also available in fixed-dose combinations with benzoyl peroxide to increase efficacy over monotherapies.

- **Tazarotene** (Tazorac) is as effective as adapalene in reducing noninflammatory and inflammatory lesion counts when applied half as frequently. Compared with tretinoin, it is as effective for comedonal and more effective for inflammatory lesions when applied once daily. The product is available as a 0.05% and 0.1% cream or gel and a 0.1% foam. Tazarotene is contraindicated in pregnancy.

- **Trifarotene** (Aklief) is approved in the United States for treatment of acne in patients aged 9 years and older. It is available as a 0.005% cream for application once daily in the evening. Trifarotene should be avoided during pregnancy.

Topical Antibacterial Agents

- **Benzoyl peroxide** is bactericidal to *C. acnes* and is also mildly comedolytic. It suppresses sebum production and reduces free fatty acids, which are comedogenic and trigger inflammation. No resistance has been reported, and addition of benzoyl peroxide to antibiotic therapy improves efficacy and may reduce resistance development.
  ✓ Benzoyl peroxide is useful for both noninflammatory and inflammatory acne. It has a rapid onset and may decrease the number of inflamed lesions within 5 days. Used alone or in combination, benzoyl peroxide is the standard of care for mild-to-moderate papulopustular acne. It is an agent of first choice when combined

with adapalene for most patients with mild-to-moderate inflammatory acne and a second-line choice for patients with noninflammatory comedonal acne. It is often combined with a topical retinoid or antibiotic. For maintenance therapy, benzoyl peroxide can be added to a topical retinoid.

✓ Topical washes, foams, creams, or gels can be used as leave-on or wash-off agents. Strengths available range from 2.5% to 10%. All single-agent preparations are available without prescription.

✓ Therapy should be initiated with the weakest concentration (2.5%) in a water-based formulation in the evening. Once tolerance is achieved, the strength may be increased to 5% or the base changed to the acetone or alcohol gels, or to paste. It is important to wash the product off in the morning. A sunscreen should be applied during the day.

✓ Side effects of benzoyl peroxide include dryness, irritation, and, rarely, allergic contact dermatitis. It may bleach hair, clothing, and towels.

- **Topical clindamycin** and **erythromycin** are macrolide antibiotics that are effective and well-tolerated acne treatments. They are recommended for use in combination with topical benzoyl peroxide (wash-off or leave-on) or retinoids, which increases efficacy and decreases development of resistant organisms. Clindamycin is preferred over erythromycin because of its better efficacy and lack of systemic absorption; it is available as a single-ingredient topical preparation or in combination with benzoyl peroxide. Erythromycin is available alone and in combination with retinoic acid or benzoyl peroxide, but it is seldom used in practice.

- **Azelaic acid** has antibacterial, anti-inflammatory, and comedolytic activity. It is used for mild-to-moderate inflammatory acne but has limited efficacy compared with other therapies. It is an alternative to first-choice therapy for comedonal and inflammatory acne, particularly in combination. It is also an alternative to topical retinoids for maintenance therapy. Azelaic acid is well tolerated, with adverse effects of pruritus, burning, stinging, and tingling occurring in 1%–5% of patients. Erythema, dryness, peeling, and irritation occur in fewer than 1% of patients. Azelaic acid is available in 20% cream (Azelex) and 15% gel (Finacea) formulations, which are usually applied twice daily (morning and evening) on clean, dry skin. Most patients experience improvement within 4 weeks, but treatment may be continued over several months if necessary.

- **Dapsone** (Aczone) is a sulfone that has antibacterial and anti-inflammatory properties and improves both inflammatory and noninflammatory acne. It may be particularly useful for patients with sensitivities or intolerance to conventional antiacne agents and may be used in sulfonamide-allergic patients. Dapsone 5% topical gel is applied twice daily; the 7.5% gel is applied once daily. Combination therapy with topical retinoids may be indicated if comedonal lesions are present. Topical dapsone 5% gel has also been used in combination with adapalene or benzoyl peroxide.

Oral Antibacterials

- Use of oral antibiotics is reserved for patients with moderate-to-severe inflammatory acne. Tetracyclines (**minocycline** and **doxycycline**) have both antibacterial and anti-inflammatory effects and are considered first-line therapy. Macrolides (**erythromycin, azithromycin**) and **trimethoprim/sulfamethoxazole** are acceptable alternative agents. Because of bacterial resistance, erythromycin should be limited to patients who cannot use a tetracycline (eg, pregnant women and children <8 years old).

- **Ciprofloxacin** and **trimethoprim** alone may be effective in cases where other antibiotics cannot be used or are ineffective.

- **Sarecycline** (Seysara) is a narrow-spectrum tetracycline derivative with anti-inflammatory properties approved for treatment of inflammatory lesions of non-nodular moderate-to-severe acne vulgaris in patients 9 years of age or older.

- Oral antibiotics should be accompanied by early use of combination therapy with retinoids. In such cases, the antibiotic may often be discontinued after 3–6 months of therapy.

- The incidence of significant adverse effects with oral antibiotic use is low. Vaginal candidiasis may complicate use of all oral antibiotics. Minocycline has been associated with pigment deposition in the skin, mucous membranes, and teeth; it may also cause dose-related dizziness, urticaria, hypersensitivity syndrome, autoimmune hepatitis, a systemic lupus erythematosus–like syndrome, and serum sickness–like reactions. Doxycycline is a photosensitizer, especially at higher doses.
- The choice of antibiotic should be determined based on the side effect profile, resistance, cost, and consensus guidelines.

Intralesional Corticosteroids

Intralesional **triamcinolone acetonide** injections are effective for large individual inflammatory nodules. Intralesional injections may produce rapid improvement and decreased pain but may also be associated with local skin atrophy.

Hormonal Agents

- **Oral contraceptives** containing estrogen can be useful for acne in some women because of their antiandrogenic properties. Agents with FDA approval for acne in women who also desire contraception include **norgestimate with ethinyl estradiol** and **norethindrone acetate with ethinyl estradiol**; other estrogen-containing products may also be effective. They may be used alone or in combination with other acne treatments.
- **Spironolactone** is an antiandrogen and has been shown to be effective for acne in select women. It may cause hyperkalemia, especially in higher doses and in patients with cardiac or renal compromise. Spironolactone is not FDA approved for this use and should not be used in males.
- **Clascoterone** 1% cream (Winlevi) is an androgen receptor inhibitor approved for acne treatment in male and female patients 12 years of age and older. It is applied twice daily (morning and evening). Common adverse effects include erythema, edema, and scaling/dryness.
- **Oral corticosteroids** in high doses used for short courses may provide temporary benefit in patients with severe inflammatory acne. Low-dose **prednisone** (5–15 mg daily) given alone or with high estrogen-containing combination oral contraceptives has shown efficacy for acne and seborrhea. Long-term adverse effects preclude oral corticosteroid use as a primary therapy for acne.

Isotretinoin

- **Isotretinoin** is a metabolite of vitamin A that decreases sebum production, inhibits *C. acnes* growth, and reduces inflammation. It is approved for treatment of severe recalcitrant nodular acne in non-pregnant patients 12 years of age and older with multiple inflammatory nodules with a diameter of 5 mm or greater. It has also been used for moderate acne that is treatment resistant, relapses quickly after discontinuation of oral antibiotic therapy, or produces physical scarring or significant psychosocial distress. Isotretinoin is the only drug treatment for acne that produces prolonged remission.
  - ✓ The approved isotretinoin dose range is 0.5–2 mg/kg/day, usually given over a 20-week course. Drug absorption is greater when taken with food.
  - ✓ Initial flares can be minimized by Guidelines that recommend initiation at 0.5 mg/kg/day or less when appropriate, subsequently increasing to 1 mg/kg/day after the first month as tolerated, with a goal cumulative dose between 120 and 150 mg/kg.
  - ✓ Side effects include those of the mucocutaneous (most common), musculoskeletal, and ophthalmic systems, as well as headaches and central nervous system effects. Most adverse effects, such as cheilitis and dry nose, eyes, and mouth, are temporary and resolve after discontinuation. Laboratory monitoring during therapy should include triglycerides, cholesterol, transaminases, and complete blood counts. Mood disorders, depression, suicidal ideation, and suicides have been reported sporadically, but a causal relationship has not been established. The

issue is complex because depression and suicidal ideation occur with severe acne in the absence of isotretinoin.

✓ Because of teratogenicity, two different forms of contraception must be started in female patients of childbearing potential beginning 1 month before therapy, continuing throughout treatment, and for up to 4 months after discontinuation of therapy. All patients receiving isotretinoin must participate in the iPLEDGE program, which requires pregnancy tests and assurances by prescribers and pharmacists that they will follow required procedures.

EVALUATION OF THERAPEUTIC OUTCOMES

- Provide patients with acne with a monitoring framework that includes specific parameters and frequency of monitoring. Have them record the objective response to treatment in a diary. Contact patients within 2–3 weeks after the start of therapy to assess progress and then every 4–8 weeks thereafter.
- Good adherence to therapy is the key to treatment success.
- Lesion counts should decrease by 10%–15% within 4–8 weeks or by more than 50% within 2–4 months. Inflammatory lesions should resolve within a few weeks, and comedones should resolve in 3–4 months. If anxiety or depression is present at the outset, control or improvement should be achieved within 2–4 months.
- Long-term parameters should include no progression of severity, lengthening of acne-free periods throughout therapy, and no further scarring or pigmentation throughout therapy.
- Monitor patients regularly for adverse treatment effects with appropriate dose reduction, alternative therapy, preventative measures, or drug discontinuation as appropriate.

See Chapter 117, Acne Vulgaris, authored by Debra J. Sibbald and Cathryn Sibbald, for a more detailed discussion of this topic.

Dermatologic Drug Reactions and Common Skin Conditions

CHAPTER 16

- *Drug-induced skin reactions* can be irritant or allergic in origin. Allergic drug reactions are classified into exanthematous, urticarial, blistering, and pustular eruptions.
- Severe cutaneous adverse reactions to drugs (SCARs) include Stevens–Johnson syndrome (SJS), toxic epidermal necrolysis (TEN), and drug reaction with eosinophilia and systemic symptoms (DRESS).
- Skin disorders discussed in this chapter include contact dermatitis, diaper dermatitis, and atopic dermatitis.

PATHOPHYSIOLOGY

- *Exanthematous* drug reactions include maculopapular rashes and drug hypersensitivity syndrome. *Urticarial* reactions include urticaria, angioedema, and serum sickness-like reactions. *Blistering* reactions include fixed drug eruptions, Stevens–Johnson syndrome, and toxic epidermal necrolysis. *Pustular* eruptions include acneiform drug reactions and acute generalized exanthematous pustulosis (AGEP) (Fig. 16-1).
- Drug-induced *hyperpigmentation* may be related to increased melanin (eg, hydantoins), direct deposition (eg, silver, mercury, tetracyclines, and antimalarials), or other mechanisms (eg, fluorouracil).
- Drug-induced photosensitivity reactions may be *phototoxic* (a nonimmunologic reaction) or *photoallergic* (an immunologic reaction). Medications associated with phototoxicity include amiodarone, tetracyclines, sulfonamides, psoralens, and coal tar. Common causes of photoallergic reactions include sulfonamides, sulfonylureas, thiazides, nonsteroidal anti-inflammatory drugs (NSAIDs), chloroquine, and carbamazepine.
- *Contact dermatitis* is skin inflammation caused by irritants or allergic sensitizers. In *allergic contact dermatitis* (ACD), an antigenic substance triggers an immunologic response, sometimes several days later. *Irritant contact dermatitis* (ICD) is caused by an organic substance that usually results in a reaction within a few hours of exposure.
- *Diaper dermatitis* (diaper rash) is an acute, inflammatory dermatitis of the buttocks, genitalia, and perineal regions that are covered by the diaper. It is a type of contact dermatitis resulting from direct fecal and moisture contact with the skin in an occlusive environment.
- *Atopic dermatitis* (eczema) is an inflammatory condition with genetic, environmental, and immunologic mechanisms. Neuropeptides, irritation, or pruritus-induced scratching may cause release of proinflammatory cytokines from keratinocytes.

CLINICAL PRESENTATION

- *Maculopapular skin reaction* presents with erythematous macules and papules that may be pruritic. Lesions usually begin within 7–10 days after starting the offending medication and generally resolve within 7–14 days after drug discontinuation. Because of the delayed reaction, the offending agent could be discontinued (eg, a 7-day antibiotic treatment course) before the lesions appear. Lesions may spread and become confluent. Common culprits include penicillins, cephalosporins, sulfonamides, and some anticonvulsants.
- *Drug hypersensitivity syndrome* (also known as drug reaction with eosinophilia and systemic symptoms or DRESS) is an exanthematous eruption accompanied by fever, lymphadenopathy, and multiorgan involvement (kidneys, liver, lung, bone marrow, heart, and brain). Signs and symptoms begin 1–4 weeks after starting the offending drug, and the reaction may be fatal if not promptly treated. Drugs implicated include allopurinol, sulfonamides, some anticonvulsants (barbiturates, phenytoin, carbamazepine, and lamotrigine), and dapsone.

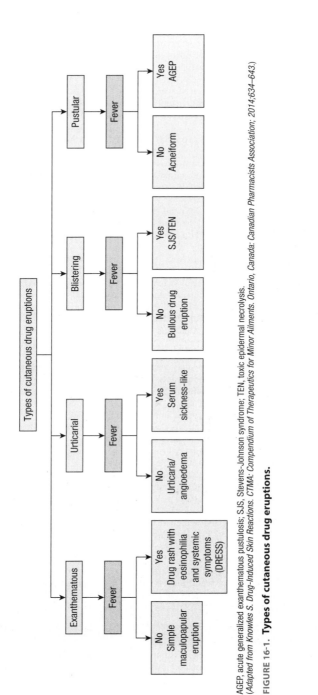

AGEP, acute generalized exanthematous pustulosis; SJS, Stevens–Johnson syndrome; TEN, toxic epidermal necrolysis.
(*Adapted from Knowles S. Drug-Induced Skin Reactions. CTMA: Compendium of Therapeutics for Minor Ailments. Ontario, Canada: Canadian Pharmacists Association; 2014;634–643.*)

FIGURE 16-1. Types of cutaneous drug eruptions.

- *Urticaria* and *angioedema* are simple eruptions that are caused by drugs in 5%–10% of cases. Other causes are foods (most common) and physical factors such as cold or pressure, infections, and latex exposure. Urticaria may be the first sign of an emerging anaphylactic reaction characterized by hives, extremely pruritic red raised wheals, angioedema, and mucous membrane swelling that typically occurs within minutes to hours. Offending drugs include penicillins and related antibiotics, aspirin, sulfonamides, radiograph contrast media, and opioids.

- *Serum sickness-like reactions* are complex urticarial eruptions presenting with fever, rash (usually urticarial), and arthralgias usually within 1–3 weeks after starting the offending drug.

- *Fixed drug eruptions* present as pruritic, red, raised lesions that may blister. Symptoms can include burning or stinging. Lesions may evolve into plaques. These so-called fixed eruptions recur in the same area each time the offending drug is given. Lesions appear and disappear within minutes to days, leaving hyperpigmented skin for months. Usual offenders include tetracyclines, barbiturates, sulfonamides, codeine, phenolphthalein, and NSAIDs.

- *Stevens–Johnson syndrome* (SJS) and *toxic epidermal necrolysis* (TEN) are blistering eruptions that are rare but severe and life-threatening. They are considered variants of the same disorder and are often discussed together as SJS/TEN. Onset occurs within 7–14 days after drug exposure. Patients present with generalized tender/painful bullous formation with fever, headache, and respiratory symptoms leading to rapid clinical deterioration. Lesions show rapid confluence and spread, resulting in extensive epidermal detachment and sloughing. This may result in marked fluid loss, hypotension, electrolyte imbalances, and secondary infections. Usual offending drugs include sulfonamides, penicillins, some anticonvulsants (hydantoins, carbamazepine, barbiturates, and lamotrigine), NSAIDs, and allopurinol.

- *Acneiform drug reactions* are pustular eruptions that induce acne. Onset is within 1–3 weeks. Common culprits include corticosteroids, androgenic hormones, some anticonvulsants, isoniazid, and lithium.

- *Acute generalized exanthematous pustulosis* (AGEP) has an acute onset (within days after starting the offending drug), fever, diffuse erythema, and many pustules. Generalized desquamation occurs 2 weeks later. Common offending drugs include β-lactam antibiotics, macrolides, and calcium channel blockers.

- *Sun-induced skin reactions* appear similar to a sunburn and present with erythema, papules, edema, and sometimes vesicles. They appear in areas exposed to sunlight (eg, ears, nose, cheeks, forearms, and hands).

- *Diaper dermatitis* results in an erythematous rash, and severe cases may have vesicles and oozing erosions. The rash may be infected by *Candida* species and present with confluent red plaques, papules, and pustules.

- *Atopic dermatitis* presents differently depending on age. In infancy, an erythematous, patchy, pruritic, papular skin rash may first appear on the cheeks and chin and progress to red, scaling, oozing lesions. The rash affects the malar region of the cheeks, forehead, scalp, chin, and behind the ears while sparing the nose and paranasal creases. Over several weeks, lesions may spread to extensor surfaces of the lower legs (due to the infant's crawling), and eventually, the entire body may be involved except for the diaper area and nose. In childhood, the skin is often dry, flaky, rough, and cracked. Pruritus is a quintessential feature, and a diagnosis cannot be made if there is no history of itching. Scratching and rubbing itchy skin may result in bleeding and lichenification. In adulthood, lesions are more diffuse with underlying erythema. The face is commonly involved and may be dry and scaly. Lichenification may be seen.

DIAGNOSIS

- A comprehensive patient history is important to obtain the following information:
  - ✓ Signs and symptoms (onset, progression, timeframe, lesion location and description, presenting symptoms, and previous occurrence)

✓ Urgency (severity, area, and extent of skin involvement; signs of a systemic/generalized reaction or disease condition)
✓ Medication history (temporal correlation, previous exposure, and nonprescribed products)
✓ Differential diagnosis

- Lesion assessment includes identifying macules, papules, nodules, blisters, plaques, and lichenification. Some skin conditions cause more than one type of lesions.
- Inspect lesions for color, texture, size, and temperature. Areas that are oozing, erythematous, and warm to the touch may be infected.

TREATMENT

- <u>Goals of Treatment</u>: Relieve bothersome symptoms, remove precipitating factors, prevent recurrences, avoid adverse treatment effects, and improve quality of life.

DRUG-INDUCED SKIN REACTIONS

- If a drug-induced skin reaction is suspected, the most important treatment is discontinuing the suspected drug as quickly as possible and avoiding use of potential cross-sensitizers.
- The next step is to control symptoms (eg, pruritus). Signs or symptoms of a systemic or generalized reaction may require additional supportive therapy. For high fevers, acetaminophen is more appropriate than aspirin or another NSAID, which may exacerbate some skin lesions.
- Most maculopapular reactions disappear within a few days after discontinuing the agent, so symptomatic control of the affected area is the primary intervention. Topical corticosteroids and oral antihistamines can relieve pruritus. In severe cases, a short course of systemic corticosteroids may be warranted.
- Treatment of fixed drug reactions involves removal of the offending agent. Other therapeutic measures include topical corticosteroids, oral antihistamines to relieve itching, and perhaps cool water compresses on the affected area.
- Photosensitivity reactions typically resolve with drug discontinuation. Some patients benefit from topical corticosteroids and oral antihistamines, but these are relatively ineffective. Systemic corticosteroids (eg, oral prednisone 1 mg/kg/day tapered over 3 weeks) are more effective.
- For life-threatening SJS/TEN, supportive measures such as maintenance of adequate blood pressure, fluid and electrolyte balance, broad-spectrum antibiotics and vancomycin for secondary infections, and IV immunoglobulin (IVIG) may be appropriate. Corticosteroid use is controversial; if used, employ relatively high doses initially, followed by rapid tapering as soon as disease progression stops.
- Inform patients about the suspected drug, potential drugs to avoid in the future, and which drugs may be used instead. Give patients with photosensitivity reactions information about preventive measures, such as use of sunscreens and sun avoidance.

CONTACT DERMATITIS

- The first intervention involves identification, withdrawal, and avoidance of the offending agent.
- The second treatment is symptomatic relief while decreasing skin lesions. Cold compresses help soothe and cleanse the skin; they are applied to wet or oozing lesions, removed, remoistened, and reapplied every few minutes for a 20- to 30-minute period. If affected areas are already dry or hardened, wet dressings applied as soaks (without removal for up to 20–30 minutes) will soften and hydrate the skin; soaks should not be used on acute exudating lesions. **Calamine lotion** or **Burow solution (aluminum acetate)** may also be soothing.
- **Topical corticosteroids** help resolve the inflammatory process and are the mainstay of treatment. ACD responds better to topical corticosteroids than does ICD. Generally, use higher potency corticosteroids initially, switching to medium or lower

potency corticosteroids as the condition improves (see Chapter 17, Table 17–1, for topical corticosteroid potencies).

- **Oatmeal baths** or oral **first-generation antihistamines** may provide relief for excessive itching.
- **Moisturizers** may be used to prevent dryness and skin fissuring.

DIAPER DERMATITIS

- Management involves frequent diaper changes, air drying (removing the diaper for as long as practical), gentle cleansing (preferably with nonsoap cleansers and lukewarm water), and use of barrier products. **Zinc oxide** has astringent and absorbent properties and provides an effective barrier. **Petrolatum** also provides a water-impermeable barrier but has no absorbent ability and may trap moisture.
- Candidal (yeast) diaper rash should be treated with a topical antifungal agent and then covered by a barrier product. **Imidazoles** are the treatment of choice. The antifungal agents should be stopped once the rash subsides and the barrier product continued to prevent recurrence.
- In severe inflammatory diaper rashes, a very low potency topical corticosteroid **(hydrocortisone 0.5%–1%)** may be used for short periods (1–2 weeks).
- Medical referral is indicated if the rash does not respond after a week of treatment, if pain or inflammation increases during therapy, if ulcerations develop, or if systemic signs or symptoms are present (eg, fever, diarrhea, skin lesions elsewhere).

ATOPIC DERMATITIS

- Nonpharmacologic measures for infants and children include the following:
  - ✓ Apply moisturizers frequently throughout the day
  - ✓ Give lukewarm baths
  - ✓ Apply lubricants/moisturizers immediately after bathing
  - ✓ Use nonsoap cleansers (which are neutral to low pH, hypoallergenic, fragrance-free)
  - ✓ Use wet-wrap therapy (with or without topical corticosteroid) during flare-ups for patients with moderate-to-severe disease. Wet-wrap involves applying damp tubular elasticized bandages and occlusive dressing to the limbs to promote skin hydration and absorption of emollients and topical corticosteroids.
  - ✓ Keep fingernails filed short
  - ✓ Select clothing made of soft cotton fabrics
  - ✓ Consider sedating oral antihistamines to reduce scratching at night
  - ✓ Keep the child cool; avoid situations that cause overheating
  - ✓ Learn to recognize skin infections and seek treatment promptly
  - ✓ Identify and remove irritants and allergens
- Topical corticosteroids are the drug treatment of choice. Low-potency agents (eg, **hydrocortisone 1%**) are suitable for the face, and medium-potency products (eg, **betamethasone valerate 0.1%**) may be used for the body. For longer-duration maintenance therapy, low-potency corticosteroids are recommended. Use mid-strength and high-potency corticosteroids for short-term management of exacerbations. Reserve ultra-high and high-potency agents (eg, **betamethasone dipropionate 0.05%** and **clobetasone propionate 0.05%**) for short-term treatment (1–2 weeks) of lichenified lesions in adults. After lesions have improved significantly, use a lower-potency corticosteroid for maintenance when necessary. Avoid potent fluorinated corticosteroids on the face, genitalia, and intertriginous areas and in infants.
- The topical immunomodulators **tacrolimus** (Protopic) and **pimecrolimus** (Elidel) inhibit calcineurin, which normally initiates T-cell activation. Both agents are approved for atopic dermatitis in adults and children older than age 2. Tacrolimus ointment 0.03% (for moderate-to-severe atopic dermatitis in patients ages 2 and older) and 0.1% (for ages 16 and older) is applied twice daily. Pimecrolimus cream 1% is applied twice daily for mild-to-moderate atopic dermatitis in patients older than age 2. The most common adverse effect is transient burning at the site of application. Both drugs are recommended as second-line treatments due to concerns about a

possible risk of cancer. For this reason, sun protection factor (SPF) 30 or higher is recommended on all exposed skin areas.

- **Coal tar preparations** (**crude coal tar**, **liquor carbonis detergens**) have been widely used, but few controlled trials support their efficacy. These products are also staining and malodorous, although newer products may be more cosmetically acceptable. They are not recommended on acutely inflamed skin, since this may result in additional skin irritation.

- **Crisaborole** (Eucrisa) 2% ointment is a phosphodiesterase (PDE) 4 inhibitor approved for treatment of mild-to-moderate AD in adults and children 2 years of age or older. A thin layer of ointment is applied twice daily to affected areas. Burning or stinging may occur at the site of application.

- Phototherapy may be recommended when the disease is not controlled by topical corticosteroids and calcineurin inhibitors. It may also be steroid sparing, allowing for use of lower-potency corticosteroids, or even eliminating the need for corticosteroids in some cases.

- **Dupilumab** (Dupixent) subcutaneous (SC) injection is an interleukin-4 receptor alpha antagonist FDA approved for treatment of patients aged 12 years and older with moderate-to-severe atopic dermatitis whose disease is not adequately controlled with topical prescription therapies or when those therapies are not advisable. It can be used with or without topical corticosteroids. Topical calcineurin inhibitors may be used but should be reserved for problem areas such as the face, neck, intertriginous, and genital areas. The recommended adult dose is 600 mg initially (given as two 300-mg SC injections), followed by 300-mg SC every other week. The dose for patients 12–17 years of age is based on body weight: <60 kg, 400 mg (two 200-mg injections) then 200 mg every other week; >60 kg, 600 mg (two 300-mg injections) then 300 mg every other week. The most common adverse reactions (≥1%) are injection site reactions, conjunctivitis, blepharitis, oral herpes, keratitis, eye pruritus, other herpes simplex virus infection, and dry eye.

- **Upadacitinib** (Rinvoq) and **abrocitinib** (Cibinqo) are oral Janus kinase (JAK) inhibitors approved for refractory, moderate to severe atopic dermatitis not adequately controlled with other systemic drugs, including biologics. Upadacitinib is approved for use in adults and children age 12 and older, whereas abrocitinib is approved for use only in adults. The initial upadacitinib dose is 15 mg orally once daily, which can be increased to 30 mg once daily if an adequate response is not achieved. The abrocitinib dose is 100 mg orally once daily; 200 mg daily is recommended for patients not responding to the 100-mg dose. Both products carry a warning of increased risk of serious infections, mortality, malignancy, major cardiovascular events, and thrombosis.

- Other systemic therapies that have been used (but not FDA approved) for atopic dermatitis include other biologic agents, corticosteroids, cyclosporine, interferon-γ, azathioprine, methotrexate, mycophenolate mofetil, and IVIG.

EVALUATION OF THERAPEUTIC OUTCOMES

- Provide patients with information regarding causative factors, avoidance of substances that trigger skin reactions, and potential benefits and limitations of nondrug and drug therapy.

- Evaluate patients with chronic skin conditions periodically to assess disease control, the efficacy of current therapy, and the presence of possible adverse effects.

See Chapter e17, Skin Care and Minor Dermatologic Conditions, by Rebecca M. Law and Howard I. Maibach; Chapter 119, Atopic Dermatitis, by Rebecca M. Law Wayne P. Gulliver; and Chapter e121, Dermatologic Drug Reactions, Contact Dermatitis, and Common Skin Conditions, by Rebecca M. Law, David T.S. Law, and Howard I. Maibach, for more detailed discussions of these topics.

Psoriasis

- *Psoriasis* is a chronic T-lymphocyte–mediated systemic inflammatory disease characterized by recurrent exacerbations and remissions of thickened, erythematous, and scaling plaques and multiple comorbidities, including psoriatic arthritis.

PATHOPHYSIOLOGY

- Genetic predisposition coupled with an unknown precipitating factor triggers an abnormal immune response mediated via T-lymphocytes, resulting in keratinocyte proliferation and the initial psoriatic skin lesions. Precipitating factors implicated in the development of psoriasis include skin injury, infection, drugs, smoking, alcohol consumption, obesity, and psychogenic stress.
- Psoriasis susceptibility genes and variants reside on various chromosomes. The psoriasis susceptibility locus 1 (*PSORS1*) on chromosome 6p is a key gene locus, accounting for up to 50% of disease heritability. The major histocompatibility complex antigen HLA-Cw6 and tumor necrosis factor (TNF)-α are major psoriasis susceptibility genes, along with interleukin (IL)-23 and many other loci. There appears to be a general role for T lymphocytes and a specific role for TH17 lymphocytes in psoriasis pathogenesis and as indicators of psoriasis risk.
- Interactions between dermal dendritic cells and activated Th-1 and Th-17 cells in concert with numerous growth factors and cytokines (eg, TNF-α, interferon gamma, IL-1) cause epidermal hyperplasia and dermal inflammation.

CLINICAL PRESENTATION

- Skin lesions in plaque psoriasis (psoriasis vulgaris) are erythematous, red-violet in color, at least 0.5 cm in diameter, well-demarcated, and typically covered with silver flaking scales. They may appear as single lesions on predisposed areas (eg, knees and elbows) or generalized over a wide body surface area (BSA).
- Pruritus may be severe and require treatment to minimize excoriations from frequent scratching. Lesions may be physically debilitating or socially isolating.
- Preexisting psoriasis can be exacerbated by drugs (eg, lithium, nonsteroidal anti-inflammatory drugs [NSAIDs], antimalarials, β-adrenergic blockers, fluoxetine, and withdrawal of corticosteroids), times of stress, and seasonal changes.
- Potential comorbidities include psoriatic arthritis, depression, anxiety, hypertension, obesity, diabetes mellitus, Crohn's disease, and alcoholism.
- Psoriatic arthritis develops in about 30% of patients with plaque psoriasis. It most commonly presents as polyarticular peripheral arthritis but can vary widely with peripheral and/or axial, monoarticular, or polyarticular patterns.

DIAGNOSIS

- Diagnosis is based on physical examination findings of characteristic lesions. Skin biopsies are not diagnostic of psoriasis.
- Classification of psoriasis as mild, moderate, or severe is based on BSA and Psoriasis Area and Severity Index (PASI) measurements. A 2011 European classification system defines severity of plaque psoriasis as either mild or moderate-to-severe.

TREATMENT

- <u>Goals of Treatment</u>: Minimize or eliminate skin lesions, alleviate pruritus, reduce frequency of flare-ups, treat comorbid conditions, screen for and manage lifestyle factors that may trigger exacerbations, avoid adverse treatment effects, provide

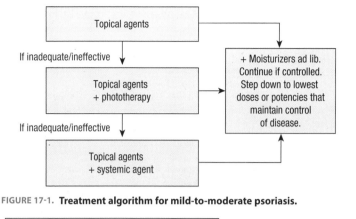

FIGURE 17-1. Treatment algorithm for mild-to-moderate psoriasis.

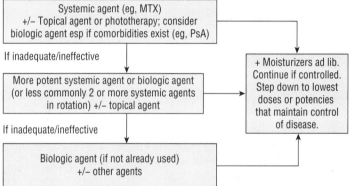

MTX, methotrexate; PsA, psoriatic arthritis.

FIGURE 17-2. Treatment algorithm for moderate-to-severe psoriasis.

cost-effective treatment, provide appropriate counseling (eg, stress reduction), and maintain or improve quality of life.
- See **Figs. 17-1** and **17-2** for psoriasis treatment algorithms based on disease severity.

NONPHARMACOLOGIC THERAPY

- Nonmedicated moisturizers help maintain skin moisture, reduce skin shedding, control scaling, and reduce pruritus.
- Oatmeal baths further reduce pruritus, and regular use may decrease need for systemic antipruritic drugs. Harsh soaps and detergents should be avoided. Cleansing should involve tepid water, preferably with lipid- and fragrance-free cleansers.
- Sunscreens (preferably sun protection factor [SPF] 30 or higher) should be used when outdoors.
- Stress management can improve extent and severity of psoriasis.

PHARMACOLOGIC THERAPY

Topical Therapies

- **Corticosteroids** (Table 17-1) have anti-inflammatory, antiproliferative, immunosuppressive, and vasoconstrictive effects. They are recommended in U.S. treatment guidelines as first-line treatment for limited psoriasis either as monotherapy or with

TABLE 17-1	Topical Corticosteroid Potency Chart
Potency Rating	**Topical Corticosteroid**
Class 1: Superpotent	Betamethasone dipropionate 0.05% ointment (Diprolene and Diprosone ointment)
	Clobetasol propionate 0.05% lotion/spray/shampoo/foam (Clobex lotion/spray/shampoo, OLUX and OLUX-E foam)
	Clobetasol propionate 0.05% cream, gel, solution (scalp), ointment (Cormax, Temovate, Dermovate)
	Diflorasone diacetate 0.05% ointment (Florone, Psorcon, ApexiCon)
	Flurandrenolide tape 4 mcg/cm^2 (Cordran)
	Halobetasol propionate 0.05% cream, lotion, ointment (Ultravate)
Class 2: Potent	Amcinonide 0.1% ointment (Cyclocort, Amcort)
	Betamethasone dipropionate 0.05% cream/gel (Diprolene cream, gel, and Diprosone cream)
	Desoximetasone 0.25% cream, gel, ointment (Topicort)
	Diflorasone diacetate 0.05% ointment (ApexiCon, Florone, Psorcon)
	Fluocinonide 0.05% cream, gel, ointment (Lidex)
	Halcinonide 0.1% cream (Halog)
Class 3: Upper mid-strength	Amcinonide 0.1% cream (Cyclocort)
	Betamethasone valerate 0.1% ointment (Betnovate/Valisone)
	Diflorasone diacetate 0.05% cream (Psorcon, Florone, ApexiCon)
	Fluticasone propionate 0.005% ointment (Cutivate)
	Mometasone furoate 0.1% ointment (Elocon)
	Triamcinolone acetonide 0.5% cream and ointment (Aristocort)
Class 4: Mid-strength	Betamethasone dipropionate 0.05% spray (Sernivo)
	Betamethasone valerate 0.12% foam (Luxiq)
	Clocortolone pivalate 0.1% cream (Cloderm)
	Desoximetasone 0.05% cream and gel (Topicort LP)
	Fluocinolone acetonide 0.025% ointment (Synalar)
	Fluocinolone acetonide 0.2% cream (Synalar-HP)
	Hydrocortisone valerate 0.2% ointment (Westcort)
	Mometasone furoate 0.1% cream, lotion, solution (Elocon)
	Triamcinolone acetonide 0.1% ointment (Kenalog)
Class 5: Lower mid-strength	Betamethasone dipropionate 0.05% lotion (Diprosone)
	Betamethasone valerate 0.1% cream and lotion (Betnovate/Valisone)
	Desonide 0.05% lotion, ointment, gel (DesOwen, Tridesilon)
	Fluocinolone acetonide 0.01% shampoo (Capex)
	Fluocinolone acetonide 0.01%, 0.025%, 0.03% cream (Synalar)
	Flurandrenolide 0.05% cream and lotion (Cordran)
	Fluticasone propionate 0.05% cream and lotion (Cutivate)
	Hydrocortisone butyrate 0.1% ointment, lotion, cream (Locoid, Locoid Lipocream)
	Hydrocortisone probutate 0.1% cream (Pandel)
	Hydrocortisone valerate 0.2% cream (Westcort)
	Prednicarbate 0.1% cream and ointment (Dermatop)
	Triamcinolone acetonide 0.1% cream, ointment, and lotion (Kenalog)
Class 6: Mild (low potency)	Alclometasone dipropionate 0.05% cream and ointment (Aclovate)
	Betamethasone valerate 0.05% cream and ointment (Valisone)
	Desonide 0.05% cream, ointment, gel (DesOwen, Desonate, Tridesilon)
	Desonide 0.05% foam (Verdeso)
	Fluocinonide acetonide 0.01% cream and solution (Synalar)
	Fluocinonide acetonide 0.01% FS oil (Derma-Smoothe)
Class 7: Least Potent	Hydrocortisone 0.5%, 1%, 2%, 2.5% cream, lotion, spray, and ointment (various brands)

nonsteroidal topical agents; potency can be enhanced with different vehicles, and as needed by occlusion.

✓ Lower-potency products should be used for infants and for lesions on the face, intertriginous areas, and areas with thin skin. Mid- to high-potency agents are recommended as initial therapy for other body areas in adults. Reserve the highest potency corticosteroids for patients with very thick plaques or recalcitrant disease, such as plaques on the palms and soles. Use potency class I corticosteroids for only 2–4 weeks.

✓ Ointments are the most occlusive and most potent formulations because of enhanced penetration into the dermis. Patients may prefer less greasy creams or lotions for daytime use.

✓ Cutaneous adverse effects include skin atrophy, acne, contact dermatitis, hypertrichosis, folliculitis, hypopigmentation, perioral dermatitis, striae, telangiectasias, and traumatic purpura. Systemic adverse effects may occur with superpotent agents or with extended or widespread use of mid-potency agents. Such effects include hypothalamic–pituitary–adrenal axis suppression and less commonly Cushing syndrome, osteonecrosis of the femoral head, cataracts, and glaucoma.

- **Calcipotriene** (Dovonex) and **calcitriol** (Vectical) are vitamin D_3 analogs that bind to vitamin D receptors, which inhibit keratinocyte proliferation and enhance keratinocyte differentiation. They also inhibit T-lymphocyte activity. These agents can be used as first-line monotherapy or in combination with a topical corticosteroid for mild plaque psoriasis. Calcipotriene 0.005% cream, ointment, foam, or gel is applied to affected areas twice daily. Calcitriol ointment 3 mcg/g is applied to affected areas twice daily. Adverse effects include mild irritant contact dermatitis, burning, pruritus, edema, peeling, dryness, and erythema.

- **Tazarotene** (Tazorac) is a topical retinoid that normalizes keratinocyte differentiation, diminishes keratinocyte hyperproliferation, and clears the inflammatory infiltrate in psoriatic plaques. It is available as a 0.05% or 0.1% gel and cream and is applied once daily (usually in the evening). It may be combined with a topical corticosteroid to enhance efficacy and reduce irritation. Adverse effects of tazarotene include a high incidence of dose-dependent irritation at application sites, resulting in burning, stinging, and erythema. Irritation may be reduced by using the cream formulation, lower concentration, alternate-day applications, or short-contact (30–60 minutes) treatment. Tazarotene is contraindicated in pregnancy and should not be used in women of childbearing potential unless effective contraception is being used.

- **Anthralin** has a direct antiproliferative effect on epidermal keratinocytes, normalizing keratinocyte differentiation. Short-contact anthralin therapy (SCAT) is the preferred regimen, with ointment applied only to the thick plaque lesions for 2 hours or less and then wiped off. Zinc oxide ointment or nonmedicated stiff paste should be applied to the surrounding normal skin to protect it from irritation. Use anthralin with caution, if at all, on the face and intertriginous areas due to potential for severe irritation. Anthralin concentrations for SCAT range from 1% to 4% or as tolerated. Concentrations for continuous therapy vary from 0.05% to 0.4%. Anthralin may cause severe skin irritation, folliculitis, and allergic contact dermatitis.

- **Coal tar** is keratolytic and may have antiproliferative and anti-inflammatory effects. Formulations include crude coal tar and tar distillates (liquor carbonis detergens) in ointments, creams, and shampoos. Coal tar is used infrequently due to limited efficacy and poor patient adherence and acceptance. It has a slower onset of action than calcipotriene, has an unpleasant odor, and stains clothing. Adverse effects include folliculitis, acne, local irritation, and phototoxicity. Risk of teratogenicity is low when used in pregnancy.

- **Salicylic acid** has keratolytic properties and has been used in shampoos or bath oils for scalp psoriasis. It enhances penetration of topical corticosteroids, thereby increasing corticosteroid efficacy. Systemic absorption and toxicity can occur, especially when applied to >20% BSA or in patients with renal impairment. Salicylic acid should not be used in children. It may be used for limited and localized plaque psoriasis in pregnancy.

- **Pimecrolimus** 1% cream (Elidel) is a calcineurin inhibitor shown to be effective for plaque psoriasis when used under occlusion and for patients with moderate-to-severe inverse psoriasis (involving intertriginous areas). It may be a useful alternative for patients with intertriginous or facial lesions because it is less irritating than calcipotriene and does not have the topical adverse effects of corticosteroids (eg, skin atrophy).

Phototherapy and Photochemotherapy

- Phototherapy consists of nonionizing electromagnetic radiation, either ultraviolet A (UVA) or ultraviolet B (UVB), as light therapy for psoriatic lesions. UVB is given alone as either broadband or narrowband (NB-UVB). UVB is also given as photochemotherapy with topical agents such as crude coal tar (Goeckerman regimen) or anthralin (Ingram regimen) for enhanced efficacy. UVA is generally given with a photosensitizer such as an oral psoralen to enhance efficacy; this regimen is called PUVA (psoralen + UVA treatment). Adverse effects of phototherapy include erythema, pruritus, xerosis, hyperpigmentation, and blistering. Patients must be provided with eye protection during and for 24 hours after PUVA treatments. PUVA therapy may also cause nausea or vomiting, which may be minimized by taking the oral psoralens with food or milk. Long-term PUVA use can lead to photoaging and cataracts. PUVA is also associated with a dose-related risk of carcinogenesis.

Systemic Nonbiologic Agents

- **Acitretin** (Soriatane) is a retinoic acid derivative and the active metabolite of etretinate. Retinoids may be less effective than methotrexate or cyclosporine when used as monotherapy. Acitretin is more commonly used in combination with topical calcipotriene or phototherapy. Although low-dose acitretin (25 mg/day) is safer and better tolerated than higher-dose (50 mg/day) therapy, low-dose acitretin is not recommended as monotherapy. Therapy is continued until lesions have resolved. It is better tolerated when taken with meals. Adverse effects include hypertriglyceridemia and mucocutaneous effects such as dryness of the eyes, nasal and oral mucosa; chapped lips; cheilitis; epistaxis; xerosis; brittle nails; and burning skin. Ophthalmologic changes include photosensitivity, decreased color vision, and impaired night vision. Hepatitis and jaundice are rare and liver enzyme elevations are usually transient. All retinoids are teratogenic and are contraindicated in pregnancy. Acitretin should not be used in women of childbearing potential unless they use effective contraception for the duration of therapy and for at least 2 years after drug discontinuation. Blood donation (men and women) is not permitted during and for at least 1 year after treatment.

- **Cyclosporine** is a systemic calcineurin inhibitor that is effective for inducing remission and for maintenance therapy of moderate-to-severe plaque psoriasis. Intermittent short-course therapy (<12 weeks) is preferable to continuous therapy because it appears to reduce the risk of nephrotoxicity. Cyclosporine is significantly more effective than etretinate and has similar or slightly better efficacy than methotrexate. The usual oral dose is 2.5–5 mg/kg/day given in two divided doses. After inducing remission, maintenance therapy using low doses (1.25–3 mg/kg/day) may prevent relapse. When discontinuing cyclosporine, a gradual taper of 1 mg/kg/day each week may prolong the time before relapse compared to abrupt discontinuation. Because more than half of patients stopping cyclosporine relapse within 4 months, patients should be given appropriate alternative treatments shortly before or after discontinuing cyclosporine. Adverse effects include nephrotoxicity, hypertension, hypomagnesemia, hyperkalemia, hypertriglyceridemia, hypertrichosis, and gingival hyperplasia. The risk of skin cancer increases with the duration of treatment and with prior PUVA treatments.

- **Methotrexate** has anti-inflammatory effects due to its effects on T-cell gene expression and also has cytostatic effects. It is more effective than acitretin and has similar or slightly less efficacy than cyclosporine. Methotrexate can be administered orally, subcutaneously (SC), or intramuscularly. The starting dose is 7.5–15 mg once weekly, increased incrementally by 2.5 mg every 2–4 weeks until response; maximal doses are 25 mg weekly. Adverse effects include nausea, vomiting, stomatitis, macrocytic anemia, and hepatic and pulmonary toxicity. Nausea and macrocytic anemia may be reduced by giving oral folic acid 1–5 mg daily. It is an abortifacient and teratogenic and is contraindicated in pregnancy.

- **Tofacitinib** (Xeljanz, Xeljanz XR) is a small-molecule Janus Kinase (JAK) inhibitor that blocks signaling through common receptors for cytokines including IL-2, IL-4, IL-7, IL-9, IL-15, and IL-21. It is indicated for the treatment of adults with active psoriatic arthritis who have had an inadequate response or intolerance to methotrexate or other disease-modifying antirheumatic drugs (DMARDs). The recommended dose (in combination with nonbiologic DMARDs) is 5 mg orally twice daily or 11 mg (extended-release) once daily. The recommended dose is 5 mg once daily in patients with moderate-to-severe renal impairment or moderate hepatic impairment. Tofacitinib should not be used in combination with biologic DMARDs or potent immunosuppressants such as azathioprine and cyclosporine.

- **Apremilast** (Otezla) is a small-molecule inhibitor of phosphodiesterase 4 (PDE4), which increases intracellular cyclic AMP (cAMP) and reduces production of pro-inflammatory mediators. It is indicated for treatment of adults with active psoriatic arthritis and patients with moderate-to-severe plaque psoriasis who are candidates for phototherapy or systemic therapy. Recommended dosing is 10 mg orally on day 1, 10 mg twice daily on day 2, 10 mg in the morning and 20 mg in the evening on day 3, 20 mg twice daily on day 4, 20 mg in the morning and 30 mg in the evening on day 5, then 30 mg twice daily thereafter. The dosage regimen should be reduced in severe renal impairment. The most common adverse reactions ($\geq$5%) are diarrhea, nausea, and headache.

Systemic Biologic Agents

- Biologic agents are considered for moderate-to-severe psoriasis when other systemic agents are inadequate or contraindicated or when comorbidities exist. Cost considerations tend to limit their use as first-line therapy.

TNF Inhibitors

- **Adalimumab** (Humira) is a monoclonal TNF-α antibody that provides rapid control of psoriasis. It is indicated for psoriatic arthritis and treatment of adults with moderate-to-severe chronic plaque psoriasis who are candidates for systemic therapy or phototherapy. The recommended dose for psoriatic arthritis is 40-mg SC every other week. The recommended dose for adults with plaque psoriasis is an initial dose of 80-mg SC, followed by 40 mg every other week starting 1 week after the initial dose. The most common adverse reactions are infections (eg, upper respiratory and sinusitis), injection site reactions, headache, and rash.

- **Etanercept** (Enbrel) is a fusion protein that binds TNF-α, competitively interfering with its interaction with cell-bound receptors. Unlike the chimeric infliximab, etanercept is fully humanized, minimizing the risk of immunogenicity. Etanercept is FDA approved for reducing signs and symptoms and inhibiting the progression of joint damage in patients with psoriatic arthritis; it can be used alone or in combination with methotrexate. It is also indicated for patients 4 years or older with chronic moderate-to-severe plaque psoriasis who are candidates for systemic therapy or phototherapy. The recommended dose for psoriatic arthritis is 50-mg SC once weekly. For plaque psoriasis, the dose is 50-mg SC twice weekly (administered 3 or 4 days apart) for 3 months, followed by a maintenance dose of 50 mg once weekly. Adverse effects include local reactions at the injection site (20% of patients), respiratory tract and GI infections, abdominal pain, nausea and vomiting, headaches, and rash.

- **Infliximab** (Remicade) is a chimeric monoclonal antibody directed against TNF-α. It is indicated for psoriatic arthritis and chronic severe plaque psoriasis. The recommended dose is 5 mg/kg by IV infusion at weeks 0, 2, and 6, then every 8 weeks thereafter. For psoriatic arthritis, it may be used with or without methotrexate. Adverse effects include headaches, fever, chills, fatigue, diarrhea, pharyngitis, and upper respiratory and urinary tract infections. Hypersensitivity reactions (urticaria, dyspnea, and hypotension) and lymphoproliferative disorders have been reported.

- **Certolizumab pegol** (Cimzia) is a humanized antigen-binding fragment of a monoclonal antibody that is further conjugated with a polyethylene glycol moiety. This binds to TNF-α, blocking its interaction with TNF receptors. It is indicated for treatment of adults with psoriatic arthritis or moderate-to-severe plaque psoriasis who are candidates for systemic therapy or phototherapy. Recommended dosing is 400 mg (as 2 × 200-mg SC injections) every 2 weeks, with a dose-reduced regimen for patients <90 kg: 400 mg (as 2 × 200-mg SC injections) initially and at weeks 2 and 4, followed by 200-mg SC every other week.

Interleukin-12/23 Inhibitors

- **Ustekinumab** (Stelara) is an IL-12/23 monoclonal antibody approved for the treatment of psoriasis in adults 18 years or older with moderate-to-severe plaque psoriasis. The recommended dose for patients weighing ≤100 kg is 45-mg SC initially and 4 weeks later, followed by 45-mg SC every 12 weeks. For patients weighing >100 kg, the dose is 90-mg SC initially and 4 weeks later, followed by 90-mg SC every 12 weeks. Common adverse effects include upper respiratory infections, headache, and tiredness. Serious adverse effects include those seen with other biologics, including tubercular, fungal, and viral infections and cancers. Reversible posterior leukoencephalopathy syndrome (RPLS) has also been reported.

Interleukin-17A Inhibitors

- **Secukinumab** (Cosentyx), **ixekizumab** (Taltz), and **brodalumab** (Siliq) are monoclonal antibodies that inhibit IL-17A, a proinflammatory cytokine that binds to receptors on keratinocytes, leading to inflammation and recruitment of inflammatory cell types, resulting in psoriatic plaques. These agents have comparable efficacy and similar adverse effects (eg, nasopharyngitis, upper respiratory tract infections, injection site reactions).
  ✓ Secukinumab is a fully human IgG1κ monoclonal antibody that selectively binds and inhibits IL-17A. Recommended dosing for plaque psoriasis is 300-mg SC at weeks 0, 1, 2, 3, and 4 followed by 300-mg SC every 4 weeks.
  ✓ Ixekizumab is a humanized IgG4 monoclonal antibody that neutralizes IL-17A. Recommended dosing is an initial dose of 160-mg SC followed by 80 mg every 2 weeks until week 12, followed by a maintenance phase of 80-mg SC every 4 weeks thereafter. Neutralizing anti-ixekizumab antibodies develop over time and are associated with reduced drug concentrations and loss of efficacy.
  ✓ Brodalumab is a fully human IgG2 anti-IL-17RA monoclonal antibody that binds to the IL-17 receptor A and blocks the biologic activities of multiple IL-17 subtypes. The recommended dose is 210-mg SC on weeks 0, 1, and 2, then 210 mg every 2 weeks thereafter.

Interleukin-23 Inhibitors

- **Guselkumab** (Tremfya), **tildrakizumab** (Ilumya), and **risankizumab** (Skyrizi) inhibit IL-23, which induces a population of T-helper cells (TH17 cells) with a unique inflammatory gene signature important in the pathogenesis of psoriasis and other autoimmune diseases. Neutralizing antibodies to specific IL-17 inhibitors have been reported that may be associated with lower biologic serum concentrations and reduced efficacy.
  ✓ Guselkumab is a fully human IgG1 lambda monoclonal antibody that blocks the p19 subunit of IL-23. The recommended dose is 100-mg SC at weeks 0 and 4, and then every 8 weeks thereafter.
  ✓ Tildrakizumab is a humanized IgG1 monoclonal antibody designed to selectively block IL-23 by binding to the p19 subunit. The recommended dose is 100-mg

SC administered only by a healthcare provider at weeks 0 and 4, and then every 12 weeks thereafter.

✓ Risankizumab is a humanized IgG1 monoclonal antibody that selectively inhibits IL-23 by binding to the p19 subunit. The recommended dose is 150 mg (two 75-mg SC injections) at weeks 0 and 4 and then every 12 weeks thereafter.

Combination Therapies

- Combination therapy may be used to enhance efficacy or minimize toxicity. Combinations can include two topical agents, a topical agent plus phototherapy, a systemic agent plus topical therapy, a systemic agent plus phototherapy, two systemic agents used in rotation, or a biologic agent with either a nonbiologic systemic or topical agent (see Figs. 17-1 and 17-2).
- The combination of a topical corticosteroid and a topical vitamin D_3 analog is effective and safe with less skin irritation than monotherapy with either agent. The combination product containing calcipotriene and betamethasone dipropionate ointment (Taclonex) is effective for relatively severe psoriasis and may also be steroid sparing.
- The combination of retinoids with phototherapy (eg, tazarotene plus broadband UVB, acitretin plus broadband UVB or NB-UVB) also increases efficacy. Because retinoids may be photosensitizing and increase the risk of burning after UV exposure, doses of phototherapy should be reduced to minimize adverse effects. The combination of acitretin and PUVA (RE-PUVA) may be more effective than monotherapy with either treatment.
- Phototherapy has also been used with other topical agents, such as UVB with coal tar (Goeckerman regimen) to increase treatment response, because coal tar is also photosensitizing.
- Cyclosporine in combination with calcipotriene/betamethasone dipropionate is superior to cyclosporine alone. Cyclosporine may also be used with SCAT, but it should not be used with PUVA due to reduced efficacy and an increased risk of cutaneous malignancies.
- The combination of methotrexate and UVB appears to be synergistic. Low-dose methotrexate (eg, 7.5–10 mg once weekly) in combination with a biologic agent may be beneficial.

Alternative Drug Treatments

- **Mycophenolate mofetil** (CellCept) inhibits DNA and RNA synthesis and may have a lymphocyte antiproliferative effect. Although not FDA approved for psoriasis indications, oral mycophenolate mofetil may be effective in some cases of moderate-to-severe plaque psoriasis.
- **Hydroxyurea** inhibits cell synthesis in the S phase of the DNA cycle. It is occasionally used off-label for patients with recalcitrant severe psoriasis, but biologic agents may be a better option in these patients.

EVALUATION OF THERAPEUTIC OUTCOMES

- Help patients understand the general principles of therapy and the importance of medication adherence.
- A positive response involves normalization of involved areas of skin, as measured by reduced erythema and scaling, as well as reduction of plaque elevation.
- Successful management also includes control of itching and comorbid conditions such as dyslipidemia, hypertension, psoriatic arthritis, and depression.
- PASI is a uniform method to determine the extent of BSA affected, along with the degree of erythema, induration, and scaling. In the United States, severity of psoriasis is classified as mild, moderate, or severe:
  ✓ Mild: ≤5% BSA involvement
  ✓ Moderate: PASI ≥8 (higher in trials of biologics)
  ✓ Severe: PASI ≥10 or Dermatology Life Quality Index (DLQI) ≥10 or BSA ≥10%

- The Physician Global Assessment can also be used to summarize erythema, induration, scaling, and extent of plaques relative to baseline assessment.
- Achievement of efficacy by any therapeutic regimen requires days to weeks. The initial dramatic response may be achieved with some agents, such as corticosteroids. However, sustained benefit with pharmacologically specific antipsoriatic therapy may require 2–8 weeks or longer for clinically meaningful response.

See Chapter 118, Psoriasis, authored by Rebecca M. Law and Wayne P. Gulliver, for a more detailed discussion of this topic.

18 Adrenal Gland Disorders

- Hyperfunction of the adrenal glands involves excess production of the adrenal hormones cortisol (resulting in Cushing syndrome) or aldosterone (resulting in hyperaldosteronism).
- Adrenal gland hypofunction is associated with primary (Addison disease) or secondary adrenal insufficiency.

Cushing Syndrome

PATHOPHYSIOLOGY

- Cushing syndrome results from effects of supraphysiologic glucocorticoid concentrations originating from either exogenous administration or endogenous overproduction by the adrenal gland (adrenocorticotropic hormone [ACTH] dependent) or by abnormal adrenocortical tissues (ACTH independent).
- ACTH-dependent Cushing syndrome (80% of all Cushing syndrome cases) is usually caused by overproduction of ACTH by the pituitary gland, causing bilateral adrenal hyperplasia. Pituitary adenomas account for about 85% of these cases (Cushing disease). Ectopic ACTH-secreting tumors and nonneoplastic corticotropin hypersecretion cause the remaining 20% of ACTH-dependent cases.
- Ectopic ACTH syndrome refers to excessive ACTH production resulting from an endocrine or nonendocrine tumor, usually of the pancreas, thyroid, or lung (eg, small-cell lung cancer).
- ACTH-independent Cushing syndrome is usually caused by adrenal adenomas and carcinomas.

CLINICAL PRESENTATION

- The most common findings in Cushing syndrome are central obesity and facial rounding (90% of patients). Peripheral obesity and fat accumulation occur in 50% of patients. Fat accumulation in the dorsocervical area (buffalo hump) is nonspecific, but increased supraclavicular fat pads are more specific for Cushing syndrome. Patients are often described as having moon facies and a buffalo hump.
- Other findings may include myopathy or muscular weakness, abdominal striae, hypertension, glucose intolerance, psychiatric changes, gonadal dysfunction, facial plethora (reddish complexion), and amenorrhea and hirsutism in women.
- Up to 60% of patients develop Cushing-induced osteoporosis; about 40% present with back pain, and 20% progress to spinal compression fractures.

DIAGNOSIS

- Hypercortisolism can be established with one or more of the following tests: 24-hour urinary free cortisol (UFC), midnight plasma cortisol, late-night (11 PM) salivary cortisol, and/or low-dose dexamethasone suppression test (DST).
- Other tests to determine etiology are plasma ACTH; adrenal vein catheterization; metyrapone stimulation test; adrenal, chest, or abdominal computed tomography (CT);

corticotropin-releasing hormone (CRH) stimulation test; inferior petrosal sinus sampling; and pituitary magnetic resonance imaging (MRI).
- Adrenal nodules and masses are identified using high-resolution CT scanning or MRI.

TREATMENT

- <u>Goals of Treatment</u>: Limit morbidity and mortality and return the patient to a normal functional state by removing the source of hypercortisolism while minimizing pituitary or adrenal deficiencies.
- Treatment plans in Cushing syndrome based on etiology are included in Table 18-1.

NONPHARMACOLOGIC THERAPY

- Treatment of choice for both ACTH-dependent and ACTH-independent Cushing syndrome is surgical resection of offending tumors.
- Transsphenoidal resection of the pituitary tumor is the treatment of choice for Cushing disease. Radiotherapy may be preferred for tumors invading the dura or cavernous sinus and provides clinical improvement in ~50% of patients within 3–5 years but increases the risk for pituitary-dependent hormone deficiencies (hypopituitarism).
- Laparoscopic adrenalectomy is often preferred for unilateral adrenal adenomas or when transsphenoidal surgery and pituitary radiotherapy have failed or cannot be used.

PHARMACOLOGIC THERAPY

- Pharmacotherapy is generally used as second-line treatment in patients who are not surgical candidates and may also be used preoperatively or as adjunctive therapy in postoperative patients awaiting response (Table 18-1). Rarely, monotherapy is used as a palliative treatment when surgery is not indicated.

Steroidogenesis Inhibitors

- **Metyrapone** inhibits 11 β-hydroxylase, thereby inhibiting cortisol synthesis. After administration, a sudden decrease in cortisol concentration prompts a compensatory rise in plasma ACTH levels. With cortisol synthesis blocked, adrenal steroidogenesis shunts toward androgen production, resulting in androgenic side effects such as acne and hirsutism. Inhibition of aldosterone synthesis can result in natriuresis and blood pressure changes. Nausea, vomiting, vertigo, headache, dizziness, abdominal discomfort, and allergic rash have been reported after oral administration.
- **Ketoconazole** inhibits cytochrome P-450 enzymes, including 11 β-hydroxylase and 17 α-hydroxylase. It is effective in lowering serum cortisol levels after several weeks of therapy. It also has antiandrogenic activity, which may be beneficial in women but can cause gynecomastia and hypogonadism in men. The most common adverse effects are reversible elevation of hepatic transaminases, GI discomfort, and dermatologic reactions. Because of the risk of severe hepatotoxicity, monitoring should include liver function tests at baseline followed by weekly monitoring of serum ALT throughout therapy. Ketoconazole may be used concomitantly with metyrapone to achieve synergistic reduction in cortisol levels; in addition, ketoconazole's antiandrogenic actions may offset the androgenic potential of metyrapone.
- **Etomidate** is an imidazole derivative similar to ketoconazole that inhibits 11 β-hydroxylase and may have other mechanisms. Because it is only available in a parenteral formulation, use is limited to patients with acute hypercortisolemia requiring emergency treatment or in preparation for surgery. Frequent monitoring of serum cortisol is advised to prevent hypocortisolemia. Side effects include sedation, injection site pain, hypotension, myoclonus, nausea, and vomiting. The initial dose is 0.03 mg/kg by IV bolus followed by a continuous infusion of 0.1–0.3 mg/kg/h.
- **Osilodrostat** (Itsurisa) prevents cortisol synthesis via inhibition of 11βhydroxylase and is indicated for patients with Cushing disease who are either not candidates for surgery or in whom symptoms persist after surgery. Osilodrostat is available as an oral tablet taken twice daily, with or without food. Hypokalemia and hypomagnesemia should be corrected prior to use, and an ECG should be obtained at baseline

TABLE 18-1 Treatment Options in Cushing Syndrome Based on Etiology

Etiology	Nondrug	Generic (Brand) Drug Name	Dosing		
			Initial Dose	Usual Range	Maximum
Ectopic ACTH syndrome	Surgery, chemotherapy, irradiation	Metyrapone (Metopirone) 250-mg capsules	0.5–1 g/day, divided every 4–6 hours	1–2 g/day, divided every 4–6 hours	6 g/day
		Ketoconazole (Nizoral) 200-mg tablets	200 mg once or twice a day	200–1200 mg/day, divided twice daily	1600 mg/day divided four times daily
Pituitary dependent	Surgery, irradiation	Mitotane (Lysodren) 500-mg tablets	0.5–1 g/day, increased by 0.5–1 g/day every 1–4 weeks	1–4 g daily, with food to decrease GI effects	12 g/day
		Metyrapone	See above	See above	See above
		Mifepristone (Korlym) 300-mg tablets	300 mg once daily, increased by 300 mg/day every 2–4 weeks	600–1200 mg/day	1200 mg/day or 20 mg/kg/day
		Cabergoline (Dostinex) 0.5-mg tablets	0.5 mg once weekly	0.5–7 mg once weekly	7 mg/week
		Pasireotide (Signifor) 0.3-, 0.6-, and 0.9-mg/mL solution	0.6–0.9 mg twice daily	0.3–0.9 mg twice daily	1.8 mg/day
Adrenal adenoma	Surgery, postoperative replacement	Ketoconazole	See above	See above	See above
Adrenal carcinoma	Surgery	Mitotane	See above	See above	See above

ACTH, adrenocorticotropic hormone.

193

and again one week after treatment initiation to monitor possible QTc prolongation. Adverse effects are similar to other 11βhydroxylase inhibitors, including hypocortisolism, QTc prolongation, nausea, and headache.

Adrenolytic Agents

- **Mitotane** is a cytotoxic drug that inhibits the 11-hydroxylation of 11-deoxycortisol and 11-desoxycorticosterone in the adrenal cortex, reducing synthesis of cortisol and corticosterone. Similar to ketoconazole, mitotane takes weeks to months to exert beneficial effects. Sustained cortisol suppression occurs in most patients and may persist after drug discontinuation in up to one-third of patients. Mitotane degenerates cells within the zona fasciculata and reticularis, resulting in atrophy of the adrenal cortex; the zona glomerulosa is minimally affected during acute therapy but can be damaged during long-term treatment. Mitotane can cause significant neurologic and GI side effects, and patients should be monitored carefully or hospitalized when initiating therapy. Nausea and diarrhea are common at doses greater than 2 g/day and can be avoided by gradually increasing the dose and/or administering it with food. Lethargy, somnolence, and other CNS effects are also common. Reversible hypercholesterolemia and prolonged bleeding times can occur.

Neuromodulators of ACTH Release

- Pituitary secretion of ACTH is normally mediated by neurotransmitters such as serotonin, γ-aminobutyric acid (GABA), acetylcholine, and catecholamines. Although ACTH-secreting pituitary tumors (Cushing disease) self-regulate ACTH production to some degree, these neurotransmitters can still promote pituitary ACTH production. Consequently, agents that target these transmitters have been proposed for treatment of Cushing disease, including cyproheptadine, bromocriptine, cabergoline, valproic acid, octreotide, lanreotide, pasireotide, rosiglitazone, and tretinoin. With the exception of pasireotide, none of these drugs have demonstrated consistent clinical efficacy for treating Cushing disease.
- **Cyproheptadine**, a nonselective serotonin receptor antagonist and anticholinergic drug, can decrease ACTH secretion in some patients with Cushing disease. However, side effects such as sedation and weight gain significantly limit its use.
- **Pasireotide** (Signifor) is a somatostatin analog that binds and activates somatostatin receptors, thereby inhibiting ACTH secretion, leading to decreased cortisol secretion. It is approved for treatment of adults with Cushing disease for whom pituitary surgery is not an option or has not been curative. Side effects include nausea, diarrhea, cholelithiasis, increased hepatic transaminases, hyperglycemia, sinus bradycardia, and QT prolongation.

Glucocorticoid-Receptor Blocking Agents

- **Mifepristone** (Korlym) is a progesterone- and glucocorticoid-receptor antagonist that inhibits dexamethasone suppression and increases endogenous cortisol and ACTH levels in normal subjects. Evidence suggests that mifepristone is highly effective in reversing the manifestations of hypercortisolism (hyperglycemia, hypertension, and weight gain). It is FDA approved for treatment of endogenous Cushing syndrome in patients who have type 2 diabetes or glucose intolerance and who are not eligible for, or have had poor response to, surgery. Common adverse effects include fatigue, nausea, headache, arthralgia, peripheral edema, endometrial hyperplasia, and hypokalemia.

EVALUATION OF THERAPEUTIC OUTCOMES

- Close monitoring of 24-hour UFC and serum cortisol is essential to identify adrenal insufficiency in patients with Cushing syndrome. Monitor steroid secretion with all drug therapy (except mifepristone) and give corticosteroid replacement if needed.

Hyperaldosteronism

PATHOPHYSIOLOGY

- Hyperaldosteronism involves excess aldosterone secretion and is categorized as either primary (stimulus arising from within the adrenal gland) or secondary (stimulus from extra-adrenal etiologies).
- *Primary hyperaldosteronism* (PA) is usually caused by bilateral adrenal hyperplasia and aldosterone-producing adenoma (Conn syndrome). Rare causes include unilateral (primary) adrenal hyperplasia, adrenal cortex carcinoma, renin-responsive adrenocortical adenoma, and three forms of familial hyperaldosteronism (FH): Type I (glucocorticoid-remediable aldosteronism); Type II (familial occurrence of adenoma or hyperplasia type II); and Type III.
- *Secondary hyperaldosteronism* results from excessive stimulation of the zona glomerulosa by an extra-adrenal factor, usually the renin–angiotensin system. Elevated aldosterone secretion can result from excessive potassium intake, oral contraceptives, pregnancy, and menses. Heart failure, cirrhosis, renal artery stenosis, and Bartter syndrome also can lead to elevated aldosterone concentrations.

CLINICAL PRESENTATION

- Patients may complain of muscle weakness, fatigue, paresthesias, headache, polydipsia, and nocturnal polyuria.
- Signs may include hypertension, tetany/paralysis, and polydipsia/nocturnal polyuria.
- A plasma aldosterone concentration-to-plasma renin activity (PAC-to-PRA) ratio or aldosterone-to-renin ratio (ARR) >30 ng/dL per ng/(mL·h) (830 pmol/L per mcg/(L·h) and a PAC >15 ng/dL (420 pmol/L) is suggestive of PA.
- Other laboratory findings include suppressed renin activity, elevated plasma aldosterone, hypernatremia (>142 mEq/L), hypokalemia, hypomagnesemia, elevated serum bicarbonate (>31 mEq/L), and glucose intolerance.

DIAGNOSIS

- Initial diagnosis is made by screening patients with suspected PA. Any patient with a blood pressure >150/100 mm Hg measured on three separate days, and those meeting the criteria for treatment-resistant hypertension should be screened. Additional patients at risk for PA include those with diuretic-induced hypokalemia, hypertension and adrenal incidentaloma, hypertension and sleep apnea, hypertension and a family history of early onset hypertension or cerebrovascular accident at an age <40 years, and all patients with hypertension and a first-degree relative diagnosed with PA.
- Screening for PA is most often done using the PAC-to-PRA ratio (also known as the ARR). An elevated ARR is highly suggestive of PA.
- If the ARR is positive, confirmatory tests to exclude false-positives include the oral sodium-loading test, saline infusion test, fludrocortisone suppression test (FST), and captopril challenge test. A positive test indicates autonomous aldosterone secretion under inhibitory pressures and is diagnostic for PA.

TREATMENT

NONPHARMACOLOGIC THERAPY

- Aldosterone-producing adenomas are treated by laparoscopic resection of the tumor, leading to permanent cures in up to 72% of patients. Medical management with an aldosterone receptor antagonist is often effective if surgery is contraindicated.

PHARMACOLOGIC THERAPY

- Aldosterone-receptor antagonists are the treatment of choice for bilateral adrenal hyperplasia.
  - ✓ **Spironolactone** (Aldactone) is a nonselective aldosterone receptor antagonist that competes with aldosterone for binding at aldosterone receptors, thus preventing the negative effects of aldosterone receptor activation. The initial dose is 25 mg once daily titrated upward at 4- to 8-week intervals. Most patients respond to doses between 25 and 400 mg/day given in single or divided doses. Adverse effects include GI discomfort, impotence, gynecomastia, menstrual irregularities, and hyperkalemia.
  - ✓ **Eplerenone** (Inspra) is a selective aldosterone receptor antagonist with high affinity for aldosterone receptors and low affinity for androgen and progesterone receptors. Consequently, it elicits fewer sex-steroid–dependent effects than spironolactone. Dosing starts at 50 mg daily, with titration at 4- to 8-week intervals to 50 mg twice a day; some patients may require total daily doses as high as 200–300 mg.
  - ✓ **Amiloride** (Amiloride), a potassium-sparing diuretic, is less effective than spironolactone, and patients often require additional therapy to adequately control blood pressure. The initial dose is 5 mg twice daily, with a usual range of 20 mg/day given in two divided doses; doses up to 30 mg/day may be necessary.
  - ✓ Additional second-line options include calcium channel blockers, ACE inhibitors, and diuretics such as chlorthalidone, although all of these lack outcome data in PA.
- Treatment of secondary aldosteronism is dictated by etiology. Control or correction of the extra-adrenal stimulation of aldosterone secretion should resolve the disorder. Medical therapy with spironolactone is undertaken until the etiology is identified.

Adrenal Insufficiency

PATHOPHYSIOLOGY

- Primary adrenal insufficiency (Addison disease) usually involves destruction of all regions of the adrenal cortex. There are deficiencies of cortisol, aldosterone, and the various androgens, and levels of CRH and ACTH increase in a compensatory manner.
- Autoimmune dysfunction is responsible for 80%–90% of cases in developed countries, whereas tuberculosis is the predominant cause in developing countries.
- Medications that inhibit cortisol synthesis (eg, ketoconazole) or accelerate cortisol metabolism (eg, phenytoin, rifampin, phenobarbital) can also cause primary adrenal insufficiency.
- Secondary adrenal insufficiency most commonly results from exogenous corticosteroid use, leading to suppression of the hypothalamic–pituitary–adrenal axis and decreased ACTH release as well as impaired androgen and cortisol production. Mirtazapine and progestins (eg, medroxyprogesterone acetate, megestrol acetate) have also been reported to induce secondary adrenal insufficiency. Secondary disease typically presents with normal mineralocorticoid concentrations.

CLINICAL PRESENTATION

- Patients with adrenal insufficiency commonly complain of weakness, weight loss, GI symptoms, salt craving, headaches, memory impairment, depression, and postural dizziness.
- Early symptoms of acute adrenal insufficiency also include myalgias, malaise, and anorexia. As the situation progresses, vomiting, fever, hypotension, and shock develop.
- Signs of adrenal insufficiency include increased skin pigmentation, postural hypotension, fever, decreased body hair, vitiligo, amenorrhea, and cold intolerance.

DIAGNOSIS

- The short cosyntropin stimulation test can be used to assess patients with suspected hypercortisolism. An increase to a cortisol level of ≥18 mcg/dL (500 nmol/L) rules out adrenal insufficiency.
- Patients with Addison disease have an abnormal response to the short cosyntropin stimulation test. Plasma ACTH levels are usually elevated (400–2000 pg/mL or 88–440 pmol/L) in primary insufficiency versus normal to low (5–50 pg/mL or 1.1–11 pmol/L]) in secondary insufficiency. A normal cosyntropin-stimulation test does not rule out secondary adrenal insufficiency.
- Other tests include the insulin hypoglycemia test, the metyrapone test, and the CRH stimulation test.

TREATMENT

- <u>Goals of Treatment</u>: Limit morbidity and mortality, return the patient to a normal functional state, and prevent episodes of acute adrenal insufficiency.

NONPHARMACOLOGIC THERAPY

- Inform patients of treatment complications, expected outcomes, proper medication administration and adherence, and possible side effects.

PHARMACOLOGIC THERAPY

Corticosteroids

- The agents of choice are **hydrocortisone** and **cortisone acetate**, usually administered two times daily, with the goal of establishing the lowest effective dose while mimicking the normal diurnal adrenal rhythm. Once-daily **prednisolone** is an alternative when adherence to a multidose regimen is a concern.
- Recommended starting total daily doses are hydrocortisone 15–25 mg daily, which is approximately equivalent to cortisone acetate 20–35 mg daily, or prednisolone 3–5 mg daily (Table 18-2). For hydrocortisone or cortisone, two-thirds of the dose is given in the morning and one-third is given 6–8 hours later.
- Monitor the patient's symptoms every 6–8 weeks to assess proper glucocorticoid replacement. Measure body weight, postural blood pressures, subjective energy levels, and signs of glucocorticoid excess.
- In primary adrenal insufficiency, **fludrocortisone acetate** 0.05–0.2 mg orally once daily can be used to replace mineralocorticoid loss and maintain volume status. If parenteral therapy is needed, 2–5 mg of **deoxycorticosterone trimethylacetate** in oil can be administered intramuscularly every 3–4 weeks. Mineralocorticoid

TABLE 18-2	Relative Potencies of Glucocorticoids			
Glucocorticoid	Anti-inflammatory Potency	Equivalent Potency (mg)	Approximate Half-Life (min)	Sodium-Retaining Potency
Cortisone	0.8	25	30	2
Hydrocortisone	1	20	90	2
Prednisone	3.5	5	60	1
Prednisolone	4	5	200	1
Triamcinolone	5	4	300	0
Methylprednisolone	5	4	180	0
Betamethasone	25	0.6	100–300	0
Dexamethasone	30	0.75	100–300	0

replacement attenuates development of hyperkalemia, and patients on fludrocortisone therapy do not need to restrict salt intake. Mineralocorticoid therapy may be unnecessary in some cases because glucocorticoids (especially in large doses) also bind to mineralocorticoid receptors.

- Because most adrenal crises occur because of glucocorticoid dose reductions or lack of stress-related dose adjustments, patients receiving corticosteroid replacement therapy should add 5–10 mg hydrocortisone (or equivalent) to their normal daily regimen shortly before strenuous activities, such as exercise. During times of severe physical stress (eg, febrile illness, injury), patients should be instructed to double their daily dose until recovery.
- Treatment of secondary adrenal insufficiency is similar to primary disease treatment, except that mineralocorticoid replacement is usually not necessary.

PHARMACOLOGIC THERAPY OF ACUTE ADRENAL INSUFFICIENCY

- Acute adrenal insufficiency (adrenal crisis or Addisonian crisis) represents a true endocrine emergency. Major clinical features include volume depletion and hypotension that resolve within 1–2 hours after parenteral glucocorticoid administration.
- Stressful situations, surgery, infection, and trauma are potential events that increase adrenal requirements, especially in patients with some underlying adrenal or pituitary insufficiency.
- The most common cause of adrenal crisis is HPA-axis suppression brought on by abrupt withdrawal of chronic glucocorticoid use.
- **Hydrocortisone** given parenterally is the corticosteroid of choice because of its combined glucocorticoid and mineralocorticoid activity. The starting dose is 100 mg IV by rapid infusion, followed by 200 mg over 24 hours as a continuous infusion or a 50 mg intermittent bolus every 6 hours. IV administration is continued for an additional day at a reduced dose of 100 mg over 24 hours. If the patient is stable at that time, oral hydrocortisone can be started at a dose of 50 mg every 6–8 hours, followed by tapering to the individual's chronic replacement needs.
- **Fluid replacement** often is required and can be accomplished with IV dextrose 5% in normal saline solution at a rate to support blood pressure.
- If therapy is needed for hypoglycemia, dextrose 25% in water can be infused at a dose of 2–4 mL/kg (maximum single dose of 25-g dextrose).
- If hyperkalemia is present after the hydrocortisone maintenance phase, additional mineralocorticoid supplementation can be achieved with **fludrocortisone acetate** 0.1 mg daily.
- Patients with adrenal insufficiency should carry a card or wear a bracelet or necklace that contains information about their condition. They should also have easy access to injectable hydrocortisone or glucocorticoid suppositories in case of an emergency or during times of physical stress, such as febrile illness or injury.

EVALUATION OF THERAPEUTIC OUTCOMES

- The endpoint of therapy for adrenal insufficiency is difficult to assess in most patients, but a reduction in excess pigmentation is a good clinical marker. Development of features of Cushing syndrome indicates excessive replacement.

See Chapter 97, Adrenal Gland Disorders, authored by Steven M. Smith, Christopher R. Piszczatoski, and John G. Gums, for a more detailed discussion of this topic.

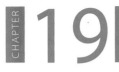
- *Diabetes mellitus* (DM) is a group of metabolic disorders characterized by chronically elevated blood glucose (BG) and abnormal carbohydrate, fat, and protein metabolism. Without effective treatment, DM can lead to acute complications such as diabetic keto-acidosis (DKA) and hyperosmolar hyperglycemic syndrome (HHS). Chronic hyperglycemia can cause microvascular, macrovascular, and neuropathic complications.

PATHOPHYSIOLOGY

- Type 1 DM (5%–10% of cases) usually results from autoimmune destruction of pancreatic β-cells, leading to absolute deficiency of insulin. It usually presents in children and adolescents but can occur at any age. The disorder is believed to be initiated by exposure to an unknown environmental trigger in a genetically susceptible individual. The autoimmune process is mediated by macrophages and T lymphocytes with autoantibodies to β-cell antigens (eg, islet cell antibody, insulin antibodies). Amylin (a hormone cosecreted from pancreatic β-cells with insulin) is also deficient in type 1 DM due to β-cell destruction. Amylin suppresses inappropriate glucagon secretion, slows gastric emptying, and causes centrally mediated satiety.
  - ✓ After the initial diagnosis, a period of transient remission called the "honeymoon" phase may occur, during which insulin doses can be reduced or withdrawn before continued β-cell destruction requires lifelong insulin replacement therapy.
- Type 2 DM (90%–95% of cases) is characterized by multiple defects:
  - ✓ *Impaired insulin secretion*: β-cell mass and function are both reduced, and β-cell failure is progressive.
  - ✓ *Reduced incretin effect*: Normally, the gut incretin hormones glucagon-like peptide-1 (GLP-1) and glucose-dependent insulinotropic peptide (GIP) are released and stimulate insulin secretion in response to a meal. Patients with type 2 DM have a reduced incretin effect due to decreased concentrations of or resistance to the effects of incretin hormones.
  - ✓ *Insulin resistance*: This is manifested by excessive hepatic glucose production, decreased skeletal muscle uptake of glucose, and increased lipolysis and free fatty acid production.
  - ✓ *Excess glucagon secretion*: This occurs because type 2 DM patients fail to suppress glucagon in response to meals because of GLP-1 resistance/deficiency and insulin resistance/deficiency, which directly suppress glucagon.
  - ✓ *Sodium-glucose cotransporter-2 (SGLT-2) upregulation in the kidney*: This increases reabsorption of glucose by proximal renal tubular cells, which further contributes to hyperglycemia.
- *Gestational diabetes* (GDM) is DM that occurs in women during pregnancy.
- Less common causes of DM (1%–2%) include maturity onset diabetes of the young (MODY), genetic syndromes (eg, Down syndrome), endocrine disorders (eg, acromegaly, Cushing syndrome), pancreatic exocrine dysfunction, infections, and medications (eg, glucocorticoids, thiazides, niacin, atypical antipsychotics).
- Microvascular complications include retinopathy, neuropathy, and nephropathy. Macrovascular complications include coronary heart disease (CHD), stroke, and peripheral vascular disease.

CLINICAL PRESENTATION

TYPE 1 DIABETES MELLITUS

- Patients often have symptoms in the days or weeks preceding the diagnosis. The most common initial symptoms are polyuria, polydipsia, polyphagia, weight loss, fatigue, and lethargy.

- Individuals are often thin and are prone to develop DKA in the absence of an adequate insulin supply; many patients initially present with DKA. Symptom onset can be triggered by infection, trauma, or psychological stress.

TYPE 2 DIABETES MELLITUS

- Most patients are asymptomatic or have only mild fatigue at the time of diagnosis. Many patients are incidentally found to have type 2 DM after routine laboratory testing (eg, plasma glucose or A1C) or development of complications (eg, myocardial infarction, stroke).
- Because mild hyperglycemia may exist for years prior to the diagnosis, microvascular and macrovascular complications are often present at the time of diagnosis.
- Most patients are overweight or obese with an elevated waist:hip ratio.

DIAGNOSIS

- Normal fasting (no caloric intake for at least 8 hours) plasma glucose (FPG) is 70–99 mg/dL (3.9–5.5 mmol/L). Impaired fasting glucose (IFG) is FPG 100–125 mg/dL (5.6–6.9 mmol/L).
- Normal glucose tolerance based on a 2-hour post-load plasma glucose using the equivalent of 75 g anhydrous glucose dissolved in water (oral glucose tolerance test or OGTT) is <140 mg/dL (7.8 mmol/L). Impaired glucose tolerance (IGT) is OGTT 140–199 mg/dL (7.8–11.0 mmol/L).
- Normal A1C is 4%–5.6% (39–46 mmol/mol Hb). Increased risk of DM (prediabetes) is A1C 5.7%–6.4% (39–46 mmol/mol Hb).
- Criteria for diagnosis of DM include any one of the following:
  1. A1C ≥6.5% (48 mmol/mol Hb)
  2. FPG ≥126 mg/dL (7.0 mmol/L)
  3. OGTT ≥200 mg/dL (11.1 mmol/L)
  4. Random plasma glucose ≥200 mg/dL (11.1 mmol/L) with classic symptoms of hyperglycemia or hyperglycemic crisis

  In the absence of unequivocal hyperglycemia, a diagnosis using criteria 1 through 3 requires two abnormal test results from the same sample or in two separate test samples.
- *Prediabetes* is a condition of abnormal BG that is not sufficiently high to meet the thresholds that define DM but often progresses to the diagnosis.
- Screening for type 1 DM in asymptomatic children or adults is not recommended due to low disease prevalence and the acute onset of symptoms. Screening for type 2 DM is recommended for asymptomatic adults who are overweight (BMI ≥25 kg/m^2 or ≥23 kg/m^2 in Asian Americans) and have at least one other risk factor for developing type 2 DM. All adults, even those without risk factors, should be screened every 3 years starting at 45 years old. Children at risk for developing type 2 DM should undergo screening every 3 years starting at age 10 years. Pregnant women should undergo risk assessment for GDM at the first prenatal visit; those with multiple risk factors for type 2 DM should be tested as soon as feasible. All women (even if the initial test was negative) should undergo testing at 24–28 weeks' gestation.

TREATMENT

- <u>Goals of Treatment</u>: The primary goal is to prevent or delay progression of long-term microvascular and macrovascular complications. Additional goals are to alleviate symptoms of hyperglycemia, minimize hypoglycemia and other adverse effects, minimize treatment burden, and maintain quality of life. General glycemic targets for most nonpregnant adults with DM are listed in Table 19-1.

INITIAL ASSESSMENT

- During the initial visit, perform a full medical evaluation to confirm the diagnosis, classify the type of diabetes, identify complications or potential comorbid conditions, and review previous treatments and risk factors in established patients.

TABLE 19-1	Glycemic Target Recommendations for Most Nonpregnant Adults with Diabetes	
Parameter	American Diabetes Association (ADA)	American Association of Clinical Endocrinologists (AACE)
A1C	<7.0% (53 mmol/mol Hb)	≤6.5% (48 mmol/mol Hb)
Fasting plasma glucose (FPG)	80–130 mg/dL (4.4–7.2 mmol/L)	<110 mg/dL (6.1 mmol/L)
Peak postprandial glucose (PPG)	<180 mg/dL (10 mmol/L)	<140 mg/dL (7.8 mmol/L)

Glycemic targets should be individualized. More stringent or less stringent goals may be appropriate for some patients.

- Review past medical, family, and social history as well as medication use, adherence, tolerability, and use of diabetes technology.
- Screen for psychosocial conditions, self-management education needs, and hypoglycemia.
- Perform a thorough physical exam (including height, weight, BMI, blood pressure, thyroid palpation, and foot exam) and laboratory evaluation (including A1C, lipid profile, liver function tests, serum creatinine, and eGFR).
- Calculate a 10-year ASCVD risk score.

NONPHARMACOLOGIC THERAPY

- Medical nutrition therapy (MNT) involves an individually tailored nutrition plan. Implement a healthy meal plan that is moderate in calories and carbohydrates and low in saturated fat with all of the essential vitamins and minerals. Target an initial weight loss goal of at least 5% in all type 2 DM patients who are overweight or obese through calorie restriction. For individuals with type 1 DM, focus on physiologically regulating insulin administration rather than the amount and type of carbohydrates ingested.
- Aerobic exercise can improve insulin sensitivity, modestly improve glycemic control, reduce cardiovascular (CV) risk, contribute to weight control, and improve well-being. Physical activity goals include at least 150 min/week of moderate (50%–70% maximal heart rate) intensity exercise spread over at least 3 days/week with no more than 2 days between activity. Resistance/strength training is recommended at least 2 times/week for patients without proliferative diabetic retinopathy.
- Reassess patients every 3–6 months, obtain an A1C, and adjust treatment as needed. Patients on intensive insulin therapy should self monitor blood glucose (SMBG) at least four times daily, before meals and at bedtime, or should use a continuous glucose monitoring (CGM) device.
- Offer access to diabetes self-management education and support (DSME/S) programs to all patients. Such programs target self-care behaviors of healthy eating, being active, monitoring glucose levels, taking medications, problem-solving, reducing risk of complications, and healthy coping. Patients must be involved in decision making and have strong knowledge of the disease and associated complications.

PHARMACOLOGIC THERAPY

Insulin

- The main advantage of insulin over other antihyperglycemic agents is that it can achieve a wide range of glucose targets and the dose can be individualized based on glycemic levels. Disadvantages include the risk of hypoglycemia, need for injections, weight gain, and treatment burden.
- All commercial insulin preparations are produced using recombinant DNA technology. "Human" insulins (NPH, regular) are recombinant DNA–derived human insulin, whereas insulin analogs have had amino acids substitutions in the insulin molecule that change the onset or duration of action.

- Most insulin products are administered subcutaneously (SC) for chronic diabetes management, except for inhaled human insulin, which is a dry powder of regular insulin that is inhaled and absorbed through pulmonary tissue.
- The most commonly used insulin concentration is 100 units/mL (U-100); more concentrated insulins (U-200, U-300, U-500) may be considered for patients requiring larger doses. U-500 regular insulin is reserved for patients with extreme insulin resistance and is usually given two or three times a day.
- The pharmacodynamics of insulin products is characterized by their onset, peak, and duration of action (Table 19-2).
- *Basal insulin* (or background insulin) refers to longer-acting insulins that regulate BG levels in between meals by suppressing hepatic glucose production and maintaining near-normal glycemic levels in the fasting state. Options include the following insulins:
  - ✓ **NPH** is the least ideal product because it has a distinct peak and a duration of action much less than 24 hours and usually requires twice-daily dosing.
  - ✓ **Detemir** also has a peak and often lasts <24 hours; it can be given once daily in some patients but should be dosed twice daily at low doses (<0.3 units/kg).
  - ✓ **Glargine U-100** is considered to be peakless and can usually be given once daily.
  - ✓ **Glargine U-300** and **degludec U-100 or U-200** are longer acting-agents that have no peak and are given once daily.

  All basal insulins can achieve similar A1C reductions if dosed and titrated properly, but the longer-acting products have a lower risk of hypoglycemia (particularly nocturnal hypoglycemia) and may result in less glucose variability. However, they are more expensive.
- *Bolus insulin* refers to short- or rapid-acting insulins that cover meals (also called prandial insulin) or glycemic excursions (also called correction insulin). Basal insulin is the preferred and most convenient initial insulin formulation for patients with type 2 DM, whereas patients with type 1 DM require a combination of basal and bolus insulin to achieve adequate glycemic control. Bolus insulin options include:
  - ✓ **Aspart**, **lispro**, and **glulisine**: the rapid-onset, short-duration insulins
  - ✓ **Inhaled human insulin, fast-acting insulin aspart (Fiasp)**, and insulin lispro aabc (Lyumjev): the ultra-rapid onset insulins

  Rapid-acting insulins offer a faster onset and shorter duration of action than **regular insulin**, and ultra-rapid acting insulins offer an even faster onset; this may more closely mimic prandial endogenous insulin release. Rapid-acting insulins have a modestly lower risk of hypoglycemia than regular insulin. All prandial insulins can be used effectively, but cost differences can be substantial.
- Various premixed insulin products containing both a basal and a prandial component are also available for patients who require fewer injections or a simpler regimen (Table 19-2). However, these products are limited by fixed mixed formulations, which can make it challenging to tailor the dosing regimen.
- The insulin dose must be individualized. In type 1 DM, the average daily requirement is 0.5–0.6 units/kg, with approximately 50% given as basal insulin and the remaining 50% dedicated to meal coverage. During the honeymoon phase, requirements may fall to 0.1–0.4 units/kg. Higher doses are often needed during acute illness or with ketosis.
- Hypoglycemia is the most common adverse effects of insulin therapy. Insulin also causes dose-dependent weight gain, which occurs predominantly in truncal fat. Injection site reactions may include redness, pain, itching, urticaria, edema, and inflammation. SC administration can result in lipoatrophy or lipohypertrophy, which can be prevented by routinely rotating injection sites. Inhaled human insulin can cause cough and upper respiratory infections, and it is contraindicated in chronic obstructive pulmonary disease and asthma due to bronchospasm risk. Because inhaled insulin has been associated with a small decline in pulmonary function, patients should have spirometry tests performed at baseline, 6 months, and annually thereafter.

TABLE 19-2 Pharmacodynamics of Insulin Preparations

Type of Insulin by Generic (Brand) Name (U-100 unless otherwise noted)	Onset	Peak[a]	Duration[a]
Ultra-rapid acting			
Insulin aspart (Fiasp)	15–20 min[b]	90–120 min	5–7 hours
Insulin lispro aabc (Lyumjev)	15–17 min[c]	120–174 min	4.6–7.3 hours
Insulin human—inhaled (Afrezza)	12 min	35–55 min	1.5–4.5 hours
Rapid-acting			
Insulin aspart (NovoLog)	10–20 min	30–90 min	3–5 hours
Insulin lispro U-100, U-200 (Humalog, Admelog)			
Insulin glulisine (Apidra)			
Short-acting			
Regular (Humulin R, Novolin R)	30–60 min	2–4 hours	5–8 hours
Intermediate-acting			
NPH (Humulin N, Novolin N)	2–4 hours	4–10 hours	10–24 hours
Regular U-500 (Humulin R 500)	15–30 min	4–8 hours	13–24 hours
Long-acting			
Insulin detemir (Levemir)	1.5–4 hours	6–14 hours[c]	16–20 hours
Insulin glargine (Lantus, Basaglar)	2–4 hours	No peak	20–24 hours
Insulin glargine U-300 (Toujeo)	6 hours	No peak	36 hours
Insulin degludec U-100, U-200 (Tresiba)	1 hour	No peak	42 hours
Combination Products			
70% NPH/30% Regular (Humulin 70/30, Novolin 70/30)	30–60 min	Dual	10–16 hours
75% NPL, 25% lispro (Humalog 75/25)	5–15 min		10–16 hours
50% NPL, 50% lispro (Humalog 50/50)	5–15 min		10–16 hours
70% insulin aspart protamine, 30% insulin aspart (NovoLog 70/30)	5–15 min		15–18 hours

[a]The peak and duration of insulin action are variable, depending on the injection site, duration of diabetes, kidney function, smoking status, and other factors.
[b]Onset of appearance is 2.5 minutes compared to 5.2 minutes for insulin aspart (NovoLog).
[c]Long-acting insulins are considered "peakless," although they have exhibited peak effects during comparative testing.
NPH, neutral protamine Hagedorn; NPL, insulin lispro protamine suspension.

Biguanides

- **Metformin** decreases hepatic glucose production and enhances insulin sensitivity in peripheral (muscle) tissues, allowing for increased glucose uptake into muscle cells.
- Metformin is recommended as first-line pharmacotherapy in patients with type 2 DM (unless a contraindication or intolerability exists) due to extensive experience, high efficacy, minimal hypoglycemia risk, positive or neutral effects on weight, potential positive impact on CV risk, manageable side-effect profile, and low cost. It reduces A1C levels by 1.5%–2% (16–22 mmol/mol Hb) and FPG levels by 60–80 mg/dL (3.3–4.4 mmol/L) in drug-naïve patients with initial A1C values of approximately 9% (75 mmol/mol Hb). It does not cause weight gain and may lead to a modest (2–3 kg) weight loss. It has a low risk of hypoglycemia because it does not directly increase

pancreatic insulin secretion. Metformin decreases plasma triglycerides and low-density lipoprotein cholesterol (LDL-C) by approximately 8%–15% and modestly increases high-density lipoprotein cholesterol (HDL-C) by 2%.

- Metformin frequently causes GI side effects (diarrhea, abdominal discomfort, stomach upset); these effects are usually dose-dependent, transient, mild, and can be minimized with slow dose titration and taking metformin with or immediately after meals. When initiating therapy, use a low dose (typically 500 mg) given with the largest meal. Then increase the dose in 500-mg increments over several weeks. Extended-release metformin may lessen some of the GI side effects, but a comparison of immediate-release vs extended-release metformin found no significant differences in rates of GI adverse effects.

- Metformin may cause a metallic taste and may lower vitamin B_{12} concentrations; B_{12} levels or methylmalonic acid should be measured annually or if a deficiency is suspected, with vitamin B_{12} supplementation given if indicated.

- Lactic acidosis occurs rarely, usually in the setting of severe illness or acute kidney injury. The risk may increase in moderate-to-severe kidney insufficiency or tissue hypoperfusion states such as acute heart failure (HF), excessive alcohol intake, and hepatic impairment. Because symptoms are often nonspecific, the diagnosis must be confirmed by laboratory measurement of high lactic acid levels and acidosis.

- Metformin is renally excreted and accumulates in kidney insufficiency; it is con-traindicated in patients with eGFR <30 mL/min/1.73 m^2 and should be used with caution in patients with milder kidney insufficiency. Metformin initiation is not recommended in patients with eGFR 30–45 mL/min/1.73 m^2 but can be continued with increased kidney function monitoring; a reduction of 50% of maximal dose may be warranted. Due to the risk of acute kidney failure with use of IV contrast dye, withhold metformin therapy starting the day of the procedure and resume it 2–3 days later if normal kidney function has been documented.

- Metformin can be used in combination with any other antihyperglycemic therapy and is often continued when insulin therapy is initiated. The target metformin dose is 1000 mg twice daily or 2000 mg daily if the extended-release product is used. The minimal effective dose is 1000 mg/day. See Table 19-3 for metformin dosing recommendations.

- Numerous combination products containing metformin as well as combinations of other drug classes are available (Table 19-4).

Sodium-Glucose Cotransporter-2 Inhibitors

- **Canagliflozin, dapagliflozin, empagliflozin**, and **ertugliflozin** reduce plasma glu-cose by preventing the kidneys from reabsorbing glucose back into the bloodstream, leading to increased glucose excretion in the urine. SGLT-2 inhibitors lower both FPG and PPG and are effective even in the absolute absence of insulin.

- SGLT-2 inhibitors reduce A1C by 0.5%–1% (6–11 mmol/mol Hb) and appear to be more effective in patients with higher baseline A1C levels. Kidney impairment decreases the efficacy of SGLT-2 inhibitors.

- SGLT-2 inhibitors can be added to metformin or other second-line agents. They can be used as monotherapy in patients who cannot tolerate or take metformin. They are recommended for patients at high risk for or with established ASCVD, heart failure, or CKD and those with a need to avoid hypoglycemia or weight gain or loss. They are unlikely to cause hypoglycemia unless combined with medications such as sulfo-nylureas, meglitinides, or insulin.

- SGLT-2 inhibitors have FDA-approved indications beyond glycemic control in adults with type 2 DM and established atherosclerotic cardiovascular disease (ASCVD), such as reducing the risk of major adverse CV events (canagliflozin) and reducing the risk of CV death (empagliflozin). Refer to textbook Table 94-9 for more details.

- The most common adverse effect is genital mycotic infections, which are more common in women and uncircumcised men. There is also a slightly increased risk of urinary tract infections. Polyuria, dehydration, dizziness, or hypotension may

TABLE 19-3 Dosing Recommendations for Oral Medications Used to Treat Type 2 Diabetes

Generic (Brand) Name	Starting Dose	Usual Recommended Dose	Maximal Dose (mg/day)	Dosing/Use Based on Kidney Function[a]
Biguanides				
Metformin (Glucophage)	500 once or twice daily or 850 mg once daily, titrate to target dose as tolerated	1000 mg twice daily	2550	Do not initiate if eGFR 30–45; Do not use if eGFR <30
Metformin XR	500–1000 mg once daily, titrate to target dose as tolerated	2000 mg once daily	2500	Do not initiate if eGFR 30–45; Do not use if eGFR <30
Sodium-glucose transporter (SGLT)-2 inhibitors				
Canagliflozin (Invokana)	100 mg once daily, taken before the first meal of the day	100–300 mg once daily	300	100 mg once daily if eGFR 30–60; Avoid if eGFR <30
Dapagliflozin (Farxiga)	5 mg once daily in the morning with or without food	5–10 mg once daily	10	Not recommended if eGFR <25; Avoid if eGFR <25
Empagliflozin (Jardiance)	10 mg once daily in the morning with or without food	10–25 mg once daily	25	Not recommended if eGFR <45
Ertugliflozin (Steglatro)	5 mg once daily in the morning with or without food	5–15 mg once daily	15	Do not initiate if eGFR<60; Avoid if eGFR <30
Dipeptidyl peptidase (DPP)-4 inhibitors				
Alogliptin (Nesina)	25 mg once daily with or without food	25 mg once daily	25	12.5 mg once daily if CrCl 30–60 mL/min (0.5–1.0 mL/sec); 6.25 mg once daily if CrCl <30 mL/min (0.5 mL/sec)
Linagliptin (Tradjenta)	5 mg once daily with or without food	5 mg once daily	5	No dose adjustment needed
Saxagliptin (Onglyza)	2.5–5 mg once daily with or without food	5 mg once daily	5	2.5 mg once daily if eGFR ≤50

(Continued)

TABLE 19-3	Dosing Recommendations for Oral Medications Used to Treat Type 2 Diabetes (*Continued*)			
Generic (Brand) Name	Starting Dose	Usual Recommended Dose	Maximal Dose (mg/day)	Dosing/Use Based on Kidney Function[a]
Sitagliptin (Januvia)	100 mg once daily with or without food	100 mg once daily	100	50 mg once daily if eGFR 30–50; 25 mg once daily if eGFR <30
Thiazolidinediones				
Pioglitazone (Actos)	15 mg once daily	30 mg once daily	45	No dose adjustment required
Rosiglitazone (Avandia)	4 mg once daily or in two divided doses	4 mg once daily or in two divided doses	8	No dose adjustment required
Sulfonylureas (first generation)				
Chlorpropamide	250 mg once daily (100 mg once daily in older adults)	100–500 mg once daily	750	Consider alternative agent or initiate conservatively at 100 mg in kidney insufficiency to avoid hypoglycemia
Tolazamide	250 mg once daily (100 mg once daily in older adults or if FPG <200 mg/dL [11.1 mmol/L])	250–500 mg once daily	1000	Consider alternative agent or initiate conservatively at 100 mg in kidney insufficiency to avoid hypoglycemia
Tolbutamide	1000–2000 mg once daily (250–500 mg once daily in older adults)	1000–2000 mg once daily	3000	Consider alternative agent or initiate conservatively in kidney insufficiency to avoid hypoglycemia
Sulfonylureas (second generation)				
Glimepiride (Amaryl)	1–2 mg once daily (1 mg once daily in older adults)	4 mg once daily	8	Initiate conservatively at 1 mg in kidney insufficiency to avoid hypoglycemia
Glipizide (Glucotrol)	5 mg once daily (2.5 mg daily in older adults)	5–10 mg once daily	40	Initiate conservatively at 2.5 mg in kidney insufficiency to avoid hypoglycemia
Glipizide XL (Glucotrol XL)	5 mg once daily (2.5 mg once daily in older adults)	5–10 mg once daily	20	Initiate conservatively at 2.5 mg in kidney insufficiency to avoid hypoglycemia
Glyburide (Diabeta)	2.5–5 mg once daily (1.25 mg once daily in older adults)	5–10 mg once daily	20	Consider alternative agent or initiate conservatively at 1.25 mg in kidney insufficiency to avoid hypoglycemia

Glyburide micronized (Glynase)	1.5–3 mg once daily (0.75 mg once daily in older adults)	3–6 mg once daily	12	Consider alternative agent or initiate conservatively at 0.75 mg in kidney insufficiency to avoid hypoglycemia
Meglitinides				
Nateglinide (Starlix)	120 mg three times daily before meals	120 mg three times daily before meals	360	No adjustment required
Repaglinide (Prandin)	1–2 mg three times daily before meals (0.5 mg before meals if A1C <8% [64 mmol/mol Hb])	2–4 mg three times daily before meals	16	Initiate conservatively at 0.5 mg before meals if CrCl 20–40 mL/min (0.33–0.67 mL/sec)
α-Glucosidase inhibitors				
Acarbose (Precose)	25 mg once to three times daily with the first bite of a meal	50 mg once to three times daily with meals	300	Avoid if CrCl <25 mL/min (0.42 mL/sec)
Miglitol (Glyset)	25 mg once to three times daily with the first bite of a meal	50 mg once to three times daily with meals	300	Avoid if CrCl <25 mL/min (0.42 mL/sec)
Bile acid sequestrants				
Colesevelam (Welchol)	1.875 g twice daily or 3.75 g once daily with meals	1.875 g twice daily or 3.75 g once daily with meals	3.75 g/day	No dose adjustment needed
Dopamine agonists				
Bromocriptine (Cycloset)	0.8 mg once daily, taken within 2 hours after waking in the morning with food	1.6–4.8 mg once daily	4.8	No dose adjustment needed

aeGFR units: mL/min/1.73 m²; CrCl units: mL/min.

TABLE 19-4	Combination Drug Products for Type 2 Diabetes	
Drug Classes	**Drug Combination**	**Brand Name**
Biguanide and sulfonylurea	Metformin	Glipizide	Metaglip[a]
	Metformin	Glyburide	Glucovance[a]
Biguanide and meglitinide	Metformin	Repaglinide	Prandimet[a]
Biguanide and thiazolidinedione	Metformin	Pioglitazone	Actoplus Met[a], Actoplus Met XR
	Metformin	Rosiglitazone	Avandamet[a]
Biguanide and DPP-4 inhibitor	Metformin	Alogliptin	Kazano
	Metformin	Linagliptin	Jentadueto, Jentadueto XR
	Metformin	Saxagliptin	Kombiglyze XR
	Metformin	Sitagliptin	Janumet, Janumet XR
Biguanide and SGLT-2 inhibitor	Metformin	Canagliflozin	Invokamet, Invokamet XR
	Metformin	Dapagliflozin	Xigduo XR
	Metformin	Empagliflozin	Synjardy, Synjardy XR
	Metformin	Ertugliflozin	Segluromet
Thiazolidinedione and sulfonylurea	Pioglitazone	Glimepiride	Duetact[a]
	Rosiglitazone	Glimepiride	Avandaryl
Thiazolidinedione and DPP-4 inhibitor	Pioglitazone	Alogliptin	Oseni
SGLT-2 inhibitor and DPP-4 inhibitor	Dapagliflozin	Saxagliptin	Qtern
	Empagliflozin	Linagliptin	Glyxambi
	Ertugliflozin	Sitagliptin	Steglujan
Basal insulin and GLP-1 receptor agonist	Insulin glargine U-100	Lixisenatide	Soliqua
	Insulin degludec U-100	Liraglutide	Xultophy

[a]Available as generic product.
XR, extended release.

occur because of the osmotic diuresis effects. Concomitant diuretic use may increase the risk of orthostatic hypotension and electrolyte abnormalities. Older adults and patients with stage 4 or 5 CKD are not optimal treatment candidates. Other potential safety concerns include ketoacidosis, amputations, fractures, and Fournier gangrene.

• The SGLT-2 inhibitors should be started at a low dose with assessment of volume status, adverse effects, and kidney function. The dose may be titrated in patients who are tolerating the drug well and require additional glucose control (Table 19-3).

Glucagon-like Peptide 1 Receptor Agonists (GLP1-RAs)

• **Dulaglutide**, **exenatide**, **exenatide XR**, **lixisenatide**, **liraglutide**, and **semaglutide** stimulate insulin secretion and suppress inappropriately high postprandial glucagon secretion, decreasing hepatic glucose output. They also slow gastric emptying, increase satiety, and cause weight loss (average 1–3 kg).

- Short-acting agents (exenatide, lixisenatide) predominantly lower postprandial glucose (PPG) levels, whereas long-acting agents (dulaglutide, liraglutide, exenatide XR, semaglutide) lower both FPG and PPG, but with larger effects on FPG. Evidence suggests that liraglutide and semaglutide have the highest A1C and weight-lowering efficacy while exenatide and lixisenatide have the lowest.

- Dulaglutide, liraglutide, and semaglutide are FDA approved to reduce the risk of major adverse CV events in adults with type 2 DM and established ASCVD (see textbook Table 94-9 for more details).

- GLP1-RAs can be used as monotherapy in patients who cannot tolerate or take first-line therapy. They are recommended for patients at high risk for or with established ASCVD or chronic kidney disease (CKD) and those with a compelling need to avoid hypoglycemia or to avoid weight gain or induce weight loss. They can be used in combination with many agents, including metformin, sulfonylureas, SGLT-2 inhibitors, and basal insulin. They should not be used in combination with DPP-4 inhibitors due to similar mechanisms of action.

- Six GLP1-RAs are administered SC (Table 19-5). Semaglutide is available as SC and oral preparations. The oral dose (Rybelsus) ranges from 3 to 14 mg once daily, taken 30 minutes before the first food, beverage, or other medication of the day with no more than 4 ounces of water.

- The most common adverse effects of GLP1-RAs are nausea, vomiting, and diarrhea. These effects are dose related, so dose titration is recommended. They usually occur early in the treatment course and are mild and transient but may require drug discontinuation in some patients. Instruct patients to eat slowly and stop eating when satiated or nausea may worsen and cause vomiting. Injection site reactions and hypersensitivity reactions (including anaphylaxis and angioedema) have been reported. GLP-1 RAs have been associated with cases of acute pancreatitis, but no causal relationship has been established.

- Because GLP1-RAs enhance insulin secretion in response to food intake, the risk of hypoglycemia is low when combined with metformin, DPP-4 inhibitors, SGLT-2 inhibitors, or a TZD. However, hypoglycemia may occur when combined with a sulfonylurea or insulin.

TABLE 19-5	Dosing Recommendations for Subcutaneous GLP-1 Receptor Agonists		
Generic (Brand) Name	Dose[a]	Interval	Dose/Use Based on Kidney Function[b]
Exenatide (Byetta)	5–10 mcg	Twice daily (30–60 min before breakfast and dinner)	Avoid if eGFR <30
Lixisenatide (Adlyxin)	10–20 mcg	Once daily (1 hour before breakfast)	Limited experience in severe kidney renal impairment; avoid if eGFR <15
Dulaglutide (Trulicity)	0.75–4.5 mg	Once weekly (at any time of day, with or without food)	Use with caution in patients with ESKD
Exenatide XR (Bydureon)	2 mg	Once weekly (at any time of day, with or without meals)	Use with caution if CrCl 30-50 (0.5–0.83 mL/sec) Avoid if eGFR <30
Liraglutide (Victoza)	0.6–1.8 mg	Once daily (with or without meals)	Limited experience in ESKD
Semaglutide (Ozempic)	0.25–1 mg	Once weekly	No dose adjustment recommended

[a]All products require subcutaneous administration into the abdomen, thigh, or upper arm.
[b]eGFR units: mL/min/1.73 m^2.

Dipeptidyl Peptidase-4 (DPP-4) Inhibitors

- **Alogliptin**, **linagliptin**, **saxagliptin**, and **sitagliptin** prolong the half-life of endogenously produced GLP-1 and GIP, thereby increasing glucose-dependent insulin secretion from the pancreas and reducing inappropriate postprandial glucagon secretion, resulting in lower glucose levels without an increase in hypoglycemia when used as monotherapy. They do not alter gastric emptying, cause nausea, have significant effects on satiety, or cause weight gain/loss.
- DPP-4 inhibitors produce average A1C reductions of 0.5%–0.9% (6–10 mmol/mol Hb) when used at maximum doses. There are no clear differences in efficacy among agents in the class.
- DPP-4 inhibitors are considered second- or third-line therapy. Advantages include once-daily dosing, oral administration, weight neutrality, low risk of hypoglycemia, and good tolerability. However, they have less A1C lowering efficacy than other medication classes and are expensive.
- Adverse effects are uncommon and include stuffy, runny nose; headache; and upper respiratory tract infections. The labeling of saxagliptin and alogliptin includes information about increased risk of hospitalizations for HF. The FDA has also issued a warning on the risk of severe joint pain with DPP-4 inhibitors. Pancreatitis appears to be an established but rare safety concern.
- There is no need to titrate the dose of DPP-4 inhibitors; however, renal dose adjustments are required for alogliptin, saxagliptin, and sitagliptin (Table 19-3).

Thiazolidinediones (TZDs)

- TZDs bind to the peroxisome proliferator activator receptor-γ (PPAR-γ) located primarily on fat and vascular cells, enhancing insulin sensitivity in muscle, liver, and fat tissues.
- At maximal doses, **pioglitazone** and **rosiglitazone** reduce A1C by 1%–1.5% (11–22 mmol/mol Hb) and FPG by 60–70 mg/dL (3.3–3.9 mmol/L), and they have high durability over time. Maximum effects may not be seen until 3–4 months of therapy.
- TZDs are considered second- or third-line agents and can be used in combination with metformin and other commonly prescribed medications for type 2 DM.
- Pioglitazone decreases plasma triglycerides by 10%–20%, whereas rosiglitazone tends to have no effect. Pioglitazone does not significantly increase LDL-C, whereas rosiglitazone may increase LDL-C by 5%–15%. Both drugs increase HDL-C, but the magnitude may be greater with pioglitazone.
- Fluid retention may occur due to peripheral vasodilation and improved insulin sensitization in the kidney with increased sodium and water retention. This may result in peripheral edema (4%–5% of patients with monotherapy; 15% or more when combined with insulin), HF, hemodilution of hemoglobin and hematocrit, and weight gain. Edema is dose related and if not severe may be managed by dose reduction in most patients. TZDs are contraindicated in patients with New York Heart Association Class III or IV HF and should be used with caution in patients with Class I or II HF.
- Weight gain is dose related and results from both fluid retention and fat accumulation; a gain of 4 kg is not uncommon, and higher gains may require drug discontinuation. TZDs have also been associated with an increased fracture rate in the upper and lower limbs of postmenopausal women. An increased risk of bladder cancer is controversial.
- See Table 19-3 for TZD dosing information.

Sulfonylureas

- Sulfonylureas enhance insulin secretion by binding to the sulfonylurea receptor SUR1 on pancreatic β-cells. First-generation agents (**chlorpropamide**, **tolazamide**, and **tolbutamide**) are lower in potency than second-generation drugs (**glyburide**, **glipizide**, and **glimepiride**), and are rarely used due to a higher risk of adverse effects.
- All sulfonylureas are equally effective in lowering BG when given in equipotent doses. On average, the A1C falls by 1.5%–2% (16–22 mmol/mol Hb) with FPG reductions of 60–70 mg/dL (3.3–3.9 mmol/L) in drug-naïve patients.

- Sulfonylureas are widely used because they have an extensive record of safety and effectiveness, are given orally, and are inexpensive. However, current treatment guidelines either discourage their use or suggest caution due to the risk of hypoglycemia and weight gain. In addition, tachyphylaxis to the insulin secretion effect occurs, leading to poor long-term durability of response in most patients.
- The most common side effect is hypoglycemia. Patients who skip meals, exercise vigorously, or lose a substantial amount of weight are more prone to hypoglycemia. Sulfonylureas with long durations of action and those with active metabolites should be used with extreme caution in older patients and those with renal insufficiency due to the high risk of hypoglycemia. Weight gain is common (typically 1–2 kg). Patients with sulfa allergy rarely experience crossreactivity with sulfonylureas.
- See Table 19-3 for sulfonylurea dosing information.

α-Glucosidase Inhibitors

- **Acarbose** and **miglitol** delay the breakdown of sucrose and complex carbohydrates in the small intestine, prolonging carbohydrate absorption. The net effect is reduction in PPG (40–50 mg/dL; 2.2–2.8 mmol/L) with relatively unchanged FBG. A1C lowering is modest, with average A1C reductions of 0.3%–1%.
- Good candidates for these drugs are patients who are near target A1C levels with near-normal FPG but high PPG levels.
- The most common side effects are flatulence, abdominal pain, and diarrhea, which can be reduced by slow dosage titration (Table 19-3).

Meglitinides

- **Nateglinide** and **repaglinide** stimulate insulin secretion from pancreatic β-cells by binding to a site adjacent to the sulfonylurea receptor. They are similar to sulfonylureas except that they have a faster onset and shorter duration of action. As monotherapy, they reduce PPG excursions and reduce A1C by 0.8%–1% (9–11 mmol/mol Hb).
- Similar to sulfonylureas, the main side effects are hypoglycemia and weight gain.
- Their role in therapy is unclear due to lack of clinical evidence. They are not included in the American Diabetes Association (ADA) treatment algorithm. They may be used in patients with kidney insufficiency and may be a good option for patients with erratic meal schedules. However, multiple daily dosing may decrease adherence.
- Meglitinides should be taken by mouth with each meal, initiated at a low dose, and titrated over time until glycemic control is achieved (Table 19-3).

Bile Acid Sequestrants

- **Colesevelam** binds bile acid in the intestinal lumen, decreasing the bile acid pool for reabsorption. Its mechanism in lowering plasma glucose levels is unknown, and its role in therapy is unclear.
- A1C lowering efficacy is modest. It reduces LDL-C in patients with type 2 DM by 12%–16% but has not been proven to reduce CV morbidity or mortality. Colesevelam is weight neutral and has a low risk of hypoglycemia. Patients with type 2 DM who need a small reduction in A1C as well as additional LDL-C lowering may be candidates for this agent.
- The most common side effects are constipation and dyspepsia; colesevelam should be taken with a large amount of water. Colesevelam has multiple absorption-related drug–drug interactions. See Table 19-3 for dosing information.

Dopamine Agonists

- **Bromocriptine mesylate** is FDA approved for treatment of type 2 DM. The mechanisms by which it improves glycemic control are unknown but may involve improved hepatic insulin sensitivity and decreased hepatic glucose output.
- The A1C lowering efficacy is modest, and its role in the treatment of type 2 DM is unclear.
- Common side effects include nausea, vomiting, constipation, fatigue, headache, dizziness, and asthenia. Somnolence and orthostatic hypotension may also occur.

Amylin Analogs

- **Pramlintide** (Symlin) is a synthetic amylin analog that reduces glucagon secretion, slows gastric emptying, and increases satiety. It was the first noninsulin agent approved for patients with type 1 DM.
- Pramlintide lowers both PPG levels and A1C. The average A1C reduction is about 0.6% (7 mmol/mol Hb) in patients with type 2 DM and 0.4%–0.5% (5–6 mmol/mol Hb) in type 1 DM.
- It is used primarily in type 1 DM as adjunctive therapy for patients who are not achieving PPG goals despite maximizing mealtime insulin doses. It can also decrease weight (average loss 1.5 kg) and may allow for lower mealtime insulin doses.
- The most common adverse effects are nausea, vomiting, and anorexia. It does not cause hypoglycemia when used alone, but hypoglycemia can occur when used with insulin. To minimize the risk of severe hypoglycemia, empirically reduce the mealtime insulin dose by 30%–50% when pramlintide is initiated.
- In type 2 DM, the starting dose is 60 mcg SC prior to meals, titrated to the maximally recommended 120-mcg SC dose as tolerated and warranted based on PPG levels. In type 1 DM, dosing starts at 15 mcg SC prior to meals and can be titrated up in 15-mcg increments to a maximum of 60 mcg SC prior to each meal, if tolerated.

TREATMENT OF TYPE 2 DIABETES

- Upon diagnosis, assess the patient's current lifestyle, existing comorbidities, A1C, age, weight, presence or absence of symptoms, motivation, cultural preferences, health literacy level, and cost limitations. Set a patient-specific A1C target and discuss it with the patient.
- Implement comprehensive lifestyle modifications with MNT, physical activity, weight loss if obese, smoking cessation, and psychologic support upon diagnosis and reinforce them at every visit. All patients should be offered access to ongoing DSME/S programs.
- Initiate metformin as first-line therapy in patients without contraindications or tolerability issues. Start with a low dose and titrate to the maximum effective dose over time to improve tolerability.
- If the initial A1C is close to goal (eg, ≤7.5% [58 mmol/mol Hb]) consider initial treatment with lifestyle modifications alone if the patient is motivated.
- Consider starting two medications (metformin plus a second agent) if the initial A1C is >1.5% (16 mmol/mol Hb) higher than the target A1C. In addition, initial combination therapy may reduce glucose faster and maintain glycemic control longer compared to a stepwise approach.
- Consider early introduction of basal insulin in patients with very high A1C levels (>10% [86 mmol/mol Hb]), symptoms of hyperglycemia, or evidence of catabolism (eg, weight loss).
- See patients at least every 3 months if they are not meeting their goals and at least every 6 months if they are meeting goals. At those times, check an A1C level, assess medication adherence, and reinforce lifestyle recommendations. Add additional therapy if glucose targets have not been met.
- Most patients eventually require combination therapy. Intensification beyond metformin monotherapy requires careful consideration of patient- and drug-related factors. Patient-specific factors to consider in medication selection include the individualized A1C target and presence of comorbidities (eg, ASCVD, HF, CKD, obesity). Drug-specific factors to consider include glucose-lowering efficacy, impact on comorbidities, effect on weight and hypoglycemia risk, side-effect profile, ease of use, and cost. Recommendations based on patient-specific comorbidities and other factors include:
  ✓ High-risk or established ASCVD: SGLT-2 inhibitor (canagliflozin, empagliflozin) or GLP1-RA (dulaglutide, liraglutide, or SC semaglutide) with proven CV benefit.
  ✓ High-risk or established ASCVD and HF: SGLT-2 inhibitor with proven benefit in reducing HF progression (empagliflozin, canagliflozin, dapagliflozin). Avoid TZDs in patients with HF.

- ✓ CKD (with or without ASCVD): SGLT-2 inhibitor with proven benefit in reducing CKD progression (canagliflozin, dapagliflozin).
- ✓ Need to minimize weight gain or promote weight loss in patients without ASCVD or CKD: GLP1-RA or SGLT-2 inhibitor. If these agents cannot be used, use a weight-neutral medication such as a DPP-4 inhibitor. Avoid sulfonylureas, insulin, and TZDs due to weight gain.
- ✓ Compelling need to minimize hypoglycemia: DPP-4 inhibitor, GLP1-RA, SGLT-2 inhibitor, or TZD could be added to metformin.

- If the A1C target is not achieved after 3 months of dual therapy or if the patient did not tolerate the selected drug(s), then triple therapy is warranted, adding a drug from another class. These recommendations are independent of baseline A1C, individualized A1C target, or metformin use.
- People with type 2 DM can often be managed with oral medications for years before injectable medications are needed. Insulin is recommended for extreme (A1C >10% [86 mmol/mol Hb]) or symptomatic hyperglycemia. Otherwise, GLP-1 RAs are preferred over insulin because they have equal or superior A1C lowering efficacy and lead to weight loss instead of weight gain with a low risk of hypoglycemia. Basal insulin can be initiated if additional glucose lowering is needed after the GLP-1 RA dose has been maximized.
- Basal insulin is started at a low dose (10 units once daily or 0.1–0.2 units/kg/day) and titrated slowly over time to a target FPG range (ie, 80–130 mg/dL [4.4-7.2 mmol/L] for patients targeting an A1C <7% [53 mmol/mol Hb]). If the A1C target is not reached by maximally titrating basal insulin, PPG levels are likely elevated and a GLP1-RA or SGLT-2 inhibitor should be considered if the patient is not already taking one. Prandial insulin is also an option, starting with 4 units or 10% of the basal dose with the largest meal of the day. If the A1C is <8% (64 mmol/mol Hb), the basal insulin dose can be decreased by the same amount to avoid hypoglycemia. Titrate the dose over time to achieve target PPG levels <180 mg/dL (10 mmol/L). A second or third injection can be added to the other meals if needed.
- Reevaluate the appropriateness of oral medications when injectable agents are started:
  - ✓ GLP-1 RAs can be used in combination with all oral agents except DPP-4 inhibitors.
  - ✓ Continue metformin when insulin is started. Stop TZDs and sulfonylureas or reduce the dose.
  - ✓ SGLT-2 inhibitors can be continued, but educate the patient about the risk of DKA.

TREATMENT OF HYPERGLYCEMIA IN TYPE 1 DIABETES

- All patients with type 1 DM require exogenous insulin. Achieving adequate glycemic control usually requires intensive insulin regimens designed to provide insulin in a manner that mimics normal physiologic insulin secretion, with consistent secretion of insulin throughout the day to manage glucose levels overnight and in between meals (ie, basal insulin), and bursts of insulin in response to glucose rises after ingestion of carbohydrates (ie, prandial insulin).
- Intensive insulin regimens can be given with either multiple daily injections (MDI) or use of continuous subcutaneous insulin infusion (CSII) via an insulin pump (**Fig. 19-1**).
- A common MDI approach is one injection of long-acting insulin (eg, insulin glargine U-100) for the basal component and three injections of rapid-acting insulin (eg, insulin lispro U-100) for the prandial component (**Fig. 19-1A**). A less expensive option consists of two injections of intermediate-acting insulin (eg, NPH insulin) and two injections of short-acting insulin (eg, regular insulin) (**Fig. 19-1B**). However, the ADA Standards of Care recommend that most patients should use rapid-acting insulins rather than regular insulin to reduce the risk of hypoglycemia.
- Insulin pump therapy or CSII infuses rapid-acting insulin to cover both the basal and prandial insulin needs (**Fig. 19-1C**). The pump infuses a basal rate constantly

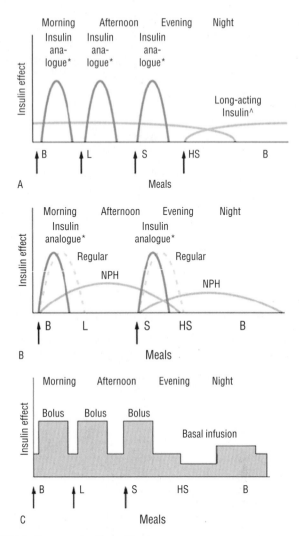

FIGURE 19-1. Common insulin regimens.
(A) Multiple-component insulin regimen consisting of one injection of long-acting insulin (^detemir, glargine degludec) to provide basal glycemic coverage and three injections of rapid-acting insulin (*aspart, lispro, glulisine) to provide glycemic coverage for each meal.
(B) Insulin regimen consisting of two injections of intermediate-acting insulin (NPH) and rapid-acting insulin (*aspart, lispro, glulisine [solid line]), or short-acting regular insulin (dashed line). Only one formulation of short-acting insulin is used.
(C) Insulin administration by insulin infusion device. The basal insulin rate is decreased during the evening and increased slightly prior to the patient awakening in the morning. Rapid-acting insulin (aspart, lispro, or glulisine) is used in the insulin pump.

throughout the day and allows the patient to give bolus doses using a bolus dose calculator based on current glucose levels, carbohydrate intake, and insulin on board. Insulin pump therapy can provide more precise glucose control and allow greater flexibility and fine-tune tailoring.

- The starting insulin dose for someone with newly diagnosed type 1 DM is typically 0.4–1 units/kg/day of total insulin. The total daily insulin dose is then divided to give 50% as basal insulin and 50% as prandial insulin (distributed across meals). For example, an 80-kg patient started on 0.5 units/kg/day would start with a total daily dose of 40 units, with 20 units given as a long-acting insulin (eg, insulin detemir, glargine) and 7 units of rapid-acting insulin (eg, insulin aspart, lispro, or glulisine) with breakfast, lunch, and dinner. The insulin doses would then be adjusted based on SMBG data.
- Ideally, patients should learn to count carbohydrates so they can match their prandial insulin doses to their carbohydrate intake. Patients should also SMBG before each meal or use continuous glucose monitoring (CGM) to evaluate the insulin regimen and make treatment decisions. Bolus insulin doses can be better individualized by using carbohydrate-to-insulin ratios (C:I ratios) and correction factors (CF); refer to the textbook chapter for more detailed information.
- Pramlintide is indicated as adjunctive treatment in patients with type 1 DM who are not achieving glycemic targets despite optimization of mealtime insulin (refer to discussion earlier in this chapter). Pramlintide may improve glycemic control and minimize weight gain caused by insulin, but its use is limited by adverse effects such as nausea and vomiting, modest glucose improvements, increased injections and cost, and increased risk of hypoglycemia.
- Assess patients every 3 months if uncontrolled and every 6 months if controlled. Obtain an A1C and adjust treatment as needed. Patients on intensive insulin therapy should SMBG at least four times daily, before meals and at bedtime. Patients should also test before exercise, prior to critical tasks such as driving, and if symptoms of hypoglycemia occur. SMBG is crucial during times of intercurrent illness or stresses for early detection and prevention of DKA.
- Continuous glucose monitors report interstitial glucose levels in real time, provide insight into glucose trends, and can reduce A1C and reduce glucose variability in patients with type 1 DM. Current guidelines recommend CGM in patients with type 1 DM who are not meeting glycemic goals. They are also recommended in patients with hypoglycemia unawareness to better detect and prevent hypoglycemic events.

HYPOGLYCEMIA

- Hypoglycemia is a common complication of some diabetes medications and is associated with falls, injury, motor vehicle accidents, decreased quality of life, and increased risk of developing dementia, CV events, arrhythmias, and death.
- The severity of hypoglycemia is classified as follows:
  ✓ *Level 1 (hypoglycemia alert value; ≤70 mg/dL [3.9 mmol/L])*: May not cause symptoms but should be treated with a fast-acting carbohydrate
  ✓ *Level 2 (clinically significant hypoglycemia; <54 mg/dL [3.0 mmol/L])*: Serious, clinically important hypoglycemia
  ✓ *Level 3 (severe hypoglycemia)*: Associated with cognitive impairment requiring external assistance for recovery and can be life threatening
- Initial autonomic symptoms include tachycardia, palpitations, sweating, tremors, and hunger. Neuroglycopenic symptoms often occur with BG <60 mg/dL (3.3 mmol/L) and can include cognitive impairment, confusion, behavioral changes, anger, irritability, blurred vision, headaches, seizures, and loss of consciousness.
- Some patients have hypoglycemia unawareness and are unable to detect the early warning symptoms of hypoglycemia; they are at increased risk for the serious sequelae associated with severe hypoglycemia.
- SMBG and CGM can be useful in preventing hypoglycemia. Patients must be educated to understand situations that increase risk of hypoglycemia (eg, delaying meals, during or after exercising, or fasting).
- Treatment of hypoglycemia requires ingestion of carbohydrates, preferably glucose. Patients should carry a source of fast-acting glucose with them at all times and use the "rule of 15" for proper treatment:

✓ First use SMBG to confirm BG <70 mg/dL (3.9 mmol/L) and then ingest 15 g of fast-acting carbohydrates such as 1/2 cup (4 oz or 125 mL) of milk, juice, or soda; 1 tablespoon of honey; hard candy; jelly beans; or glucose tablets.

✓ Repeat SMBG in 15 minutes; if the BG is <70 mg/dL (3.9 mmol/L), repeat the process.

✓ Once the BG is normalized, eat a snack or meal that includes complex carbohydrates and protein to prevent further hypoglycemic episodes.

• If the patient is unconscious, give IV glucose or glucagon injection. Glucagon increases glycogenolysis in the liver and may be given in any situation in which IV glucose cannot be rapidly administered. A glucagon kit should be prescribed and readily available to all patients on insulin who have a history of or high risk for severe hypoglycemia. It can take 10–15 minutes before glucose levels start to rise, and patients often vomit. Position the patient on the side with the head tilted slightly downward to avoid aspiration.

• Clinicians should inquire about hypoglycemia at every visit. Ask the patient about the frequency, severity, and timing of hypoglycemic events, need for assistance by others, or the need to administer glucagon. Reevaluate the treatment regimen of patients with frequent or severe hypoglycemia to minimize future episodes.

COMPLICATIONS OF DIABETES

Macrovascular Complications

• Macrovascular complications (eg, CHD, ischemic stroke) are the leading causes of death in people with diabetes.

• The ADA recommends low-dose **aspirin** therapy (75–162 mg daily) in all patients with established ASCVD. **Clopidogrel** may be used in patients allergic to aspirin. The role of antiplatelet therapy for primary CV prevention is unclear because the benefits may be offset by a higher risk of bleeding; some practice guidelines recommend aspirin if the 10-year risk of a CV event is >20% and the patient is at relatively low risk for bleeding complications.

• In patients with established ASCVD, use of a GLP1-RA or an SGLT-2 inhibitor should be strongly considered.

• For all patients whose blood pressure (BP) exceeds 120/80 mm Hg, the ADA recommends dietary changes, physical activity, and weight loss in overweight or obese patients. Drug therapy using agents proven to reduce CV events should be started for BP >140/90 mm Hg. A combination of two medications should be used for BP >160/100 mm Hg.

• Initiate high-intensity statin therapy in all patients with diabetes and preexisting ASCVD regardless of baseline lipid levels. In the absence of ASCVD, prescribe a moderate-intensity statin to all patients with type 1 or type 2 DM over the age of 40. In patients <40 years of age, a moderate-intensity statin may be appropriate for patients with multiple CV risk factors. A fibrate (eg, **fenofibrate**), **omega-3 fatty acid**, or **niacin** can be added for patients with marked hypertriglyceridemia.

• Peripheral arterial disease can lead to claudication, nonhealing foot ulcers, and limb amputation. Smoking cessation, statin therapy, good glycemic control, and antiplatelet therapy are important strategies. **Cilostazol** may be useful in select patients to reduce symptoms. Revascularization surgery can be considered in some situations. Perform foot examinations during each face-to-face patient encounter and a yearly monofilament test to assess for loss of protective sensation to identify high-risk patients.

Microvascular Complications

• Efforts to improve glucose control significantly reduce the risk of developing microvascular complications and slow their progression.

• *Nephropathy*: Albuminuria is a marker of kidney damage and can be predictive of end-stage kidney disease. The ADA recommends measuring eGFR and screening for albuminuria upon diagnosis and annually thereafter in persons with type 2 DM.

Annual screening with type 1 DM should begin with puberty or when the disease duration has been at least 5 years. Glucose and BP control are important for preventing and slowing progression of nephropathy. The SGLT2 inhibitors empagliflozin, canagliflozin, and dapagliflozin significantly reduce the decline in kidney function in patients with CKD, with or without diabetes. Angiotensin-converting enzyme (ACE) inhibitors and angiotensin receptor blockers (ARBs) can slow the progression of renal disease in patients with diabetes. Diuretics are often necessary due to volume-expanded states and are recommended second-line therapy. The ADA recommends a BP goal <140/90 mm Hg in patients with nephropathy but a lower target (eg, <130/80) if it can be achieved without undue burden or side effects. Three or more antihypertensives are often needed to reach goal BP.

- *Retinopathy*: Patients with diabetes should have routine dilated eye examinations to fully evaluate the retina. Early background retinopathy may reverse with improved glycemic control and optimal BP control. More advanced retinopathy will not fully regress with improved glycemia, and aggressive BG reductions may acutely worsen retinopathy. Laser photocoagulation has markedly improved sight preservation. Intravitreal antivascular endothelial growth factor (VEGF) therapy is also highly effective for sight preservation. **Bevacizumab** (used off-label) and **ranibizumab** are anti-VEGF monoclonal antibodies, and **aflibercept** is a VEGF decoy receptor.
- *Neuropathy*:
  - ✓ Distal symmetrical peripheral neuropathy is the most common complication in patients with type 2 DM. Paresthesias, numbness, or pain are the predominant symptoms. The feet are involved far more often than the hands. Improved glycemic control is the primary treatment and may alleviate some symptoms. Pharmacologic therapy is symptomatic and includes low-dose tricyclic antidepressants (**nortriptyline** or **desipramine**), **duloxetine**, **gabapentin**, **pregabalin**, **venlafaxine**, **topical capsaicin**, and **tramadol**.
  - ✓ Gastroparesis can be severe and debilitating. Improved glycemic control, discontinuation of medications that slow gastric motility, and use of **metoclopramide** or low-dose **erythromycin** may be helpful.
  - ✓ Diabetic diarrhea is often nocturnal and frequently responds to a 10- to 14-day course of an antibiotic such as **doxycycline** or **metronidazole**. **Octreotide** may be useful in unresponsive cases.
  - ✓ Orthostatic hypotension may require mineralocorticoids (eg, **fludrocortisone**) or adrenergic agonists (**midodrine**).
  - ✓ Erectile dysfunction is common, and initial therapy should include a trial of an oral phosphodiesterase-5 inhibitor (eg, **sildenafil, vardenafil**, or **tadalafil**).

EVALUATION OF THERAPEUTIC OUTCOMES

- Measure A1C every 3–6 months to follow long-term glycemic control for the previous 2–3 months, even in patients who are stable on a therapeutic regimen and meeting treatment goals (Table 19-1).
- SMBG provides an opportunity to adjust medications, food intake, or physical activity and enables patients to detect hypoglycemia. For patients with type 1 DM, SMBG is typically performed 4–6 times per day—prior to food intake and physical activity and at bedtime. The optimal frequency of SMBG in patients with type 2 DM on oral agents is controversial.
- CGM should be considered in adults with type 1 DM who are at least 25 years of age and those younger than 25 years of age who can demonstrate adherence to its use.
- At each visit, ask patients with type 1 DM about the frequency and severity of hypoglycemia. Document any hypoglycemic episodes requiring assistance of another person, medical attention, or hospitalization and take steps to prevent future episodes.
- Screen for complications at the time of diagnosis and thereafter as follows:
  - ✓ Obtain yearly dilated eye exams in type 2 DM and an initial exam in the first 5 years in type 1 DM, then yearly.

✓ Assess BP at each visit.

✓ Examine the feet at each visit, including palpation of distal pulses and visual inspection for skin integrity, calluses, and deformities.

✓ Screen for pedal sensory loss annually using a 10-g force monofilament.

✓ Screen for albuminuria at the time of diagnosis in patients with type 2 DM and 5 years after diagnosis in type 1 DM. At least once a year, assess urinary albumin (urine albumin-to-creatinine ratio) and eGFR in all patients with type 2 DM and in patients with type 1 DM for at least 5 years.

✓ Check fasting lipid panel annually if the patient is on lipid-lowering therapy.

• Administer an annual influenza vaccine and assess for administration of the pneumococcal vaccine and hepatitis B vaccine series along with management of other CV risk factors (eg, smoking).

See Chapter 94, Diabetes Mellitus, authored by Jennifer Trujillo and Stuart Haines, for a more detailed discussion of this topic.

20 Thyroid Disorders

- *Thyroid disorders* involve thyroid hormone production or secretion and result in alterations in metabolic stability.

THYROID HORMONE PHYSIOLOGY

- The thyroid hormones thyroxine (T_4) and triiodothyronine (T_3) are formed within thyroglobulin, a large glycoprotein synthesized in the thyroid cell. Inorganic iodide enters the thyroid follicular cell and is oxidized by thyroid peroxidase and covalently bound (organified) to tyrosine residues of thyroglobulin.
- Iodinated tyrosine residues monoiodotyrosine (MIT) and diiodotyrosine (DIT) combine (couple) to form iodothyronines in reactions catalyzed by thyroid peroxidase. Thus, two molecules of DIT combine to form T_4, and MIT and DIT join to form T_3.
- Proteolysis within thyroid cells releases thyroid hormone into the bloodstream. T_4 and T_3 are transported by thyroid-binding globulin (TBG), transthyretin, and albumin. Only the unbound (free) thyroid hormone can diffuse into cells, elicit biologic effects, and regulate thyroid-stimulating hormone (TSH) secretion from the pituitary.
- T_4 is secreted solely from the thyroid, but <20% of T_3 is produced there; most T_3 is formed from breakdown of T_4 catalyzed by the enzyme 5′-monodeiodinase in peripheral tissues. T_3 is five times more active than T_4. T_4 may also be acted on by 5′-monodeiodinase to form reverse T_3, which has no significant biologic activity.
- Thyroid hormone production is regulated by TSH secreted by the anterior pituitary, which in turn is under negative feedback control by the circulating level of free thyroid hormone and the positive influence of hypothalamic thyrotropin-releasing hormone (TRH). Thyroid hormone production is also regulated by extrathyroidal deiodination of T_4 to T_3, which can be affected by nutrition, nonthyroidal hormones, drugs, and illness.

Thyrotoxicosis (Hyperthyroidism)

PATHOPHYSIOLOGY

- Thyrotoxicosis results when tissues are exposed to excessive levels of T_4, T_3, or both. Hyperthyroidism, which is one cause of thyrotoxicosis, refers to overproduction of thyroid hormone by the thyroid gland.
- TSH-secreting pituitary tumors occur sporadically and release biologically active hormone that is unresponsive to normal feedback control. The tumors may cosecrete prolactin or growth hormone; therefore, patients may present with amenorrhea, galactorrhea, or signs of acromegaly.
- Resistance to thyroid hormone occurs rarely and can be due to various molecular defects, including mutations in the TRβ gene. Pituitary resistance to thyroid hormone (PRTH) refers to selective resistance of the pituitary thyrotrophs to thyroid hormone.
- Graves' disease is the most common cause of hyperthyroidism, which results from the action of thyroid-stimulating antibodies (TSAb) directed against the thyrotropin receptor on the surface of thyroid cells. These immunoglobulins bind to the receptor and activate the enzyme adenylate cyclase in the same manner as TSH.
- An autonomous thyroid nodule (toxic adenoma) is a benign thyroid mass that produces thyroid hormone independent of pituitary and TSH control. Hyperthyroidism usually occurs with larger nodules (>3 cm in diameter).
- In multinodular goiter, follicles with autonomous function coexist with normal or even nonfunctioning follicles. Thyrotoxicosis occurs when autonomous follicles generate more thyroid hormone than is required.

- Painful subacute (granulomatous or de Quervain) thyroiditis often develops after a viral syndrome, but rarely has a specific virus been identified in thyroid parenchyma.
- Painless (silent, lymphocytic, or postpartum) thyroiditis is a common cause of thyrotoxicosis. Its etiology is not fully understood; autoimmunity may underlie most cases.
- Thyrotoxicosis factitia is hyperthyroidism due to ingestion of exogenous thyroid hormone. This may occur when thyroid hormone is used for inappropriate indications, excessive doses are used for accepted medical indications, there is accidental ingestion, or it is used surreptitiously.
- Amiodarone may induce thyrotoxicosis (2%–3% of patients), overt hypothyroidism (5% of patients), subclinical hypothyroidism (25% of patients), or euthyroid hyperthyroxinemia. Because of amiodarone's high iodine content (37% by weight), increased thyroid hormone synthesis commonly exacerbates thyroid dysfunction in patients with preexisting thyroid disease. Amiodarone also causes a destructive thyroiditis with leakage of thyroglobulin and thyroid hormones.

CLINICAL PRESENTATION

- Symptoms of thyrotoxicosis include nervousness, anxiety, palpitations, emotional lability, easy fatigability, heat intolerance, weight loss concurrent with increased appetite, increased frequency of bowel movements, proximal muscle weakness (noted on climbing stairs or arising from a sitting position), and scanty or irregular menses in women.
- Physical signs include warm, smooth, moist skin, and unusually fine hair; separation of the ends of the fingernails from the nail beds (onycholysis); retraction of the eyelids and lagging of the upper lid behind the globe upon downward gaze (lid lag); tachycardia at rest, widened pulse pressure, and systolic ejection murmur; occasional gynecomastia in men; fine tremor of the protruded tongue and outstretched hands; and hyperactive deep tendon reflexes. Thyromegaly is usually present.
- Graves' disease is manifested by hyperthyroidism, diffuse thyroid enlargement, and extrathyroidal findings of exophthalmos, pretibial myxedema, and thyroid acropathy. In severe disease, a thrill may be felt and a systolic bruit may be heard over the gland.
- In subacute thyroiditis, patients have severe pain in the thyroid region, which often extends to the ear. Systemic symptoms include fever, malaise, myalgia, and signs and symptoms of thyrotoxicosis. The thyroid gland is firm and exquisitely tender on physical examination.
- Painless thyroiditis has a triphasic course that mimics painful subacute thyroiditis. Most patients present with mild thyrotoxic symptoms; lid retraction and lid lag are present, but exophthalmos is absent. The thyroid gland may be diffusely enlarged without tenderness.
- Thyroid storm is a life-threatening medical emergency characterized by decompensated thyrotoxicosis, high fever (often >39.4°C [103°F]), tachycardia, tachypnea, dehydration, delirium, coma, nausea, vomiting, and diarrhea. Precipitating factors include infection, trauma, surgery, radioactive iodine (RAI) treatment, and withdrawal from antithyroid drugs.

DIAGNOSIS

- Elevated 24-hour radioactive iodine uptake (RAIU) indicates true hyperthyroidism: the patient's thyroid gland is overproducing T_4, T_3, or both (normal RAIU 10%–30%). A low RAIU indicates that excess thyroid hormone is not a consequence of thyroid gland hyperfunction but is likely caused by thyroiditis, struma ovarii, follicular cancer, or exogenous thyroid hormone ingestion.
- In thyrotoxic Graves' disease, there is an increase in the overall hormone production rate with a disproportionate increase in T_3 relative to T_4 (Table 20-1). Saturation of TBG is increased due to elevated serum levels of T_4 and T_3, which is reflected in elevated T_3 resin uptake. As a result, concentrations of free T_4, free T_3, and the free T_4 and T_3 indices are increased to an even greater extent than the measured serum total

TABLE 20-1	Thyroid Function Tests in Different Thyroid Conditions			
	Total T$_4$	Free T$_4$	Total T$_3$	TSH
Normal	4.5–10.9 mcg/dL	0.8–2.7 ng/dL	60–181 ng/dL	0.5–4.7 milli-international units/L
Hyperthyroid	↑↑	↑↑	↑↑↑	↓↓[a]
Hypothyroid	↓↓	↓↓	↓	↑↑[a]
Increased TBG	↑	Normal	↑	Normal

[a]Primary thyroid disease.

T$_4$ and T$_3$ concentrations. The TSH level is undetectable due to negative feedback by elevated levels of thyroid hormone at the pituitary. In patients with symptomatic disease, measurement of serum-free T$_4$, total T$_4$, total T$_3$, and TSH will confirm the diagnosis of thyrotoxicosis. If the patient is not pregnant or lactating, an increased 24-hour RAIU indicates that the thyroid gland is inappropriately using iodine to produce more thyroid hormone when the patient is thyrotoxic.

- For toxic adenomas, because there may be isolated elevation of serum T$_3$ with autonomously functioning nodules, a T$_3$ level must be measured to rule out T$_3$ toxicosis if the T$_4$ level is normal. If autonomous function is suspected but the TSH is normal, the diagnosis can be confirmed by failure of the autonomous nodule to decrease iodine uptake during exogenous T$_3$ administration sufficient to suppress TSH.
- In multinodular goiters, a thyroid scan shows patchy areas of autonomously functioning thyroid tissue.
- TSH-induced hyperthyroidism is diagnosed by evidence of peripheral hypermetabolism, diffuse thyroid gland enlargement, elevated free thyroid hormone levels, and elevated serum immunoreactive TSH concentrations. Because the pituitary gland is extremely sensitive to even minimal elevations of free T$_4$, a "normal" or elevated TSH level in any thyrotoxic patient indicates inappropriate production of TSH.
- TSH-secreting pituitary adenomas are diagnosed by demonstrating lack of TSH response to TRH stimulation, inappropriate TSH levels, elevated TSH α-subunit levels, and radiologic imaging.
- In subacute thyroiditis, thyroid function tests typically run a triphasic course in this self-limited disease. Initially, serum T$_4$ levels are elevated due to release of preformed thyroid hormone. The 24-hour RAIU during this time is <2% because of thyroid inflammation and TSH suppression by the elevated T$_4$ level. As the disease progresses, intrathyroidal hormone stores are depleted, and the patient may become mildly hypothyroid with appropriately elevated TSH level. During the recovery phase, thyroid hormone stores are replenished, and serum TSH elevation gradually returns to normal.
- During the thyrotoxic phase of painless thyroiditis, the 24-hour RAIU is suppressed to <2%. Antithyroglobulin and antithyroid peroxidase antibody levels are elevated in more than 50% of patients.
- Thyrotoxicosis factitia should be suspected in a thyrotoxic patient without evidence of increased hormone production, thyroidal inflammation, or ectopic thyroid tissue. The RAIU is low because thyroid gland function is suppressed by exogenous thyroid hormone. Measurement of plasma thyroglobulin reveals presence of very low levels.

TREATMENT

- <u>Goals of Treatment</u>: Eliminate excess thyroid hormone; minimize symptoms and long-term consequences; and provide individualized therapy based on the type and severity of disease, patient age and gender, existence of nonthyroidal conditions, and response to previous therapy.

NONPHARMACOLOGIC THERAPY

- Surgical removal of the thyroid gland should be considered in patients with a large gland (>80 g), severe ophthalmopathy, or lack of remission on antithyroid drug treatment.
- If thyroidectomy is planned, **methimazole** is given until the patient is biochemically euthyroid (usually 6–8 weeks), followed by addition of **iodides** (500 mg/day) for 10–14 days before surgery to decrease vascularity of the gland.
- **Propranolol** has been used for several weeks preoperatively and 7–10 days after surgery to maintain pulse rate <90 beats/min. Combined pretreatment with propranolol and 10–14 days of **potassium iodide** also has been advocated.

PHARMACOLOGIC THERAPY

Thionamides

- **Methimazole** and **propylthiouracil (PTU)** block thyroid hormone synthesis by inhibiting the peroxidase enzyme system of the thyroid, preventing oxidation of trapped iodide and subsequent incorporation into iodotyrosines and ultimately iodo-thyronine ("organification"); and by inhibiting coupling of MIT and DIT to form T_4 and T_3. PTU (but not methimazole) also inhibits peripheral conversion of T_4 to T_3.
- Usual initial doses include methimazole 30–60 mg daily given in two or three divided doses or PTU 300–600 mg daily (usually in three or four divided doses). Evidence exists that both drugs can be given as a single daily dose.
- Improvement in symptoms and laboratory abnormalities should occur within 4–8 weeks, at which time a tapering regimen to maintenance doses can be started. Make dosage changes monthly because the endogenously produced T_4 will reach a new steady-state concentration in this interval. Typical daily maintenance doses are methimazole 5–30 mg and PTU 50–300 mg. Continue therapy for at least 12–24 months to induce long-term remission.
- Monitor patients every 6–12 months after remission. If a relapse occurs, alternate therapy with RAI is preferred over a second course of antithyroid drugs, but continued long-term low-dose methimazole may also be considered.
- Minor adverse reactions include pruritic maculopapular rashes, arthralgias, fever, and benign transient leukopenia (white blood cell count <4000/mm³ or 4×10^9/L). The alternate thionamide may be tried in these situations, but cross-sensitivity occurs in about 50% of patients.
- Major adverse effects include agranulocytosis (with fever, malaise, gingivitis, oro-pharyngeal infection, and granulocyte count <250/mm³ or 0.25×10^9/L), aplastic anemia, lupus-like syndrome, polymyositis, GI intolerance, hepatotoxicity, and hypoprothrombinemia. If agranulocytosis occurs, it usually develops in the first 3 months of therapy; routine WBC count monitoring is not recommended because of its sudden onset.
- Because of the risk of serious hepatotoxicity, PTU should not be considered first-line therapy in either adults or children. Exceptions to this recommendation include (1) the first trimester of pregnancy (when the risk of methimazole-induced embryopathy may exceed that of PTU-induced hepatotoxicity), (2) intolerance to methimazole, and (3) thyroid storm.

Iodides

- **Iodide** acutely blocks thyroid hormone release, inhibits thyroid hormone biosynthesis by interfering with intrathyroidal iodide use, and decreases size and vascularity of the gland.
- Symptom improvement occurs within 2–7 days of initiating therapy, and serum T_4 and T_3 concentrations may be reduced for a few weeks.
- Iodides are often used as adjunctive therapy to prepare a patient with Graves' disease for surgery, to acutely inhibit thyroid hormone release and quickly attain the euthyroid state in severely thyrotoxic patients with cardiac decompensation, or to inhibit thyroid hormone release after RAI therapy.

- **Potassium iodide** is available as a saturated solution (**SSKI**, 38 mg iodide per drop) or as **Lugol solution**, containing 6.3 mg of iodide per drop.
- Typical starting dose of SSKI is 3–10 drops daily (120–400 mg) in water or juice. When used to prepare a patient for surgery, it should be administered 7–14 days preoperatively.
- As an adjunct to RAI, SSKI should not be used before but rather 3–7 days after RAI treatment so that the RAI can concentrate in the thyroid.
- Adverse effects of iodide therapy include hypersensitivity reactions (skin rashes, drug fever, and rhinitis, conjunctivitis), salivary gland swelling, "iodism" (metallic taste, burning mouth and throat, sore teeth and gums, symptoms of a head cold, and sometimes stomach upset and diarrhea), and gynecomastia. Iodide is contraindicated in toxic multinodular goiter because the autonomous tissue utilizes the iodine for subsequent thyroid hormone synthesis.

Adrenergic Blockers

- β-Blockers are used to ameliorate symptoms such as palpitations, anxiety, tremor, and heat intolerance. They have no effect on peripheral thyrotoxicosis and protein metabolism and do not reduce TSAb or prevent thyroid storm. **Propranolol** and **nadolol** partially block conversion of T_4 to T_3, but this contribution to overall effect is small.
- β-Blockers are usually used as adjunctive therapy with antithyroid drugs, RAI, or iodides when treating Graves' disease or toxic nodules, in preparation for surgery, or in thyroid storm. The only conditions for which β-blockers are primary therapy for thyrotoxicosis are those associated with thyroiditis.
- **Propranolol** doses required to relieve adrenergic symptoms vary, but an initial dose of 20–40 mg orally four times daily is effective for most patients (goal heart rate <90 beats/min). Younger or more severely toxic patients may require 240–480 mg/day, perhaps because of increased clearance.
- β-Blockers are contraindicated in decompensated heart failure unless it is caused solely by tachycardia (high output). Other contraindications are sinus bradycardia, concomitant therapy with monoamine oxidase inhibitors or tricyclic antidepressants, and patients with spontaneous hypoglycemia. Side effects include nausea, vomiting, anxiety, insomnia, lightheadedness, bradycardia, and hematologic disturbances.
- Centrally acting sympatholytics (eg, **clonidine**) and calcium channel antagonists (eg, **diltiazem**) may be useful for symptom control when contraindications to β-blockade exist.

Radioactive Iodine

- **Sodium iodide–131** is an oral liquid that concentrates in the thyroid and initially disrupts hormone synthesis by incorporating into thyroid hormones and thyroglobulin. Over a period of weeks, follicles that have taken up RAI and surrounding follicles develop evidence of cellular necrosis and fibrosis of interstitial tissue.
- RAI is the agent of choice for Graves' disease, toxic autonomous nodules, and toxic multinodular goiters. Pregnancy is an absolute contraindication to use of RAI because radiation would be delivered to the fetal tissue.
- β-Blockers are the primary adjunctive therapy to RAI because they may be given anytime without compromising RAI therapy.
- If iodides are administered, they should be given 3–7 days after RAI to prevent interference with uptake of RAI in the thyroid gland.
- Patients with cardiac disease and elderly patients are often treated with thionamides prior to RAI ablation because thyroid hormone levels transiently increase after RAI treatment due to release of preformed thyroid hormone.
- Administering antithyroid drug therapy immediately after RAI may result in a higher rate of posttreatment recurrence or persistent hyperthyroidism.

- Use of lithium as adjunctive therapy to RAI has benefits of increased cure rate, shortened time to cure, and prevention of posttherapy increases in thyroid hormone levels.
- The goal of therapy is to destroy overactive thyroid cells, and a single dose of 4000–8000 rad results in a euthyroid state in 60% of patients at 6 months or sooner. A second dose of RAI should be given 6 months after the first RAI treatment if the patient remains hyperthyroid.
- Hypothyroidism commonly occurs months to years after RAI. The acute, short-term side effects include mild thyroidal tenderness and dysphagia. Long-term follow-up has not revealed an increased risk for development of mutations or congenital defects.

TREATMENT OF THYROID STORM

- Initiate the following therapeutic measures promptly: (1) suppression of thyroid hormone formation and secretion, (2) antiadrenergic therapy, (3) administration of corticosteroids, and (4) treatment of associated complications or coexisting factors that may have precipitated the storm (Table 20-2).
- **PTU** in large doses may be the preferred thionamide because it blocks peripheral conversion of T_4 to T_3 in addition to interfering with thyroid hormone production. However, β-blockers and corticosteroids serve the same purpose. **Methimazole** has a longer duration of action, which offers a theoretical advantage.
- **Iodides**, which rapidly block the release of preformed thyroid hormone, should be administered after a thionamide is initiated to inhibit iodide utilization by the overactive gland.
- Antiadrenergic therapy with the short-acting agent **esmolol** is preferred because it can be used in patients with pulmonary disease or at risk for cardiac failure and because its effects can be rapidly reversed.
- **Corticosteroids** are generally recommended, but there is no convincing evidence of adrenocortical insufficiency in thyroid storm; their benefits may be attributed to their antipyretic action and stabilization of blood pressure (BP).
- General supportive measures, including **acetaminophen** as an antipyretic (avoid aspirin or other nonsteroidal anti-inflammatory drugs, which may displace bound thyroid hormone), **fluid and electrolyte replacement, sedatives, digoxin, antiarrhythmics, insulin**, and **antibiotics** should be given as indicated.

TABLE 20-2	Drug Dosages Used in the Management of Thyroid Storm
Drug	**Regimen**
Propylthiouracil	900–1200 mg/day orally in four or six divided doses
Methimazole	90–120 mg/day orally in four or six divided doses
Sodium iodide	Up to 2 g/day IV in single or divided doses
Lugol solution	5–10 drops three times a day in water or juice
Saturated solution of potassium iodide	1–2 drops three times a day in water or juice
Propranolol	40–80 mg every 6 hours
Dexamethasone	5–20 mg/day orally or IV in divided doses
Prednisone	25–100 mg/day orally in divided doses
Methylprednisolone	20–80 mg/day IV in divided doses
Hydrocortisone	100–400 mg/day IV in divided doses

EVALUATION OF THERAPEUTIC OUTCOMES

- After therapy (surgery, thionamides, or RAI) for hyperthyroidism has been initiated, evaluate patients monthly until they reach a euthyroid condition.
- Assess for clinical signs of continuing thyrotoxicosis or development of hypothyroidism.
- If T_4 replacement is initiated, the goal is to maintain both the free T_4 level and the TSH concentration in the normal range. Once a stable dose of T_4 is identified, monitor the patient every 6–12 months.

Hypothyroidism

PATHOPHYSIOLOGY

- The vast majority of patients have primary hypothyroidism due to thyroid gland failure caused by chronic autoimmune thyroiditis (Hashimoto disease). Defects in suppressor T lymphocyte function lead to survival of a randomly mutating clone of helper T lymphocytes directed against antigens on the thyroid membrane. The resulting interaction stimulates B lymphocytes to produce thyroid antibodies.
- Iatrogenic hypothyroidism follows exposure to destructive amounts of radiation, after total thyroidectomy, or with excessive thionamide doses used to treat hyperthyroidism. Other causes of primary hypothyroidism include iodine deficiency, enzymatic defects within the thyroid, thyroid hypoplasia, and ingestion of goitrogens.
- Secondary hypothyroidism due to pituitary failure is uncommon. Pituitary insufficiency may be caused by destruction of thyrotrophs by pituitary tumors, surgical therapy, external pituitary radiation, postpartum pituitary necrosis (Sheehan syndrome), trauma, and infiltrative processes of the pituitary (eg, metastatic tumors, tuberculosis).

CLINICAL PRESENTATION

- Symptoms of hypothyroidism include dry skin, cold intolerance, weight gain, constipation, weakness, lethargy, depression, fatigue, exercise intolerance, loss of ambition or energy, muscle cramps, myalgia, and stiffness. Menorrhagia and infertility are common in women. In children, thyroid hormone deficiency may manifest as growth or intellectual retardation.
- Physical signs include coarse skin and hair, cold or dry skin, periorbital puffiness, bradycardia, and slowed or hoarse speech. Objective weakness (with proximal muscles affected more than distal muscles) and slow relaxation of deep tendon reflexes are common. Reversible neurologic syndromes such as carpal tunnel syndrome, polyneuropathy, and cerebellar dysfunction may also occur.
- Most patients with secondary hypothyroidism due to inadequate TSH production have clinical signs of generalized pituitary insufficiency, such as abnormal menses and decreased libido, or evidence of a pituitary adenoma, such as visual field defects, galactorrhea, or acromegaloid features.
- Myxedema coma is a rare consequence of decompensated hypothyroidism manifested by hypothermia, advanced stages of hypothyroid symptoms, and altered sensorium ranging from delirium to coma. Mortality rates of 60%–70% necessitate immediate and aggressive therapy.

DIAGNOSIS

- A rise in TSH level is the first evidence of primary hypothyroidism. Many patients have a free T_4 level within the normal range (compensated or subclinical hypothyroidism) and few, if any, symptoms of hypothyroidism. As the disease progresses, the free T_4 drops below normal. The T_3 concentration is often maintained in the normal range despite low T_4. Eventually, free and/or total T_4 and T_3 serum concentrations should be low.

- In secondary hypothyroidism in patients with pituitary disease, serum TSH concentrations are generally low or normal. A serum TSH in the normal range is inappropriate if the patient's T_4 is low.

TREATMENT OF HYPOTHYROIDISM (TABLE 20-3)

- <u>Goals of Treatment</u>: Restore thyroid hormone concentrations in tissue, provide symptomatic relief, prevent neurologic deficits in newborns and children, and reverse the biochemical abnormalities of hypothyroidism.
- **Levothyroxine** (L-thyroxine, T_4) is the drug of choice for thyroid hormone replacement and suppressive therapy because it is chemically stable, relatively inexpensive, active when given orally, free of antigenicity, and has uniform potency. Because T_3 (and not T_4) is the biologically active form, levothyroxine administration results in a pool of thyroid hormone that is readily converted to T_3.
- In patients with longstanding disease and older individuals without known cardiac disease, start therapy with levothyroxine 50 mcg daily and increase after 1 month.
- The recommended initial dose for older patients with known cardiac disease is 25 mcg/day titrated upward in increments of 25 mcg at monthly intervals to prevent stress on the cardiovascular system.
- The average maintenance dose for most adults is ~125 mcg/day, but there is a wide range of replacement doses, necessitating individualized therapy and appropriate TSH monitoring to determine an appropriate dose.
- Most patients with subclinical hypothyroidism can be observed without treatment. Treatment may be indicated for subclinical hypothyroidism and serum thyrotropin levels 10 mU/L or higher or for young and middle-aged individuals with symptoms consistent with mild hypothyroidism.
- Levothyroxine is the drug of choice for pregnant women, and the goal is to decrease TSH to the normal reference range for pregnancy.
- Cholestyramine, calcium carbonate, sucralfate, aluminum hydroxide, ferrous sulfate, soybean formula, dietary fiber supplements, and espresso coffee may impair the GI absorption of levothyroxine. Acid suppression with histamine blockers and proton pump inhibitors may also reduce levothyroxine absorption. Drugs that increase nondeiodinative T_4 clearance include rifampin, carbamazepine, and possibly phenytoin. Selenium deficiency and amiodarone may block conversion of T_4 to T_3.
- **Thyroid USP** (or desiccated thyroid) is usually derived from pig thyroid gland. It may be antigenic in allergic or sensitive patients. Inexpensive generic brands may not be bioequivalent.
- **Liothyronine** (synthetic T_3) has uniform potency but has a higher incidence of cardiac adverse effects, higher cost, and difficulty in monitoring with conventional laboratory tests. It must be administered three times a day and may require a prolonged adjustment period to achieve stable euthyroidism.
- **Liotrix** (synthetic T_4:T_3 in a 4:1 ratio) is chemically stable, pure, and has a predictable potency but is expensive. It also lacks therapeutic rationale because most T_3 is converted peripherally from T_4.
- Excessive doses of thyroid hormone may lead to heart failure, angina pectoris, and myocardial infarction (MI). Hyperthyroidism leads to reduced bone density and increased risk of fracture.

TREATMENT OF MYXEDEMA COMA

- Immediate and aggressive therapy with IV bolus **levothyroxine**, 300–500 mcg, has traditionally been used. Initial treatment with IV **liothyronine** or a combination of both hormones has also been advocated because of impaired conversion of T_4 to T_3.
- Give glucocorticoid therapy with IV **hydrocortisone** 100 mg every 8 hours until coexisting adrenal suppression is ruled out.

TABLE 20-3 Thyroid Preparations Used in the Treatment of Hypothyroidism

Drug/Dosage Form	Content	Relative Dose	Comments/Equivalency
Thyroid USP Armour Thyroid, Nature-Throid, and Westhroid (T_4:T_3 ratio approximately 4.2:1); Armour, 1 grain = 60 mg; Nature-Throid and Westhroid, 1 grain = 65 mg. Doses include 1/4, 1/2, 1, 2, 3, 4, and 5 grain tablets	Desiccated pork thyroid gland	1 grain (equivalent to 74 mcg of T_4)	High T_3:T_4 ratio; inexpensive
Levothyroxine Synthroid, Levothroid, Levoxyl, Levo-T, Unithroid, and other generics 25, 50, 75, 88, 100, 112, 125, 137, 150, 175, 200, 300 mcg tablets; Tirosint 13–150 mcg liquid in gelatin capsule; Tirosint-Sol liquid solution 13, 25, 50, 75, 88, 100, 112, 137, 150, 175, and 200 mcg in unit-dose ampules; 200 and 500 mcg per vial solution for injection	Synthetic T_4	100 mcg	Stable; predictable potency; generics may be bioequivalent; when switching from natural thyroid to L-thyroxine, lower dose by one-half grain; variable absorption between products; half-life = 7 days, so daily dosing; considered to be drug of choice
Liothyronine Cytomel 5, 25, and 50 mcg tablets	Synthetic T_3	33 mcg (~equivalent to 100 mcg T_4)	Uniform absorption, rapid onset; half-life = 1.5 days, rapid peak and troughs
Liotrix Thyrolar 1/4, 1/2, 1, 2, and 3 grain tablets	Synthetic T_4:T_3 in 4:1 ratio	Thyrolar 1 = 50 mcg T_4 and 12.5 mcg T_3	Stable; predictable; expensive; risk of T_3 thyrotoxicosis because of high ratio of T_3 relative to T_4

- Consciousness, lowered TSH concentrations, and improvement in vital signs are expected within 24 hours.
- Maintenance levothyroxine doses are typically 75–100 mcg IV until the patient stabilizes and oral therapy is begun.
- Provide supportive therapy to maintain adequate ventilation, euglycemia, BP, and body temperature. Diagnose and treat underlying disorders that may have precipitated the event, such as sepsis and MI.

EVALUATION OF THERAPEUTIC OUTCOMES

- Serum TSH concentration is the most sensitive and specific monitoring parameter for adjustment of levothyroxine dose. Concentrations begin to fall within hours and are usually normalized within 2–6 weeks.
- Check both TSH and T_4 concentrations every 6 weeks until a euthyroid state is achieved. An elevated TSH level indicates insufficient replacement. Serum T_4 concentrations can be useful in detecting noncompliance, malabsorption, or changes in levothyroxine product bioequivalence. TSH may also be used to help identify noncompliance.
- In patients with hypothyroidism caused by hypothalamic or pituitary failure, alleviation of the clinical syndrome and restoration of serum T_4 to the normal range are the only criteria available for estimating the appropriate replacement dose of levothyroxine.

See Chapter 96, Thyroid Disorders, authored by Michael P. Kane and Gary Bakst, for a more detailed discussion of this topic.

CHAPTER 21

Cirrhosis and Portal Hypertension

- Chronic liver injury causes damage to normal liver tissue, resulting in development of regenerative nodules surrounded by dense fibrotic material, which are diagnostic hallmarks of cirrhosis.

PATHOPHYSIOLOGY

- The distorted architecture of the cirrhotic liver impedes portal blood flow, interferes with hepatocyte perfusion, and disrupts hepatic synthetic functions such as the production of albumin. Clinical consequences of cirrhosis include increased intrahepatic resistance leading to portal hypertension, varices, and variceal bleeding; ascites; infection; hepatic encephalopathy (HE); and hepatocellular carcinoma.
- Primary causes of cirrhosis in developed countries include hepatitis C, excessive alcohol intake, and nonalcoholic fatty liver disease (Table 21-1).
- Cirrhosis causes changes to the splanchnic vasculature and circulation. Splanchnic vasodilation and the formation of new blood vessels contribute to increased splanchnic blood flow, formation of gastroesophageal varices, and variceal bleeding. Additionally, splanchnic vasodilation leads to hypoperfusion of the renal system, which causes activation of the renin–angiotensin–aldosterone system and, subsequently, significant fluid retention. The pathophysiologic abnormalities that cause it often result in ascites, portal hypertension and esophageal varices, HE, and coagulation disorders.

TABLE 21-1	Etiology of Cirrhosis
Alcohol use disorder	
Chronic hepatitis C	
Metabolic liver disease	
Hemochromatosis	
Wilson's disease	
Nonalcoholic fatty liver disease	
Immunologic disease	
Autoimmune hepatitis	
Primary biliary cirrhosis	
Primary biliary cholangitis	
Vascular disease	
Budd–Chiari	
Drug-induced livery injury (below list not all-inclusive)	
Isoniazid, macrolides, amoxicillin-clavulanate, nitrofurantoin, fluoroquinolones, amiodarone, nonsteroidal anti-inflammatory drugs, allopurinol, sulfasalazine, methotrexate, interferon-β, interferon-α, anti-tumor necrosis factor inhibitors, valproate, lamotrigine, phenytoin, carbamazepine, green tea extract	

- **Portal hypertension** is noted by elevated pressure gradient between the portal and central venous pressure and is characterized by hypervolemia, increased cardiac index, hypotension, and decreased systemic vascular resistance.
- Ascites is the pathologic accumulation of fluid within the abdomen. It is a common complication of cirrhosis.

PORTAL HYPERTENSION AND VARICES

- The most important sequelae of portal hypertension are the development of varices and alternative routes of blood flow resulting in acute variceal bleeding. Portal hypertension is defined by the presence of a gradient of >5 mm Hg (0.7 kPa) between the portal and central venous pressures.
- Progression to bleeding can be predicted by Child–Pugh score, size of varices, and the presence of red wale markings on the varices. First variceal hemorrhage occurs at an annual rate of about 15% and carries a mortality of 7%–15%.

HEPATIC ENCEPHALOPATHY

- HE is a functional disturbance of the brain caused by liver insufficiency or portal systemic shunting that presents on a wide spectrum of symptom severity ranging from subclinical alterations to coma.
- The symptoms of HE are thought to result from an accumulation of gut-derived nitrogenous substances in the systemic circulation as a consequence of decreased hepatic functioning. These substances then enter the central nervous system (CNS) and result in alterations of neurotransmission that affect consciousness and behavior.
- Altered ammonia, glutamate, benzodiazepine receptor agonists, and aromatic amino acids are potential causes of HE. An established correlation between blood ammonia levels and mental status does not exist.
- Type A HE is induced by acute liver failure, type B results from portal-systemic bypass without intrinsic liver disease, and type C occurs in patients with cirrhosis. HE may be classified as episodic, persistent, or minimal.

COAGULATION DEFECTS

- End-stage chronic liver disease is associated with decreased synthetic capability of the liver leading to decreased levels of most procoagulant factors as well as the naturally occurring anticoagulants: antithrombin, protein C, and protein S.
- Antithrombin and protein C are decreased, but two procoagulant factors, factor VIII and von Willebrand factor, are actually elevated. The net effect of these events could be thrombosis or clinically significant bleeding.
- Both platelet number and function may be affected in cirrhosis. Thrombocytopenia, a common finding in cirrhosis, could promote bleeding.

CLINICAL PRESENTATION

- Initial symptoms of cirrhosis may be nonspecific including fatigue, loss of appetite, and weight loss (Table 21-2). Patients may also present with much more significant symptoms secondary to decompensation related to cirrhosis complications such as ascites (abdominal distention) and HE (confusion, lethargy).
- Muscle wasting, palmar erythema, spider angiomas, parotid gland enlargement, white nails, Dupuytren contracture, asterixis, and metabolic complications including gynecomastia, testicular atrophy, and axillary hair loss are all possibly related to cirrhosis.
- A thorough history including risk factors that predispose patients to cirrhosis or nonalcoholic liver disease should be taken. Diagnostics for cirrhosis include liver function tests, coagulation tests, complete blood count, and serologic tests for viral causes including hepatitis B and C.

LABORATORY ABNORMALITIES

- There are no laboratory or radiographic tests of hepatic function that can accurately diagnose cirrhosis. Serum or plasma chemistries called "liver function tests" can

TABLE 21-2 Clinical Presentation of Cirrhosis

Signs and Symptoms
- Asymptomatic
- Splenomegaly
- Jaundice, palmar erythema, and spider nevi
- Gynecomastia
- Ascites and edema
- Malaise, anorexia, and weight loss
- Encephalopathy

Laboratory Tests
- Hypoalbuminemia
- Elevated prothrombin time (PT)
- Thrombocytopenia
- Elevated alkaline phosphatase
- Elevated aspartate transaminase (AST), alanine transaminase (ALT), and γ-glutamyl transpeptidase (GGT)

be grouped into two broad categories: (1) markers of liver injury such as aspartate transaminase (AST), alanine aminotransferase (ALT), γ-glutamyl transpeptidase (GGT), and alkaline phosphatase, and (2) markers of hepatocellular function such as prothrombin time (PT), bilirubin, and albumin.

- The aminotransferases, AST and ALT, are enzymes that have increased concentrations in plasma after acute or chronic hepatocellular injury. The highest elevations ($>10,000$ units per liter [167 ukat/L]) are most likely to occur in shock liver and drug- or toxin-induced hepatitis. The ratio of AST to ALT with AST>ALT is more likely when cirrhosis of any etiology exists but also occurs in alcoholic and ischemic liver disease.

- Elevated serum alkaline phosphatase and GGT occur in cases of liver injury with a cholestatic pattern and therefore often accompany conditions such as primary biliary cirrhosis, primary sclerosing cholangitis, drug-induced cholestasis, and bile duct obstruction.

- Elevations in serum conjugated (or direct) bilirubin indicate hepatocellular dysfunction or cholestasis. Indirect bilirubin elevations occur due to overproduction (as seen with hemolysis), decreased uptake, or decreased hepatic conjugation of bilirubin. Direct hyperbilirubinemia is the result of liver injury or biliary obstruction and is associated with a number of hepatic diseases including cirrhosis.

- Albumin and coagulation factors are markers of hepatic synthetic activity and are used to estimate hepatocyte function in cirrhosis. Reduction in albumin usually indicates a disease duration of more than 3 weeks whereas severe liver disease can cause PT elevation in less than 24 hours. Thrombocytopenia is a common feature in chronic liver disease.

- The Child–Pugh classification system uses a combination of physical and laboratory findings to assess and define the severity of cirrhosis and is a predictor of patient survival, surgical outcome, and risk of variceal bleeding (Table 21-3).

- The model for end-stage liver disease (MELD-Na) is a newer scoring system:

$$\text{MELD score} = 9.57 \times \log_e(\text{serum creatinine}[\text{mg/dL}]) + 3.78$$
$$\times \log_e(\text{bilirubin}[\text{mg/dL}]) + 11.20 \times \log_e(\text{INR}) + 6.43$$

or using SI units:

$$\text{MELD score} = 9.57 \times \log_e(\text{creatinine}[\mu\text{mol/L}]) + 3.78$$
$$\times \log_e(\text{bilirubin}[\mu\text{mol/L}]) \times 0.05848) + 11.20 \times \log_e(\text{INR}) + 6.43$$

where international normalized ratio (INR) is TK.

$$\text{MELD-Na score} = \text{MELD} - (\text{sodium}[\text{mEq/L}]) - (0.025 \times \text{MELD}$$
$$\times (140 - \text{sodium}[\text{mEq/L}])) + 140$$

TABLE 21-3	Criteria and Scoring for the Child–Pugh Grading of Chronic Liver Disease		
Score	**1**	**2**	**3**
Total bilirubin (mg/dL)	<2 (34.2 μmol/L)	2–3 (34.2–51.3 μmol/L)	>3 (51.3 μmol/L)
Albumin (g/dL)	>3.5 (35 g/L)	2.8–3.5 (28–35 g/L)	<2.8 (28 g/L)
Ascites	None	Mild	Moderate
Encephalopathy (grade)	None	1 and 2	3 and 4
Prothrombin time (seconds prolonged)	<4	4-6	>6

Grade A, <7 points; grade B, 7–9 points; grade C, 10–15 points.

or using SI units:

$$\text{MELD-Na score} = \text{MELD} - (\text{sodium[mmol/L]}) - (0.025 \times \text{MELD} \\ \times (140 - \text{sodium[mmol/L]})) + 140$$

- In MELD, laboratory values less than 1 are rounded up to 1. The formula's score is multiplied by 10 and rounded to the nearest whole number.

TREATMENT

- <u>Goals of Treatment</u>: *Resolution of acute complications* such as tamponade of bleeding and resolution of hemodynamic instability for an episode of acute variceal hemorrhage and *prevention of complications* through lowering of portal pressure with medical therapy using nonselective β-adrenergic blocker therapy or supporting abstinence from alcohol.

GENERAL APPROACH TO TREATMENT

- Approaches to treatment include the following:
  ✓ Identify and eliminate the causes of cirrhosis (eg, alcohol abuse).
  ✓ Assess the risk for variceal bleeding and begin pharmacologic prophylaxis where indicated, reserving endoscopic therapy for high-risk patients or acute bleeding episodes as well as patients with contraindications or intolerance to nonselective β-adrenergic blockers.
  ✓ Evaluate for clinical signs of ascites and manage with pharmacologic treatment (eg, diuretics) and paracentesis. Spontaneous bacterial peritonitis (SBP) should be carefully monitored in patients with ascites who undergo acute deterioration.
  ✓ HE is a common complication of cirrhosis and requires clinical vigilance and treatment with dietary restriction, elimination of CNS depressants, and therapy to lower ammonia levels.
  ✓ Frequent monitoring for signs of hepatorenal syndrome, pulmonary insufficiency, and endocrine dysfunction is necessary.

MANAGEMENT OF PORTAL HYPERTENSION AND VARICEAL BLEEDING

- The management of varices involves three strategies: (1) primary prophylaxis to prevent first bleeding episode, (2) treatment of variceal hemorrhage, and (3) secondary prophylaxis to prevent rebleeding in patients who have already bled.

Primary Prophylaxis

- All patients with cirrhosis and portal hypertension should be screened for varices on diagnosis.
- The mainstay of primary prophylaxis is the use of a nonselective β-adrenergic blocking agent such as **propranolol, nadolol,** or **carvedilol**. These agents reduce portal

pressure by reducing portal venous inflow via two mechanisms: decrease in cardiac output and decrease in splanchnic blood flow.

- β-Adrenergic blocker therapy is not indicated in patients without varices to prevent the formation of varices.
- Patients with small varices plus risk factors for variceal hemorrhage including red wale marks or Child–Pugh grade C should receive prophylactic therapy with a non-selective β-adrenergic blocker.
- Therapy for medium or large varices that have not bled should be initiated with pro-pranolol 20 mg twice daily, nadolol 20–40 mg once daily and titrate every 2–3 days to maximal tolerated dose or to a heart rate of 55–60 beats/min, or, rather than pro-pranolol or nadolol, carvedilol could be chosen and started at 3.125 mg twice daily with titration to 6.25 mg twice daily after 3 days.
- Carvedilol may be considered in patients unable to tolerate propranolol or nadolol due to side effects like fatigue, weakness, and shortness of breath as it is perceived to be better tolerated than the pure nonselective β-adrenergic blockers.
- β-Adrenergic blocker therapy should be continued indefinitely.
- Endoscopic vein ligation (EVL) is an alternative to β-adrenergic blockers. If EVL is chosen, it will be performed every 2–4 weeks until the obliteration of varices.
- Monitor patients for development of contraindications to β-adrenergic blockers such as renal impairment and hypotension that may accompany end-stage liver disease.

ACUTE VARICEAL HEMORRHAGE

- Figure 21-1 presents an algorithm for managing variceal hemorrhage. Evidence-based recommendations for select treatments are presented in Tables 21-4 and 21-5.
- Treatment of acute variceal bleeding includes general stabilizing and assessment measures as well as specific measures to control the acute hemorrhage and prevent complications.
- Initial treatment goals include: (1) adequate blood volume resuscitation, (2) protec-tion of the airway from aspiration of blood, (3) prophylaxis against SBP and other infections, (4) control of bleeding, (5) prevention of rebleeding, (6) preservation of liver function of HE, and (7) prevention of acute kidney injury.
- Prompt stabilization of blood volume to maintain hemoglobin of 7 g/dL (70 g/L; 4.34 mmol/L) to 8 g/dL (80 g/L; 4.97 mmol/L) is recommended.
- Combination pharmacologic therapy plus EVL (preferred) or sclerotherapy (when EVL is not technically feasible) is the most rational approach to treatment of acute variceal bleeding.
- Vasoactive drug therapy is used to stop or slow bleeding as soon as a diagnosis of variceal bleeding is suspected and is started before endoscopy. Treatment with **octreotide** should be initiated early to control bleeding and facilitate endoscopy. Octreotide is administered as an IV bolus of 50 mcg followed by a continuous infu-sion of 50 mcg/h. It should be continued for 2–5 days after acute variceal bleeding. Vasoactive therapy discontinuation can be considered once the patient is free of bleeding for at least 24 hours.
- Prophylactic antibiotic therapy to prevent SBP and other infections should be imple-mented upon admission. For all patients with cirrhosis and acute variceal bleeding, intravenous ceftriaxone 1 g/24 hours is recommended. A 250-mg dose of **erythro-mycin** intravenously prior to endoscopy may be used to accelerate gastric emptying of clots and improve visibility during the endoscopic procedure.
- Child–Pugh Class C patients and those in Class B with active hemorrhage at the time of diagnostic endoscopy are at high risk for failing standard therapy with EVL plus octreotide. In these patients early transjugular intrahepatic portosystemic shunt (TIPS) may be considered instead of standard therapy. The TIPS procedure involves the placement of one or more stents between the hepatic vein and the portal vein.

Prevention of Rebleeding

- A nonselective β-adrenergic blocker along with EVL is the best treatment option for variceal bleeding—secondary prophylaxis.

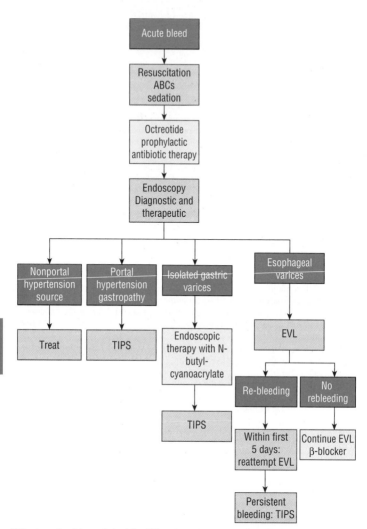

ABCs, airway, breathing, and circulation; EVL, endoscopic variceal ligation; TIPS, transjugular intrahepatic portosystemic shunt.

FIGURE 21-1. Management of acute variceal hemorrhage.

- **Propranolol** may be given at 20 mg twice daily (or **nadolol** 40 mg once daily) and titrated weekly to achieve a goal of heart rate 55–60 beats/min or the maximal tolerated dose. Patients should be monitored for evidence of bradycardia, bronchospasm, and hypoglycemia, particularly in patients with insulin-dependent diabetes, as well as symptoms of heart failure and excessive sodium and water retention. Maximum doses of propranolol 320 mg/day for patients without ascites and 160 mg/day for patients with ascites, and nadolol 160 mg/day for patients without ascites and 80 mg/day for patients with ascites are recommended.
- Patients who cannot tolerate or who fail pharmacologic and endoscopic interventions can be considered for tips to prevent bleeding.

TABLE 21-4	Evidence-Based Table of Select Treatment Recommendations: Variceal Bleeding in Portal Hypertension	
Recommendation		**Grade**
Prevention of variceal bleeding		
Nonselective β-blocker therapy should be initiated in:		
Patients with small varices and criteria for increased risk of hemorrhage		1b
Patients with medium/large varices		1a
EVL may be recommended for prevention in patients with medium/large varices at high risk of hemorrhage instead of nonselective β-blocker therapy		1a
Treatment of variceal bleeding		
Short-term antibiotic prophylaxis should be instituted on admission		1a
Vasoactive drugs should be started as soon as possible, prior to endoscopy, and maintained for up to 5 days		1a
Endoscopy should be performed to diagnose variceal bleeding and treat bleeding with EVL		1b
Endoscopy should be performed within 12 hours of presentation		5
Unless contraindicated, erythromycin 250 mg IV should be administered 30–120 minutes prior to endoscopy		1b
Secondary prophylaxis of variceal bleeding		
Nonselective β-blocker therapy plus EVL is the best therapeutic option for prevention of recurrent variceal bleeding		1a

Recommendation grading:
1a: Systematic review (with homogeneity) of randomized controlled trials.
1b: Individual randomized controlled trial with narrow confidence interval.
1c: All or none.
2a: Systematic review (with homogeneity) of cohort studies.
2b: Individual cohort study (including low-quality randomized controlled trial).
2c: Outcomes research; ecological studies.
3a: Systematic review (with homogeneity) of case-controlled studies.
3b: Individual case-control study.
4: Case-series (and poor quality cohort and case-control studies).
5: Expert opinion.

ASCITES

- The therapeutic goals for patients with ascites are to control the ascites, prevent or relieve ascites-related symptoms (dyspnea, abdominal pain, and distention), and prevent SBP and hepatorenal syndrome.
- For patients with ascites, a serum–ascites albumin gradient should be determined. If the gradient is ≥1.1 g/dL (11 g/L), the patient almost certainly has portal hypertension.
- The treatment of ascites secondary to portal hypertension includes abstinence from alcohol, sodium restriction (to 2 g/day), and diuretic therapy. Fluid loss and weight change depend directly on sodium balance in these patients. A goal of therapy is to increase urinary excretion of sodium to >78 mmol/day.
- Diuretic therapy should be initiated with single morning doses of **spironolactone** 100 mg and **furosemide** 40 mg, titrated every 3–5 days (or spironolactone alone), using the 100:40 mg dose ratio (spironolactone to furosemide) with a goal of 0.5 kg maximum daily weight loss. The dose of each can be increased together, maintaining the 100:40 mg ratio, to a maximum daily dose of 400 mg spironolactone and 160 mg furosemide.

TABLE 21-5	Evidence-Based Table of Selected Treatment Recommendations: Ascites and Spontaneous Bacterial Peritonitis	
Recommendation		**Grade**

Ascites

Paracentesis should be performed in patients with apparent new-onset ascites	IC
Sodium restriction of 2000 mg/day should be instituted as well as oral diuretic therapy with spironolactone and furosemide	IIaA
Diuretic-sensitive patients should be treated with sodium restriction and diuretics rather than serial paracentesis	IIaC

Refractory ascites

Serial therapeutic paracenteses may be performed	IC
Postparacentesis albumin infusion of 6–8 g/L of fluid removed can be considered if more than 5 L is removed during paracentesis	IIaA

Treatment of SBP

If ascitic fluid polymorphonuclear leukocytes (PMN) counts are >250 cells/mm³ (0.25 × 10⁹/L), empiric antibiotic therapy should be instituted (cefotaxime 2 g every 8 hours)	IA
If ascitic fluid PMN counts are <250 cells/mm³ (0.25 × 10⁹/L), but signs or symptoms of infection exist, empiric antibiotic therapy should be initiated while awaiting culture results	IB
If ascitic fluid polymorphonuclear leukocyte counts are >250 cells/mm³ (0.25 × 10⁹/L), clinical suspicion of SBP is present, and the patient has a serum creatinine >1 mg/dL (88 μmol/L), blood urea nitrogen >30 mg/dL (10.7 mmol/L), or total bilirubin over 4 mg/dL (68.4 μmol/L), 1.5 g/kg albumin should be infused within 6 hours of detection and 1 g/kg albumin infusion should also be given on day 3	IIaB

Prophylaxis against SBP

Short-term antibiotic prophylaxis should be used for 7 days to prevent SBP in cirrhosis patients with GI hemorrhage	IA
Patients who survive an episode of SBP should receive long-term prophylaxis with either daily ciprofloxacin or trimethoprim–sulfamethoxazole	IA
Patients with low-protein ascites (<1.5 g/dL [15 g/L]) plus at least one of the following: serum creatinine ≥1.2 mg/dL (106 μmol/L), blood urea nitrogen ≥25 mg/dL (8.9 mmol/L), serum sodium ≤130 mEq/L (mmol/L), or Child-Pugh score of ≥9 with bilirubin ≥3 mg/dL (51.3 μmol/L) may also justifiably receive long-term ciprofloxacin or sulfamethoxazole/trimethoprim as prophylaxis	IA

Recommendation grading: Class I—conditions for which there is evidence and/or general agreement; Class II—conditions for which there is conflicting evidence and/or a divergence of opinion; Class IIa—weight of evidence/opinion is in favor of efficacy; Class IIb—efficacy less well established; Class III—conditions for which there is evidence and/or general agreement that treatment is not effective and/or potentially harmful; Level A—data from multiple randomized trials or meta-analyses; Level B—data derived from single randomized trial or nonrandomized studies; Level C—only consensus opinion, case studies, or standard of care.

- Diuretic therapy should be discontinued in patients who experience uncontrolled or recurrent encephalopathy, severe hyponatremia (serum sodium <120 mEq/L [mmol/L]) despite fluid restriction, or renal insufficiency (serum creatinine >2 mg/dL [177 μmol/L]).
- If tense ascites is present, paracentesis should be performed prior to institution of diuretic therapy and salt restriction.
- Liver transplant should be considered in patients with refractory ascites.

SPONTANEOUS BACTERIAL PERITONITIS

- Patients with documented or suspected SBP should receive broad-spectrum antibiotic therapy to cover *Escherichia coli, Klebsiella pneumoniae,* and pneumococci. Patients with ascitic fluid PMN counts greater than or equal to 250 cells/mm^3 (0.25 × 10^9/L) should receive empiric antibiotic therapy.
- **Cefotaxime** 2 g every 8 hours IV or a similar third-generation cephalosporin for 5 days is recommended. Ceftriaxone or piperacillin/tazobactam is an alternative for community-acquired SBP.
- Patients who survive an episode of SBP should receive long-term antibiotic prophylaxis with daily ciprofloxacin 500 mg.

HEPATIC ENCEPHALOPATHY

- The general approach to the management of HE is four pronged and includes the following: care for patients with altered consciousness, identify and treat any other causes besides HE for altered mental status, identify and treat any precipitating factors, and begin empirical HE treatment.
- The grading system for HE is provided in **Table 21-6**.
- Treatment approaches include: reduction in blood ammonia concentrations by protein withdrawal, with drug therapy aimed at inhibiting ammonia production or enhancing its removal (nonabsorbable disaccharides such as lactulose and antibiotics).
- To reduce blood ammonia concentrations in patients with episodic HE, protein intake is limited or withheld (while maintaining caloric intake) until the clinical situation improves. Once successful reversal of HE symptoms is achieved, protein intake can be titrated back up based on tolerance to a total of 1.2–1.5 g/kg/day. Vegetable-source and dairy-source protein may be preferable to meat-source protein because the latter contains a higher calorie-to-nitrogen ratio.
- In episodic HE, lactulose is initiated at a dose of 30 mL (20 g) orally every 1 to 2 hours until catharsis begins and the patient experiences one to two bowel movements. The

TABLE 21-6	Grading System for Hepatic Encephalopathy		
Grade	Level of Consciousness	Personality/Intellect	Neurologic Abnormalities
Unimpaired	Normal	Normal	Normal
Minimal	No clinical evidence of change	No clinical evidence of change/alterations identified on psychometric or neuropsychological testing	No clinical evidence of change
I	Trivial lack of awareness; shortened attention span	Euphoria or anxiety; impairment of addition or subtraction	Altered sleep rhythm
II	Lethargic	Obvious personality changes; inappropriate behavior; apathy	Asterixis; dyspraxia; disoriented for time
III	Somnolent but arousable	Bizarre behavior	Responsive to stimuli; confused; gross disorientation to time and space
IV	Coma/unarousable	None	Does not respond to stimuli

dose is then adjusted to produce two to three soft stools per day for chronic therapy. Patients are monitored for changes to their electrolytes periodically as well as for changes in mental status. Polyethylene glycol may be considered for patients suffering an acute HE episode.

- **Rifaximin** 550 mg twice daily plus lactulose is effective in the treatment of HE.
- Other adjunctive therapies include zinc replacement in patients with zinc deficiency and flumazenil in cases of refractory HE with the possibility of benzodiazepine use.

EVALUATION OF THERAPEUTIC OUTCOMES

- Table 21-7 summarizes the drug monitoring guidelines for patients with cirrhosis and portal hypertension, including monitoring parameters and therapeutic outcomes.

TABLE 21-7	Drug Monitoring Guidelines		
Drug	**Adverse Drug Reaction**	**Monitoring Parameter**	**Comments**
Nonselective β-adrenergic blocker	Heart failure, bronchospasm, glucose intolerance	BP, HR Goal HR: 55–60 beats/min or maximal tolerated dose	Nadolol, propranolol
Nonselective β-adrenergic blocker; alpha-blocker	Similar to nonselective β-adrenergic blocker, but potentially better tolerated	Goal BP: Systolic > 90 mm Hg	Carvedilol
Octreotide	Bradycardia, hypertension, arrhythmia, abdominal pain	BP, HR, EKG, abdominal pain	
Spironolactone/ furosemide	Electrolyte disturbances, dehydration, renal insufficiency, hypotension	Serum electrolytes (especially potassium), SCr, blood urea nitrogen, BP Goal sodium excretion: >78 mmol/day	Spot urine sodium concentration greater than potassium concentration correlates well with daily sodium excretion >78 mmol/day
Lactulose	Electrolyte disturbances	Serum electrolytes Goal number of soft stools per day: 2–3	
Neomycin	Ototoxicity, nephrotoxicity	SCr, annual auditory monitoring	
Metronidazole	Neurotoxicity	Sensory and motor neuropathy	
Rifaximin	Nausea, diarrhea		

BP, blood pressure; beats/min, beats per minute; EKG, electrocardiogram; HR, heart rate; SCr, serum creatinine; mmol, millimole.

See Chapter 55, Portal Hypertension and Cirrhosis, authored by Julie M. Sease for a more detailed discussion of this topic.

22 Constipation

- *Constipation* is the difficult or infrequent passage of stool, at times associated with straining or a feeling of incomplete defecation. The condition is considered chronic if symptoms last for at least 3 months.

PATHOPHYSIOLOGY

- Constipation may be primary (occurs without an underlying identifiable cause) or secondary (the result of constipating drugs, lifestyle factors, or medical disorders).
- Constipation commonly results from a diet low in fiber, inadequate fluid intake, decreased physical activity, or from use of constipating drugs such as opioids.
- Diseases or conditions that may cause constipation include the following:
  - ✓ Gastrointestinal (GI) disorders: Irritable bowel syndrome (IBS), diverticulitis, upper and lower GI tract diseases, hemorrhoids, anal fissures, ulcerative proctitis, tumors, hernia, volvulus of the bowel, syphilis, tuberculosis, lymphogranuloma venereum, and Hirschsprung disease.
  - ✓ Metabolic and endocrine disorders: Diabetes mellitus with neuropathy, hypothyroidism, panhypopituitarism, pheochromocytoma, hypercalcemia, and enteric glucagon excess.
  - ✓ Pregnancy: Depressed gut motility, increased fluid absorption from colon, use of iron salts.
  - ✓ Cardiac disorders (eg, heart failure).
  - ✓ Lifestyle factors: Dietary changes, inadequate fluid intake, low dietary fiber, decreased physical activity.
  - ✓ Neurogenic constipation: Head trauma, CNS tumors, spinal cord injury, cerebrospinal accidents, and Parkinson disease.
  - ✓ Psychogenic causes such as ignoring or postponing the urge to defecate and psychiatric diseases.

- Causes of drug-induced constipation are listed in Table 22-1. All opioid derivatives are associated with constipation, but the degree of intestinal inhibitory effects seems

TABLE 22-1	Drugs Causing Constipation

Analgesics
   Inhibitors of prostaglandin synthesis
   Opioids
Anticholinergics
   Antihistamines
   Antiparkinsonian agents (eg, benztropine or trihexyphenidyl)
   Phenothiazines
   Tricyclic antidepressants
Antacids containing calcium carbonate or aluminum hydroxide
Barium sulfate
Calcium channel antagonists
Clonidine
Diuretics (non–potassium-sparing)
Ganglionic blockers
Iron preparations
Muscle blockers (D-tubocurarine, succinylcholine)
Nonsteroidal anti-inflammatory agents
Polystyrene sodium sulfonate

to differ among agents. Orally administered opioids appear to have a greater inhibitory effect than parenterally administered agents.

CLINICAL PRESENTATION

- The general clinical presentation of constipation is shown below. According to the Rome IV criteria, patients should have at least two of the signs and symptoms listed below which apply to a minimum of 25% of bowel movements.
- A complete and thorough history should be obtained from the patient, including the frequency of bowel movements and duration of symptoms. The patient should also be carefully questioned about usual diet and laxative regimens.
- General health status, signs of underlying medical illness (ie, hypothyroidism), and psychological status (eg, depression or other psychological illness) should be assessed.
- Patients with "alarm symptoms," a family history of colon cancer, or those older than 50 years with new symptoms may need further diagnostic evaluation.
- **Signs and symptoms**:
  ✓ Infrequent bowel movements (<3 per week).
  ✓ Stools that are hard, small, or dry.
  ✓ Straining.
  ✓ Feeling of incomplete evacuation.
  ✓ Feeling of anorectal obstruction or blockage.
  ✓ Physical tactics needed for defecation.
  ✓ Loose stools rarely occur without laxative use.

- **Alarm signs and symptoms**:
  ✓ Hematochezia.
  ✓ Melena.
  ✓ Family history of colon cancer.
  ✓ Family history of inflammatory bowel disease.
  ✓ Anemia.
  ✓ Weight loss.
  ✓ Anorexia.
  ✓ Nausea and vomiting.
  ✓ Severe, persistent constipation that is refractory to treatment.
  ✓ New-onset or worsening constipation in elderly without evidence of primary cause.

- **Physical examination**:
  ✓ Perform rectal exam to check for the presence of anatomical abnormalities (such as fistulas, fissures, hemorrhoids, rectal prolapse) or abnormalities of perianal descent.
  ✓ Digital examination of rectum to check for fecal impaction, anal stricture, or rectal mass.

- **Laboratory and other diagnostic tests**:
  ✓ No routine recommendations for lab testing—as indicated by clinical discretion.
  ✓ In patients with signs and symptoms suggestive of organic disorder, specific testing may be performed (ie, thyroid function tests, electrolytes, glucose, complete blood count) based on clinical presentation.
  ✓ In patients with alarm signs and symptoms or when structural disease is a possibility, select appropriate diagnostic studies: rectal balloon expulsion test (BET), anorectal manometry, colonoscopy, barium enema.

TREATMENT

- Goals of Treatment: The major goals of treatment are to: (a) relieve symptoms; (b) reestablish normal bowel habits; and (c) improve quality of life by minimizing adverse effects of treatment.

GENERAL APPROACH

- If an underlying disease is recognized as the cause of constipation, attempts should be made to correct it. GI malignancies may be removed through a surgical resection. Endocrine and metabolic derangements are corrected by the appropriate methods.
- If a patient is consuming medications known to cause constipation, consideration should be given to alternative agents. If no reasonable alternatives exist to the medication thought to be responsible for constipation, consideration should be given to lowering the dose. If a patient must remain on constipating medications, more attention must be given to general measures for prevention of constipation.
- The proper management of constipation requires a combination of nonpharmacologic and pharmacologic therapies.

NONPHARMACOLOGIC THERAPY

- The most important aspect of the therapy for constipation is dietary modification to increase the amount of fiber consumed. Gradually increase daily fiber intake to 20–30 g, either through dietary changes or through fiber supplements. Fruits, vegetables, and cereals have the highest fiber content.
- A trial of dietary modification with high-fiber content should be continued for at least 1 month. Most patients begin to notice effects on bowel function 3–5 days after beginning a high-fiber diet.
- Patients with constipation due to pelvic floor dysfunction/disordered defecation may have a less favorable response to fiber therapy than other constipation subtypes. Many adult patients with functional defecatory disorders appear to benefit from pelvic floor retraining with biofeedback therapy.
- Abdominal distention and flatus may be particularly troublesome in the first few weeks, particularly with high bran consumption.

PHARMACOLOGIC THERAPY

- The laxatives are divided into three classifications: (1) those causing softening of feces in 1–3 days (bulk-forming laxatives, **docusates**, and low-dose **polyethylene glycol [PEG], lactulose, and lactitol**), (2) those resulting in soft or semifluid stool in 6–12 hours (**bisacodyl, senna, and magnesium sulfate**), and (3) those causing water evacuation in 1–6 hours (**magnesium salts, rectal bisacodyl**, and **PEG—electrolyte lavage solution**).
- Other agents include the calcium channel activator **lubiprostone**, the guanylate cyclase C agonists, **linaclotide, plecanatide**, and **naldemedine**, as well as opioid receptor antagonists **alvimopan, methylnaltrexone, naloxegol**, and **naldemedine**, and the prokinetic agent, **prucalopride**.
- Dosage recommendations for laxatives and cathartics are provided in Table 22-2.

Recommendations

- A constipation treatment algorithm is presented in Fig. 22-1.
- Osmotic laxative therapy is considered the preferred first line for the treatment of constipation, in addition to increasing dietary fiber or using fiber supplementation.
- Patients are often encouraged to increase daily fluid intake and physical activity as well as dedicate time to respond to the urge to defecate, although efficacy data are conflicting for these measures.

Emollient Laxatives (Docusates)

- **Docusates** are surfactant agents that increase water and electrolyte secretion in the small and large bowel and result in a softening of stools within 1–3 days.
- Emollient laxatives are not effective in treating constipation but are used mainly to prevent constipation. They may be helpful in situations where straining at stool should be avoided, such as after recovery from myocardial infarction, with acute perianal disease, or after rectal surgery.

TABLE 22-2 Dosage Recommendations for Pharmacologic Therapy

Agent	Recommended Adult Dose
Agents that Cause Softening of Feces in 1–3 Days	
Bulk-forming agents	
Methylcellulose	Varies with product
Polycarbophil	4–6 g/day
Psyllium	Varies with product
Emollients	
Docusate sodium	50–360 mg/day
Docusate calcium	50–360 mg/day
Docusate potassium	100–300 mg/day
Osmotic laxatives	
Polyethylene glycol 3350	17 g/dose
Lactulose	15–30 mL orally
Lactitol	20 g/day orally
Sorbitol	30–50 g/day orally
Agents that Result in Soft or Semifluid Stool in 6–12 Hours	
Bisacodyl (oral)	5–15 mg orally
Senna	Dose varies with formulation
Magnesium sulfate (low dose)	<10 g orally
Agents that Cause Watery Evacuation in 1–6 Hours	
Magnesium citrate	18 g in 300 mL water
Magnesium hydroxide	2.4–4.8 g orally
Magnesium sulfate (high dose)	10–30 g orally
Sodium phosphates	Varies with salt used
Bisacodyl	10 mg rectally
Polyethylene glycol–electrolyte preparations	4 L for bowel cleansing
Intestinal Secretagogues	
Lubiprostone	24 mcg orally twice daily
Linaclotide	145 mcg orally daily
Plecanatide	3 mg orally daily
Opioid Antagonists	
Methylnaltrexone	450 mg orally daily or 12 mg subcutaneously daily
Naloxegol	25 mg daily
Naldemedine	0.2 mg daily
Prokinetics	
Prucalopride	2 mg daily

• It is unlikely that these agents are effective in preventing constipation if major causative factors (eg, heavy opiate use, uncorrected pathology, and inadequate dietary fiber) are not concurrently addressed.

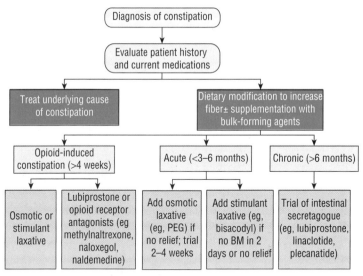

BM, bowel movement; PEG, polyethylene glycol.

FIGURE 22-1. A general treatment algorithm for constipation.

Lactulose

- **Lactulose** is generally not recommended as a first-line agent for the treatment of constipation because it is costly and may cause flatulence, nausea, and abdominal discomfort or bloating. It may be justified as an alternative for acute constipation or in patients with an inadequate response to increased dietary fiber and bulking agents.

Magnesium Salts

- Magnesium salts, including hydroxide, phosphate, and citrate, and sodium phosphate are categorized as saline cathartics. These agents are frequently used as bowel preparations prior to diagnostic procedures such as colonoscopy.
- Milk of magnesia (an 8% suspension of magnesium hydroxide) may be used occasionally to treat constipation in otherwise healthy adults, but efficacy data are limited.
- Saline cathartics should not be used on a routine basis. These agents may cause fluid and electrolyte depletion. Also, magnesium or sodium accumulation may occur in patients with renal dysfunction or congestive heart failure. These risks increase with long-term use.
- **Glycerin** is usually administered as a suppository and with an onset of action usually less than 30 minutes. Glycerin is considered a safe laxative, although it may occasionally cause rectal irritation. Its use is acceptable on an intermittent basis for constipation, particularly in children.

PEG–Electrolyte Lavage Solution

- For bowel cleansing 4 L is administered 240 mL every 10 minutes beginning the evening before colonoscopy.
- Low doses of PEG solution (10–30 g or 17–34 g per 120–240 mL) once or twice daily may be used for treatment of constipation. Daily use in low dose (17 g) may be safe and effective for up to 6 months.
- The most common adverse effects are GI-related and include nausea, vomiting, flatulence, and abdominal cramping.

Stimulant Laxatives

- Stimulant laxatives such as diphenylmethane (bisacodyl) and anthraquinone (senna and others) derivates are expected to cause a bowel movement within 8–12 hours of administration.
- They are typically reserved for intermittent use or in patients who fail to respond adequately to bulking and osmotic laxatives. Some patients with severe chronic constipation and nonmodifiable risk factors may use these agents on a more regular basis.

Lubiprostone and Linaclotide

- **Lubiprostone** (Amitiza) is approved for chronic idiopathic constipation as well as for opioid-induced constipation (OIC). The dose is one 24-mg capsule twice daily with food. It appears safe for long-term treatment (up to 48 weeks). Lubiprostone may cause nausea, headache, and diarrhea.
- Lubiprostone is reserved for patients with chronic constipation who fail conventional first-line agents such as osmotic laxatives and fiber supplementation, or for those with OIC.
- **Linaclotide** (Linzess) is approved for the treatment of constipation and IBS with constipation (IBS-C). It is approved in a 145-mcg dose to be taken on an empty stomach at least 30 minutes before the first meal of the day. It should not be used in patients younger than 18 years of age.
- Plecanatide is approved for chronic idiopathic constipation in an adult dose of 3 mg given once daily without regard to food. It should not be used in patients under the age of 18.

Opioid-Receptor Antagonists and Prucalopride

- Alvimopan is an oral GI-specific μ-receptor antagonist for short-term use in hospitalized patients to accelerate recovery of bowel function after large or small bowel resection. It is given as one 12-mg (capsule) 30 minutes–5 hours before surgery and then 12 mg twice daily for up to 7 days or until hospital discharge (maximum 15 doses). It is contraindicated in patients receiving therapeutic doses of opioids for more than 7 consecutive days prior to surgery.
- Methylnaltrexone is another μ-receptor antagonist approved for OIC in patients with advanced disease receiving palliative care or when response to laxative therapy has been insufficient for OIC with chronic noncancer pain.
- Other opioid-receptor antagonists include naloxegol and nalemedine.
- Prucalopride is a selective 5-hydroxytryptamine-4 (5-HT4) receptor agonist used for chronic constipation.

See Chapter 53, Diarrhea, Constipation, and Irritable Bowel Syndrome, authored by Patricia H. Fabel and Kayce M. Shealy, for a more detailed discussion of this topic.

CHAPTER 23

Diarrhea

- Diarrhea is an increased frequency and decreased consistency of fecal discharge as compared with an individual's normal bowel pattern. Diarrhea can be thought of as both a symptom and a sign of systemic disease.
- Acute diarrhea is commonly defined as shorter than 14 days' duration, persistent diarrhea as longer than 14 days' duration, and chronic diarrhea as longer than 30 days' duration. Most cases of acute diarrhea are caused by infections with viruses, bacteria, or protozoa, and are generally self-limited.

PATHOPHYSIOLOGY

- Although viruses are more commonly associated with acute gastroenteritis, bacteria are responsible for more cases of acute diarrhea. Common causative bacterial organisms include *Shigella*, *Salmonella*, *Campylobacter*, *Staphylococcus*, and *Escherichia coli*. Acute viral infections are attributed mostly to the Norwalk and rotavirus groups.
- Diarrhea is an imbalance in absorption and secretion of water and electrolytes. It may be associated with a specific disease of the gastrointestinal (GI) tract or with a disease outside the GI tract.
- Four general pathophysiologic mechanisms disrupt water and electrolyte balance, leading to diarrhea: (1) a change in active ion transport by either decreased sodium absorption or increased chloride secretion, (2) a change in intestinal motility, (3) an increase in luminal osmolarity, and (4) an increase in tissue hydrostatic pressure. These mechanisms have been related to four broad clinical diarrheal groups: secretory, osmotic, exudative, and altered intestinal transit.
- Secretory diarrhea occurs when a stimulating substance (eg, vasoactive intestinal peptide [VIP] from a pancreatic tumor, unabsorbed dietary fat in steatorrhea, laxatives, hormones [such as secretion], bacterial toxins, and excessive bile salts) increases secretion or decreases absorption of large amounts of water and electrolytes.
- Inflammatory diseases of the GI tract can cause exudative diarrhea by discharge of mucus, proteins, or blood into the gut. With altered intestinal transit, intestinal motility is altered by reduced contact time in the small intestine, premature emptying of the colon, or bacterial overgrowth.

CLINICAL PRESENTATION

- Acute diarrhea is usually self-limiting and subsides within 72 hours of onset, whereas chronic diarrhea involves frequent attacks over extended time periods. However, infants, young children, the elderly, and debilitated persons are at risk for morbid and mortal events in prolonged or voluminous diarrhea.
- Signs and symptoms include the following:
  - ✓ Abrupt onset of nausea, vomiting, abdominal pain, headache, fever, chills, and malaise
  - ✓ Bowel movements are frequent and never bloody, and diarrhea lasts 12–60 hours.
  - ✓ Intermittent periumbilical or lower right quadrant pain with cramps and audible bowel sounds is characteristic of small intestinal disease.
  - ✓ When pain is present in large intestinal diarrhea, it is a gripping, aching sensation with tenesmus (straining, ineffective, and painful stooling).
  - ✓ In chronic diarrhea, a history of previous bouts, weight loss, anorexia, and chronic weakness are important findings.
- Physical examination typically demonstrates hyperperistalsis with borborygmi and generalized or local tenderness.

- Laboratory tests:
  - ✓ Stool analysis studies include examination for microorganisms, blood, mucus, fat, osmolality, pH, electrolyte and mineral concentration, and cultures.
  - ✓ Stool test kits are useful for detecting GI viruses, particularly rotavirus.
  - ✓ Antibody serologic testing shows rising titers over a 3- to 6-day period, but this test is not practical and is nonspecific.
  - ✓ Occasionally, total daily stool volume is also determined.
  - ✓ Direct endoscopic visualization and biopsy of the colon may be undertaken to assess for the presence of conditions such as colitis or cancer.
- Radiographic studies are helpful in neoplastic and inflammatory conditions.
- Many agents, including antibiotics and other drugs, cause diarrhea (Table 23-1). Laxative abuse for weight loss may also result in diarrhea.

TREATMENT

- Goals of Treatment: To manage the diet, prevent excessive water, electrolyte, and acid–base disturbances; provide symptomatic relief; treat curable causes of diarrhea; and manage secondary disorders causing diarrhea. Diarrhea, like a cough, may be a body's defense mechanism for ridding itself of harmful substances or pathogens. The correct therapeutic response is not necessarily to stop diarrhea at all costs. If diarrhea is secondary to another illness, controlling the primary condition is necessary.

GENERAL APPROACH

- Management of the diet is a first priority for treatment of diarrhea (Figs. 23-1 and 23-2). Most clinicians recommend stopping solid foods for 24 hours and avoiding dairy products.
- Dietary management is a first priority in the treatment of diarrhea. Feeding should continue in children with acute bacterial diarrhea.
- If vomiting is present and is uncontrollable with antiemetics, nothing is taken by mouth. As bowel movements decrease, a bland diet is begun.
- Rehydration and maintenance of water and electrolytes are the primary treatment measures until the diarrheal episode ends. If vomiting and dehydration are not severe, enteral feeding is the less costly and preferred method. In the United States, many commercial oral rehydration preparations are available (Table 23-2). The WHO now recommends an oral rehydration solution (ORS) with a lower osmolarity, sodium content, and glucose load (see Table 23-2).
- Oral supplementation of zinc 20 mg daily for 10 days in addition to ORS significantly reduces the severity and duration of acute diarrhea in developing countries.

PHARMACOLOGIC THERAPY

- Drugs used to treat diarrhea (Table 23-3) are grouped into several categories: antimotility, adsorbents, antisecretory compounds, antibiotics, enzymes, and intestinal microflora. Usually, these drugs are not curative but palliative.
- Opiates and opioid derivatives delay the transit of intraluminal content or increase gut capacity, prolonging contact and absorption. The limitations of the opiates are addiction potential (a real concern with long-term use) and worsening of diarrhea in selected infectious diarrheas.
- **Loperamide** is often recommended for managing acute (including traveler's diarrhea) and chronic diarrhea. Diarrhea lasting 48 hours beyond initiating loperamide warrants medical attention.
- **Diphenoxylate and difenoxin (a diphenoxylate derivative)** are combined with **atropine** and have the same uses, precautions, and side effects.
- **Bismuth subsalicylate** is often used for treatment or prevention of diarrhea (traveler's diarrhea) and has antisecretory, anti-inflammatory, and antibacterial effects.

TABLE 23-1	Drugs Causing Diarrhea	
Laxatives		Guanadrel
Antacids containing magnesium		Angiotensin-converting enzyme inhibitors
Antineoplastics		Cholinergics
Auranofin (gold salt)		Bethanechol
Antibiotics		Neostigmine
Clindamycin		Cardiac agents
Tetracyclines		Quinidine
Sulfonamides		Digitalis
Any broad-spectrum antibiotic		Digoxin
Antihypertensives		Nonsteroidal anti-inflammatory drugs
Reserpine		Misoprostol
Guanethidine		Colchicine
Methyldopa		Proton pump inhibitors
Guanabenz		H2-receptor blockers

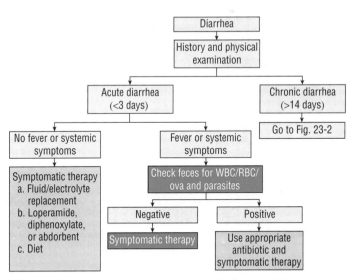

FIGURE 23-1. Recommendations for treating acute diarrhea. Follow these steps: (1) Perform a complete history and physical examination. (2) Is the diarrhea acute or chronic? If chronic diarrhea, go to Fig. 23-2. (3) If acute diarrhea, check for fever and/or systemic signs and symptoms (ie, toxic patient). If systemic illness (fever, anorexia, or volume depletion), check for an infectious source. If positive for infectious diarrhea, use the appropriate antibiotic/anthelmintic drug and symptomatic therapy. If negative for infectious cause, use only symptomatic treatment. (4) If no systemic findings, use symptomatic therapy based on severity of volume depletion, oral or parenteral fluid/electrolytes, antidiarrheal agents (see Table 23-3), and diet.

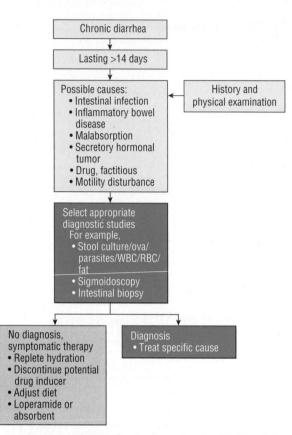

FIGURE 23-2. Recommendations for treating chronic diarrhea. Follow these steps: (1) Perform a careful history and physical examination. (2) The possible causes of chronic diarrhea are many. These can be classified into intestinal infections (bacterial or protozoal), inflammatory disease (Crohn's disease or ulcerative colitis), malabsorption (lactose intolerance), secretory hormonal tumor (intestinal carcinoid tumo r or vasoactive intestinal peptide [VIP]–secreting tumors), drug (antacid), factitious (laxative abuse), or motility disturbance (diabetes mellitus, irritable bowel syndrome, or hyperthyroidism). (3) If the diagnosis is uncertain, appropriate diagnostic studies should be ordered. (4) Once diagnosed, treatment is planned for the underlying cause with symptomatic antidiarrheal therapy. (5) If no specific cause can be identified, symptomatic therapy is prescribed.

Bismuth subsalicylate contains multiple components that might be toxic if given in excess to prevent or treat diarrhea.

- **Probiotics**, including microorganisms such as *Saccharomyces boulardii*, *Lactobacillus* GG, and *Lactobacillus acidophilus* decrease the duration of infectious and antibiotic-induced diarrhea in adults and children. The dosage of probiotic preparations varies depending on the brand used. Intestinal flatus is the primary patient complaint experienced with this modality.

| TABLE 23-2 | Oral Rehydration Solutions |

	WHO-ORSYT[a]	Pedialyte[b] (Ross)	CeraLyte (Cera Products)	Enfalyte (Mead Johnson)
Osmolality (mOsm/ kg or mmol/kg)	245	250	220	167
Carbohydrates[b] (g/L)	13.5	25	40[c]	30[c]
Calories (cal/L [J/L])	65 (272)	100 (418)	160 (670)	126 (527)
Electrolytes (mEq/L; mmol/L)				
Sodium	75	45	50–90	50
Potassium	20	20	20	25
Chloride	65	35	40–80	45
Citrate	—	30	30	34
Bicarbonate	30	—	—	—
Calcium	—	—	—	—
Magnesium	—	—	—	—
Sulfate	—	—	—	—
Phosphate	—	—	—	—

[a]World Health Organization reduced osmolarity oral rehydration solution.
[b]Carbohydrate is glucose.
[c]Rice syrup solids are carbohydrate source.

| TABLE 23-3 | Selected Antidiarrheal Preparations |

	Dose Form	Adult Dose
Antimotility		
Diphenoxylate	2.5 mg/tablet 2.5 mg/5 mL	5 mg four times daily; do not exceed 20 mg/day
Loperamide	2 mg/capsule	Initially 4 mg, and then 2 mg after each loose stool; do not exceed 16 mg/day
Paregoric	2 mg/5 mL (morphine)	5–10 mL one to four times daily
Opium tincture	10 mg/mL (morphine)	0.6 mL four times daily
Difenoxin	1 mg/tablet	Two tablets, and then one tablet after each loose stool; up to eight tablets per day
Antisecretory		
Bismuth subsalicylate	1050 mg/30 mL 262 mg/15 mL 524 mg/15 mL 262 mg/tablet	Two tablets or 30 mL every 30 minutes to 1 hour as needed up to eight doses per day

(Continued)

TABLE 23-3	Selected Antidiarrheal Preparations *(Continued)*	
	Dose Form	**Adult Dose**
Enzymes (lactase)		
	1250 neutral lactase units/4 drops	Three to four drops taken with milk or dairy product
	3300 FCC lactase units per tablet	
Bacterial replacement (*Lactobacillus acidophilus, Lactobacillus bulgaricus*)		Two tablets or one granule packet three to four times daily; give with milk, juice, or water
Octreotide	0.05 mg/mL	Initial: 50 mcg subcutaneously
	0.1 mg/mL	One to two times per day
	0.5 mg/mL	and titrate dose based on indication up to 600 mcg/day in two to four divided doses

- **Octreotide**, a synthetic octapeptide analog of endogenous somatostatin, is prescribed for the symptomatic treatment of carcinoid tumors and other peptide- secreting tumors, dumping syndrome, and chemotherapy-induced diarrhea. The dosage range for managing diarrhea associated with carcinoid tumors is 100–600 mcg daily in two to four divided doses, subcutaneously, for 2 weeks. Octreotide is associated with adverse effects such as cholelithiasis, nausea, diarrhea, and abdominal pain.
- Vaccines. An oral vaccine for cholera (Vaxchora') is licensed and available in the United States. The Advisory Committee for Immunization Practices (ACIP) recommends the vaccine for adults aged 18–64 years old who are traveling to an endemic area. Two orally administered rotavirus vaccines (RotaTeq and Rotarix) prevent gastroenteritis due to rotavirus infection in infants and children.

EVALUATION OF THERAPEUTIC OUTCOMES

- Therapeutic outcomes are directed to key symptoms, signs, and laboratory studies. The constitutional symptoms usually improve within 24–72 hours. Monitoring for changes in the frequency and character of bowel movements on a daily basis in conjunction with vital signs and improvement in appetite are of utmost importance.
- Monitor body weight, serum osmolality, serum electrolytes, complete blood cell count, urinalysis, and cultures (if appropriate). With an urgent or emergency situation, any change in the volume status of the patient is the most important outcome.
- In the urgent/emergent situation, restoration of the patient's volume status is the most important outcome. Toxic patients (fever dehydration, hematochezia, or hypotension) require hospitalization, IV fluids and electrolyte administration, and empiric antibiotic therapy while awaiting culture and sensitivity results. With timely management, these patients usually recover within a few days.

See Chapter 54, Diarrhea, Constipation, and Irritable Bowel Syndrome, authored by Patricia H. Fabel and Kayce M. Shealy, for a more detailed discussion of this topic.

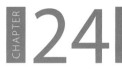

CHAPTER 24

Gastroesophageal Reflux Disease

- *Gastroesophageal reflux disease* (GERD) is defined as the symptoms or complications resulting from refluxed stomach contents into the esophagus, oral cavity (including the larynx), or lungs. Episodic heartburn that is not frequent or painful enough to be bothersome is not included in the definition.

PATHOPHYSIOLOGY

- In some cases, reflux is associated with defective lower esophageal sphincter (LES) pressure or function. Patients may have decreased LES pressure from spontaneous transient LES relaxations, transient increases in intra-abdominal pressure, or an atonic LES. Some foods and medications decrease LES pressure (Table 24-1).
- Problems with other normal mucosal defense mechanisms may contribute to development of GERD, including abnormal esophageal anatomy, improper esophageal clearance of gastric fluids, reduced mucosal resistance to acid, delayed or ineffective gastric emptying, inadequate production of epidermal growth factor, and reduced salivary buffering of acid.
- Esophagitis occurs when the esophagus is repeatedly exposed to refluxed gastric contents for prolonged periods. This can progress to erosion of the squamous epithelium of the esophagus (erosive esophagitis).
- Substances that promote esophageal damage upon reflux into the esophagus include gastric acid, pepsin, bile acids, and pancreatic enzymes. Composition and volume of the refluxate and duration of exposure are the primary determinants of the consequences of gastroesophageal reflux.
- An "acid pocket" is thought to be an area of unbuffered acid in the proximal stomach that accumulates after a meal and may contribute to GERD symptoms postprandially. GERD patients are predisposed to upward migration of acid from the acid pocket, which may also be positioned above the diaphragm in patients with hiatal hernia, increasing the risk for acid reflux.
- Reflux and heartburn are common in pregnancy because of hormonal effects on LES tone and increased intra-abdominal pressure from an enlarging uterus.
- Obesity is a risk factor for GERD due to increased intra-abdominal pressure. Transient LES relaxations, an incompetent LES, and impaired esophageal motility have also been attributed to obesity.
- Complications from long-term acid reflux include esophagitis, esophageal strictures, Barrett esophagus, and esophageal adenocarcinoma.

CLINICAL PRESENTATION

- *Symptom-based GERD* (with or without esophageal tissue injury) typically presents with heartburn, usually described as a substernal sensation of warmth or burning rising up from the abdomen that may radiate to the neck. It may wax and wane in character and be aggravated by activities that worsen reflux (eg, recumbent position, bending-over, eating a high-fat meal). Other symptoms are water brash (hypersalivation), belching, and regurgitation. Alarm symptoms that may indicate complications include dysphagia, odynophagia, bleeding, and weight loss. The absence of tissue injury or erosions is termed nonerosive reflux disease (NERD).
- *Tissue injury–based GERD* (with or without esophageal symptoms) may present with esophagitis, esophageal strictures, Barrett esophagus, or esophageal carcinoma. Alarm symptoms may also be present.
- Extraesophageal symptoms may include chronic cough, laryngitis, wheezing, and asthma.

251

TABLE 24-1	Foods and Medications That May Worsen GERD Symptoms	
Foods/Beverages	**Medications**
Decreased lower esophageal sphincter pressure	
Fatty meal	Anticholinergics
Carminatives (peppermint, spearmint)	Barbiturates
Chocolate	Caffeine
Coffee, cola, tea	Dihydropyridine calcium channel blockers
Garlic	Dopamine
Onions	Estrogen
Chili peppers	Nicotine
Alcohol	Nitrates
	Progesterone
	Tetracycline
	Theophylline
Direct irritants to the esophageal mucosa	
Spicy foods	Aspirin
Orange juice	Bisphosphonates
Tomato juice	Nonsteroidal anti-inflammatory drugs (NSAIDs)
Coffee	Iron
Tobacco	Quinidine
	Potassium chloride

DIAGNOSIS

- Clinical history is sufficient to diagnose GERD in patients with typical symptoms.
- Perform diagnostic tests in patients who do not respond to therapy or who present with alarm symptoms. Endoscopy is preferred for assessing mucosal injury and identifying strictures, Barrett esophagus, and other complications.
- Ambulatory pH monitoring, combined impedance–pH monitoring, high-resolution esophageal pressure topography (HREPT), impedance manometry, and an empiric trial of a proton pump inhibitor (PPI) may be useful in some situations.

TREATMENT

- <u>Goals of Treatment</u>: The goals are to reduce or eliminate symptoms, decrease frequency and duration of gastroesophageal reflux, promote healing of injured mucosa, prevent complications, and improve quality of life.

GENERAL APPROACH

- Therapy is directed toward decreasing acidity of the refluxate, decreasing the gastric volume available to be refluxed, improving gastric emptying, increasing LES pressure, enhancing esophageal acid clearance, and protecting the esophageal mucosa.
- Treatment is determined by disease severity and includes the following:
  - ✓ Lifestyle changes and patient-directed therapy with **antacids** and/or nonprescription acid suppression therapy (**histamine 2–receptor antagonists [H₂RAs]** and/ or **PPIs**)
  - ✓ Pharmacologic treatment with prescription-strength acid suppression therapy
  - ✓ Antireflux surgery
  - ✓ Endoscopic therapies

- The initial intervention depends in part on the patient's condition (symptom frequency, degree of esophagitis, and presence of complications). A step-down approach is most often advocated, starting with a PPI instead of an H_2RA, and then stepping down to the lowest dose of acid suppression needed to control symptoms (**Table 24-2**).
- Patient-directed therapy (self-treatment with nonprescription medication) is appropriate for mild, intermittent symptoms. Patients with continuous symptoms for longer than 2 weeks should seek medical attention; such patients are generally started on empiric acid-suppression therapy. Patients not responding satisfactorily or those with alarm symptoms (eg, dysphagia) should undergo endoscopy.

NONPHARMACOLOGIC THERAPY

- Potential lifestyle changes depending on the patient situation:
  - ✓ Elevate head of the bed by placing 6- to 8-in blocks under the headposts. Sleep on a foam wedge.
  - ✓ Weight reduction for overweight or obese patients.
  - ✓ Avoid foods that decrease LES pressure (eg, fats, chocolate).
  - ✓ Include protein-rich meals to augment LES pressure.
  - ✓ Avoid foods with irritant effects on the esophageal mucosa (eg, citrus juices, coffee, pepper).
  - ✓ Eat small meals and avoid eating immediately prior to sleeping (within 3 hours if possible).
  - ✓ Stop smoking.
  - ✓ Avoid alcohol.
  - ✓ Avoid tight-fitting clothes.
  - ✓ For mandatory medications that irritate the esophageal mucosa, take in the upright position with plenty of liquid or food (if appropriate).

- Antireflux surgery (eg, laparoscopic Nissen fundoplication) should be considered when long-term pharmacotherapy is undesirable or when patients have complications. Bariatric surgery, specifically Roux-en-Y gastric bypass, should be considered in obese patients (BMI >35 kg/m²) contemplating surgery.
- Two endoscopic therapies are (1) radiofrequency ablation (for managing Barrett esophagus primarily when dysplasia is present), and (2) transoral incisionless fundoplication (for select patients with chronic GERD).
- Magnetic sphincter augmentation can improve lower esophageal resistance and reduce GERD symptoms. Its long-term effectiveness is uncertain.

PHARMACOLOGIC THERAPY

Antacids and Antacid-Alginic Acid Products

- Antacids provide immediate symptomatic relief for mild GERD and are often used concurrently with acid suppression therapies. Patients who require frequent use for chronic symptoms should receive prescription-strength acid suppression therapy instead.
- Some antacid products are combined with alginic acid, which is not a potent acid-neutralizing agent and does not enhance LES pressure, but it forms a viscous solution that floats on the surface of gastric contents. This serves as a protective barrier for the esophagus against reflux of gastric contents and reduces frequency of reflux episodes. The combination product may be superior to antacids alone in relieving GERD symptoms, but efficacy data indicating endoscopic healing are lacking.
- Antacids have a short duration, which necessitates frequent administration throughout the day to provide continuous acid neutralization. Taking antacids after meals can increase duration from approximately 1 hour to 3 hours; however, nighttime acid suppression cannot be maintained with bedtime doses. Antacids may cause diarrhea or constipation depending on the magnesium or aluminum content. These agents have significant drug interactions with tetracycline, ferrous sulfate, isoniazid, sulfonylureas, and quinolone antibiotics.

TABLE 24-2 Therapeutics Approach to GERD in Adults

Recommended Treatment Regimen	Brand Name	Oral Dose	Comments
Intermittent, mild heartburn (individualized lifestyle modifications + patient-directed therapy with antacids and/or nonprescription H₂RAs or nonprescription PPI)			
Individualized lifestyle modifications			Lifestyle modifications should be individualized for each patient.
Patient-directed therapy with antacids (≥12 years old)			
Magnesium hydroxide/Aluminum hydroxide with simethicone	Maalox	10–20 mL as needed or after meals and at bedtime	If symptoms are unrelieved with lifestyle modifications and nonprescription medications after 2 weeks, patient should seek medical attention; do not exceed 16 teaspoonfuls per 24 hours.
Antacid/Alginic acid	Gaviscon	2–4 tablets or 10–20 mL after meals and at bedtime	Note: Content of alginic acid varies greatly among products; the higher the alginic acid the better (at least 500 mg).
Calcium carbonate	Tums	500 mg, 2–4 tablets as needed	
Patient-directed therapy with nonprescription H₂RAs (up to twice daily) (≥12 years old)			
Cimetidine	Tagamet HB	200 mg	If symptoms are unrelieved with lifestyle modifications and nonprescription medications after 2 weeks, patient should seek medical attention.
Famotidine	Pepcid AC	10–20 mg	
Nizatidine	Axid AR	75 mg	
Patient-directed therapy (>18 years old) with nonprescription PPIs (taken once daily)			
Esomeprazole	Nexium 24HR	20 mg	If symptoms are unrelieved with lifestyle modifications and nonprescription medications after 2 weeks, patient should seek medical attention.
Lansoprazole	Prevacid 24HR	15 mg	
Omeprazole	Prilosec OTC	20 mg	
Omeprazole/sodium bicarbonate	Zegerid OTC	20 mg/1100 mg	

Symptomatic relief of GERD (individualized lifestyle modifications + prescription-strength H₂RAs or prescription-strength PPIs)

Individualized lifestyle modifications

Lifestyle modifications should be individualized for each patient.

Prescription-strength H₂RAs (for 6–12 weeks)

Cimetidine (off-label use)	Tagamet	400 mg four times daily or 800 mg twice daily	For typical symptoms, treat empirically with prescription-strength acid suppression therapy.
Famotidine	Pepcid	20 mg twice daily	If symptoms recur, consider maintenance therapy. Note: Most
Nizatidine	Axid	150 mg twice daily	patients will require standard doses for maintenance therapy.

Prescription-strength PPIs (for 4–8 weeks)

Dexlansoprazole	Dexilant	30 mg once daily for 4 weeks	For typical symptoms, treat empirically with prescription-strength acid suppression therapy
Esomeprazole	Nexium	20–40 mg once daily	Patients with moderate-to-severe symptoms should receive a PPI as
Lansoprazole	Prevacid	15 mg once daily	initial therapy.
Omeprazole	Prilosec	20 mg once daily	
Omeprazole/Sodium bicarbonate	Zegerid	20 mg once daily	If symptoms recur, consider maintenance therapy.
Pantoprazole (off-label use)	Protonix	40 mg once daily	
Rabeprazole	Aciphex	20 mg once daily	

Healing of erosive esophagitis or treatment of patients with moderate-to-severe symptoms or complications (individualized lifestyle modifications + high-dose H₂RAs or PPIs or antireflux surgery)

Individualized lifestyle modifications

Lifestyle modifications should be individualized for each patient.

(Continued)

TABLE 24-2 Therapeutics Approach to GERD in Adults (*Continued*)

Recommended Treatment Regimen	Brand Name	Oral Dose	Comments
PPIs (up to twice daily for up to 8 weeks)			
Dexlansoprazole	Dexilant	60 mg daily	For extraesophageal or alarm symptoms, obtain endoscopy with biopsy to evaluate mucosa.
Esomeprazole	Nexium	20–40 mg daily	If symptoms are relieved, consider maintenance therapy. PPIs are the most effective maintenance therapy for patients with extraesophageal symptoms, complications, and erosive disease.
Lansoprazole	Prevacid	30 mg once or twice daily	
Omeprazole	Prilosec	20 mg once or twice daily	
Rabeprazole	Aciphex	20 mg once or twice daily	Start with twice-daily PPI therapy if reflux chest syndrome present
Pantoprazole	Protonix	40 mg once or twice daily	Patients not responding to pharmacologic therapy, including those with persistent extraesophageal symptoms, should be evaluated via manometry and/or ambulatory reflux monitoring.
High-dose H$_2$RAs (for 8–12 weeks)			
Cimetidine	Tagamet	400 mg four times daily or 800 mg twice daily	If high-dose H$_2$RA is needed, one may consider using PPI to lower cost, increase convenience, and increase tolerability.
Famotidine	Pepcid	20–40 mg twice daily	Four times daily H$_2$RA is considered off-label use for nizatidine.
Nizatidine	Aciphex	150 mg two to four times daily	
Interventional therapy			
Antireflux surgery			
Bariatric surgery			
Endoscopic therapies			

H$_2$RA, histamine$_2$-receptor antagonist; PPI, proton pump inhibitor.

Proton Pump Inhibitors

- **Dexlansoprazole, esomeprazole, lansoprazole, omeprazole, pantoprazole**, and **rabeprazole** block gastric acid secretion by inhibiting hydrogen potassium adenosine triphosphatase in gastric parietal cells, resulting in profound and long-lasting antisecretory effects.

- PPIs provide more rapid symptom relief and higher healing rates than H_2RAs in patients with moderate-to-severe GERD and should be given empirically to patients with troublesome symptoms. Twice-daily use is indicated in patients not responding to standard once-daily therapy.

- Adverse effects include headache, diarrhea, nausea, and abdominal pain. Community-acquired pneumonia may occur with short-term use. Potential long-term adverse effects include enteric infections, vitamin B_{12} deficiency, hypomagnesemia, and bone fractures. PPIs can decrease the absorption of **ketoconazole** and **itraconazole**, which require an acidic environment for absorption. Although some PPIs (especially omeprazole) inhibit cytochrome P450 2C19 and may reduce conversion of clopidogrel to its active metabolite and decrease effectiveness of clopidogrel.

- PPIs degrade in acidic environments and are therefore formulated in delayed-release capsules or tablets. Dexlansoprazole, esomeprazole, lansoprazole, and omeprazole contain enteric-coated (pH-sensitive) granules in capsules. For patients unable to swallow the capsules, the contents can be mixed in applesauce or orange juice. In patients with nasogastric tubes, the contents can be mixed in 8.4% sodium bicarbonate solution. Esomeprazole granules can be dispersed in water. Esomeprazole, omeprazole, and pantoprazole are also available in a delayed-release oral suspension powder packet, and lansoprazole is available as a delayed-release, orally disintegrating tablet. Patients taking delayed-release tablets of pantoprazole or rabeprazole should be instructed not to crush, chew, or split them. Dexlansoprazole is available in a dual delayed-release capsule, with the first release occurring 1–2 hours after the dose, and the second release occurring 4–5 hours after the dose.

- **Zegerid** is a combination product containing omeprazole 20 or 40 mg with 1100 mg sodium bicarbonate in immediate-release oral capsules and powder for oral suspension. It should be taken on an empty stomach at least 1 hour before a meal. The capsules should be swallowed whole and not opened, sprinkled on food, or administered via nasogastric tube. The powder for oral suspension offers an alternative to delayed-release capsules or IV formulation in adults with nasogastric tubes.

- **Esomeprazole** and **pantoprazole** are available in IV formulations for patients who cannot take oral medications, but they are not more effective than oral preparations and are significantly more expensive.

- Patients should take oral PPIs in the morning 30–60 minutes before breakfast or their largest meal of the day to maximize efficacy. Dexlansoprazole can be taken without regard to meals. If dosed twice daily, the second PPI dose should be taken approximately 10–12 hours after the morning dose and prior to a meal or snack.

Histamine 2–Receptor Antagonists

- **Cimetidine, ranitidine**, and **famotidine** in divided doses are effective for treating mild-to-moderate GERD. Low-dose nonprescription H_2RAs or standard doses given twice daily may be beneficial for symptomatic relief of mild GERD. Patients not responding to standard doses may be hypersecretors of gastric acid and require higher doses (**Table 24-2**). However, when standard doses of H_2RAs do not adequately relieve symptoms, it is more cost-effective and clinically effective to switch to a PPI. The efficacy of H_2RAs for GERD treatment is highly variable and frequently less than desired. Prolonged courses are frequently required.

- The most common adverse effects include headache, fatigue, dizziness, and either constipation or diarrhea. Cimetidine may inhibit the metabolism of theophylline, warfarin, phenytoin, nifedipine, and propranolol, among other drugs.

- Because all H_2RAs are equally effective, selection of the specific agent should be based on differences in pharmacokinetics, safety profile, and cost.

Promotility Agents

- Promotility agents may be useful adjuncts to acid-suppression therapy in patients with a known motility defect (eg, LES incompetence, decreased esophageal clearance, delayed gastric emptying). However, these agents are not as effective as acid suppression therapy and have undesirable adverse effects.
- **Metoclopramide**, a dopamine antagonist, increases LES pressure in a dose-related manner and accelerates gastric emptying. However, it does not improve esophageal clearance. Metoclopramide provides symptomatic improvement for some patients, but evidence supporting endoscopic healing is lacking. Common adverse reactions include somnolence, nervousness, fatigue, dizziness, weakness, depression, diarrhea, and rash. In addition, extrapyramidal effects, tardive dyskinesia, and other CNS effects limit its usefulness.
- **Bethanechol** has limited value because of side effects (eg, urinary retention, abdominal discomfort, nausea, flushing). It is not routinely recommended for treatment of GERD.

Mucosal Protectants

- **Sucralfate** is a nonabsorbable aluminum salt of sucrose octasulfate. It has limited value for treatment of GERD but may be useful for management of radiation esophagitis and bile or nonacid reflux GERD.

Combination Therapy

- Combination therapy with an acid-suppressing agent and a promotility agent or mucosal protectant seems logical, but data supporting such therapy are limited. This approach is not recommended unless a patient has GERD with motor dysfunction. Using the omeprazole-sodium bicarbonate immediate-release product in addition to once-daily PPI therapy offers an alternative for nocturnal GERD symptoms.

Maintenance Therapy

- Many patients with GERD relapse after medication is withdrawn, so maintenance treatment may be required. Consider long-term therapy to prevent complications and worsening of esophageal function in patients who have symptomatic relapse after discontinuation of therapy or dosage reduction.
- Most patients require standard doses to prevent relapses. PPIs are the drugs of choice for maintenance treatment of moderate-to-severe esophagitis or symptoms. Usual once-daily doses are omeprazole 20 mg, lansoprazole 30 mg, rabeprazole 20 mg, or esomeprazole 20 mg. Low doses of a PPI or alternate-day regimens may be effective in some patients with milder symptoms. H_2RAs may be effective maintenance therapy in patients with mild disease.
- "On-demand" maintenance therapy, by which patients take their PPIs only when they have symptoms, may be effective for patients with endoscopy-negative GERD.

EVALUATION OF THERAPEUTIC OUTCOMES

- Monitor frequency and severity of GERD symptoms, and educate patients on symptoms that suggest presence of complications requiring immediate medical attention, such as dysphagia. Evaluate patients with persistent symptoms for presence of strictures or other complications.
- Monitor patients for adverse drug effects and the presence of extraesophageal symptoms such as laryngitis, asthma, or chest pain. These symptoms require further diagnostic evaluation.

See Chapter 50, Gastroesophageal Reflux Disease, authored by Dianne May, Devin L. Lavender, and Satish S.C. Rao, for a more detailed discussion of this topic.

CHAPTER 25

Hepatitis, Viral

- Viral hepatitis refers to the clinically important hepatotropic viruses responsible for hepatitis A (HAV), hepatitis B (HBV), delta hepatitis, hepatitis C (HCV), and hepatitis E.

HEPATITIS A

- HAV infection usually produces a self-limited disease and acute viral infection, with a low fatality rate, and confers lifelong immunity. Outbreaks occur each year in the United States.
- HAV infection primarily occurs through transmission by the fecal-oral route, person-to-person, or by ingestion of contaminated food or water. HAV's prevalence is linked to resource-limited regions and specifically to those with poor sanitary conditions and overcrowding. Rates of HAV infection are increased among international travelers, persons who inject drugs, persons unhoused, and men who have sex with men.
- The disease exhibits three phases: (1) incubation (averaging 28 days, range 15–50 days), (2) acute hepatitis (generally lasting 2 months), and (3) convalescence. Acute hepatitis is marked by an abrupt onset of nonspecific symptoms; some very mild. Some patients may experience symptoms for up to 9 months. Nearly all individuals have a clinical resolution within 6 months of the infection, and a majority have resolution within 2 months. HAV does not lead to chronic infections.
- The clinical presentation of HAV infection is given in Table 25-1. There are no specific symptoms unique to HAV. Children younger than 6 years of age are typically asymptomatic.
- The diagnosis of acute HAV is made through the IgM anti-HAV which is detectable 5 to 10 days prior to symptomatic HAV infections in the majority of patients. Clinical criteria consist of acute onset of fatigue, abdominal pain, loss of appetite, intermittent nausea and vomiting, jaundice or elevated serum aminotransferase levels, and serologic testing for immunoglobulin (Ig) M anti-HAV.

PREVENTION

- The spread of HAV can be best controlled by avoiding exposure. The most important measures to avoid exposure include good handwashing techniques and personal hygiene practices.
- The current vaccination strategy in the United States includes vaccinating all children at 1 year of age. Groups who should receive HAV vaccine are shown in Table 25-2. Persons at risk for worse outcomes with HAV infection are also recommended to receive vaccination and include persons over the age of 40, persons with immuno-compromising conditions, persons with chronic liver disease planning on traveling, and persons with HIV.
- Three inactivated virus vaccines are licensed in the United States: Havrix, Vaqta, and Twinrix. Approved dosing recommendations are shown in Table 25-3. Seroconversion rates of 94% or greater are achieved with the first dose.
- Common vaccine side effects include soreness and warmth at the injection site, headache, malaise, and pain.
- Ig is used when pre- or postexposure prophylaxis against HAV infection is needed in persons for whom vaccination is not an option. It is most effective if given during the incubation phase of infection. A single dose of Ig 0.02 mL/kg is given intramuscularly for postexposure prophylaxis or short-term (≤5 months) preexposure prophylaxis. For lengthy stays, a single dose of 0.06 mL/kg is used. HAV vaccine may also be given with Ig.
- For people recently exposed to HAV and not previously vaccinated, Ig is indicated for patients older than 40 years or with underlying medical conditions, when vaccine

TABLE 25-1	Clinical Presentation of Acute Hepatitis		
	Hepatitis A (HAV)	**Hepatitis B (HBV)**	**Hepatitis C (HCV)**
Signs and symptoms	>70% of patients are symptomatic with fever, jaundice, scleral icterus, hepatomegaly. Less common: splenomegaly, skin rash, arthralgia.	Approximately 70% of patients are anicteric or subclinical. Younger patients are most likely to be asymptomatic. If symptoms occur, jaundice, dark urine, white stool, abdominal pain, fatigue, fever, chills, loss of appetite, and pruritus are possible.	Approximately 70% of patients are asymptomatic. If symptoms occur, jaundice, dark urine, white stool, abdominal pain, fatigue, fever, chills, loss of appetite, and pruritus are possible.
Laboratory Findings in the Acute Phase of Infection			
Aminotransferase (ALT, AST) elevations	>1000 IU/L (6.7 μkat/L) ALT>AST	1000–2000 IU/L (16.7–33.3 μkat/L) ALT>AST	Highly variable, can be approximately 1000 IU/L (16.7 μkat/L) ALT>AST
Bilirubin	Elevated and preceded by aminotransferase elevations	Can be within normal or elevated	Elevated and preceded by aminotransferase elevations
Virus-specific tests	IgM anti-HAV	IgM anti-HBc (+), HBsAg (+)	HCV RNA (+) or quantifiable; HCV antibody reactive within 12 weeks of exposure

ALT, alanine aminotransferase; AST, aspartate aminotransferase; anti-, antibody to; HBc, hepatitis B core; HBsAg, hepatitis B surface antigen; IgM, immunoglobulin; IU, international units; L, liter; RNA, ribonucleic acid.

experience is limited, or the vaccine is contraindicated. Combined vaccine and immunoglobulin may be preferred for optimal protection.

• Ig is recommended with vaccination if travel to an HAV high or intermediate-risk country will begin in ≤2 weeks and the individual is an older adult, immunocompromised, or has chronic liver disease or other chronic medical condition.

• Anaphylaxis to Ig has been reported in patients with IgA deficiency.

TREATMENT

• No specific treatment options exist for HAV. Management of HAV infection is primarily supportive. Corticosteroid use is not recommended.

HEPATITIS B

• HBV is a leading cause of chronic hepatitis, cirrhosis, and hepatocellular carcinoma (HCC).

• Transmission of HBV occurs sexually, parenterally, and perinatally. In areas of high HBV prevalence, perinatal transmission from mother to child at birth is the most common. In the United States, perinatal transmission and sexual contact continue to be key routes of transmission.

| **TABLE 25-2** | Recommendations for Hepatitis A Virus Vaccination |

All children at 1 year of age

Any unvaccinated children ages 2–18 years

Persons traveling to or working in countries that have high or intermediate endemicity of infection[a]

Men who have sex with men

Users of injection and noninjection drugs

Persons with occupational risk for infection (eg, persons who work with HAV-infected primates or with HAV in a research laboratory)

Persons with chronic liver disease, including persons with hepatitis B virus infection, Hepatitis C virus infection.

All previously unvaccinated persons anticipating close personal contact (eg, household contact or regular babysitter) with an international adoptee from a country of high or intermediate endemicity within the first 60 days after the arrival of the adoptee

Anyone who would like to obtain immunity

[a]Travelers to Canada, Western Europe, Japan, Australia, or New Zealand are at no greater risk for infection than they are in the United States. All other travelers should be assessed for HAV risk.
HAV, hepatitis A virus.
Data from Centers for Disease Control and Prevention.

| **TABLE 25-3** | Recommended Dosing of Hepatitis A Vaccines |

Vaccine	Age (Years)	Dose of Hepatitis A Antigen (Volume)	No. of Doses	Schedule[a]
HAVRIX	1–18	720 ELISA units (0.5 mL)	2	0, 6–12 months
	≥19	1440 ELISA units (1 mL)	2	0, 6–12 months
VAQTA	1–18	25 units (0.5 mL)	2	0, 6–18 months
	≥19	50 units (1 mL)	2	0, 6–18 months
TWINRIX[b]	≥18	720 ELISA units (1 mL)	3	0, 1, 6 months
	≥18 (accelerate schedule)	720 ELISA units (1 mL)	4	0, 7 days, 21–30 days, + 12 months

[a]Zero (0) denotes initial dose, subsequent numbers denote time after initial dose for timing of additional doses.
[b]Combination of hepatitis A and B vaccines, also contains 20 mcg of hepatitis B surface antigen, and requires a three-dose schedule for adequate HBV response.
ELISA, enzyme-linked immunosorbent assay.
Data from Centers for Disease Control and Prevention.

- The hepatitis B surface antigen (HBsAg) is the most abundant of the three surface antigens and is detectable at the onset of clinical symptoms. Its persistence past 6 months after initial detection corresponds to chronic infection and indicates an increased risk for cirrhosis, hepatic decompensation, and hepatocellular carcinoma.
- The interpretation of serologic markers for HBV is given in Table 25-4.
- The clinical presentation of HBV infection is given in Table 25-1.

TABLE 25-4	Interpretation of Serologic Tests in Hepatitis B Virus	
Tests	**Result**	**Interpretation**
HBsAg	(−)	Susceptible
Anti-HBc	(−)	
Anti-HBs	(−)	
HBsAg	(−)	Past HBV infection, resolved
Anti-HBc	(+)	No further management is needed unless undergoing
Anti-HBs	(+)	immunosuppressive therapy or chemotherapy
HBsAg	(−)	Immune because of vaccination (valid only if test
Anti-HBc	(−)	performed 1–2 months after third vaccine dose)
Anti-HBs	(+)	
HBsAg	(+)	Acute infection
Anti-HBc	(+)	
IgM anti-HBc	(+)	
Anti-HBs	(−)	
HBsAg	(+)	Chronic infection. Further evaluation needed
Anti-HBc	(+)	
IgM anti-HBc	(−)	
Anti-HBs	(−)	
HBsAg	(−)	Possible interpretations: Resolved infection or false
Anti-HBc	(+)	positive. If patient is immunocompromised, check
Anti-HBs	(−)	HBV DNA

Anti-, antibody to; HBsAg, hepatitis B surface antigen; HBc, hepatitis B core; HBs, hepatitis B surface; IgM, immunoglobulin M.

Note: Anti-HBc includes both IgM anti-HBc and IgG anti-HBc. IgM is present during acute phase of infection.

Data from Hepatitis B Serology, Centers for Disease Control and Prevention. https://www.cdc.gov/hepatitis/hbv/interpretationofhepbserologicresults.htm.

PREVENTION

- Prophylaxis of HBV can be achieved by vaccination (HBV vaccine) or by passive immunity in postexposure cases with HBV Ig which provides temporary passive immunity.
- The goal of immunization against viral hepatitis is prevention of the short-term viremia that can lead to transmission of infection, clinical disease, and chronic HBV infection.
- Vaccination is the most effective strategy to prevent HBV infection, and a comprehensive vaccination strategy was implemented in the United States. Persons who should receive HBV vaccine are listed in Table 25-5.
- The most commonly reported adverse events for single-antigen vaccine are nausea/dizziness and fever/headache; for combination vaccines, fever, injection site erythema, and vomiting. For Heplisav-B, the most common adverse reactions reported within 7 days of vaccination included injection site pain, fatigue, and headache.

TREATMENT

- <u>Goals of treatment:</u> The goals of therapy are to suppress HBV replication and prevent disease progression to cirrhosis and HCC. Another important goal is preventing HBV reactivation in patients with inactive HBV infections.

| **TABLE 25-5** | Recommendations for Hepatitis B Virus Vaccination |

All infants

All unvaccinated adults aged 19–59 with diabetes; those aged >60 should be vaccinated at the discretion of treating clinician

Sex partners of persons who are HBsAg positive

Sexually active persons not in a long-term monogamous relationship (>1 partner/6 months)

Men who have sex with men

STD clinic patients

Persons with HIV

Current or recent injection drug use

Household contacts of persons with chronic hepatitis B infection

Household contacts of persons with chronic hepatitis B infection; clients and staff of institutions for the developmentally disabled

Healthcare and public safety workers with anticipated risk for exposure to blood or blood-contaminated fluid in the workplace

Chronic dialysis/ESRD patients including predialysis, peritoneal dialysis, and home dialysis patients

Correctional facilities inmates

International travelers to regions with high or intermediate levels (HBsAg prevalence ≥2%) of endemic HBV infection

Persons with chronic HCV infection

Persons with chronic liver disease (eg, patients with alcoholic liver disease, cirrhosis, fatty liver disease, autoimmune hepatitis)

All unvaccinated adults seeking vaccination (specific risk factor not required)

ESRD, end-stage renal disease; HBsAg, hepatitis B surface antigen; HBV, hepatitis B virus; HIV, human immunodeficiency virus; STDs, sexually transmitted diseases.

- Some patients with chronic HBV infection should be treated. Recommendations for treatment consider the patient's age, serum HBV DNA and ALT levels, and whether or not the patient has cirrhosis. All patients with cirrhosis require HBV treatment, irrespective of DNA or ALT levels. Generally accepted criteria for treatment of HBV are given in Table 25-6.
- All patients with chronic HBV infection should be counseled on preventing disease transmission, avoiding alcohol, and on being immunized against HAV. Sexual and household contacts should be vaccinated against HBV.
- The immune-mediating agents approved for HBV treatment are interferon (**IFN**)-**alfa** and **pegylated (peg) IFN-alfa**. The nucleos(t)ide antiviral agents **lamivudine**, **telbivudine**, **adefovir**, **entecavir**, and **tenofovir** diproxoxil and tenofovir alafenamide are approved treatment options for chronic HBV.

HEPATITIS C

- HCV infection is prevalent in high-risk populations such as prisoners, persons who inject drugs, and homeless individuals. Less common routes of transmission include sexual transmission and infants born to HCV-infected women. Screening for HCV infection is recommended in groups who are at high risk for infection (Table 25-7).
- Multiple sexual partners and coinfection with sexually transmitted diseases, including HIV, increase the risk for HCV sexual transmission.
- HCV is differentiated into seven major genotypes (GT), numbered 1–6. GTs are further classified into subtypes (a, b, c, etc.). In the United States, GT1a and GT1b, followed by GT2 and GT3, cause most infections.

TABLE 25-6 Generally Accepted Criteria for Treatment of HBV

Characteristics

Anyone with HBeAg (+) or HBeAg (−) active HBV defined as:

HBV DNA >2000 IU/mL (kIU/L)

ALT 2 × upper limit of normal[a] and/or with evidence of histological disease[b]

Anyone with compensated or decompensated cirrhosis with HBV DNA >2000 IU/mL (kIU/L)[c]

Anyone not fulfilling the above criteria with ALT <2 × ULN and any detectable HBV DNA (<2000 IU/mL [kIU/L]), consider:

    Patient's age

    Family history of HCC

    Prior history of HBV treatment

    Extrahepatic manifestations of HBV

[a]Per European guidelines, any elevations in ALT.
[b]Moderate or greater fibrosis as determined by biopsy or noninvasive measures.
[c]Per European guidelines, any detectable HBV DNA.

TABLE 25-7 Recommendations for Hepatitis C Virus Screening

All adults ≥18 years

All pregnant females during each pregnancy

Routine periodic testing for persons with ongoing risk factors:

    Persons who inject drugs, share needles, syringes, or other drug preparation equipment

    Persons undergoing maintenance hemodialysis

    Sexually active MSM with HIV

    MSM at initiation of HIV pre-exposure prophylaxis

HIV, human immunodeficiency virus, MSM, men who have sex with men.

- The initial test for HCV infection is the anti-HCV or antibody test. Patients who are antibody positive for HCV require confirmatory testing for HCV RNA to verify current HCV infection.
- In an acute HCV infection, most patients are asymptomatic and undiagnosed. HCV RNA is detectable within 1–2 weeks of exposure and levels rise quickly during the initial weeks.
- Patients with acute HCV are often asymptomatic and undiagnosed. One-third of adults will experience some mild and nonspecific symptoms, including fatigue, anorexia, weakness, jaundice, abdominal pain, or dark urine.
- Up to 85% of acutely infected patients go on to develop chronic HCV infection, defined as persistently detectable HCV RNA for 6 months or more. Most patients will have few, if any, specific symptoms of chronic HCV infection.
- HCV cirrhosis poses a 30% risk of developing the end-stage liver disease over 10 years as well as a 1%–2% risk per year of developing hepatocellular carcinoma.

TREATMENT

- Goals of Treatment: The goal is to eradicate HCV infection, which prevents the development of chronic HCV infection, end-stage liver disease, HCC, and death.
- Virologic cure, or sustained virologic response (SVR), is defined as a nondetectable HCV RNA at least 12 weeks after completing HCV therapy. Patients who achieve SVR will continue to have detectable HCV antibody, though this does not imply HCV immunity.

| TABLE 25-8 | AASLD/IDSA Recommended Treatment Regimens for Treatment-Naive Patients with No Cirrhosis (NC) or Compensated Cirrhosis (CC) and Hepatitis C Genotypes 1-6 |

	GT1a NC	GT1a CC	GT1b NC or CC	GT2 NC or CC	GT3 NC	GT3 CC	GT4 NC or CC	GT5, 6 NC or CC
DAA Therapy								
Glecaprevir/ Pibrentasvir	Yes	Yes	Yes	Yes	Yes	Yes	Yes	Yes
Ledipasvir/ Sofosbuvir	Yes	Yes	Yes	No	No	No	Yes	Yes
Sofosbuvir/ Velpatasvir	Yes	Yes	Yes	Yes	Yes	Yes[a]—but with RAS testing	Yes	Yes
Elbasvir/Grazoprevir	No[b]	No	Yes	No	No	No	Yes	No

[a]Considered an alternative regimen because NS5A resistance testing is required prior to treatment start.
[b]Pre-treatment resistance testing for NS5A resistance-associated substitutions (RAS) should be done; if the Y93 RAS is identified, an alternative therapy is recommended. AASLD/IDSA. Recommendations for testing, managing, and treating hepatitis C. Available at: http://www.hcvguidelines.org.

- Treatment is recommended for all HCV-infected persons. Patients with a short life expectancy (<12 months) are currently the only populations for whom treatment is not recommended.
- Patients without cirrhosis may be candidates for a much more simplified treatment approach if the patient is HCV treatment naïve, has no history or suspicion of HCC, has not received a liver transplant, and has no evidence of HIV or active HBV infection. Patients with cirrhosis will likely require on-treatment monitoring as well as additional post-treatment follow-up to manage the complications.
- The following laboratory tests are suggested prior to treatment: HCV RNA, complete blood count, liver function tests, INR, GFR, HIV antigen/antibody, Hep B serologies, Anti-HAV.
- The simplified treatment regimen for treatment-naïve patients with hepatitis C (all genotypes) is glecaprevir/pibrentasvir 3 tabs orally daily with food × 8 weeks, or sofosbuvir/velpatasvir 1 tab orally daily with or without food × 12 weeks. HCV RNA and LFTs should be repeated 12 weeks after completing HCV therapy to assess for cure (SVR) and resolution of hepatic inflammation. See Table 25-8 for treatment exclusions.
- Patients without cirrhosis or those with compensated cirrhosis are treated similarly with no difference in treatment duration.
- Patients with decompensated cirrhosis (CTP class B or C) often require concomitant ribavirin and have fewer treatment options due to the underlying level of liver disease and concerns for safety. The only therapies recommended for use in decompensation include ledipasvir/sofosbuvir and sofosbuvir/velpatasvir.
- Adherence to therapy is a crucial component in response, especially among genotype 1–infected patients.
- Clinically significant drug–drug interactions are expected with carbamazepine, phenobarbital, phenytoin, oxcarbazepine, rifampin, and St. John's wort and concurrent use of these agents with any of the HCV therapies is expected to result in HCV treatment failure.
- All patients with chronic HCV infection should be vaccinated for HAV and HBV.
- No HCV vaccine is currently available.

See Chapter 58, Viral Hepatitis, authored by Paulina Deming, for a more detailed discussion of this topic.

Inflammatory Bowel Disease

- There are two forms of idiopathic *inflammatory bowel disease* (IBD): ulcerative colitis (UC), a mucosal inflammatory condition confined to the rectum and colon, and Crohn's disease (CD), a transmural inflammation of gastrointestinal (GI) mucosa that may occur in any part of the GI tract. The etiologies of both conditions are unknown, but they may have a common pathogenic mechanism.

ETIOLOGY AND PATHOPHYSIOLOGY

- Factors that cause IBD include infectious agents, genetics, the environment, and the immune system. This may involve abnormal regulation of the innate immune response or a reaction to various antigens. The microflora of the GI tract may provide an environmental trigger to activate inflammation in genetically susceptible individuals and is highly implicated in the development of IBD.
- Suspect infectious agents include viruses, protozoans, mycobacteria such as *Mycobacterium paratuberculosis* or *avium*, and other bacteria such as *Ruminococcus gnavus, Ruminococcus torques, Listeria monocytogenes, Fusobacterium varium, Chlamydia trachomatis*, and *Escherichia coli*. Patients with CD typically have circulating antibodies to *Saccharomyces cerevisiae*, which demonstrates some immunologic response to intestinal organisms.
- Genetic factors play a significant role in the predisposition to IBD. First-degree relatives of patients with IBD may have up to a 20-fold increase in the risk of disease and risk is extended to second- and third-degree relatives.
- Th1 cytokine activity is excessive in CD, and increased expression of interferon-γ in the intestinal mucosa and excess production of IL-12, IL-17A, and IL-22 are features of the immune response in CD. In contrast, Th2 cytokine activity is excessive with UC. Tumor necrosis factor-α (TNF-α) is a pivotal proinflammatory cytokine that is increased in the mucosa and intestinal lumen of patients with CD and UC.
- Antineutrophil cytoplasmic antibodies are found in a high percentage of patients with UC and less frequently with CD.
- Smoking appears to be protective for UC but is associated with increased frequency and severity of CD. Use of nonsteroidal anti-inflammatory drugs (NSAIDs) may trigger disease occurrence or lead to disease flares.
- UC and CD differ in two general respects: anatomical sites and depth of involvement within the bowel wall. There is, however, overlap between the two conditions, with a small fraction of patients showing features of both diseases (Table 26-1).

ULCERATIVE COLITIS

- UC is confined to the colon and rectum and affects primarily the mucosa and the submucosa. The primary lesion occurs in the crypts of the mucosa (crypts of Lieberkühn) in the form of a crypt abscess.
- Local complications (involving the colon) occur in the majority of patients with UC. Relatively minor complications include hemorrhoids, anal fissures, and perirectal abscesses.
- A major complication is toxic megacolon, a severe condition that occurs in up to 7.9% of UC patients admitted to hospitals. Patients with toxic megacolon usually have a high fever, tachycardia, distended abdomen, elevated white blood cell count, and a dilated colon.
- The risk of colonic carcinoma is much greater in patients with UC than in the general population.
- Patients with UC may have hepatobiliary complications, including fatty liver, pericholangitis, chronic active hepatitis, cirrhosis, sclerosing cholangitis, cholangiocarcinoma, and gallstones.

TABLE 26-1	Comparison of the Clinical and Pathologic Features of Crohn's Disease and Ulcerative Colitis	
Feature	**Crohn's Disease**	**Ulcerative Colitis**
Clinical		
Malaise, fever	Common	Uncommon
Rectal bleeding	Common	Common
Abdominal tenderness	Common	May be present
Abdominal mass	Common	Absent
Abdominal pain	Common	Unusual
Abdominal wall and internal fistulas	Common	Absent
Distribution	Discontinuous	Continuous
Aphthous or linear ulcers	Common	Rare
Pathologic		
Rectal involvement	Rare	Common
Ileal involvement	Very common	Rare
Strictures	Common	Rare
Fistulas	Common	Rare
Transmural involvement	Common	Rare
Crypt abscesses	Rare	Very common
Granulomas	Common	Rare
Linear clefts	Common	Rare
Cobblestone appearance	Common	Absent

- Arthritis commonly occurs in patients with IBD and is typically asymptomatic and migratory. Arthritis typically involves one or a few large joints, such as the knees, hips, ankles, wrists, and elbows.
- Ocular complications including dry eye, blepharitis, iritis, uveitis, episcleritis, and conjunctivitis occur in up to 29% of patients with IBD occur in some patients. Skin and mucosal lesions associated with IBD include erythema nodosum, pyoderma gangrenosum, aphthous ulceration, and Sweet syndrome.

CROHN'S DISEASE

- CD is a transmural inflammatory process. The terminal ileum is the most common site, but it may occur in any part of the GI tract. Most patients have some colonic involvement. Patients often have normal bowel separating segments of diseased bowel; that is, the disease is often discontinuous.
- Complications of CD may involve the intestinal tract or organs unrelated to it. Small bowel stricture with subsequent obstruction is a complication that may require surgery. Fistula formation is common and occurs much more frequently than with UC.
- Systemic complications of CD are common and similar to those found with UC. Arthritis, iritis, skin lesions, and liver disease often accompany CD.
- Nutritional deficiencies are common with CD (including deficiencies of folate, vitamin B_{12}, vitamins A to D, calcium, magnesium, iron, and zinc).

CLINICAL PRESENTATION AND DIAGNOSIS

ULCERATIVE COLITIS

- There is a wide range of presenting symptoms in UC, from mild abdominal cramping with frequent small-volume bowel movements to profuse diarrhea. Many patients have disease confined to the rectum (proctitis).
- Most patients with UC experience intermittent bouts of illness after varying intervals of no symptoms.
- Mild disease, which afflicts two-thirds of patients, has been defined as fewer than four stools daily, with or without blood, with no systemic disturbance and a normal erythrocyte sedimentation rate (ESR <30 mm/h).
- Patients with moderate disease have more than four stools per day but with minimal systemic disturbance.
- With severe disease, the patient has more than six stools per day with blood, with systemic manifestations of fever, tachycardia, anemia, or ESR greater than 30 mm/h (8.3 μm/sec). With fulminant disease, there are more than 10 bowel movements per day with continuous bleeding, toxicity, abdominal tenderness, requirement for transfusion, and colonic dilation.

- **Signs and symptoms**

  ✓ Abdominal cramping
  ✓ Frequent bowel movements, often with blood in the stool
  ✓ Weight loss
  ✓ Fever and tachycardia in severe disease.
  ✓ Blurred vision, eye pain, and photophobia with ocular involvement
  ✓ Arthritis
  ✓ Raised, red, tender nodules that vary in size from 1 cm to several centimeters

- **Physical examination**

  ✓ Hemorrhoids, anal fissures, or perirectal abscesses may be present
  ✓ Iritis, uveitis, episcleritis, and conjunctivitis with ocular involvement
  ✓ Dermatologic findings with erythema nodosum, pyoderma gangrenosum, or aphthous ulceration

- **Laboratory Tests**

  ✓ Decreased hematocrit/hemoglobin
  ✓ Increased ESR, CRP, and fecal calprotectin
  ✓ Leukocytosis and hypoalbuminemia with severe disease
  ✓ (+) perinuclear antineutrophil cytoplasmic antibodies

CROHN'S DISEASE

- As with UC, the presentation of CD is highly variable. A patient may present with diarrhea and abdominal pain or a perirectal or perianal lesion. Patients with mild-to-moderate CD are typically ambulatory and have no evidence of dehydration, systemic toxicity, less than 10% loss of body weight, or abdominal tenderness, mass, or obstruction.
- The course of CD is characterized by periods of remission and exacerbation. Some patients may be free of symptoms for years, whereas others experience chronic problems despite medical therapy.
- The Crohn's Disease Activity Index (CDAI) is used to gauge response to therapy and determine remission. Disease activity may be assessed and correlated by evaluation of serum C-reactive protein concentrations.

- **Signs and Symptoms**

  ✓ Malaise and fever
  ✓ Abdominal pain
  ✓ Frequent bowel movements

✓ Hematochezia
✓ Fistula
✓ Weight loss and malnutrition
✓ Arthritis

- **Physical examination**
  ✓ Abdominal mass and tenderness
  ✓ Perianal fissure or fistula

- **Laboratory tests**
  ✓ Increased white blood cell count, ESR, CRP, and fecal calprotectin
  ✓ (+) anti–*Saccharomyces cerevisiae* antibodies

TREATMENT

- <u>Goals of Treatment</u>: Resolution of acute inflammatory processes, resolution of attendant complications (eg, fistulas or abscesses), alleviation of systemic manifestations (eg, arthritis), maintenance of remission from acute inflammation, or surgical palliation or cure.
- Treatment often involves use of specific targets, such as mucosal healing and endoscopic remission, or resolution of symptoms such as abdominal pain and diarrhea, as the main indicators of treatment efficacy (referred to as "Treat to Target").

NONPHARMACOLOGIC TREATMENT

- Patients with IBD have a five-fold higher risk of malnutrition compared to those without IBD. Patients should be screened for malnutrition upon diagnosis and assessed intermittently for the presence of micronutrient deficiencies.
- Elimination of specific foods that appear to exacerbate symptoms can be tried; however, exclusion diets are generally not endorsed, even in the setting of severe disease.
- Parenteral nutrition is generally reserved for patients with severe malnutrition or those who fail enteral therapy or have a contraindication to receiving enteral therapy, such as perforation, protracted vomiting, short bowel syndrome, or severe intestinal stenosis.
- While probiotics are considered to be generally safe in patients with IBD, the added cost and requirement to often take multiple doses per day, coupled with the lack of quality data to support their use, should weigh into the decision to use them in IBD.
- Colectomy may be necessary for UC patients with disease uncontrolled by maximum medical therapy or when there are disease complications such as colonic perforation, toxic megacolon, uncontrolled colonic hemorrhage, or colonic strictures.
- Surgery in patients with CD is usually reserved for patients with intractable hemorrhage, perforation, persistent or recurrent obstruction, abscess, dysplasia, cancer, or medically refractory disease. CD has a high recurrence rate after surgery.

PHARMACOLOGIC THERAPY

- The major drug therapies used in IBD are **aminosalicylates; corticosteroids**; immunomodulators (**azathioprine, mercaptopurine,** and **methotrexate**); immunosuppressive agents (**cyclosporine** and **tacrolimus**); antimicrobials (**metronidazole** and **ciprofloxacin**); and agents to inhibit TNF-α (anti–TNF-α antibodies), leukocyte adhesion and migration (**natalizumab** and **vedolizumab**), interleukin function (**ustekinumab**), or Janus kinase function (**tofacitinib**).
- **Sulfasalazine** combines a sulfonamide (sulfapyridine) antibiotic and mesalamine (5-aminosalicylic acid) in the same molecule. Oral **mesalamine** derivatives are alternatives to sulfasalazine for treatment of mild-to-moderate UC with similar rates of efficacy. Mesalamine-based products are listed in **Table 26-2**.

TABLE 26-2   Agents for the Treatment of Inflammatory Bowel Disease

Drug	Brand Name	Initial Dose (g)	Usual Range
Sulfasalazine	Azulfidine	500 mg–1 g	4–6 g/day
	Azulfidine EN	500 mg–1 g	4–6 g/day
Mesalamine suppository	Canasa	1 g	1 g daily to three times weekly
Mesalamine enema	Rowasa	4 g	4 g daily to three times weekly
Mesalamine (oral)	Asacol HD	1.6 g/day	2.8–4.8 g/day
	Apriso	1.5 g/day	1.5 g/day once daily
	Lialda	1.2–2.4 g/day	1.2–4.8 g/day once daily
	Pentasa	2 g/day	2–4 g/day
	Delzicol	1.2 g/day	2.4–4.8 g/day
Olsalazine	Dipentum	1.5 g/day	1.5–3 g/day
Balsalazide	Colazal	2.25 g/day	2.25–6.75 g/day
Azathioprine	Imuran, Azasan	50–100 mg	1–2.5 mg/kg/day
Cyclosporine	Gengraf	2–4 mg/kg/day IV	2–4 mg/kg/day IV
	Neoral, Sandimmune	2–8 mg/kg/day oral	
Mercaptopurine	Purinethol	50–100 mg	1–2.5 mg/kg/day
Methotrexate	No branded IM injection	15–25 mg IM weekly	15–25 mg IM weekly
Adalimumab	Humira	160 mg SC day 1	80 mg SC 2 (day 15), and then 40 mg every 2 weeks
Adalimumab-atto	Amjevita		
Adalimumab-abdm	Cyltezo		
Adalimumab-adaz	Hyrimoz[a]		
Adalimumab-afzb	Adrilada[a]		
Adalimumab-bwwd	Adalimumab-bwwd Hadlima[a]		
Certolizumab	Cimzia	400 mg SC	400 mg SC weeks 2 and 4, and then 400 mg SC monthly
Infliximab	Remicade	5 mg/kg IV	5 mg/kg weeks 2 6, 5–10 mg/kg every 8 weeks
Infliximab-dyyb	Inflectra		
Infliximab-abda	Renflexis		
Infliximab-qbtx	IXIFI		
Infliximab-axxq	AVSOLA		
Natalizumab	Tysabri	300 mg IV	300 mg IV every 4 weeks
Budesonide	Entocort EC capsule, Uceris tablet	9 mg orally once daily	6–9 mg daily
	Uceris rectal foam	2 mg twice daily	2 mg daily

(Continued)

TABLE 26-2	Agents for the Treatment of Inflammatory Bowel Disease (*Continued*)		
Drug	**Brand Name**	**Initial Dose (g)**	**Usual Range**
Vedolizumab	Entyvio	300 mg IV	300 mg IV weeks 2 and 6 and then every 8 weeks
Golimumab	Simponi	200 mg SC	100 mg SC weeks 2 and 4
Ustekinumab	Stelara	Weight-based initial IV dose <55 kg (260 mg), 55–85 kg (390 mg), >85 kg (520 mg)	90 mg SC every 8 weeks
Tofacitinib	Xeljanz	10 mg twice daily for 8 weeks; may continue for maximum of 16 weeks	5 mg twice daily
Ozanimod	Zeposia	0.23 mg orally once daily days 1–4, then 0.46 mg once daily days 5–7	0.92 mg orally once daily starting day 8 of therapy

[a]Not available until 2023
IM, intramuscular; SC, subcutaneous.

- Oral corticosteroids in doses of 40–60 mg/day **prednisone** equivalent can be used for patients with moderate-to-severe active disease who are refractory to oral aminosalicylates or require more rapid control of symptoms.
- Immunomodulators such as azathioprine, mercaptopurine (a metabolite of azathioprine), methotrexate, or cyclosporine are used in the long-term treatment of IBD. These agents are generally reserved for patients who fail aminosalicylate therapy or are refractory to or dependent on corticosteroids.
- Cyclosporine has a short-term benefit in the treatment of acute, severe UC to avoid colectomy in patients failing corticosteroids but has little efficacy in CD.
- Methotrexate 15–25 mg intramuscularly or subcutaneously once weekly is useful for treatment and maintenance of CD and may be steroid sparing.
- Antimicrobial agents have limited roles as adjunctive therapies in IBD. Metronidazole can be used as adjunctive therapy for simple perianal fistulae and may be combined with infliximab.
- **Infliximab** is an anti-TNFα antibody that is useful in moderate-to-severe active CD and UC as well as steroid-dependent or fistulizing disease, both as induction and maintenance therapy. **Adalimumab** is another anti-TNFα (fully humanized) antibody that is an option for patients with moderate-to-severe active CD or UC previously treated with infliximab who have lost response.
- Natalizumab and vedolizumab are leukocyte adhesion and migration inhibitors that are used for patients with CD who are unresponsive to other therapies.

Ulcerative Colitis

Mild-to-Moderate Active Disease

- Most patients with mild-to-moderate active UC can be managed on an outpatient basis with oral and/or topical aminosalicylates (Fig. 26-1). For patients with extensive disease, oral once-daily mesalamine is generally preferred in doses of 2–3 g/day. Doses greater than 3 g/day can be used in patients who are unresponsive to standard doses and generally should be combined with a rectal mesalamine formulation at a dose of 1 g/day.

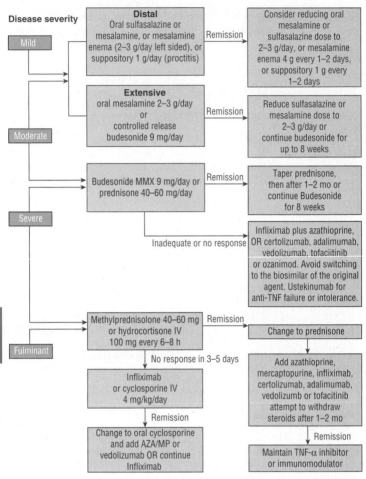

AZA, Azathioprine; MMX, Multi-matrix system; MP, mercaptopurine, and TNF, tumor necrosis factor.

FIGURE 26-1. Treatment approaches for ulcerative colitis.

- Oral mesalamine derivatives (see **Table 26-2**) are reasonable alternatives to sulfasalazine for treatment of UC because they are better tolerated. Topical mesalamine in an enema or suppository formulation is more effective than oral mesalamine or topical steroids for distal disease.
- **Budesonide** 9 mg/day is preferred for patients who are unresponsive to optimized doses of mesalamine.

Moderate-to-Severe Active Disease

- While oral mesalamine products may be effective for moderately severe UC, oral budesonide MMX is the preferred alternative prior to use of more systemic corticosteroids and for moderate disease.

- Steroids have a place in the treatment of moderate-to-severe UC or in patients who are unresponsive to maximal doses of oral and topical mesalamine. Oral corticosteroids in doses of 40–60 mg prednisone equivalent daily are recommended for adults.
- TNF-α inhibitors are an option for patients with moderate-to-severe disease who are unresponsive to aminosalicylates or corticosteroids, or are corticosteroid dependent, and are more effective than immunomodulator monotherapy for induction of remission. For treatment-naive patients, infliximab or vedolizumab in combination with an immunomodulator (eg, azathioprine) is recommended preferentially.

Active Severe or Fulminant Disease

- Patients with uncontrolled acute severe UC or incapacitating symptoms require hospitalization for effective management. Most medications are given parenterally. Patients should be tested for *Clostridoidies difficile* infection and receive venous thromboembolism (VTE) prophylaxis.
- Methylprednisolone IV at a dose of 40–60 mg daily is considered a first-line agent. A trial of corticosteroids is warranted in most patients before proceeding to colectomy, unless the condition is grave or rapidly deteriorating.
- Patients who are unresponsive to parenteral corticosteroids can receive cyclosporine or infliximab. A continuous IV infusion of cyclosporine 2–4 mg/kg/day is the typical dose range used and may delay the need for colectomy.

Maintenance of Remission

- Once remission from active disease has been achieved, the goal of therapy is to maintain the remission for as long as possible.
- For patients with previously mildly active extensive or left-side disease, the oral aminosalicylate agents are preferred for maintenance therapy at a dose of at least 2 g/day. The newer mesalamine derivatives are generally better tolerated than sulfasalazine and are associated with fewer adverse effects, making them a preferred choice.
- The TNF-α inhibitors, vedolizumab, ustekinumab, or tofacitinib are all options for maintenance in patients with moderate-to-severe UC following successful induction of remission, and in those who are steroid-dependent or have failed azathioprine.
- Steroids do not have a role in the maintenance of remission with UC because they are ineffective. Steroids should be withdrawn gradually over 2–4 weeks after remission is induced.

Crohn's Disease

- Sulfasalazine has marginal efficacy in mild-to-moderate CD. The newer mesalamine derivatives are generally considered to have minimal efficacy.
- Mesalamine derivatives that release mesalamine in the small bowel (eg, Pentasa) may be more effective than sulfasalazine for ileal involvement.
- Systemic corticosteroids are frequently used for treating moderate-to-severe active CD; however, controlled-release budesonide (Entocort) 9 mg daily is a preferred first-line option for patients with mild-to-moderate ileal or right-sided (ascending colonic) disease.
- Oral corticosteroids, such as prednisone 40–60 mg/day, are generally considered first-line therapy and are frequently used for moderate-to-severe active CD unresponsive to aminosalicylates.
- Metronidazole 10–20 mg/kg/day orally in divided doses may be useful in some patients with CD, particularly for patients with colonic or ileocolonic involvement, those with perineal disease, or those who are unresponsive to sulfasalazine.
- Azathioprine, mercaptopurine, and methotrexate are not recommended to induce remission in moderate-to-severe CD; however, they are effective in maintaining steroid-induced remission and are generally limited to use for patients not achieving adequate response to standard medical therapy or in the setting of steroid dependency.

- Clinical response to azathioprine and mercaptopurine may be related to whole-blood concentrations of the metabolite 6-thioguanine (TGN). Concentrations of TGN greater than 230–450 pmol/8 × 10⁸ erythrocytes have beneficial effects, but monitoring is not routinely performed or may not be available at some sites.
- Methotrexate given weekly intramuscularly or subcutaneously in doses of 15–25 mg is effective in reducing steroid dependency and maintaining remission, and may be considered as an alternative to azathioprine or mercaptopurine.
- The TNF-α inhibitors are the most effective and thus the preferred agents in managing moderate-to-severe CD. All agents in this class, with the exception of golimumab, which is not approved for use in CD in the United States, have similar rates of efficacy. The use of TNF-α inhibitors in combination with thiopurines has quickly become the preferred approach to treatment of moderate-to-severe CD.
- The integrin antagonists are options for patients who do not respond to steroids or TNF-α inhibitors, and vedolizumab is also considered a first-line alternative to TNF-α inhibitors for moderate-to-severe disease.

Maintenance of Remission

- Prevention of recurrence of disease is more difficult with CD than with UC. There is minimal evidence that sulfasalazine and oral mesalamine derivatives are effective for maintenance of CD remission following medically induced remission, and therefore these agents are not preferred (Fig. 26-2).
- Systemic steroids have no role in the maintenance of remission or prevention of recurrence of CD; these agents do not appear to alter the long-term course of the disease. Budesonide can be considered for maintenance therapy for up to 4 months.
- All of the TNF-α inhibitors currently approved for use in CD are viable options for maintenance of remission. Combination therapy with a thiopurine should be highly considered to further improve efficacy and to extend the duration of TNF-α inhibitor efficacy by reducing immunogenicity.
- Methotrexate may be considered as an alternative to thiopurines to maintain corticosteroid-induced remission.

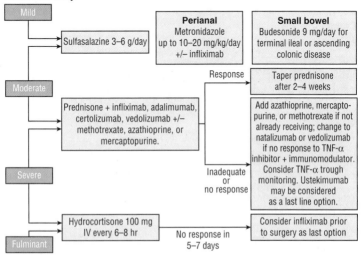

FIGURE 26-2. **Treatment approaches for Crohn's disease.**

SELECT COMPLICATIONS

Toxic Megacolon

- The treatment required for toxic megacolon includes general supportive measures to maintain vital functions, consideration for early surgical intervention, and drug therapy.
- Aggressive fluid and electrolyte management are required for dehydration. When the patient has lost significant amounts of blood (through the rectum), blood transfusion may be necessary.
- Steroids in high doses (eg, hydrocortisone 100 mg every 8 hours) should be administered IV to reduce acute inflammation.
- Broad-spectrum antimicrobials that include coverage for gram-negative bacilli and intestinal anaerobes should be used as preemptive therapy if perforation occurs.

Extraintestinal Manifestations

- For arthritis, **aspirin** or another NSAID may be beneficial, as are corticosteroids. However, NSAID use may exacerbate the underlying IBD and predispose patients to GI bleeding.
- Anemia secondary to blood loss from the GI tract can be treated with oral **ferrous sulfate**. **Vitamin B$_{12}$** or **folic acid** may also be required.
- If the patient is deemed high risk for osteoporosis or exhibits a reduced serum vitamin D concentration, **vitamin D** and **calcium** should be administered. If osteoporosis is present, then calcium, vitamin D, and a **bisphosphonate** or possibly **teriparatide** are recommended.

EVALUATION OF THERAPEUTIC OUTCOMES

- See Table 26-3 for drug monitoring guidelines.
- Patients receiving sulfasalazine should receive oral **folic acid** supplementation because sulfasalazine inhibits folic acid absorption.
- The success of therapeutic regimens to treat IBDs can be measured by patient-reported complaints, signs and symptoms, direct physician examination (including endoscopy), history and physical examination, select laboratory tests, and quality of life measures.
- Adverse effects of corticosteroids include hyperglycemia, hypertension, osteoporosis, acne, fluid retention, electrolyte disturbances, myopathies, muscle wasting, increased appetite, psychosis, infection, and adrenocortical suppression. To minimize corticosteroid effects, clinicians may use alternate-day steroid therapy; however, some patients do not do well clinically on the days when no steroid is given.
- To create more objective measures, disease-rating scales or indices have been created. CDAI is a commonly used scale, particularly for evaluation of patients during clinical trials. The scale incorporates eight elements: (1) number of stools in the past 7 days, (2) sum of abdominal pain ratings from the past 7 days, (3) rating of general well-being in the past 7 days, (4) use of antidiarrheals, (5) body weight, (6) hematocrit, (7) finding of abdominal mass, and (8) a sum of symptoms present in the past week.
- Standardized assessment tools have also been constructed for UC. Elements in these scales include: (1) stool frequency; (2) presence of blood in the stool; (3) mucosal appearance (from endoscopy); and (4) physician's global assessment based on physical examination, endoscopy, and laboratory data.

See Chapter 52, Inflammatory Bowel Disease, authored by Brian A. Hemstreet, for a more detailed discussion of this topic.

TABLE 26-3	Drug Monitoring Guidelines		
Drug(s)	Adverse Drug Reaction	Monitoring Parameters	Comments
Sulfasalazine	Nausea, vomiting, headache	Folate, complete blood count	Increase the dose slowly, over 1–2 weeks
	Rash, anemia, pneumonitis	Liver function tests, Scr, BUN	
	Hepatotoxicity, nephritis		
	Thrombocytopenia, lymphoma		
Mesalamine	Nausea, vomiting, headache	GI disturbances	
Corticosteroids	Hyperglycemia, dyslipidemia	Blood pressure, fasting lipid panel	Avoid long-term use if possible or consider budesonide
	Osteoporosis, hypertension, acne	Glucose, vitamin D, bone density	
	Edema, infection, myopathy, psychosis		
Azathioprine/Mercaptopurine	Bone marrow suppression, pancreatitis, Lymphoma	Complete blood count	Check TPMT activity or NUDT15 phenotype
	Liver dysfunction, rash, arthralgia	Scr, BUN, liver function tests, genotype/phenotype	May monitor TGN
Methotrexate	Bone marrow suppression, pancreatitis	Complete blood count, Scr, BUN	Check baseline pregnancy test
	Pneumonitis, pulmonary fibrosis, hepatitis	Liver function tests	Chest x-ray
Infliximab	Infusion-related reactions (infliximab), infection	Blood pressure/heart rate (infliximab)	Need negative PPD and viral serologies
Adalimumab		Neurologic exam, mental status	
Certolizumab	Heart failure, optic neuritis, demyelination, injection site reaction, signs of infection	Trough concentrations (infliximab)	
Golimumab		Antidrug antibodies (all agents)	
Natalizumab	Infusion-related reactions	Brain MRI, mental status, progressive multifocal leukoencephalopathy	Vedolizumab not associated with PML
Vedolizumab			

Drug			
Ustekinumab	Infections, skin cancers	Signs/symptoms of infection, annual skin exam	Rare instances of reversible posterior leukoencephalopathy syndrome (RPLS) Avoid live vaccines
Tofacitinib	Infection, thrombosis, lymphoma, elevated cholesterol, CK, LFTs, lymphopenia, neutropenia, anemia	Symptoms of infection or thrombosis	Avoid live vaccines Screen for baseline TB Do not initiate in patients with lymphocytes <500/mm³, ANC <1000/mm³, or hemoglobin <9 g/dL Monitor lipids and LFTs every 4–8 weeks Gastrointestinal perforation has been reported with use of the XR formulation Drug interactions with CYP3A4 and 2C19 inhibitors
Ozanimod	Infection, heart rate, blood pressure, LFTs, respiratory rate, fetal abnormalities, macular edema, headache	Symptoms of infection or respiratory dysfunction, changes in vision	Need baseline ECG, WBC, LFTs, ophthalmic assessment, and testing for varicella zoster antibodies. Contraindicated if patient has experienced MI, unstable angina, stroke, TIA, decompensated heart failure, or Mobitz type II second- or third-degree AV block, sick sinus syndrome in the last 6 months, presence of sleep apnea, and concomitant use of MAOI. Women of childbearing age should use effective contraception during and for 3 months after use

ANC, absolute neutrophil count; BUN, blood urea nitrogen; CK, creatine kinase; GI, gastrointestinal; LFTs, liver function tests; MRI, magnetic resonance imaging; PML, progressive multifocal leukoencephalopathy; PPD, purified protein derivative; SCr, serum creatinine; TGN, thioguanine; TPMT, thiopurine methyltransferase; XR, extended-release.

Nausea and Vomiting

- Nausea is usually defined as the inclination to vomit or as a feeling in the throat or epigastric region alerting an individual that vomiting is imminent. Vomiting is defined as the ejection or expulsion of gastric contents through the mouth, often requiring a forceful event.

ETIOLOGY AND PATHOPHYSIOLOGY

- Specific etiologies associated with nausea and vomiting are presented in Table 27-1.
- Table 27-2 presents cytotoxic agents categorized by their emetogenic potential. Although some agents may have greater emetogenic potential than others, combinations of agents, high doses, clinical settings, psychological conditions, prior treatment experiences, and unusual stimuli to sight, smell, or taste may alter a patient's response to a drug treatment.

TABLE 27-1	Etiologies of Nausea and Vomiting

Intraperitoneal

Mechanical obstruction
    Gastric outlet obstruction
    Small-bowel obstruction
Altered sensorimotor function
    Gastroparesis
    Gastroesophageal reflux
    Intestinal pseudo-obstruction
    Irritable bowel syndrome
    Chronic idiopathic nausea
    Functional vomiting
    Cyclic vomiting syndrome
    Cannabinoid hyperemesis syndrome
    Rumination syndrome
Inflammatory diseases
    Pancreatitis
    Pyelonephritis
    Cholecystitis
    Appendicitis
    Hepatitis
Acute gastroenteritis
    Viral
    Bacterial
Biliary colic
Liver failure

Cardiovascular diseases

    Myocardial infarction
    Cardiomyopathy

(Continued)

| TABLE 27-1 | Etiologies of Nausea and Vomiting (*Continued*) |

Neurologic processes

    Increased intracranial pressure

    Migraine headache

    Vestibular disorders

    Intracerebral hemorrhage

    Intracerebral malignancy

Metabolic disorders

    Diabetes mellitus (diabetic ketoacidosis)

    Addison's disease

    Renal disease (uremia)

Psychiatric causes

    Depression

    Anxiety disorders

    Anorexia and bulimia nervosa

Therapy-induced causes

    Antineoplastic agents

    Radiation therapy

    Anticonvulsant preparations

    Digoxin, cardiac antiarrhythmics

    Opioids

    Oral hypoglycemics

    Oral contraceptives

    Antibiotics

    Volatile general anesthetics

Drug withdrawal

    Opioids

    Benzodiazepines

Miscellaneous causes

    Pregnancy

    Noxious odors

    Postoperative vomiting

- The three consecutive phases of emesis are nausea, retching, and vomiting. Nausea, the imminent need to vomit, is associated with gastric stasis. Retching is the labored movement of abdominal and thoracic muscles before vomiting. The final phase of emesis is vomiting, the forceful expulsion of gastric contents due to GI retroperistalsis.

- Vomiting is triggered by afferent impulses to the vomiting center, a nucleus of cells in the medulla. Impulses are received from sensory centers, such as the chemoreceptor trigger zone, cerebral cortex, and visceral afferents from the pharynx and GI tract. The vomiting center integrates the afferent impulses, resulting in efferent impulses to the salivation center, respiratory center, and the pharyngeal, GI, and abdominal muscles, leading to vomiting.

TABLE 27-2	Emetic Risk of Agents Used in Oncology and Treatment Options	
Antiemetic Agent	**Antiemetic Dose on Day 1 of Chemotherapy**	**Antiemetic Dose on Subsequent Days**

High Risk (>90%): Anthracycline/Cyclophosphamide combination, Carmustine, Cisplatin, Cyclophosphamide >1500 mg/m², Dacarbazine, Mechlorethamine, Streptozocin

NK-1 Antagonist		
Aprepitant	125 mg oral or 130 mg IV	80 mg oral on days 2-3
Fosaprepitant	150 mg IV	
Netupitant-palonosetron	300 mg/0.5 mg oral	
Fosnetupitant-palonosetron	235 mg fosnetupitant/0.25 mg palonosetron IV	
Rolapitant	180 mg oral	
5-HT₃ Antagonist[a]		
Granisetron	2 mg oral or 1 mg IV or 10 mcg/kg IV or 1 patch or 10 mg SQ	
Ondansetron	24 mg oral or 8 mg IV or 0.15 mg/kg IV	
Palonosetron	0.5 mg oral	
Ramosetron	0.3 mg IV	
Tropisetron	5 mg oral OR 5 mg IV	
Dexamethasone[b]	12 mg or 20 mg oral/IV	8 mg oral/IV daily or twice daily on days 2–4
Olanzapine	5 mg or 10 mg oral	5 mg or 10 mg oral on days 2–4

Moderate Risk (30%–90%): Aldesleukin, Alemtuzumab, Arsenic trioxide, Azacitidine, Bendamustine, Busulfan, Carboplatin, Clofarabine, Cyclophosphamide <1500 mg/m², Cytarabine >1000 mg/m², Daunorubicin, Daunorubicin and cytarabine liposomal, Doxorubicin, Epirubicin, Fam-trastuzumab deruxtecan-nxki, Idarubicin, Ifosfamide, Irinotecan, Irinetecan liposomal injection, Oxaliplatin, Romidepsin, Temozolomide, Thiotepa, Trabectidin

5-HT₃ Antagonist		
Granisetron	2 mg oral or 1 mg IV or 10 mcg/kg IV or 1 patch or 10 mg SQ	
Ondansetron	8 mg oral twice daily or 8 mg IV or 0.15 mg/kg IV	
Palonosetron	0.5 mg oral or 0.25 mg IV	
Ramosetron	0.3 mg IV	
Tropisetron	5 mg oral or 5 mg IV	
Dexamethasone	8 mg oral/IV	8 mg oral/IV on days 2–3[c]

Low Risk (10%–30%): Aflibercept, Axicabtogene ciloleucel, Belinostat, Blinatumomab, Bortezomib, Brentuximab, Cabazitaxel, Carfilzomib, Cetuximab, Copanlisib, Cytarabine <1000 mg/m², Decitabine, Docetaxel, Elotuzumab, Enfortumab vedotin-ejfv, Eribulin, Etoposide, Fluorouracil, Gemcitabine, Gemcitabine ozogamicin, Inotuzumab ozogamicin, Ixabepilone, Methotrexate, Mitomycin, Mitoxantrone, Moxetumomab pasudotox, Nab-paclitaxel, Necitumumab, Nelarabine, Paclitaxel (conventional and albumin-bound), Panitumumab, Pegylated liposomal doxorubicin, Prmetrexed, Pertuzumab, Tagraxofusp-erzs, Topotecan, Trastuzumab emtansine, Vinflunine

(Continued)

TABLE 27-2	Emetic Risk of Agents Used in Oncology and Treatment Options *(Continued)*	
Antiemetic Agent	**Antiemetic Dose on Day 1 of Chemotherapy**	**Antiemetic Dose on Subsequent Days**
Choose One:		
5-HT$_3$ Antagonist		
Granisetron	2 mg oral or 1 mg IV or 10 /kg IV or 1 patch or 10 mg SQ	
Ondansetron	8 mg oral or IV	
Palonosetron	0.5 mg oral or 0.25 mg IV	
Ramosetron	0.3 mg IV	
Tropisetron	5 mg oral or IV	
OR		
Dexamethasone	8 mg oral or IV	

Minimal Risk (<10%): Avelumab, Atezolizumab, Bevacizumab, Bleomycin, Cemiplimab, 2-Chlorodeoxyadenosine, Cladribine, Daratumumab, Durvalumab, Emapalumab, Fludarabine, Ipilimumab, Nivolumab, Obinutuzumab, Ofatumumab, Pembrolizumab, Pralatrexate, Ramucirumab, Rituximab (IV and SQ), Trastuzumab, Vinblastine, Vincristine (conventional and liposomal), Vinorelbine

No routine prophylactic antiemetics are needed

[a]No additional 5-HT3-RA is needed if netupitant/palonosetron is used.
[b]Dexamethasone dose on day 1 should be reduced to 12 mg when given with aprepitant, fosaprepitant, and netupitant/palonosetron due to drug interactions. Dexamethasone dose on days 2–4 should be omitted when used as antiemetic with anthracycline/cyclophosphamide combination regimen or carboplatin AUC ≥4.
[c]Only if regimen is known to cause delayed nausea/vomiting (eg, cyclophosphamide, doxorubicin, oxaliplatin).

CLINICAL PRESENTATION

- The clinical presentation of nausea and vomiting is given below in Table 27-3. Nausea and vomiting may be classified as either simple or complex.
- **General**
  ✓ Depending on severity of symptoms, patients may present in mild-to-severe distress
- **Symptoms**
  ✓ *Simple:* Self-limiting, resolves spontaneously, and requires only symptomatic therapy
  ✓ *Complex:* Not relieved after administration of antiemetics; progressive deterioration of patient secondary to fluid-electrolyte imbalances; usually associated with noxious agents or pyschogenic events
- **Signs**
  ✓ *Simple:* Patient complaint of queasiness or discomfort
  ✓ *Complex:* Weight loss, fever, abdominal pain
- **Laboratory tests**
  ✓ *Simple:* None
  ✓ *Complex:* Serum electrolyte concentrations, upper/lower GI evaluation
- **Other information**
  ✓ Fluid input and output
  ✓ Medication history
  ✓ Recent history of behavioral or visual changes, headache, pain, or stress
  ✓ Family history positive for psychogenic vomiting

TABLE 27-3	Risk Factors for Postoperative Nausea and Vomiting (PONV)

Patient-related factors

Age less than 50 years old

Female gender (two to three times greater incidence of PONV vs males)

Nonsmoker

History of PONV or motion sickness (threefold increase in incidence of PONV)

Hydration status

Factors related to anesthesia

Use of general anesthesia

Use of volatile anesthetics

Nitrous oxide

Use of opioids (intraoperative or postoperative)

Factors related to surgery

Type of surgical procedure (laparoscopic, gynecological, cholecystectomy)

Duration of surgery

TREATMENT

- **Goal of treatment**: Prevent or eliminate nausea and vomiting; ideally accomplished without adverse effects or with clinically acceptable adverse effects.

GENERAL APPROACH

- Treatment options for nausea and vomiting include drug and nondrug modalities. For patients who are suffering due to excessive or disagreeable food or beverage consumption, avoidance or moderation in dietary intake may lead to symptom resolution.

- Patients with symptoms of systemic illness may quickly improve as their underlying condition resolves. Patients in whom these symptoms result from labyrinthine changes produced by motion may benefit quickly by assuming a stable physical position.

- Nonpharmacologic interventions include relaxation, biofeedback, hypnosis, cognitive distraction, optimism, guided imagery, acupuncture, yoga, transcutaneous electrical stimulation, chewing gum, and systematic desensitization.

- Changes in diet such as restricting oral intake, eating smaller meals, avoiding spicy or fried foods and instead eating bland foods such as with the BRAT diet (Bananas, Rice, Applesauce, and Toast) can help alleviate symptoms.

PHARMACOLOGIC MANAGEMENT

- Information concerning commonly available antiemetic preparations is compiled in Table 27-4. The treatment of simple nausea and vomiting often involves self-care from a list of nonprescription products. Nonprescription and prescription drugs are useful in the treatment of simple nausea and vomiting in small, infrequently administered doses and are associated with minimal side effects. As the symptoms persist or become worse, prescription medications may be chosen, either as single-agent therapy or in combination.

- Factors that enable the clinician to choose the appropriate regimen include: (a) the suspected etiology of the symptoms; (b) the frequency, duration, and severity of the episodes; (c) the ability of the patient to use oral, rectal, injectable, or transdermal medications; and (d) the success of previous antiemetic medications.

- The management of complex nausea and vomiting, such as in patients who are receiving antineoplastic agents, may require initial combination therapy. In combination regimens, the goal is to achieve symptomatic control through administration of agents with different pharmacologic mechanisms of action.

TABLE 27-4 Common Antiemetic Preparations and Adult Dosage Regimens[a]

Drug	Adult Dosage Regimen	Dosage Form/ Route	Availability
Antacids: Useful with simple nausea/vomiting			
Adverse drug reactions: Magnesium products—diarrhea; Aluminum or calcium products— constipation			
Antacids (various)	15–30 mL every 2–4 hours prn	Liquid/Oral	Nonprescription
Antihistaminic–Anticholinergic Agents: Especially problematic in the elderly; increased risk of complications in patients with BPH, narrow angle glaucoma, or asthma			
Adverse drug reactions: Drowsiness, confusion, blurred vision, dry mouth, urinary retention			
Dimenhydrinate (Dramamine)	50–100 mg every 4–6 hours prn	Tab, chew tab, cap	Nonprescription
Diphenhydramine (Benadryl)	25–50 mg every 4–6 hours prn 10–50 mg every 2–4 hours prn	Tab, cap, liquid IM, IV	Prescription/ nonprescription
Hydroxyzine (Vistaril, Atarax)	25–100 mg every 4–6 hours prn	Tab (unlabeled use)	Prescription
Meclizine (Bonine, Antivert)	12.5–25 mg 1 hour before travel; repeat every 12–24 hours prn	Tab, chew tab	Prescription/ nonprescription
Scopolamine (Transderm Scop)	1.5 mg every 72 hours	Transdermal patch	Prescription
Trimethobenzamide (Tigan)	300 mg three to four times daily 200 mg three to four times daily	Cap IM	Prescription
Benzodiazepine: Used for ANV but is contraindicated with olanzapine			
Adverse drug reactions: Dizziness, sedation, appetite changes, memory impairment; observe for additive sedation especially if used with narcotic analgesics			
Lorazepam (Ativan)	0.5–2 mg on night before and morning of chemotherapy	Tab, IV	Prescription (C-IV)
Butyrophenones: Used for breakthrough CINV; droperidol has limited use			
Adverse drug reactions: Haloperidol—sedation, constipation, hypotension, EPS; droperidol—QTc prolongation and/or torsade de pointes, 12-lead electrocardiogram prior to administration, followed by cardiac monitoring for 2–3 hours after administration			
Haloperidol (Haldol)	0.5–2 mg every 4–6 hours prn	Tab, liquid, IM, IV	Prescription
Droperidol (Inapsine)[b]	2.5 mg; additional 1.25 mg may be given	IM, IV	Prescription
Cannabinoids: Used for breakthrough CINV			
Adverse drug reactions: Eurphoria, somnolence, xerostomia			

(Continued)

TABLE 27-4	Common Antiemetic Preparations and Adult Dosage Regimens[a] *(Continued)*		
Drug	**Adult Dosage Regimen**	**Dosage Form/ Route**	**Availability**
Dronabinol (Marinol)	5–15 mg/m² every 2–4 hours prn	Cap	Prescription (C-III)
	4.2–12.6 mg/m² every 2–4 hours prn	Oral solution	
Nabilone (Cesamet)	1–2 mg twice daily	Cap	Prescription (C-II)
Corticosteroids: Useful as a single agent or in combination therapy for prophylaxis of CINV or PONV			
Adverse drug reactions: Insomnia, GI symptoms, agitation, appetite stimulation, hypertension, and hyperglycemia			
Dexamethasone	See Table 27-2 for CINV dosing and Table 27-3 for PONV dosing	Tab, IV	Prescription
Histamine (H2) Antagonists: Useful with nausea secondary to heartburn or GERD			
Adverse drug reactions: Headache, constipation, or diarrhea			
Cimetidine (Tagamet HB)	200 mg twice daily prn	Tab	Nonprescription
Famotidine (Pepcid AC)	10 mg twice daily prn	Tab	Nonprescription
Nizatidine (Axid AR)	75 mg twice daily prn	Tab	Nonprescription
5-Hydroxytryptamine-3 Receptor Antagonists: Useful as a single-agent or combination therapy for prophylaxis of CINV or PONV			
Adverse drug reactions: Asthenia, constipation, headache			
	See **Table 27-2** for CINV dosing and Table 27-3 for PONV dosing	Tab, IV	Prescription
Miscellaneous Agents			
Metoclopramide: Prokinetic activity useful in diabetic gastroparesis.			
Adverse drug reactions: Asthenia, headache, somnolence, EPS			
Amisulpride: Mainly used in PONV; avoid use in severe renal impairment.			
Adverse drug reactions: Increased serum prolactin, prolonged QTc interval			
Olanzapine: Use with caution in elderly; contraindicated with benzodiazepines.			
Adverse drug reactions: Sedation, prolonged QTc interval, EPS			
Pyridoxine: Used in NVP. May be used alone or in combination with doxylamine 12.5 mg. Combination product available as prescription.			
Adverse drug reactions: Drowsiness, headache			
Metoclopramide (Reglan)	10–20 mg (0.5–2 mg/kg) four times daily	Tab, IV	Prescription
Olanzapine (Zyprexa)	5–10 mg daily	Tab	Prescription
Pyridoxine (vitamin B₆)	10–25 mg orally three to four times daily	Tab, cap	Nonprescription

(Continued)

TABLE 27-4	Common Antiemetic Preparations and Adult Dosage Regimens[a] (Continued)		
Drug	**Adult Dosage Regimen**	**Dosage Form/ Route**	**Availability**
Amisulpride	5–10 mg once either before or after surgery	Tab	Prescrription

Phenothiazines: Useful in simple nausea/vomiting or breakthrough CINV

Adverse drug reactions: Prolonged QTc interval, constipation, dizziness, tachycardia, tardive dyskinesia, drowsiness

Chlorpromazine (Thorazine)	10–25 mg every 4–6 hours prn	Tab, liquid	Prescription
	25–50 mg every 4–6 hours prn	IM, IV	
Prochlorperazine (Compazine)	5–10 mg every 4–6 hours prn	Tab, liquid	Prescription
	5–10 mg every 3–4 hours prn	IM	
	2.5–10 mg every 3–4 hours prn	IV	Prescription
	25 mg twice daily prn	Supp	Prescription
Promethazine (Phenergan)	12.5–25 mg every 4–6 hours prn	Tab, liquid, IM, IV, supp	Prescription

Substance P/Neurokinin-1 Receptor Antagonist: Useful in combination therapy for prophylaxis of CINV and PONV

Adverse drug reactions: Constipation, diarrhea, headache, hiccups, dyspepsia, and fatigue

Aprepitant	See Table 27-2 for CINV dosing and Table 27-5 for PONV dosing	Cap, IV	Prescription
Fosaprepitant		IV	Prescription
Fosnetupitant-palonosetron		IV	Prescription
Netupitant/ Palonosetron		Cap	Prescription
Rolapitant		Cap	Prescription

[a]All regimens should be monitored for resolution or occurrence of nausea and vomiting as well as maintaining an adequate hydration status.
[b]See text for warnings.
ANV, anticipatory nausea and vomiting; C-II, C-III, and C-IV, controlled substance schedule 2, 3, and 4, respectively; cap, capsule; chew tab, chewable tablet; CINV, chemotherapy-induced nausea and vomiting; GERD, gastroesophageal reflux disease; liquid, oral syrup, concentrate, or suspension; PONV, postoperative nausea and vomiting; prn, as needed; supp, rectal suppository; tab, tablet.

CHEMOTHERAPY-INDUCED NAUSEA AND VOMITING (CINV)

- There are five categories of CINV: acute, delayed, anticipatory, breakthrough, and refractory. Nausea or vomiting that occurs within 24 hours of chemotherapy administration is defined as acute CINV, whereas when it starts more than 24 hours after chemotherapy administration, it is defined as delayed CINV.

- Nausea or vomiting that occurs prior to receiving chemotherapy is termed anticipatory nausea and vomiting (ANV). Breakthrough nausea and vomiting is defined as emesis occurring despite prophylactic administration of antiemetics and requiring the use of rescue antiemetics. Breakthrough emesis occurs in 10%–40% treated with antiemetics.
- Refractory nausea and vomiting is evident when there is a poor response to antiemetic regimens in prior cycles of chemotherapy.
- The emetogenic potential of the chemotherapeutic agent or regimen (see Table 27-2) is the primary factor to consider when selecting an antiemetic for prophylaxis of CINV. Recommendations for antiemetics in patients receiving chemotherapy are presented in Table 27-2.

Prophylaxis of CINV

- The primary goal of emesis prevention is no nausea and/or vomiting throughout the period of emetic risk.
- The duration of emetic risk is 2 days for patients receiving moderately emetogenic chemotherapy and 3 days for highly emetogenic chemotherapy. Emetic prophylaxis should be provided through the entire period of risk.
- The selection of the antiemetic regimen should be based on the chemotherapy drug with highest emetogenicity (see Table 27-2). Prior emetic experience and patient-specific factors should also be considered.
- When given in equipotent doses, oral and IV 5-HT3-RAs are equivalent in efficacy.
- The toxicities of antiemetics should be considered and managed appropriately.

RADIATION-INDUCED NAUSEA AND VOMITING

- RINV occurs in approximately one-third of patients, is site dependent, and can have a substantial impact on a patient's quality of life. Risk factors associated with the development of RINV include combination chemoradiotherapy, prior CINV, upper abdomen RT, and field size.
- For information on treatment options for the prevention of RINV, see Chapter 150, "Supportive Care" in Pharmacotherapy: A Pathophysiologic Approach, 12th edition.

POSTOPERATIVE NAUSEA AND VOMITING (PONV)

- Risk factors for PONV are listed in Table 27-3. Patients with multiple risk factors are at highest risk for PONV. In adults with 0, 1, 2, 3, and 4 of the risk factors the incidence of PONV is 10%, 20%, 40%, 60%, and 80%, respectively. Those who are found to have 0 to one risk factors are considered low risk, those with two risk factors are considered medium risk, and those with three or more risk factors are considered high risk.
- A variety of pharmacologic approaches are available and may be prescribed as single or combination therapy for prophylaxis of PONV. See Table 27-3 for doses of specific agents.
- Patients at highest risk of vomiting (>2 risk factors) should receive three or four prophylactic antiemetics from different pharmacologic classes, while those at moderate risk (1–2 risk factors) should receive a two-drug regimen. For prophylaxis of PONV **scopolamine patches** must be initiated the evening before the surgery or at least 2 hours prior, whereas NK1 antagonists should be given during the induction of anesthesia; all other agents are recommended to be given at the end of the surgery.
- Patients who experience PONV after receiving prophylactic treatment with a combination of 5-HT3-RA plus **dexamethasone** should be given rescue therapy from a different drug class such as a phenothiazine, metoclopramide, or droperidol. If no prophylaxis was given initially, the recommended treatment is **ondansetron** 4 mg orally or IV or **ramosetron** 0.3 mg IV.

TABLE 27-5	Recommended Prophylactic Doses of Selected Antiemetics for Postoperative Nausea and Vomiting in Adults and Postoperative Vomiting in Children		
Drug	**Adult Dose**	**Pediatric Dose (IV)**	**Timing of Dose**[a]
Amisulpride	5 mg	Not included in consensus guidelines	At induction
Aprepitant	40 mg orally	3 mg/kg up to 125 mg	At induction
Dexamethasone	4–8 mg IV	150 mcg/kg up to 5 mg	At induction
Dimenhydrinate	1 mg/kg IV	0.5 mg/kg up to 25 mg	Not specified
Droperidol[b]	0.625 mg IV	10–15 mcg/kg up to 1.25 mg	At end of surgery
Granisetron	0.35–3 mg IV	40 mcg/kg up to 0.6 mg	At end of surgery
Haloperidol	0.5–2 mg (IM or IV)	Not included in consensus guidelines	Not specified
Methylprednisolone	40 mg IV	Not included in consensus guidelines	Not specified
Metoclopramide	10 mg	Not included in consensus guidelines	Not specified
Ondansetron	4 mg IV, 8 mg orally or orally disintegrating tablet	50–100 mcg/kg up to 4 mg	At end of surgery
Palonosetron	0.075 mg IV	0.5–1.5 mcg/kg	At induction
Promethazine[b]	6.25 mg IV	Not included in consensus guidelines	At induction
Ramosetron	0.3 mg IV	Not included in consensus guidelines	At end of surgery
Rolapitant	70–200 mg orally	Not included in consensus guidelines	At induction
Scopolamine	Transdermal patch	Not included in consensus guidelines	Prior evening or 24 hr before surgery
Tropisetron	2 mg IV	0.1 mg/kg up to 2 mg	At end of surgery

[a]Based on recommendations from consensus guidelines.
[b]See FDA "black box" warning.

DISORDERS OF BALANCE

• Beneficial therapy for patients with nausea and vomiting associated with disorders of balance can reliably be found among the antihistaminic–anticholinergic agents. Oral regimens of antihistaminic–anticholinergic agents given one to several times each day may be effective, especially when the first dose is administered prior to motion.
• **Scopolamine** (usually administered as a patch) is effective for the prevention of motion sickness and is considered first line for this indication.

ANTIEMETIC USE DURING PREGNANCY

• A prenatal vitamin started 1 month prior to becoming pregnant may help reduce the incidence and severity of nausea and vomiting of pregnancy (NVP). Eating smaller, more frequent meals every 1–2 hours, and avoiding foods or odors that trigger symptoms is recommended.

- **Pyridoxine** (10–25 mg one to four times daily) is recommended as first-line therapy with or without doxylamine (12.5–20 mg one to four times daily). **Dimenhydrinate, diphenhydramine, prochlorperazine**, or **promethazine** may also be considered in the treatment of NVP.
- Patients with persistent NVP or who show signs of dehydration should receive IV fluid replacement with thiamine then dextrose.
- **Ondansetron, promethazine**, and **metoclopramide** have similar effectiveness for hyperemesis gravidarum, although ondansetron may be better tolerated due to less adverse effects.

See Chapter 53, Nausea and Vomiting, authored by Leigh Anne Hylton Gravatt, Krista L. Donohoe, and Mandy L. Gatesman, for a more detailed discussion of this topic.

- *Acute pancreatitis* (AP) is an inflammatory disorder of the pancreas characterized by upper abdominal pain and pancreatic enzyme elevations.
- *Chronic pancreatitis* (CP) is a progressive disease characterized by long-standing pancreatic inflammation leading to loss of pancreatic exocrine and endocrine function.

Acute Pancreatitis:

PATHOPHYSIOLOGY

- Gallstones and alcohol abuse account for most cases in the United States. Diabetes mellitus and autoimmune disorders such as inflammatory bowel disease are also associated with an increase in AP. A cause cannot be identified in some patients (idiopathic pancreatitis).
- Many medications have been implicated (Table 28-1), but drug-induced AP is rare. A causal association is difficult to confirm because ethical and practical considerations preclude rechallenge.
- AP is initiated by premature activation of trypsinogen to trypsin within the pancreas, leading to activation of other digestive enzymes and autodigestion of the gland.
- Activated pancreatic enzymes within the pancreas and surrounding tissues produce damage and necrosis to pancreatic tissue, surrounding fat, vascular endothelium, and adjacent structures. Lipase damages fat cells, producing noxious substances that cause further pancreatic and peripancreatic injury.
- Release of cytokines by acinar cells injures those cells and enhances the inflammatory response. Injured acinar cells liberate chemoattractants that attract neutrophils, macrophages, and other cells to the area of inflammation, causing systemic inflammatory response syndrome (SIRS). Vascular damage and ischemia cause release of kinins, which make capillary walls permeable and promote tissue edema.
- Pancreatic infection may result from increased intestinal permeability and translocation of colonic bacteria.
- Local complications in severe AP include acute fluid collection, pancreatic necrosis, infection, abscess, pseudocyst formation, and pancreatic ascites.
- Systemic complications include respiratory failure and cardiovascular, renal, metabolic, hemorrhagic, and CNS abnormalities.

CLINICAL PRESENTATION

- Clinical presentation depends on severity of the inflammatory process and whether damage is confined to the pancreas or involves local and systemic complications.
- The initial presentation ranges from moderate abdominal discomfort to excruciating pain, shock, and respiratory distress. Abdominal pain occurs in 95% of patients and is usually epigastric, often radiating to the upper quadrants or back. Onset is usually sudden, and intensity is often described as "knife-like" or "boring." Pain usually reaches maximum intensity within 30 minutes and may persist for hours or days. Nausea and vomiting occur in 85% of patients and usually follow onset of pain.
- Signs include marked epigastric tenderness on palpation with rebound tenderness and guarding in severe cases. The abdomen is often distended and tympanic with decreased or absent bowel sounds in severe disease.

TABLE 28-1	Medications Associated with Acute Pancreatitis		
Well-Supported Association	**Probable Association**	**Possible Association**	
5-Aminosalicylic acid	Acetaminophen	Aldesleukin	Indinavir
Asparaginase	Hydrochlorothiazide	Amiodarone	Indomethacin
Azathioprine	Itraconazole	Atorvastatin	Infliximab
Bortezomib	Ifosfamide	Calcium	Ketoprofen
Carbamazepine	Interferon α2b	Ceftriaxone	Ketorolac
Cimetidine	Maprotiline	Capecitabine	Lipid emulsion
Corticosteroids	Methyldopa	Carboplatin	Liraglutide
Cisplatin	Oxaliplatin	Celecoxib	Lisinopril
Cytarabine		Clozapine	Mefenamic acid
Didanosine		Cholestyramine	Metformin
Enalapril		Ciprofloxacin	Metolazone
Erythromycin		Clarithromycin	Metronidazole
Estrogens		Clonidine	Nitrofurantoin
Furosemide		Cyclosporine	Omeprazole
Mercaptopurine		Danazol	Ondansetron
Mesalamine		Diazoxide	Paclitaxel
Octreotide		Etanercept	Pravastatin
Olsalazine		Ethacrynic acid	Propofol
Opioids		Exenatide	Propoxyphene
Pentamidine		Famciclovir	Rifampin
Pentavalent antimonials		Glyburide	Sertraline
Sulfasalazine		Gold salts	Simvastatin
Sulfamethoxazole and trimethoprim		Granisetron	Sorafenib
		Ibuprofen	Sulindac
Sulindac		Imatinib	Zalcitabine
Tamoxifen			
Tetracyclines			
Valproic acid/Salts			

- Vital signs may be normal, but hypotension, tachycardia, and low-grade fever are often observed, especially with widespread pancreatic inflammation and necrosis. Dyspnea and tachypnea are signs of acute respiratory complications.
- Jaundice and altered mental status may be present; other signs of alcoholic liver disease may be present in patients with alcoholic pancreatitis.

DIAGNOSIS

- Diagnosis of AP requires two of the following: (1) upper abdominal pain, (2) serum lipase or amylase at least three times the upper limit of normal, and (3) characteristic findings on imaging studies.
- Transabdominal ultrasound should be performed in all patients to detect dilated biliary ducts and gallstones. Contrast-enhanced computed tomography (CECT) is

used if the diagnosis cannot be made from clinical and laboratory findings. Magnetic resonance imaging is used to grade severity of AP, identify bile duct problems not seen on CECT, or if there are contraindications to CECT.

- AP may be associated with leukocytosis, hyperglycemia, and hypoalbuminemia. Hepatic transaminases, alkaline phosphatase, and bilirubin are usually elevated in gallstone pancreatitis and in patients with intrinsic liver disease. Marked hypocalcemia indicates severe necrosis and is a poor prognostic sign.
- Serum amylase usually rises 4–8 hours after symptom onset, peaks at 24 hours, and returns to normal over the next 8–14 days. Concentrations greater than three times the upper limit of normal are highly suggestive of AP.
- Serum lipase is specific to the pancreas, and concentrations are elevated and parallel the serum amylase elevations. Increases persist longer than serum amylase elevations and can be detected after the amylase has returned to normal.
- Hematocrit may be normal, but hemoconcentration results from multiple factors (eg, vomiting). Hematocrit >47% predicts severe AP, and hematocrit <44% predicts mild disease.
- C-reactive protein levels >190 mg/dL at 48 hours predict severe AP.
- Thrombocytopenia and increased international normalized ratio (INR) occur in some patients with severe AP and associated liver disease.

TREATMENT (FIG. 28-1)

- Goals of Treatment: Relieve abdominal pain and nausea; replace fluids; correct electrolyte, glucose, and lipid abnormalities; minimize systemic complications; and manage pancreatic necrosis and infection.

NONPHARMACOLOGIC THERAPY

- Endoscopic retrograde cholangiopancreatography (ERCP) may be performed to remove biliary tract stones.
- Patients with alcohol-related pancreatitis should receive abstinence interventions during the inpatient stay.
- Nutritional support is important because AP creates a catabolic state that promotes nutritional depletion. Patients with mild to moderate AP should begin oral feeding as soon as tolerated, regardless of serum lipase concentrations, usually within 24 hours of admission. In severe disease, oral or enteral nutrition is recommended within 24–72 hours of admission. Enteral nutrition via nasogastric or nasojejunal tube is preferred over parenteral nutrition (PN) in severe AP, if tolerated. If enteral feeding is not possible or is inadequate, PN should be implemented before protein and calorie depletion become advanced.

PHARMACOLOGIC THERAPY

- Patients with AP often require IV antiemetics for nausea.
- Patients requiring ICU admission should be treated with antisecretory agents if they are at risk of stress-related mucosal bleeding.
- Vasodilation from the inflammatory response, vomiting, and nasogastric suction contribute to hypovolemia and fluid and electrolyte abnormalities, necessitating replacement. Patients should receive goal-directed fluid management to reduce the risks of persistent SIRS and organ failure. Guidelines generally recommend lactated Ringer's 5–10 mL/kg/h or 250–500 mL/h in the first 12-24 hours.
- Intravenous potassium, calcium, and magnesium are used to correct electrolyte deficiency, and insulin is used to treat hyperglycemia.
- Parenteral opioid analgesics are used to control abdominal pain, although high-quality supporting evidence is lacking. Parenteral **morphine** is often used, and patient-controlled analgesia should be considered in patients who require frequent opioid dosing (eg, every 2–3 hours). Nonsteroidal anti-inflammatory agents (NSAIDs) may be sufficient in patients with mild-to-moderate pain if not contraindicated.

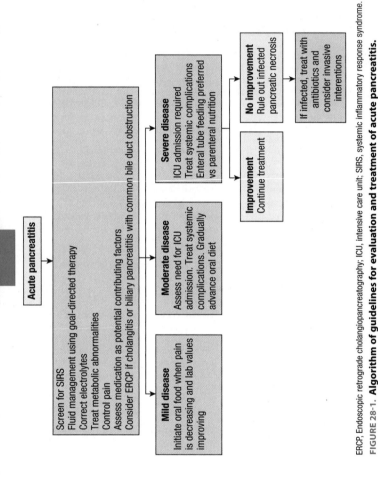

ERCP, Endoscopic retrograde cholangiopancreatography; ICU, intensive care unit; SIRS, systemic inflammatory response syndrome.

FIGURE 28–1. Algorithm of guidelines for evaluation and treatment of acute pancreatitis.

- Prophylactic antibiotics are not recommended in patients with AP without signs or symptoms of infection, including those predicted to develop severe AP or necrotizing pancreatitis.
- Patients with known or suspected infected AP should receive broad-spectrum antibiotics that cover the range of enteric aerobic gram-negative bacilli and anaerobic organisms. **Imipenem–cilastatin** (500 mg IV every 8 hours) has been widely used but has been replaced on many formularies by newer carbapenems (eg, **meropenem**). A fluoroquinolone (eg, **ciprofloxacin** or **levofloxacin**) combined with **metronidazole** should be considered for penicillin-allergic patients.

EVALUATION OF THERAPEUTIC OUTCOMES

- In patients with mild AP, assess pain control, fluid and electrolyte status, and nutrition periodically depending on the degree of abdominal pain and fluid loss.
- Goals for fluid therapy include one or more of the following: heart rate <120 bpm, mean arterial pressure 65–85 mm Hg, urinary output >0.5–1 mL/kg/h, or hematocrit 35%–44% with blood transfusion.
- Transfer patients with severe AP to an intensive care unit for close monitoring of vital signs, fluid and electrolyte status, white blood cell count, blood glucose, lactate dehydrogenase, aspartate aminotransferase, serum albumin, hematocrit, blood urea nitrogen, serum creatinine, and INR. Continuous hemodynamic and arterial blood gas monitoring is essential. Serum lipase, amylase, and bilirubin require less frequent monitoring. Monitor for signs of infection, relief of abdominal pain, and adequate nutritional status. Assess severity of disease and patient response using evidence-based methods.

Chronic Pancreatitis:

PATHOPHYSIOLOGY

- CP results from long-standing pancreatic inflammation and leads to irreversible destruction of pancreatic tissue with fibrin deposition and loss of exocrine and endocrine function.
- Chronic ethanol consumption accounts for about two-thirds of cases in Western society. Most of the remaining cases are idiopathic, and a small percentage is due to rare causes such as autoimmune, hereditary, and tropical pancreatitis.
- The exact pathogenesis is unknown. Activation of pancreatic stellate cells by toxins, oxidative stress, and/or inflammatory mediators appears to be the cause of fibrin deposition.
- Abdominal pain may be caused by abnormal pain processing in the central nervous system and sensitization of visceral nerves. This may explain the hyperalgesia that CP patients often experience with the need for various methods of pain management. Impaired inhibition of somatic and visceral pain pathways may also cause pain in areas distant to the pancreas.

CLINICAL PRESENTATION

- The main features of CP are abdominal pain, malabsorption with steatorrhea, weight loss, and diabetes. Jaundice occurs in ~10% of patients.
- Patients typically report deep, penetrating epigastric or abdominal pain that may radiate to the back. Pain often occurs with meals and at night and may be associated with nausea and vomiting.
- Steatorrhea and azotorrhea occur in most patients. Steatorrhea is often associated with diarrhea and bloating. Weight loss may occur.
- Pancreatic diabetes is a late manifestation commonly associated with pancreatic calcification.

DIAGNOSIS

- Diagnosis is based primarily on clinical presentation and either imaging or pancreatic function studies. Noninvasive imaging includes abdominal ultrasound, CT, and MRI. Invasive imaging includes endoscopic ultrasonography (EUS) and ERCP.
- Serum amylase and lipase are usually normal or only slightly elevated but may be increased in acute exacerbations.
- Total bilirubin, alkaline phosphatase, and hepatic transaminases may be elevated with ductal obstruction. Serum albumin and calcium may be low with malnutrition.
- Pancreatic function tests include:
  - ✓ Serum trypsinogen (<20 ng/mL is abnormal)
  - ✓ Fecal elastase (<200 mcg/g of stool is abnormal)
  - ✓ Fecal chymotrypsin (<3 units/g of stool is abnormal)
  - ✓ Fecal fat estimation (>7 g/day is abnormal; stool must be collected for 72 hours)
  - ✓ ^{13}C-mixed triglyceride breath test (not available in the United States)
  - ✓ Secretin stimulation (evaluates duodenal bicarbonate secretion)
  - ✓ Cholecystokinin stimulation (evaluates pancreatic lipase secretion)

TREATMENT

- Goals of Treatment: Major goals for uncomplicated CP are to relieve abdominal pain, treat complications of malabsorption and glucose intolerance, and improve quality of life. Secondary goals are to delay development of complications and treat associated disorders such as depression and malnutrition.

NONPHARMACOLOGIC THERAPY

- Lifestyle modifications should include abstinence from alcohol and smoking cessation.
- Advise patients with steatorrhea to eat smaller, more frequent meals and reduce dietary fat intake.
- Reduction in dietary fat may be needed if symptoms are uncontrolled with enzyme supplementation. Enteral nutrition via a feeding tube is recommended for patients with malnutrition who do not have an adequate response to oral nutrition support.
- Invasive procedures and surgery are used primarily to treat uncontrolled pain and the complications of CP.

PHARMACOLOGIC THERAPY

- Pain may initially be treated with **acetaminophen** (eg, 500–650 mg every 4–6 hours) with or without NSAIDs (eg, **ibuprofen** 200–400 mg every 6–8 hours initially), with adjuvant agents added for inadequate pain relief or as the disease progresses.
- Analgesic regimens should be individualized and start with the lowest effective dose, with titration to maximum recommended or tolerated doses before adding or substituting agents. Schedule analgesics around the clock (rather than as needed) to maximize efficacy. Scheduling short-acting analgesics prior to meals may decrease postprandial pain.
- **Pregabalin** (75 mg twice daily initially; maximum 300 mg twice daily) has the best evidence as an adjuvant agent. Consider selective serotonin reuptake inhibitors (eg, **paroxetine**), serotonin/norepinephrine reuptake inhibitors (eg, **duloxetine**), and tricyclic antidepressants in patients with pain that is difficult to manage.
- **Tramadol** (50–100 mg every 4–6 hours, maximum 400 mg/day) may be tried before adding more potent opioid analgesics.
- Opioids should be reserved for severe or refractory pain:
  - ✓ **Codeine:** 30–60 mg every 6 hours
  - ✓ **Hydrocodone:** 5–10 mg every 4–6 hours
  - ✓ **Morphine sulfate (extended-release):** 30–60 mg every 8–12 hours
  - ✓ **Oxycodone:** 5–10 mg every 6 hours
  - ✓ **Methadone:** 2.5–10 mg every 8–12 hours
  - ✓ **Hydromorphone:** 0.5–1 mg every 4–6 hours
  - ✓ **Fentanyl patch:** 25–100 /h every 72 hours

- Adding pancreatic enzyme supplements for pain control has been studied but is not recommended based on available evidence.
- Pancreatic enzyme supplementation is required for most patients with malabsorption to achieve adequate nutritional status and reduction in steatorrhea (Fig. 28-2). The enzyme dose required to minimize malabsorption is 20,000–50,000 units of lipase administered with each meal initially. Half of the necessary mealtime dose is recommended with snacks. The mealtime dose may be increased to a maximum of 90,000 units. Products containing enteric-coated microspheres are preferred (Table 28-2). Ideally, patients should eat 3–5 meals/day, and those who require more than one capsule/tablet per meal should distribute the doses throughout the meal.
- An antisecretory agent (ie, histamine-2 receptor antagonist or proton pump inhibitor) should be added when there is an inadequate response to enzyme therapy alone.
- Adverse effects from pancreatic enzyme supplements are generally benign, but high doses can cause nausea, diarrhea, and intestinal upset. A more serious but uncommon adverse effect is fibrosing colonopathy, which has been reported mostly in children with cystic fibrosis who received high enzyme doses for prolonged periods.
- Assess patients with CP for deficiencies in fat-soluble vitamins and provide supplementation as required.
- Exogenous insulin is the primary means for treating diabetes mellitus associated with CP. Metformin may be initiated in early CP and has the added benefit of reducing the risk of pancreatic cancer.

EVALUATION OF THERAPEUTIC OUTCOMES

- Assess the severity and frequency of abdominal pain periodically using a standardized scale to determine analgesic efficacy. Patients receiving opioids should be prescribed laxatives on an as-needed or scheduled basis and be monitored for constipation.

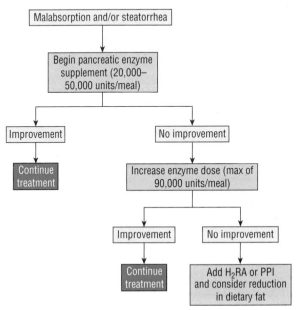

H_2RA, histamine-2 receptor antagonist; PPI, proton pump inhibitor.

FIGURE 28-2. Algorithm for the treatment of malabsorption and steatorrhea in chronic pancreatitis.

TABLE 28-2	Commercially Available Pancreatic Enzyme (Pancrelipase) Preparations		
	Enzyme Content Per Unit Dose (USP Units)		
Product	**Lipase**	**Amylase**	**Protease**
Tablets			
Viokace 10,440 lipase units	10,440	39,150	39,150
Viokace 20,880 lipase units	20,880	78,300	78,300
Enteric-coated beads			
Zenpep 3000 lipase units	3000	16,000	10,000
Zenpep 5000 lipase units	5000	27,000	17,000
Zenpep 10,000 lipase units	10,000	55,000	34,000
Zenpep 15,000 lipase units	15,000	82,000	51,000
Zenpep 20,000 lipase units	20,000	109,000	68,000
Zenpep 25,000 lipase units	25,000	136,000	85,000
Zenpep 40,000 lipase units	40,000	218,000	136,000
Enteric-coated microspheres with bicarbonate buffer			
Pertzye 4000 lipase units	4000	15,125	14,375
Pertzye 8000 lipase units	8000	30,250	28,750
Pertzye 16,000 lipase units	16,000	60,500	57,500
Enteric-coated microspheres			
Creon 3000 lipase units	3000	15,000	9500
Creon 6000 lipase units	6000	30,000	19,000
Creon 12,000 lipase units	12,000	60,000	38,000
Creon 24,000 lipase units	24,000	120,000	76,000
Creon 36,000 lipase units	36,000	180,000	114,000
Enteric-coated minitablets/microtablets			
Pancreaze 2600	2600	10,850	6200
Pancreaze 4200 lipase units	4200	17,500	10,000
Pancreaze 10,500 lipase units	10,500	43,750	25,000
Pancreaze 16,800 lipase units	16,800	70,000	40,000
Pancreaze 21,000 lipase units	21,000	61,000	37,000
Ultresa 4000 lipase units	4000	8000	8000
Ultresa 13,800 lipase units	13,800	27,600	27,600
Ultresa 20,700 lipase units	20,700	41,400	41,400
Ultresa 23,000 lipase units	23,000	46,000	46,000

USP, United States Pharmacopeia.

- For patients receiving pancreatic enzymes for malabsorption, monitor body weight and stool frequency and consistency periodically.
- Monitor blood glucose carefully in diabetic patients.

See Chapter 57 Pancreatitis, authored by Scott Bolesta, for a more detailed discussion of this topic.

29   **Peptic Ulcer Disease**

- *Peptic ulcer disease* (PUD) refers to ulcerative disorders of the upper gastrointestinal (GI) tract that require acid and pepsin for their formation. The three common etiologies include (1) *Helicobacter pylori* (*H. pylori*) infection, (2) nonsteroidal anti-inflammatory drug (NSAID) use, and (3) stress-related mucosal damage (SRMD).

PATHOPHYSIOLOGY

- Benign gastric ulcers, erosions, and gastritis can occur anywhere in the stomach, but the antrum and lesser curvature are the most common locations. Most duodenal ulcers occur in the first part of the duodenum (duodenal bulb).
- Pathophysiology is determined by the balance between aggressive factors (gastric acid and pepsin) and protective factors (mucosal defense and repair). Gastric acid, *H. pylori* infection, and NSAID use are independent factors that contribute to disruption of mucosal integrity. Increased acid secretion may be involved in duodenal ulcers, but patients with gastric ulcers usually have normal or reduced acid secretion (hypochlorhydria).
- Mucus and bicarbonate secretion, intrinsic epithelial cell defense, and mucosal blood flow normally protect the gastroduodenal mucosa from noxious endogenous and exogenous substances. Endogenous prostaglandins (PGs) facilitate mucosal integrity and repair. Disruptions in normal mucosal defense and healing mechanisms allow acid and pepsin to reach the gastric epithelium.
- *H. pylori* infection causes gastric mucosal inflammation in all infected individuals, but only a minority develops an ulcer or gastric cancer. Bacterial enzymes (urease, lipases, and proteases), bacterial adherence, and *H. pylori* virulence factors produce gastric mucosal injury. *H. pylori* induces gastric inflammation by altering the host inflammatory response and damaging epithelial cells.
- Nonselective NSAIDs (including aspirin) cause gastric mucosal damage by two mechanisms: (1) direct or topical irritation of the gastric epithelium, and (2) systemic inhibition of endogenous mucosal PG synthesis (the primary mechanism). COX-2 selective inhibitors have a lower risk of ulcers and related GI complications than nonselective NSAIDs. Addition of aspirin to a selective COX-2 inhibitor reduces its ulcer-sparing benefit and increases ulcer risk.
- Use of corticosteroids alone does not increase risk of ulcer or complications, but ulcer risk is doubled in corticosteroid users taking NSAIDs concurrently.
- Cigarette smoking has been linked to PUD, impaired ulcer healing, and ulcer recurrence. Risk is proportional to amount smoked per day.
- Psychological stress has not been shown to cause PUD, but ulcer patients may be adversely affected by stressful life events.
- Carbonated beverages, coffee, tea, beer, milk, and spices may cause dyspepsia but do not appear to increase PUD risk. Ethanol ingestion in high concentrations is associated with acute gastric mucosal damage and upper GI bleeding but is not clearly the cause of ulcers.

CLINICAL PRESENTATION

- Abdominal pain is the most frequent PUD symptom. Pain is often epigastric and described as burning but can present as vague discomfort, abdominal fullness, or cramping. Nocturnal pain may awaken patients from sleep, especially between 12 AM and 3 AM.
- Pain from duodenal ulcers often occurs 1–3 hours after meals and is usually relieved by food, whereas food may precipitate or accentuate ulcer pain in gastric ulcers. Antacids provide rapid pain relief in most ulcer patients.

- Heartburn, belching, and bloating often accompany pain. Nausea, vomiting, and anorexia are more common in gastric than duodenal ulcers and may be signs of an ulcer-related complication.
- Severity of symptoms varies among patients and may be seasonal, occurring more frequently in spring or fall.
- Presence or absence of epigastric pain does not define an ulcer, and ulcer healing does not necessarily render the patient asymptomatic. Conversely, absence of pain does not preclude an ulcer diagnosis, especially in older persons, who may present with a "silent" ulcer complication.
- Ulcer complications include upper GI bleeding, perforation into the peritoneal cavity, penetration into an adjacent structure (eg, pancreas, biliary tract, or liver), and gastric outlet obstruction. Bleeding may be occult or present as melena or hematemesis. Perforation is associated with sudden, sharp, severe pain, beginning first in the epigastrium but quickly spreading over the entire abdomen. Symptoms of gastric outlet obstruction typically occur over several months and include early satiety, bloating, anorexia, nausea, vomiting, and weight loss.

DIAGNOSIS

- Physical examination may reveal epigastric tenderness between the umbilicus and the xiphoid process that sometimes radiates to the back.
- Routine blood tests are not helpful in establishing a diagnosis of PUD. Hematocrit, hemoglobin, and stool guaiac tests are used to detect bleeding.
- Diagnosis of PUD depends on visualizing the ulcer crater; upper GI endoscopy has replaced radiography as the procedure of choice because it provides a more accurate diagnosis and permits direct visualization of the ulcer and implementation of maneuvers to control bleeding.
- Diagnosis of *H. pylori* infection can be made using endoscopic or nonendoscopic (urea breath test [UBT], serologic antibody detection, and fecal antigen) tests. Testing for *H. pylori* is only recommended if eradication therapy is planned. If endoscopy is not planned, serologic antibody testing is reasonable to determine *H. pylori* status. Endoscopic biopsy-based tests, UBT, and fecal antigen tests are the recommended tests to verify *H. pylori* eradication but must be delayed until at least 4 weeks after completion of antibiotic treatment and after proton pump inhibitor (PPI) therapy has been discontinued for 2 weeks to avoid confusing bacterial suppression with eradication.

TREATMENT

- <u>Goals of Treatment</u>: Overall goals are to relieve ulcer pain, heal the ulcer, prevent ulcer recurrence, and reduce ulcer-related complications. In *H. pylori*–positive patients with an active ulcer, previously documented ulcer, or history of an ulcer-related complication, goals are to eradicate *H. pylori*, heal the ulcer, and cure the disease with a cost-effective drug regimen. The primary goal for a patient with an NSAID-induced ulcer is to heal the ulcer as rapidly as possible.

NONPHARMACOLOGIC TREATMENT

- Lifestyle modifications including stress reduction and smoking cessation should be implemented. NSAIDs should be avoided if possible, and alternative agents such as acetaminophen or a nonacetylated salicylate (eg, salsalate) should be used for pain relief when feasible.
- There is no specific recommended diet, but patients should avoid foods and beverages that cause dyspepsia or exacerbate ulcer symptoms (eg, spicy foods, caffeine, and alcohol).
- Emergent surgery may be required for patients with ulcer-related complications (eg, bleeding, perforation, or obstruction).

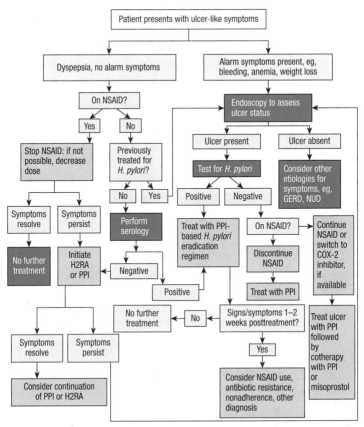

FIGURE 29-1. Guidelines for the evaluation and management of a patient who presents with dyspeptic or ulcer-like symptoms.

PHARMACOLOGIC TREATMENT

- Figure 29-1 depicts an algorithm for evaluation and management of a patient with dyspeptic or ulcer-like symptoms.
- Established indications for treatment of *H. pylori* infection include active PUD, past history of PUD (unless eradication was previously documented), mucosa-associated lymphoid tissue (MALT) lymphoma, and postendoscopic resection of gastric cancer. Treatment should be effective, well-tolerated, convenient, and cost-effective. Drug regimens to eradicate *H. pylori* are shown in Table 29-1.
- *Clarithromycin triple therapy* (PPI, clarithromycin, amoxicillin) is no longer recommended in areas where *H. pylori* resistance exceeds 15%, which includes all of North America. This regimen given for 14 days remains an option in regions where clarithromycin resistance is <15% and no prior macrolide exposure is documented.
- *Bismuth quadruple therapy* (PPI or H2RA, bismuth subsalicylate, metronidazole, tetracycline) for 10–14 days is the preferred first-line therapy to eradicate *H. pylori* infection. PPIs generally produce higher *H. pylori* eradication rates and are preferred

TABLE 29-1 Drug Regimens Used to Eradicate *Helicobacter pylori*

Regimen	Duration	Drug #1	Drug #2	Drug #3	Drug #4
Proton pump inhibitor–based triple therapy[a]	14 days	PPI once or twice daily[b]	Clarithromycin 500 mg twice daily	Amoxicillin 1 g twice daily or metronidazole 500 mg twice daily	
Bismuth quadruple therapy[a]	10—14 days	PPI or H2RA once or twice daily[b,c]	Bismuth subsalicylate[d] 525 mg four times daily	Metronidazole 250—500 mg four times daily	Tetracycline 500 mg four times daily
Non-bismuth quadruple or "concomitant" therapy[e]	10—14 days	PPI once or twice daily on days 1—10[b]	Clarithromycin 250—500 mg twice daily on days 1—10	Amoxicillin 1 g twice daily on days 1—10	Metronidazole 250—500 mg twice daily on days 1—10
Sequential therapy[e]	10 days	PPI once or twice daily on days 1—10[b]	Amoxicillin 1 g twice daily on days 1—5	Metronidazole 250—500 mg twice daily on days 6—10	Clarithromycin 250—500 mg twice daily on days 6—10
Hybrid therapy[e]	14 days	PPI once or twice daily on days 1—14[b]	Amoxicillin 1 g twice daily on days 1—14	Metronidazole 250—500 mg twice daily on days 7—14	Clarithromycin 250—500 mg twice daily on days 7—14
Levofloxacin triple	10—14 days	PPI twice daily	Levofloxacin 500 mg daily	Amoxicillin 1 g twice daily	
Levofloxacin sequential	10 days	PPI twice daily on days 1—10	Amoxicillin 1 g twice daily on days 1—10	Levofloxacin 500 mg once daily on days 6—10	Metronidazole 500 mg twice daily on days 6—10
LOAD	7—10 days	Levofloxacin 250 mg once daily	Omeprazole (or other PPI) at high dose once daily	Nitazoxanide (Alinia) 500 mg twice daily	Doxycycline 100 mg once daily
Rifabutin-based triple therapy	14 days	Omeprazole 40 mg every 8 hours	Amoxicillin 1 g every 8 hours	Rifabutin 50 mg every 8 hours	

H2RA, Histamine-2-receptor antagonist; PPI, proton pump inhibitor.

[a]Although treatment is minimally effective if used for 7 days, 10—14 days is recommended. The antisecretory drug may be continued beyond antimicrobial treatment for patients with a history of a complicated ulcer, for example, bleeding, or in heavy smokers.

[b]Standard PPI peptic ulcer healing dosages given once or twice daily.

[c]Standard H2RA peptic ulcer healing dosages may be used in place of a PPI.

[d]Bismuth subcitrate potassium (biskalcitrate) 140 mg, as the bismuth salt, is contained in a prepackaged capsule (Pylera), along with metronidazole 125 mg and tetracycline 125 mg; three capsules are taken with each meal and at bedtime; a standard PPI dosage is added to the regimen and taken twice daily. All medications are taken for 10 days.

[e]Requires validation as first-line therapy in the United States.

over H2RA. All medications except the PPI should be taken with meals and at bedtime. The PPI should be taken 30–60 minutes before a meal. The mean eradication rate for a 10-day course is ~90%, but limitations include the need for four-times-daily therapy (which can impair adherence), and frequent minor side effects.

- *Non-bismuth quadruple (or "concomitant") therapy* (PPI, clarithromycin, amoxicillin, metronidazole) for 10–14 days is another recommended first-line therapy. "Concomitant" therapy means that all four drugs are given at the same time twice daily for the entire duration of therapy. There is a lack of evidence in North America for this regimen.

- *Sequential therapy* involves a PPI plus antibiotics given in sequence rather than together. The rationale is to treat initially with antibiotics that rarely promote resistance (eg, amoxicillin) to reduce bacterial load and preexisting resistant organisms and then to follow with different antibiotics (eg, clarithromycin and metronidazole) to kill any remaining organisms. The potential advantage of high eradication rates requires validation in the United States and is only conditionally recommended within guidelines as a first-line *H. pylori* eradication therapy.

- *Hybrid therapy* combines the strategies of concomitant and sequential therapy; it involves 7 days of dual therapy (PPI and amoxicillin) followed by 7 days of quadruple therapy (PPI, amoxicillin, clarithromycin, metronidazole). There is lack of evidence in North America with this regimen.

- *Levofloxacin-based regimens* include (1) triple therapy with amoxicillin and a PPI, (2) modified sequential therapy with 5–7 days of amoxicillin plus a PPI followed by 5–7 days of levofloxacin, and (3) quadruple therapy with levofloxacin, omeprazole or another PPI, nitazoxanide (Alinia), and doxycycline ("LOAD" therapy). The LOAD regimen is not currently recommended due to high cost and lack of efficacy data. In addition, concerns with fluoroquinolone use include development of resistance and adverse effects (eg, tendonitis, hepatotoxicity).

- If initial treatment fails to eradicate *H. pylori*, second-line (salvage) treatment should: (1) use antibiotics that were not included in the initial regimen, (2) be guided by region-specific or individual antibiotic resistance testing, and (3) use an extended treatment duration of 10–14 days. Patients failing clarithromycin triple therapy can be treated with either bismuth quadruple therapy or the levofloxacin triple regimen for 14 days. Other salvage regimens may also be successful. Penicillin allergy testing is recommended for patients who report penicillin allergy because many patients are not truly allergic.

- Patients with NSAID-induced ulcers should be tested to determine *H. pylori* status. If they are *H. pylori* positive, start treatment with a recommended first-line regimen (Table 29-1). If patients are *H. pylori* negative, discontinue the NSAID and treat with a PPI, H2RA, or sucralfate (Table 29-2). PPIs are generally preferred due to more rapid symptom relief and ulcer healing. If the NSAID must be continued, implement cotherapy with a PPI or misoprostol. Patients at highest risk of recurrent ulcers or ulcer-related complications should be switched to a COX-2 inhibitor.

- Limit maintenance therapy with a PPI or H2RA to high-risk patients with ulcer complications, patients who fail *H. pylori* eradication, and those with *H. pylori*–negative ulcers.

- Patients with ulcers refractory to treatment should undergo upper endoscopy to confirm a nonhealing ulcer, exclude malignancy, and assess *H. pylori* status. *H. pylori*–positive patients should receive eradication therapy. Refractory ulcers despite a complete standard PPI course should be retreated with double dose of PPI, or consideration can be given to using a different PPI.

EVALUATION OF THERAPEUTIC OUTCOMES

- Monitor patients for symptomatic relief of ulcer pain, potential adverse drug effects, and drug interactions.
- Ulcer pain typically resolves in a few days when NSAIDs are discontinued and within 7 days upon initiation of antiulcer therapy. Patients with uncomplicated PUD

TABLE 29-2	Drug Dosing Table		
Drug	**Brand Name**	**Initial Dose**	**Usual Range**
Proton pump inhibitors			
Omeprazole	Prilosec, various	40 mg daily	20–40 mg/day
Omeprazole + sodium bicarbonate	Zegerid	40 mg daily	20–40 mg/day
Lansoprazole	Prevacid, various	30 mg daily	15–30 mg/day
Rabeprazole	Aciphex	20 mg daily	20–40 mg/day
Pantoprazole	Protonix, various	40 mg daily	40–80 mg/day
Esomeprazole	Nexium	40 mg daily	20–40 mg/day
Dexlansoprazole	Dexilant	30–60 mg daily	30–60 mg/day
H$_2$-receptor antagonists			
Cimetidine	Tagamet, various	300 mg four times daily, 400 mg twice daily, or 800 mg at bedtime	800–1600 mg/day in divided doses
Famotidine	Pepcid, various	20 mg twice daily, or 40 mg at bedtime	20–40 mg/day
Nizatidine	Axid, various	150 mg twice daily, or 300 mg at bedtime	150–300 mg/day
Ranitidine[a]	Zantac, various	150 mg twice daily, or 300 mg at bedtime	150–300 mg/day
Mucosal protectants			
Sucralfate	Carafate, various	1 g four times daily, or 2 g twice daily	2–4 g/day
Misoprostol	Cytotec	100–200 mcg four times daily	400–800 mcg/day

[a]Ranitidine products are no longer available in the United States.

are usually symptom-free after treatment with any of the recommended antiulcer regimens.
• Persistent or recurrent symptoms within 14 days after the end of treatment suggest failure of ulcer healing or *H. pylori* eradication or presence of an alternative diagnosis such as gastroesophageal reflux disease.
• Eradication of *H. pylori* should be confirmed after treatment in all patients, particularly those who are at risk for complications.
• Monitor patients taking NSAIDs closely for signs and symptoms of bleeding, obstruction, penetration, and perforation.
• Follow-up endoscopy is justified in patients with frequent symptomatic recurrence, refractory disease, complications, or suspected hypersecretory states.

See Chapter 51, Peptic Ulcer Disease and Related Disorders, authored by Bryan L. Love, for a more detailed discussion of this topic.

CHAPTER

30

Contraception

- *Contraception* is the prevention of pregnancy by inhibiting sperm from reaching a mature ovum or by preventing a fertilized ovum from implanting in the endometrium.
- While cis-women are the primary use of hormonal contraception, these agents are also used by transgender individuals and this chapter has been written to reflect this.

MENSTRUAL CYCLE PATHOPHYSIOLOGY

- The median menstrual cycle length is 28 days (range 21–40 days). Day 1 is the first day of menses and marks the beginning of the follicular phase. Ovulation usually occurs on day 14, followed by the luteal phase that lasts until the beginning of the next cycle.
- The hypothalamus secretes gonadotropin-releasing hormone, which stimulates the anterior pituitary to secrete the gonadotropins follicle-stimulating hormone (FSH) and luteinizing hormone (LH).
- In the follicular phase, FSH levels increase and cause recruitment of a small group of follicles for continued growth. Between days 5 and 7, one of these becomes the dominant follicle, which later ruptures to release the oocyte. The dominant follicle develops increasing amounts of estradiol and inhibin, providing a negative feedback on the secretion of gonadotropin-releasing hormone and FSH.
- The dominant follicle continues to grow and synthesizes estradiol, progesterone, and androgen. Estradiol stops the menstrual flow from the previous cycle, thickens the endometrial lining, and produces thin, watery cervical mucus. FSH regulates aromatase enzymes that induce conversion of androgens to estrogens in the follicle.
- The pituitary releases a midcycle LH surge that stimulates the final stages of follicular maturation and ovulation. Ovulation occurs 24–36 hours after the estradiol peak and 10–16 hours after the LH peak.
- The LH surge is the most clinically useful predictor of approaching ovulation. Conception is most successful when intercourse takes place from 2 days before ovulation to the day of ovulation.
- After ovulation, the remaining luteinized follicles become the corpus luteum, which synthesizes androgen, estrogen, and progesterone (Fig. 30-1).
- If pregnancy occurs, human chorionic gonadotropin prevents regression of the corpus luteum and stimulates continued production of estrogen and progesterone. If pregnancy does not occur, the corpus luteum degenerates, progesterone declines, and menstruation occurs.

TREATMENT

- <u>Goal of Treatment</u>: The prevention of pregnancy from sexual intercourse. Additional benefits include prevention of sexually transmitted infections [STIs] and menstrual cycle regulation.

NONPHARMACOLOGIC THERAPY

- A comparison of methods of nonhormonal contraception is shown in Table 30-1.
- The fertility awareness-based method includes avoiding intercourse when contraception is likely to occur. It is associated with relatively high pregnancy rates.
- **Diaphragms** and the **cervical cap** are effective barriers that should be used with spermicide and inserted up to 6 hours before intercourse. They must be left in place

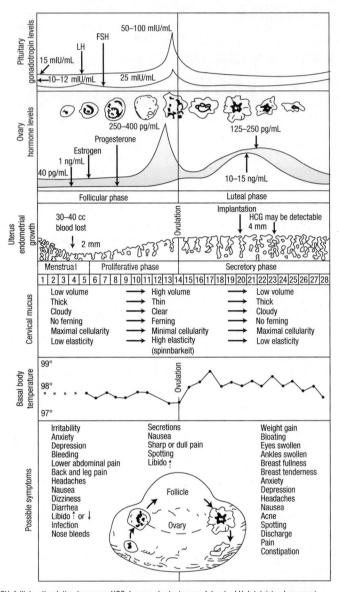

(FSH, follicle-stimulating hormone; HCG, human chorionic gonadotropin; LH, luteinizing hormone.)
LH: 15 mIU/mL = 15 IU/L; 50–100 mIU/mL = 50–100 IU/L.
FSH: 10–12 mIU/mL = 10–12 IU/L; 25 mIU/mL = 25 IU/L. Estrogen: 40 pg/mL = ~150 pmol/L;
250–400 pg/mL = ~920–1470 pmol/L; 125–250 pg/mL = ~460–920 pmol/L.
Progesterone: 1 ng/mL = 3 nmol/L; 10–15 ng/mL = ~30–50 nmol/L.
Temperatures: 99°F = 37.2°C; 98°F = 36.7°C; 97°F = 36.1°C.

FIGURE 30-1. Menstrual cycle events, idealized 28-day cycle. (Reprinted with permission from Hatcher RA, Trussell J, Nelson AL, et al. *Contraceptive Technology*. 21st ed. Ardent, NY: Median, Inc.; 2015.)

TABLE 30-1 Comparison of Methods of Nonhormonal Contraception

Method	Absolute Contraindications	Advantages	Disadvantages	Pregnancy Risk with Use[a]	
				Perfect Use	Typical Use
Internal condoms, male	Allergy to latex or rubber	Inexpensive STI/STD protection, including HIV (latex only)	High failure rate Poor acceptance Possibility of breakage Efficacy decreased by oil-based lubricants Possible allergic reactions to latex in either partner	2	13
External condoms, female	Allergy to polyurethane History of TSS	Inserted just before intercourse or ahead of time STI/STD protection, including HIV	High failure rate Dislike ring hanging outside vagina Cumbersome	5	21
Diaphragm with spermicide	Allergy to latex, rubber, or spermicide Recurrent UTIs History of TSS Abnormal gynecologic anatomy	Low cost Decreased incidence of cervical neoplasia Some protection against STIs/STDs	High failure rate Decreased efficacy with increased intercourse frequency Increased incidence of vaginal yeast UTIs, TSS Efficacy decreased by oil-based lubricants Cervical irritation	16	17
Cervical cap (FemCap)	Allergy to spermicide History of TSS Abnormal gynecologic anatomy Abnormal papanicolaou smear	Low cost Latex-free Some protection against STIs/STDs Reusable for up to 1 years	High failure rate Decreased efficacy with parity Cannot be used during menses	13.5	4–29[b]

(Continued)

TABLE 30-1 Comparison of Methods of Nonhormonal Contraception (*Continued*)

Method	Absolute Contraindications	Advantages	Disadvantages	Pregnancy Risk with Use[a] Perfect Use	Pregnancy Risk with Use[a] Typical Use
Spermicides alone (Phexxi)	Allergy to spermicide	Inexpensive	High failure rate Must be reapplied before each act of intercourse May enhance HIV transmission No protection against STI/STDs Risk of cystitis	16	21–28[c]
Sponge (Today)	Allergy to spermicide Recurrent UTIs History of TSS Abnormal gynecologic anatomy	Inexpensive	High user failure rate Decreased efficacy with parity Cannot be used during menses No protection against STIs/STDs	9[d]	14[e]

HIV, human immunodeficiency virus; STI/STD, sexually transmitted infection/disease; TSS, toxic shock syndrome; UTI, urinary tract infection.

[a]Failure rate in the United States during the first year of use.
[b]Failure rate with FemCap reported to be 8% per package insert.
[c]Failure rate with Phexxi reported to be 27.5% per package insert.
[d]Failure rate with Today sponge reported to be 20% in parous individuals.
[e]Failure rate with Today sponge reported to be 27% in parous individuals.

for at least 6 hours after. A diaphragm should not be left in place for more than 24 hours due to the risk of toxic shock syndrome (TSS), while the cervical cap should not remain in place for longer than 48 hours to reduce TSS risk. These do not protect against STIs including human immunodeficiency virus (HIV).

- Most **external condoms** (also known as male condoms) are made from latex, which is impermeable to viruses. A small percentage are made from lamb intestine, which are not impermeable to viruses. Water-soluble lubricants (ie, Astroglide and K-Y Jelly) are preferred to prevent condom breakdown. Condoms with spermicides are not recommended, as they provide no additional protection against pregnancy or STIs, and may increase vulnerability to HIV.
- The **internal condom** (also known as the female condom) covers the labia and the cervix. Its pregnancy rate is higher than with external condoms, but it protects against many viruses, including HIV. Do not use external and internal condoms together.
- Most spermicides contain **nonoxynol-9**, a surfactant that destroys sperm cell walls and blocks entry into the cervical os. They offer no protection against STIs, and when used more than twice daily, nonoxynol-9 may increase HIV transmission.
- **Phexxi** is a prescription non-oxynol-9-free spermicide. It should be used within 1 hour before each act of intercourse. It reduces vaginal pH to reduce sperm motility but carries a risk of cystitis.
- The **vaginal contraceptive sponge** is available over the counter and contains nonoxynol-9 and provides protection for 24 hours. After intercourse, it must be left in place for at least 6 hours but no more than 24–30 hours to reduce the risk of TSS. It should not be reused after removal.

PHARMACOLOGIC THERAPY

- Table 30-2 compares unintended pregnancy rates and continuation rates for pharmacologic contraceptive methods.

Hormonal Contraceptives

- Hormonal contraceptives contain a combination of estrogen and progestin or progestin alone. They may be administered as oral contraception (OC), transdermal patch, vaginal ring, long-acting injection, subdermal implant, and intrauterine device (IUD).
- **Combined Hormonal Contraceptive** (CHC) contain both estrogen and progestin and work primarily before fertilization to prevent conception.
- Estrogens suppress FSH release (contributing to blocking the LH surge) and also stabilize the endometrial lining and provide cycle control. **Ethinyl estradiol** (EE) is the most common synthetic estrogen; however, estetrol (E4) and estradiol valerate are also used.
- **Progestins** thicken cervical mucus, delay sperm transport, and induce endometrial atrophy, while also blocking the LH surge and inhibiting ovulation. They vary in their progestational activity and differ in their inherent estrogenic, antiestrogenic,

TABLE 30-2	Pregnancy and Continuation Rates for Various Hormonal Contraceptive Methods		
Method	**Pregnancy Typical Use**	**Pregnancy Ideal Use**	**Continuation After 1 Year**
Combined oral contraceptive	7%	<1%	67%
Drospirenone-only oral contraceptive	4%	—	—
Combined transdermal contraceptive patch	3%-7%	<1%	—
Combined vaginal contraceptive ring	3%-7%	<1%	—
Depot medroxyprogesterone acetate	4%	<1%	56%
Copper IUD	<1%	<1%	78%
Levonorgestrel IUD	<1%	<1%	80%
Progestin-only implant	<1%	<1%	89%

and androgenic effects. Androgenic activity depends on the presence of sex hormone (testosterone)–binding globulin and the androgen-to-progesterone activity ratio. If sex hormone–binding globulin decreases, free testosterone levels increase, and androgenic adverse effects are more prominent.

- Table 30-3 lists available OCs by brand name and hormonal composition.
- With perfect use, CHC efficacy is more than 99%, but with typical use, up to 7% of individuals experience unintended pregnancy.
- Monophasic CHCs contain a constant amount of estrogen and progestin for 21 days, while biphasic and triphasic pills contain variable amounts of estrogen and progestin for 21 days. All are followed by a 7-day placebo phase.
- Extended-cycle pills and continuous combination regimens may reduce adverse effects and are more convenient as the number of hormone-containing pills increases from 21 to 84 days, followed by a 7-day placebo phase, resulting in four menstrual cycles per year.
- The progestin-only "minipills" are less effective than CHCs and are associated with irregular and unpredictable menstrual bleeding. They must be taken every day at approximately the same time of day to maintain efficacy and are associated with more ectopic pregnancies than other hormonal contraceptives.
- The first-day start method starts on the first day of the menstrual cycle. The Sunday start method starts on the first Sunday after the menstrual cycle starts. The quick start method starts the day of the office visit. A second contraceptive method should be used for 7−30 days after CHC initiation and hormonal contraception should resume no sooner than 5 days after the use of emergency contraception (ie, ulipristal acetate).
- Provided guidance about what to do if a pill is missed or if vomiting and diarrhea occur.
- CHCs lack protection against STIs, and condoms should be used.
- The choice of an initial CHC is based on hormonal content and dose, preferred formulation, and coexisting medical conditions.
- A complete medical examination and papanicolaou (Pap) smear are not necessary before a CHC is prescribed. Obtain a medical history and blood pressure measurement, and discuss the risks, benefits, and adverse medication effects before prescribing a CHC.
- Fig. 30-2 shows graded eligibility criteria for contraceptive use.
- Noncontraceptive benefits of CHCs include decreased menstrual cramps and ovulatory pain; decreased menstrual blood loss; improved menstrual regularity; decreased iron deficiency anemia; reduced risk of ovarian and endometrial cancer; and reduced risk of ovarian cysts, ectopic pregnancy, pelvic inflammatory disease, endometriosis, uterine fibroids, and benign breast disease.
  - ✓ Serious symptoms associated with CHCs are given in Table 30-4.
  - ✓ Adverse medication effects occurring in the first cycle of CHC use (eg, breakthrough bleeding, nausea, and bloating) improve by the third cycle of use. Table 30-5 shows monitoring for CHCs.
  - ✓ Immediately discontinue if any warning signs referred to by the mnemonic ACHES (Abdominal pain, Chest pain, Headaches, Eye problems, and Severe leg pain) occur.

Transdermal Contraceptives

- Two combination contraceptives are available as a **transdermal patch**. Xulane delivers 35-mcg EE and 150-mcg norgestimate daily. Twirla provides 120 mcg of levonorgestrel and 30 mcg of EE daily. They are effective as CHCs in individuals weighing less than 90 kg (198 lb) or having a BMI less than 30 kg/m^2 with failure rates between 3% and 7%.
  - ✓ Apply patch to the abdomen, buttocks, upper torso, or upper arm at the beginning of the menstrual cycle and replace every week for 3 weeks. The fourth week is patch-free. Individuals should be counseled on the steps to follow should the patch detach or is forgotten.
  - ✓ Approved labeling includes a warning regarding VTE risk.

TABLE 30-3 Composition of Commonly Prescribed Oral Contraceptives[a]

Common Brand Names	Estrogen	Micrograms[a] (Number of Days)	Progestin	Milligrams[a] (Number of Days)	Spotting and Breakthrough Bleeding by Third Cycle (Up to Tenth Decimal)
Monophasic Preparations					
Kelnor 1/50	Ethinyl estradiol	50	Ethynodiol diacetate	1	13.9
Zovia 1/35E, Kelnor 1/35	Ethinyl estradiol	35	Ethynodiol diacetate	1	37.4
Apri, Cyred, Cyred EQ, Emoquette, Enskyce, Isibloom, Juleber, Kalliga, Reclipsen	Ethinyl estradiol	30	Desogestrel	0.15	13.1
Azurette, Bekyree, Kariva, Mircette, Pimtrea, Similya, Viorele, Volnea	Ethinyl estradiol	20 (21) 10 (5)	Desogestrel	0.15	19.7
Nextstellis	Estetrol	14.2 (mg)	Drospirenone	3	N/A
Ocella, Safyral, Syeda, Tydemy, Yasmin, Zarah, Zumandimine	Ethinyl estradiol	30	Drospirenone	3	14.5
Beyaz, Gianvi, Jasmiel, Lo-Zumandimine, Loryna, Nikki, Rajani, Vestura, Yaz[b]	Ethinyl estradiol	20	Drospirenone	3	13.8[c]
Altavera, Ayuna, Chateal, Chateal EQ, Kurvelo, Levora 0.15/30, Lillow, Marlissa, Portia-28	Ethinyl estradiol	30	Levonorgestrel	0.15	14
Iclevia, Introvale, Jolessa, Setlakin[d]	Ethinyl estradiol	30	Levonorgestrel	0.15	15.1[c]
Amethia, Ashlyna, Camrese Daysee, Jaimiess, Seasonique, Simpesse	Ethinyl estradiol	30 (84) 10 (7)	Levonorgestrel	0.15	14.3[e]
Afirmelle, Aubra, Aubra EQ, Aviane, Balcoltra, Delyla, Falmina, Larissia, Lessina, Lutera, Orsythia, Sronyx, Tyblume, Vienva	Ethinyl estradiol	20	Levonorgestrel	0.1	26.5
Camrese Lo, LoJaimiess, LoSeasonique	Ethinyl estradiol	20/10	Levonorgestrel	0.1	21.5[e]

(Continued)

TABLE 30-3 Composition of Commonly Prescribed Oral Contraceptives[a] (*Continued*)

Common Brand Names	Estrogen	Micrograms[a] (Number of Days)	Progestin	Milligrams[a] (Number of Days)	Spotting and Breakthrough Bleeding by Third Cycle (Up to Tenth Decimal)
Amethyst, Dolishale	Ethinyl estradiol	20	Levonorgestrel	0.09	N/A[c]
Estarylla, Femynor, Mili, Mono-Linyah, Mononessa, NymyoPrevifem, Sprintec, VyLibra	Ethinyl estradiol	35	Norgestimate	0.25	14.3
—	Ethinyl estradiol	50	Norgestrel	0.5	N/A
Cryselle, Elinest, Low-Ogestrel	Ethinyl estradiol	30	Norgestrel	0.3	9.6
Balziva, Briellyn, Gildagia, Philith, Vyfemla, Wymzya Fe chewable	Ethinyl estradiol	35	Norethindrone	0.4	11
Necon 0.5/35, Nortrel 0.5/35, Norminest Fe, Wera	Ethinyl estradiol	35	Norethindrone	0.5	24.6
Alyacen 1/35, Cyclafem 1/35, Dasetta 1/35, Nortrel 1/35, Pirmella 1/35	Ethinyl estradiol	35	Norethindrone	1	14.7
Generess Fe chewable, Kaitlib Fe chewable, Layolis Fe chewable	Ethinyl estradiol	25	Norethindrone	0.8	19.0
Aurovela 1.5/30-21, Aurovela 1.5/30-28, Aurovela Fe 1.5/30, Blisovi Fe 1.5/30, Hailey Fe 1/20, Gildess Fe 1.5/30, Junel 1.5/30, Junel Fe 1.5/30, Larin 1.5/30, LarinFe 1.5/30, Loestrin Fe 1.5/30, Microgestin 1.5/30	Ethinyl estradiol	30	Norethindrone acetate	1.5	25.2
Aurovela 1/20, Aurovela Fe 1/20, Blisovi 1/20, Hailey Fe 1/20, Junel Fe 1/20, Junel 1/20, Larin (Fe) 1/20, Loestrin 1/20; Fe 1/20, Microgestin 1/20; Microgestin Fe 1/20, Tarina Fe 1/20, Tarina Fe 1/20 EQ	Ethinyl estradiol	20	Norethindrone acetate	1	29.7
Aurovela 24 Fe, Blisovi 24 Fe, Gemmily (capsules), Junel Fe 24, Hailey Fe, Larin 24 Fe, Minastrin 24 Fe chewable, Merzee (capsules), Melodetta 24 Fe (chewable), Microgestin 24 Fe, Tarina 24 Fe, Taytulla (capsules)	Ethinyl estradiol	20	Norethindrone acetate	1	23.2[c]

	Ethinyl estradiol	10	Norethindrone acetate	1	52.0ᶜ
Lo Loestrin-24 Feᵇ					

Multiphasic Preparations (Biphasic, Triphasic, and Quadriphasic)

—	Ethinyl estradiol	35 (10) 35 (11)	Norethindrone	0.5 (10) 1 (11)	N/A
Caziant, Cyclessa, Velivet	Ethinyl estradiol	25 (7) 25 (7) 25 (7)	Desogestrel	0.1 (7) 0.125 (7) 0.15 (7)	11.1
Enpresse, Trivora, Levonest Myzilra	Ethinyl estradiol	30 (6) 40 (5) 30 (10)	Levonorgestrel	0.05 (6) 0.075 (5) 0.125 (10)	15.1
Ortho Tri-Cyclen, Tri-Estarylla, Tri-Femynor, Tri-Linyah, TriNessa, Tri-Previfem, Tri-Sprintec	Ethinyl estradiol	35 (7) 35 (7) 35 (7)	Norgestimate	0.18 (7) 0.215 (7) 0.25 (7)	17.7
Tri-Lo Estarylla, Tri-Lo-Marzia, Tri-Lo-Mili, Tri-Lo-Sprintec, Tri-VyLibra Lo	Ethinyl estradiol	25 (7) 25 (7) 25 (7)	Norgestimate	0.18 (7) 0.215 (7) 0.25 (7)	11.5
Alyacen 7/7/7, Cyclafem 7/7/7, Dasetta 7/7/7, Nortrel 7/7/7, Nylia 7/7/7, Pirmella 7/7/7	Ethinyl estradiol	35 (7) 35 (7) 35 (7)	Norethindrone	0.5 (7) 0.75 (7) 1 (7)	14.5
Aranelle, Leena	Ethinyl estradiol	35 (7) 35 (9) 35 (5)	Norethindrone	0.5 (7) 1 (9) 0.5 (5)	25.5

(Continued)

311

TABLE 30-3 Composition of Commonly Prescribed Oral Contraceptives[a] (*Continued*)

Common Brand Names	Estrogen	Micrograms[a] (Number of Days)	Progestin	Milligrams[a] (Number of Days)	Spotting and Breakthrough Bleeding by Third Cycle (Up to Tenth Decimal)
Estrostep Fe, Tilia Fe, Tri-Legest Fe	Ethinyl estradiol	20 (5) 30 (7) 35 (9)	Norethindrone acetate	1 (5) 1 (7) 1 (9)	21.7
Fayosim, Quartette, Rivelsa	Ethinyl estradiol	20 (42) 25 (21) 30 (21) 10 (7)	Levonorgestrel	0.15	N/A[e]
Natazia	Estradiol valerate	3 (2) 2 (5) 2 (17) 1 (2)	Dienogest	0 (2) 2 (5) 3 (17) 0 (4)	14
Progestin-Only Oral Contraceptives					
Camila, Deblitane Errin, Heather, Incassia, Jencycla Lyleq, Lyza, Ortho Micronor, Nora-BE, Norlyda, Norlyroc, Orthor Micronor, Sharobel, Tulana	Ethinyl estradiol	—	Norethindrone	0.35 (28)	42.3
Slynd	Ethinyl estradiol	—	Drospirenone	4 (24)	N/A

[a]28-day regimens (21-day active pills, then 7-day pill-free interval) unless otherwise noted.
[b]Number in parentheses refers to the number of days the dose is received in multiphasic oral contraceptives.
[c]28-day regimen (24-day active pills, then 4-day pill-free interval).
[d]91-day regimen (84-day active pills, then 7-day pill-free interval).
[e]Percent reporting after 6 to 12 months of use.
N/A—Data not available per references.

Vaginal Rings

- There are two vaginal rings available. Over a 3-week period **NuvaRing** releases ~ 15 mcg/day of EE and 120 mcg/day of etonogestrel and **Annovera** releases 13 mcg of EE and 150 mcg of segesterone acetate. On first use, the ring should be inserted on or prior to the fifth day of the cycle, remain in place for 3 weeks, and then be removed. One week should lapse before the new ring is inserted on the same day of the week as it was for the last cycle. A second form of contraception should be used for the first 7 days of ring use or if the ring has been expelled for more than 3 hours for NuvaRing or 2 hours for Annovera.

- If the Annovera is not removed after 4 weeks, no backup contraception is needed, but 1 week should lapse before a new ring is inserted. If the NuvaRing is left in place for 4 weeks, a pregnancy test should be taken, followed by new ring insertion with 7 days of nonhormonal contraception.

Condition	Sub-Condition	Cu-IUD		LNG-IUD		Implant		DMPA		POP		CHC	
		I	C	I	C	I	C	I	C	I	C	I	C
Age		Menarche to <20 yrs:2		Menarche to <20 yrs:2		Menarche to <18 yrs:1		Menarche to <18 yrs:1		Menarche to <18 yrs:1		Menarche to <40 yrs:1	
		≥ 20 yrs:1		≥ 20 yrs:1		18-45 yrs:1 >45 yrs:1		18-45 yrs:1 >45 yrs:2		18-45 yrs:1 >45 yrs:1		≥ 40 yrs:2	
Anatomical abnormalities	a) Distorted uterine cavity	4		4									
	b) Other abnormalities	2		2									
Anemias	a) Thalassemia	2	1	1		1		1		1			
	b) Sickle cell disease‡	2	1	1		1		1		2			
	c) Iron-deficiency anemia	2	1	1		1		1		1			
Benign ovarian tumors	(including cysts)	1	1	1		1		1		1			
Breast disease	a) Undiagnosed mass	1	2	2*		2*		2*		2*			
	b) Benign breast disease	1	1	1		1		1		1			
	c) Family history of cancer	1	1	1		1		1		1			
	d) Breast cancer‡												
	i) Current	1	4	4		4		4		4			
	ii) Past and no evidence of current disease for 5 years	1	3	3		3		3		3			
Breastfeeding	a) <21 days postpartum					2*		2*		2*		4*	
	b) 21 to <30 days postpartum												
	i) With other risk factors for VTE					2*		2*		2*		3*	
	ii) Without other risk factors for VTE					2*		2*		2*		3*	
	c) 30-42 days postpartum												
	i) With other risk factors for VTE					1*		1*		1*		3*	
	ii) Without other risk factors for VTE					1*		1*		1*		2*	
	d) >42 days postpartum					1*		1*		1*		2*	
Cervical cancer	Awaiting treatment	4	2	4	2	2		2		1		2	
Cervical ectropion		1	1	1		1		1		1			
Cervical intraepithelial neoplasia		1	2	2		1		1		1		2	
Cirrhosis	a) Mild (compensated)	1	1	1		1		1		1			
	b) Severe‡ (decompensated)	1	3	3		3		3		3		4	
Cystic fibrosis‡		1*	1*	1*		1*		2*		1*		1*	
Deep venous thrombosis (DVT)/Pulmonary embolism (PE)	a) History of DVT/PE, not receiving anticoagulant therapy												
	i) Higher risk for recurrent DVT/PE	1	2	2		2		2		2		4	
	ii) Lower risk for recurrent DVT/PE	1	2	2		2		2		2		3	
	b) Acute DVT/PE	2	2	2		2		2		2		4	
	c) DVT/PE and established anticoagulant therapy for at least 3 months												
	i) Higher risk for recurrent DVT/PE	2	2	2		2		2		2		4*	
	ii) Lower risk for recurrent DVT/PE	2	2	2		2		2		2		3*	
	d) Family history (first-degree relatives)	1	1	1		1		1		1		2	
	e) Major surgery												
	i) With prolonged immobilization	1	2	2		2		2		2		4	
	ii) Without prolonged immobilization	1	1	1		1		1		1		2	
	f) Minor surgery without immobilization	1	1	1		1		1		1		1	
Depressive disorders		1*	1*	1*		1*		1*		1*		1*	

Key:

1 No restriction (method can be used)	3 Theoretical or proven risks usually outweigh the advantages
2 Advantages generally outweigh theoretical or proven risks	4 Unacceptable health risk (method not to be used)

FIGURE 30-2. Summary chart of U.S. medical eligibility criteria for contraceptive use.

Condition	Sub-Condition	Cu-IUD (I / C)	LNG-IUD (I / C)	Implant	DMPA	POP	CHC
Diabetes	a) History of gestational disease	1	1	1	1	1	1
	b) Nonvascular disease						
	i) Non-insulin dependent	1	2	2	2	2	2
	ii) Insulin dependent	1	2	2	2	2	2
	c) Nephropathy/retinopathy/neuropathy‡	1	2	2	3	2	3/4*
	d) Other vascular disease or diabetes of >20 years' duration‡	1	2	2	3	2	3/4*
Dysmenorrhea	Severe	2	1	1	1	1	1
Endometrial cancer‡		4 / 2	4 / 2	1	1	1	1
Endometrial hyperplasia		1	1	1	1	1	1
Endometriosis		2	1	1	1	1	1
Epilepsy‡	(see also Drug Interactions)	1	1	1*	1*	1*	1*
Gallbladder disease	a) Symptomatic						
	i) Treated by cholecystectomy	1	2	2	2	2	2
	ii) Medically treated	1	2	2	2	2	3
	iii) Current	1	2	2	2	2	3
	b) Asymptomatic	1	2	2	2	2	2
Gestational trophoblastic disease‡	a) Suspected GTD (immediate postevacuation)						
	i) Uterine size first trimester	1*	1*	1*	1*	1*	1*
	ii) Uterine size second trimester	2*	2*	1*	1*	1*	1*
	b) Confirmed GTD						
	i) Undetectable/non-pregnant β-hCG levels	1* / 1*	1* / 1*	1*	1*	1*	1*
	ii) Decreasing β-hCG levels	2* / 1*	2* / 1*	1*	1*	1*	1*
	iii) Persistently elevated β-hCG levels or malignant disease, with no evidence or suspicion of intrauterine disease	2* / 1*	2* / 1*	1*	1*	1*	1*
	iv) Persistently elevated β-hCG levels or malignant disease, with evidence or suspicion of intrauterine disease	4* / 2*	4* / 2*	1*	1*	1*	1*
Headaches	a) Nonmigraine (mild or severe)	1	1	1	1	1	1*
	b) Migraine						
	i) Without aura (includes menstrual migraine)	1	1	1	1	1	2*
	ii) With aura	1	1	1	1	1	4*
History of bariatric surgery‡	a) Restrictive procedures	1	1	1	1	1	1
	b) Malabsorptive procedures	1	1	1	1	3	COCs: 3 / P/R: 1
History of cholestasis	a) Pregnancy related	1	1	1	1	1	2
	b) Past COC related	1	2	2	2	2	3
History of high blood pressure during pregnancy		1	1	1	1	1	2
History of Pelvic surgery		1	1	1	1	1	1
HIV	a) High risk for HIV	1* / 1*	1* / 1*	1	1*	1	1
	b) HIV infection			1*	1*	1*	1*
	i) Clinically well receiving ARV therapy	1 / 1	1 / 1	If on treatment, see Drug Interactions			
	ii) Not clinically well or not receiving ARV therapy‡	2 / 1	2 / 1	If on treatment, see Drug Interactions			

Abbreviations: ARV = antiretroviral; C=continuation of contraceptive method; CHC=combined hormonal contraception (pill, patch, and, ring); COC=combined oral contraceptive; Cu-IUD=copper-containing intrauterine device; DMPA = depot medroxyprogesterone acetate; I=initiation of contraceptive method; LNG-IUD=levonorgestrel-releasing intrauterine device; NA=not applicable; POP=progestin-only pill; P/R=patch/ring; SSRI=selective serotonin reuptake inhibitor; ‡ Condition that exposes a woman to increased risk as a result of pregnancy. *Please see the complete guidance for a clarification to this classification: https://www.cdc.gov/reproductivehealth/contraception/contraception_guidance.htm

FIGURE 30-2. (Continued)

Condition	Sub-Condition	Cu-IUD		LNG-IUD		Implant		DMPA		POP		CHC	
		I	C	I	C	I	C	I	C	I	C	I	C
Hypertension	a) Adequately controlled hypertension	1*		1*		1*		2*		1*		3*	
	b) Elevated blood pressure levels (*properly taken measurements*)												
	i) Systolic 140-159 or diastolic 90-99	1*		1*		1*		2*		1*		3*	
	ii) Systolic ≥160 or diastolic ≥100‡	1*		2*		2*		3*		2*		4*	
	c) Vascular disease	1*		2*		2*		3*		2*		4*	
Inflammatory bowel disease	(*Ulcerative colitis, Crohn's disease*)	1		1		1		2		2		2/3*	
Ischemic heart disease‡	Current and history of	1		2	3	2	3	3		2	3	4	
Known thrombogenic mutations‡		1*		2*		2*		2*		2*		4*	
Liver tumors	a) Benign												
	i) Focal nodular hyperplasia	1		2		2		2		2		2	
	ii) Hepatocellular adenoma‡	1		3		3		3		3		4	
	b) Malignant‡ (hepatoma)	1		3		3		3		3		4	
Malaria		1		1		1		1		1		1	
Multiple risk factors for atherosclerotic cardiovascular disease	(e.g., older age, smoking, diabetes, hypertension, low HDL, high LDL, or high triglyceride levels)	1		2		2*		3*		2*		3/4*	
Multiple sclerosis	a) With prolonged immobility	1		1		1		2		1		3	
	b) Without prolonged immobility	1		1		1		2		1		1	
Obesity	a) Body mass index (BMI) ≥30 kg/m²	1		1		1		1		1		2	
	b) Menarche to <18 years and BMI ≥ 30 kg/m²	1		1		1		2		1		2	
Ovarian cancer‡		1		1		1		1		1		1	
Parity	a) Nulliparous	2		2		1		1		1		1	
	b) Parous	1		1		1		1		1		1	
Past ectopic pregnancy		1		1		1		1		2		1	
Pelvic inflammatory disease	a) Past												
	i) With subsequent pregnancy	1	1	1	1	1		1		1		1	
	ii) Without subsequent pregnancy	2	2	2	2	1		1		1		1	
	b) Current	4	2*	4	2*	1		1		1		1	
Peripartum cardiomyopathy‡	a) Normal or mildly impaired cardiac function												
	i) <6 months	2		2		1		1		1		4	
	ii) ≥6 months	2		2		1		1		1		3	
	b) Moderately or severely impaired cardiac function	2		2		2		2		2		4	
Postabortion	a) First trimester	1*		1*		1*		1*		1*		1*	
	b) Second trimester	2*		2*		1*		1*		1*		1*	
	c) Immediate postseptic abortion	4		4		1*		1*		1*		1*	
Postpartum (*nonbreastfeeding women*)	a) <21 days							1		1		4	
	b) 21 days to 42 days												
	i) With other risk factors for VTE							1		1		3*	
	ii) Without other risk factors for VTE							1		1		2	
	c) >42 days							1		1		1	
Postpartum (*in breastfeeding or non-breastfeeding women, including cesarean delivery*)	a) <10 minutes after delivery of the placenta												
	i) Breastfeeding	1*		2*									
	ii) Nonbreastfeeding	1*		1*									
	b) 10 minutes after delivery of the placenta to <4 weeks	2*		2*									
	c) ≥4 weeks	1*		1*									
	d) Postpartum sepsis	4		4									

FIGURE 30-2. (*Continued*)

Condition	Sub-Condition	Cu-IUD		LNG-IUD		Implant		DMPA		POP		CHC	
		I	C	I	C	I	C	I	C	I	C	I	C
Pregnancy		4*		4*		NA*		NA*		NA*		NA*	
Rheumatoid arthritis	a) On immunosuppressive therapy	2	1	2	1	1		2/3*		1		2	
	b) Not on immunosuppressive therapy	1		1		1		2		1		2	
Schistosomiasis	a) Uncomplicated	1		1		1		1		1		1	
	b) Fibrosis of the liver‡	1		1		1		1		1		1	
Sexually transmitted diseases (STDs)	a) Current purulent cervicitis or chlamydial infection or gonococcal infection	4	2*	4	2*	1		1		1		1	
	b) Vaginitis (including trichomonas vaginalis and bacterial vaginosis)	2	2	2	2	1		1		1		1	
	c) Other factors relating to STDs	2*	2	2*	2	1		1		1		1	
Smoking	a) Age <35	1		1		1		1		1		2	
	b) Age ≥35, <15 cigarettes/day	1		1		1		1		1		3	
	c) Age ≥35, ≥15 cigarettes/day	1		1		1		1		1		4	
Solid organ transplantation‡	a) Complicated	3	2	3	2	2		2		2		4	
	b) Uncomplicated	2		2		2		2		2		2*	
Stroke‡	History of cerebrovascular accident	1		2		2	3	3		2	3	4	
Superficial venous disorders	a) Varicose veins	1		1		1		1		1		1	
	b) Superficial venous thrombosis (acute or history)	1		1		1		1		1		3*	
Systemic lupus erythematosus‡	a) Positive (or unknown) antiphospholipid antibodies	1*	1*	3*		3*		3*	3*	3*		4*	
	b) Severe thrombocytopenia	3*	2*	2*		2*		2*	3*	2*		2*	
	c) Immunosuppressive therapy	2*	1*	2*		2*		2*	2*	2*		2*	
	d) None of the above	1*	1*	2*		2*		2*	2*	2*		2*	
Thyroid disorders	Simple goiter/ hyperthyroid/hypothyroid	1		1		1		1		1		1	
Tuberculosis‡ (see also Drug Interactions)	a) Nonpelvic	1	1	1	1	1*		1*		1*		1*	
	b) Pelvic	4	3	4	3	1*		1*		1*		1*	
Unexplained vaginal bleeding	(suspicious for serious condition) before evaluation	4*	2*	4*	2*	3*		3*		2*		2*	
Uterine fibroids		2		2		1		1		1		1	
Valvular heart disease	a) Uncomplicated	1		1		1		1		1		2	
	b) Complicated‡	1		1		1		1		1		4	
Vaginal bleeding patterns	a) Irregular pattern without heavy bleeding	1		1		2		2		2		1	
	b) Heavy or prolonged bleeding	2*		1*	2*	2*		2*		2*		1*	
Viral hepatitis	a) Acute or flare	1		1		1		1		1		3/4*	2
	b) Carrier/Chronic	1		1		1		1		1		1	1
Drug Interactions													
Antiretrovirals used for prevention (PrEP) or treatment of HIV	Fosamprenavir (FPV)	1/2*	1*	1/2*	1*	2*		2*		2*		3*	
	All other ARVs are 1 or 2 for all methods.												
Anticonvulsant therapy	a) Certain anticonvulsants (phenytoin, carbamazepine, barbiturates, primidone, topiramate, oxcarbazepine)	1		1		2*		1*		3*		3*	
	b) Lamotrigine	1		1		1		1		1		3*	
Antimicrobial therapy	a) Broad spectrum antibiotics	1		1		1		1		1		1	
	b) Antifungals	1		1		1		1		1		1	
	c) Antiparasitics	1		1		1		1		1		1	
	d) Rifampin or rifabutin therapy	1		1		2*		1*		3*		3*	
SSRIs		1		1		1		1		1		1	
St. John's wort		1		1		2		1		2		2	

Updated in 2020. This summary sheet only contains a subset of the recommendations from the U.S. MEC. For complete guidance, see: https://www.cdc.gov/reproductivehealth/contraception/contraception_guidance.htm. Most contraceptive methods do not protect against sexually transmitted diseases (STDs). Consistent and correct use of the male latex condom reduces the risk of STDs and HIV.

CS314239-A

FIGURE 30-2. (Continued)

Injectable Progestins

- Individuals who particularly benefit from progestin-only methods, including mini-pills, are those who are lactating, intolerant of estrogens, and those with concomitant medical conditions in which estrogen is not recommended (Table 30-4).
- Injectable and implantable contraceptives are also beneficial for individuals with adherence issues as failure rates are lower than with CHC.
- **Depot medroxyprogesterone acetate (DMPA)** 150 mg is administered by deep intramuscular injection in the gluteal or deltoid muscle within 5 days of onset of menstrual bleeding, and repeated every 12 weeks. Another formulation contains 104 mg of DMPA (Depo-SubQ Provera 104), which is injected subcutaneously into the thigh or abdomen. Exclude pregnancy if more than 1 week late for repeat injection of the intramuscular formulation or 2 weeks late for repeat injection of the subcutaneous formulation. Return of fertility may be delayed after discontinuation.
- DMPA can be given immediately postpartum in individuals not breastfeeding, and at 6 weeks postpartum if breastfeeding. The median time to conception from the first omitted dose is 10 months.

TABLE 30-4	Serious or Potentially Serious Symptoms Associated with Combined Hormonal Contraception

SERIOUS: Stop immediately

Loss of vision, proptosis, diplopia, papilledema	Hemoptysis
Unilateral numbness, weakness, or tingling	Severe pain, tenderness or swelling, warmth or palpable cord in legs
Severe pain in chest, left arm, or neck	
	Hepatic mass or tenderness
	Slurring of speech

POTENTIALLY SERIOUS: May continue with caution while being evaluated

Absence of menses	Severe nonvascular headache
Spotting or breakthrough bleeding	Galactorrhea
Breast mass, pain, or swelling	Jaundice, pruritus
Right upper-quadrant pain	Depression, sleepiness
Mid-epigastric pain	Uterine size increase
Migrane headache	

✓ DMPA is contraindicated with a current breast cancer diagnosis and used cautiously with a history of breast cancer, cardiovascular disease, or lupus.

✓ The most frequent adverse medication effect is menstrual irregularity, which decreases after the first year. Breast tenderness, weight gain, and depression occur less frequently.

✓ DMPA has a black box warning for reduced bone mineral density (BMD) but not increased fracture risk. BMD loss seems to be greater with increasing duration of use, and for the majority it is reversible. DMPA should not be continued beyond 2 years unless other contraceptive methods are inadequate.

Subdermal Progestin Implants

• **Etonogestrel implant** (Nexplanon) is a radiopaque, 4-cm implant containing 68 mg of etonogestrel that is placed under the skin of the upper arm. It releases 60 mcg daily for the first month, decreasing gradually to 30 mcg/day at the end of the 3 years of recommended use. Efficacy exceeds 99%, but it may be less in individuals who weigh more than 130% of their ideal body weight.

• Its contraceptive effects are quickly reversible upon removal.

• Need for backup contraception varies based on prior contraceptive use and where in the menstrual cycle the implant is inserted. Fertility returns 30 days after removal.

✓ Irregular menstrual bleeding is common followed by headache, vaginitis, weight gain, acne, and breast and abdominal pain. It does not appear to decrease BMD. Fertility returns within 30 days of removal.

✓ There is potential for interactions in the presence of potent CYP450 inducers (eg, rifampin, phenytoin, and carbamazepine).

Intrauterine Devices (IUDs)

• The contraceptive activity occurs before implantation. Endometrial suppression is caused by progestin-releasing IUDs. Efficacy rates are greater than 99% and their contraceptive effects are reversible upon removal.

• Consideration of an IUD is appropriate in nulliparous and adolescent individuals, given high efficacy and low complication rates. Need for backup contraception varies based on prior contraceptive use and when in the menstrual cycle the implant is inserted.

• The risk of pelvic inflammatory disease among users is low with no long-term effects on fertility.

TABLE 30-5	Monitoring for Hormonal Contraception	
Adverse Medication Effect	**Monitoring Parameter**	**Comments**
Combined hormonal Contraception		
Nausea/vomiting Breast tenderness Weight gain	Patient symptoms and Weight	Typically improves after two to three cycles; consider changing to lower estrogenic
Acne, oily skin	Visual inspection	Consider changing to lower androgenic
Depression, fatigue	Depression screening	Data are limited and conflicting
Breakthrough bleeding/ spotting	Menstrual symptoms	Consider changing to higher estrogenic
Application site reaction (transdermal)	Visual inspection	
Vaginal irritation (vaginal ring)	Patient symptoms	
Depot medroxyprogesterone acetate		
Menstrual irregularities[a]	Menstrual symptoms	Typically improves after 6 months
Weight gain Acne Hirsutism Depression	Weight, Visual inspection, and Depression Screening	Data are limited and conflicting
Decreased bone density	BMD	Do not routinely screen with DXA
Levonorgestrel IUD		
Menstrual irregularities[a]	Menstrual symptoms	Typically spotting, amenorrhea Typically heavier menses with copper IUD
Insertion-related complications	Cramping, pain	Prophylactic nonsteroidal anti-inflammatory drugs (NSAIDs) or local anesthetic may reduce occurrence
Expulsion	Cramping, pain, spotting, dyspareunia, missing strings	IUD strings should be checked regularly to ensure IUD properly placed
Pelvic inflammatory disease	Lower abdominal pain, unusual vaginal discharge, fever	Overall risk of developing is rare, but counseling on STI prevention is important
Progestin-only implant		
Menstrual irregularities[a]	Menstrual symptoms	Typically well-tolerated and resolve without treatment; infection is rare
Insertion-site reactions	Pain, bruising, skin irritation, erythema, pus, fever	

[a]Suggested management of irregular bleeding may include use of NSAIDs for 5–7 days; hormonal treatment (if medically eligible) with CHC or estrogen therapy for 10–20 days of treatment.

- ParaGard (copper) can be left in place for 10 years. Mirena, Liletta, Skyla, and Kyleena release levonorgestrel and must be replaced after 6 years (Mirena, Liletta, and Kyleena) and 3 years (Skyla).

  ✓ Major adverse medication effects include increased menstrual blood flow and dysmenorrhea with ParaGard, while levonorgestrel IUDs are associated with reduced menstrual blood loss and possible amenorrhea.

Special Consideration for Contraceptive Use

Over 35 Years of Age

- Use of CHCs containing less than 50-mcg estrogen may be considered in healthy nonsmoking individuals older than 35 years.
- CHCs are not recommended for individuals older than 35 years with migraine, uncontrolled hypertension, smoking, or diabetes with vascular disease.
- Studies have not demonstrated an increased risk of cardiovascular disease with low-dose CHCs in healthy, nonobese individuals.
- Smoking 15 or more cigarettes per day by individuals over 35 years is a contraindication to the use of CHCs, and progestin-only methods should be considered.

Smoking

- Use of a CHC with less than 50-mcg EE should be used in individuals younger than 35 who smoke to reduce the risk of myocardial infarction (MI).

Hypertension

- CHCs, regardless of estrogen dose, can cause small increases in blood pressure (6–8 mm Hg). Use of low-dose CHCs is acceptable in those younger than 35 years with well-controlled and monitored hypertension to reduce the risk of MI and stroke.
- Individuals with a systolic blood pressure of 140−159 or a diastolic blood pressure of 90−99 mm Hg should avoid CHCs. Their use is contraindicated with blood pressures ≥160/100 mm Hg.
- Monitor potassium with potassium-sparing diuretics, angiotensin-converting enzyme inhibitors, angiotensin-receptor blockers, or aldosterone antagonists if also using a product containing drospirenone.

Diabetes

- Nonsmoking individuals younger than 35 years with diabetes but no vascular disease can safely use CHCs. Individuals with diabetes for >20 years or with vascular disease should not use CHCs.

Dyslipidemia

- Generally, synthetic progestins decrease high-density lipoprotein (HDL) and increase low-density lipoprotein (LDL). Estrogens decrease LDL but increase HDL and may moderately increase triglycerides. Most low-dose CHCs have no significant impact on HDL, LDL, triglycerides, or total cholesterol.
- The mechanism for the increased cardiovascular disease in CHC users is believed to be thromboembolic and thrombotic changes, not atherosclerosis.
- CHCs use in individuals with dyslipidemia as a single cardiovascular risk factor is generally acceptable. An alternative method of contraception is recommended in individuals with dyslipidemia and other cardiovascular risk factors.

Thromboembolism

- The risk of venous thromboembolism (VTE) in individuals using combined oral contraceptives (COCs) is three times that of nonusers, but is less than the risk of thromboembolic events during pregnancy.
- Estrogens increase hepatic production of factors involved in the coagulation cascade. Risk for thromboembolic events is increased in those with underlying

hypercoagulable states or with acquired conditions (eg, obesity, pregnancy, immobility, trauma, surgery, and certain malignancies) that predispose to coagulation abnormalities.

- COCs containing the newer progestins (eg, drospirenone, desogestrel, norgestimate) carry a slightly increased risk of thrombosis compared to other progestins due to unknown mechanisms.
- The transdermal patch and vaginal ring provide continuous higher exposure to estrogen and have an increased thromboembolic risk.
- For individuals at increased risk of thromboembolism (older than 35 years, obesity, smoking, personal or family history of venous thrombosis, prolonged immobilization), consider low-dose oral estrogen contraceptives containing older progestins or progestin-only methods.

Obesity

- COCs have lower efficacy in obesity, and low-dose COCs may be especially problematic. IUDs, implants, and DMPA have very low failure rates, and progestin-only contraceptives are considered safe in obese individuals.
- Obese individuals have increased VTE risk, and progestin-only contraception may be better for those over 35 years.

Migraine Headache

- CHCs may decrease or increase migraine frequency.
- CHCs may be considered for healthy, nonsmoking individuals (less than 35 years old) with migraines without aura. Discuss continued use of CHC risks and benefits with individuals developing migraines without aura.
- individuals of any age who have migraine with aura should not use CHCs due to the risk of stroke. individuals who develop migraines with aura while receiving CHCs should discontinue their use and consider a progestin-only option.

Breast Cancer

- There is a small increase in the relative risk of having breast cancer while CHCs are taken and for up to 10 years following discontinuation.
- For individuals over the age of 40 or those with elevated breast cancer risk due to family history or other factors, alternatives may be considered.
- The choice to use CHCs should not be influenced by the presence of benign breast disease or a family history of breast cancer. For individuals with either BRCA1 or BRCA2 mutation, CHC use is controversial, and individuals with a current or past history of breast cancer should not use CHCs.

Systemic Lupus Erythematosus (SLE)

- COCs with less than 50-mcg EE do not increase the risk of flare in those with stable SLE and without antiphospholipid/anticardiolipin antibodies.
- CHCs and progestin-only products should be avoided in individuals with SLE and antiphospholipid antibodies or vascular complications. The copper IUD may be the best.
- For those with SLE without antiphospholipid antibodies or vascular complications, progestin-only contraceptives or the copper IUD may be an alternative.
- A copper IUD and DMPA injection should be avoided in those with SLE and severe thrombocytopenia.

Postpartum

- In the first 21 days postpartum (when the risk of thrombosis is higher), estrogen-containing hormonal contraceptives should be avoided due to increased VTE risk. Progestin-only methods should be used if contraception is necessary.
- CHC should be avoided in the first 42 days postpartum in individuals with VTE risk factors and for 30 days for those without VTE risk factors who are breastfeeding.

Medication Interactions

- Tell patients to use an alternative method of contraception if a possible medication interaction may compromise OC efficacy.
- There is a small interaction risk with antimicrobials, and additional nonhormonal contraceptives should be considered, especially when receiving an antimicrobial for more than 2 months.
- Rifampin reduces the efficacy of CHCs. Additional nonhormonal contraception should be used for at least 7−28 days after rifampin therapy.
- Phenobarbital, carbamazepine, and phenytoin potentially reduce the efficacy of CHCs, and many anticonvulsants are known teratogens. IUDs, injectable medroxy-progesterone, or nonhormonal options should be used instead.
- CHCs may decrease the efficacy of lamotrigine and increase seizure risk.
- Certain antiretroviral therapies and St. John's Wort may decrease the efficacy of CHCs.
- Monitor potassium in patients taking drospirenone and concomitant medications that increase potassium levels or those taking strong CYP3A4 inhibitors.

Return of Fertility After Discontinuation

- There is no evidence that hormonal contraception use decreases subsequent fertility and there is no greater chance of miscarriage or a birth defect in the first month after discontinuation.

Emergency Contraception (EC)

- EC is used to prevent unintended pregnancy after unprotected or inadequately protected sexual intercourse.
- FDA-approved progestin-only and progesterone receptor modulator products are recommended as first-line EC options. They will not disrupt the fertilized egg if implantation has already occurred.
- Progestin-only EC formulations containing one 1.5-mg tablet of levonorgestrel are available without a prescription in the United States. They may be less effective in individuals weighing greater than 75 kg.
- **Ulipristal** (Ella) is a prescription selective progesterone receptor modulator. It is taken as a single dose of 30 mg within 120 hours (5 days) of unprotected intercourse. It is considered noninferior to levonorgestrel-containing ECs and is not recommended in breastfeeding individuals.
- Common adverse medication effects of EC include nausea, vomiting, and irregular bleeding.
- Insertion of a copper IUD or prescribing higher doses of CHCs (Yuzpe method) are other EC options.
- EC should be given within 72 hours (3 days) of unprotected intercourse, but the sooner it is taken, the greater the efficacy. There is some evidence that it may be effective for up to 5 days after unprotected intercourse, but in this situation ulipristal or a copper IUD may be a better option.
- Backup nonhormonal contraceptive methods should be used after EC for at least 7 days.

Pregnancy Termination

- Medications used in early pregnancy (≤70 days) termination include **mifepristone** and **misoprostol**. Misoprostol can be used alone or more effectively in combination with mifepristone. The FDA has approved mifepristone 200 mg orally on day 1 and then misoprostol 800 mcg buccally 24–48 hours after the mifepristone dose. This regimen has a 98% efficacy in pregnancies up to 49 days.
- Mifepristone binds progesterone receptors to block progesterone, resulting in cervical softening and an increase in prostaglandin sensitivity, leading to contraction stimulation. Mifepristone is usually administered orally, and prescribing is limited to trained prescribers who also dispense the medication. It is contraindicated in patients with bleeding disorders or those on anticoagulants. It is a major substrate for CYP3A4, so medication interactions need to be considered.

- Misoprostol is a prostaglandin 1 analog that has good absorption when given vaginally, buccally, or sublingually resulting in cervical ripening and contractions. Oral administration is not recommended.

    ✓ Adverse medication effects of misoprostol include stomach upset, diarrhea, headache, dizziness, and fever. Mifepristone has a boxed warning regarding infection and excessive bleeding may occur and could be a sign of incomplete termination or other complications and needs prompt medical attention.

EVALUATION OF THERAPEUTIC OUTCOMES

- Monitor blood pressure annually in all CHC users.
- Monitor glucose levels closely when CHCs are started or stopped in individuals with a history of glucose intolerance or diabetes mellitus.
- Contraceptive users should have an annual exam that may include cytologic screening, and pelvic and breast examination. Regularly evaluate for problems that may relate to the CHCs (eg, breakthrough bleeding, amenorrhea, weight gain, and acne). These screenings do not have to occur before prescribing hormonal contraceptives.
- Monitor Nexplanon users annually for menstrual cycle disturbances, weight gain, local inflammation or infection at the implant site, acne, breast tenderness, headaches, and hair loss.
- Evaluate individuals using DMPA every 3 months for weight gain, menstrual cycle disturbances, and fractures.
- Monitor IUD users at 1- to 3-month intervals for proper IUD positioning, changes in menstrual bleeding patterns, and upper genital tract infection.
- Clinicians should monitor and when indicated screen for HIV and STIs. Counsel about healthy sexual practices, including the use of condoms to prevent transmission of STIs when necessary.

See Chapter 19, Contraception, authored by Shareen Y. El-Ibiary, for a more detailed discussion of this topic.

CHAPTER 31

Hormone Therapy

- *Perimenopause* begins with the onset of menstrual irregularity and ends 12 months after the last menstrual period, which marks the beginning of menopause. *Menopause* is the permanent cessation of menses caused by the loss of ovarian follicular activity. Females spend about 40% of their lives in postmenopause.
- Discussions around menopause and its treatment are primarily framed around cisgender women. However, any individual with a female reproductive system who has not undergone medical intervention may experience menopause. Therefore, the use of the term *female* is specifically meant to refer to biology.

PATHOPHYSIOLOGY

- The hypothalamic–pituitary–ovarian axis controls reproductive physiology. Follicle-stimulating hormone (FSH) and luteinizing hormone (LH), produced by the pituitary in response to gonadotropin-releasing hormone from the hypothalamus, regulate ovarian function. Gonadotropins are also influenced by negative feedback from the sex steroids estradiol (produced by the dominant follicle) and progesterone (produced by the corpus luteum). Other sex steroids are androgens, primarily testosterone and androstenedione, secreted by the ovarian stroma.
- As females age, circulating FSH progressively rises, and ovarian inhibin-B and anti-Mullerian hormone decline. In menopause, there is a 10- to 15-fold increase in circulating FSH, a 4- to 5-fold increase in LH, and a greater than 90% decrease in circulating estradiol concentrations.

CLINICAL PRESENTATION

- Symptoms of perimenopause and menopause include vasomotor symptoms (hot flushes and night sweats), sleep disturbances, depression, anxiety, poor concentration and memory, vaginal dryness and dyspareunia, headache, sexual dysfunction, and arthralgia. Individuals of different races/ethnicity experience vasomotor symptoms differently.
- Signs include urogenital atrophy in menopause and dysfunctional uterine bleeding in perimenopause. Rule out other potential causes of dysfunctional uterine bleeding.
- Additionally, loss of estrogen production results in metabolic changes; increase in central abdominal fat; and effects on lipids, vascular function, and bone metabolism.

DIAGNOSIS

- Menopause is determined retrospectively after 12 consecutive months of amenorrhea. FSH on day 2 or 3 of the menstrual cycle greater than 10–12 IU/L indicates diminished ovarian reserve.
- The diagnosis should include a comprehensive medical history and physical examination, complete blood count, and measurement of serum FSH. Altered thyroid function and pregnancy must be excluded.

TREATMENT

- <u>Goals of Treatment</u>: The goals are to relieve symptoms, improve quality of life, and minimize medication adverse effects.

NONPHARMACOLOGIC THERAPY

- Mild vasomotor and/or vaginal symptoms can often be alleviated by lowering the room temperature; decreasing intake of caffeine, spicy foods, and hot beverages; smoking cessation; exercise; and a healthy diet.
- Mild vulvovaginal symptoms may be adequately managed with nonhormonal lubricants and moisturizers.

PHARMACOLOGIC THERAPY

- Food and Drug Administration (FDA)-approved indications and contraindications for menopausal hormone therapy (MHT) are shown in Table 31-1. Figure 31-1 outlines the pharmacologic treatment of menopausal symptoms.
- The decision to use MHT and the type of formulation used must be individualized based on several factors, including personal preference, age, menopause onset, the severity of menopausal symptoms, and MHT-associated risks.
- MHT remains the most effective treatment for moderate and severe vasomotor symptoms, impaired sleep quality, and vulvovaginal symptoms of menopause.

TABLE 31-1	FDA-Approved Indications and Contraindications for Menopausal Hormone Therapy with Estrogens and Progestins
Indications	
For systemic use	Treatment of moderate-to-severe vasomotor symptoms (ie, moderate-to-severe hot flashes)
For intravaginal use (low systemic exposure)	Treatment of moderate-to-severe symptoms of vulvar and vaginal atrophy (ie, moderate-to-severe vaginal dryness, dyspareunia, and atrophic vaginitis)
Contraindications	
Absolute contraindications	Undiagnosed abnormal genital bleeding
	Known, suspected, or history of cancer of the breast
	Known or suspected estrogen- or progesterone-dependent neoplasia
	Active deep vein thrombosis, pulmonary embolism, or a history of these conditions
	Active or recent (eg, within the past year) arterial thromboembolic disease (eg, stroke, myocardial infarction)
	Liver dysfunction or disease
Relative contraindications	Elevated blood pressure
	Hypertriglyceridemia
	Impaired liver function and past history of cholestatic jaundice
	Hypothyroidism
	Fluid retention
	Severe hypocalcemia
	Ovarian cancer
	Exacerbation of endometriosis
	Exacerbation of asthma, diabetes mellitus, migraine, systemic lupus erythematosus, epilepsy, porphyria, and hepatic hemangioma

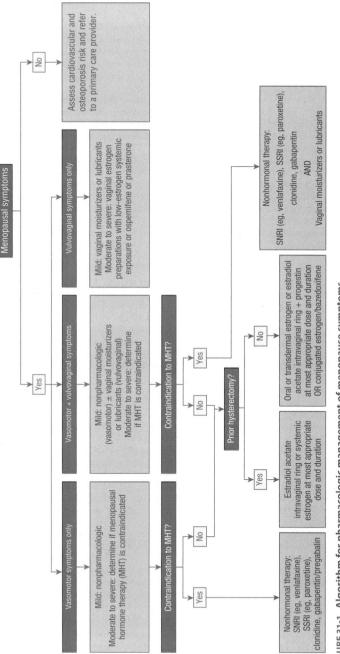

FIGURE 31-1. Algorithm for pharmacologic management of menopause symptoms.

Menopausal symptoms

No → Assess cardiovascular and osteoporosis risk and refer to a primary care provider.

Yes

Vasomotor symptoms only
- Mild: nonpharmacologic
- Moderate to severe: determine if menopausal hormone therapy (MHT) is contraindicated

Contraindication to MHT?
- No → Estradiol acetate intravaginal ring or systemic estrogen at most appropriate dose and duration
- Yes → Nonhormonal therapy: SNRI (eg, venlafaxine), SSRI (eg, paroxetine), clonidine, gabapentin/pregabalin

Vasomotor + vulvovaginal symptoms
- Mild: nonpharmacologic (vasomotor) ± vaginal moisturizers or lubricants (vulvovaginal)
- Moderate to severe: determine if MHT is contraindicated

Contraindication to MHT?
- No
- Yes

Prior hysterectomy?
- Yes → Estradiol acetate intravaginal ring or systemic estrogen at most appropriate dose and duration
- No → Oral or transdermal estrogen or estradiol acetate intravaginal ring + progestin at most appropriate dose and duration OR conjugated estrogen/bazedoxifene

(Contraindication to MHT? Yes) → Nonhormonal therapy: SNRI (eg, venlafaxine), SSRI (eg, paroxetine), clonidine, gabapentin AND Vaginal moisturizers or lubricants

Vulvovaginal symptoms only
- Mild: vaginal moisturizers or lubricants
- Moderate to severe: vaginal estrogen preparations with low-estrogen systemic exposure or ospemifene or prasterone

- Several national and international guidelines and consensus statements on menopause management are available.
- When urogenital symptoms, such as vaginal dryness and dyspareunia, are the only menopausal complaint, **intravaginal estrogen cream, tablet**, or **ring** should be considered before oral therapy. Intravaginal estrogen minimizes systemic absorption and is more effective for vaginal symptoms than oral therapy. **Ospemifene**, a selective estrogen receptor modulator, is another option. Intravaginal estrogen reduces the risk of recurrent urinary tract infections and may improve urge incontinence and overactive bladder.
- MHT is the most effective treatment for moderate-to-severe vasomotor symptoms, and impaired sleep quality. **Estrogen-only** therapy may decrease heart disease and all-cause mortality in 50- to 59-year-old females with a history of hysterectomy.
- MHT is effective and appropriate for prevention of osteoporosis-related fractures in recently menopausal individuals at risk.
- In patients with an intact uterus, MHT consists of an **estrogen plus a progestogen** or **estrogen agonist/antagonist** (eg, **bazedoxifene,** see Fig. 31-1). In patients who have undergone hysterectomy, estrogen therapy is given unopposed by a progestogen. Concomitant progestogen therapy is unnecessary when low-dose vaginal estrogen is used, with the exception of Femring, which delivers systemic estrogen.
- Individuals with vasomotor symptoms taking MHT have better mental health and fewer depressive symptoms compared with those receiving placebo, but MHT may worsen the quality of life in individuals without vasomotor symptoms.

Estrogens

- Estrogen products and doses for MHT are shown in Table 31-2. The oral and transdermal routes are used most frequently and are considered equally effective.
- **Conjugated equine estrogens** are composed of estrone sulfate (50%–60%) and other estrogens such as equilin and 17α-dihydroequilin.
- **Estradiol** is the predominant and most active form of endogenous estrogens. Given orally, it is metabolized by the intestinal mucosa and liver, and resultant estrone concentrations are three to six times those of estradiol.
- **Ethinyl estradiol** is a semisynthetic estrogen that has similar activity following oral or parenteral administration.
- **Nonoral estrogens**, including transdermal, intranasal, and vaginal products, avoid first-pass metabolism and result in a more physiologic estradiol:estrone ratio (ie, estradiol concentrations greater than estrone concentrations). Transdermal estrogen is also less likely to increase sex hormone–binding globulin, triglycerides, blood pressure, or C-reactive protein levels. Transdermal dosage forms may also have a lower risk for deep vein thrombosis, stroke, and myocardial infarction.
- Variability in absorption is common with percutaneous preparations (ie, gels, creams, and emulsions).
- **Vaginal creams**, **tablets**, and **rings** are used for treatment of urogenital atrophy. Most tablets and rings provide local estrogen, but Femring is designed to achieve systemic estrogen concentrations and is indicated for moderate-to-severe vasomotor symptoms.
- New evidence indicates that lower doses of estrogens are effective in controlling postmenopausal symptoms and reducing bone loss. Low-dose estrogen regimens include 0.3−0.45 mg conjugated estrogens, 0.5 mg micronized 17β-estradiol, and 0.014−0.0375 mg transdermal 17β-estradiol patch. Topical gels, creams, and sprays are also available in low doses. Lower doses typically have fewer adverse effects, and may have better benefit to risk profiles than standard doses. The lowest effective dose should be used.

  ✓ Adverse effects of estrogen include nausea, headache, breast tenderness, and heavy bleeding. More serious adverse effects include increased risk for stroke, venous thromboembolism (VTE), and gallbladder disease. Transdermal estrogen is less likely to cause breast tenderness, gallbladder disease, and deep vein thrombosis.

TABLE 31-2 FDA-Approved Estrogen Products for Menopausal Hormone Therapy

Medication	Brand Name[a]	Initial Dose/Low Dose	Usual Dose Range
Systemic Estrogen Products (for the treatment of moderate and severe vasomotor symptoms ± urogenital symptoms)			
Oral estrogens[b]			
Conjugated equine estrogens	Premarin	0.3 or 0.45 mg once daily	0.3–1.25 mg once daily
Esterified estrogens (75%–85% estrone + 6%–15% equilin)	Menest	0.3 mg once daily	0.3–1.25 mg once daily - Administer 3 weeks on and 1 week of
Micronized 17β-estradiol	Estrace Generics	1 mg once daily	1 or 2 mg once daily - Administer 3 weeks on and 1 week off
Transdermal estrogens patches			
17β-estradiol	Alora	0.025 mg/day (patch applied twice weekly)[c]	0.025–0.1 mg/day (patch applied twice weekly)[c]
	Climara	0.025 mg/day (patch applied once weekly)[c]	0.025–0.1 mg/day (patch applied once weekly)[c]
	Menostar	0.014 mg/day (patch applied once weekly)[c,d]	0.014 mg/day (patch applied once weekly)[c,d]
	Minivelle, Vivelle, Vivelle Dot	0.025 mg/day (patch applied twice weekly)[c]	0.025–0.1 mg/day, 0.05 is standard dose (patch applied twice weekly)[c]
Other topical forms of estrogen			
17β-estradiol topical emulsion	Estrasorb 0.25% emulsion	—	Two pouches once daily (which delivers 0.05 mg of estradiol per day)
17β-estradiol topical gel	EstroGel 0.06% metered-dose pump	—	1.25 g/day once daily (contains 0.75 mg estradiol)—Apply from wrist to shoulder
	Elestrin 0.06% metered-dose pump	—	1–2 unit doses once daily (1 unit dose: 0.87 g, which contains 0.52-mg estradiol)—Apply to upper arm

(Continued)

TABLE 31-2 FDA-Approved Estrogen Products for Menopausal Hormone Therapy (Continued)

Medication	Brand Name[a]	Initial Dose/Low Dose	Usual Dose Range
	Divigel 0.1% (topical once daily)	0.25 g once daily	0.25–1 g (provides 0.25–1 mg of estradiol)—Apply to upper thigh
17β-estradiol transdermal spray	Evamist	1 spray once daily	1–3 sprays once daily (1.53 mg of estradiol per spray)—Apply to inner surface of forearm
Vaginal estrogens			
Estradiol acetate vaginal ring	Femring	12.4 mg every 3 months	12.4-, 24.8-mg ring (delivers 0.05- or 0.1-mg estradiol/day)
Intravaginal Estrogen Products (for the treatment of urogenital symptoms only/low systemic exposure)			
Conjugated equine estrogens (CEE) vaginal cream	Premarin		0.5–2 g/day (contains 0.625 mg CEE per g)—Administer 21 days on and 7 days off
17β-estradiol vaginal cream	Estrace	500 mg to 1 gm daily for 2 weeks, then 500 mg to 1 gm one to three times weekly, or 2–4 g daily for 1 or 2 weeks then gradually reduced to ½ initial dosage for a similar period	Maintenance dose of 0.5–1 g, one to three times weekly
17β-estradiol vaginal ring	Estring	2 mg ring replaced every 90 days	2 mg ring (delivers 0.0075 mg/day) replaced every 90 days
17β-estradiol vaginal insert	Imvexxy	1 vaginal insert (4 mcg) daily for 2 weeks, then reduce to 1 insert twice weekly	4 or 10 mcg twice weekly, every 3–4 days
Estradiol hemihydrate vaginal tablet	Vagifem Yuvafem Generics	10 mcg once weekly for 2 weeks, then twice weekly	10 mcg twice weekly

aUS brand names.

bOrally administered estrogens stimulate synthesis of hepatic proteins and increase circulating concentrations of sex hormone-binding globulin, which in turn may compromise the bioavailability of androgens and estrogens. Patients with elevated triglyceride concentrations or significant liver function abnormalities are candidates for nonoral estrogen therapy.

cDo not apply estrogen patches on or near breasts. Avoid waistline as patch may rub off with tight-fitting clothing.

dFDA-approved for prevention of postmenopausal osteoporosis only.

✓ The Early versus Late Intervention Trial with Estradiol (ELITE) trial suggests that the benefits of hormone therapy are dependent on the timing of initiation. Hormone therapy may be cardioprotective if started around the time of menopause (within 6 years) and may be harmful when initiated in late postmenopause (after 10 years). MHT should not be initiated or continued solely for prevention of cardiovascular disease.

✓ Risk of VTE and stroke increases with oral MHT containing estrogen, but the absolute risk is low below 60 years of age. Transdermal MHT and low-dose oral estrogen therapy appear to have a lower risk of VTE and stroke compared to standard-dose oral estrogen regimens. The norpregnane progestogens also appear to be thrombogenic. MHT should be avoided in those at high risk for thromboembolic events (eg, those with Factor V Leiden mutation, obesity, or history of previous thromboembolic events).

✓ MHT is contraindicated in individuals with a personal history of breast cancer. The risk of MHT-related breast cancer appears to be associated with the addition of progestogen to estrogen after 3 years of combined use.

✓ Combined oral MHT does not increase endometrial cancer risk compared with placebo, but estrogen-alone given to individuals with an intact uterus significantly increases uterine cancer risk.

✓ Recent research now suggests that MHT is associated with an increased risk of ovarian cancer regardless of the type or the regimen used. More research is needed.

✓ Postmenopausal individuals 65 years or older taking estrogen plus progestogen therapy had twice the rate of dementia, including Alzheimer disease, than those taking placebo. Combined therapy did not prevent mild cognitive impairment. The estrogen-alone arm showed similar findings.

Progestogens

• In individuals who have not undergone hysterectomy, a **progestogen** or tissue-selective estrogen complex (estrogen/bazedoxifene) should be added for endometrial protection.

• Several progestogen regimens to prevent endometrial hyperplasia are shown in **Table 31-3**. **Combination estrogen–progestogen** regimens are shown in **Table 31-4**.

Methods of administration include the following:

• **Cyclic (Sequential) estrogen-progestogen** results in scheduled vaginal withdrawal bleeding in approximately 80%–90% of patients. The progestogen is administered 12−14 days of the 28-day cycle.

• **Continuous-combined estrogen-progestogen** causes endometrial atrophy but prevents monthly bleeding, which is preferable, although it may initially cause unpredictable spotting or bleeding. Use of conjugated equine estrogens (0.625 mg/day) plus medroxyprogesterone acetate (2.5 mg/day) lead to a decreased risk of endometrial cancer.

• **Intermittent-combined estrogen-progestogen (continuous pulsed)** consists of 3 days of estrogen therapy alone, followed by 3 days of combined estrogen and progestogen, repeated without interruption. It causes fewer adverse effects than regimens with higher progestogen doses and lowers the incidence of uterine bleeding.

✓ Adverse effects of progestogens include irritability, headache, mood swings, fluid retention, and sleep disturbance. See previous estrogen section for additional adverse effects associated with estrogen and progesterone in combination.

TABLE 31-3	Progestogen Dosing for Endometrial Protection (Cyclic Administration)
Progestogen	**Dosage**
Medroxyprogesterone acetate	5−10 mg/day for 12−14 days per calendar month
Micronized progesterone	200 mg/day for 12−14 days per calendar month
Norethindrone acetate	5 mg/day for 12−14 days per calendar month

TABLE 31-4	Common Combination Menopausal Hormone Therapy Regimens	
Regimen	**Brand name**	**Dosage**
Oral Regimens		
Conjugated equine estrogen (CEE) + medroxyprogesterone acetate (MPA)	Prempro (continuous)	0.625 mg CEE/2.5 mg MPA, 0.625 mg CEE/5 mg MPA daily
		Low-dose: 0.3 mg CEE/1.5 mg MPA, 0.45 mg CEE/1.5 mg MPA daily
	Premphase (continuous cyclic)	0.625 mg CEE daily only in the first 2 weeks of a 4-week cycle, then 0.625 mg daily, CEE + 5 mg MPA daily in the last 2 weeks of a 4-week cycle
Conjugated equine estrogen (CEE) + bazedoxifene	Duavee (continuous)	0.45/20 mg daily
Ethinyl estradiol (EE) + norethindrone acetate (NETA)	Generic, Femhrt (continuous)	Femhrt: 2.5 mcg EE/0.5 mg NETA daily
	Fayvolv (continuous)	Fyavolv: 2.5 mcg EE/0.5 mg NETA daily, 5 mcg EE/1 mg NETA daily
Estradiol (E) + drospirenone (DRSP)	Angeliq (continuous)	1 mg E/0.5 mg DRSP daily
		Low dose: 0.5 mg E/0.25 mg DRSP daily
Estradiol (E) + norgestimate	Prefest (estrogen/intermittent progestogen)	1 mg E daily for first 3 days, then 1 mg E/0.09 mg norgestimate daily for next 3 days; this pattern is repeated continuously
Estradiol (E) + norethindrone acetate (NETA)	Activella (continuous)	1 mg E/0.5 mg NETA daily
	Mimvey (continuous)	Low-dose: 0.5 mg E/0.1 mg NETA daily
	Mimvey Lo (continuous)	
	Amabelz (continuous)	
	Lopreeza (continuous)	
Estradiol (E) + progesterone	Bijuva (continuous)	1 mg E/100 mg progesterone daily
Transdermal Regimens		
Estradiol + norethindrone acetate patch	CombiPatch (continuous) CombiPatch (continuous cyclic)	Continuous: 0.05/0.14 mg, 0.05/0.25 mg (apply one patch twice weekly)
		Continuous cyclic: 0.05 mg of an estradiol-only patch (apply one patch twice weekly) in the first 2 weeks of a 4-week cycle, then either dose of the CombiPatch (apply one patch twice weekly) in the last 2 weeks of a 4-week cycle
Estradiol (E) + levonorgestrel patch	Climara Pro (continuous)	0.045 mg E/0.015 mg/day (apply 1 patch once weekly)

CEE, conjugated equine estrogen; DRSP, drospirenone; E, estradiol; EE, ethinyl estradiol; NETA, norethindrone acetate; MPA, medroxyprogesterone acetate.

Compounded Bioidentical Hormone Therapy (CBHT)

- CBHTs are hormone therapy formulations custom-prepared (ie, compounded) for individual patients, often involving the use of measuring and monitoring hormone levels in blood and/or other body fluids such as saliva. Hormones commonly used in CBHT include estrone, estradiol, estriol, progesterone, testosterone, DHEA, and thyroid hormone. Bioidentical hormones appear to carry the same risks as traditional hormone therapy products. Use is only recommended only when there is a medical need for an unusual dosing regimen or ingredients or when patients have allergies to FDA-approved therapies.

Estrogen Alternatives for the Treatment of Hot Flashes

- For those with contraindications to or who cannot tolerate estrogens and/or progestogens, other treatment options for hot flashes can be considered (Table 31-5). Some clinicians consider **selective serotonin reuptake inhibitors** (eg, paroxetine, fluoxetine, citalopram, escitalopram) or serotonin-norepinephrine reuptake inhibitors (eg, venlafaxine and desvenlafaxine) to be first-line agents. **Clonidine** can be effective, but adverse effects are often problematic (eg, sedation, dry mouth, hypotension). **Gabapentin** has beneficial effects for reducing the frequency and severity of vasomotor symptoms but adverse effects may limit dosing. It may be a reasonable option for those with disrupted sleep and hot flashes when administered in the evening.

Androgens

- **Testosterone** use is controversial, but use with or without estrogen, may improve the quality of the sexual experience in postmenopausal individuals.
- Absolute contraindications to androgen therapy include pregnancy or lactation and known or suspected androgen-dependent neoplasia.
  - ✓ Adverse effects include virilization, fluid retention, and adverse lipoprotein lipid effects, which are more likely with oral administration. Evidence on the efficacy and safety of testosterone in females is lacking.
- **Dehydroepiandrosterone** (DHEA) is a precursor hormone in the synthesis of estrone, estradiol, and testosterone. Intravaginal DHEA (Prasterone) has FDA approval for the treatment of moderate-to-severe dyspareunia at a dose of 6.5 mg once daily at bedtime, which does not appear to convey the same systemic risks seen from other oral hormonal products.

Selective Estrogen Receptor Modulators (SERMs)

- SERMs are nonsteroidal compounds that act as estrogen agonists in some tissues such as bone and as estrogen antagonists in other tissues such as breast through high-affinity binding to the estrogen receptor.
- **Tamoxifen** is an antagonist in breast tissue and an agonist on the bone and endometrium (see Chapter 61).
- **Raloxifene** is approved for prevention and treatment of postmenopausal osteoporosis and reduction in risk of invasive breast cancer. The dose is 60 mg once daily.
- The third-generation SERM, **bazedoxifene**, is used in conjunction with **conjugated estrogen**, and is FDA-approved for moderate-to-severe vasomotor symptoms and prevention of osteoporosis.
- **Ospemifene** is approved for moderate-to-severe dyspareunia from menopausal vulvar and vaginal atrophy. It has a boxed warning for increased risk of endometrial cancer in patients with a uterus who use ospemifene (an estrogen agonist in the endometrium) without a progestogen to reduce endometrial hyperplasia. It also has a boxed warning about the possible risk of stroke and VTE.
  - ✓ Depending on tissue selectively, the SERMs are associated with hot flashes and leg cramps. They can also increase the risk of VTE and stroke similar to oral estrogen, but the degree of risk is agent specific. Additional adverse effects of

TABLE 31-5 Alternatives to Estrogen for Treatment of Hot Flashes[a]

Medication	Brand Name[b]	Initial Dose	Usual Dose Range	Adverse Effects
Venlafaxine	Effexor, Effexor XR	37.5 mg	37.5–75 mg/day	Nausea, headache, somnolence, dizziness, insomnia, nervousness, xerostomia, anorexia, constipation, diaphoresis, weakness, and hypertension
Desvenlafaxine	Pristiq	50 mg	50–100 mg/day	Nausea, headache, somnolence, dizziness, insomnia, xerostomia, anorexia, constipation, diaphoresis, and weakness
Paroxetine[c]	Brisdelle,[d] Paxil, Paxil CR, Pexeva	7.5 mg/day (Brisdelle),[d] 10 mg/day (paroxetine), or 12.5 mg/day (paroxetine CR)	7.5 mg/day,[d] 10[d]–20 mg/day or 12.5–25 mg/day	Nausea, somnolence, insomnia, headache, dizziness, xerostomia, constipation, diarrhea, weakness, and diaphoresis
Citalopram		10 mg/day	10–20 mg/day	Drowsiness, insomnia, diaphoresis, nausea, xerostomia, dose-dependent QTc prolongation
Escitalopram		10 mg/day, start with 5 mg/day in sensitive or older individuals and titrate up	10–20 mg/day	Headache, insomnia, nausea, increased sweating, fatigue, and somnolence; decreased libido and anorgasmia
Clonidine patch	Catapres-TTS (transdermal)	0.1 mg/day (0.1 mg/24-hour period)	0.1 mg/day	Drowsiness, dizziness, hypotension, and dry mouth, especially with higher doses
Pregabalin	Lyrica	50 mg/day	75–150 mg twice/day	Drowsiness, dizziness, dry mouth, edema, blurred vision, weight gain, impaired concentration
Gabapentin	Gralise, Neurontin, generics	300 mg at bedtime	900 mg/day (divided in three daily doses), doses up to 2400 mg/day (divided in three daily doses) have been studied	Somnolence and dizziness; these symptoms often can be obviated with a gradual increase in dosing

[a]Treatment of postmenopausal hot flashes is an off-label indication in the United States for all medications listed except for one formulation of paroxetine (paroxetine mesylate).
[b]US brand names.
[c]Other selective serotonin reuptake inhibitors (eg, citalopram, escitalopram, fluoxetine, and sertraline) have also been studied and may be used for the treatment of hot flashes.
[d]The brand Brisdelle contains 7.5 mg of paroxetine and is FDA-approved to treat moderate-to-severe vasomotor symptoms of menopause. This specific product is not FDA-approved for treating psychiatric conditions.

bazedoxifene include muscle spasms, nausea, diarrhea, dyspepsia, upper abdominal pain, oropharyngeal pain, dizziness, and neck pain. Adverse effects of ospemifene include hot flashes, vaginal discharge, muscle spasm, genital discharge, and hyperhidrosis.

Complementary and Alternative Agents

- **Phytoestrogens** are plant compounds with estrogen-like biologic activity and relatively weak estrogen receptor-binding properties, resulting in physiologic effects in humans.
- Although some data support their use, clarity regarding, dosing, biological activity, safety, and efficacy is needed before they can be considered as an alternative to MHT in postmenopause.

  ✓ Common adverse effects include constipation, bloating, and nausea.

- Other herbals and alternative treatments that may be used include **black cohosh, dong quai, red clover leaf** (contains phytoestrogens), and **ginseng**. Complementary and alternative therapies should not be recommended to treat menopausal symptoms as their efficacy and safety have not been completely established.

EVALUATION OF THERAPEUTIC OUTCOMES

- Management of patients taking hormone therapy is summarized in Table 31-6.
- In order to adequately assess treatment effect, individuals should be encouraged to continue their MHT regimen for at least 1 month with dosages being modified to balance adverse effects and efficacy. Those receiving MHT should be seen annually for monitoring.
- Many individuals have no difficulty stopping MHT, while some develop vasomotor symptoms after discontinuation, regardless of discontinuation rate (ie, gradual or sudden withdrawal).

| TABLE 31-6 | Management of Patients Taking Hormone Therapy Regimens |

Initiation of Hormone Therapy

Hormone therapy should be used only as long as vasomotor symptom control is necessary.

Six-Week Follow-up Visit

To discuss patient concerns about hormone therapy.

To evaluate the patient for symptom relief, adverse effects, and patterns of withdrawal bleeding (if continuous sequential hormone therapy is given).

Medication	Common Adverse Medication Effects	Monitoring Parameter	Suggested Change
Estrogen		Persistence of hot flashes	Increase estrogen dose.
Estrogen	Breast tenderness		Reduce estrogen dose; switch to a transdermal regimen.
Progestogen	Bloating Premenstrual-like symptoms		Switch to another progestogen or bazedoxifene.
			(Continued)

TABLE 31-6	Management of Patients Taking Hormone Therapy Regimens (*Continued*)

Annual Follow-up Visit

Annual monitoring: Medical history, physical examination (including pelvic examination), blood pressure measurement, and routine endometrial cancer surveillance (as indicated). Additional follow-up is determined based on the patient's initial response to therapy and the need for any modification of the regimen.

Breast examinations: Annual mammograms (scheduled based on patient's age and risk factors).

Osteoporosis prevention: BMD should be measured in those 65 years and older and in those younger than 65 years with risk factors for osteoporosis. Repeat testing should be performed as clinically indicated.

For sequential hormone therapy	Transvaginal ultrasound and where indicated an endometrial biopsy should be performed if vaginal bleeding occurs at any time other than the expected time of withdrawal bleeding or when heavier or more prolonged withdrawal bleeding occurs (if endometrial pathology cannot be excluded by endovaginal ultrasonography, further evaluation may be required, such as hysteroscopy).
For continuous combined hormone therapy	Endometrial evaluation should be considered when irregular bleeding persists for more than 6 months after initiating therapy.

BMD, bone mineral density.

See Chapter 102, Post Menopausal Hormone Therapy, authored by Devra K. Dang and Judy T. Chen, for a more detailed discussion of this topic.

CHAPTER 32

Pregnancy and Lactation

- Resources on the use of *medications in pregnancy and lactation* include the Food and Drug Administration (FDA) product labeling, the primary literature, tertiary compendia, textbooks, and computerized databases (eg, www.motherisk.org and www.toxnet.nlm.nih.gov).
- The American College of Obstetricians and Gynecologists (ACOG) and the International Lactation Consultants Association recommend the use of nongendered terms to be more inclusive of transgender individuals. All included gendered terms refer to biological sex and not gender.

PREGNANCY PHYSIOLOGY

PREGNANCY PHYSIOLOGY

- The duration of pregnancy is approximately 280 days (measured from the first day of the last menstrual period to birth). Pregnancy is divided into three periods of three calendar months (ie, trimesters).
- Medication absorption during pregnancy may be altered by delayed gastric emptying and vomiting, and increased gastric pH may affect absorption of weak acids and bases. Hepatic perfusion increases during pregnancy and higher estrogen and progesterone levels may alter liver enzyme activity and increase elimination of some medications or cause accumulation of others.
- In pregnant individuals, increases are seen in plasma volume (50%), cardiac output (30%–50%), and glomerular filtration (50%–80%) possibly lowering the plasma concentration of renally cleared medications. Body fat increases; thus, the volume of distribution of fat-soluble medications may increase. Plasma albumin concentrations decrease; thus, the volume of distribution of highly protein-bound medications may increase. However, there may be little change in serum concentration, as these unbound medications are more rapidly cleared by the liver and kidneys.
- The placenta is the organ of exchange for medications between the fetus and the pregnant individual. Those with molecular weights less than 500 Dalton (Da) transfer readily, those weighing 600–1000 Da cross more slowly, and those with molecular weights greater than 1000 Da (eg, insulin and heparin) do not cross in significant amounts.
- Lipophilic medications (eg, opiates and antibiotics) cross more easily than do water-soluble ones. Certain protein-bound medications may achieve higher plasma concentrations in the fetus than in the pregnant individual.

MEDICATION SELECTION DURING PREGNANCY

- The incidence of congenital malformation is approximately 3%–5%, with less than 1% of all birth defects caused by medication exposure.
- Principles for medication use during pregnancy include: (1) selecting those with strong safety data; (2) prescribing doses at the lower end of the range; (3) eliminating nonessential medication and discouraging self-medication; and (4) avoiding medications known to be harmful.
- Medication adverse effects on the fetus depend on dosage, route of administration, and stage of pregnancy when the exposure occurred.
- Fetal exposure to a teratogen in the first 2 weeks after conception may have an "all or nothing" effect (ie, could destroy the embryo or have no ill effect). Exposure during organogenesis (18–60 days postconception) may cause structural anomalies (eg, **methotrexate, cyclophosphamide, diethylstilbestrol, lithium, retinoids, thalidomide**, some **antiseizure medications [ASMs]**, and **coumarin derivatives**).
- Exposure after this point may result in growth retardation, central nervous system (CNS) or other abnormalities, or death. **Nonsteroidal anti-inflammatory drugs**

335

(NSAIDs) and **tetracycline derivatives** are more likely to exhibit effects in the second or third trimester.

- Also consider other factors that can influence pregnancy outcomes, such as exposure to tobacco, alcohol, recreational substances, environmental factors, and infection and uncontrolled disease states in the pregnant individual, as these are not always accounted for in literature and each can impact pregnancy outcomes.

PRECONCEPTION PLANNING

- **Folic acid** supplementation of at least 0.4 mg daily is recommended throughout the reproductive years to reduce the risk for neural tube defects (NTDs) in offspring. Folic acid 4 mg daily starting 3 months prior to conception and continued until 12-week gestation is recommended for those at high risk for NTDs, which includes those with a personal, partner, or previous pregnancy history of NTDs.
- Reduced alcohol, tobacco, and other substance use prior to pregnancy improve outcomes. For smoking cessation, behavioral interventions are preferred. Pharmacotherapy for smoking cessation may be effective but should be closely monitored as safety data is limited.

ACUTE PREGNANCY ISSUES

GASTROINTESTINAL TRACT

- Constipation commonly occurs during pregnancy. Institute education, physical exercise, and increased intake of dietary fiber and fluid. If additional therapy is warranted, give **supplemental fiber** and/or a stool softener. **Polyethylene glycol**, **lactulose**, and **sorbitol**, can be used intermittently. **Senna** and **bisacodyl** can also be used occasionally. Magnesium and sodium salts can cause electrolyte imbalance. Avoid **castor oil** and **mineral oil**.
- Therapy for gastroesophageal reflux disease includes nonpharmacologic therapy with lifestyle and dietary modifications (ie, small, frequent meals; alcohol, tobacco, and caffeine avoidance; food avoidance before bedtime; and elevation of the head of the bed) alone or with medication therapy. If necessary, initiate **aluminum**, **calcium**, or **magnesium antacids**; **sucralfate**; **cimetidine**; or **ranitidine**. Proton pump inhibitors are options if response to histamine 2 (H_2)–receptor blockers is inadequate. Avoid **sodium bicarbonate** and **magnesium trisilicate**.
- Therapy for hemorrhoids includes high intake of dietary fiber, adequate oral fluid intake, and use of sitz baths. If response is inadequate, laxatives and stool softeners can be used. Topical anesthetics, skin protectants, and astringents may help irritation and pain. Topical hydrocortisone may reduce inflammation and pruritus.
- Nonpharmacologic treatments for nausea and vomiting are the same as for reflux as well as acupressure and trigger avoidance. Pharmacotherapy may include ginger, antihistamines (eg, **doxylamine**), and **pyridoxine**. The ACOG considers pyridoxine alone or in combination with doxylamine to be first line. Second-line therapies include dimenhydrinate, diphenhydramine, prochlorperazine, and promethazine and third-line options are metoclopramide, ondansetron, and trimethobenzamide. Metoclopramide and phenothiazines may cause sedation and extrapyramidal effects and **ondansetron** may cause oral clefts.
- **Corticosteroids** may be effective for hyperemesis gravidarum (ie, severe nausea and vomiting causing weight loss >5% of prepregnancy weight, dehydration, and ketonuria), but are reserved until after 10 weeks due to the risk of oral clefts.

DIABETES IN PREGNANCY

- All pregnant individuals, not previously diagnosed with type 1 or 2 diabetes should be screened between 24 and 48 weeks gestation. Those considered at high risk should be screened early in pregnancy at the first visit.

- Table 32-1 summarizes the screening and diagnosis of gestational diabetes mellitus (GDM) using a two-step approach.
- First-line therapy for GDM includes exercise, dietary modification, and caloric restrictions for obese individuals. Daily self-monitoring of blood glucose is required. If lifestyle interventions fail to achieve glycemic control, medication therapy is indicated under the following parameters: fasting glucose concentrations consistently greater than 95 mg/dL, 1-hour postprandial concentrations consistently greater than 140 mg/dL, or 2-hour postprandial concentrations consistently greater than 120 mg/dL. **Human insulin** is the first-line choice for diabetes management during pregnancy, as it does not cross the placenta. **Glyburide** and **metformin** are alternatives, but long-term safety data are limited and they may not be as effective as insulin.
- Screening with a 2-hour oral glucose tolerance test (OGTT) between 4 and 12 weeks postpartum is recommended for those diagnosed with GDM to diagnose type 2 diabetes not recognized prior to pregnancy.

HYPERTENSION (HTN)

- Hypertensive disorders of pregnancy (HDP) include: (1) chronic HTN; pre-existing HTN or developing before 20 weeks of gestation; (2) gestational HTN (HTN without proteinuria developing after 20 weeks of gestation); (3) preeclampsia (HTN with proteinuria) with gestational HTN; may present as the first symptoms of HTN disorder during pregnancy; and (4) chronic HTN with superimposed preeclampsia.
- Eclampsia, a medical emergency, is preeclampsia with seizures. HTN in pregnancy is either systolic blood pressure (SBP) above 140 mm Hg or diastolic blood pressure (DBP) above 90 mm Hg based on two or more measurements at least 4 hours apart. Severe HTN is two measurements of SBP >160 mm Hg and/or DBP >110 mm Hg at least 15 minutes apart.

TABLE 32-1	Screening and Diagnosis of Gestational Diabetes Mellitus
One-Step Method	
Complete a 75-g OGTT. Plasma glucose is assessed at fasting, and after 1 and 2 hours. The test should be performed in the morning following an overnight fast of at least 8 hours.	GDM diagnosis is confirmed when one or more of the plasma glucose levels are met or exceeded: Fasting: 92 mg/dL 1 hour: 180 mg/dL 2 hour: 153 mg/dL
Two-Step Method	
Step 1: Complete a 50-g oral glucose loading test. This is typically completed nonfasting. Plasma glucose is assessed after 1 hour.	If the plasma glucose level is greater than or equal to 140 mg/dL[a], the patient moves to step 2.
Step 2: Complete a 100-g OGTT. Plasma glucose is assessed at fasting, after 1, 2, and 3 hours.	GDM diagnosis is confirmed when at least two of the following plasma glucose levels are met or exceeded: Fasting: 95 mg/dL 1 hour: 180 mg/dL 2 hour: 155 mg/dL 3 hour: 140 mg/dL

GDM, gestational diabetes mellitus; OGTT, oral glucose tolerance test.
[a]A lower threshold of 130 or 135 mg/dL may be utilized by some providers; the American Diabetes Association recommends 140 mg/dL.

- Nonpharmacologic management of HDP includes stress reduction and light exercise or activity restriction. Exercise >50 minutes 3 days a week can reduce the incidence of HTN threefold over individuals who are more sedentary.
- For those at risk for preeclampsia, **aspirin** (81–162 mg/day) beginning weeks 12–28 of gestation reduces the risk for preeclampsia. Aspirin also reduces the risk of preterm birth, intrauterine growth restriction, and perinatal mortality.
- **Magnesium sulfate** started during active labor and continued 12–24 hours postpartum decreases the risk of progression to eclampsia and also treats eclamptic seizures. **Benzodiazepines** and **phenytoin** could be considered in those with contraindications to magnesium.
- Pharmacologic therapy for HTN is recommended once the patient has persistent blood pressures greater or equal to 160 mm Hg and/or DBP 110 mm Hg. Chronic HTN can cause complications in the pregnant individual, fetal growth restriction, and hospital admission.
- When antihypertensive therapy is used, maintenance of SBP between 120 and 160 mm Hg and DBP between 80 and 105 mm Hg is recommended. If there is no evidence of end-organ damage, and SBP is below 160 mm Hg and DBP is below 105 mm Hg, pharmacologic therapy is not suggested.
- Severe HTN in pregnancy requires treatment, and lowering of BP should occur over a period of hours to prevent compromise of uteroplacental blood flow. Recommended agents are **labetalol** and **nifedipine**. Labetalol may be limited due to its potential for bronchoconstriction and nifedipine needs to be dosed twice a day. **Hydrochlorothiazine** is considered second or third line. **Clonidine** and **prazosin** use is generally reserved for patients being closely followed by a medical specialist. **Atenolol, angiotensin-converting enzyme inhibitors, angiotensin receptor blockers, renin inhibitors,** and **mineralocorticoid receptor antagonists** are not recommended. Limited evidence supports the use of **magnesium sulfate,** except when it is being used concomitantly for preeclampsia. Intravenous **labetalol,** intravenous or intramuscular **hydralazine,** or immediate-release oral nifedipine should be reserved for severe HTN needing urgent blood pressure control.

THYROID DISORDERS

- Gestational transient thyrotoxicosis may occur but antithyroid medication is usually not needed.
- For hypothyroidism in pregnancy, initiate **levothyroxine** 0.1 mg/day. Those receiving thyroid replacement therapy before pregnancy may require increased dosage during pregnancy. Monitor thyroid-stimulating hormone (TSH) levels every 4–6 weeks during pregnancy to allow for dose titration according to TSH levels.
- Hyperthyroidism therapy includes thioamides (eg, **methimazole, propylthiouracil**). The goal of therapy is to attain free thyroxine concentrations near the upper limit of normal.

THROMBOEMBOLIC DISORDERS

- For treatment and prophylaxis of acute venous thromboembolism (VTE) during pregnancy, **low-molecular-weight heparin (LMWH)** is preferred over **unfractionated heparin** or **warfarin**. Continue treatment throughout pregnancy and for 6 weeks after delivery. The duration of therapy should be not less than 3 months. Consider **fondaparinux** if heparin cannot be used. **Dabigatran, rivaroxaban, and apixaban** are not recommended due to limited data. Avoid **warfarin** because it may cause fetal bleeding, nasal hypoplasia, stippled epiphyses, or CNS anomalies.
- For individuals at intermediate or high risk for recurrent VTE, provide antepartum therapy with LMWH or heparin plus 6-week postpartum therapy with LMWH or warfarin. For individuals with prosthetic heart valves, thrombophilias, and those at very high risk for VTE, consult current guidelines.

ACUTE CARE ISSUES IN PREGNANCY

HEADACHE

- For tension and migraine headaches during pregnancy, first-line therapies are non-pharmacologic, including relaxation, stress management, and biofeedback.
- For tension headaches, **acetaminophen** is the treatment of choice. All **NSAIDs** and **aspirin** are not recommended and contraindicated after 20 weeks of gestation due to their inhibition of prostaglandins. Antiemetics may be used in those with nausea and vomiting. **Opioids** are rarely used.
- For migraine headaches, acetaminophen and antiemetics (ie, promethazine, prochlorperazine, and metoclopramide) are commonly used. Opioids have been used, but they can contribute to nausea, and long-term use can cause neonatal withdrawal. For nonresponsive migraines, **triptans** (ie, sumatriptan) can be used. **Ergotamine** and **dihydroergotamine** are contraindicated.
- For pregnant individuals with severe headaches (usually migraine) not responsive to other treatments, **propranolol**, at the lowest effective dose, can be used as a preventive treatment. Alternatives include **amitriptyline** or **nortriptyline**, 10–25 mg daily by mouth.

URINARY TRACT INFECTION

- The principal infecting organism is *Escherichia coli*. Untreated bacteriuria may result in pyelonephritis, preterm birth, and low birth weight.
- Treatment of asymptomatic bacteriuria is necessary to reduce the risk of pyelonephritis and premature delivery. Treatment of asymptomatic bacteriuria and cystitis for 3–7 days is common.
- The most commonly used antibiotics for asymptomatic bacteriuria and cystitis are the β-lactams (penicillins and cephalosporins) and nitrofurantoin. *E. coli* resistance to ampicillin and amoxicillin is problematic. **Nitrofurantoin** is not active against *Proteus* and should not be used after week 37 in patients with glucose-6-phosphate dehydrogenase deficiency due to concern for hemolytic anemia in the newborn. **Sulfa-containing medications** may increase the risk for kernicterus in the newborn and should be avoided during the last weeks of gestation. **Folate antagonists**, such as **trimethoprim**, are relatively contraindicated during the first trimester because of their association with cardiovascular malformations. Regionally, increased rates of *E. coli* resistance to trimethoprim-sulfa limit its use. Single-dose **fosfomycin** may also be considered. **Fluoroquinolones** and **tetracyclines** are contraindicated.
- Inpatient therapy for pyelonephritis includes parenteral administration of broad spectrum beta-lactam antibiotics, (eg, **cefazolin, ceftriaxone, cefuroxime, ampicillin plus gentamicin**) as preferred treatment. Switching to oral antibiotics can occur after the patient is afebrile for 48 hours, but avoid nitrofurantoin, fosfomycin, and fluroquinolines. The total duration of antibiotic therapy for pyelonephritis is 7–14 days.

SEXUALLY TRANSMITTED INFECTIONS (STIs)

- Pharmacotherapy for selected STIs is shown in Table 32-2.
- Screening for STIs should occur at the first prenatal visit, with selected repeat testing for some diseases.
- *Chlamydia trachomatis* infection can be transmitted at birth to the neonate and cause conjunctivitis and a subacute, afebrile pneumonia.
- **Benzathine penicillin G** is the medication of choice for all stages of syphilis except neurosyphilis, which is treated with **aqueous penicillin G**. Penicillin is effective for preventing transmission to the fetus and treating the already infected fetus.
- *Neisseria gonorrhoeae* symptoms in the neonate (eg, rhinitis, vaginitis, urethritis, ophthalmia neonatorum, and sepsis) usually start 2–5 days of age. Blindness can occur, thus all neonates receive ocular erythromycin ointment as prophylaxis within 24 hours after delivery. Coinfection with *Chlamydia* is common, so usually treatment of gonorrhea includes treatment for *Chlamydia*.

TABLE 32-2	Management of STIs in Pregnancy	
STI	**Recommended Therapy**	**Alternative Therapy**
Bacterial vaginosis	• Metronidazole 500 mg by mouth twice daily for 7 days • Metronidazole 0.75% gel 5 g intravaginally once daily for 5 days • Clindamycin 2% cream 5 g intravaginally at bedtime for 7 days	• Clindamycin 300 mg by mouth twice daily for 7 days • Clindamycin ovules 100 mg intravaginally at bedtime for 3 days
Chlamydia	• Azithromycin 1 g by mouth for 1 dose	• Amoxicillin 500 mg by mouth three times a day for 7 days
Genital herpes	• Acyclovir 400 mg by mouth three times a day • Valacyclovir 500 mg by mouth twice daily	
Gonorrhea	• Ceftriaxone 500 mg IM for 1 dose; if chlamydia has not been excluded, treat for chlamydia as well	• Consult with infectious disease specialists or STI clinical expert if patient has a cephalosporin allergy or other reasons to not use the preferred treatment.
Syphilis[a]		
Primary, secondary, early latent	• Benzathine penicillin G 2.4 million units IM for 1 dose; a second dose can be given 1 week after initial dose to help reduce the risk for congenital syphilis	
Tertiary[b], late latent[c]	• Benzathine penicillin G 2.4 million units IM for 3 doses at 1-week intervals	
Neurosyphilis, ocular syphilis, otosyphilis	• Aqueous crystalline penicillin G 3–4 million units IV every 4 hours or 18–24 million units IV continuously for 10–14 days	• Procaine penicillin 2.4 million units IM daily for 10–14 day PLUS Probenecid 500 mg by mouth four times daily for 10–14 days
Trichomoniasis	• Metronidazole 500 mg by mouth twice daily for 7 days	

CSF, cerebrospinal fluid; g, grams; IM, intramuscular; IV, intravenous; mg, milligrams; STI, sexually transmitted infection.
[a] Pregnant individuals with history of penicillin allergy should undergo penicillin desensitization as no proven alternatives exist.
[b] With normal cerebrospinal fluid examination.
[c] If a patient misses a dose (ie, greater than 9 days between doses), series needs to be restarted.

- The overriding concern with genital herpes is transmission of the virus to the neonate during birth. Both **acyclovir** and **valacyclovir** are recommended as therapy; however, they require more frequent dosing due to increased renal elimination.
- Bacterial vaginosis is caused by anaerobic bacteria, mycoplasmas, and *Gardnerella vaginalis,* but is not an STI. Untreated it is a risk factor for premature rupture of membranes, preterm labor, preterm birth, intra-amniotic infection, and postpartum endometritis.
- Trichomoniasis is associated with an increased risk of premature rupture of membranes, premature delivery, and low birth weight. Treatment may prevent respiratory or genital infection in the neonate.

CHRONIC ILLNESSES IN PREGNANCY

ALLERGIC RHINITIS AND ASTHMA

- Diagnosis and staging of asthma during pregnancy is the same as in nonpregnant individuals, but more frequent follow-up is necessary. The risks of medication use to the fetus are lower than the risks of untreated asthma.
- **Inhaled corticosteroids** should be continued for those planning to become or are currently pregnant, as these reduce risk for exacerbations. Step down therapy should be a low priority until the patient is postpartum. All pregnant patients with asthma should have access to a short-acting inhaled β_2-agonist (**albuterol** is the preferred agent). Long-acting β_2-agonists are safe. **Cromolyn, leukotriene receptor antagonists**, and **theophylline** are considered alternative agents, but they are not preferred. For patients with the most severe disease, systemic corticosteroids are recommended.
- First-line medications for allergic rhinitis during pregnancy include **intranasal corticosteroids, nasal cromolyn**, and first-generation antihistamines (eg, **chlorpheniramine, diphenhydramine**, and **hydroxyzine**). Intranasal corticosteroids are the most effective treatment and have a low risk for systemic effect. **Beclomethasone** and **budesonide** have been used most. **Loratadine** and **cetirizine** do not appear to increase fetal risk, but they have not been extensively studied.
- Immunotherapy is not contraindicated, but should not be initiated for the first time in pregnancy due to anaphylaxis.

EPILEPSY

- Major malformations are two to three times more likely in children born to individuals taking antiseizure medications (ASMs) than to those who do not, but the risks of untreated epilepsy to the fetus are considered to be greater than those associated with the ASMs.
- ASM monotherapy is recommended. When possible, avoid **valproic acid, phenytoin, carbamazepine, phenobarbital**, and polytherapy during the first trimester; however, if used, the lowest effective dose should be taken. **Topiramate** and **zonisamide** have been associated with lower birth weights and length.
- Pharmacologic therapy should be optimized prior to conception. If medication withdrawal is planned, it should be fully completed prior to conception.
- Experts recommend supplemental folic acid, 0.4–4 mg daily, starting before pregnancy and continuing through at least the first trimester and preferably through the entire pregnancy for those receiving ASMs.

HUMAN IMMUNODEFICIENCY VIRUS (HIV) INFECTION

- In individuals newly diagnosed with HIV, or who have not previously received **antiretroviral therapy** (ART), it should be initiated as soon as pregnancy is determined, since risk of perinatal transmission is lower with earlier viral suppression. ART therapy is selected from those recommended for nonpregnant adults (with consideration given to the teratogenic profiles of each medication). Individuals already taking ART therapy should continue their regimen provided that viral suppression below the level of detection is documented.

- Recommendations regarding combination ART change frequently and the most recent clinical guidelines can be found at https://aidsinfo.nih.gov.
- Pregnant individuals with HIV RNA levels above 1000 copies/mL (1000 × 10^3/L) approaching delivery should have a cesarean section at 38 weeks of gestation to reduce the risk of perinatal HIV transmission. Cesarean section is not recommended if HIV RNA levels are at or below that level. If the viral load is greater than that level or unknown, IV zidovudine should be initiated with a 1-hour load (2 mg/kg) followed by a continuous infusion (1 mg/kg/h) for 2 hours (cesarean) with a minimum of 3 hours total. Those with a viral load at or below 1000 copies/mL (1000 × 10^3/L) near delivery do not require zidovudine IV, but should continue their ART.

DEPRESSION

- Symptoms of depression are often overlooked as they overlap with pregnancy symptoms. All patients should be screened prenatally and postpartum. Antidepressants should be used at the lowest possible dose for the shortest possible time to minimize adverse outcomes. Monotherapy is preferred over polytherapy even if higher doses are required.
- The risks and benefits of antidepressant use during pregnancy and the risks of untreated depression must be discussed with all patients in order to increase understanding.
- The **selective serotonin reuptake inhibitors (SSRIs)** are not considered major teratogens; however, paroxetine has been associated with cardiovascular malformations in the fetus. The **serotonin/norepinephrine reuptake inhibitors (SNRIs)** are less well defined. The use of SSRIs and SNRIs in the latter part of pregnancy is associated with persistent pulmonary HTN of the newborn and poor neonatal adaptation syndrome, which is usually mild. **Second-generation antipsychotics** can be used for treatment-resistant depression, but they can cause weight gain, gestational diabetes, and metabolic syndrome which have implications for poorer obstetric outcomes. **Tricyclic antidepressants** are not considered major teratogens but have been associated with neonatal withdrawal syndrome when used late in pregnancy. **Buspirone** can be used for anxiety symptoms, as **benzodiazepine** use is not recommended.

LABOR AND DELIVERY

PRETERM LABOR

- Preterm labor is labor that occurs before 37 weeks of gestation when changes in cervical dilations and/or effacement happen along with regular uterine contractions or when the initial presentation includes regular contractions and cervical dilation of at least 2 cm.

Tocolytic Therapy

- Tocolytic therapy is used to postpone delivery long enough to allow for maximum effect of antenatal steroids, for transportation of the mother to a facility equipped to deal with high-risk deliveries, and to prolong pregnancy when there are underlying self-limited conditions that can cause labor. Tocolytics can be started when there are regular uterine contractions with cervical change. They are not generally used before neonatal viability or beyond 34 weeks of gestation.
- There are four classes of tocolytics in the United States: **β-agonists**, **magnesium sulfate**, **NSAIDs**, and **calcium channel blockers**. Prolongation of pregnancy with tocolytics is not associated with significant reduction in rates of respiratory distress syndrome, neonatal death, or birth before 37 weeks of gestation.
- The β-Agonist **terbutaline** has a higher risk for adverse medication effects for the pregnant individual. A common dose of terbutaline is 250 mcg subcutaneously which may be repeated in 15–30 minutes for inadequate response, with a maximum of 500 mcg given in a 4-hour period.
  - ✓ An FDA black box warning cautions against oral dosing or prolonged parenteral use (beyond 48–72 hours) because of cardiotoxicity and death for the pregnant individual.

- Intravenous **magnesium sulfate** is primarily used for fetal neuroprotection and reducing the incidence of cerebral palsy. It may need to be used in combination with another short-term tocolytic if the patient still experiences short-term labor.
  - ✓ Adverse effects are common in the pregnant patient and include a general feeling of warmth, flushing, diaphoresis, nausea, loss of deep tendon reflexes, and respiratory depression.
- **Nifedipine** is associated with fewer adverse medication effects than magnesium or β-agonist therapy and decreases risk of delivery within 7 days compared to β-agonist.
  - ✓ It can cause dizziness, flushing, and hypotension.
- **Indomethacin** is the preferred agent in patients receiving magnesium sulfate. It can be dosed 50–100 mg orally or rectally, followed by 25–50 mg orally every 6 hours for 48 hours has been used.
  - ✓ Premature constriction of the ductus arteriosus has been reported.

Antenatal Glucocorticoids

- Antenatal **corticosteroids** are used for fetal lung maturation to prevent respiratory distress syndrome, intraventricular hemorrhage, and infant mortality in those delivered prematurely.
- Current recommendations are **betamethasone**, 12 mg IM every 24 hours for two doses, or **dexamethasone**, 6 mg IM every 12 hours for four doses, to pregnant individuals between 24 and 34 weeks of gestation who are at risk for preterm delivery within the next 7 days. Benefits from antenatal glucocorticoid administration are believed to begin within 24 hours.

GROUP B *STREPTOCOCCUS* INFECTION

- Prenatal screening (vaginal/rectal cultures) for group B *Streptococcus* colonization of all pregnant individuals at 36–38 weeks of gestation is recommended. Antibiotics are given if cultures are positive, or if the patient had a previous infant with invasive group B *Streptococcus* disease, or had group B *Streptococcus* bacteriuria.
- The currently recommended regimen for group B *Streptococcus* disease is **penicillin G** and is given IV every 4 hours until delivery. Alternatives include **ampicillin** IV every 4 hours; **cefazolin** every 8 hours; **clindamycin** IV every 8 hours; or **erythromycin** every 6 hours. In penicillin-allergic individuals in whom sensitivity testing shows resistance to clindamycin and erythromycin, **vancomycin** IV every 8 hours until delivery, can be used.

CERVICAL RIPENING AND LABOR INDUCTION

- Prostaglandin E$_2$ analogues (eg, **dinoprostone** [Prepidil Gel and Cervidil Vaginal Insert]) are commonly used for cervical ripening. Fetal heart rate monitoring is required when Cervidil Vaginal Insert is used and for 15 minutes after its removal. **Misoprostol**, a prostaglandin E$_1$ analogue, is effective and inexpensive that can be administered intravaginally, orally, sublingually, and buccally.
  - ✓ It has been associated with uterine hyperstimulation, meconium-stained amniotic fluid, and uterine rupture.
- **Oxytocin** is the most commonly used agent for labor induction after cervical ripening.

LABOR ANALGESIA

- Massage, water immersion during the first stage of labor, acupuncture, relaxation, and hypnotherapy have all been utilized for pain management during pregnancy. Additionally, the use of visualization and breathing techniques, yoga postures, massage, acupressure, and facilitated partner support leads to more vaginal deliveries and reduced epidural use.
- The IV or IM administration of opioids (ie, **fentanyl, morphine, butorphanol**) are commonly used for pain associated with labor. They are less effective than epidural analgesia, and possibly produce less pain response.

- Epidural analgesia involves administering an opioid and/or an anaesthetic (eg, **fentanyl** and/or **bupivacaine**) through a catheter into the epidural space to provide pain relief. Patient-controlled epidural analgesia results in a lower total dose of local anaesthetic.
  - ✓ Epidural analgesia is associated with longer stages of labor, more instrumental deliveries, and fever in the pregnant patient compared to parenteral narcotic analgesia. Complications of epidural analgesia include hypotension, itching, and urinary retention.
- Other options for labor analgesia include spinal analgesia, combined spinal-epidural analgesia, and nerve blocks.

POSTPARTUM HEMORRHAGE (PPH)

- PPH is an obstetrical emergency and is a major cause of morbidity and mortality worldwide.
- A stepwise approach to the treatment is advised starting with the exclusion of retained products of contraception.
- **Oxytocin** administration results in reduced blood loss, fewer cases of PPH, and a shorter third stage of labor for the pregnant patient. Other agents to use include **methylergonovine, carboprost**, and **tranexamic acid**.

MEDICATION USE DURING LACTATION

- Medications enter human milk via passive diffusion of nonionized and non–protein-bound medication. Medications with high molecular weights, lower lipid solubility, and higher protein binding are less likely to cross into human milk, or they transfer more slowly or in smaller amounts. The higher the serum concentration of medication for the lactating individual, the higher the concentration in the milk. Medications with longer half-lives are more likely to maintain higher human milk levels. The timing and frequency of feedings and the amount of milk ingested by the infant are also important.
- Strategies for reducing infant risk from medication transferred into human milk include selecting medications for the lactating individual that would be considered safe for use in the infant, and choosing medications with shorter half-lives, higher protein binding, lower bioavailability, and lower lipid solubility.
- The use of a galactogogue (ie, **metoclopramine** or **domperidone**) is not recommended as a first-line agent to increase milk production due to the inconclusive evidence and potential for adverse medication effects. Nonpharmacologic measures (ie, work with a lactation consultant) should be tried first.
- Penicillin-resistant *Staphylococcus aureus* is the most common bacterial cause of mastitis. Treatment with penicillinase-resistant penicillins or first-generation **cephalosporins** may be indicated. Application of heat and direct massage along with NSAIDs may be used for pain relief.

POSTPARTUM DEPRESSION

- Postpartum depression affects up to 13% of individuals, with almost 5% experiencing major depression.
- Nonpharmacologic treatment may include interpersonal psychotherapy, cognitive behavioral therapy, and group/family therapy.
- Sertraline, paroxetine, fluoxetine, and nortriptyline are the most studied in the postpartum period and the selection of medication with low transfer to human milk is desirable.

See Chapter 99, Pregnancy and Lactation, authored by Alicia B. Forinash and Kylie Barnes, for a more detailed discussion of this topic.

33 · Anemias

- *Anemia* is a group of diseases characterized by a decrease in either hemoglobin (Hb) or the volume of red blood cells (RBCs), resulting in decreased oxygen-carrying capacity of blood. The World Health Organization defines anemia as Hb less than 13 g/dL (130 g/L; 8.07 mmol/L) in men or less than 12 g/dL (120 g/L; 7.45 mmol/L) in women.

PATHOPHYSIOLOGY

- The functional classification of anemias is found in Fig. 33-1. The most common anemias are included in this chapter.
- Morphologic classifications are based on cell size. Macrocytic cells are larger than normal and are associated with deficiencies of vitamin B_{12} or folic acid. Microcytic cells are smaller than normal and are associated with iron deficiency, whereas normocytic anemia may be associated with recent blood loss or chronic disease.
- Iron-deficiency anemia (IDA), characterized by decreased levels of ferritin (most sensitive marker) and serum iron, and decreased transferrin saturation, can be caused by inadequate dietary intake, inadequate gastrointestinal (GI) absorption, increased iron demand (eg, pregnancy), blood loss, and chronic diseases.
- Vitamin B_{12}– and folic acid–deficiency anemias, macrocytic in nature, can be caused by inadequate dietary intake, malabsorption syndromes, and inadequate utilization. Deficiency of intrinsic factor causes decreased absorption of vitamin B_{12} (ie, pernicious anemia). Folic acid–deficiency anemia can be caused by hyperutilization due to pregnancy, hemolytic anemia, malignancy, chronic inflammatory disorders, long-term dialysis, burn patients, or adolescents and infants during growth spurts. Drugs can cause anemia by reducing absorption of folate (eg, phenytoin) or through folate antagonism (eg, methotrexate).
- Anemia of inflammation (AI) is a term used to describe both anemia of chronic disease and anemia of critical illness. A diagnosis of exclusion, AI is an anemia that traditionally has been associated with malignant, infectious, or inflammatory processes, tissue injury, and conditions associated with release of proinflammatory cytokines. Serum iron is decreased but in contrast to IDA, the serum ferritin concentration is normal or increased. For information on anemia of chronic kidney disease, see Chapter 75.
- Age-related reductions in bone marrow reserve can render elderly patients more susceptible to anemia caused by multiple minor and often unrecognized diseases (eg, nutritional deficiencies) that negatively affect erythropoiesis.
- Pediatric anemias are often due to a primary hematologic abnormality. The risk of IDA is increased by rapid growth spurts and dietary deficiency.

CLINICAL PRESENTATION

- Signs and symptoms depend on rate of development and age and cardiovascular status of the patient. Acute-onset anemia is characterized by cardiopulmonary symptoms such as palpitations, angina, light-headedness, and shortness of breath. Chronic anemia is characterized by weakness, fatigue, headache, orthopnea, dyspnea on exertion, vertigo, faintness, cold sensitivity, and pallor.

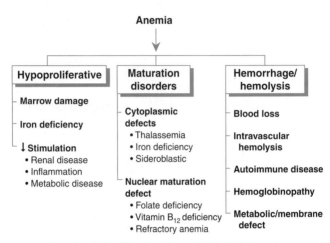

FIGURE 33-1. Functional classification of anemia. Each of the major categories of anemia (hypoproliferative, maturation disorders, and hemorrhage/hemolysis) can be further subclassified according to the functional defect in the several components of normal erythropoiesis.

- IDA is characterized by glossal pain, smooth tongue, reduced salivary flow, pica (compulsive eating of nonfood items), and pagophagia (compulsive eating of ice).
- Neurologic effects (eg, numbness and parasthesisas) of vitamin B_{12} deficiency may precede hematologic changes. Psychiatric findings, including irritability, depression, and memory impairment, may also occur with vitamin B_{12} deficiency. Anemia with folate deficiency is not associated with neurologic symptoms.

DIAGNOSIS

- Rapid diagnosis is essential because anemia is often a sign of underlying pathology. Severity of symptoms does not always correlate with the degree of anemia.
- Initial evaluation of anemia involves a complete blood cell count (CBC), reticulocyte index, and examination of the stool for occult blood. Figure 33-2 shows a broad, general algorithm for the diagnosis of anemia based on laboratory data.
- The earliest and most sensitive laboratory change for IDA is decreased serum ferritin (storage iron), which should be interpreted in conjunction with decreased transferrin saturation and increased total iron-binding capacity (TIBC). Hb, hematocrit (Hct), and RBC indices usually remain normal until later stages of IDA.
- In macrocytic anemias, mean corpuscular volume is usually elevated to greater than 100 fL. Vitamin B_{12} and folate concentrations can be measured to differentiate between the two deficiency anemias. A vitamin B_{12} value less than 200 pg/mL (148 pmol/L), together with appropriate peripheral smear and clinical symptoms, is diagnostic of vitamin B_{12}–deficiency anemia. A decreased RBC folate concentration (less than 150 ng/mL [340 nmol/L]) appears to be a better indicator of folate-deficiency anemia than a decreased serum folate concentration (less than 2 ng/mL [4.5 nmol/L]).
- The diagnosis of AI is usually one of exclusion, with consideration of coexisting iron and folate deficiencies. Serum iron is usually decreased, but, unlike IDA, serum ferritin is normal or increased, and TIBC is decreased. The bone marrow reveals an abundance of iron; the peripheral smear reveals normocytic anemia.

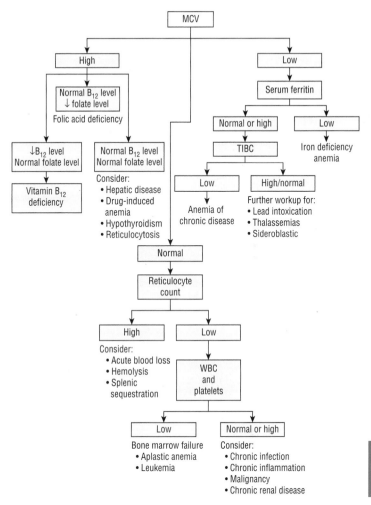

FIGURE 33-2. General algorithm for diagnosis of anemias based on laboratory data.

- Elderly patients with symptoms of anemia should undergo a CBC with peripheral smear and reticulocyte count and other laboratory studies as needed to determine the etiology of anemia.
- The diagnosis of anemia in pediatric populations requires use of age- and sex-adjusted norms for laboratory values.

TREATMENT

- <u>Goals of Treatment</u>: The goals are to return hematologic parameters to normal, restore normal function and quality of life, and prevent long-term complications.

IRON-DEFICIENCY ANEMIA

- **Oral iron** therapy with soluble ferrous iron salts, which are not enteric coated and not slow or sustained release, is recommended at a daily dosage of 150–200 mg elemental iron in two or three divided doses (see Table 33-1). Continue therapy for 3–6 months after resolution of anemia to replete iron stores and prevent relapse.
- Iron is best absorbed from meat, fish, and poultry. Administer iron at least 1 hour before meals because food interferes with absorption, but administration with food may be needed to improve tolerability.
- Consider **parenteral iron** for patients with iron malabsorption, intolerance of oral iron therapy, or nonadherence. The following formula can be used to estimate the total dose of parenteral iron needed to correct anemia:

Dose of iron (mg) = whole blood hemoglobin deficit (g/L) × body weight (kg) × 0.22

- **Iron dextran**, **sodium ferric gluconate**, **iron sucrose**, **ferumoxytol**, **ferric derisomaltose**, **ferric pyrophosphate citrate**, and **ferric carboxymaltose** are available parenteral iron preparations with similar efficacy but different molecular size, pharmacokinetics, bioavailability, and adverse effect profiles (see Table 75–2).

VITAMIN B$_{12}$–DEFICIENCY ANEMIA

- Oral vitamin B$_{12}$ supplementation is as effective as parenteral, even in patients with pernicious anemia, because the alternate vitamin B$_{12}$ absorption pathway is independent of intrinsic factor. Initiate oral **cobalamin** at 1 mg daily.
- Parenteral therapy acts more rapidly than oral therapy and is recommended if neurologic symptoms are present. A popular regimen is IM **cyanocobalamin**, 1000 mcg daily for 1 week, then weekly for 1 month, and then monthly for maintenance therapy. Initiate daily oral cobalamin administration after symptoms resolve.
- Continue vitamin B$_{12}$ for life in patients with pernicious anemia.

FOLATE-DEFICIENCY ANEMIA

- Oral **folic acid**, 1 mg daily for 4 months, is usually sufficient for treatment of folic acid–deficiency anemia, unless the etiology cannot be corrected. If malabsorption is present, a dose of 1–5 mg daily may be necessary. Parenteral folic acid is available but rarely necessary.

ANEMIA OF INFLAMMATION

- Treatment of AI is less specific than that of other anemias and should focus on correcting reversible causes. Reserve iron therapy for an established IDA; iron is not effective when inflammation is present. RBC transfusions are effective but should be limited to episodes of inadequate oxygen transport and Hb of 7–8 g/dL (70–80 g/L; 4.34–4.97 mmol/L).

TABLE 33-1	Oral Iron Products	
Iron Salt	**Percent Elemental Iron**	**Common Formulations and Elemental Iron Provided**
Ferrous sulfate	20	60–65 mg/324–325 mg tablet
		44 mg/5 mL elixir
		15 mg/1 mL solution
Ferrous gluconate	12	38 mg/325 mg tablet
		28–29 mg/240–246 mg tablet
Ferrous fumarate	33	66 mg/200 mg tablet
		106 mg/324–325 mg tablet
Ferric maltol	100	30 mg/30 mg

- **Erythropoiesis-stimulating agents (ESAs)** can be considered, but response can be impaired in patients with AI. The initial dosage for **epoetin alfa** is 50–100 units/kg three times weekly and **darbepoetin alfa** 0.45 mcg/kg once weekly. Iron, cobalamin, and folic acid supplementation may improve response to ESA treatment.
- Potential toxicities of exogenous ESA administration include increases in blood pressure, nausea, headache, fever, bone pain, and fatigue. Hb must be monitored during ESA therapy. An increase in Hb greater than 12 g/dL (120 g/L; 7.45 mmol/L) with treatment or a rise of greater than 1 g/dL (10 g/L; 0.62 mmol/L) every 2 weeks has been associated with increased mortality and cardiovascular events.
- In patients with anemia of critical illness, parenteral iron is often used but is associated with a theoretical risk of infection.

ANEMIA IN PEDIATRIC POPULATIONS

- Infants aged 9–12 months: Administer ferrous sulfate 3–6 mg/kg/day (elemental iron) divided once or twice daily between meals for 4 weeks. Continue for two additional months in responders to replace storage iron pools. The dose and schedule of vitamin B_{12} should be titrated according to clinical and laboratory response. The daily dose of folic acid is 1 mg.

EVALUATION OF THERAPEUTIC OUTCOMES

- IDA: Positive response to oral iron therapy is characterized by modest reticulocytosis in a few days with an increase in Hb seen at 2 weeks. Reevaluate the patient if reticulocytosis does not occur. Hb should return to normal after 2 months; continue iron therapy until iron stores are replenished and serum ferritin normalized (up to 12 months).
- Megaloblastic anemia: Signs and symptoms usually improve within a few days after starting vitamin B_{12} or folic acid therapy. Neurologic symptoms can take longer to improve or can be irreversible, but should not progress during therapy. Reticulocytosis should occur within 3–5 days. Hb begins to rise a week after starting vitamin B_{12} therapy and should normalize in 1–2 months. Hct should rise within 2 weeks after starting folic acid therapy and should normalize within 2 months.
- ESAs: Reticulocytosis should occur within a few days. Monitor iron, TIBC, transferrin saturation, and ferritin levels at baseline and periodically during therapy. The optimal form and schedule of iron supplementation are unknown. Discontinue ESAs if a clinical response does not occur after 8 weeks.
- Pediatrics: Monitor Hb, Hct, and RBC indices 4–8 weeks after initiation of iron therapy. Monitor Hb or Hct weekly in premature infants.

See Chapter 122, Anemias, authored by Kristen M. Cook and Devon M. Greer, for a more detailed discussion of this topic.

Sickle Cell Disease

- *Sickle cell syndromes*, which can be divided into sickle cell trait (SCT) and sickle cell disease (SCD), are hereditary conditions characterized by the presence of sickle hemoglobin (HbS) in red blood cells (RBCs).
- SCT is the heterozygous inheritance of one normal β-globin gene-producing hemoglobin A (HbA) and one sickle gene-producing HbS (HbAS) gene. Individuals with SCT are asymptomatic.
- SCD can be of homozygous or compounded heterozygous inheritance. Homozygous HbS (HbSS) has historically been referred to as sickle cell anemia (SCA), which now also includes HbSβ⁰-thal due to similarities in clinical severity. The heterozygous inheritance of HbS with another qualitative or quantitative β-globin mutation results in sickle cell hemoglobin C (HbSC), sickle cell β-thalassemia (HbSβ⁺-thal and HbSβ⁰-thal), and some other rare phenotypes.

PATHOPHYSIOLOGY

- Clinical manifestations of SCD are due to impaired circulation, RBC destruction, and stasis of blood flow and ongoing inflammatory responses. These changes result from disturbances in RBC polymerization and membrane damage. In addition to sickling, other factors contributing to the clinical manifestations include functional asplenia (and increased susceptibility to infection by encapsulated organisms), deficient opsonization, and coagulation abnormalities.
- Polymerization allows deoxygenated hemoglobin to exist as a semisolid gel that protrudes into the cell membrane, distorting RBCs into sickle shapes. Sickled RBCs increase blood viscosity and encourage sludging in the capillaries and postcapillary venules, leading to local tissue hypoxia that accentuates the pathologic process.
- Repeated cycles of sickling, upon deoxygenation, and unsickling, upon oxygenation, damage the RBC membrane and cause irreversibly sickled cells (ISC). Rigid ISCs are easily trapped, resulting in shortened circulatory survival and chronic hemolysis.

CLINICAL PRESENTATION

- SCD is usually identified by routine neonatal screening programs using isoelectric focusing, high-performance liquid chromatography, or electrophoresis.
- Laboratory findings include low hemoglobin; increased reticulocyte, platelet, and white blood cell counts; and sickled red cell forms on the peripheral smear.
- SCD involves multiple organ systems. Clinical manifestations depend on the genotype (Table 34-1).
- Cardinal features of SCD are hemolytic anemia and vasoocclusion. Symptoms are delayed until 4–6 months of age when HbS replaces fetal hemoglobin (HbF). Common findings include pain with fever, pneumonia, splenomegaly, and, in infants, pain and swelling of the hands and feet (eg, hand-and-foot syndrome or dactylitis).
- Usual clinical signs and symptoms of SCD include chronic anemia and pallor; fever; arthralgia; scleral icterus; abdominal pain; weakness; anorexia; fatigue; enlarged liver, spleen, and heart; and hematuria.
- Acute complications of SCD include fever and infection (eg, sepsis caused by encapsulated pathogens such as *Streptococcus pneumoniae*), stroke, acute chest syndrome, and priapism. Acute chest syndrome is characterized by pulmonary infiltration with fever and/or respiratory symptoms. Hypoxia is a predictor of severity and outcome.
- Microvascular occlusion in the bone marrow is the usual cause of sickle cell pain. Acute episodes can be precipitated by fever, infection, dehydration, hypoxia, acidosis, and sudden temperature changes. Acute splenic sequestration is the sudden massive enlargement of the spleen due to sequestration of sickled RBCs. The trapping

TABLE 34-1	Clinical Features of Sickle Cell Trait and Common Types of Sickle Cell Disease
Type	**Clinical Features**
Sickle cell trait (SCT)	Rare painless hematuria; heavy exercise under extreme conditions can provoke gross hematuria and complications (normal Hb)
Sickle cell anemia (SCA-HbSS)	Pain episodes, microvascular disruption of organs (spleen, liver, bone marrow, kidney, brain, and lung), gallstones, priapism, leg ulcers; anemia (Hb 6–9 g/dL [60–90 g/L; 3.72–5.59 mmol/L])
Sickle cell hemoglobin C (HbSC)	Painless hematuria and rare aseptic necrosis of bone; pain episodes are less common and occur later in life; other complications are ocular disease and pregnancy-related problems; mild anemia (Hb 9–14 g/dL [90–140 g/L; 5.59–8.69 mmol/L])
Sickle cell β^{+}-thalassemia (HbSβ^{+}-thal)	Rare pain; milder severity than HbSS because of the production of some HbA; Hb 9–12 g/dL [90–120 g/L; 5.59–7.45 mmol/L] with microcytosis
Sickle cell β^{0}-thalassemia (HbSβ^{0}-thal)	No HbA production; severity similar to SCA; Hb 7–9 g/dL [70–90 g/L; 4.34–5.59 mmol/L] with microcytosis

of sickled RBCs by the spleen leads to hypotension and shock; it can cause sudden death in young children. Repeated infarctions lead to autosplenectomy; therefore, incidence declines as adolescence approaches. There is increased susceptibility to venous thromboembolism due to a hypercoagulable state, endothelial dysfunction, and impaired blood flow.

- Chronic complications involve many organs and include pulmonary hypertension, airway inflammation and hyperresponsiveness, bone and joint destruction, ocular problems, cholelithiasis, cardiovascular abnormalities, and renal manifestations.

TREATMENT

- Goals of Treatment: The goals are to reduce hospitalizations, complications, and mortality as well as to improve quality of life.

GENERAL PRINCIPLES

- Patients with SCD require lifelong interprofessional care that combines general symptomatic supportive care, preventative medical therapies, and specific disease-modifying therapies.
- Routine immunizations plus influenza, meningococcal, and pneumococcal vaccinations are recommended.

PHARMACOLOGIC THERAPY

- Prophylactic **penicillin** is recommended until at least 5 years of age. An effective regimen is penicillin V potassium, 125 mg orally twice daily until 3 years of age and then 250 mg orally twice daily until age 5 years.
- HbF reduces polymer formation of HbS. Increases in HbF correlate with decreased RBC sickling and adhesion. Patients with low HbF levels have more frequent pain and higher mortality. HbF levels of 20% or greater reduce the risk of acute sickle cell complications. **Hydroxyurea**, a chemotherapeutic agent, stimulates HbF production and increases the number of HbF-containing reticulocytes and intracellular HbF. It is indicated for patients 2 years of age and older with recurrent moderate to severe painful crises to reduce the frequency of pain crises and the need for blood transfusions. The recommended single daily dose for adults is 15 mg/kg and 20 mg/kg for children (**Fig. 34-1**).
- L-**Glutamine** is approved for patients with SCD age 5 and older to reduce the acute complications of SCD. Dose is weight-based: 5 g twice a day for <30 kg; 10 g twice a day for 30–65 kg and 15 g twice a day for >65 kg.

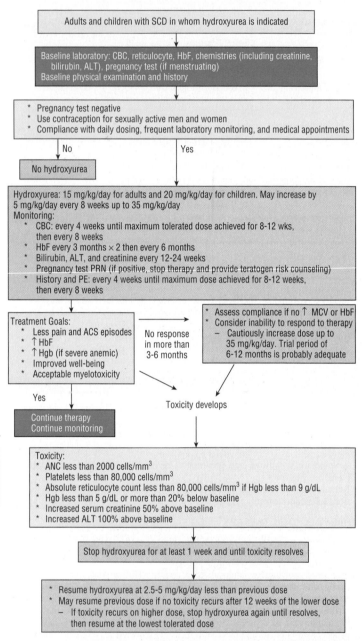

FIGURE 34-1 Hydroxyurea use in sickle cell disease. Blood test results expressed in SI units that are consistent with toxicity are <2 × 10⁹/L for ANC; <80 × 10⁹/L for platelets; <80 × 10⁹/L for absolute reticulocyte count if Hb <90 g/L (5.59 mmol/L); and Hb <50 g/L (3.10 mmol/L). ALT, alanine aminotransferase; ANC, absolute neutrophil count; PE, physical examination; PRN, as needed.

- **Crizanlizumab** is a monoclonal antibody against the adhesion molecule P-selectin. It is an IV solution approved for patients with SCD age 16 and older at a dose of 5 mg/kg every 2 weeks for 2 doses, followed by 5 mg/kg every 4 weeks.
- **Voxelotor** inhibits HbS polymerization, a major contributor to SCD-related complications. It is approved for patients with SCD age 21 and older at a dose of 1500 mg once daily. Dose is decreased with severe hepatic impairment (Child Pugh class C). Avoid use with strong CYP3A4 inducers or inhibitor since voxelotor is a CYP3A4 substrate.

OTHER THERAPIES

- Chronic RBC transfusions are indicated for primary and secondary stroke prevention and amelioration of organ damage. Transfusions are usually given every 3–4 weeks or as needed to maintain desired HbS levels. The optimal duration of primary prophylactic transfusion therapy in children is unknown. Risks include alloimmunization, hyperviscosity, transfusion-transmitted viral infections (requiring hepatitis A and B vaccination), volume and iron overload, and nonhemolytic transfusion reactions.
- Allogeneic hematopoietic stem cell transplantation is a curative therapy for SCD. The best candidates are younger than 16 years, have severe complications, and have human leukocyte antigen–matched donors. Risks must be carefully considered and include mortality, graft rejection, and secondary malignancies.

TREATMENT OF COMPLICATIONS

- Educate patients to recognize signs and symptoms of complications and conditions that require urgent evaluation. Balanced fluid status and oxygen saturation of at least 92% are important to avoid exacerbation during acute illness.
- RBC transfusions are indicated for (1) acute exacerbation of baseline anemia (eg, aplastic crisis, hepatic or splenic sequestration, or severe hemolysis); (2) acute chest syndrome, stroke, intrahepatic cholestasis, or acute multisystem organ failure; and (3) preparation for procedures requiring general anesthesia.
- Hydration and analgesics are mainstays of treatment for vasoocclusive (painful) crisis. Administer fluids IV or orally at 1–1.5 times the maintenance requirement; monitor closely to avoid volume overload. Consider an infectious etiology and initiate empiric therapy if indicated.
- Tailor analgesic therapy to the individual because of the variable frequency and severity of pain. Pain scales should be used to quantify the degree of pain.
- Use **nonsteroidal anti-inflammatory drugs (NSAIDs)** or **acetaminophen** for mild to moderate pain. Consider adding an opioid if mild to moderate pain persists. (eg, **codeine** or **hydrocodone**).
- Treat severe pain aggressively with an opioid, such as **morphine**, **hydromorphone**, **fentanyl**, or **methadone**. Avoid **meperidine** due to accumulation of the normeperidine metabolite, which can cause neurotoxicity, especially in patients with impaired renal function. Consider **ketamine** for opioid-dependent or -tolerant patients with acute or chronic sickle cell pain. Titrate IV opioids to pain relief and then administer as a scheduled dose or continuous infusion with as-needed dosing for breakthrough pain. Patient-controlled analgesia is commonly utilized.
- Treatment of chronic pain in SCD requires an interprofessional team approach. Guidelines for chronic pain management are available.
- Promptly evaluate fever of 38.5°C (101.3°F) or higher. Empiric antibiotic therapy should provide coverage against encapsulated organisms (eg, **ceftriaxone** for outpatients [unless if used in previous 8 weeks, give ampicillin], **clindamycin** for cephalosporin-allergic patients). Add a macrolide antibiotic if *M. pneumoniae* is suspected.
- For acute chest syndrome, initiate incentive spirometry; appropriate fluid therapy; broad-spectrum antibiotics, including a **macrolide** or **quinolone**; and, for hypoxia or acute distress, oxygen therapy. Other potential therapies include steroids and nitric oxide.
- Priapism has been treated with analgesics, antianxiety agents, and vasoconstrictors to force blood out of the corpus cavernosum (eg, **phenylephrine** and **epinephrine**), and vasodilators to relax smooth muscle (eg, **terbutaline** and **hydralazine**).

- Treatment of aplastic crisis is primarily supportive. Blood transfusions may be indicated for severe or symptomatic anemia.
- Hydration and blood transfusions are indicated to treat hypovolemia associated with splenic sequestration. Manage recurrent episodes with observation and splenectomy. Consider chronic transfusions in children younger than 2 years of age to delay splenectomy until the age of 2 years. Splenectomy is an option for chronic hypersplenism.

EVALUATION OF THERAPEUTIC OUTCOMES

- Evaluate patients on a regular basis to establish baseline symptoms, monitor changes, and provide age-appropriate education.
- Evaluate CBC and reticulocyte counts every 3–6 months up to 2 years of age, then every 6–12 months. Screen HbF level annually until 2 years of age. Evaluate renal, hepatobiliary, and pulmonary function annually. Screen patients for retinopathy.
- Assess efficacy of hydroxyurea by monitoring the number, severity, and duration of sickle cell crises.

See Chapter 124, Sickle Cell Disease, authored by Jin Han, Santosh L. Saraf, and Victor R. Gordeuk, for a more detailed discussion of this topic.

35 Antimicrobial Regimen Selection

- A systematic approach to the selection and evaluation of an antimicrobial regimen is provided in Table 35-1. An *empiric* antimicrobial regimen is begun before the offending organism is identified and sometimes before documentation of the presence of infection, whereas a *definitive* regimen is instituted when the causative organism is known.

CONFIRMING THE PRESENCE OF INFECTION

FEVER

- *Fever* is defined as a controlled elevation of body temperature above the expected 37°C (98.6°F) (measured orally) and is a manifestation of many disease states other than infection.
- Many drugs have been identified as causes of fever. Drug-induced fever is defined as persistent fever in the absence of infection or other underlying condition. The fever must coincide temporally with the administration of the offending agent and disappear promptly upon its withdrawal, after which the temperature remains normal.

WHITE BLOOD CELL COUNT

- Most infections result in elevated white blood cell (WBC) counts (leukocytosis) because of the mobilization of granulocytes and/or lymphocytes to destroy invading microbes. Normal values for WBC counts are between 4000 and 10,000 cells/mm^3 (4×10^9 and 10×10^9/L).

TABLE 35-1	Systematic Approach for Selection of Antimicrobials

Confirm the presence of infection
    Careful history and physical examination
    Signs and symptoms
    Predisposing factors
Identification of the pathogen (see Pharmacotherapy textbook Chapter e126)
    Collection of infected material
    Stains
    Serologies
    Culture and sensitivity
Selection of presumptive therapy considering every infected site
    Host factors
    Drug factors
Monitor therapeutic response
    Clinical assessment
    Laboratory tests
    Assessment of therapeutic failure

- Bacterial infections are associated with elevated granulocyte counts (neutrophils and basophils), often with increased numbers of immature forms (band neutrophils) seen in peripheral blood smears. With infection, peripheral leukocyte counts may be high, but they are rarely higher than 30,000 to 40,000 cells/mm³ (30 × 10⁹/L to 40 × 10⁹/L). Low neutrophil counts (neutropenia) after the onset of infection indicate an abnormal response and are generally associated with a poor prognosis for bacterial infection.
- Relative lymphocytosis, even with normal or slightly elevated total WBC counts, is generally associated with tuberculosis and viral or fungal infections. Many types of infections, however, may be accompanied by a completely normal WBC count and differential.

LOCAL SIGNS

- Pain and inflammation may accompany infection and are sometimes manifested by swelling, erythema, tenderness, and purulent drainage. Unfortunately, these signs may be apparent only if the infection is superficial or in a bone or joint.
- The manifestations of inflammation with deep-seated infections such as meningitis, pneumonia, endocarditis, and urinary tract infection must be ascertained by examining tissues or fluids. For example, the presence of polymorphonuclear leukocytes (neutrophils) in spinal fluid, lung secretions (sputum), and urine is highly suggestive of bacterial infection.

IDENTIFICATION OF THE PATHOGEN

- Identification and antimicrobial susceptibility of a suspected pathogen are the most important factors in determining the choice of antimicrobial therapy.
- Infected body materials must be sampled, if at all possible or practical, before the institution of antimicrobial therapy. A Gram stain of the material may reveal bacteria, or an acid-fast stain may detect mycobacteria or actinomycetes. Premature use of antimicrobials can suppress the growth of pathogens that might result in false-negative culture results or alterations in the cellular and chemical composition of infected fluids.
- Blood cultures should be performed in the acutely ill, febrile patient. Infected materials produced by the patient (eg, blood, sputum, urine, stool, and wound or sinus drainage) and less accessible fluids or tissues are obtained when needed to assess localized signs or symptoms. Abscesses and cellulitic areas should also be aspirated.
- After a positive Gram stain, culture results, or both are obtained, the clinician must be cautious in determining whether the organism recovered is a true pathogen, a contaminant, or a part of the normal flora. Cultures of specimens from purportedly infected sites that are obtained by sampling from or through contaminated areas might contain significant numbers of the normal flora.

SELECTION OF PRESUMPTIVE THERAPY

- A variety of factors must be considered to select rational antimicrobial therapy for a given clinical situation. These include the severity and acuity of the disease, local epidemiology and antibiogram, patient history, host factors, factors related to the drugs used, and the necessity for using multiple agents. Choice of antimicrobial is influenced by local antimicrobial susceptibility data rather than information published by other institutions or national compilations.
- The drugs of choice for the treatment of most pathogens are compiled from a variety of sources and are intended as guidelines rather than specific rules for antimicrobial use (Table 35-2).
- Important considerations when selecting empiric antimicrobial therapy include: (1) prior knowledge of colonization or infections, (2) previous antimicrobial use, (3) the site of infection and the organisms most likely pathogens, and (4) local antibiogram and resistance patterns for important pathogens.

TABLE 35-2 Drug(s) of Choice, *Alternative(s)*

Gram-Positive Cocci

Organism	Drug(s) of Choice	*Alternatives*
Enterococcus faecalis Serious infections	Ampicillin, penicillin G (± gentamicin or ceftriaxone)	*Vancomycin, daptomycin,[a] linezolid*
Enterococcus faecalis Urinary tract infection	Ampicillin, amoxicillin	*Fosfomycin, nitrofurantoin*
Enterococcus faecium *Recommend consultation with ID specialist*	Vancomycin, linezolid, daptomycin[a]	*Eravacycline, omadacycline*
Methicillin-susceptible *Staphylococcus aureus* (MSSA)	Nafcillin, oxacillin, cefazolin	*Daptomycin,[a] trimethoprim/ sulfamethoxazole, clindamycin,[b] BL/BLI*
Methicillin-resistant *Staphylococcus aureus* (MRSA) Serious infections	Vancomycin, daptomycin[a]	*Linezolid, ceftaroline*
Methicillin-resistant *Staphylococcus aureus* (MRSA) SSTIs, CAP	Doxycycline, trimethoprim/ sulfamethoxazole	*Clindamycin, linezolid, oritavancin, tedizolid, telavancin, dalbavancin*
Group A *Streptococcus* (*S. pyogenes*)	Penicillin G (± clindamycin or linezolid[c])	*Erythromycin, azithromycin, clarithromycin*
Group B *Streptococcus* (*S. agalactiae*)	Penicillin G, ampicillin, amoxicillin	*Cephalexin, clindamycin,[b] vancomycin, azithromycin*
Group C, F, G *Streptococcus*	Penicillin G, penicillin V, ampicillin	*Daptomycin,[a] clindamycin,[b] cefazolin*
Viridans group *Streptococcus*	Penicillin G	*Ceftriaxone, cefotaxime, vancomycin, doxycycline*
Penicillin-susceptible *Streptococcus pneumoniae*	Penicillin G, ampicillin, amoxicillin	*Ceftriaxone, doxycycline*
Penicillin-resistant *Streptococcus pneumoniae*	Ceftriaxone, vancomycin	*Levofloxacin, moxifloxacin, vancomycin, linezolid, ceftaroline*

Gram-Negative Cocci

Organism	Drug(s) of Choice	*Alternatives*
Moraxella catarrhalis	Ampicillin/sulbactam, amoxicillin/clavulanate	*Trimethoprim/ sulfamethoxazole, doxycycline, azithromycin, ceftriaxone*
Neisseria gonorrhoeae	Ceftriaxone	*Gentamicin + azithromycin*
Neisseria meningitides	Penicillin G, ceftriaxone	*Moxifloxacin, ampicillin*

(Continued)

TABLE 35-2 Drug(s) of Choice, *Alternative(s)* *(Continued)*

Gram-Positive Bacilli

Organism	Drug(s) of Choice	Alternatives
Clostridium perfringes	Penicillin G (± clindamycin)	*Metronidazole, ceftriaxone, ampicillin, piperacillin/ tazobactam, meropenem, imipenem/cilastatin*
Clostridioides difficile (formerly *Clostridium difficile*)	PO vancomycin, fidaxomicin	*Metronidazole*

Gram-Negative Bacilli

Organism	Drug(s) of Choice	Alternatives
Acinetobacter spp.	Cefepime, meropenem, imipenem/cilastatin, ampicillin/sulbactam	*Amikacin, fluoroquinolone, minocycline, piperacillin/ tazobactam, tigecycline, trimethoprim/ sulfamethoxazole*
Bacteroides spp.	Metronidazole	*BL/BLI[d] meropenem, imipenem, cefoxitin*
Enterobacter spp.	Cefepime, meropenem, imipenem/cilastatin	*Trimethoprim/sulfamethoxazole, amikacin, piperacillin/ tazobactam, fluoroquinolone,[e] tigecycline*
Escherichia coli	Ceftriaxone	*Cefepime, BL/BLI, fluoroquinolone,[e] trimethoprim/ sulfamethoxazole, cephalexin, nitrofurantoin (cystitis), carbapenem[f]*
Haemophilus influenzae	Ampicillin/sulbactam, ceftriaxone *If β-lactamase-negative, may use ampicillin*	*Trimethoprim/sulfamethoxazole, azithromycin, fluoroquinolone,[e] carbapenem[f]*
Klebsiella pneumoniae	Ceftriaxone, BL/BLI	*Cefepime, carbapenem,[f] fluoroquinolone[e]*
Legionella spp.[g]	Levofloxacin, moxifloxacin, azithromycin	*Erythromycin, ciprofloxacin*
Pasteurella multocida	Ampicillin/sulbactam	*Penicillin G, doxycycline, trimethoprim/ sulfamethoxazole*
Proteus mirabilis	Ceftriaxone	*Penicillin G, BL/BLI,[d] cefepime*
Indole-positive *Proteus* (ie, *Providencia spp., Morganella morganii*)	Cefepime, meropenem, imipenem/cilastatin	*Trimethoprim/sulfamethoxazole, amikacin, piperacillin/ tazobactam, fluoroquinolone,[e] minocycline, tigecycline*

(Continued)

TABLE 35-2 Drug(s) of Choice, *Alternative(s)* *(Continued)*

Gram-Negative Bacilli *(Continued)*

Organism	Drug(s) of Choice	Alternatives
Pseudomonas aeruginosa	Cefepime, meropenem, amikacin, tobramycin, imipenem/cilastatin, piperacillin/tazobactam	*Ceftazidime, ciprofloxacin, levofloxacin, aztreonam*
Salmonella typhi	Ceftriaxone	*Ciprofloxacin, levofloxacin, sulfamethoxazole/ trimethoprim, carbapenem[f]*
Serratia marcescens	Cefepime, meropenem, imipenem/cilastatin	*Trimethoprim/sulfamethoxazole, amikacin, piperacillin/ tazobactam, fluoroquinolone[e]*
Stenotrophomonas maltophilia	Trimethoprim/ sulfamethoxazole	*Minocycline, levofloxacin[h]*

Miscellaneous Microorganisms

Organism	Drug(s) of Choice	Alternatives
Chlamydia pneumoniae	Azithromycin, clarithromycin, doxycycline	*Levofloxacin, moxifloxacin*
Mycoplasma pneumoniae	Azithromycin, clarithromycin, doxycycline	*Levofloxacin, moxifloxacin*
Treponema pallidum	Penicillin G	*Ceftriaxone*

Multidrug Resistant (MDR) Gram-Negative Organisms

Organism	Drug(s) of Choice	Alternatives
Any ESBL-positive *Enterobacterales* Infections outside the urinary tract	Carbapenem[f]	*Trimethoprim/ sulfamethoxazole,[i] fluoroquinolone[e, i]*
Any ESBL-positive *Enterobacterales* Pyelonephritis	Trimethoprim/ sulfamethoxazole	*Carbapenem,[f] levofloxacin, ciprofloxacin*
Any ESBL-positive *Enterobacterales* Cystitis	Nitrofurantoin	*Trimethoprim/ sulfamethoxazole, levofloxacin, ciprofloxacin*
Any *Enterobacterales* positive for KPC carbapenemase	Meropenem/vaborbactam, ceftazidime/avibactam, imipenem/cilastatin/ relebactam	*Cefiderocol*
Any *Enterobacterales* positive for ametallo- β-lactamase (ie, VIM, NDM, or IMP)	Ceftazidime/avibactam + aztreonam	*Cefiderocol*

(Continued)

TABLE 35-2	Drug(s) of Choice, *Alternative(s)* *(Continued)*	

Multidrug Resistant (MDR) Gram-Negative Organisms *(Continued)*

Organism	Drug(s) of Choice	*Alternatives*
Any *Enterobacterales* positive for OXA-48 carbapenemase	Ceftazidime/avibactam	*Cefiderocol*
***Pseudomonas aeruginosa* resistant to all routinely tested β-lactams**	Ceftolozane/tazobactam	*Ceftazidime/avibactam, imipenem/cilastatin/ relebactam, cefiderocol*

Recommendations in chart are assuming in vitro susceptibility.
BL/BLI, β-Lactam/β-lactamase inhibitor; CAP, community acquired pneumonia; ESBL, extended-spectrum β-lactamase; GAS, Group A Streptococcus; SSTIs, skin and soft tissue infections.
[a]Daptomycin does not achieve appreciable CNS concentrations and therefore would not be recommended for treatment of meningitis.
[b]Clindamycin is not an appropriate alternative for treatment of bloodstream or CNS infections.
[c]Both clindamycin and linezolid provide antitoxin activity against GAS and selection of agent dependent upon patient-specific factors.
[d]May consider the addition of rifampin for serious *Legionella* infections.
[e]Fluoroquinolones: ciprofloxacin, levofloxacin, moxifloxacin.
[f]β-Lactam/β-lactamase inhibitor combination: ampicillin–sulbactam, piperacillin–tazobactam, ticarcillin–clavulanate, amoxicillin–clavulanate.
[g]Carbapenem: meropenem, imipenem/cilastatin, ertapenem.
[h]Levofloxacin should not be used as monotherapy for treatment of *Stenotrophomonas maltophilia*.
[i]Oral step-down therapy to trimethoprim/sulfamethoxazole, levofloxacin, or ciprofloxacin may be considered after (1) susceptibility to the oral agent is demonstrated, (2) patients are afebrile and hemodynamically stable, (3) appropriate source control is achieved, and (4) there are no issues with intestinal absorption.

HOST FACTORS

- When a patient for initial or empiric therapy is evaluated, the following factors should be considered:
  ✓ Allergy or history of adverse drug reactions.
  ✓ Age of patient.
  ✓ Pregnancy.
  ✓ Metabolic or genetic variation.
  ✓ *Renal and hepatic function*: Patients with diminished renal and/or hepatic function will accumulate certain drugs unless the dosage is adjusted.
  ✓ *Concomitant drug therapy*: Any concomitant therapy the patient is receiving may influence the selection of drug therapy, the dose, and monitoring. A list of selected drug interactions involving antimicrobials is provided in **Table 35-3**.
  ✓ Concomitant disease states.

DRUG FACTORS

- Integration of both pharmacokinetic and pharmacodynamic properties of an agent is important when choosing antimicrobial therapy to ensure efficacy and prevent resistance. Antibiotics may demonstrate concentration-dependent (aminoglycosides and fluoroquinolones) or time-dependent (β-lactams) bactericidal effects.
- The importance of tissue penetration varies with the site of infection. The central nervous system (CNS) is one body site where the importance of antimicrobial penetration is relatively well defined, and correlations with clinical outcomes are established. Drugs that do not reach significant concentrations in CSF should either be avoided or instilled directly when treating meningitis.
- Apart from the bloodstream, other body fluids in which drug concentration data are clinically relevant are cerebrospinal fluid, urine, synovial fluid, and peritoneal fluid.

TABLE 35-3 Major Drug Interactions with Antimicrobials

Antimicrobial	Other Agent(s)	Mechanism of Action/Effect	Clinical Management
Aminoglycosides	Neuromuscular blocking agents	Additive adverse effects	Avoid
	Nephrotoxins (N) or ototoxins (O) (eg, amphotericin B [N], cisplatin [N/O], cyclosporine [N], furosemide [O], NSAIDs [N], radiocontrast [N], vancomycin [N])	Additive adverse effects	Monitor aminoglycoside SDC and renal function
Amphotericin B	Nephrotoxins (eg, aminoglycosides, cidofovir, cyclosporine, foscarnet, pentamidine)	Additive adverse effects	Monitor renal function
Azoles	See Chapter 38		
Chloramphenicol	Phenytoin, tolbutamide, ethanol	Decreased metabolism of other agents	Monitor phenytoin SDC, blood glucose
Foscarnet	Pentamidine IV	Increased risk of severe nephrotoxicity/ hypocalcemia	Monitor renal function/serum calcium
Isoniazid	Carbamazepine, phenytoin	Decreased metabolism of other agents (nausea, vomiting, nystagmus, ataxia)	Monitor drug SDC
Macrolides/ Azalides	Digoxin	Decreased digoxin bioavailability and metabolism	Monitor digoxin SDC; avoid if possible
	Theophylline	Decreased metabolism of theophylline	Monitor theophylline SDC
Metronidazole	Ethanol (drugs containing ethanol)	Disulfiram-like reaction	Avoid
Penicillins and cephalosporins	Probenecid, aspirin	Blocked excretion of β-lactams	Use if prolonged high concentration of β-lactam desirable
Ciprofloxacin/ Norfloxacin	Theophylline	Decreased metabolism of theophylline	Monitor theophylline

(Continued)

TABLE 35-3 Major Drug Interactions with Antimicrobials (*Continued*)

Antimicrobial	Other Agent(s)	Mechanism of Action/Effect	Clinical Management
Quinolones	Classes Ia and III antiarrhythmics	Increased Q-T interval	Avoid
	Multivalent cations (antacids, iron, sucralfate, zinc, vitamins, dairy, citric acid), didanosine	Decreased absorption of quinolone	Separate by 2 hours
Rifampin	Azoles, cyclosporine, methadone propranolol, PIs, oral contraceptives, tacrolimus, warfarin	Increased metabolism of other agent	Avoid if possible
Sulfonamides	Sulfonylureas, phenytoin, warfarin	Decreased metabolism of other agent	Monitor blood glucose, SDC, PT
Tetracyclines	Antacids, iron, calcium, sucralfate	Decreased absorption of tetracycline	Separate by 2 hours
	Digoxin	Decreased digoxin bioavailability	Monitor digoxin SDC; avoid if possible

PI, protease inhibitor; PT, prothrombin time; SDC, serum drug concentrations.
Azalides: azithromycin; azoles: fluconazole, itraconazole, ketoconazole, and voriconazole; macrolides: erythromycin and clarithromycin; protease inhibitors: amprenavir, indinavir, lopinavir/ritonavir, nelfinavir, ritonavir, and saquinavir; quinolones: ciprofloxacin, gemifloxacin, levofloxacin, and moxifloxacin.

- Pharmacokinetic parameters such as area under the drug concentration-time curve (AUC) and maximal plasma concentration can be predictive of treatment outcome when specific ratios of AUC or maximal plasma concentration to the minimum inhibitory concentration (MIC) are achieved. For some agents, the ratio of AUC to MIC, peak-to-MIC ratio, or the time that the drug concentration is above the MIC (T > MIC) may predict efficacy.
- The most important pharmacodynamic relationship for antimicrobials that display time-dependent bactericidal effects (such as penicillins and cephalosporins) is the duration that drug concentrations exceed the MIC.

COMBINATION ANTIMICROBIAL THERAPY

- Combinations of antimicrobials are generally used to broaden the spectrum of coverage for empiric therapy, achieve synergistic activity against the infecting organism, and prevent the emergence of resistance.
- Increasing the coverage of antimicrobial therapy is generally necessary in mixed infections in which multiple organisms are likely to be present, such as intra-abdominal and female pelvic infections in which a variety of aerobic and anaerobic bacteria may produce disease. Combination antimicrobial therapy is also used in critically ill patients with presumed healthcare-associated infections in which an increased spectrum of activity is desirable.

Synergism

- The achievement of synergistic antimicrobial activity is advantageous for infections caused by gram-negative bacilli in immunosuppressed patients.

- Traditionally, combinations of aminoglycosides and β-lactams have been used because these drugs together generally act synergistically against a wide variety of bacteria. However, the data supporting superior efficacy of synergistic over nonsynergistic combinations are weak.
- Synergistic combinations may produce better results in infections.
- The use of combinations to prevent the emergence of resistance is widely applied but not often realized. The only circumstance in which this has been clearly effective is in the treatment of tuberculosis.

Disadvantages of Combination Therapy

- Although there are potentially beneficial effects from combining drugs, there are also potential disadvantages, including increased cost, greater risk of drug toxicity, and superinfection with even more resistant bacteria.
- Some combinations of antimicrobials are potentially antagonistic. For example, the effect of antagonism may be evident when one drug induces β-lactamase production and another drug is β-lactamase unstable.

MONITORING THERAPEUTIC RESPONSE

- After antimicrobial therapy has been instituted, the patient must be monitored carefully for a therapeutic response. Culture and sensitivity reports from specimens sent to the microbiology laboratory must be reviewed and the therapy changed accordingly.
- Use of agents with the narrowest spectrum of activity against identified pathogens is recommended.
- Patient monitoring should include a variety of parameters, including WBC count, body temperature, signs and symptoms of infection, appetite, radiologic studies as appropriate, and determination of antimicrobial concentrations in body fluids.
- As the patient improves, the route of antibiotic administration should be reevaluated. Streamlining therapy from parenteral to oral (switch therapy) has become an accepted practice for many infections. Criteria favoring the switch to oral therapy include the following:

  ✓ Overall clinical improvement
  ✓ Lack of fever for 8–24 hours
  ✓ Decreased WBC
  ✓ A functioning gastrointestinal (GI) tract

FAILURE OF ANTIMICROBIAL THERAPY

- A variety of factors may be responsible for the apparent lack of response to therapy. It is possible that the disease is not infectious or nonbacterial in origin, or there is an undetected pathogen in a polymicrobial infection. Other factors include those directly related to drug selection, the host, or the pathogen. Laboratory error in identification and/or susceptibility testing errors are rare.

Failures Caused by Drug Selection

- Factors directly related to the drug selection include an inappropriate selection of drug, dosage, or route of administration. Malabsorption of a drug product due to GI disease (eg, short-bowel syndrome) or a drug interaction (eg, complexation of fluoroquinolones with multivalent cations resulting in reduced absorption) may lead to potentially subtherapeutic serum concentrations.
- Accelerated drug elimination is also a possible reason for failure and may occur in patients with cystic fibrosis or during pregnancy, when more rapid clearance or larger volumes of distribution may result in low serum concentrations, particularly for aminoglycosides.
- A common cause of failure of therapy is poor penetration into the site of infection. This is especially true for the so-called privileged sites, such as the CNS, the eye, and the prostate gland.

Failures Caused by Host Factors

- Patients who are immunosuppressed (eg, granulocytopenia from chemotherapy and acquired immunodeficiency syndrome) may respond poorly to therapy because their own defenses are inadequate to eradicate the infection despite seemingly adequate drug regimens.
- Other host factors are related to the necessity for surgical drainage of abscesses or removal of foreign bodies and/or necrotic tissue. If these situations are not corrected, they result in persistent infection and, occasionally, bacteremia, despite adequate antimicrobial therapy.

Failures Caused by Microorganisms

- Factors related to the pathogen include the development of drug resistance during therapy. Primary resistance refers to the intrinsic resistance of the pathogens producing the infection. However, acquisition of resistance during treatment has become a major problem as well.
- The increase in resistance among pathogenic organisms is believed to be due, in large part, to continued overuse of antimicrobials in the community, as well as in hospitals, and the increasing prevalence of immunosuppressed patients receiving long-term suppressive antimicrobials for the prevention of infections.

See Chapter 123, Antimicrobial Regimen Selection, authored by Katie B. Olney and David S. Burgess, for a more detailed discussion of this topic.

Central Nervous System Infections

- *Central nervous system* (CNS) infections include a wide variety of clinical conditions and etiologies: meningitis, meningoencephalitis, encephalitis, brain and meningeal abscesses, and shunt infections. The focus of this chapter is meningitis.
- CNS infections may be caused by a variety of bacteria, fungi, viruses, and parasites. The most common causes of bacterial meningitis are *Streptococcus pneumoniae,* group B Streptococcus, *Neisseria meningitidis, Haemophilus influenzae,* and *Listeria monocytogenes.*

PATHOPHYSIOLOGY

- The development of bacterial meningitis involves four main processes: (1) mucosal colonization and bacterial invasion of the host and CNS; (2) bacterial replication in the subarachnoid space; (3) pathophysiologic alterations resulting in progressive inflammation; and (4) increased intracranial pressure (ICP) and cerebral edema leading to neuronal damage.
- The critical first step in the acquisition of acute bacterial meningitis is nasopharyngeal colonization of the host by the bacterial pathogen. Most cases of acute bacterial meningitis probably occur following bacteremia, but the high incidence of pneumococcal meningitis in patients with sinusitis and otitis media suggests that direct spread to the CNS can also occur.
- A common characteristic of most CNS bacterial pathogens (eg, *H. influenzae, Escherichia coli, N. meningitidis*) is the presence of an extensive polysaccharide capsule that is resistant to neutrophil phagocytosis and complement opsonization.
- The neurologic sequelae of meningitis occur due to the activation of host inflammatory pathways. Bacterial cell lysis causes the release of cell wall components such as lipopolysaccharide, lipid A (endotoxin), lipoteichoic acid, teichoic acid, and peptidoglycan, depending on whether the pathogen is gram-positive or gram-negative.
- These cell wall components cause capillary endothelial cells and CNS macrophages to release cytokines (interleukin-1, tumor necrosis factor, and other inflammatory mediators). Proteolytic products and toxic oxygen radicals cause an alteration of the blood–brain barrier, whereas platelet-activating factor activates coagulation, and arachidonic acid metabolites stimulate vasodilation. These events lead to cerebral edema, elevated ICP, cerebrospinal fluid (CSF) pleocytosis, decreased cerebral blood flow, cerebral ischemia, and death.
- Passive and active exposure to cigarette smoke and the presence of a cochlear implant that includes a positioner both increase the risk of bacterial meningitis.

CLINICAL PRESENTATION

- Signs and symptoms of acute bacterial meningitis include fever, nuchal rigidity, altered mental status, chills, vomiting, photophobia, and severe headache. Up to 95% of patients exhibit at least two of the following symptoms: fever, nuchal rigidity, headache, and altered mental status. Kernig and Brudzinski signs may be present but are poorly sensitive and frequently absent in children.
- Clinical signs and symptoms in young children may include bulging fontanelle, apnea purpuric rash, and convulsions.
- Purpuric and petechial skin lesions typically indicate meningococcal involvement, although the lesions may be present with *H. influenzae* meningitis. Rashes rarely occur with pneumococcal meningitis.
- Meningitis causes changes in CSF fluid, and these changes can be used as diagnostic markers of infection (Table 36-1).

TABLE 36-1	Mean Values of the Components of Normal and Abnormal Cerebrospinal Fluid				
Type	**Normal**	**Bacterial**	**Viral**	**Fungal**	**Tuberculosis**
WBC (cells/ mm³ or 10⁶/L)	<5 (<30 in newborns)	1000–5000	50–1000	20–500	25–500
Differentialª	Monocytes	Neutrophils	Lymphocytes	Lymphocytes	Lymphocytes
Protein (mg/dL)	<50 (<500 mg/L)	Elevated	Mild elevation	Elevated	Elevated
Glucose (mg/dL)	45–80 (2.5–4.4 mmol/L)	Low	Normal	Low	Low
CSF/blood glucose ratio	50%–60%	Decreased	Normal	Decreased	Decreased

ªInitial cerebrospinal fluid (CSF), while blood cell (WBC) count may reveal a predominance of polymorphonuclear neutrophils (PMNs). In CNS infection due to tuberculosis, "therapeutic paradox" may occur in which a lymphocytic predominance becomes neutrophilic during antituberculous treatment.

- CSF examination is essential for establishing diagnosis of bacterial meningitis, identifying the pathogen, and performing susceptibility testing. CSF polymorphonuclear pleocytosis, an elevated CSF protein of >50 mg/dL (500 mg/L), and a CSF glucose concentration of <50% of the simultaneously obtained peripheral value suggest bacterial meningitis.
- CSF culture is the gold standard for diagnosis of bacterial meningitis and is positive in 80%–90% of patients with community-acquired bacterial meningitis if the CSF sample is obtained before the start of antimicrobial therapy.
- Gram stain is a rapid, inexpensive, and accurate method to assess the presence of bacteria in CSF. However, prior antibiotic therapy may cause the Gram stain and CSF culture to be negative, but the antibiotic therapy rarely affects CSF protein or glucose. The sensitivity of the Gram stain depends on the causative microorganism, so that its aggregate diagnostic yield is 90% in pneumococcal, 70%–90% in meningococcal, 50% in *H. influenzae*, and only 25%–35% in *L. monocytogenes* meningitis.
- Polymerase chain reaction techniques can rapidly diagnose CNS infections and may be particularly useful in patients who have received antimicrobial therapy before lumbar puncture, have negative cultures, or when the organism is fastidious or fails to grow in conventional culture.

TREATMENT

- Goals of Treatment: Effective eradication of infection, amelioration of signs and symptoms, and reduction of morbidity and mortality.
- Key elements include initiating appropriate antimicrobials, providing supportive care, and preventing disease through timely introduction of vaccination and chemoprophylaxis.
- Administration of fluids, electrolytes, antipyretics, and analgesics may be indicated for patients presenting with a possible CNS infection. Additionally, venous thromboembolism prophylaxis, antiepileptic therapy, and ICP monitoring may be needed.

PHARMACOLOGIC TREATMENT

- Empiric antimicrobial therapy should be instituted as soon as possible to eradicate the causative organism (Table 36-2). Antimicrobial therapy should last at least 48–72 hours or until the diagnosis of bacterial meningitis can be ruled out. The first dose of antibiotic should not be withheld even when lumbar puncture is delayed

TABLE 36-2	Bacterial Meningitis: Most Likely Etiologies and Empiric Therapy by Age Group	
Age	**Most Likely Organisms**	**Empirical Therapy**[a]
<1 month	S. agalactiae Gram-negative enterics[b] L. monocytogenes	Ampicillin + cefotaxime or ampicillin + aminoglycoside
1–23 months	S. pneumoniae N. meningitidis H. influenzae S. agalactiae	Vancomycin[c] + third generation cephalosporin (cefotaxime or ceftriaxone)
2–50 years	N. meningitidis S. pneumoniae	Vancomycin[c] + third generation cephalosporin (cefotaxime or ceftriaxone)
>50 years	S. pneumoniae N. meningitidis Gram-negative enterics[b] L. monocytogenes	Vancomycin[c] + ampicillin + third generation cephalosporin (cefotaxime or ceftriaxone)

[a]All recommendations are A-III.
[b]E. coli, Klebsiella spp., Enterobacter spp. common.
[c]Vancomycin use should be based on local incidence of penicillin-resistant S. pneumoniae and until
cefotaxime or ceftriaxone minimum inhibitory concentration results are available.
Strength of recommendation: (A) Good evidence to support a recommendation for use; should
always be offered. (B) Moderate evidence to support a recommendation for use; should generally
be offered.
Quality of evidence: (I) Evidence from one or more properly randomized, controlled trial.
(II) Evidence from one or more well-designed clinical trial, without randomization; from cohort or
case-controlled analytic studies (preferably from one or more center) or from multiple time-series.
(III) Evidence from opinions of respected authorities, based on clinical experience, descriptive
studies, or reports of expert committees.

or neuroimaging is being performed. The time period from suspected diagnosis to
initiation of antibiotic treatment should not exceed 1 hour.

- Continued therapy should be based on the assessment of clinical improvement,
cultures, and susceptibility testing results. Once a pathogen is identified, antibiotic
therapy should be tailored to the specific pathogen.
- With increased meningeal inflammation, there will be greater antibiotic penetration
(Table 36-3). Problems of CSF penetration can be overcome by direct instillation of
antibiotics intrathecally or intraventricularly. The advantages of direct instillation,
however, must be weighed against the risks of invasive CNS procedures and adverse
effects. Intraventricular delivery may be necessary in patients who have shunt infections that are difficult to eradicate or who cannot undergo the surgical management.
- See Table 36-4 for antimicrobial agents of first choice and alternatives for treatment
of meningitis caused by gram-positive and gram-negative microorganisms.
- Meningitis caused by S. pneumoniae has been treated successfully with 10–14 days of
antibiotic therapy, while cases caused by N. meningitidis or H. influenzae usually can
be treated with a 7-day course. In contrast, a longer duration (21 days or more) has
been recommended for patients with L. monocytogenes, Gram-negative or pseudomonal meningitis. Nonetheless, antibiotic treatments for bacterial meningitis should
be individualized, and some patients may require enduring courses.

Dexamethasone as an Adjunctive Treatment for Meningitis

- In addition to antibiotics, dexamethasone is a commonly used adjunctive therapy in the
treatment of acute bacterial meningitis to immunomodulate the inflammatory response.

TABLE 36-3 Penetration of Anti-infective Agents into the CSF[a]

Therapeutic Levels in CSF with or without Inflammation of Meninges

Acyclovir	Levofloxacin
Chloramphenicol	Linezolid
Ciprofloxacin	Metronidazole
Fluconazole	Moxifloxacin
Flucytosine	Pyrazinamide
Foscarnet	Rifampin
Fosfomycin	Sulfonamides
Ganciclovir	Trimethoprim
Isoniazid	Voriconazole

Therapeutic Levels in CSF with Inflammation of Meninges

Ampicillin ± sulbactam	Imipenem
Aztreonam	Meropenem
Cefepime	Nafcillin
Cefotaxime	Ofloxacin
Ceftazidime	Penicillin G
Ceftriaxone	Piperacillin/Tazobactam[b]
Cefuroxime	Pyrimethamine
Colistin	Quinupristin/Dalfopristin
Daptomycin	Ticarcillin ± clavulanic acid[b]
Ethambutol	Vancomycin

Nontherapeutic Levels in CSF with or without Inflammation of Meninges

Aminoglycosides	Cephalosporins (second generation)[d]
Amphotericin B	Doxycycline[e]
β-Lactamase inhibitors[c]	Itraconazole[f]
Cephalosporins (first generation)	

[a]Using recommended CNS dosing and compared to minimum inhibitory concentration (MIC) of target pathogens.
[b]May not achieve therapeutic levels against organisms with higher MIC, as in *P. aeruginosa*. Tazobactam does not penetrate the blood-brain barrier.
[c]Includes clavulanic acid, sulbactam, and tazobactam.
[d]Cefuroxime is an exception.
[e]Documented effectiveness for *B. burgdorferi*.
[f]Achieves therapeutic concentrations for *Cryptococcus neoformans* therapy.

- Recommendations call for the use of adjunctive dexamethasone in infants and children (6 weeks of age and older) with *H. influenzae* meningitis. The recommended intravenous dose is 0.15 mg/kg every 6 hours for 2–4 days, initiated 10–20 minutes prior to or concomitant with the first dose of antibiotics. In infants and children with pneumococcal meningitis, adjunctive dexamethasone may be considered after weighing the potential benefits and possible risks. If pneumococcal meningitis is suspected or proven, adults should receive dexamethasone 0.15 mg/kg (up to 10 mg) every 6 hours for 2–4 days with the first dose administered 10–20 minutes prior to first dose of antibiotics.

TABLE 36-4	Antimicrobial Agents of First Choice and Alternative Choice for Treating Meningitis Caused by Gram-Positive and Gram-Negative Microorganisms		
Organism	**Antibiotics of First Choice**	**Alternative Antibiotics**	**Recommended Duration of Therapy**
Gram-Positive Organisms			
Streptococcus pneumoniae[a]			10–14 days
Penicillin susceptible MIC ≤0.06 mcg/mL (mg/L)	Penicillin G or ampicillin (A-III)	Cefotaxime (A-III), ceftriaxone (A-III), cefepime (B-II), or meropenem (B-II)	
Penicillin resistant MIC >0.06 mcg/mL (mg/L)	Vancomycin[b,c] + cefotaxime or ceftriaxone (A-III)	Moxifloxacin (B-II)	
Ceftriaxone resistant MIC >0.5 mcg/mL (mg/L)	Vancomycin[b,c] + cefotaxime or ceftriaxone (A-III)	Moxifloxacin (B-II)	
Staphylococcus aureus			14–21 days
Methicillin susceptible	Nafcillin or oxacillin (A-III)	Vancomycin (A-III) or meropenem (B-III)	
Methicillin resistant	Vancomycin[b,c] (A-III)	Trimethoprim-sulfamethoxazole or linezolid (B-III)	
Group B *Streptococcus*	Penicillin G or ampicillin (A-III) ± gentamicin[b,c]	Ceftriaxone or cefotaxime (B-III)	14–21 days
S. epidermidis	Vancomycin[b,c] (A-III)	Linezolid (B-III)	14–21 days[d]
L. monocytogenes	Penicillin G or ampicillin ± gentamicin[b,c,e] (A-III)	Trimethoprim-sulfamethoxazole (A-III), meropenem (B-III)	≥21 days
Gram-Negative Organisms			
Neisseria meningitis			7–10 days
Penicillin susceptible	Penicillin G or ampicillin (A-III)	Cefotaxime or ceftriaxone (A-III)	
Penicillin resistant	Cefotaxime or ceftriaxone (A-III)	Meropenem or moxifloxacin (A-III)	
Haemophilus influenzae			7–10 days
β-lactamase negative	Ampicillin (A-III)	Cefotaxime (A-III), ceftriaxone (A-III), cefepime (A-III) or moxifloxacin (A-III)	

(Continued)

TABLE 36-4	Antimicrobial Agents of First Choice and Alternative Choice for Treating Meningitis Caused by Gram-Positive and Gram-Negative Microorganisms (*Continued*)

Organism	Antibiotics of First Choice	Alternative Antibiotics	Recommended Duration of Therapy
β-lactamase positive	Cefotaxime or ceftriaxone (A-I)	Cefepime (A-I) or moxifloxacin (A-III)	
Enterobacteriaceae[f]	Cefotaxime or ceftriaxone (A-II)	Cefepime (A-III), moxifloxacin (A-III), meropenem (A-III) or aztreonam (A-III)	21 days
Pseudomonas aeruginosa	Cefepime or ceftazidime (A-II) ± tobramycin[b,c] (A-III)	Ciprofloxacin (A-III), meropenem (A-III), piperacillin plus tobramycin[a,b] (A-III), colistin sulfomethate[g] (B-III), aztreonam (A-III)	21 days

[a]European Guidelines recommend considering the addition of rifampin to vancomycin therapy.
[b]Direct CNS administration may be considered if failed conventional treatment.
[c]Monitor serum drug levels.
[d]Based on clinical experience; no clear recommendations.
[e]European guidelines recommend adding gentamicin for the first 7 days of treatment.
[f]Includes *E. coli* and *Klebsiella* spp.
[g]Should be reserved for multidrug-resistant pseudomonal or *Acinetobacter* infections for which all other therapeutic options have been exhausted.
See Table 36-2 footnotes for rating scale of evidence.

Neisseria meningitidis (Meningococcus)

- *N. meningitidis* is a leading cause of bacterial meningitis among children and young adults in the United States and around the world. It is spread by direct person-to-person close contact, including respiratory droplets and pharyngeal secretions.
- The presence of petechiae may be the primary clue that the underlying pathogen is *N. meningitidis*. Patients may also have an obvious or subclinical picture of disseminated intravascular coagulation (DIC).
- Deafness unilaterally, or more commonly bilaterally, may develop early or late in the disease course.
- Third-generation cephalosporins (ie, cefotaxime and ceftriaxone) are the recommended empiric treatment for meningococcal meningitis. Penicillin G or ampicillin is recommended for penicillin-susceptible isolates. The recommended duration of therapy is typically 7 days if there is a good clinical response.
- Antimicrobial chemoprophylaxis of close contacts should be started as soon as possible (ideally <24 hours after identification of the index patient). Ciprofloxacin and rifampin are the two most used chemoprophylactic agents.
- For full details on vaccine availability and vaccination recommendations in various age groups and for those with significant risk factors, readers are referred to in Chapter 147 of *Pharamcotherapy: A Pathophysiologic Approach*, 12th edition.

Streptococcus pneumoniae (Pneumococcus or Diplococcus)

- *Streptococcus* group B is a leading cause of community-acquired bacterial meningitis in patients 2 months of age or older.
- Coma, hearing impairment, and seizures are common neurologic complications.
- Penicillin should not be used as empiric therapy if *S. pneumoniae* is suspected. Ceftriaxone and cefotaxime have served as alternatives to penicillin in the treatment of penicillin-nonsusceptible pneumococci. Therapeutic approaches to cephalosporin-resistant pneumococci include the addition of vancomycin or, to a lesser extent, rifampin. The combination of vancomycin and ceftriaxone can be used as empirical treatment until antimicrobial susceptibility data are available.
- Intravenous linezolid, daptomycin, and ceftaroline have also emerged as viable therapeutic options for treating multidrug-resistant gram-positive infections.
- Refer to Chapter 52 for information on pneumococcal vaccines.

Haemophilus influenzae Type b

- Widespread vaccination of infants and children has effectively decreased the incidence of bacterial meningitis due to Hib in children between the ages of 1 month and 5 years, resulting in a significant decline in all cases of bacterial meningitis.
- Third-generation cephalosporins (cefotaxime and ceftriaxone) are the drugs of choice for empirical therapy for *H. influenzae* type b meningitis as they are active against β-lactamase–producing and non-β-lactamase–producing strains. Cefepime and fluoroquinolones are suitable alternatives regardless of β-lactamase activity.
- Recommended duration of treatment is 7 days (adults) or 7–10 days (children).
- Dexamethasone is beneficial for treatment of infants and children with Hib meningitis to diminish the risk of hearing loss, if given before or concurrently with the first dose of antimicrobial agent(s).
- Chemoprophylaxis with rifampin is indicated to reduce the risk of secondary invasive Hib disease in close contacts by eliminating nasopharyngeal and oropharyngeal carriages of *H. influenzae*. Rifampin should be administered orally, once a day for 4 days (20 mg/kg/dose; maximum, 600 mg). For information on who should receive prophylaxis (adults and children), refer to the recommendations of the American Academy of Pediatrics.
- Refer to Chapter 52 for information on *H. influenzae* vaccination.

Listeria monocytogenes

- *L. monocytogenes* is implicated in approximately 10% of meningitis cases in patients older than 65 years of age and carries a case-fatality rate of approximately 18% in the United States.
- Treatment of *L. monocytogenes* meningitis should consist of penicillin G or ampicillin. The addition of aminoglycoside is also recommended in proven infection in both children and adults. Patients should be treated for a minimum of 21 days.
- **Trimethoprim–sulfamethoxazole** and **meropenem** may be effective alternatives because adequate CSF penetration is achieved with these agents.

See Chapter 128, Central Nervous System Infections, authored by Delaney E. Hart, Christina Koutsari, Michael A. Wankum and Ramy H. Elshaboury, and John C. Rotschafer, for a more detailed discussion of this topic.

37 Coronavirus Disease 2019 (COVID-19)

This chapter is current as of August 1, 2022. Refer to the National Institutes of Health (NIH) and Infectious Diseases Society of America (IDSA)'s COVID-19 Treatment Guidelines, and the Centers for Disease Control and Prevention (CDC) COVID-19 Vaccination site for the most current treatment and prevention recommendations.

- *Coronavirus disease 2019 (COVID-19)* is a widespread, life-threatening infection caused by Severe Acute Respiratory Syndrome Coronavirus 2 (SARS-CoV-2).

PATHOPHYSIOLOGY

- With continuing COVID-19 spread, the evolving virus led to the emergence of SARS-CoV-2 variants and lineages. The Omicron variant consists of at least seven lineages to date: B.1.1.529, BA.1, BA.1.1, BA.2, BA.3, BA.4, and BA.5.
- The risk of severe disease or mortality increases significantly with factors such as older age, presence of at least one underlying medical condition, and disabilities (including intellectual disabilities).
- The primary route of transmission is direct person-to-person respiratory transmission via infected particles (ie, droplets and aerosols). Risk of transmission is greatest for individuals in close contact (less than 6 ft apart), especially while indoors.
- COVID-19 disease progression occurs in three phases of increasing severity: (1) early infection, (2) pulmonary phase, and (3) hyperinflammation.
  - ✓ Early infection is characterized by inoculation, incubation, viral replication, and mild symptoms (eg, fever, cough, shortness of breath).
  - ✓ The pulmonary phase is characterized by localized lung inflammation with continued viral replication and moderate symptoms. Development of hypoxia (oxygen saturation 94% or less), is associated with a poorer prognosis. The pulmonary phase can be subdivided into phase IIa (without hypoxia) and phase IIb (with hypoxia).
  - ✓ Monocytes and neutrophils are recruited to the site of infection, and potent cytokines such as interleukin-6 (IL-6) are released by activated macrophages and other immune cells. Pulmonary infiltration is often recognized as bilateral ground glass opacities and/or consolidations on chest radiograph or computed tomography.
  - ✓ Hyperinflammation is characterized by marked systemic inflammation and severe symptoms. High cytokine levels (cytokine storm) lead to dilation of the pulmonary vascular bed with vascular permeability and leakage, thickening and fibrosis of alveolar walls, edema filling alveolar sacs, and thrombus formation, which all contribute to pulmonary ischemia and damage.
  - ✓ Cytokine storm in critically ill patients involves elevated blood concentrations of interleukin-1 (IL-1), IL-2, IL-6, granulocyte colony-stimulating factor (G-CSF), and tumor necrosis factor-alpha (TNF-α), and other inflammatory markers.
- Most COVID-19 deaths result from this cascade leading to acute respiratory distress syndrome (ARDS) with hypoxic respiratory failure. Many critically ill patients also experience significant injury to one or more additional organ systems, such as the heart, brain, liver, kidneys, and gastrointestinal tract.
- Coagulopathy in critically ill patients can appear similar to disseminated intravascular coagulation (DIC). Other manifestations of end-organ damage include acute complications of the cardiac and cardiovascular system (eg, dysrhythmias, myocardial infarction, heart failure, cardiogenic shock) as well as thromboembolic (eg, pulmonary embolism, deep venous thromboembolism) and neurologic complications (eg, encephalopathy).
- Long-term sequelae from COVID-19 can include permanent lung injury or other end-organ damage. Theorized causes of long COVID include: (1) persistence of SARS-CoV-2 in tissues due to immune evasion, (2) damage from ongoing inflammation, and (3) ongoing microvascular blood clots.

- Children and adolescents are at risk of a serious complication termed multisystem inflammatory syndrome in children (MIS-C). MIS-C occurs after acute infection with SARS-CoV-2 and is similar in presentation to Kawasaki disease.

CLINICAL PRESENTATION

- The time from virus exposure to symptom onset (the incubation period) ranges from 2 to 14 days with a median of 4–5 days.
- There is a wide range in clinical presentation and severity from asymptomatic, pre-symptomatic, mild illness, moderate illness, severe illness, to critical illness that can result in death.
- Signs and Symptoms:
  ✓ Severity of the case may take days to weeks to become fully evident.
  ✓ 40% of patients progress to feeling short of breath with a median of 7 days after initial symptom onset.
  ✓ 14% of patients progress to severe disease and 5% progress to critical illness with a median of 10 days after initial symptom onset.
- Most common symptoms, often presenting together: runny nose, headache, sore throat, sneezing, and cough.
- Less common symptoms: fever and/or chills, fatigue, sputum production, muscle or body aches, shortness of breath, diarrhea, nausea or vomiting, abdominal pain, and new loss of taste or smell.
- In children, MIS-C is characterized by fever, elevated laboratory markers for inflammation (eg, IL-6, TNF-α), and involvement of two or more organ systems in the presence of current or recent COVID-19 infection or exposure within four weeks and in the absence of alternative plausible diagnoses.
  ✓ Other presenting signs and symptoms include abdominal pain, vomiting, diarrhea, skin rash, mucocutaneous lesions, and, in severe cases, hypotension and shock.
  ✓ Organ involvement may include cardiac dysfunction (eg, myocarditis, cardiogenic shock) and renal dysfunction (eg, acute kidney injury).
- While symptoms of acute COVID-19 infection usually resolve in a matter of weeks, some patients experience prolonged symptoms for more than 4 weeks and potentially for months or years. This is commonly referred to as *long COVID*, *post-COVID conditions*, *long-haul COVID*, *post-acute sequelae of COVID-19 (PASC)*, and *chronic COVID*.
  ✓ The most common symptoms of long COVID include fatigue, self-reported "brain fog" which is also described as sluggish or fuzzy cognition, dyspnea, headache, chest tightness, numbness/tingling, dysgeusia, myalgia, anosmia, depression/anxiety, chest pain, and variation in heart rate and blood pressure.

DIAGNOSIS

- Nucleic acid amplification tests (NAATs), such as real-time reverse transcription polymerase chain reaction (RT-PCR), to detect genetic material of SARS-CoV-2 are the gold standard diagnostic tests for COVID-19 infection.
- SARS-CoV-2 antigen immunoassay tests are alternative methods that indicate active or recent infection.
- Specimens for NAATs or antigen tests include nasopharyngeal, oropharyngeal, sputum, bronchoalveolar, or saliva samples. Acceptable specimens may vary by the specific test.
- Serologic tests for antibody against SARS-CoV-2 are complementary diagnostics that indicate past infection and/or vaccination. Blood specimens for analysis are typically collected via fingerstick or venipuncture.
- Probable COVID-19 can be diagnosed by presence of a compatible syndrome in either the absence of viral testing or a negative test. False negative tests are most common early in infection.

LABORATORY TESTS

- Comprehensive metabolic panel test results (eg, liver function tests) may be elevated.
- Peripheral blood cell counts are often low (eg, lymphopenia, leukopenia, thrombocytopenia).
- Inflammatory markers are often elevated (eg, C-reactive protein lactate dehydrogenase, ferritin, creatine kinase).
- Coagulation studies are often abnormal (eg, elevated D-dimer).
- Abnormalities become more numerous and pronounced with more severe disease.

OTHER DIAGNOSTIC TESTS

- Chest radiograph is typically performed for patients presenting to the emergency department; computed tomography (CT) is typically reserved for hospitalized patients with severe disease.

PREVENTION

- Vaccination is the best way to decrease morbidity and mortality associated with COVID-19. Face masks, social distancing, and increased ventilation are also effective prevention strategies; hand washing and disinfectants may also be important to minimize spread of infection.
- Monoclonal antibodies are effective for primary prevention or post-exposure prophylaxis of SARS-CoV-2 infection but are only available for pre-exposure prophylaxis in immunosuppressed patients.
- As of August 1, 2022, four vaccines are available in the United States under either full Food and Drug Administration (FDA) approval or Emergency Use Authorization (EUA): two as a two-dose primary series using mRNA technology (Pfizer [BNT162b2]), Moderna [mRNA1273], one as a one-dose primary series using an adenovirus vector platform (Johnson & Johnson [Ad26.CoV2S]), and one as a two-dose primary series using an adjuvanted recombinant spike protein platform (Novavax [NVX-CoV2373]).
- An additional dose (a third dose of an mRNA vaccine or a second dose of adenovirus vector vaccine) is recommended as part of the primary series for patients with moderate or severe immunocompromise who are less likely to respond to vaccination.
- mRNA vaccines are preferred over viral vector vaccines for both the primary series and booster doses due to increased efficacy against infection and severe disease, a broadened immune response, and a more favorable safety profile.
- Because the Novavax vaccine was approved in July 2022 and there are no data on the safety or efficacy of additional doses, there is currently no recommendation for additional doses in any patient population.
- A booster vaccine dose is recommended for most people ≥5 months after completion of the primary series. A second booster is recommended for adults ≥50 years of age, to be given ≥4 months after the first booster (Table 37-1). All current booster recommendations from the CDC prefer use of mRNA vaccines regardless of what was used for the primary series.
- Reports of allergic reactions with administration of both mRNA vaccines surfaced soon after the global vaccination campaign commenced. Anaphylaxis was reported in 4.7 cases per million doses with Pfizer/BNT162b2 and 2.5 cases per million doses of Moderna/mRNA1273.
- A delayed (median onset 8 days), large rash at the injection site has been observed following receipt of mRNA1273.
- An association between mRNA vaccines (both BNT162b2 and mRNA1273) and myocarditis has been demonstrated and is more frequently seen with the second dose and in younger males.
- With viral vector vaccine (Ad26.CoV2S), the most common adverse events were injection site pain, headache, fatigue, and myalgia.
- A potentially life-threatening thrombosis with thrombocytopenia syndrome (TTS) can occur in women aged 18–49 years, estimated at 7 cases per 1 million vaccinations.

TABLE 37-1 CDC Recommended Vaccine Schedule as of July 2022

Immunocompetent Patients

	Age Range	Dose	Primary Series	1st Booster[a]	2nd Booster[a]
Moderna (mRNA1273)	6 months – 5 years	25 mcg	Two doses, 4–8 weeks apart	Not currently recommended	
	6–11	50 mcg		Not currently recommended	
	12–17	100 mcg		Not currently recommended	
	18–49	100 mcg		≥5 months after dose 2	Not currently recommended
	≥50	100 mcg		≥5 months after dose 2	≥4 months after dose 3
Pfizer (BNT162b2)	6 months – 4 years	3 mcg	Three-dose series, second dose 3–8 weeks after first, third dose ≥8 weeks after second	Not currently recommended	
	5–11	10 mcg	Two doses, 3–8 weeks apart	≥5 months after dose 2	Not currently recommended
	12–49	30 mcg			
	≥50	30 mcg		≥5 months after dose 2	≥4 months after dose 3
Johnson & Johnson (Ad26.CoV2S)	18–49	0.5 mL	One dose	≥2 months after dose 1	Not currently recommended
	50+	0.5 mL	One dose	≥2 months after dose 1	≥4 months after dose 2
Novavax (NVX-CoV2373)	≥18	0.5 mL	Two doses, 3–8 weeks apart	Not currently recommended[b]	

Patients with moderate to severe immunocompromise

	Age range	Dose	Primary Series	1st booster[a]	2nd booster[a]
Moderna (mRNA1273)	6 months – 5 years	25 mcg	Three-dose series, second dose 4 weeks after first, third dose ≥4 weeks after second	Not currently recommended	
	6–11	50 mcg		Not currently recommended	
	12–17	100 mcg		Not currently recommended	
	18–49	100 mcg		≥3 months after dose 2	Not currently recommended
	≥50	100 mcg			≥4 months after dose 3

(Continued)

| TABLE 37-1 | CDC Recommended Vaccine Schedule as of July 2022 (*Continued*) |

Immunocompetent Patients

	Age Range	Dose	Primary Series	1st Booster[a]	2nd Booster[a]
Pfizer (BNT162b2)	6 months – 4 years	3 mcg	Three-dose series, second dose 3 weeks after first, third dose $\geq$ 8 weeks after second	Not currently recommended	
	5–11	10 mcg	Three-dose series, second dose 3 weeks after first, third dose $\geq$4 weeks after second	$\geq$3 months after dose 3	$\geq$4 months after dose 4
	12–49	30 mcg			
	$\geq$50	30 mcg		$\geq$3 months after dose 3	$\geq$4 months after dose 4
Johnson & Johnson (Ad26.CoV2S)	$\geq$18	0.5 mL	Two doses; dose 2 should be an mRNA vaccine $\geq$4 weeks after the first dose	$\geq$2 months after dose 2	$\geq$4 months after dose 3
Novavax (NVX-CoV2373)	$\geq$18	0.5 mL	Two doses, 3–8 weeks apart	Not currently recommended[b]	

[a]Can mix and match between mRNA boosters; if possible, mRNA vaccines are recommended for booster doses for patients with primary series of Johnson & Johnson given increase breadth of immune response and safety.

[b]Authorized July 2022 as two-dose series; at time of chapter writing, no one is eligible for booster doses. Recommendations may change in fall of 2022.

[a]Can mix and match between mRNA boosters; if possible, mRNA vaccines are recommended for booster doses for patients with primary series of Johnson & Johnson given increase breadth of immune response and safety.

[b]Authorized July 2022 as two-dose series with no data available supporting an extra dose as part of primary series in patients with moderate to severe immunocompromise; at time of chapter writing, there is no recommendation for additional doses. Recommendations may change in the fall of 2022.

TREATMENT

<u>Goals of Treatment</u>: For outpatients, the treatment goals are to prevent progression to severe disease requiring hospitalization or death and hasten symptom resolution. For those treated in an inpatient setting, the primary goals are survival, prevention of the need for mechanical ventilation or intensive care unit admission, and shortening the length of hospital stay.

GENERAL APPROACH

- Pharmacotherapy early in the course of illness is focused on minimizing viral replication by either supplementing the immune response to eradicate the virus (ie, monoclonal antibodies) or directly inhibiting viral replication (ie, **remdesivir**, **nirmatrelvir/ritonavir, molnupiravir**).

- Table 37-2 outlines treatments to be considered for each severity stage of COVID-19, and Tables 37-3 and 37-4 summarize dosing, monitoring, and counseling considerations for drugs recommended for outpatient and inpatient remdesivir treatment.
- Other agents that have demonstrated efficacy for COVID-19 include monoclonal antibodies, oral antivirals (ie, ritonavir-boosted nirmatrelvir, molnupiravir), and immunomodulatory therapies (eg, corticosteroids, **tocilizumab, baricitinib**).
- For patient progressing to more severe stages, pharmacotherapy is focused on immune modulation (ie, corticosteroids, IL-6 inhibitors, Janus kinase inhibitors) to blunt the hyperinflammatory phase that could otherwise cause significant end-organ damage, morbidity, and mortality.

NONPHARMACOLOGIC THERAPY

- Patients infected with SARS-CoV-2 with mild to moderate symptoms should isolate at home for at least 5 days, where day 0 is the first day of symptoms or a positive test. Day 1 is the first full day after symptoms developed or test specimen was collected.
- Isolation can end after 5 full days in patients who are fever-free for 24 hours and whose symptoms are improving or those who were asymptomatic. Patients should wear a well-fitting mask and avoid travel until day 10.
- Wherever possible, separate rooms, bathrooms, and household items should be used by the infected patient during this time, and everyone in the household should wear a well-fitting mask. During isolation, patients are encouraged to monitor their blood oxygen saturation using a home pulse oximeter and seek medical care if oxygen saturation falls to 94% or lower.
- Symptom control with cough/throat lozenges, warm tea, soup, and nonprescription nonsteroidal anti-inflammatory drugs (NSAIDs) or antipyretics (ie, acetaminophen) are appropriate as needed.

PHARMACOLOGIC THERAPY

OUTPATIENT TREATMENT

- Three anti-SARS-CoV-2 antiviral therapies are available for outpatient use, two as a 5-day oral course (nirmatrelvir/ritonavir and molnupiravir) and one as a 3-day intravenous regimen (remdesivir). Both oral antivirals are authorized for use within 5 days of symptom onset, whereas remdesivir is authorized for use within 7 days from symptom onset in outpatients with mild to moderate COVID-19 at high risk for progression to severe disease.
- Outpatient treatment options are summarized in Table 37-3.
- The FDA has authorized pharmacist prescribing of nirmatrelvir/ritonavir to patients who qualify for therapy per the EUA if no drug interactions requiring therapy modification are present and renal and hepatic function can be assessed.
- **Bebtelovimab** is the only anti-SARS-CoV-2 monoclonal antibody available under EUA for outpatient use for mild to moderate SARS-CoV-2 infection in patients at high risk for progression of disease.
- Outpatient therapies that should not be used: ivermectin, hydroxychloroquine or chloroquine, azithromycin, inhaled corticosteroids, and supplements (vitamin D, vitamin C, vitamin K, zinc, and melatonin).

INPATIENT TREATMENT

- Remdesivir is recommended for hospitalized patients requiring supplemental oxygen or non-invasive ventilation only (ie, it is not recommended for mechanically ventilated patients) for a duration of 5 days.
- Remdesivir is FDA approved for all hospitalized adults and children, including neonates. Dosing by age and weight is described in Table 37-2. Use in pregnant patients

TABLE 37-2   Treatment Recommendations by Disease Severity and Patient Location

Severity of Illness	Nirmatrelvir/ ritonavir	Bebtelovimab	Remdesivir	Corticosteroids	Tocilizumab	Baricitinib	Therapeutic Anticoagulation	Notes
Mild to Moderate, Not Hospitalized Outpatient or Emergency Department Not requiring supplemental oxygen above baseline needs	Patients at high risk of hospitalization per FDA EUA criteria	Patients at high risk of hospitalization per FDA EUA criteria.	Patients at high risk of hospitalization per FDA EUA criteria (3-day therapy).	No	No	No	No	Patients breathing ambient air should not receive corticosteroids. Patients should not receive more than one EUA therapy, and choice between those available is based on patient characteristics and preferences, drug interactions, and drug availability. Molnupiravir may be considered if ninrmaltrevir/ritonavir, remdesivir, and bebtelovimab are all unavailable. There is an unclear benefit to fluvoxamine, and it should not be routinely recommended. Colchicine, ivermectin, hydroxychloroquine, azithromycin, and inhaled corticosteroids are not recommended.

Moderate Hospitalized Not requiring supplemental oxygen above baseline needs Radiographic evidence of pneumonia	No	Patients hospitalized for reasons other than COVID-19 and incidentally found to have COVID-19 may be eligible.	No	Not routinely recommended; consider in high-risk patients (3–5 day therapy).	No	No	Avoid unless otherwise indicated for thrombosis treatment	Patients breathing ambient air should not receive corticosteroids. High-risk patients include those with profound immunosuppression.
Severe Hospitalized Requiring supplemental oxygen above baseline needs or non-invasive ventilation	No	No	Low-flow O₂: Yes (5-day therapy) HFNC or NIV: No	Yes	Yes (see notes)	Yes (see notes)	Low-flow O₂: Yes HFNC or NIV: Avoid therapeutic anticoagulation unless indicated for thrombosis treatment	Discontinue corticosteroid if supplemental oxygen is no longer required. Administer tocilizumab or baricitinib only in combination with corticosteroids. Patients should not receive both tocilizumab and baricitinib. Tocilizumab or baricitinib is recommended in patients who have rapidly increasing oxygen needs and require HFNC or NIV and/or who have significantly increased markers of inflammation (eg, CRP ≥75 mg/L). *(Continued)*

TABLE 37-2 Treatment Recommendations by Disease Severity and Patient Location *(Continued)*

Severity of Illness	Nirmatrelvir/ritonavir	Bebtelovimab	Remdesivir	Corticosteroids	Tocilizumab	Baricitinib	Therapeutic Anticoagulation	Notes
Severe-Critical Hospitalized Mechanically ventilated, ECMO, septic shock, and/or multiple organ dysfunction	No	No	No	Yes	Yes (see notes)	Yes (see notes)	Avoid unless otherwise indicated for thrombosis treatment	Large, randomized trials demonstrated no benefit of remdesivir and possible harm of therapeutic anticoagulation in patients requiring mechanical ventilation. Discontinue corticosteroid if supplemental oxygen is no longer required. Administer either tocilizumab or baricitinib only in combination with corticosteroids. Benefit has not been established in patients not receiving corticosteroids. Patients should not receive both tocilizumab and baricitinib. Tocilizumab or baricitinib are recommended for recently intubated patients who have not already received one of these agents during their admission.

TABLE 37-3 Dosing, Monitoring, and Counseling for Drugs Recommended for Outpatients with Mild-Moderate COVID-19 at High Risk for Progression to Severe Disease

Drug	Dose	Duration	Drug Interactions	Adverse Events	Treatment Pearls
Preferred					
Bebtelovimab	175 mg IV	Once	None	Infusion-related reactions	Can be infused as rapidly as over 30 seconds; authorized for use within 7 days of symptom onset
Nirmatrelvir/ Ritonavir	300 mg / 100 mg orally twice daily	Five Days	Strong CYP3A4 and PGP inhibitor – many interactions, utilize interaction checker and work closely with providers to optimize treatment plan	Dysgeusia Diarrhea	Requires renal dose adjustments and not authorized for use if estimated GFR <30 mL/min; authorized for use within 5 days of symptom onset
Remdesivir	200 mg IV on day 1, then 100 mg IV once daily Pediatric patients 3–40 kg: 5 mg/kg/dose IV on day 1 (max dose = 200 mg), followed by 2.5 mg/kg/dose IV once daily (max dose = 100 mg)	Three Days	Chloroquine and hydroxychloroquine may theoretically diminish therapeutic effect of remdesivir	Elevated LFTs Infusion reaction Bradycardia Hypotension	Authorized for use within 7 days of symptom onset
Alternative					
Molnupiravir	800 mg orally twice daily	Five days	None	Diarrhea Nausea Dizziness	Do not use in pregnancy/breastfeeding; Counsel patients with reproductive potential about need to use effective contraception; authorized for use within 7 days of symptom onset

TABLE 37-4	Dosing, Monitoring, and Counseling for Drugs Recommended for Inpatients with COVID-19			
Drug	**Dose**	**Duration**	**Drug Interactions**	**Adverse Events**	**Treatment Pearls**
Remdesivir	Adults: 200 mg IV on day 1, followed by 100 mg IV once daily Pediatrics: 3–40 kg: 5 mg/kg/dose IV on day 1 (max dose = 200 mg), followed by 2.5 mg/kg/dose IV once daily (max dose = 100 mg)	5 days or until hospital discharge. Guidelines state may extend to 10 days if no substantial improvement by day 5, although data are lacking, and this is not routinely done in clinical practice.	Chloroquine and hydroxychloroquine may theoretically diminish therapeutic effect of remdesivir	Elevated LFTs Infusion reaction Bradycardia, Hypotension	Patients should not be kept in the hospital to complete remdesivir therapy. Discharge patients when medically ready. Use lyophilized powder product only for pediatrics (less SBECD, see text).
Dexamethasone	Adults: 6 mg IV or orally once daily Pediatrics: 0.15 mg/kg orally or IV once daily (max dose = 6 mg)	10 days or until hospital discharge or until patient is no longer requiring oxygen support	Moderate CYP3A4 inducer	Hyperglycemia Fluid retention Leukocytosis Dermatologic Adrenal suppression Gastrointestinal hemorrhage or perforation Amyotrophy, Myopathy	Higher doses of 10–20 mg per day were evaluated in smaller trials of severe ARDS but are not currently recommended.
Tocilizumab	8 mg/kg IV once based on actual body weight (max dose = 800 mg)	Once	May increase metabolism of CYP3A4 substrates Caution with other immunosuppressive therapies	Bacterial infection Hypersensitivity	Gastrointestinal, hepatic, and hematologic effects with prolonged therapy (when used for rheumatoid arthritis)
Baricitinib	4 mg orally daily	14 days or until hospital discharge	Caution with other immunosuppressive therapies	Bacterial infection Increased aminotransferases Venous thromboembolism	Renal dose adjustment needed

appears to be safe and should be based on clinical judgment if benefit is deemed to outweigh risk.

- Treatment guidelines recommend **dexamethasone** 6 mg for up to 10 days for hospitalized patients requiring oxygen support. Corticosteroids are not recommended if patients do not require supplemental oxygen because of concern for potential harm.
- **Tocilizumab** (or **baricitinib**) is recommended in addition to dexamethasone for patients with rapidly increasing oxygen requirements and significantly increased inflammatory markers.
- Therapeutic heparin or low-molecular-weight heparin is recommended in nonpregnant, hospitalized patients with COVID-19 requiring supplemental oxygen, elevated D-dimer levels, and who are not at increased bleeding risk. Prophylactic-dose heparin is recommended for patients requiring high-flow supplemental oxygen, noninvasive or mechanical ventilation, or who do not require oxygen support.

EVALUATION OF THERAPEUTIC OUTCOMES

- Monitor for resolution of signs and symptoms (eg, hypoxia, fever, cough, shortness of breath). Also, monitor for adverse events while on therapy (eg, transaminitis while on remdesivir; hyperglycemia, neurologic side effects, secondary infections while on corticosteroids).
- Report any adverse events while on medication therapy to FDA MedWatch program and any adverse events following vaccine administration to FDA Vaccine Adverse Event Reporting System (VAERS), especially if serious or previously unreported.
- If patient improves such that they are no longer eligible for a specific therapy (eg, on dexamethasone, yet no longer requiring supplemental oxygen), be sure to modify or discontinue therapy as needed.
- Upon resolution of illness, encourage preventive measures such as vaccination, wearing a mask, social distancing, increased ventilation, and handwashing for the patient, their family, and/or other members of their household.

See Chapter e132, Coronavirus Disease (COVID-19), authored by Jason M. Pogue, Erin K. McCreary, and Julie Ann Justo for a more detailed discussion of this topic.

Endocarditis and Bacteremia

- *Endocarditis* is an inflammation of the endocardium, the membrane lining the chambers of the heart and covering the cusps of the heart valves. *Infective endocarditis* (IE) refers to infection of the heart valves by microorganisms, primarily bacteria.
- Endocarditis is often referred to as either acute or subacute depending on the clinical presentation. Acute bacterial endocarditis is a fulminating infection associated with high fevers, systemic toxicity, and possibly death within days to weeks if untreated. Subacute infectious endocarditis is a more indolent infection, usually occurring in a setting of prior valvular heart disease.
- Bacteremia reflects the presence of bacteria in the bloodstream, an otherwise sterile environment, which is identified based on the detection of any true-positive blood culture.

ETIOLOGY

- Most patients with IE have risk factors, such as preexisting cardiac valve abnormalities. Many types of structural heart disease resulting in turbulence of blood flow will increase the risk for IE. Some of the most important risk factors include the following:
  ✓ Highest risk: The presence of a prosthetic valve or previous IE.
  ✓ Congenital heart disease (CHD), advanced age, chronic intravenous (IV) access, diabetes mellitus, acquired valvular dysfunction (eg, rheumatic heart disease), cardiac implantable device, chronic heart failure, mitral valve prolapse with regurgitation, IV drug abuse (IVDA), HIV infection, and poor dentition and/or oral hygiene.
- Three groups of organisms cause most cases of IE: staphylococci, streptococci, and enterococci (**Table 38-1**). Staphylococci (*Staphylococcus aureus* and coagulase-negative staphylococci) are the most common cause of prosthetic valve endocarditis (PVE) within the first year after valve surgery, and *S. aureus* is common in those with a history of IVDA.
- *Escherichia coli*, *Klebsiella spp.*, *Pseudomonas aeruginosa*, *S. aureus*, *Enterococcus* spp., and *Streptococcus pneumoniae* are most often identified in patients with bacteremia from high-income countries with the addition of *Salmonella* spp. in developing regions.
- Risk factors for bacteremia include: advanced age, chronic liver disease, diabetes mellitus, end-stage renal disease on hemodialysis, functional or anatomic asplenia HIV infection, immunosuppressive medications, indwelling prostheses (eg, vascular catheters, surgically implanted materials, and orthopedic prostheses), IV drug use, malignancies, malnutrition and hypoalbuminemia (less than 3 g/dL [30 g/L]), neutropenia, peripheral vascular disease, corticosteroids use, recent procedures (eg, urogenital surgery, prostate biopsy, endoscopic retrograde cholangiopancreatography), solid organ or stem cell transplant, trauma or loss of skin integrity, urinary retention.

CLINICAL PRESENTATION AND DIAGNOSIS

- The clinical presentation of patients with IE is highly variable and nonspecific. Fever is the most common finding (more than 90% of patients). The mitral and aortic valves are most often affected.
- IE usually begins insidiously and worsens gradually. Patients may present with nonspecific findings such as fever, chills, weakness, dyspnea, cough, night sweats, weight loss, or malaise.
- Important clinical signs, especially prevalent in subacute illness, may include the following peripheral manifestations ("stigmata") of endocarditis: Osler nodes, Janeway lesions, splinter hemorrhages, petechiae, clubbing of the fingers, Roth spots, and emboli. The patient may also have a heart murmur (sometimes new or changing).

TABLE 38-1	Etiologic Organisms in Infective Endocarditis[a]
Agent	**Percentage of Cases**
Staphylococci	30–70
Coagulase-positive *S. aureus*	20–68
Coagulase-negative	3–26
Streptococci	9–38
Viridans streptococci	10–28
Other streptococci	3–14
Enterococci	5–18
Gram-negative aerobic bacilli	1.5–13
Fungi	1–9
Miscellaneous bacteria	<5
Polymicrobial infections	1–2
Culture negative	<5–17

[a]Values encompass community-acquired, healthcare-associated, native valve, and prosthetic valve infective endocarditis.

- Without appropriate antimicrobial therapy and surgery, IE is usually fatal. With proper management, recovery can be expected in most patients.
- Factors associated with increased mortality include: heart failure, increasing age, endocarditis caused by resistant organisms, such as gram-negative bacteria, or fungi, left-sided endocarditis caused by *S. aureus*, paravalvular complications, healthcare-acquired infection, and PVE.
- The hallmark of infective endocarditis is a continuous bacteremia caused by bacteria shedding from the vegetation into the bloodstream; 90%–95% of patients with infective endocarditis have positive blood cultures. The patient's white blood cell count may be normal or only slightly elevated.
- Nonspecific findings include anemia (normochromic, normocytic), thrombocytopenia, an elevated erythrocyte sedimentation rate or C-reactive protein, and altered urinalysis (proteinuria/microscopic hematuria). Urinalysis may reveal proteinuria and microscopic hematuria.
- Echocardiography plays an important role in the diagnosis and management of infective endocarditis and should be performed for all patients suspected of this infection. Transesophageal echocardiography is more sensitive for detecting vegetations (90%–100%), compared with transthoracic echocardiography (40%–65%).
- The Modified Duke criteria, encompassing major findings of persistent bacteremia and echocardiographic findings and other minor findings, are used to categorize patients as "definite IE" or "possible IE."
- Clinical manifestations of bacteremia vary but may involve fever, chills, rigors, altered hemodynamics, shock, coagulation disorders, cutaneous findings (eg, ulcerations), and a documented or suspected primary source of infection. Patients with bacteremia may be normothermic with a normal white blood cell count as neither leukocytosis nor fever ($\geq$38°C) alone or in combination predict the presence of bacteremia.

TREATMENT

GENERAL APPROACH

- <u>Goals of Treatment</u>: For infective endocarditis, relieve the signs and symptoms of disease and decrease morbidity and mortality associated with infection. Eradicate the causative organism with minimal drug exposure. Provide cost-effective antimicrobial therapy. Prevent IE from occurring or recurring in high-risk patients with appropriate prophylactic antimicrobials.

- For bacteremia: Eradicate the causative organism with optimal therapy while minimizing therapeutic failure and potential for resistance; identify and manage the focal (primary) source of infection as well as any secondary foci (metastatic) of infections; relieve the signs and symptoms associated with the infection including the bacteremia, primary source of infection, and if present, secondary metastatic infections; decrease morbidity and mortality associated with the bacteremia and primary source of infection; and provide cost-effective antimicrobial therapy.
- The most important approach to the treatment of IE is isolation of the infecting pathogen and determination of antimicrobial susceptibilities, followed by high-dose bactericidal antibiotics for an extended period.
- Treatment usually is started in the hospital, but in selected patients, it may be completed in the outpatient setting.
- Large doses of parenteral antimicrobials as opposed to oral antimicrobials are currently recommended to achieve bactericidal concentrations within vegetations. An extended duration of therapy is required, even for susceptible pathogens, because microorganisms are enclosed within valvular vegetations and fibrin deposits.
- For bacteremia, empirical parenteral therapy should be based on the usual pathogens at the site(s) of presumptive primary source(s) of infection. In the case of an unknown primary source of infection or primary bacteremia (those without an obvious source), the selection of empirical parenteral antibacterial therapy should provide a broad spectrum of activity while additional diagnostic testing is performed to determine the site(s) of infection.
- Drug dosing for treatment of IE is given in Table 38-2. β-Lactam antibiotics, such as penicillin G (or ceftriaxone), nafcillin (or oxacillin), and ampicillin, remain the drugs of choice for streptococcal, staphylococcal, and enterococcal endocarditis, respectively.

NONPHARMACOLOGIC THERAPY

- Surgical intervention to remove the infectious foci and repair valves and/or valvular structures is an important adjunct in the management of both native valve endocarditis (NVE) and PVE. In most cases, valvectomy and valve replacement are performed to remove infected tissues and restore hemodynamic function. Indications for surgery include heart failure, persistent bacteremia, persistent vegetation, an increase in vegetation size, or recurrent emboli despite prolonged antibiotic treatment, valve dysfunction, paravalvular extension (eg, abscess), or endocarditis caused by resistant organisms.

STREPTOCOCCAL ENDOCARDITIS

- Streptococci are a common cause of IE, with most isolates being viridans group streptococci.
- Most viridans group streptococci are highly sensitive to penicillin G with minimum inhibitory concentrations (MICs) of 0.12 mcg/mL (mg/L) or less. The MIC should be determined for all viridans streptococci and the results used to guide therapy. Approximately 10%–20% are moderately susceptible (MIC 0.12–0.5 mcg/mL [mg/L]).
- Recommended therapy in the uncomplicated case caused by fully susceptible strains in native valves is 4 weeks of either high-dose **penicillin G** or **ceftriaxone**, or 2 weeks of combined penicillin G or ceftriaxone therapy plus **gentamicin** (Table 38-3).
- Shorter-course antimicrobial regimens are advocated when possible. With susceptible streptococcal endocarditis (MICs ≤0.12 mcg/mL [mg/L]), a 2-week regimen of high-dose parenteral penicillin G or ceftriaxone in combination with an aminoglycoside is as effective as 4 weeks of penicillin alone.
- When a patient has a history of immediate-type hypersensitivity to penicillin, vancomycin should be chosen for IE caused by viridans group streptococci. When vancomycin is used, the addition of gentamicin is not recommended.

TABLE 38-2 Drug Dosing Table for Treatment of Infective Endocarditis[a]

Drug	Brand Name	Recommended Dose	Pediatric (Ped) Dose[b]	Additional Information
Ampicillin	NA	2 g IV every 4 hours	50 mg/kg every 4 hours or 75 mg/kg every 6 hours	24-hour total dose may be administered as a continuous infusion: 12 g IV every 24 hours
Ampicillin–sulbactam	Unasyn*	3 g IV every 6 hours	50 mg/kg every 4 hours or 75 mg/kg every 6 hours	
Aqueous crystalline penicillin G sodium	NA			
• MIC <0.12 mcg/mL (mg/L) (native valve only)		3 million units IV every 4 hours or every 6 hours	50,000 units/kg IV every 6 hours	24-hour total dose may be administered as a continuous infusion: 12–18 million units IV every 24 hours (Ped: 200,000 units/kg IV/24 hours)
• All other indications		4 million units IV every 4 hours or 6 million units IV every 6 hours	50,000 units/kg IV every 4 hours or 75,000 units/kg IV every 6 hours	24 million units IV every 24 hours (Ped: 300,000 units/kg IV every 24 hours)
Cefazolin	N/A	2 g IV every 8 hours	33 mg/kg IV every 8 hours	
Cefepime	Maxipime*	2 g IV every 8 hours	50 mg/kg IV every 8 hours	
Ceftriaxone sodium	N/A	2 g IV or IM every 24 hours	100 mg/kg IV or IM every 24 hours	
		2 g IV or IM every 12 hours (E. faecalis only)		
Ciprofloxacin	Cipro*	400 mg IV every 12 hours or 500 mg orally every 12 hours	20–30 mg/kg IV or orally every 12 hours	Avoid use if possible in patients <18 years of age

(Continued)

TABLE 38-2	Drug Dosing Table for Treatment of Infective Endocarditis[a] (Continued)			
Drug	Brand Name	Recommended Dose	Pediatric (Ped) Dose[b]	Additional Information
Daptomycin	Cubicin*	≥8 mg/kg IV every 24 hours	6 mg/kg IV every 24 hours	Doses as high as 10–12 mg/kg IV every 24 hours have been used in adults with enterococcus resistant to penicillin, aminoglycosides, and vancomycin; doses should be calculated using actual body weight
Doxycycline	Vibramycin*	100 mg IV or orally every 12 hours	1–2 mg/kg IV or orally every 12 hours	
Gentamicin sulfate	NA	3 mg/kg IV or IM every 24 hours or 1 mg/kg IV or IM every 8 hours[c]	1 mg/kg IV or IM every 8 hours	Once-daily dosing is only recommended for treatment of streptococcal infections
Linezolid	Zyvox*	600 mg IV or orally every 12 hours	10 mg/kg IV every 8 hours	
Nafcillin or oxacillin	NA	2 g IV every 4 hours	50 mg/kg IV every 6 hours	24-hour total dose may be administered as a continuous infusion: 12 g IV every 24 hours
Rifampin	Rifadin*	300 mg IV or orally every 8 hours	5–7 mg/kg IV or orally every 8 hours	
Streptomycin	NA	7.5 mg/kg IV or IM every 12 hours		
Vancomycin	Vancocin*	15–20 mg/kg IV every 8 hours or every 12 hours	15 mg/kg IV every 6 hours	A loading dose of 25–30 mg/kg may be administered in adults; doses should be calculated using actual body weight; single doses should not exceed 2 g

IM, intramuscular; IV, intravenous; MIC, minimum inhibitory concentration.

[a]All doses assume normal renal function.

[b]Should not exceed adult dosage.

[c]Actual body weight should be used when the full aminoglycoside dose is administered once daily; when administered in three divided doses, use ideal body weight or adjusted body weight when actual body weight is > 120% ideal body weight.

TABLE 38-3 Treatment Options for NVE by Causative Organism

Agent[a]	Duration	Strength of Recommendation	Comments
Highly Penicillin-Susceptible (MIC ≤0.12 mcg/mL [mg/L]) Viridans Group Streptococci and S. gallolyticus			
Aqueous crystalline penicillin G sodium[b]	4 weeks	IIaB	2-week regimens are not intended for the following patients:
Ceftriaxone	4 weeks	IIaB	• Most patients >65 years of age
			• Children
Aqueous crystalline penicillin G sodium[b] plus gentamicin	2 weeks	IIaB	• Impairment of the eighth cranial nerve function • Renal function with a creatinine clearance <20 mL/min (0.33 mL/sec)
Ceftriaxone plus gentamicin	2 weeks	IIaB	• Known cardiac or extracardiac abscess • Infection with *Abiotrophia*, *Granulicatella*, or *Gemella* species
Vancomycin	4 weeks	IIaB	Recommended only for patients unable to tolerate penicillin or ceftriaxone
Viridans Group Streptococci and S. Gallolyticus Relatively Resistant to Penicillin (MIC >0.12 to ≤0.5 mcg/mL [mg/L])			
Aqueous crystalline penicillin G sodium[b]	4 weeks	IIaB	
plus gentamicin	2 weeks		
Ceftriaxone	4 weeks	IIbC	
plus gentamicin	2 weeks		
Vancomycin	4 weeks	IIaB	Recommended only for patients unable to tolerate penicillin or ceftriaxone
Oxacillin-Susceptible Staphylococci[c]			
Nafcillin or oxacillin	6 weeks	IC	
Cefazolin	6 weeks	IB	For use in patients with nonanaphylactoid-type penicillin allergies; patients with an unclear history of immediate-type hypersensitivity to penicillin should be considered for skin testing

(Continued)

TABLE 38-3	Treatment Options for NVE by Causative Organism (Continued)		
Agent[a]	Duration	Strength of Recommendation	Comments
Vancomycin	6 weeks	IB	For use in patients with anaphylactoid-type hypersensitivity to penicillin and/or cephalosporins
Daptomycin	6 weeks	IIaB	For use in patients with immediate-type hypersensitivity reactions to penicillin
Oxacillin-Resistant Staphylococci			
Vancomycin	6 weeks	IB	
Daptomycin	6 weeks	IIbB	

[a]See Table 38-2 for appropriate dosing, administration, and monitoring information.

[b]May use ampicillin in the event of a penicillin shortage.

[c]Regimens indicate treatment for left-sided endocarditis or complicated right-sided endocarditis; uncomplicated right-sided endocarditis may be treated for shorter durations and is described in the text.

Please refer to Table 38-5 for treatment of NVE caused by enterococci.

- For patients with complicated infection (eg, extracardiac foci) or when the organism is relatively resistant (MIC = 0.12–0.5 mcg/mL [mg/L]), combination therapy with an aminoglycoside and penicillin (higher dose) or ceftriaxone for the first 2 weeks is recommended followed by penicillin or ceftriaxone alone for an additional 2 weeks.
- In patients with endocarditis of prosthetic valves or other prosthetic material caused by viridans streptococci and *Streptococcus bovis*, treatment courses are extended to 6 weeks (Table 38-4).

STAPHYLOCOCCAL ENDOCARDITIS

- Endocarditis is most commonly caused by staphylococci, in particular *S. aureus*, mainly because of increased IVDA, more frequent use of peripheral and central venous catheters, and increased frequency of valve replacement surgery. Coagulase-negative staphylococci (usually *S. epidermidis*) are prominent causes of PVE.
- The recommended therapy for patients with left-sided IE caused by methicillin-susceptible *S. aureus* (MSSA) is 6 weeks of **nafcillin** or **oxacillin** (see Table 38-3).
- If a patient has a mild, delayed allergy to penicillin, first-generation cephalosporins (such as **cefazolin**) are effective alternatives but should be avoided in patients with an immediate-type hypersensitivity reaction.
- In a patient with a positive penicillin skin test or a history of immediate hypersensitivity to penicillin, **vancomycin** is an option. Vancomycin, however, kills *S. aureus* slowly and is generally regarded as inferior to penicillinase-resistant penicillins for MSSA. Penicillin-allergic patients who fail on vancomycin therapy should be considered for penicillin desensitization. **Daptomycin** (at a dose of 6 mg/kg/day) is a recommended alternative.
- **Vancomycin** is the drug of choice for methicillin-resistant staphylococci because most methicillin-resistant *S. aureus* (MRSA) and most coagulase-negative staphylococci are susceptible. Reports of *S. aureus* strains resistant to vancomycin are increasing. Daptomycin (at a dose of 6 mg/kg/day) is now a recommended alternative.

Treatment of *Staphylococcus* Endocarditis in IV Drug Abusers

- IE in IV drug abusers is most frequently (60%–70%) caused by *S. aureus*, although other organisms may be more common in certain geographic locations.
- A 2-week course of **nafcillin, oxacillin**, or **daptomycin** without an aminoglycoside is recommended. If vancomycin is selected, the standard 6-week regimen should therefore be used.

Treatment of Staphylococcal Prosthetic Valve Endocarditis

- PVE that occurs within 2 months of cardiac surgery is usually caused by staphylococci implanted at the time of surgery. Methicillin-resistant organisms are common. Vancomycin is the cornerstone of therapy.
- Because of the high morbidity and mortality associated with PVE and refractoriness to therapy, combinations of antimicrobials are usually recommended.
- For methicillin-resistant staphylococci (both MRSA and coagulase-negative staphylococci), **vancomycin** is used with rifampin for 6 weeks or more (see Table 38-4). An **aminoglycoside** is added for the first 2 weeks if the organism is susceptible. Due to the risk of developing on therapy resistance, rifampin should not be started until blood cultures have cleared.
- For methicillin-susceptible staphylococci, **penicillinase-resistant penicillin** is used in place of vancomycin. If an organism is identified other than staphylococci, the treatment regimen should be guided by susceptibilities and should be at least 6 weeks in duration.

ENTEROCOCCAL ENDOCARDITIS

- Enterococci are the third leading cause of endocarditis and are noteworthy for the following reasons: (1) no single antibiotic is bactericidal; (2) MICs to penicillin are relatively high (1–25 mcg/mL [mg/L]); (3) they are intrinsically resistant to all

| TABLE 38-4 | Treatment Options for PVE by Causative Organism |

Agent[a]	Duration	Strength of Recommendation	Comments
Highly Penicillin-Susceptible (MIC ≤0.12 mcg/mL [mg/L]) Viridans Group Streptococci and *S. gallolyticus*			
Aqueous crystalline penicillin G sodium[b] with or without gentamicin	6 weeks / 2 weeks	IIaB	Combination therapy with gentamicin has not demonstrated superior cure rates compared with monotherapy with penicillin or cephalosporin and should be avoided in patients with CrCl <30 mL/min (0.50 mL/sec)
Ceftriaxone with or without gentamicin	6 weeks / 2 weeks	IIaB	
Vancomycin	6 weeks	IIaB	Recommended only for patients unable to tolerate penicillin or ceftriaxone
Relatively Resistant or Fully Resistant (MIC >0.12 mcg/mL [mg/L]) Viridans Group Streptococci and *S. gallolyticus*			
Aqueous crystalline penicillin G sodium[b] plus gentamicin	6 weeks	IIaB	
Ceftriaxone plus gentamicin	6 weeks	IIaB	
Vancomycin[c]	6 weeks	IIaB	Recommended only for patients unable to tolerate penicillin or ceftriaxone
Oxacillin-Susceptible Staphylococci			
Nafcillin or oxacillin plus rifampin plus gentamicin	≥6 weeks / ≥6 weeks / 2 weeks	IB	Cefazolin may be substituted for nafcillin or oxacillin in patients with nonimmediate-type hypersensitivity
Vancomycin plus rifampin plus gentamicin	≥6 weeks / ≥6 weeks / 2 weeks	IB	Recommended only for patients with anaphylactoid-type hypersensitivity to penicillin and/or cephalosporins
Oxacillin-Resistant Staphylococci			
Vancomycin plus rifampin plus gentamicin	≥6 weeks / ≥6 weeks / 2 weeks	IB	

[a]See Table 38-2 for appropriate dosing, administration, and monitoring information.
[b]May use ampicillin in the event of a penicillin shortage.
[c]The ESC 2015 guidelines recommend gentamicin (3 mg/kg/day) be administered with vancomycin for the initial 2 weeks of therapy in patients with relatively resistant strains to penicillin.
Please refer to Table 38-5 for treatment of PVE caused by enterococci.

cephalosporins and relatively resistant to aminoglycosides (ie, "low-level" aminoglycoside resistance); (4) combinations of a cell wall–active agent, such as penicillin or vancomycin, plus an aminoglycoside are necessary for killing; and (5) resistance to all available drugs is increasing.

- Enterococcal endocarditis ordinarily requires 4–6 weeks of high-dose **penicillin G** or **ampicillin**, plus **gentamicin** for cure (Table 38-5). Ampicillin plus ceftriaxone is as effective as ampicillin plus gentamicin and should be considered as a treatment option. A 6-week course is recommended for patients with symptoms lasting longer than 3 months and those with PVE. Relatively low serum concentrations of aminoglycosides appear adequate for successful therapy, such as a gentamicin peak concentration of approximately 3–4 mcg/mL (mg/L; 6.3–8.4 μmol/L).

- In addition to isolates with high-level aminoglycoside resistance, β-lactamase–producing enterococci (especially *Enterococcus faecium*) are increasingly reported. If these organisms are discovered, use of vancomycin or ampicillin–sulbactam in combination with gentamicin should be considered.

TABLE 38-5 Treatment Options for NVE or PVE Caused by Enterococci

Agent[a]	Duration[b]	Strength of Recommendation	Comments
Ampicillin-, Penicillin-, and Vancomycin-Susceptible Strains			
Ampicillin plus gentamicin	4–6 weeks	IIaB	Native valve plus symptoms present for <3 months: use 4-week regimen
Aqueous crystalline penicillin G sodium plus gentamicin	4–6 weeks	IIAB	Prosthetic valve or native valve plus symptoms present for >3 months: use 6-week regimen
Ampicillin plus ceftriaxone	6 weeks	IIaB	Recommended regimen if creatinine clearance is <50 mL/min (0.83 mL/sec; at baseline or due to therapy with a gentamicin-containing regimen)
Vancomycin plus gentamicin	6 weeks	IIaB	Recommended only for patients unable to tolerate penicillin or ampicillin
Gentamicin-Resistant Strains			
If susceptible, use streptomycin in place of gentamicin in the regimens listed above if creatinine clearance is >50 mL/min (0.83 mL/sec), cranial nerve VIII function is intact, and there is laboratory capability for rapid streptomycin serum concentrations.			
Penicillin-Resistant Strains			
Ampicillin–sulbactam plus gentamicin (β-lactamase–producing strain)	6 weeks	IIbC	
Vancomycin plus gentamicin (intrinsic penicillin resistance[c])	6 weeks	IIbC	May also use in patients with β-lactamase–producing strains who have known intolerance to ampicillin–sulbactam

(Continued)

TABLE 38-5	Treatment Options for NVE or PVE Caused by Enterococci *(Continued)*		
Agent[a]	**Duration**[b]	**Strength of Recommendation**	**Comments**
Enterococcus faecium Strains Resistant to Penicillin, Aminoglycosides, and Vancomycin[d]			
Linezolid	>6 weeks	IIbC	Antimicrobial cure rates may be <50%; bacteriologic cure may only be achieved with cardiac valve replacement
Daptomycin	>6 weeks	IIbC	

[a]See Table 38-2 for appropriate dosing, administration, and monitoring information.
[b]All patients with prosthetic valves should be treated for at least 6 weeks.
[c]Infectious diseases consult highly recommended.
[d]Patients should be managed by a multidisciplinary team that includes specialists in cardiology, cardiovascular surgery, infectious diseases, and clinical pharmacy.

EVALUATION OF THERAPEUTIC OUTCOMES

- The evaluation of patients treated for IE includes assessment of signs and symptoms, blood cultures, microbiologic tests (eg, MIC, minimum bactericidal concentration [MBC], or serum bactericidal titers), serum drug concentrations, and other tests to evaluate organ function.
- Persistence of fever beyond 1 week may indicate ineffective antimicrobial therapy, emboli, infections of intravascular catheters, or drug reactions. In some patients, fever may persist even with appropriate antimicrobial therapy.
- With effective therapy, blood should sterilize with negative cultures within a few days, although the microbiologic response to vancomycin may be unusually slower. After the initiation of therapy, blood cultures should be rechecked until they are negative. During the remainder of the therapy, frequent blood culturing is not necessary.
- If bacteria continue to be isolated from blood beyond the first few days of therapy, it may indicate that the antimicrobials are inactive against the pathogen or that the doses are not producing adequate concentrations at the site of infection.
- For all isolates from blood cultures, MICs (not MBCs) should be determined.

PREVENTION OF ENDOCARDITIS

- Antimicrobial prophylaxis is used to prevent IE in patients believed to be at high risk.
- The use of antimicrobials for this purpose requires consideration of the types of patients who are at risk; the procedures causing bacteremia; the organisms that are likely to cause endocarditis; and the pharmacokinetics, spectrum, cost, and ease of administration of available agents. The objective of prophylaxis is to diminish the likelihood of IE in high-risk individuals who are undergoing procedures that cause transient bacteremia.
- The literature lacks adequate evidence to prove the effectiveness or ineffectiveness of antibiotic prophylaxis, and the common practice of using antimicrobial therapy in this setting remains controversial.
- IE prophylaxis should be recommended only for patients with underlying cardiac conditions associated with the highest risk, which includes the presence of a prosthetic heart valve, prosthetic material used for cardiac valve repair, prior diagnosis of IE, cardiac transplantation with subsequent valvulopathy, CHD, for dental procedures involving manipulation of gingival tissue or the periapical region of teeth or perforation of the oral mucosa, invasive respiratory procedures involving an incision or biopsy, or invasive procedures involving infected skin, skin structures, or musculoskeletal tissues.
- Antibiotic regimens for a dental procedure are given in Table 38-6.

TABLE 38-6	Prophylaxis of Infective Endocarditis

Highest Risk Cardiac Conditions	Presence of a prosthetic heart valve
	Prosthetic material used for cardiac valve repair
	Prior diagnosis of infective endocarditis
	Cardiac transplantation with subsequent valvulopathy
	Congenital heart disease[a]
Types of Procedures	Dental procedures that require perforation of the oral mucosa or manipulation of the periapical region of the teeth of gingival tissue
	Invasive respiratory procedures involving an incision or biopsy
	Invasive procedures involving infected skin, skin structures, or musculoskeletal tissue

Antimicrobial Options	Adult Doses[b]	Pediatric Doses[b] (mg/kg)
Oral amoxicillin	2 g	50
IM or IV ampicillin[c]	2 g	50
IM or IV cefazolin or ceftriaxone[c,d,e]	1 g	50
Oral cephalexin[d,e,f]	2 g	50
Oral azithromycin or clarithromycin[e]	500 mg	15
IV or IM clindamycin[c,e]	600 mg	20

IM, intramuscular; IV, intravenous.
[a]Includes only the following: unrepaired cyanotic CHD, prophylaxis within the first 6 months of implanting prosthetic material to repair a congenital heart defect, and repaired CHD with residual defects at or adjacent to prosthetic material.
[b]All one-time doses administered 30–60 minutes prior to initiation of the procedure.
[c]For patients unable to tolerate oral medication.
[d]Should be avoided in patients with immediate-type hypersensitivity reaction to penicillin or ampicillin (eg, anaphylaxis, urticaria, or angioedema).
[e]Option for patients with nonimmediate hypersensitivity reaction to penicillin or ampicillin.
[f]May substitute with an alternative first- or second-generation cephalosporin at an equivalent dose.

See Chapter 134, Infective Endocarditis, authored by Daniel B. Chastain for a more detailed discussion of this topic.

Fungal Infections, Invasive 39

Histoplasmosis

- *Histoplasmosis* is primarily a pulmonary infection caused by inhalation of dust-borne microconidia of the dimorphic fungus *Histoplasma capsulatum*. Disseminated histoplasmosis may occur in those who are immunocompromised. In the United States, most disease is localized along the Ohio and Mississippi river valleys.

CLINICAL PRESENTATION AND DIAGNOSIS

- In the vast majority of patients, low-inoculum exposure to *H. capsulatum* results in mild or asymptomatic pulmonary histoplasmosis. The course of disease is generally benign, and symptoms usually abate within a few weeks of onset. Patients exposed to a higher inoculum during a primary infection or reinfection may experience an acute, self-limited illness with flu-like pulmonary symptoms, including fever, chills, headache, myalgia, and nonproductive cough.
- Chronic pulmonary histoplasmosis generally presents as an opportunistic infection imposed on a preexisting structural abnormality, such as lesions resulting from emphysema. Patients demonstrate chronic pulmonary symptoms and apical lung lesions that progress with inflammation, calcified granulomas, and fibrosis. Progression of disease over a period of years, seen in 25%–30% of patients, is associated with cavitation, bronchopleural fistulas, extension to the other lung, pulmonary insufficiency, and often death.
- In patients exposed to a large inoculum and in immunocompromised hosts, progressive illness, disseminated histoplasmosis, may occur. The clinical severity of the diverse forms of disseminated histoplasmosis (Table 39-1) generally parallels the degree of macrophage parasitization observed.
- Acute (infantile) disseminated histoplasmosis is seen in infants and young children and (rarely) in adults with Hodgkin disease or other lymphoproliferative disorders. It is characterized by unrelenting fever; anemia; leukopenia or thrombocytopenia; enlargement of the liver, spleen, and visceral lymph nodes; and GI symptoms, particularly nausea, vomiting, and diarrhea.
- If untreated it is uniformly fatal in 1–2 months. A less severe "subacute" form of the disease, which occurs in both infants and immunocompetent adults, is characterized by focal destructive lesions in various organs, weight loss, weakness, fever, and malaise.
- Most adults with disseminated histoplasmosis demonstrate a mild, chronic form of the disease. Untreated patients are often ill for 10–20 years, with long asymptomatic periods interrupted by relapses characterized by weight loss, weakness, and fatigue.
- Adult patients with acquired immunodeficiency syndrome (AIDS) demonstrate an acute form of disseminated disease that resembles the syndrome seen in infants and children. Progressive disseminated histoplasmosis can occur as the direct result of initial infection or because of reactivation of dormant foci.
- In most patients, serologic evidence (complement fixation test or immunodiffusion testing) remains the primary method in the diagnosis of histoplasmosis. Detection of histoplasma antigen by enzyme immunoassay (EIA) in the urine, blood, or bronchoalveolar lavage fluid of infected patients provides rapid diagnostic information and is particularly useful in patients who are severely ill.

TREATMENT

- <u>Goals of Treatment:</u> Resolution of clinical abnormalities, prevention of relapse, and eradication of infection whenever possible, although chronic suppression of infection can be adequate in immunosuppressed patients, including those with HIV disease.
- Recommended therapy for the treatment of histoplasmosis is summarized in Table 39-1.

TABLE 39-1	Clinical Manifestations and Therapy of Histoplasmosis
Type of Disease and Common Clinical Manifestations	**Therapy/Comments**
Acute pulmonary histoplasmosis	
Asymptomatic or mild-to-moderate disease	*Asymptomatic, mild, or symptoms <4 weeks:* No therapy is generally required; itraconazole[a] orally (200 mg three times daily for 3 days and then 200 mg once or twice daily for 6–12 weeks) is recommended for patients who continue to have symptoms for greater than 1 month[a]
Moderately severe to severe diffuse pulmonary disease	Lipid amphotericin B 3–5 mg/kg/day IV for 1–2 weeks followed by itraconazole[a] orally 200 mg orally three times daily for 3 days then twice daily for a total of 12 weeks of therapy; methylprednisolone (0.5–1 mg/kg daily IV) during the first 1–2 weeks of antifungal therapy is recommended for patients who develop respiratory complications, including hypoxemia or significant respiratory distress
CNS histoplasmosis	Amphotericin B should be used as initial therapy (lipid formulations at 5 mg/kg/day IV, for a total dosage of 175 mg/kg for 4–6 weeks, followed by itraconazole[a] orally 200 mg orally two or three times daily for at least a year; some patients may require lifelong therapy; response to therapy should be monitored by repeat lumbar punctures to assess *Histoplasma* antigen levels, WBC, and CSF antibody titers
Progressive histoplasmosis	*Moderately severe to severe:* Liposomal amphotericin B (3 mg/kg daily) IV, amphotericin B lipid complex (ABLC, 5 mg/kg daily) IV, or deoxycholate amphotericin B (0.7–1 mg/kg daily) for 1–2 weeks IV, followed by itraconazole[a] orally (200 mg orally twice daily for at least 12 months)
	Mild to moderate: Itraconazole[a] orally (200 mg orally twice daily for at least 12 months); immunosuppressed patients may require lifelong suppressive therapy with itraconazole[a] orally 200 mg daily

CNS, central nervous system; CSF, cerebrospinal fluid; IV, intravenous; WBC, white blood cell.
[a]Itraconazole plasma concentrations should be measured during the second week of therapy to ensure that detectable concentrations have been achieved. If the concentration is below 1 mcg/mL (mg/L; 1.4 μmol/L), the dose may be insufficient or drug interactions can be impairing absorption or accelerating metabolism, requiring a change in dosage. If plasma concentrations are greater than 10 mcg/mL (mg/L; 14 μmol/L), the dosage can be reduced.

- Response to therapy should be measured by resolution of radiologic, serologic, and microbiologic parameters and improvement in signs and symptoms of infection.
- After the initial course of therapy for histoplasmosis is completed, lifelong suppressive therapy with oral azoles is recommended, because of the frequent recurrence of infection.
- Relapse rates in AIDS patients not receiving preventive maintenance are 50%–90%.

Blastomycosis

- North American *blastomycosis* is a systemic fungal infection caused by *Blastomyces dermatitidis*. Pulmonary disease can be acute or chronic and can mimic infection with tuberculosis, pyogenic bacteria, other fungi, or malignancy.

CLINICAL PRESENTATION AND DIAGNOSIS

- Pulmonary blastomycosis is the most common manifestation and can range from asymptomatic infection to acute pneumonia, with or without respiratory failure, to chronic disease. Typical symptoms of acute pulmonary infection include fever, shaking chills, and a productive, purulent cough, with or without hemoptysis in immunocompetent individuals.
- Sporadic pulmonary blastomycosis may present as a more chronic or subacute disease, with low-grade fever, night sweats, weight loss, and a productive cough resembling that of tuberculosis rather than bacterial pneumonia. Chronic pulmonary blastomycosis is characterized by fever, malaise, weight loss, night sweats, chest pain, and productive cough.
- The simplest and most successful method of diagnosing blastomycosis is by direct microscopic visualization of the large, multinucleated yeast with single, broad-based buds in sputum or other respiratory specimens, following staining.

TREATMENT

- In the immunocompetent host, acute pulmonary blastomycosis can be mild and self-limited and may not require treatment. However, consideration should be given to treating all infected individuals to prevent extrapulmonary dissemination. All individuals with moderate-to-severe pneumonia, disseminated infection, or those who are immunocompromised require antifungal therapy (Table 39-2).
- Some authors recommend azole therapy for the treatment of self-limited pulmonary disease, with the hope of preventing late extrapulmonary disease.
- In patients with mild-to-moderate pulmonary blastomycosis, **itraconazole** is effective; however, in patients with moderately severe to severe pulmonary disease, the clinical presentation of the patient, the immune competence of the patient, and the toxicity of the antifungal agents are the main determinants of the choice of antifungal therapy.
- All patients with disseminated blastomycosis, as well as those with extrapulmonary disease, require therapy.

TABLE 39-2	Therapy of Blastomycosis
Type of Disease	**Preferred Treatment**
Pulmonary[a]	
Moderately severe to severe disease	Lipid formulation of amphotericin B 3–5 mg/kg IV daily or amphotericin B[b] 0.7–1 mg/kg IV daily (total dose 1.5–2.5 g) × 1–2 weeks or until improvement is noted, followed by itraconazole[c,d] 200 mg orally three times daily for 3 days, then 200 mg twice daily, × total of 6–12 months
Mild-to-moderate disease	Itraconazole[b,d] 200 mg orally three times daily for 3 days, then 200 mg twice daily, for a total of 6 months[b]
CNS Disease	*Induction:* Lipid formulation of amphotericin B 5 mg/kg IV daily × 4–6 weeks, followed by an oral azole as consolidation therapy
	Consolidation: Fluconazole[d] 800 mg orally daily, or itraconazole[d] 200 mg two or three times orally daily, or voriconazole[d] 200–400 mg orally twice daily, for ≥12 months and until resolution of CSF abnormalities

(Continued)

TABLE 39-2	Therapy of Blastomycosis (*Continued*)
Type of Disease	**Preferred Treatment**
Disseminated or Extrapulmonary Disease	
Moderately severe to severe disease	Lipid formulation of amphotericin B 3–5 mg/kg IV daily or amphotericin B[b] 0.7–1 mg/kg IV daily × 1–2 weeks or until improvement is noted, followed by itraconazole[c,d] 200 mg orally three times daily for 3 days, then 200 mg twice daily × 6–12 months; treat osteoarticular disease with 12 months of antifungal therapy
	Most clinicians prefer to step-down to itraconazole[d] therapy once the patient's condition improves
Mild to moderate	Itraconazole[c,d] 200 mg orally three times daily for 3 days, then 200 mg once or twice daily × ≥12 months; treat osteoarticular disease with 12 months of antifungal therapy
Immunocompromised Host (Including Patients with AIDS, Transplants, or Receiving Chronic Glucocorticoid Therapy)	
Acute disease	Lipid formulation of amphotericin B 3–5 mg/kg IV daily or amphotericin B[a] 0.7–1 mg/kg IV daily × 1–2 weeks or until improvement is noted, then give suppressive therapy for a total of at least 12 months of therapy
Suppressive therapy	Itraconazole[c,d] 200 mg orally three times daily for 3 days, then 200 mg twice daily for a total of at least 12 months of therapy; lifelong suppressive therapy with oral itraconazole[d] 200 mg daily may be required for immunosuppressed patients in whom immunosuppression cannot be reversed, and in patients who experience relapse despite appropriate therapy

CNS, central nervous system; CSF, cerebrospinal fluid; IV, intravenous.
[a]In the immunocompetent host, acute pulmonary blastomycosis can be mild and self-limited and may not require treatment.
[b]Desoxycholate amphotericin B.
[c]Serum levels of itraconazole should be determined after the patient has received itraconazole for ≥2 weeks to ensure adequate drug exposure.
[d]Azoles should not be used during pregnancy.

Coccidioidomycosis

- *Coccidioidomycosis* is caused by infection with *Coccidioides immitis* and *C. posadasii*. The endemic regions encompass the semiarid areas of the southwestern United States from California to Texas, known as the Lower Sonoran Zone.

CLINICAL PRESENTATION AND DIAGNOSIS

- Approximately 60% of infected patients have an asymptomatic, self-limited infection without clinical or radiological manifestations. The remaining 40% of patients exhibit nonspecific symptoms that are often indistinguishable from ordinary upper respiratory infections, including fever, cough, headache, sore throat, myalgias, and fatigue that occur 1–3 weeks after exposure to the pathogen. A fine, diffuse rash may appear during the first few days of illness.
- Chronic, persistent pneumonia or persistent pulmonary coccidioidomycosis (primary disease lasting >6 weeks) is complicated by hemoptysis, pulmonary scarring, and the formation of cavities or bronchopleural fistulas.
- Disseminated infection occurs in less than 1% of infected patients. Dissemination may occur to the skin, lymph nodes, bone, meninges, spleen, liver, kidney,

and adrenal gland. CNS infection occurs in ~16% of patients with disseminated infection.

- The diagnoses of coccidioidomycosis generally include identification or recovery of *Coccidioides* spp. from clinical specimens and detection of specific anticoccidioidal antibodies in serum or other body fluids.

TREATMENT

- Goals of Treatment: Desired outcomes of treatment are resolution of signs and symptoms of infection, reduction of serum concentrations of anticoccidioidal antibodies, and return of function of involved organs.
- Therapy of coccidioidomycosis is difficult, and the results are unpredictable. Only 5% of infected persons require therapy.
- Azole antifungals, primarily fluconazole and itraconazole, are initially recommended therapy for most chronic pulmonary or disseminated infections. Specific antifungals (and their usual dosages) for the treatment of coccidioidomycosis include IV lipid formulations of **amphotericin B** (3–5 mg/kg/day), IV or oral **fluconazole** (usually 400–800 mg/day, although dosages as high as 1200 mg/day have been used without complications), and **itraconazole** (200–300 mg orally twice daily or three times daily, as capsules or solution). If itraconazole is used, measurement of serum concentrations can be helpful to ascertain whether oral bioavailability is adequate.
- Therapy often ranges from many months to years in duration, and in some patients, lifelong suppressive therapy is needed to prevent relapses.
- Amphotericin B is now usually reserved for patients with respiratory failure because of infection with *Coccidioides* spp., those with rapidly progressive coccidioidal infections, or women during pregnancy. Lipid formulations of amphotericin B have not been extensively studied for coccidioidomycosis but can offer a means of giving more drugs with less toxicity.
- Patients with disease outside the lungs should be treated with 400 mg/day of an oral azole. For meningeal disease, fluconazole 400 mg/day orally should be used; however, some clinicians initiate therapy with 800 or 1000 mg/day, and itraconazole doses of 400–600 mg/day are comparable.

Cryptococcosis

- *Cryptococcosis* is a noncontagious, systemic mycotic infection caused by the ubiquitous encapsulated soil yeast *Cryptococcus neoformans*.

CLINICAL PRESENTATION AND DIAGNOSIS

- Primary cryptococcosis in humans almost always occurs in the lungs. Symptomatic infections are usually manifested by cough, rales, and shortness of breath that generally resolve spontaneously. Infection is acquired by inhalation of the organism.
- Disease may remain localized in the lungs or disseminate to other tissues, particularly the central nervous system (CNS), although the skin can also be affected.
- In the non-AIDS patient, the symptoms of cryptococcal meningitis are nonspecific. Symptomatic infections usually are manifested by cough, rales, and shortness of breath that generally resolve spontaneously. Headache, fever, nausea, vomiting, mental status changes, and neck stiffness are generally observed. In AIDS patients, fever and headache are common, but meningismus and photophobia are much less common than in non-AIDS patients.
- Examination of cerebrospinal fluid (CSF) in patients with cryptococcal meningitis generally reveals an elevated opening pressure, CSF pleocytosis (usually lymphocytes), leukocytosis, a decreased CSF glucose, an elevated CSF protein, and a positive cryptococcal antigen by latex agglutination.
- *C. neoformans* can be detected in ~60% of patients by India ink smear of CSF and cultured in more than 96% of patients.

TREATMENT

- The management of cryptococcosis includes systemic antifungal therapy, control of elevated intracranial pressure (ICP), and supportive care. Treatment of cryptococcosis is detailed in Table 39-3. For asymptomatic, immunocompetent persons with isolated pulmonary disease and no evidence of CNS disease, careful observation may be warranted. With symptomatic infection, **fluconazole** for 6–12 months is warranted.
- The use of intrathecal **amphotericin B** is not recommended for the treatment of cryptococcal meningitis except in very ill patients or in those with recurrent or progressive disease despite aggressive IV amphotericin B therapy. Lipid formulations of amphotericin B are preferred because they increase the likelihood of completing the full course of therapy.
- Immunocompromised patients with CNS infection require more prolonged therapy; treatment regimens are based on those used in the HIV-infected population and follow induction therapy with amphotericin B and consolidation therapy with 6–12 months of suppressive therapy with fluconazole.
- Relapse of *C. neoformans* meningitis occurs in ~50% of AIDS patients after completion of primary therapy. After the completion of induction/consolidation phases of therapy, long-term chronic suppression with fluconazole (200 mg orally daily) should be continued for a minimum of 1 year.

Candida Infections

- Eight species of *Candida* are regarded as clinically important pathogens in human disease: *C. albicans, C. tropicalis, C. parapsilosis, C. krusei, C. stellatoidea, C. guilliermondii, C. lusitaniae*, and *C. glabrata. C. albicans* is a normal commensal of the skin, female genital tract, and entire gastrointestinal (GI) tract of humans.

TABLE 39-3	Therapy of Cryptococcosis[a,b]
Type of Disease and Common Clinical Manifestations	**Therapy/Comments**
Non-immunocompromised Patients (Non–HIV-Infected, Nontransplant)	
Meningoencephalitis *without* neurological complications, in patients in whom CSF yeast cultures are negative after 2 weeks of therapy	*Induction:* Amphotericin B[c,d] IV 0.7–1 mg/kg/day *plus* flucytosine 100 mg/kg/day orally in four divided doses × ≥4 weeks
Meningoencephalitis with neurological complications	*Induction:* Same as for patients without neurologic complications, but consider extending the induction therapy for a total of 6 weeks.
Follow all regimens with suppressive therapy	*Consolidation:* Fluconazole 400–800 mg orally daily × 8 weeks
	Maintenance: Fluconazole 200 mg orally daily × 6–12 months
Mild-to-moderate pulmonary disease (Nonmeningeal disease)	Fluconazole 400 mg orally daily × 6–12 months
Severe pulmonary cryptococcosis	*Same as CNS disease × 12 months*
Cryptococcemia (non-meningeal, non-pulmonary disease)	*Same as CNS disease × 12 months*

(Continued)

TABLE 39-3	Therapy of Cryptococcosis[a,b] (Continued)
Type of Disease and Common Clinical Manifestations	**Therapy/Comments**
HIV-Infected Patients	
Primary therapy; induction and consolidation[e]	*Preferred regimen:* *Induction:* Amphotericin B[c,d] IV 0.7–1 mg/kg IV daily *plus* flucytosine 100 mg/kg/day orally in four divided doses for ≥2 weeks. *Alternative regimens, in order of preference:* Amphotericin B[c,e] IV 0.7–1 mg/kg IV daily × 4–6 weeks *or* liposomal amphotericin B 3–4 mg/kg IV daily[f] × 4–6 weeks *or* ABLC 5 mg/kg IV daily × 4–6 weeks *or* Amphotericin B[c] IV 0.7 mg/kg IV daily, *plus* fluconazole 800 mg (12 mg/kg) orally daily × 2 weeks, followed by fluconazole 800 mg (12 mg/kg) orally daily × ≥8 weeks *or* Fluconazole ≥800 mg (1200 mg/day is preferred) orally daily *plus* flucytosine 100 mg/kg/day orally in four divided doses × 6 weeks *or* fluconazole 800–1200 mg/day orally daily × 10–12 weeks (a dosage ≥1200 mg/day is preferred when fluconazole is used alone)[g]
Follow all regimens with suppressive therapy	*Consolidation:* Fluconazole 400 mg (6 mg/kg) orally daily × ≥8 weeks *Maintenance:* Fluconazole 200 mg orally daily × ≥1 year[h,i]
Organ Transplant Recipients	
Mild-to-moderate non-CNS disease or mild-to-moderate symptoms without diffuse pulmonary infiltrates	Fluconazole 400 mg (6 mg/kg) orally daily × 6–12 months
CNS disease, moderately severe or severe CNS disease or disseminated disease without CNS disease, or severe pulmonary disease without evidence of extrapulmonary or disseminated disease	*Induction:* Liposomal amphotericin B 3–4 mg/kg IV daily,[f] or ABLC 5 mg/kg IV daily *plus* flucytosine 100 mg/kg/day orally in four divided doses × ≥2 weeks If induction therapy does not include flucytosine, consider a lipid formulation of amphotericin B for ≥4–6 weeks of induction therapy. Consider the use of a lipid formulation of amphotericin B lipid formulation (6 mg/kg IV daily) in patients with a high-fungal burden disease or relapse of disease *Consolidation:* Fluconazole 400–800 mg (6–12 mg/kg) per day orally for 8 weeks *Maintenance:* Fluconazole 200–400 mg per day orally for 6–12 months

(Continued)

TABLE 39-3	Therapy of Cryptococcosis[a,b] (Continued)
Type of Disease and Common Clinical Manifestations	**Therapy/Comments**
Follow all regimens with suppressive therapy	*Consolidation:* Fluconazole 400–800 mg (6–12 mg/kg) per day orally for 8 weeks *Maintenance:* Fluconazole 200–400 mg per day orally for 6–12 months

CNS, central nervous system; CSF, cerebrospinal fluid; HIV, human immunodeficiency virus; IV, intravenous.

[a]When more than one therapy is listed, they are listed in order of preference.

[b]See Chapter 144, "Invasive Fungal Infections," *Dipiro's Pharmacotherapy: A Pathophysiologic Approach*, 12th ed., for definitions of induction, consolidation, suppressive/maintenance therapy, and prophylactic therapy.

[c]Deoxycholate amphotericin B.

[d]In patients with, or at risk of renal disease, lipid formulations of amphotericin B can be substituted for deoxycholate amphotericin B. Doses are liposomal amphotericin B 3–4 mg/kg IV daily, or amphotericin B lipid complex (ABLC) 5 mg/kg IV daily.

[e]Initiate HAART therapy 2–10 weeks after commencement of initial antifungal treatment.

[f]Liposomal amphotericin B has been given safely up to 6 mg/kg daily; could be considered in treatment failure or in patients with a high fungal burden.

[g]Or until CSF cultures are negative.

[h]Consider discontinuing suppressive therapy during HAART in patients with a CD4 cell count ≥100 cells/μL (0.1 × 10⁹/L) and an undetectable or very low HIV RNA level sustained for ≥3 months (with a minimum of 12 months of antifungal therapy). Consider reinstitution of maintenance therapy if the CD4 cell count decreases to <100 cells/μL (0.1 × 10⁹/L).

[i]Drug level monitoring is strongly advised.

HEMATOGENOUS CANDIDIASIS

- Dissemination of *C. albicans* can result in infection in single or multiple organs, particularly the kidney, brain, myocardium, skin, eye, bone, and joints.
- *Candida* is generally acquired via the GI tract, although organisms may also enter the bloodstream via indwelling IV catheters.
- Immunosuppressed patients, including those with lymphoreticular or hematologic malignancies, diabetes, immunodeficiency diseases, or those receiving immunosuppressive therapy with high-dose corticosteroids, immunosuppressants, antineoplastic agents, or broad-spectrum antimicrobial agents are at high risk for invasive fungal infections.
- Major risk factors for hematogenous candidiasis include the use of central venous catheters, total parenteral nutrition, receipt of multiple antibiotics, extensive surgery and burns, renal failure and hemodialysis, mechanical ventilation, and prior fungal colonization.
- Treatment of candidiasis is presented in Table 39-4.

Aspergillus Infections

- *Aspergillus fumigatus* is the most commonly observed pathogen, followed by *A. flavus*.
- Invasive aspergillosis commonly affects immunocompromised patients and patients with acute myeloid leukemia (AML) and those who undergo allogeneic HSCT who have prolonged durations (more than 10 days) of neutropenia. Aspergillosis is generally acquired by inhalation of airborne conidia that are small enough (2.5–3 mm) to reach the alveoli or the paranasal sinuses.
- Superficial or locally invasive infections of the ear, skin, or appendages can often be managed with topical antifungal therapy.

TABLE 39-4	Antifungal Therapy of Invasive Candidiasis
Type of Disease and Common Clinical Manifestations	**Therapy/Comments**
Prophylaxis of Candidemia	
Non-neutropenic patients	Not recommended except for severely ill/high-risk patients in whom fluconazole IV/oral 400 mg daily should be used (see Chapter 144, "Invasive Fungal Infections," *Dipiro's Pharmacotherapy: A Pathophysiologic Approach,* 12th ed.)
Neutropenic patients[a]	Fluconazole IV/oral 400 mg daily *or* itraconazole solution 2.5 mg/kg every 12 hours orally *or* micafungin 50 mg (1 mg/kg in patients under 50 kg) IV daily; the optimal duration of therapy is unclear but at a minimum should include the period at risk for neutropenia
Solid-organ transplantation, liver transplantation	*Patients with key risk factors*[b]: Fluconazole 400 mg orally daily is preferred
Empirical (Preemptive) Antifungal Therapy	
Suspected disseminated candidiasis in febrile non-neutropenic patients	None recommended; data are lacking defining subsets of patients who are appropriate for therapy (see Chapter 144, "Invasive Fungal Infections," *Dipiro's Pharmacotherapy: A Pathophysiologic Approach,* 12th ed.)
Suspected candidiasis in febrile neutropenic patients	A lipid formulation of amphotericin B, caspofungin, micafungin, voriconazole, isavuconazole, posaconazole, or itraconazole for duration of neutropenia
Initial Antifungal Therapy of Documented Candidemia and Acute Hematogenously Disseminated Candidiasis, Unknown Species	
Patients who are less critically ill and who have had no recent azole exposure	*Remove existing central venous catheters when feasible plus fluconazole IV (loading dose of 800 mg [12 mg/kg], then 400 mg [6 mg/kg] daily) or an echinocandin;* treatment duration: 2 weeks after the last positive blood culture and resolution of signs and symptoms of infection
Patients with recent azole exposure, moderately severe or severe illness, or who are at high risk of infection due to *C. glabrata* or *C. krusei*	An echinocandin Transition from an echinocandin to fluconazole IV/oral is recommended for patients who are clinically stable and have isolates (eg, *C. albicans*) likely to be susceptible to fluconazole
Antifungal Therapy of Specific Pathogens	
C. albicans, C. tropicalis, and *C. parapsilosis*	Fluconazole IV/oral 6 mg/kg/day *or* an echinocandin; transition to fluconazole is recommended in patients who are clinically stable and whose isolates are likely to be susceptible to fluconazole (eg, *C. albicans*); voriconazole IV (400 mg [6 mg/kg] twice daily × two doses then 200 mg [3 mg/kg] twice daily thereafter) is efficacious, but offers little advantage over fluconazole; it may be utilized as step-down oral therapy for selected cases of candidiasis due to *C. krusei* or voriconazole-susceptible *C. glabrata*

(Continued)

TABLE 39-4   Antifungal Therapy of Invasive Candidiasis (*Continued*)

Type of Disease and Common Clinical Manifestations	Therapy/Comments
	Patients intolerant or refractory to other therapy: Amphotericin B lipid complex IV 3–5 mg/kg/day Liposomal amphotericin B IV 3–5 mg/kg/day
C. krusei	An echinocandin[c]
C. lusitaniae	Fluconazole IV/orally 6 mg/kg/day
C. glabrata	An echinocandin[c] (transition to fluconazole or voriconazole therapy is not recommended without confirmation of isolate susceptibility)
Urinary candidiasis	*Asymptomatic disease:* Generally no therapy is required *Symptomatic or high-risk patients[d]:* Removal of urinary tract instruments, stents, and Foley catheters, +7–14 days therapy with fluconazole 200 mg orally daily *or* amphotericin B IV 0.3–1 mg/kg/day

IV, intravenous.

[a]Patients at significant risk for invasive candidiasis include those receiving standard chemotherapy for acute myelogenous leukemia, allogeneic bone marrow transplants, or high-risk autologous bone marrow transplants. However, among these populations, chemotherapy or bone marrow transplant protocols do not all produce equivalent risk, and local experience should be used to determine the relevance of prophylaxis.

[b]Risk factors include re-transplantation, re-operation, renal failure requiring hemodialysis, transfusion of ≥40 units of cellular blood products including platelets, packed red blood cells, and auto transfusion; choledochojejunostomy, and Candida colonization in the perioperative period.

[c]Echinocandin = caspofungin 70 mg loading dose, then 50 mg IV daily maintenance dose, or micafungin 100 mg daily, or anidulafungin 200 mg loading dose, then 100 mg daily maintenance dose.

[d]Patients at high risk for dissemination include neutropenic patients, low-birth-weight infants, and patients who will undergo urologic manipulation.

ALLERGIC BRONCHOPULMONARY ASPERGILLOSIS

- Allergic manifestations of *Aspergillus* range in severity from mild asthma to allergic bronchopulmonary aspergillosis characterized by severe asthma with wheezing, fever, malaise, weight loss, chest pain, and a cough productive of blood-streaked sputum.
- Therapy is aimed at minimizing the quantity of antigenic material released in the tracheobronchial tree.
- Antifungal therapy is generally not indicated in the management of allergic manifestations of aspergillosis, although some patients have demonstrated a decrease in their glucocorticoid dose following therapy with itraconazole.

INVASIVE ASPERGILLOSIS

- Patients with invasive aspergillosis generally have blunted or nonspecific signs and symptoms of infection due to impaired inflammatory responses. Patients often present with classic signs and symptoms of acute pulmonary embolus: pleuritic chest pain, fever, hemoptysis, and friction rubs.
- Demonstration of *Aspergillus* by repeated culture and microscopic examination of tissue provides the most firm diagnosis.

TREATMENT

- **Voriconazole** is the drug of choice for primary therapy of most patients with invasive aspergillosis as it provided improved survival and fewer side effects.
- In patients who cannot tolerate voriconazole, amphotericin B can be used. Full doses (1–1.5 mg/kg/day) are generally recommended, with response measured by defervescence and radiographic clearing. The lipid-based formulations may be preferred as initial therapy in patients with marginal renal function or in patients receiving other nephrotoxic drugs. The optimal duration of treatment is unknown.
- **Caspofungin** is indicated for treatment of invasive aspergillosis in patients who are refractory to or intolerant of other therapies such as amphotericin B; however, response rates are lower. the use of prophylactic antifungal therapy (voriconazole) to prevent primary infection or reactivation of aspergillosis during subsequent courses of chemotherapy is recommended.

See Chapter 144, Invasive Fungal Infections, authored by Peggy L. Carver and Gregory A. Eschenauer, for a more detailed discussion of this topic.

CHAPTER 40

Fungal Infections, Superficial

Vulvovaginal Candidiasis

- *Vulvovaginal candidiasis* (VVC) refers to infections in individuals with or without symptoms who have positive vaginal cultures for *Candida* species. It may be sporadic or recurrent.
- Fifty to 72% of females would have had at least one episode of VVC.

PATHOPHYSIOLOGY

- *C. albicans* is the major pathogen responsible for VVC, accounting for 80%–92% of symptomatic episodes. The remainder are caused by non–*C. albicans* species, with *C. glabrata* dominating.
- Changes in the host's vaginal environment or response are necessary to induce a symptomatic infection. In most cases of symptomatic VVC, no precipitating factor can be identified.
- There is a dramatic increase in the frequency of VVC when women become sexually active.
- Antibiotic use can increase the risk of VVC, but it is significant in only a small number of women.

CLINICAL PRESENTATION

- Symptoms include intense vulvar itching, soreness irritation, burning on urination, and dyspareunia.
- Signs include erythema, fissuring, curdy "cheese"-like discharge, satellite lesions, and edema.
- Laboratory tests: Vaginal pH—normal saline, and 10% potassium hydroxide (KOH) microscopy for blastospores or pseudohyphae.
- *Candida* cultures are not recommended unless classic signs and symptoms with normal vaginal pH and microscopy are inconclusive or recurrence is suspected.
- The diagnosis should be based on both clinical presentation and investigations, including vaginal pH, saline microscopy, and 10% KOH microscopy of vaginal discharge.

TREATMENT

- <u>Goals of Treatment:</u> Complete resolution of symptoms in patients who have symptomatic VVC.

GENERAL APPROACH

- Remove or improve any predisposing factors if they can be identified.
- Avoid harsh soaps and perfumes that can cause or worsen vulvar irritation. The genital area must be kept clean and dry by avoiding constrictive clothing and frequent or prolonged exposure to hot tub use. Douching is not recommended for either prevention or treatment.

NONPHARMACOLOGIC THERAPY

- The value of oral use of lactobacillus remains unclear.

PHARMACOLOGIC THERAPY

- Effective antimycotic agents should have limited local and systemic side effects, a high cure rate, and easy administration.

- **Table 40-1** lists treatments for uncomplicated VVC. No product route or duration of treatment is superior to any other. Oral azoles (such as **fluconazole** or **itraconazole**) are therapeutically equivalent to topical therapies.
- In the treatment of uncomplicated VVC, the duration of therapy is not critical. Cure rates with different lengths of treatment have not demonstrated that one duration of therapy is significantly better.
- Patients with complicated VVC (immunocompromised or uncontrolled diabetes mellitus) should be treated for 10–14 days.
- Pregnant females with VVC should be treated with topical imidazole therapy for 7 days. Oral therapy is not recommended as larger doses of fluconazole have been linked to birth defects.
- Patients with recurrent VVC should receive a 10-day initial treatment (such as with oral **fluconazole** 150 mg daily) followed by 6 months of prolonged treatment (with oral fluconazole once weekly 150 mg).
- Treatment of VVC is considered to have positive outcomes if the symptoms are resolved within 24–48 hours and no adverse medication events are experienced. Self-assessment of symptom relief is appropriate for most cases of VVC. If symptoms remain unresolved or recur, then further testing and treatment can be required.

TABLE 40-1	Treatment for Uncomplicated VVC	
Active Ingredient	**Preparation**	**Regimen**
Nonprescription/Topical vaginal products		
Butoconazole	2% cream	One applicator × 3 days
Clotrimazole	1% cream	One applicator × 1 day
	100 mg tablet	One 100 mg tablet × 7 days
	2% cream	One applicator × 1 day
	200 mg tablet	One 200 mg tablet × 3 days
	10% cream	One applicator × 1 day
	500 mg tablet	One 500 mg tablet × 1 day
Miconazole[a]	2% cream	One applicator × 1 day
	100 mg suppository	One 100 mg suppository × 7 days
	200 mg suppository	One 200 mg suppository × 3 days
	1200 mg ovule	One ovule × 1 day
Ticonazole	2% cream	One applicator × 3 days
	6.5% cream	One applicator × 1 day
Prescription/Topical		
Nystatin	100,000 unit tablet	One tablet × 14 days
Terconazole	0.4% cream	One applicator × 7 days
	0.8% cream	One applicator × 3 days
Oral products		
Fluconazole	150 mg	One tablet × 1 day

[a]The FDA warns of the possible increase in the anticoagulant effects of warfarin with concomitant use.

Orophyryngeal and Esophageal Candidiasis

- *Oropharyngeal candidiasis* (OPC), often referred to as thrush, is caused by the yeast *Candida*, most often *C. albicans*.

PATHOPHYSIOLOGY

- A variety of host and exogenous factors can lead to the transformation of asymptomatic colonization to symptomatic disease, such as oropharyngeal and esophageal candidiasis, including use of steroids, antibiotics and immunosuppressive drugs, dentures, xerostomia, smoking, chemotherapy and radiotherapy, HIV infection, malignancies.
- Diabetes and other endocrine disorders, such as hypothyroidism, hypoparathyroidism, and hypoadrenalism, also can predispose patients to *Candida* species overgrowth.
- Patients with primary immune deficiencies such as lymphocytic abnormalities, phagocytic dysfunction, immunoglobulin A (IgA) deficiency, viral-induced immune paralysis, and severe congenital immunodeficiencies are also at risk for OPC as well as disseminated candidiasis.
- OPC remains the most common opportunistic infection in patients with human immunodeficiency virus (HIV) disease. The absolute CD4 T-cell count is the primary risk factor for development of OPC with the greatest risk at CD4 T-cell levels 10,000 copies/mL (10×106/L).

CLINICAL PRESENTATION

- Various classifications of OPC are given in **Table 40-2**. The clinical presentation of OPC and esophageal candidiasis is presented in **Table 40-3**.
- A presumptive diagnosis of OPC usually is made by the characteristic appearance on the oral mucosa, with resolution of signs and symptoms after antifungal therapy.

TABLE 40-2	Clinical Classification of OPC	
Types	**Population at Risk**	**Clinical Signs and Appearance**
Pseudomembranous (thrush)	Neonates, patients with HIV or cancer, the debilitated elderly, patients on broad-spectrum antibiotics or steroid inhalers, patients with dry mouth from various causes, and smokers	Classic "cottage cheese" appearance, yellowish white, soft plaques (or milk curds) overlying areas of erythema on the buccal mucosa, tongue, gums, and throat; plaques are easily removed by vigorous rubbing but can leave red or bleeding sites when removed; lesions on the tongue dorsum give it a bald, depapillated appearance
Erythematous (atrophic)	Patients with HIV, patients on broad-spectrum antibiotics or steroid inhalers	Sensitive and painful erythematous mucosa with few, if any, white plaques; lesions are generally on the dorsal surface of the tongue or the hard palate, occasionally on the soft palate, but any part of the mucosa can be involved; appear as flat red patches on the palate or atrophic patches on the tongue dorsum with loss of papillae; can be acute or chronic

(Continued)

TABLE 40-2	Clinical Classification of OPC *(Continued)*	
Types	**Population at Risk**	**Clinical Signs and Appearance**
Hyperplastic (candidal leukoplakia)	People who smoke; uncommon in patients with HIV	Thick white and adherent keratotic plaques commonly seen on the buccal mucosa and lateral border of the tongue; can also be seen on the lips and the bottom of the mouth; plaques cannot be easily scraped off or only partially removed; this condition is distinct from oral hairy leukoplakia, and it can progress to severe dysplasia or malignancy
Angular cheilitis	Patients with HIV, denture wearers	Painful red, ulcerative, cracking, or fissuring lesion at one or both corners of the mouth because of an inflammatory reaction; usually lesions are small and rather punctate, but occasionally they can extend in a linear fashion from the angles onto the facial skin
Denture stomatitis (chronic atrophic)	Denture wearers who tend to be elderly and have poor oral hygiene	Red, flat lesions on the mucosa beneath the denture and extend right up to the denture border; more commonly located beneath a maxillary denture, although they can be encountered beneath a mandibular denture
Central papillary atrophy (median rhomboid glossitis)	Uncommon (<1% prevalence), men more commonly infected than women (3:1)	Rhomboid-shaped hypertrophic or atrophic plaque in the mid-dorsal tongue; lesions may not resolve completely

HIV, human immunodeficiency virus.

TABLE 40-3	Clinical Presentation of OPC and Esophageal Candidiasis
Oropharyngeal Candidiasis	**Esophageal Candidiasis**
General	**General**
The clinical features can be quite diverse (see Table 40-2)	This usually occurs as an extension of OPC; however, the esophagus can be the only site involved; the distal two-thirds, rather than the proximal one-third, is the most common site
Symptoms	**Symptoms**
Symptoms are diverse and range from none to a sore, painful mouth, burning tongue, metallic taste, and dysphagia and odynophagia with involvement of the hypopharynx	Typically, the symptoms are dysphagia, odynophagia, and retrosternal chest pain but can be asymptomatic in some patients; although rare, epigastric pain can be the dominant symptom
Signs	**Signs**
Signs are variable and can include diffuse erythema and white patches on the surfaces of the buccal mucosa, throat, tongue, or gums; constitutional signs are absent	Constitutional signs, including fever, occasionally occur; physical findings can range from a few to numerous white or beige plaques of variable size
	Plaques can be hyperemic or edematous, with ulceration in more severe cases

(Continued)

TABLE 40-3	Clinical Presentation of OPC and Esophageal Candidiasis *(Continued)*
Oropharyngeal Candidiasis	**Esophageal Candidiasis**
	Most advanced cases can occur with increased mucosal friability and narrowing of lumen
	Uncommon complications include perforation and aortic–esophageal fistula formation
Laboratory tests	**Laboratory tests**
Scraping of an active lesion for microscopic examination can help confirm the diagnosis (presence of pseudohyphae and budding yeast) but is usually not necessary	The best test is upper GI endoscopy (more useful than barium swallow); helps exclude other causes of esophagitis (eg, viral, aphthous ulcers); diagnosis is confirmed by the histologic presence of *Candida* species in biopsy lesions taken during endoscopy
Cultures are not necessary because isolation of *Candida* species does not distinguish between colonization and true infection; cultures can be taken in patients responding poorly to therapy to determine the infecting species and to predict likely drug resistance	Cultures to look for drug-resistant *Candida* species are warranted in patients who require endoscopy

GI, gastrointestinal; OPC, oropharyngeal candidiasis.

TREATMENT

- <u>Goals of Treatment:</u> The primary desired outcome in the management of OPC is a clinical cure; that is, elimination of clinical signs and symptoms. Efficacy end points for oropharyngeal and esophageal candidiasis include rapid relief of symptoms and prevention of complications without early relapse after completion of the course of therapy. Preventing or minimizing the number of future recurrences of both types of candidiasis is an equally important outcome.
- Minimizing toxicities and drug–drug interactions of systemic antifungal agents, as well as maximizing adherence by ensuring that the patient understands the importance of therapy and the directions to take the medication appropriately, are important secondary outcomes of therapy.

GENERAL APPROACH

- Whenever feasible, it is desirable to minimize all predisposing factors, such as administration of corticosteroids, chemotherapeutic agents, and antimicrobials, as well as to institute proper oral hygiene and resolve concurrent conditions, such as denture stomatitis.
- Selection of an appropriate antifungal agent for treatment of candidiasis requires consideration of several factors, including the patient's drug adherence, adequate saliva for dissolution of solid topical medications, risk of caries from sucrose- or dextrose-containing preparations, potential drug interactions, coexisting medical conditions (eg, liver disease), location and severity of the infection, and the need for long-term maintenance therapy.

PHARMACOLOGIC THERAPY

- Topical agents, such as **nystatin** and **clotrimazole**, are the standard treatment for uncomplicated OPC and generally are effective for treatment in otherwise healthy adults and infants with no underlying immunodeficiencies (Table 40-4).
- Systemic therapy is necessary in patients with OPC that is refractory to topical treatment, those who cannot tolerate topical agents, have moderate-to-severe disease, and those at high risk for disseminated systemic or invasive candidiasis.

TABLE 40-4 Therapeutic Options for Mucosal Candidiasis

Initial Episodes of OPCa: Treat for 7–14 Days (Strength of Recommendation and Level of Evidence)	Common/Significant Side Effects
Clotrimazole 10 mg troche: hold 1 troche in mouth for 15–20 minutes for slow dissolution 5 times daily (B-2)[b]	Altered taste, mild nausea, vomiting
Nystatin 100,000 units/mL suspension: 5 mL swish and swallow orally four times daily (B-2)	Mild nausea, vomiting, diarrhea
Miconazole 50 mg mucoadhesive buccal tablets 50 mg orally daily (A-1)	Diarrhea, headache, nausea, dysgeusia, upper abdominal pain, and vomiting
Fluconazole 100 mg tablets:[c] 100–200 mg orally daily (A-1)	GI upset, hepatitis not common
Itraconazole 10 mg/mL solution:[d] 200 mg orally daily (A-2)	GI upset, not common: hepatotoxicity, CHF, pulmonary edema with long-term use[e]
Posaconazole 40 mg/mL suspension: 400 mg orally daily with a full meal (A-2)	GI upset, fever, headache, increased hepatic transaminases not common
Fluconazole-Refractory OPC: Treat for ≥14 Days	
Itraconazole 10 mg/mL solution: 200 mg orally daily (A-3)	See above
Voriconazole 200 mg tablets: 200 mg orally twice daily (>40 kg), taken on empty stomach (A-3)	GI upset, rash, reversible visual disturbance (altered light perception, photopsia, chromatopsia, photophobia), increased hepatic transaminases, hallucinations, or confusion
Posaconazole 40 mg/mL suspension: 400 mg orally twice daily × 3 days, then 400 mg daily × 28 days (A-2)	See above
Amphotericin B 100 mg/mL suspension[f]: 1–5 mL swish and swallow orally 4 times daily (B-2)	Oral: nausea, vomiting, diarrhea with higher dose
Amphotericin B deoxycholate 50 mg injection: 0.3–0.7 mg/kg/day IV daily (B-2)	IV: fever, chills, sweats, nephrotoxicity, electrolyte disturbances, bone marrow suppression
Caspofungin 50 mg IV daily (B-2)	Fever, headache, infusion-related reactions (<5%) (eg, rash, facial swelling, pruritus, vasodilation), hypokalemia, increased hepatic transaminases, anemia, neutropenia
Micafungin 150 mg IV daily (B-2)	Similar to caspofungin
Anidulafungin 200 mg IV daily (B-2)	Similar to caspofungin
Esophageal Candidiasis[a]: Treat for 14–21 Days	
Fluconazole 100 mg tablets: 200–400 mg orally (3–6 mg/kg) daily (A-1)	See above
Echinocandin: see above (B-2)	See above
Amphotericin B deoxycholate 50 mg injection: 0.3–0.7 mg/kg/day IV daily (B-2)	See above

(Continued)

TABLE 40-4 Therapeutic Options for Mucosal Candidiasis *(Continued)*

Initial Episodes of OPCa: Treat for 7–14 Days (Strength of Recommendation and Level of Evidence)	Common/Significant Side Effects
Posaconazole 40 mg/mL suspension: 400 mg orally twice daily (A-3)	See above
Itraconazole 10 mg/mL solution:d 200 mg orally daily (A-3)	See above
Voriconazole 200 mg tablets: 200 mg orally twice daily (>40 kg) (A-3)	See above
Voriconazole IV and echinocandins (A-1): generally reserved for refractory cases	See above
Fluconazole-Refractory EC: Treat for 21–28 Days	
Itraconazole 10 mg/mL solution: 200 mg orally daily (A-2)	See above
Posaconazole 40 mg/mL suspension: 400 mg orally twice daily (A-3)	See above
Voriconazole 200 mg tablets: 200 mg orally twice daily (>40 kg), taken on empty stomach (A-3)	See above
Caspofungin 50 mg IV daily (B-2)	See above
Micafungin 150 mg IV daily (B-2)	Similar to caspofungin
Anidulafungin 100 mg IV on day 1, then 50 mg IV daily (B-2)	Similar to caspofungin
Amphotericin B deoxycholate: 0.3–0.7 mg/kg/day IV, or lipid-based amphotericin 3–5 mg/kg/day IV (B-2)	See above

CHF, congestive heart failure; EC, esophageal candidiasis; GI, gastrointestinal; IV, intravenous; OPC, oropharyngeal candidiasis.

aInitial episodes of OPC can be adequately treated first with topical agents before resorting to systemic therapy (B-2), but systemic therapy is required for effective treatment of esophageal candidiasis (A-2). Suppressive therapy is recommended for patients with frequent or severe recurrences (A-1).

bFluconazole is more effective than ketoconazole (A-1).

cStrength of Recommendation and Level of Evidence.

dSolution is more effective than capsule (A-1); solution is better taken on an empty stomach.

eSuspension is not marketed; can be prepared extemporaneously by pharmacy.

fSee discussion under onychomycosis.

Recommendation grades: Strength of recommendation: **A**—Both strong evidence for efficacy and substantial clinical benefit to support recommendation for use. *Should always be offered.* **B**—Moderate evidence for efficacy but only limited clinical benefit, to support recommendation for use. *Should generally be offered.* **C**—Evidence for efficacy is insufficient to support recommendation for or against use; or evidence for efficacy might not outweigh adverse consequences or cost of the treatment under consideration. *Optional.* **D**—Moderate evidence for lack of efficacy or adverse outcome supports a recommendation against use. *Should generally not be offered.* Quality of evidence: 1—Evidence from at least one properly designed randomized, controlled trial. 2—Evidence from at least one well-designed trial without randomization, from cohort or case-controlled analytic studies (preferably from more than one center), or from multiple time-series studies, or dramatic results from uncontrolled experiments. 3—Evidence from opinions of respected authorities based on clinical experience, descriptive studies, or reports of expert committees. UR—Evidence currently unrated.

EVALUATION OF THERAPEUTIC OUTCOMES

- Patient counseling tips for managing OPC are given in Table 40-5.

TABLE 40-5	Patient Counseling Tips for Managing Oropharyngeal Candidiasis

1. Clean the oral cavity prior to administering the topical antifungal agent. Daily fluoride rinses can help reduce the risk of caries when using an agent containing sucrose or dextrose.

2. Use the topical antifungal agent after meals, as saliva flow and mouth movements can reduce the contact time.

3. Troches should be slowly dissolved in the mouth, not chewed or swallowed whole, over 15–20 minutes, and the saliva swallowed.

4. Suspension should be swished around the mouth in the oral cavity to cover all areas for as long as possible, ideally at least 1 minute, then gargled and swallowed.

5. Remove dentures while medication is being applied to the oral tissues.

6. Use a suspension or buccal mucoadhesive tablet instead of a troche if xerostomia is present; if a troche is preferred, rinse or drink water prior to dosing. For xerostomia, you may use nonpharmacologic measures for symptomatic relief (eg, ice chips, sugarless gum or hard candy, citrus beverages).

7. Dentures should be removed and disinfected overnight using an antiseptic solution (eg, chlorhexidine 0.12%–0.2%). Disinfect oral tissues in addition to dental prosthesis.

8. Complete treatment course even though symptomatic improvement can occur in 48–72 hours.

9. Maintain good oral hygiene. Brush teeth daily (twice daily) and floss, rinse mouth, or brush teeth after eating sweets.

10. Stop smoking; avoid alcohol.

Mycotic Infections of the Skin, Hair, and Nails

PATHOPHYSIOLOGY

- Superficial cutaneous mycoses affect up to 20%–25% of the population globally. The usual pathogens are the dermatophytes classified by genera: *Trichophyton, Epidermophyton*, and *Microsporum*.
- Dermatophytes have the ability to penetrate keratinous structures of the body and therefore infections are limited to hair, nails, and skin. These infections affect both male and female genders and all races. Reservoirs of mycotic infections include humans, animals, and soil.
- Risk factors for the development of an infection include prolonged exposure to sweat or soaking in water, maceration, intertriginous folds, sharing personal belongings such as combs, close living quarters (dormitories, barracks).

CLINICAL PRESENTATION

- Mycotic infections of the skin have a classic appearance that consists of a central clearing surrounded by an advancing red, scaly, elevated border, also referred to as an "active" border.
- Diagnosis usually is based on patient history, as well as the physical examination. Diagnostic tests include direct microscopic examination of a specimen after the addition of KOH or fungal cultures. The KOH test is quick, inexpensive, and easy to perform.

TREATMENT

GENERAL APPROACH

- <u>Goals of Treatment:</u> A general approach to treatment of superficial mycotic infections includes keeping the infected area dry and clean and limiting exposure to the infected reservoir. Topical agents generally are considered to be first-line therapy for infections of the skin. Oral therapy is preferred when the infection is extensive or severe or when treating *tinea capitis* or onychomycosis.
- Treatment of mycoses of the skin, hair, and nails is given in **Table 40-6**.

TABLE 40-6	Treatment of Mycoses of the Skin, Hair, and Nails	
Type of Mycoses	**Topical**[a,b]	**Oral Regimen**[c]
Tinea pedis	Butenafine, daily	Fluconazole 150 mg 1 per week × 1–4 weeks
	Sertaconazole, twice daily	
	Luliconazole, daily	
	Naftifine cream daily, gel daily	
Tinea manuum	Ciclopirox, twice daily	Ketoconazole 200 mg daily × 4 weeks
Tinea cruris	Clotrimazole, twice daily	Itraconazole 200–400 mg/day × 1 week
	Luliconazole, daily	
	Naftifine cream, daily	
Tinea corporis	Econazole, daily	Terbinafine 250 mg/day × 2 weeks
	Haloprogin, twice daily	
	Ketoconazole cream, daily	
	Luliconazole, daily	
	Miconazole, twice daily	
	Naftifine cream, daily	
	Oxiconazole, twice daily	
	Sulconazole, twice daily	
	Terbinafine, twice daily	
	Tolnaftate, twice daily	
	Triacetin cream, solution, three times daily	
	Undecylenic acid, various preparations: apply as directed	
Tinea capitis	Shampoo only in conjunction with oral therapy **or** for treatment of asymptomatic carriers	Terbinafine 250 mg/day × 4–8 weeks
Tinea barbae	Ketoconazole twice weekly × 4 weeks	Ketoconazole 200 mg daily × 4 weeks
	Selenium sulfide daily × 2 weeks	Itraconazole 100–200 mg/day × 4–6 weeks
		Griseofulvin 500 mg/day × 4–6 weeks

(Continued)

TABLE 40-6	Treatment of Mycoses of the Skin, Hair, and Nails (Continued)	
Type of Mycoses	**Topical[a,b]**	**Oral Regimen[c]**
Pityriasis versicolor	Clotrimazole, twice daily Econazole, daily Haloprogin, twice daily Ketoconazole, daily Miconazole, twice daily Oxiconazole cream only, twice daily Sulconazole, twice daily Tolnaftate, three times daily	Ketoconazole, fluconazole, itraconazole 200 mg daily × 3–7 days
Onychomycosis	Ciclopirox 8% nail lacquer: apply solution at night for up to 48 weeks (fingernails and toenails) Efinaconazole 10% topical solution daily for 48 weeks (toenails) Tavaborole 5% topical solution daily for 48 weeks (toenails)	Terbinafine 250 mg/day × 6 weeks (fingernail), 12 weeks (toenail) Itraconazole 200 mg twice daily × 1 week/month for 2 months (fingernail); 200 mg daily × 12 weeks (toenail) Fluconazole 50 mg daily or 300 mg once weekly for ≥6 months (fingernail) or 12 months (toenail)

[a]Other products are available, including combination products.
[b]Length of therapy depends on mycotic sensitivity and severity of infection.
[c]Only capsule formulation studied; give with food for increased absorption.

See Chapter 143, Superficial Fungal Infections, authored by Thomas E.R. Brown and Linda Dresser, for a more detailed discussion of this topic.

- Dehydration resulting from *gastrointestinal infections* such as acute infectious diarrhea is the second leading cause of mortality in children younger than 5 years, killing 525,000 annually. Globally, 1.7 billion cases of infectious diarrhea occur yearly and cause over 1.39 million deaths.
- The highest mortality risk from infectious diarrhea in the United States occurs in the elderly, which contrasts to the developing world where the risk of death is highest among young children. In the United States, there are 179 million episodes of acute gastroenteritis each year, causing nearly 500,000 hospitalizations and over 5000 deaths.
- Viruses are now the leading global cause of infectious diarrhea. Noroviruses, previously known as Norwalk-like viruses, account for greater than 90% of viral gastroenteritis among all age groups, and 50% of outbreaks worldwide. Characteristics of agents responsible for viral gastroenteritis are given in Table 41-1. GI infections and enterotoxigenic poisonings can be caused by a wide variety of viruses, bacteria, and parasites.
- Public health measures such as clean water supply and sanitation facilities, as well as quality control of commercial products, are important for the control of most enteric infections. Sanitary food handling and preparation practices significantly decrease the incidence of enteric infections.
- Common pathogens responsible for watery diarrhea in the United States are norovirus and enterotoxigenic *Escherichia coli* (ETEC), while those most commonly associated bacteria with dysentery diarrhea are *Campylobacter* spp., enterohemorrhagic *E. coli* (EHEC), *Salmonella* spp., and *Shigella* spp. ETEC is also the most common cause of traveler's diarrhea and a common cause of food- and water-associated outbreaks. Cholera is caused by toxigenic *V. cholera*.

Rehydration, Antimotility, And Probiotic Therapy

- The cornerstone of management for all gastrointestinal (GI) infections and enterotoxigenic poisonings is to prevent dehydration by correcting fluid and electrolyte imbalances. In mild, self-limiting acute gastroenteritis, a diet of oral fluids and easily digestible foods is recommended. In patients with severe dehydrating watery diarrhea and dysenteric diarrhea, IV rehydration therapy, antibiotics, and/or antimotility treatments are needed.
- Initial assessment of fluid loss is essential for successful rehydration therapy and should include acute weight loss, as it is the most reliable means of determining the extent of water loss. Clinical signs can be helpful in determining approximate deficits (Table 41-2).
- The necessary components of **oral rehydration solution** (ORS) include glucose, sodium, potassium chloride, and water (Table 41-3). ORS should be given in small frequent volumes (5 mL every 2–3 minutes) in a teaspoon or oral syringe.
- Severely dehydrated patients should be resuscitated initially with lactated Ringer's solution or normal intravenous (IV) saline. Guidelines for rehydration therapy based on the degree of dehydration and replacement of ongoing losses are outlined in Table 41-2. After rehydration, maintenance fluid is given based on accurate recording of intake and output volumes. ORS should be instituted as soon as it can be tolerated.
- Early refeeding with age-appropriate unrestricted diet is recommended in children and shortens the course of diarrhea. Initially, easily digested foods, such as bananas, applesauce, and cereal may be added as tolerated. Foods high in fiber, sodium, and sugar should be avoided.
- Antimotility drugs such as **diphenoxylate** and **loperamide** offer symptomatic relief in patients with watery diarrhea by reducing the number of stools. Antimotility drugs should be avoided if possible and are not recommended in patients with

TABLE 41-1	Characteristics of Agents Responsible for Acute Viral Gastroenteritis				
Virus	**Peak Age of Onset**	**Time of Year**	**Duration**	**Mode of Transmission**	**Common Symptoms**
Rotavirus	6 months to 2 years	October to April	3–7 days	Fecal–oral, water, food	Nausea, vomiting, diarrhea, fever, abdominal pain, lactose intolerance
Norovirus	All age groups	Peak in winter	2–3 days	Fecal–oral, food, water, environment	Nausea, vomiting, diarrhea, abdominal cramps, myalgia
Astrovirus	<7 years	Winter	1–4 days	Fecal–oral, water, shellfish	Diarrhea, headache, malaise, nausea
Enteric adenovirus	<2 years	Year-round	7–9 days	Fecal–oral	Diarrhea, respiratory symptoms, vomiting, fever
Pestivirus	<2 years	NR	3 days	NR	Mild
Coronavirus-like particles	<2 years	Fall and early winter	7 days	NR	Respiratory disease
Enterovirus	NR	NR	NR	NR	Mild diarrhea, secondary organ damage

NR, not reported.

TABLE 41-2	Clinical Assessment of Degree of Dehydration in Children Based on Percentage of Body Weight Loss[a]		
Variable	**Minimal or No Dehydration (<3% Loss of Body Weight)**	**Mild-to-Moderate (3%–9% Loss of Body Weight)**	**Severe (≥10% Loss of Body Weight)**
Blood pressure	Normal	Normal	Normal to reduced
Quality of pulses	Normal	Normal or slightly decreased	Weak, thready, or not palpable
Heart rate	Normal	Normal to increased	Increased (bradycardia in severe cases)
Breathing	Normal	Normal to fast	Deep
Mental status	Normal	Normal to listless	Apathetic, lethargic, or comatose
Eyes	Normal	Sunken orbits/ decreased tears	Deeply sunken orbits/ absent tears
Mouth and tongue	Moist	Dry	Parched
Thirst	Normal	Eager to drink	Drinks poorly; too lethargic to drink

(Continued)

	Minimal or No Dehydration (<3% Loss of Body Weight)	Mild-to-Moderate (3%–9% Loss of Body Weight)	Severe (≥10% Loss of Body Weight)
TABLE 41-2	Clinical Assessment of Degree of Dehydration in Children Based on Percentage of Body Weight Loss[a] (*Continued*)		
Variable			
Skin fold	Normal	Recoil in <2 seconds	Recoil in >2 seconds
Extremities	Warm, normal capillary refill	Cool, prolonged capillary refill	Cold, mottled, cyanotic, prolonged capillary refill
Urine output	Normal to decreased	Decreased	Minimal
Hydration therapy	None	ORS 50–100 mL/kg over 3–4 hours	Lactated Ringer's solution or normal saline 20 mL/kg over 15–30 minutes IV until mental status or perfusion improves
			Followed by 5% dextrose/0.45% sodium chloride IV at higher maintenance rates or ORS 100 mL/kg over 4 hours
Replacement of ongoing losses	For each diarrheal stool or emesis <10 kg body weight: 60–120 mL ORS >10 kg body weight: 120–240 mL ORS	Same as minimal dehydration	If unable to tolerate ORS, administer through nasogastric tube or administer 5% dextrose/0.45% sodium chloride with 20 mEq/L (mmol/L) potassium chloride IV

IV, intravenous; ORS, oral rehydration solution.
[a]Percentages vary among patients for each dehydration category; hemodynamic and perfusion status is most important; when unsure of category, therapy for more severe category is recommended.

TABLE 41-3	Comparison of Common Solutions Used in Oral Rehydration and Maintenance				
Product	**Na (mEq/L)[a]**	**K (mEq/L)[a]**	**Base (mEq/L)**	**Carbohydrate (mmol/L)**	**Osmolarity (mOsm/L)**
WHO/UNICEF (2002)	75	20	30	75	245
Pedialyte	45	20	30	140	250
Infalyte	50	25	30	70	200
Oralyte	60	20	0	90	260
Rehydralyte	75	20	30	140	250
Cola[b]	2	0	13	700	750
Apple juice[b]	5	32	0	690	730
Chicken broth[b]	250	8	0	0	500
Sports beverage[b]	20	3	3	255	330

[a]Concentration of monovalent ions expressed in mEq/L is numerically equivalent to mmol/L concentration.
[b]These solutions should be avoided in dehydration.

many toxin-mediated dysenteric diarrheas (ie, EHEC, pseudomembranous colitis, shigellosis).
- Individual studies have not shown significant benefit from probiotics, and meta-analyses have shown conflicting results.
- Oral zinc supplementation of 20 mg/day for 1–2 weeks may have an additional benefit over ORS alone in reducing childhood mortality in developing countries.

Bacterial Infections

- Antibiotic therapy is recommended in severe cases of diarrhea, moderate-to-severe cases of traveler's diarrhea, most cases of febrile dysenteric diarrhea, and culture-proven bacterial diarrhea. Antimicrobial therapy is not recommended in EHEC diarrhea as it may increase risk of hemolytic uremic syndrome (HUS); however, it is recommended in severe cases of cholera and ETEC diarrhea. Antibiotic choices for bacterial infections are given in **Table 41-4**.

TABLE 41-4	Recommendations for Antibiotic Therapy	
Pathogen	**Children**	**Adults**
Watery Diarrhea		
Enterotoxigenic *Escherichia coli*	Azithromycin 10 mg/kg/day given orally once daily × 3 days; ceftriaxone 50 mg/kg/day given IV once daily × 3 days	Ciprofloxacin 750 mg orally once daily × 1–3 days; alternatives: rifaximin 200 mg orally three times daily × 3 days; azithromycin 1000 mg orally × 1 day *or* 500 mg orally daily × 3 days
Vibrio cholerae O1	Erythromycin 30 mg/kg/day divided every 8 hours orally × 3 days; azithromycin 10 mg/kg/day given orally once daily × 3 days	Doxycycline 300 mg orally × 1 day Alternatives: azithromycin 500 mg orally once daily × 3 days; ciprofloxacin 750 mg orally once daily × 3 days; ceftriaxone IV
Dysenteric Diarrhea		
Campylobacter species[a]	Azithromycin 10 mg/kg/day given orally once daily × 3–5 days; erythromycin 30 mg/kg/day divided into two to four doses orally × 3–5 days	Azithromycin 500 mg orally once daily × 3 days Alternatives: ciprofloxacin 750 mg orally once daily × 7 days
Salmonella Nontyphoidal[a]	Ceftriaxone 100 mg/kg/day divided IV every 12 hours × 7–10 days; azithromycin 20 mg/kg/day orally once daily × 7 days	Ceftriaxone 2 g IV/IM once; ciprofloxacin 750 mg orally once daily × 7–10 days Alternatives: ampicillin 250–500 mg orally every 6 hours × 7 days; azithromycin 500 mg orally once daily × 7 days; trimethoprim-sulfamethoxazole 160/800 mg twice daily × 7 days For immunocompromised patients, duration should be increased to 14 days for both fluoroquinolones and azithromycin
		(Continued)

TABLE 41-4 Recommendations for Antibiotic Therapy (*Continued*)		
Pathogen	Children	Adults
Shigella species[a]	Azithromycin 10 mg/kg/day given orally once daily × 3 days; ceftriaxone 50 mg/kg/day given IV once daily × 3 days	Azithromycin 500 mg orally once daily × 3 days; ceftriaxone 2 g IV/IM once; ciprofloxacin 750 mg orally once daily × 3 days Alternatives: ampicillin 250–500 mg orally every 6 hours × 7 days; trimethoprim–sulfamethoxazole 160/800 mg twice daily × 7 days
Yersinia species[a]	Treat as children with shigellosis	Trimethoprim-sulfamethoxazole 160/800 mg twice daily × 7 days Alternatives: cefotaxime IV or ciprofloxacin 750 mg orally once daily × 7 days
Traveler's Diarrhea		
Prophylaxis[a]		None recommended
Treatment		Azithromycin 1000 mg orally × 1 day or 500 mg orally daily × 3 days; ciprofloxacin 750 mg orally × 1 day or 500 mg orally every 12 hours × 3 days; levofloxacin 500 mg orally daily × 3 days; ofloxacin 400 mg twice daily × 1–3 days; rifamycin SV 388 mg twice daily × 3 days; rifaximin 200 mg three times daily × 3 days

[a]For high-risk patients only. See the preceding text for the high-risk patients in each infection.

- Antibiotic therapy is indicated in at-risk and febrile patients with dysenteric diarrhea. In shigellosis, antibiotics shorten the period of fecal shedding and attenuate the clinical illness. Antibiotic therapy is reserved for the elderly, those who are immunocompromised, children in daycare centers, malnourished children, and healthcare workers.

TRAVELER'S DIARRHEA

- Traveler's diarrhea describes the clinical syndrome caused by contaminated food or water that is manifested by malaise, anorexia, and abdominal cramps followed by the sudden onset of diarrhea that incapacitates many travelers.
- Traveler's diarrhea is caused by contaminated food or water. The most common pathogens are bacterial and include ETEC, *Campylobacter* spp., *Shigella* spp., and *Salmonella* spp.
- Patient education in avoiding high-risk food and beverages should be the best method for minimizing the risk. High-risk foods and beverages include raw or undercooked meat and seafood, moist foods served at room temperature, fruits that cannot be peeled, vegetables, milk from a questionable source, hot sauces on the table, tap water, unsealed bottled water, iced drinks, and food from street vendors.
- Bismuth subsalicylate 524 mg (two chewable tablets or 2 ounces) orally four times daily for up to 3 weeks is a commonly recommended prophylactic regimen. Prophylactic antibiotic use is not recommended for most travelers due to the potential side effects of antibiotics, predisposition to other infections such as *Clostridioides difficile* infection or vaginal candidiasis, the increased risk of selection of drug-resistant organisms, cost, lack of data on the safety and efficacy of antibiotics given for more than 2 or 3 weeks, and availability of rapidly effective antibiotics for treatment.

- Prophylactic antibiotics are recommended only in high-risk individuals or in situations in which short-term illness could ruin the purpose of the trip, such as a military mission. A fluoroquinolone is the drug of choice when traveling to most areas of the world. Azithromycin can be considered when traveling to South and Southeast Asia. Rifaximin 200 mg once, twice, or three times daily with meals for 2 weeks should be reserved for travel regions where *E. coli* predominates, such as Latin America and Africa.

TREATMENT

- The goals of treatment of traveler's diarrhea are to avoid dehydration, reduce the severity and duration of symptoms, and prevent interruption to planned activities.
- Fluid and electrolyte replacement should be initiated at the onset of diarrhea. ORS is generally not required in otherwise healthy individuals; flavored mineral water offers a good source of sodium and glucose. In infants and young children, elderly, and those with chronic debilitating medical conditions, ORS is recommended.
- Antibiotics used for treatment are found in Table 41-4. A single dose of fluoroquinolone is recommended initially, and if diarrhea is improved within 12–24 hours, antibiotics should be discontinued.
- For symptom relief, **loperamide** (preferred because of its quicker onset and longer duration of relief relative to bismuth) may be taken (4 mg orally initially and then 2 mg with each subsequent loose stool to a maximum of 16 mg/day in patients without bloody diarrhea and fever). Loperamide should be discontinued if symptoms persist for more than 48 hours.

CLOSTRIDIOIDES DIFFICILE

- *C. difficile* is the most commonly recognized cause of infectious diarrhea in healthcare settings with high rates of disease in the elderly and those exposed to antibiotic agents. The antibiotics most commonly associated with *C. difficile* infection (CDI) include fluoroquinolones, clindamycin, carbapenems, and third-/fourth-generation cephalosporins.
- Other risk factors for acquisition of *C. difficile* include recent healthcare exposure, chemotherapy, patients undergoing GI surgery or receiving tube feeding, and potentially those receiving acid suppressive medications.
- The spectrum of disease ranges from mild diarrhea to fulminant disease and toxic megacolon. The diarrhea is typically watery and nonbloody, and is often associated with abdominal discomfort, fever, and leukocytosis.
- Diagnosis of CDI is confirmed by identification of *C. difficile* organisms/toxin in stool or by colonoscopic or histopathologic findings revealing pseudomembranous colitis.
- Supportive care of CDI includes fluid and electrolyte replacement therapy, in addition to discontinuation of the offending antimicrobial if possible.

TREATMENT

- Once determination of disease severity has been made, treatment should be initiated with an antibiotic effective against *C. difficile*. **Vancomycin** and **fidaxomicin** are the most commonly prescribed agents and fidaxomicin is the preferred therapy. The recommended treatment course is 10 days and repeat stool testing is not recommended as a test of cure. The patient should be supported with fluid and electrolyte replacement.
- Antimotility agents (such as diphenoxylate/atropine and loperamide) and exchange resins (such as cholestyramine and colestipol) have been used in CDI; however, their use is discouraged.
- Classification of CDI severity and recommended treatment for adults is given in Table 41-5. In patients with severe/complicated or fulminant CDI the preferred regimen is combination therapy with IV **metronidazole** and **vancomycin**.

TABLE 41-5	*Clostridioides difficile* Infection Severity and Treatment	
Severity	**Markers of Disease Severity**	**Recommended Treatment**
Nonsevere	WBC ≤15,000 cells/mm³ (15 × 10⁹/L) SCr <1.5 mg/dL (133 μmol/L)	Vancomycin 125 mg orally 4 times daily for 10 days, OR fidaxomicin 200 mg orally twice daily for 10 days, OR metronidazole 500 mg orally every 8 hours for 10 days[a]
Severe	WBC >15,000 cells/mm³ (15 × 10⁹/L) SCr >1.5 mg/dL (133 μmol/L)	Vancomycin 125 mg orally 4 times daily for 10 days, OR fidaxomicin 200 mg orally twice daily for 10 days
Fulminant	Hypotension or shock Ileus and/or megacolon	Metronidazole 500 mg IV every 8 hours *PLUS* vancomycin 500 mg every 6 hours via NG or orally (if ileus present use rectally)

NG, nasogastric; SCr, serum creatinine; WBC, white blood cell.
[a]Metronidazole is an alternative therapy if other agents are unavailable or too costly.

- Recurrence of CDI can occur in 25%–35% of patients. If metronidazole was used initially, then a standard vancomycin course can be utilized for the first recurrence. For patients with multiple recurrences fidaxomicin remains the preferred agent; however, pulsed/tapered vancomycin, vancomycin followed by rifaximin, or fecal microbiota transplantation (FMT) are acceptable alternative.
- The American College of Gastroenterology recommends FMT by colonoscopy or capsule formulation oral ingestion with recurrent *C. difficile* infection (rCDI).
- For patients with rCDI within 6 months, bezlotoxumab (10 mg/kg IV as a single dose during antibacterial treatment) may be used during the administration of standard of care antibiotics.

See Chapter 136, Gastrointestinal Infections and Enterotoxigenic Poisonings, authored by Andrew Roecker and Brittany Bates, for a more detailed discussion of this topic.

Human Immunodeficiency Virus Infection

- A retrovirus, human immunodeficiency virus type 1 (HIV-1), is the major cause of HIV infection and AIDS.
- The natural history of HIV infection exhibits three general phases: acute, chronic, and terminal (AIDS).
- Persons with HIV infection are broadly categorized as those living with HIV and those with an AIDS diagnosis.

ETIOLOGY AND PATHOGENESIS

- Infection with HIV occurs through three primary modes: sexual, parenteral, and perinatal. Sexual intercourse, primarily anal and vaginal intercourse, is the most common vehicle for transmission. The highest risk appears to be from receptive ano-rectal intercourse at about 1.4 transmissions per 100 sexual acts. Condom use reduces the risk of transmission by approximately 80%.
- Transmission is significantly higher when the index partner has early or late HIV compared with asymptomatic HIV. Individuals with genital ulcers or sexually transmitted diseases are at great risk for contracting HIV.
- The risk of HIV transmission from sharing needles is approximately 0.67 per 100 episodes.
- Healthcare workers have a small but definite occupational risk of contracting HIV through accidental exposure, mostly the result of a percutaneous needle stick injury (estimated 0.3% risk of transmitting HIV). Mucocutaneous exposures (eg, tainted blood splash in eyes, mouth, or nose) carry a transmission risk of approximately 0.09%.
- Perinatal infection, or vertical transmission, is the most common cause of pediatric HIV infection. The risk of mother-to-child transmission is ~25% in the absence of antiretroviral therapy (ART). Breastfeeding can also transmit HIV.
- Initial rounds of HIV replication during acute infection take place largely in the mucosal CD4+, CCR5+ T-cell pools in the gut, resulting in a massive CD4 T-cell depletion in these tissues.

CLINICAL PRESENTATION AND DIAGNOSIS

- An AIDS diagnosis is made when the presence of HIV is laboratory-confirmed and the CD4 (T-helper cell) count drops below 200 cells/mm^3 (0.2×10^9/L) for those aged 6 years or older, or after an AIDS indicator condition is diagnosed.
- Primary infection is associated with a high viral load (more than 10^6 copies/mL [10^9/L]) and a precipitous drop in CD4 cells.
- The most common signs and symptoms of primary HIV infection are fever, headache, sore throat, fatigue, gastrointestinal (GI) upset (diarrhea, nausea, vomiting), weight loss, myalgia, morbilliform or maculopapular rash usually involving the trunk, lymphadenopathy, and night sweats. Less common signs and symptoms are aseptic meningitis, oral ulcers, and leukopenia.
- Clinical presentations of primary HIV infection vary, but patients often have a viral syndrome or mononucleosis-like illness with fever, headache, pharyngitis, fatigue, and lymphadenopathy. Symptoms may last for 2 weeks.
- Most children born with HIV are asymptomatic. On physical examination, they often present with unexplained physical signs such as lymphadenopathy, hepatomegaly, splenomegaly, failure to thrive, weight loss or unexplained low birth weight, and fever of unknown origin. Laboratory findings include anemia, hypergammaglobulinemia, altered mononuclear cell function, and altered T-cell subset ratios. The normal range for CD4 cell counts in children is much different than for adults.
- **Table 42-1** presents the case definitions for adult, adolescent, and children, respectively, for *HIV* infection.

TABLE 42-1 Surveillance Case Definition for HIV Infection Stage Based on CD4+ T-Lymphocyte Counts, United States, 2014

	Age on Date of CD4+ T-Lymphocyte Test[a]					
	<1 year		1–5 years		≥6 years	
Stage	Cells/μL (×10⁶/L)	%	Cells/μL (×10⁶/L)	%	Cells/μL (×10⁶/L)	%
1	≥1500	≥34	≥1000	≥30	≥500	≥26
2	750–1499	26–33	500–999	22–29	200–499	14–25
3 (AIDS)	<750	<26	<500	<22	<200	<14

AIDS Indicator Conditions

Bacterial infections, multiple or recurrent (specific to children <6 years)

Candidiasis of bronchi, trachea, or lungs

Candidiasis, esophageal

Cervical cancer, invasive (specific to adults, adolescents, children >6 years)

Coccidioidomycosis, disseminated or extrapulmonary

Cryptococcosis, extrapulmonary

Cryptosporidiosis, chronic intestinal (duration >1 month)

Cytomegalovirus disease (other than liver, spleen, or nodes), onset at age >1 month

Cytomegalovirus retinitis (with loss of vision)

Encephalopathy, HIV-related

Herpes simplex: chronic ulcer[a](s) (duration >1 month); or bronchitis, pneumonitis, or esophagitis, onset at age >1 month

Histoplasmosis, disseminated or extrapulmonary isosporiasis, chronic intestinal (duration >1 month) Kaposi's sarcoma

Lymphoma, Burkitt

Lymphoma, immunoblastic

Lymphoma, primary, or brain

Mycobacterium avium complex or *Mycobacterium kansasii*, disseminated or extrapulmonary

Mycobacterium tuberculosis, any site (pulmonary or extrapulmonary)

Mycobacterium, other species or unidentified species, disseminated or extrapulmonary

Pneumocystis jirovecii pneumonia (PCP)

Pneumonia, recurrent (specific to adults, adolescents, children >6 years)

Progressive multifocal leukoencephalopathy

Salmonella septicemia, recurrent

Toxoplasmosis of brain, onset at age >1 month

Wasting syndrome due to HIV

[a]Age-specific CD4+ T-lymphocyte count or CD4+ T-lymphocyte percentage of total lymphocytes

- The presence of HIV infection is screened with an enzyme-linked immunosorbent assay (ELISA), which detects antibodies against HIV-1. ELISA tests are generally highly sensitive (greater than 99%) and highly specific (greater than 99%), but rare false-positive results can occur particularly in those with autoimmune disorders. Positive screening tests are confirmed with another enzyme immunoassay to specify if the antibodies are to HIV-1 versus HIV-2. False-negative results also occur and may be attributed to the "window-period" before adequate production of antibodies or antigen (approximately 2–3 weeks).
- Once diagnosed, HIV disease is monitored primarily by two surrogate biomarkers, viral load and CD4 cell count. The viral load test quantifies viremia by measuring the amount of viral RNA. Methods for determining HIV-RNA include

reverse-transcription polymerase chain reaction (RT-PCR), branched-chain DNA, transcription-mediated amplification, and nucleic acid sequence-based assay.

- The number of CD4 lymphocytes in the blood is a surrogate marker of disease progression. The normal adult CD4 lymphocyte count ranges from 500 to 1600 cells/mm^3 (0.5×10^9–1.6×10^9/L), or 40% to 70% (0.4–0.7) of total lymphocytes.

TREATMENT

- <u>Goals of Treatment</u>: The central goal of ART is to decrease morbidity and mortality, improve quality of life, restore and preserve immune function, and prevent further transmission through maximum and durable suppression of HIV replication (HIV RNA level that is less than the lower limit of quantitation (ie, undetectable; usually less than 20 or 50 copies/mL [20×10^3 or 50×10^3/L]).

GENERAL APPROACH

- Contemporary combinations of three active antiretroviral agents from two pharmacologic classes potently inhibit HIV replication to undetectable plasma levels, prevent and reverse immune deficiency, and substantially decrease morbidity and mortality constitutes the modern ART era.
- Regular, periodic measurement of plasma HIV RNA levels and CD4 cell counts is necessary to determine the risk of disease progression in an HIV-infected individual and to determine when to initiate or modify antiretroviral treatment regimens.
- The use of potent combination ART to suppress HIV replication to below the levels of detection of sensitive plasma HIV RNA assays limits the potential for selection of antiretroviral-resistant HIV variants, the major factor limiting the ability of antiretroviral drugs to inhibit virus replication and delay disease progression. Maximum achievable suppression of HIV replication should be the goal of therapy.
- The most effective means to accomplish durable suppression of HIV replication is the simultaneous initiation of combinations of effective anti-HIV drugs with which the patient has not been treated previously and that are not cross-resistant with antiretroviral agents with which the patient has been treated.
- Each of the antiretroviral drugs used in combination therapy regimens should always be used according to optimum schedules and dosages.
- People of child-bearing potential should receive optimal ART regardless of pregnancy status.
- The same principles of ART apply to both HIV-infected children and adults, although the treatment of HIV-infected children involves unique pharmacologic, virologic, and immunologic considerations.
- Persons with acute primary HIV infections should be treated with combination ART to suppress virus replication to levels below the limit of detection of sensitive plasma HIV RNA assays.
- For all HIV-infected persons, even those with viral loads below detectable limits, immediate ART regardless of CD4 count is recommended.
- An excellent source for information on treatment guidelines can be found at https://clinicalinfo.hiv.gov/en/guidelines.

PHARMACOLOGIC THERAPY

Antiretroviral Agents

- Systemic delivery of antiretroviral agents for direct inhibition of viral replication has been the most clinically successful strategy for both treatment and prophylaxis.
- Inhibiting viral replication with a combination of potent ART has been the most clinically successful strategy in the treatment of HIV infection. Five general classes of drugs are available: entry inhibitors (fusion inhibitors, CD4 post-attachment inhibitors, gp120 attachment inhibitors, and chemokine receptor antagonists), nucleos(t)ide reverse transcriptase inhibitors (N(t)RTIs), non-nucleoside reverse transcriptase inhibitors (NNRTIs), integrase strand transfer inhibitors (InSTIs), and HIV PIs (Table 42-2).

TABLE 42-2	Treatment of HIV Infection: Antiretroviral Regimens Recommended as Initial Therapy for Persons with HIV
Regimen	**Selected Limitations**

Recommended Initial Regimens for Most Persons with HIV

InSTI based	Bictegravir + tenofovir alafenamide fumarate + emtricitabine (coformulated) (AI)	Not recommended if CrCl <30 mL/min (0.5 mL/s); interactions with polyvalent cations; bictegravir inhibits creatinine secretion increasing serum creatinine (distinguish vs renal dysfunction); CNS/psychiatric side effects (primarily in those with preexisting conditions)
	Dolutegravir + abacavir + lamivudine (coformulated) (AI)	Only if HLA-B*5701 negative; do not use in chronic hepatitis B infection; interactions with polyvalent cations; dolutegravir inhibits creatinine secretion increasing SCr (distinguish vs renal dysfunction); CNS/psychiatric side effects (primarily in those with preexisting conditions)
	Dolutegravir + (tenofovir disoproxil fumarate or tenofovir alafenamide fumarate)[a] + (emtricitabine or lamivudine)[b] (AI)	Same as above without HLA-B*5701 negative requirement
	Dolutegravir + lamivudine (AI)	Do not use if HIV VL ≥500,000 copies/mL (500 × 10^6/L), chronic hepatitis B infection or hepatitis B infection status is unknown, or if HIV genotype is unavailable or shows resistance to either component

Recommended initial regimens in certain clinical situations (some potential disadvantages vs previous category)

InSTI based	Elvitegravir + cobicistat + tenofovir disoproxil fumarate + emtricitabine (coformulated) (BI)	Initiation not recommended if CrCl <70 mL/min (1.17 mL/s); food requirement; interactions with polyvalent cations; CYP3A4 drug interactions; cobicistat inhibits creatinine secretion increasing SCr (distinguish vs renal dysfunction); CNS/psychiatric side effects (primarily in those with preexisting conditions)
	Elvitegravir + cobicistat + tenofovir alafenamide fumarate + emtricitabine (coformulated) (BI)	Not recommended if CrCl <30 mL/min (0.5 mL/s); otherwise, same as above
	Raltegravir + (tenofovir disoproxil fumarate or tenofovir alafenamide) + (emtricitabine or lamivudine) (BI for tenofovir disoproxil fumarate+ (emtricitabine or lamivudine)[b]; BII for tenofovir alafenamide + emtricitabine)	Raltegravir can be dosed once or twice daily depending on the formulation; interactions with polyvalent cations; creatine kinase increases; TDF/FTC not recommended if CrCl <50 mL/min (0.83 mL/s) and TAF/FTC not recommended if CrCl <30 mL/min (0.5 mL/s); CNS/psychiatric side effects (primarily in those with preexisting conditions)

(Continued)

427

TABLE 42-2 Treatment of HIV Infection: Antiretroviral Regimens Recommended as Initial Therapy for Persons with HIV *(Continued)*

Regimen		Selected Limitations
HIV PI based[c]	Atazanavir + ritonavir (or cobicistat) + (tenofovir disoproxil fumarate or tenofovir alafenamide fumarate)[a] + (emtricitabine or lamivudine) (BI)	GI side effects; food requirement; CYP3A4 drug interactions; hyperbilirubinemia leading to drug discontinuation, especially in those with Gilbert's syndrome; use of cobicistat with TDF/FTC not recommended if CrCl <70 mL/min (1.17 mL/s); use of TAF/FTC not recommended if CrCl <30 mL/min (0.5 mL/s); cobicistat inhibits creatinine secretion increasing SCr (distinguish vs renal dysfunction)
	Darunavir + (ritonavir or cobicistat) + (tenofovir disoproxil fumarate or tenofovir alafenamide)[a] + (emtricitabine or lamivudine)[b] (AI)	Rash (darunavir has sulfonamide moiety); GI side effects; food requirement; CYP3A4 drug interactions; use of cobicistat with TDF/FTC not recommended if CrCl <70 mL/min (1.17 mL/s); use of TAF/FTC not recommended if CrCl <30 mL/min (0.5 mL/s); cobicistat inhibits creatinine secretion increasing serum creatinine (distinguish vs renal dysfunction)
	Darunavir + ritonavir (or cobicistat) + abacavir + lamivudine (BII)	Only if HLA-B*5701 negative; see issues above
NNRTI based	Doravirine + tenofovir disoproxil fumarate + lamivudine (coformulated) (BI)	Not recommended if CrCl <50 mL/min (0.83 mL/s); CNS side effects
	Doravirine + tenofovir alafenamide + emtricitabine (BIII)	TAF/FTC not recommended if CrCl <30 mL/min (0.5 mL/s); CNS side effects
	Efavirenz + tenofovir disoproxil fumarate + (emtricitabine or lamivudine)[b] (coformulated) (BI)	CNS side effects with efavirenz; CYP450 drug interactions; empty stomach dosing before bed; not recommended if CrCl <50 mL/min (0.83 mL/s)
	Efavirenz + tenofovir alafenamide + emtricitabine (BII)	CNS side effects with efavirenz; CYP450 drug interactions; empty stomach dosing before bed; TAF/FTC not recommended if CrCl <30 mL/min (0.5 mL/s)
	Rilpivirine + (tenofovir disoproxil fumarate or tenofovir alafenamide)[a] + emtricitabine (coformulated) (BI for TDF and BII for TAF)	Not recommended when HIV-RNA >100,000 copies/mL (100 × 10^6/L) or CD4 <200 cells/μL (0.2 × 10^9/L); no proton-pump inhibitors (rilpivirine); food requirement; antacid interactions

(Continued)

TABLE 42-2	Treatment of HIV Infection: Antiretroviral Regimens Recommended as Initial Therapy for Persons with HIV (*Continued*)
Regimen	**Selected Limitations**
If abacavir and tenofovir cannot be used — Dolutegravir + lamivudine (AI)	Do not use if HIV VL ≥500,000 copies/mL (500 × 10⁶/L), chronic hepatitis B infection or hepatitis B infection status is unknown, or if HIV genotype is unavailable or shows resistance to either component
Darunavir + ritonavir + raltegravir (CI)	Only if HIV-RNA <100,000 copies/mL (100 × 10⁶/L) and CD4 >200 cells/mm³ (0.2 × 10⁹/L); raltegravir must be dosed twice daily; do not use in chronic hepatitis B infection
Darunavir + ritonavir + lamivudine (CI)	Do not use in chronic hepatitis B infection

Selected regimens or components that should not be used at any time

Regimen or component	Comment
Monotherapy with any single agent (AI)	Inferior virologic efficacy; risk of virologic rebound and resistance
Any NRTI only regimen (AI)	Inferior virologic efficacy
Unboosted PIs (ie, darunavir) (AII)	Inadequate bioavailability
Etravirine + unboosted PIs (AII)	Possible induction of PI metabolism, doses not established
Nevirapine in ARV naïve with higher CD4 counts (>250 cells/μL [0.25 × 10⁹/L] for women, >400 cells/μL [0.4 × 10⁹/L] for men) (BI)	High incidence of symptomatic hepatotoxicity

ᵃTAF and TDF are prodrugs of tenofovir with differing pharmacology and safety profiles. Safety, cost, and access should be considered when deciding between which form to use.
ᵇEmtricitabine and lamivudine are interchangeable.
ᶜBoosted darunavir is generally preferred over boosted atazanavir.
Evidence-based rating definition. Rating strength of recommendation—**A:** Strong recommendation. **B:** Moderate recommendation. **C:** Optional recommendation. Rating Quality of Evidence Supporting the Recommendation—I: Evidence from randomized, controlled trials. II: Evidence from at least one well-designed clinical trial without randomization or observational cohorts with long-term clinical outcomes. III: Expert opinion. Lamivudine and emtricitabine are considered interchangeable endpoints.

- Significant drug interactions can occur with many antiretroviral agents. The latest information on drug interactions of antiretroviral drugs should be consulted. Many clinically significant antiretroviral-associated drug interactions involve CYP3A-mediated first-pass metabolism and clearance.

  ✓ **Eefavirenz, etravirine,** and nevirapine are inducers of CYP3A, whereas the PIs and their pharmacoenhancers inhibit CYP3A. **Ritonavir** is a potent mechanism-based inhibitor of CYP3A-mediated metabolism and is now used exclusively at lower doses as a pharmacokinetic enhancer of other HIV protease inhibitors (PIs).

  ✓ Rifampin and rifapentine, potent inducers of CYP3A metabolism and conjugation enzymes, are contraindicated with the use of HIV PIs, most NNRTIs, bictegravir, cabotegravir (oral and injectable), elvitegravir, and **maraviroc** because concentrations are reduced substantially even with ritonavir enhancement.

  ✓ Websites are available that catalog and regularly update HIV drug-interaction information (http://www.hiv-druginteractions.org/).

TREATMENT DURING PREGNANCY

- Generally, pregnant people should be treated as would nonpregnant people, with the goal of maximally suppressing HIV RNA. Preferred initial regimens for HIV treatment during pregnancy include a dual NRTI backbone (abacavir/lamivudine or **tenofovir disoproxil fumarate/emtricitabine** or lamivudine) with either an InSTI (**dolutegravir** or **raltegravir**) or boosted PI (**atazanavir/ritonavir** or **darunavir/ritonavir**).

- **Cobicistat**-containing regimens should be avoided in pregnancy as exposures to cobicistat and co-formulated medications (ie, atazanavir, darunavir, and elvitegravir) are significantly reduced during pregnancy, which may increase the risk of treatment failure and perinatal HIV transmission.

- **Zidovudine** is recommended intrapartum depending on the mother's viral load (more than 1000 copies/mL [1×10^6/L] or unknown). Infants considered low risk for perinatal HIV transmission (ie, maternal viral load suppressed at delivery and no adherence concerns) should receive zidovudine prophylaxis for 4 weeks after birth. Infants considered high risk (ie, mother received either no antepartum or intrapartum ART, only intrapartum ART, or antepartum ART but did not achieve viral suppression) should receive presumptive HIV treatment with zidovudine/lamivudine and either nevirapine or raltegravir from birth through 6 weeks of age.

PREVENTING HIV TRANSMISSION

- Undetectable equals untransmittable ("U=U," or Treatment as Prevention [TasP]) refers to the concept that people with HIV who achieve and maintain suppressed or undetectable viral loads (meaning viral loads <200 copies/mL [200×10^3/L]) do not sexually transmit HIV to others.

- Postexposure prophylaxis (PEP) initiated as soon as possible and within a maximum of 72 hours of the potential exposure with regimens shown in Table 42-3.

- Preexposure prophylaxis (PrEP) involves the use of one of three FDA-approved antiretroviral medication options to prevent HIV. These include oral emtricitabine with tenofovir (either tenofovir disoproxil fumarate or tenofovir alafenamide) and long-acting injectable cabotegravir (Table 42-4).

TABLE 42-3	Recommended Regimens for Occupational and Nonoccupational PEP	
Population	**Ranking**	**Regimen**
Occupational postexposure prophylaxis (oPEP)		
Healthcare workers	Preferred	Tenofovir disoproxil fumarate 300 mg/emtricitabine 200 mg once daily + raltegravir 400 mg twice daily
	Alternative	Consult guidelines
Nonoccupational postexposure prophylaxis (nPEP)		
Adults and adolescents ≥13 years, including pregnant persons, and normal renal function (CrCl ≥60 mL/min [1.0 mL/s])	Preferred	Tenofovir disoproxil fumarate 300 mg/emtricitabine 200 mg once daily + raltegravir 400 mg twice daily *OR* dolutegravir 50 mg once daily
	Alternative	Tenofovir disoproxil fumarate 300 mg/emtricitabine 200 mg once daily + darunavir 800 mg/ritonavir 100 mg once daily
Adults and adolescents ≥13 years, including pregnant persons, and renal dysfunction (CrCl <60 mL/min [1.0 mL/s])	Preferred	Zidovudine/lamivudine (dose-adjusted per CrCl) + raltegravir 400 mg twice daily *OR* dolutegravir 50 mg once daily
	Alternative	Zidovudine/lamivudine (dose-adjusted per CrCl) + darunavir 800 mg/ritonavir 100 mg once daily

TABLE 42-4	Recommended Regimens for PrEP		
PrEP Option	Emtricitabine with Tenofovir Disoproxil Fumarate	Emtricitabine with Tenofovir Alafenamide	Cabotegravir
Initial FDA approval	2012	2019	2021
Administration route	Oral	Oral	IM injection
Indication	Persons at risk through sex or injection drug use[a]	Persons weighing at least 35 kg (77 lb) who are at risk through sex, excluding people at risk through receptive vaginal sex.	Persons at-risk through sex
Dosing	Emtricitabine 200 mg/ tenofovir disoproxil fumarate 300 mg	Emtricitabine 200 mg/ enofovir alafenamide fumarate 25 mg	Oral: 30 mg IM injection: 600 mg (3 mL)
	On-demand strategy also possible ("2-1-1")[b]	On-demand strategy not recommended (no data)	On-demand strategy not recommended (no data)
Dosing frequency	Once daily	Once daily	Oral lead-in: once daily IM injection: once monthly × first 2 months then every 2 months thereafter
HIV monitoring[c]	Every 3 months	Every 3 months	Month 1 visit and every 2 months thereafter
Safety monitoring	Renal[d] Optional: bone density	Renal,[d] lipids Optional: bone density	None
Side effects	"Start-up syndrome" during first month; headache, abdominal pain, weight loss	"Start-up syndrome" during first month; diarrhea, weight gain	Injection site reactions, headache, fever, fatigue, myalgia, rash
Use in renal impairment	CrCl ≥60 mL/min (1.0 mL/s)	CrCl ≥30 mL/min (0.5 mL/s)	Can be used; no restrictions

FDA, Food and Drug Administration; IM, intramuscularly.[a]Only TDF has been studied in persons who inject drugs, but this population is expected to benefit from all systemic PrEP forms.
[b]Only MSM: 2 pills 2–24 hours before sex (closer to 24 hours preferred), 1 pill 24 hours after first dose, 1 pill 48 hours after first dose. If sex occurs the day after completing the 2-1-1 series, continue taking 1 pill daily until 48 hours after the last sexual event. If sex occurs <7 days from the last 2-1-1 dose, resume 1 pill daily. If sex occurs ≥7 days between the last pill and next sexual event, reinitiate with 2 pills.
[c]Consists of laboratory testing (antigen, antibody, and HIV-1 RNA [PCR]) and assess for signs/ symptoms of acute HIV infection.
[d]Renal function should be assessed every 6 months for persons ≥50 years of age or with CrCl <90 mL/min (1.5 mL/s) and every 12 months in all other patients.

EVALUATION OF THERAPEUTIC OUTCOMES

- Following the initiation of therapy, patients are generally monitored at 3-month intervals with plasma HIV-RNA and CD4 cell counts until HIV RNA reaches undetectable levels. An assessment at 2–8 weeks is warranted to document early response. Monitoring may be increased to every 6 months in stabilized patients.
- There are two general indications to change therapy: significant toxicity and treatment failure.
- The following events should prompt consideration for changing therapy: the inability to achieve less than 200 copies/mL (200×10^3/L) HIV RNA by 24 weeks of therapy initiation (repeat testing is suggested to confirm), or, after HIV RNA suppression, repeated detection of greater than 200 copies/mL (200×10^3/L) of HIV RNA.

THERAPEUTIC FAILURE

- The most important measure of therapeutic failure is suboptimal suppression of viral replication.
- Therapeutic failure may be the result of factors such as pre-ART disease factors (eg, high viral load or preexisting drug resistance), nonadherence to medication, development of new drug resistance, intolerance to one or more medications, adverse drug–drug or drug–food interactions, or pharmacokinetic–pharmacodynamic variability.
- Drug-resistance testing is recommended while the patient is undergoing the failing regimen or within 4 weeks after stopping the regimen as long as the HIV RNA count is greater than 500 copies/mL (500×10^3/L), which is the threshold for resistance assays (~500–1000 copies/mL [~500×10^3–1000×10^3/L]). Patients should be treated with at least two (preferably three) fully active antiretroviral drugs based on medication history and resistance tests. The goal of therapy is to suppress HIV RNA to undetectable levels. In cases when undetectable HIV RNA) cannot be attained, maintenance on the regimen is preferred over drug discontinuation so as to prevent rapid immunological and clinical decline.

INFECTIOUS COMPLICATIONS OF HUMAN IMMUNODEFICIENCY VIRUS

- The probability of developing specific opportunistic infections (OIs) is closely related to CD4 count thresholds. The principle in the management of OIs is treating HIV infection to enable CD4 cells to recover and be maintained above protective levels. Other important principles are:
  ✓ Preventing exposure to opportunistic pathogens.
  ✓ Vaccinate to prevent first-episode of disease (consult HIV-specific guidelines).
  ✓ Use primary chemoprophylaxis at certain CD4 thresholds to prevent first-episode of disease.
  ✓ Treating emergent OIs.
  ✓ Use secondary chemoprophylaxis to prevent disease recurrence.
  ✓ Discontinuing prophylaxis with sustained immune recovery.
- Selected OIs and recommended first-line therapies are shown in Table 42-5.

PNEUMOCYSTIS JIROVECII PNEUMONIA

- *P. jirovecii* pneumonia (PCP) is the most common life-threatening OI in patients with AIDS. *P. jirovecii* is a fungus that has protozoan characteristics as well.
- Ninety percent of PCP cases in AIDS patients occurred in those with CD4 counts less than 200 cells/mm³ (0.2×10^9/L).

Clinical Presentation

- Characteristic symptoms include fever and dyspnea. Clinical signs are tachypnea with or without rales or rhonchi and a nonproductive or mildly productive cough occurring over a period of weeks, although more fulminant presentations can occur.

TABLE 42-5	Selected Therapies for Common Opportunistic Pathogens in HIV-Infected Individuals	
Clinical Disease	**Preferred Initial Therapies for Acute Infection in Adults (Strength of Recommendation in Parentheses)**	**Common Drug- or Dose-Limiting Adverse Reactions**
Fungi		
Candidiasis, oral	Fluconazole 100 mg orally for 7–14 days (AI)	Elevated liver function tests, hepatotoxicity, nausea, and vomiting
	or	
	Nystatin 500,000 units oral swish (~5 mL) four times daily for 7–14 days (BII)	Taste, patient acceptance
Candidiasis, esophageal	Fluconazole 100–400 mg orally or IV daily for 14–21 days (AI)	Same as above
	or	
	Itraconazole 200 mg/day orally for 14–21 days (AI)	Elevated liver function tests, hepatotoxicity, nausea, and vomiting
Pneumocystis jirovecii pneumonia	*Moderate-to-severe episodes*	Skin rash, fever, leucopenia, thrombocytopenia
	Trimethoprim-sulfamethoxazole IV or orally 15–20 mg/kg/day as trimethoprim component in three to four divided doses for 21 days[a] (AI) moderate or severe therapy should be started IV	
	Mild-to-moderate episodes	
	Trimethoprim–sulfamethoxazole 15–20 mg/kg/day as trimethoprim component orally in three divided doses or trimethoprim–sulfamethoxazole double strength tablets, two tablets three times daily	
Cryptococcal meningitis	Liposomal amphotericin B 3–4 mg/kg/day IV with flucytosine 100 mg/kg/day orally in four divided doses for a minimum of 2 weeks (AI) *followed by*	Nephrotoxicity, hypokalemia, anemia, fever, chills
	Fluconazole 400 mg/day, orally for 8 weeks or until CSF cultures are negative (AI)[a]	Same as above
Histoplasmosis	Liposomal amphotericin B 3 mg/kg/day IV for 2 weeks (AI) *followed by*	Same as above
	Itraconazole 200 mg orally thrice daily for 3 days then twice daily, for 12 months (AII)[a]	
Coccidioidomycosis	Amphotericin B deoxycholate 0.7–1.0 mg/kg IV daily (AII) or lipid formulation amphotericin B 4–6 mg/kg IV daily (AIII) until clinical improvement, then switch to an azole (BIII)	Same as above
	or	

(Continued)

TABLE 42-5	Selected Therapies for Common Opportunistic Pathogens in HIV-Infected Individuals (*Continued*)	
Clinical Disease	**Preferred Initial Therapies for Acute Infection in Adults (Strength of Recommendation in Parentheses)**	**Common Drug- or Dose-Limiting Adverse Reactions**
	Fluconazole 400–800 mg once daily (meningeal disease) (AII)[a]	Same as above
Protozoa		
Toxoplasmic encephalitis	Pyrimethamine 200 mg orally once, then 50–75 mg/day	Bone marrow suppression
	·If <60 kg, pyrimethamine 50 mg orally once daily	
	·If >60 kg, pyrimethamine 75 mg orally once daily	
	plus	
	Sulfadiazine 1–1.5 g orally four times daily	Rash, drug fever
	-If <60 kg, sulfadiazine 1 g orally four times daily	
	·If >60 kg, sulfadiazine 1.5 g orally four times daily	
	and	
	Leucovorin 10–25 mg orally daily for 6 weeks (AI)[a]	
Isosporiasis	Trimethoprim and sulfamethoxazole: 160 mg trimethoprim and 800 mg sulfamethoxazole orally or IV four times daily for 10 days (AII)[a]	Same as above
Bacteria		
Mycobacterium avium complex	Clarithromycin 500 mg orally twice daily, *plus* ethambutol 15 mg/kg/day orally (AI) for at least 12 months	GI intolerance, optic neuritis, peripheral neuritis, elevated liver tests
Salmonella enterocolitis or bacteremia	Ciprofloxacin 500–750 mg orally (or 400 mg IV) twice daily for 14 days (longer duration for bacteremia or advanced HIV) (AIII)	GI intolerance, headache, dizziness
Campylobacter enterocolitis (mild-to-moderate)	Ciprofloxacin 500–750 mg orally (or 400 mg IV) twice daily for 7–10 days (or longer with bacteremia) (BIII)	Same as above
Shigella enterocolitis	Ciprofloxacin 500–750 mg orally (or 400 mg IV) twice daily for 7–10 days (or 14 days for bacteremia) (AIII)	Same as above
Viruses		
Mucocutaneous herpes simplex	Acyclovir 5 mg/kg IV every 8 hours until lesions regress, then acyclovir 400 mg orally three times daily until complete healing (famciclovir or valacyclovir is alternative) (AIII)	GI intolerance, crystalluria

(Continued)

TABLE 42-5	Selected Therapies for Common Opportunistic Pathogens in HIV-Infected Individuals	
Clinical Disease	**Preferred Initial Therapies for Acute Infection in Adults (Strength of Recommendation in Parentheses)**	**Common Drug- or Dose-Limiting Adverse Reactions**
Primary varicella-zoster	Acyclovir 10–15 mg/kg every 8 hours IV for 7–10 days (severe cases), then switch to oral valacyclovir 1 g three times daily after defervescence (famciclovir or acyclovir is alternative) (AIII)	Obstructive nephropathy, CNS symptoms
Cytomegalovirus (retinitis)	Intravitreal ganciclovir (2 mg) or foscarnet (2.4 mg) for 1–4 doses over 7–10 days (for sight-threatening lesions) **plus** valganciclovir 900 mg twice daily for 14–21 days then once daily until immune recovery from ART (AIII)[a]	Neutropenia, thrombocytopenia
Cytomegalovirus esophagitis or colitis	Ganciclovir 5 mg/kg IV every 12 hours for 21–42 days; may switch to valganciclovir 900 mg orally every 12 hours when oral therapy can be tolerated (BI)	Same as above

ART, antiretroviral therapy; CSF, cerebrospinal fluid; GI, gastrointestinal; HIV, human immunodeficiency virus; IV, intravenous.
[a]Maintenance therapy is recommended.
See Table 42-2 for levels of evidence-based recommendations.

Chest radiographs may show florid or subtle infiltrates or may occasionally be normal, although infiltrates are usually interstitial and bilateral. Arterial blood gases may show minimal hypoxia (partial pressure of oxygen [PaO_2] 80–95 mm Hg [10.6–12.6 kPa]) but in more advanced disease may be markedly abnormal.

• The presentation of PCP is often insidious, occurring over a period of weeks. Clinical signs are tachypnea with or without rales or rhonchi and a nonproductive or mildly productive cough occurring over a period of weeks, although more fulminant presentations can occur. The diagnosis of PCP usually is made by identification of the organism in induced sputum or in specimens obtained from bronchoalveolar lavage.

Treatment

• The treatment of choice is **trimethoprim–sulfamethoxazole,** which is associated with a 60%–100% response rate. Parenteral **pentamidine** is equally efficacious but significantly more toxic.

• Trimethoprim–sulfamethoxazole is given in doses of 15–20 mg/kg/day (based on the trimethoprim component) as three or four divided doses for the treatment of PCP. Treatment duration is typically 21 days but must be based on clinical response.

• Trimethoprim–sulfamethoxazole is usually initiated by the IV route, although oral therapy (as oral absorption is high) may suffice in mildly ill and reliable patients or to complete a course of therapy after a response has been achieved with IV administration.

• Patients with moderate-to-severe PCP (eg, PaO_2 more than 70 mm Hg [9.3 kPa]) should be treated with corticosteroids as soon as possible after starting PCP therapy and certainly within 72 hours, in order to blunt the deterioration seen just after initiation of PCP therapy.

• The more common adverse reactions seen with trimethoprim–sulfamethoxazole are rash (including Stevens–Johnson syndrome), fever, leukopenia, elevated serum transaminases, and thrombocytopenia. The incidence of these adverse reactions is higher in HIV-infected individuals than in those not infected with HIV. Mild rashes should be watched closely for progression to more severe reactions but are not an absolute contraindication to continuing therapy.

Prophylaxis

- Primary prophylaxis of PCP is recommended for any HIV-infected person who has a CD4 lymphocyte count less than 200 cells/mm³ (200×10^6/L) (or CD4 percentage of total lymphocytes <14%) or a history of oropharyngeal candidiasis. Secondary prophylaxis is recommended for all HIV-infected individuals who have had a previous episode.

- Trimethoprim–sulfamethoxazole is the preferred therapy for both primary and secondary prophylaxis of PCP in adults and adolescents. The recommended dose in adults and adolescents is one double-strength tablet daily, although one double-strength tablet thrice weekly or one single-strength tablet daily and gradual dose escalation using liquid trimethoprim–sulfamethoxazole may improve adherence.

See Chapter 148, Human Immunodeficiency Virus Infection, authored by Peter L. Anderson, Kristina M. Brooks, and Courtney V. Fletcher, for a more detailed discussion of this topic.

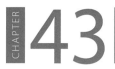

43 Influenza

- *Influenza* is a viral illness associated with high mortality and high hospitalization rates. The highest rates of severe illness, hospitalization, and death occur among those older than age 65 years, young children (younger than 2 years old), and those who have underlying medical conditions, including pregnancy and cardiopulmonary disorders.
- The route of influenza transmission is person-to-person via inhalation of respiratory droplets, which can occur when an infected person coughs or sneezes. The incubation period for influenza ranges between 1 and 7 days, with an average incubation of 2 days. Adults are considered infectious from the day before their symptoms begin through 7 days after the onset of illness, whereas children can be infectious for longer than 10 days after the onset of illness. Viral shedding can persist for weeks to months in severely immunocompromised people.

CLINICAL PRESENTATION

- The presentation of influenza is similar to a number of other respiratory illnesses.
- The clinical course and outcome are affected by age, immunocompetence, viral characteristics, smoking, comorbidities, pregnancy, and the degree of preexisting immunity.
- Complications of influenza may include exacerbation of underlying comorbidities, primary viral pneumonia, secondary bacterial pneumonia or other respiratory illnesses (eg, sinusitis, bronchitis, and otitis), encephalopathy, transverse myelitis, myositis, myocarditis, pericarditis, and Reye's syndrome.

SIGNS AND SYMPTOMS

- Classic signs and symptoms of influenza include rapid onset of fever, myalgia, headache, malaise, nonproductive cough, sore throat, and rhinitis.
- Nausea, vomiting, and otitis media are also commonly reported in children.
- Signs and symptoms typically resolve in 3–7 days, although cough and malaise may persist for more than 2 weeks.
- Primary viral pneumonia, occurring predominantly in pregnant females and those with underlying cardiovascular disease, usually begins with fever and dry cough, which changes to a productive cough of bloody sputum. This rapidly progresses to dyspnea, hypoxemia, and cyanosis with radiologic evidence of bilateral interstitial infiltrates.
- Chest radiograph should be obtained if pneumonia is suspected.

LABORATORY TESTS

- Complete blood count and chemistry panels should be obtained to assess the overall status of the patient. The gold standard for diagnosis of influenza is reverse-transcription polymerase chain reaction (RT-PCR) or viral culture.
- Influenza diagnostic tests include:
  ✓ Rapid influenza molecular assays (RIMAs) that detect influenza viral RNA in upper respiratory tract specimens with a high sensitivity (90%-95%) and high specificity (55%-99%) and produce results in approximately 15–30 minutes.
  ✓ RT-PCR is a nucleic acid amplification test that can identify the presence of influenza viral RNA or nucleic acids in respiratory specimens with high sensitivity and specificity. Results are available in approximately 45 minutes to several hours (1–6 hours).

- Rapid influenza diagnostic tests (RIDTs), also known as point-of-care (POC) tests, direct (DFA) or indirect (IFA) fluorescence antibody tests, and the RT-PCR assay may be used for rapid detection of virus.

PREVENTION

- The best means to decrease the morbidity and mortality associated with influenza is to prevent infection through vaccination. Appropriate infection control measures, such as hand hygiene, basic respiratory etiquette (cover your cough and throw tissues away), and contact avoidance, are also important in preventing the spread of influenza. Additionally, chemoprophylaxis is useful in certain situations.
- Annual vaccination is recommended for all persons age 6 months or older and caregivers (eg, parents, teachers, babysitters, nannies) of children less than 6 months of age.
- Vaccination is also recommended for those who live with and/or care for people who are at high risk, including household contacts and healthcare workers.
- The Advisory Committee on Immunization Practices (ACIP) has made the following recommendations regarding the vaccinations of persons with reports of egg allergy: (1) for persons with a history of severe allergic reaction (eg, anaphylaxis) to any egg-based inactivated influenza vaccine (IIV) or live-attenuated influenza vaccine (LAIV) of any valency, the provider can consider administering ccIIV4 or RIV4; (2) for persons with a history of severe allergic reaction (eg, anaphylaxis) to any ccIIV of any valency, the provider can consider administering RIV4; and (3) for persons with a history of severe allergic reaction (eg, anaphylaxis) to any RIV of any valency, the provider can consider administering ccIIV4.
  - ✓ The ideal time for vaccination is October or November to allow for the development and maintenance of immunity during the peak of the influenza season.
  - ✓ The two vaccines currently available for prevention of influenza are the inactivated vaccine IIV and the LAIV. The specific strains included in the vaccine each year change based on antigenic drift.
  - ✓ Intramuscular IIV is FDA-approved for use in people over 6 months of age, regardless of their immune status. Several commercial products are available and are approved for different age groups (Table 43-1). Because the vaccine content can change each year, vaccination providers should consult the most recent recommendations of the ACIP regarding use of seasonal influenza vaccines in the United States.
  - ✓ Two doses of IIVs are important for children under the age of 9 years, supporting the rationale for the recommendation of a booster dose of IIV at least 4 weeks after the initial dose in children between 6 months and less than 9 years of age if no previous vaccination.
  - ✓ Adults older than 65 years benefit from influenza vaccination, including prevention of complications and decreased risk of influenza-related hospitalization and death. However, people in this population may not generate a strong antibody response to the vaccine and may remain susceptible to infection.
  - ✓ The most frequent adverse effect associated with IIV is soreness at the injection site that lasts for less than 48 hours. IIV may cause fever and malaise in those who have not previously been exposed to the viral antigens in the vaccine. Allergic-type reactions (hives and systemic anaphylaxis) rarely occur after influenza vaccination and are likely a result of a reaction to residual egg protein in the vaccine.
  - ✓ Vaccination should be avoided in persons who are not at high risk for influenza complications and who have experienced Guillain–Barré syndrome within 6 weeks of receiving a previous influenza vaccine.
  - ✓ Some individuals are concerned about thimerosal exposure, particularly among children, because of the unfounded belief that thimerosal exposure is linked to the development of autism. No scientifically persuasive evidence exists to suggest harm from thimerosal exposure from a vaccine. Conversely, accumulating evidence reports the lack of harm from such exposure

TABLE 43-1 Approved Influenza Vaccines for Different Age Groups—United States, 2021–2022 Season

Vaccine	Trade Name	Manufacturer	Dose/Presentation	Thimerosal Mercury Content (µg Hg/0.5 mL dose)	Age Group	Number of Doses
Quadrivalent IIV (IIV4)						
IIV4	Afluria Quadrivalent	Seqirus	0.25-mL prefilled syringe	0	≥6–35 months	1 or 2[a]
			0.5-mL prefilled syringe	0	≥3 years	1 or 2[a]
			5-mL multidose vial	24.5	≥6 months (needle/syringe) or 18–64 years via jet injector	1 or 2[a]
IIV4	Fluarix Quadrivalent	GlaxoSmithKline	0.5-mL prefilled syringe	0	≥6 months	1 or 2[a]
IIV4	FluLaval Quadrivalent	GlaxoSmithKline	0.5-mL prefilled syringe	0	≥6 months	1 or 2[a]
			5-mL multidose vial	<25	≥6 months	1 or 2[a]
IIV4	Fluzone Quadrivalent[b]	Sanofi Pasteur	0.25-mL prefilled syringe	0	≥6–35 months	1 or 2[a]
			0.5-mL prefilled syringe	0	≥6 months	1 or 2[a]
			0.5-mL single-dose vial	0	≥6 months	1 or 2[a]
			5-mL multi-dose vial	25	≥6 months	1 or 2[a]
Quadrivalent IIV high dose (IIV4-HD)						
aIIV4 high dose	Fluad Quadrivalent	Seqirus	0.5-mL prefilled syringe	0	≥65 years	1
IIV4 high dose	Fluzone HD Quadrivalent	Sanofi Pasteur	0.7-mL prefilled syringe	0	≥65 years	1

(Continued)

TABLE 43-1 Approved Influenza Vaccines for Different Age Groups—United States, 2021–2022 Season (*Continued*)

Vaccine	Trade Name	Manufacturer	Dose/Presentation	Thimerosal Mercury Content (µg Hg/0.5 mL dose)	Age Group	Number of Doses
Cell culture-based quadrivalent IIV (ccIIV4)						
ccIIV4	Flucelvax Quadrivalent	Seqirus	0.5-mL prefilled syringe	0	≥6 months	1 or 2[a]
			5-mL multidose vial	25	≥6 months	1 or 2[a]
Recombinant quadrivalent IIV (RIV4)						
RIV4	Flublok Quadrivalent	Sanofi Pasteur	0.5-mL prefilled syringe	0	≥18 years	1
LAIV quadrivalent (LAIV4)						
LAIV	FluMist Quadrivalent	AstraZeneca	0.2-mL sprayer	0	2–49 years	1 or 2[c]

IIV, inactivated influenza vaccine; aIIV, adjuvanted inactivated influenza vaccine, quadrivalent, high dose; IIV4, inactivated influenza quadrivalent vaccine; ccIIV4, cell culture-based quadrivalent influenza vaccine; IIV4-HD, inactivated influenza quadrivalent vaccine – high dose; ccIIV4, cell culture-based quadrivalent influenza vaccine; RIV4, recombinant quadrivalent influenza vaccine; LAIV, live-attenuated influenza vaccine.

[a]Two doses administered at least 4 weeks apart are recommended for children aged 6 months to less than 9 years who are receiving influenza vaccine for the first time or received one dose in the first year of vaccination during the previous influenza season.

[b]Fluzone quadrivalent may be given to children aged 6 to 35 months as either 0.25 mL per dose or 0.5 mL per dose. No preference is expressed for one or the other dose volume for this age group. Persons aged ≥3 years should receive 0.5-mL dose volume.

[c]Two doses administered 4 weeks apart are recommended for children aged 2 years to less than 9 years who are receiving influenza vaccine for the first time.

Note: IIVs and RIV4 may be administered concomitantly or sequentially with other inactivated vaccines or live vaccines. LAIV4 may be given simultaneously with other live or inactivated vaccines. However, after administration of a live vaccine (such as LAIV4), at least 4 weeks should elapse before another live vaccine is administered.

Influenza antiviral medications might reduce the effectiveness of LAIV4 if given within 48 hours before to 14 days after administration of LAIV4. Persons who receive influenza antiviral medications within this period of LAIV4 vaccination can be revaccinated with another appropriate influenza vaccine (eg, IIV or RIV4).

✓ LAIV is made with live, attenuated viruses and is approved for intranasal administration in healthy people between 2 and 49 years of age (**Table 43-2**). Advantages of LAIV include its ease of administration, intranasal rather than intramuscular administration, and the potential induction of broad mucosal and systemic immune response.

✓ The adverse effects typically associated with LAIV administration include runny nose, congestion, sore throat, and headache.

✓ LAIV should not be given to immunosuppressed patients or given by healthcare workers who are severely immunocompromised. LAIV is not recommended in several populations, including persons with a history of Guillain–Barre syndrome (GBS) or hypersensitivity to eggs, those older than 50 years and pregnant females.

POSTEXPOSURE PROPHYLAXIS

• Antiviral drugs available for prophylaxis of influenza should be considered adjuncts but are not replacements for annual vaccination.

• **Amantadine** and **rimantadine** are no longer recommended for prophylaxis or treatment in the United States because of widespread resistance among influenza viruses.

• The neuraminidase inhibitors **oseltamivir** and **zanamivir** are approximately 70%–90% effective in preventing influenza against susceptible influenza viruses and are useful adjuncts to influenza vaccination. They are effective in preventing laboratory-confirmed influenza when used for seasonal prophylaxis and preventing influenza illness among persons exposed to a household contact who were diagnosed with influenza. **Table 43-3** gives dosing recommendations. **Peramivir** is not approved for chemoprophylaxis.

• **Baloxavir**, when administered within 24 hours of the onset of symptoms in persons 12 years of age and older, reduced the risk of household transmission of influenza by 86%.

• In those patients who did not receive the influenza vaccination and are receiving an antiviral drug for prevention of disease during the influenza season, the medication should optimally be taken for the entire duration of influenza activity in the community.

• Prophylaxis should be considered for seasonal influenza for the following groups of patients:

✓ Persons at high risk of serious illness and/or complications who are exposed to an infectious person and cannot be vaccinated.

✓ Persons at high risk of serious illness and/or complications who are vaccinated but exposed to an infectious person during the first 2 weeks following vaccination, because the development of sufficient antibody titers after vaccination takes ~2 weeks.

TABLE 43-2	Comparison of IIV and LAIV	
Characteristic	**IIV (IIV3/IIV4)**	**LAIV**
Age groups approved for use	≥6 months	2–49 years
Immune status requirements	Immunocompetent or immunocompromised	Immunocompetent
Viral properties	Inactivated (killed) influenza A (H3N2), A (H1N1), and B viruses	Live-attenuated influenza A (H3N2), A (H1N1), and B viruses
Route of administration	Intramuscular	Intranasal
Immune system response	High serum IgG antibody response	Lower IgG response and high serum IgA mucosal response

✓ Persons with severe immune deficiency or who may have an inadequate response to vaccination (eg, advanced human immunodeficiency virus [HIV] disease, persons receiving immunosuppressive medications), after exposure to an infectious person.

✓ Long-term care facility residents, regardless of vaccination status, when an outbreak has occurred in the institution.

- LAIV should not be administered until 48 hours after influenza antiviral therapy has stopped, and influenza antiviral drugs should not be administered for 2 weeks after the administration of LAIV because the antiviral drugs inhibit influenza virus replication.
- Postexposure prophylaxis should not be given if >48 hours has elapsed since exposure.
- Pregnant females, regardless of trimester, should receive annual influenza vaccination with IIV but not with LAIV.
- The adamantanes and neuraminidase inhibitors are not recommended during pregnancy because of concerns regarding the effects of the drugs on the fetus.
- Immunocompromised hosts should receive annual influenza vaccination with IIV but not with LAIV.

TREATMENT

- <u>Goals of Treatment</u>: To control symptoms, prevent complications, decrease work and/or school absenteeism, and prevent the spread of infection.
- Antiviral drugs are most effective if started within 48 hours of the onset of illness. Adjunct agents, such as acetaminophen for fever or an antihistamine for rhinitis, may be used concomitantly with the antiviral drugs.
- Patients suffering from influenza should get adequate sleep and maintain a low level of activity. They should stay home from work and/or school in order to rest and prevent the spread of infection. Appropriate fluid intake should be maintained. Cough/throat lozenges, warm tea, or soup may help with symptom control (cough and sore throat).

PHARMACOLOGIC THERAPY

- The cap-dependent endonuclease inhibitor, **baloxavir** and NA inhibitors, **oseltamivir**, **zanamivir**, and **peramivir**) are the only antiviral drugs available for treatment and prophylaxis of influenza. Peramivir is the only intravenous formulation commercially available. The adamantanes (**amantadine** and **rimantadine**) are no longer recommended due to high resistance among influenza viruses.
- Baloxavir is approved for use within 48 hours of illness onset, in people aged 12 years and older, for the treatment of acute, uncomplicated influenza in patients who are at high risk for developing serious influenza-related complications, for example, those with chronic conditions like asthma, heart disease, and diabetes.
- Oseltamivir, zanamivir, and peramivir are NA inhibitors that have activity against both influenza A and influenza B viruses. When administered within 48 hours of the onset of illness, NA inhibitors may reduce the duration of illness by ~1 day versus placebo. Benefits are highly dependent on the timing of initiation of treatment, ideally being within 12 hours of illness onset, up to 48 hours after onset of illness.
- Oseltamivir is approved for treatment in those older than 14 days, zanamivir is approved for treatment in those older than 7 years, and peramivir for those 2 years and older. The recommended dosages vary by agent and age (see **Table 43-3**), and the recommended duration of treatment for both agents is 5 days for oseltamivir and zanamivir and one dose for 1 day for peramivir.
- Neuropsychiatric complications consisting of delirium, seizures, hallucinations, and self-injury in pediatric patients have been reported following treatment with oseltamivir and peramivir.

TABLE 43-3 Recommended Daily Dosage of Influenza Antiviral Medications for Treatment and Prophylaxis—United States

Drug	Adult Treatment	Adult Prophylaxis[a]	Pediatric Treatment	Pediatric Prophylaxis[a]
CAP-dependent endonuclease inhibitor				
Baloxavir[b,c]	12 years and older: 40–<80 kg: One 40 mg dose >80 kg: One 80 mg dose	None	FDA-approved and recommended for use in children 12 years or older weighing at least 40 kg; see adult dosage	None
Neurominidase inhibitors				
Oseltamivir[d,e,f]	75-mg capsule twice daily × 5 days	75-mg capsule daily × 10 days	Term infants 0–8 months: 3 mg/kg/dose twice daily 9–11 months[g]: 3.5 mg/kg/dose twice daily or 3 mg/kg/dose twice daily ≥1 year: ≤15 kg: 30 mg twice daily >15–23 kg: 45 mg twice daily >23–40 kg: 60 mg twice daily >40 kg: 75 mg twice daily Duration: All for 5 days	Not recommended if <3 months 3–<12 months: 3 mg/kg/dose daily 9–11 months: 3.5 mg/kg/dose daily ≥1 year: ≤15 kg: 30 mg daily >15–23 kg: 45 mg daily >23–40 kg: 60 mg daily >40 kg: 75 mg daily Duration: All for 10 days
Zanamivir	10 mg (2 of 5 mg inhalations) twice daily × 5 days	10 mg (2 of 5 mg inhalations) daily × 10 days	10 mg (2 of 5 mg inhalations) twice daily × 5 days for ≥7 years old	10 mg (2 of 5 mg inhalations) daily for ≥5 years old × 10 days

(Continued)

TABLE 43-3	Recommended Daily Dosage of Influenza Antiviral Medications for Treatment and Prophylaxis—United States *(Continued)*			
Drug	Adult Treatment	Adult Prophylaxis[a]	Pediatric Treatment	Pediatric Prophylaxis[a]
Peramivir[c,e]	13 years and older: One 600 mg dose via intravenous infusion for 15–30 minutes	None	2–12 years of age: One 12 mg/kg dose, up to 600 mg maximum, via intravenous infusion for a minimum of 15–30 minutes	None

[a]If influenza vaccine is administered, prophylaxis can generally be stopped 14 days after vaccination for noninstitutionalized persons. When prophylaxis is being administered following an exposure, prophylaxis should be continued for 10 days after the last exposure. In persons at high risk for complications from influenza for whom vaccination is contraindicated or expected to be ineffective, chemoprophylaxis should be continued for the duration that influenza viruses are circulating in the community during influenza season.

[b]Time to peak = 4 hours. Food and cations (calcium, aluminum, magnesium, iron) can decrease peak concentration by 48%. Long half-life (79.1 hours) and is metabolized by UDP-glucuronosyltransferase (UGT1A3) and CYP3A4.

[c]For the treatment of uncomplicated influenza with oral baloxavir or intravenous peramivir, a single dose is recommended. Longer daily dosing (oral oseltamivir or intravenous peramivir) can be considered for patients who remain severely ill after 5 days of treatment.

[d]Oseltamivir dosing for preterm infants using their postmenstrual age (ie, gestational age + chronological age): <38 weeks: 1.0 mg/kg/dose twice daily; 38–40 weeks: 1.5 mg/kg/dose twice daily; >40 weeks: 3.0 mg/kg/dose twice daily.

[e]In patients with renal insufficiency, the dose should be adjusted on the basis of creatinine clearance. See https://www.cdc.gov/flu/professionals/antivirals/summary-clinicians.htm.

[f]Some experts recommend 150 mg twice daily for severe illness in pregnant women. Optimal dosing for prophylaxis in pregnant women is unknown.

[g]The American Academy of Pediatrics recommends 3.5 mg/kg per dose twice daily; CDC and US Food and Drug Administration (FDA)–approved dosing is 3 mg/kg per dose twice daily for children aged 9–11 months.

Note: Although amantadine and rimantadine have been used historically for the treatment and prophylaxis of influenza A viruses, due to high resistance, the CDC no longer recommends the use of these agents for the treatment and/or prophylaxis of influenza.

- Oseltamivir and zanamivir have been used but lack solid safety clinical data in pregnant females. Pregnancy should not be considered a contraindication to oseltamivir or zanamivir use. Oseltamivir is preferred for the treatment of pregnant females because of its systemic activity; however, the drug of choice for chemoprophylaxis is not yet defined.
- Both the adamantanes and the NA inhibitors are excreted in breast milk and should be avoided by mothers who are breastfeeding their infants.

EVALUATION OF THERAPEUTIC OUTCOMES

- Patients should be monitored daily for resolution of signs and symptoms associated with influenza, such as fever, myalgia, headache, malaise, nonproductive cough, sore throat, and rhinitis. These signs and symptoms will typically resolve within ~1 week. If the patient continues to exhibit signs and symptoms of illness beyond 10 days or a worsening of symptoms after 7 days, a physician visit is warranted, as this may be an indication of a secondary bacterial infection.

See Chapter 131, Influenza, authored by Jessica C. Njoku, for a more detailed discussion of this topic.

Acute Bronchitis

- *Bronchitis* is frequently classified as either acute or chronic. Acute bronchitis is characterized by inflammation of the epithelium of the large airways resulting from infection or exposure to irritating environmental triggers (eg, air pollution and cigarette smoke).
- Acute bronchitis occurs year-round, but more commonly during the winter months. Acute (viral) infection and/or smoking are the most common precipitants of attacks, which usually manifest initially as a persistent cough.
- Respiratory viruses are the predominant infectious agents associated with acute bronchitis. The most common infecting agents include influenza A and B, respiratory syncytial virus (RSV), and parainfluenza virus. Bacterial pathogens are involved in a minority of cases and involve pathogens often associated with community-acquired pneumonia (CAP).
- Infection of the trachea and bronchi causes hyperemic and edematous mucous membranes and an increase in bronchial secretions. Destruction of respiratory epithelium can range from mild to extensive and may affect bronchial mucociliary function. In addition, the increase in desquamated epithelial cells and bronchial secretions, which can become thick and tenacious, further impairs mucociliary activity.

CLINICAL PRESENTATION AND DIAGNOSIS

- Acute bronchitis usually begins as an upper respiratory infection with nonspecific complaints. Cough is the hallmark of acute bronchitis and occurs early. The onset of cough may be insidious or abrupt, and the symptoms persist despite resolution of nasal or nasopharyngeal complaints; cough may persist for up to 3 or more weeks. Frequently, the cough initially is nonproductive, but then progresses, yielding mucopurulent sputum.
- Fever, when present, rarely exceeds 39°C (102.2°F) and appears most commonly with adenovirus, influenza virus, and *Mycoplasma pneumoniae* infections.
- The diagnosis typically is made based on the characteristic history and physical examination and should be differentiated from asthma or bronchiolitis as these latter diseases are usually associated with wheezing, shortness of breath, and hypoxemia.
- Bacterial cultures of expectorated sputum are generally of limited utility because of the inability to avoid normal nasopharyngeal flora by the sampling technique. For the vast majority of affected patients, an etiologic diagnosis is unnecessary and will not change the prescribing of routine supportive care for the management of these patients.

TREATMENT

- <u>Goals of Treatment</u>: The goal is to provide comfort to the patient and, in the unusually severe case, to treat associated dehydration and respiratory compromise.
- The treatment of acute bronchitis is symptomatic and supportive. Reassurance and antipyretics alone are often sufficient. Bedrest for comfort may be instituted as desired. Patients should be encouraged to drink fluids to prevent dehydration and possibly to decrease the viscosity of respiratory secretions.
- **Aspirin** or **acetaminophen** (650 mg in adults or 10–15 mg/kg per dose in children with a maximum daily adult dose of <4 g and 60–75 mg/kg for children) or **ibuprofen** (200–800 mg in adults or 10 mg/kg per dose in children with a maximum daily dose of 3.2 g for adults and 40 mg/kg for children) is administered every 6–8 hours.
- In children under 19 years of age, aspirin should be avoided and acetaminophen used as the preferred agent because of the possible association between aspirin use and the development of Reye syndrome.

- In otherwise healthy patients, no meaningful benefits have been described with the use of oral or aerosolized β_2-receptor agonists and/or oral or aerosolized corticosteroids.
- Persistent, mild cough, which may be bothersome, may be treated with **dextromethorphan**; more severe coughs may require intermittent **codeine** or other similar agents. Codeine is no longer recommended for use in pediatric patients.
- Routine use of antibiotics in the treatment of acute bronchitis is strongly discouraged; however, in patients who exhibit persistent fever or respiratory symptomatology for more than 5–7 days, the possibility of a concurrent bacterial infection should be suspected.
- When possible, antibiotic therapy is directed toward anticipated respiratory pathogen(s) (ie, *Streptococcus pneumoniae* and *Haemophilus influenzae*).
- *M. pneumoniae*, if suspected by history or if confirmed by culture, serology, or PCR may be treated with **azithromycin**. Also, a fluoroquinolone with activity against these pathogens (**levofloxacin** or **moxifloxacin**) may be used empirically, but reserved for patients not responding adequately to supportive care and deemed at risk of associated complications.
- See Chapter 42 for recommendations to treat influenza.

Chronic Bronchitis

- *Chronic bronchitis* is defined clinically as the presence of a chronic cough productive of sputum lasting more than 3 consecutive months of the year for 2 consecutive years without an underlying etiology of bronchiectasis or tuberculosis.
- Chronic bronchitis is a result of several contributing factors, including cigarette smoking; exposure to occupational dusts, fumes, and environmental pollution; host factors (eg, genetic factors); and bacterial or viral infections.

CLINICAL PRESENTATION

- The hallmark of chronic bronchitis is a cough that may range from a mild-to-severe, incessant coughing productive of purulent sputum. Expectoration of the largest quantity of sputum usually occurs upon arising in the morning, although many patients expectorate sputum throughout the day. The expectorated sputum is usually tenacious and can vary in color from white to yellow-green.
- The diagnosis of chronic bronchitis is based primarily on clinical assessment and history. On physical examination, patients with advanced disease may have cyanosis and clubbing of digits.
- Chest auscultation usually reveals inspiratory and expiratory rales, rhonchi, and mild wheezing with an expiratory phase that is often prolonged. There may be hyperresonance on percussion with obliteration of the area of cardiac dullness. Normal vesicular breathing sounds are diminished.
- Chest radiograph may show increased anteroposterior diameter of the thoracic cage (barrel chest) and depressed diaphragm with limited mobility.
- Laboratory findings may include erythrocytosis (ie, increased hematocrit).
- Pulmonary function tests may reveal decreased vital capacity and prolonged expiratory flow.
- The most common bacterial isolates (expressed in percentages of total cultures) identified from sputum culture in patients experiencing an acute exacerbation of chronic bronchitis are given in Table 44-1.

TREATMENT

- Goals of Treatment: The goals are to reduce the severity of symptoms, ameliorate acute exacerbations, and achieve prolonged infection-free intervals.
- A complete occupational/environmental history for the determination of exposure to noxious and irritating gases, as well as cigarette smoking must be assessed.
- Attempts must be made to reduce the patient's exposure to known bronchial irritants (eg, reduce smoking and workplace pollution).

TABLE 44-1	Common Bacterial Pathogens Isolated from Sputum of Patients with Acute Exacerbation of Chronic Bronchitis
Pathogen	**Percent of Cultures**
H. influenzae[a,b]	45
M. catarrhalis[a]	30
S. pneumoniae[c]	20
E. coli, *Enterobacter* species, *Klebsiella* species, *P. aeruginosa*	5

[a]Often β-lactamase positive.
[b]Vast majority are nontypeable strains.
[c]More than 25% of strains may have intermediate or high resistance to penicillin.

- Pulmonary rehabilitation programs (including exercise-training program with resistance and aerobic exercise) individualized for patients with chronic respiratory impairment can improve quality of life by optimizing each patient's physical and social performance and autonomy.
- Chest physiotherapy (pulmonary toilet) can be instituted. Humidification of inspired air may promote the hydration (liquefaction) of tenacious secretions, allowing for more effective sputum production. The use of mucolytic aerosols (eg, *N*-acetylcysteine and deoxyribonuclease) is of questionable therapeutic value.
- For patients with moderate-to-severe chronic obstructive pulmonary disease (COPD), combination therapy with a long-acting β_2-agonist and inhaled corticosteroid led to decreased exacerbations and rescue medication use while it also improved quality of life, lung function, and symptom scores compared with long-acting β_2-agonist monotherapy.

PHARMACOLOGIC THERAPY

- Patients should be up-to-date with vaccinations, particularly pneumococcal and an annual influenza vaccine.
- For patients who consistently demonstrate clinical limitation in airflow, a therapeutic challenge of a short-acting β_2-agonist bronchodilator (eg, as **albuterol** aerosol) should be considered. Regular use of a long-acting β-receptor agonist (LABA) aerosol (eg, **salmeterol** and **formoterol**) in responsive patients is more effective and probably more convenient than short-acting β_2-receptor agonists. Chronic inhalation of a combination LABA and a corticosteroid (eg, **salmeterol-fluticasone** and **formoterol-mometasone**) improved pulmonary function and quality of life.
- Long-term use of aerosolized corticosteroid is associated with increased side effects including hoarseness, sore throat, thrush, pneumonia, and osteoporosis; however, caution should be exercised in withdrawing inhaled glucocorticoid administration in patients with severe COPD receiving triple inhalation therapy.
- Long-term inhalation of **ipratropium** (or **tiotropium**) decreases the frequency of cough, severity of cough, and volume of expectorated sputum.
- Inhaled long-acting muscarinic antagonists (LAMAs) alone or more frequently, in combination with a LABA, improve lung function and symptom control and reduce the number of acute exacerbations.
- Long-acting **theophylline** remains an effective "add on" therapy, particularly for severe chronic bronchitis/COPD, due to the drug's beneficial effects of bronchodilation, improved ciliary function and increased beat frequency, possibly increased mucus hydration, and low cost.
- **Roflumilast** is a highly specific (second generation) PDE-4 inhibitor that is most often reserved for use in patients with moderate to severe COPD.
- Use of antimicrobials for treatment of chronic bronchitis has been controversial but is becoming more accepted in specific circumstances. The goal is to select the most effective antibiotic drug for the patient based on their history of previous exacerbations and response to drug therapy (see **Fig. 44-1**).

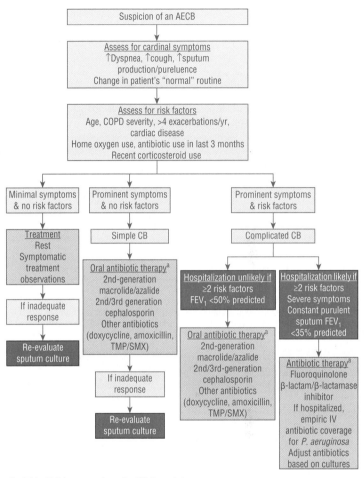

[a]See Table 44–2 for commonly used antibiotics and doses.

FIGURE 44-1. Clinical algorithm for the diagnosis and treatment of chronic bronchitic patients with an acute exacerbation incorporating the principles of the clinical classification system. AECB, acute exacerbation of chronic bronchitis; COPD, chronic obstructive pulmonary disease; CB, chronic bronchitis; TMP/SMX, trimethoprim/sulfamethoxazole.

- The Anthonisen criteria can be used to determine if antibiotic therapy is indicated. The patient will most likely benefit from antibiotic therapy if two or three of the following are present: (1) increase of shortness of breath, (2) increase in sputum volume, or (3) production of purulent sputum.
- Selection of antibiotics should consider that up to 30%–40% of *H. influenzae* and 95%–100% of *Moraxella catarrhalis* are β-lactamase producers; up to 40% of *S. pneumoniae* demonstrate intermediate susceptibility or resistance to penicillin, with 20% being highly resistant.
- Antibiotics commonly used in the treatment of these patients and their respective adult starting doses are outlined in **Table 44-2**. Duration of symptom-free periods

may be enhanced by antibiotic regimens using the upper limit of the recommended daily dose for 5–7 days.

Bronchiolitis

- *Bronchiolitis* is an acute viral infection of the lower respiratory tract of infants that affects ~50% of children during the first year of life and 100% by 2 years.
- RSV is the most common cause of bronchiolitis, accounting for up to 75% of all cases. Other detectable viruses include parainfluenza, adenovirus, and influenza. Bacteria serve as secondary pathogens in a minority of cases.

CLINICAL PRESENTATION

- The clinical presentation of bronchiolitis is often preceded by 1–4 days of symptoms (eg, nasal congestion, rhinorrhea, cough, and low-grade fever) indicative of an upper respiratory tract infection. As a result of limited oral intake due to coughing combined with fever, vomiting, and diarrhea, infants are frequently dehydrated.
- The diagnosis of bronchiolitis is based primarily on history and clinical findings. Identification of *RSV* by PCR should be available routinely from most clinical laboratories, but its relevance to the clinical management of bronchiolitis remains obscure and routine testing is not recommended.

SIGNS AND SYMPTOMS

- Prodrome with irritability, restlessness, and mild fever.
- Cough and coryza.
- Vomiting, diarrhea, noisy breathing, and increased respiratory rate as symptoms progress.
- Labored breathing with retractions of the chest wall, nasal flaring, and grunting.

TABLE 44-2	Oral Antibiotics Commonly Used for the Treatment of Acute Respiratory Exacerbations in Chronic Bronchitis		
Antibiotic	**Brand Name**	**Usual Adult Oral Dose (mg)**	**Dose Schedule (Doses/Day)**
Preferred drugs			
Ampicillin	–	250–500	3–4
Amoxicillin	–	500–875	2–3
Amoxicillin–clavulanate	Augmentin®	500–875	2–3
Ciprofloxacin	Cipro®	500–750	2
Levofloxacin	Levaquin®	500–750	1
Moxifloxacin	Avelox®	400	1
Doxycycline	Monodox®	100	2
Minocycline	Minocin®	100	2
Tetracycline HCl	–	500	4
Trimethoprim–sulfamethoxazole	Bactrim DS®/Septra DS®	1 DS	2
Supplemental drugs			
Azithromycin	Zithromax®	250–500	1
Erythromycin	Ery-Tab®/Erythrocin®	500	4
Clarithromycin	Biaxin®	250–500	2
Cephalexin	Keflex®	500	4

DS, double-strength tablet (160-mg trimethoprim/800-mg sulfamethoxazole).

PHYSICAL EXAMINATION

- Tachycardia and respiratory rate of 40–80 per minute in hospitalized infants.
- Wheezing and inspiratory rales.
- Mild conjunctivitis in one-third of patients.
- Otitis media in 5%–10% of patients.

LABORATORY TESTS

- Peripheral white blood cell (WBC) count normal or slightly elevated.
- Abnormal arterial blood gases (hypoxemia and, rarely, hypercarbia).

TREATMENT

- In the well infant, bronchiolitis usually is a self-limiting illness, and reassurance, antipyretics, and adequate fluid intake usually are all that are necessary while waiting for resolution of the underlying viral infection.
- In severely affected children, the mainstays of therapy for bronchiolitis are oxygen therapy and intravenous (IV) fluids.
- Aerosolized β2-adrenergic therapy appears to offer little benefit for most patients and may even be detrimental. The routine use of systemically administered corticosteroids is not recommended.
- The American Academy of Pediatrics guidelines support the use of nebulized hypertonic saline (eg, 3% saline) for the treatment of bronchiolitis in hospitalized infants and children.
- The American Academy of Pediatrics does not recommend the routine use of **ribavirin** in children with bronchiolitis and most experts recommend reserving use of ribavirin for severely ill patients.
- For infants with underlying pulmonary or cardiovascular disease, prophylaxis against RSV may be warranted during the RSV season, both RSV immune globulin and palivizumab (a monoclonal antibody for RSV) may decrease the number of RSV episodes and the need for hospitalization. Palivizumab is preferred, given its ease of administration, lack of administration-related adverse effects, and noninterference with select immunizations.

Pneumonia

- *Pneumonia* remains one of the most common causes of severe sepsis and infectious cause of death in children and adults in the United States, with a mortality rate as high as 50%. **Table 44-3** presents the classification of pneumonia and risk factors.

PATHOPHYSIOLOGY

- Respiratory pathogens enter the lower respiratory tract by one of three routes: (1) direct inhalation of infectious droplets, (2) aspiration of oropharyngeal contents, or (3) hematogenous spread from another infection site.
- Pneumonia is caused by a variety of viral and bacterial pathogens.
- Pneumonia is categorized as either CAP or hospital-acquired pneumonia (HAP). Pneumonia onset outside of the hospital or within 48 hours of hospital admission have CAP. Pneumonia onset in the hospital after at least 48 hours of hospitalization has HAP. Pneumonia onset following 48 hours of endotracheal intubation have ventilator-associated pneumonia (VAP).
- The causative pathogen in CAP in adult patients is most commonly viral, with human rhinovirus and influenza most common. The most prominent bacterial pathogen causing CAP in otherwise healthy adults is *S. pneumoniae* accounting for up to 35% of all acute cases. Other common bacterial causes are *H. influenzae*, the "atypical" pathogens including *M. pneumoniae*, *Legionella* species, *C. pneumoniae*.

TABLE 44-3	Pneumonia Classifications and Risk Factors	
Type of Pneumonia	**Definition**	**Risk Factors**
CAP	Pneumonia developing outside the hospital or <48 hours after hospital admission	• Age >65 years • Diabetes mellitus • Asplenia • Chronic cardiovascular, pulmonary, renal, and/or liver disease • Smoking and/or alcohol abuse
HAP	Pneumonia developing >48 hours after hospital admission	• Witnessed aspiration • COPD, ARDS, or coma • Administration of antacids, H_2-antagonists, or proton pump inhibitor • Supine position • Enteral nutrition, nasogastric tube • Reintubation, tracheostomy, or patient transport • Head trauma, ICP monitoring • Age >60 years • MDR risk (eg, MRSA, MDR *Pseudomonas*) if IV antibiotic use within 90 days
VAP	Pneumonia developing >48 hours after endotracheal intubation	• Same as hospital acquired • MDR risk with IV antibiotics in past 90 days, septic shock, ARDS preceding VAP, acute renal replacement therapy preceding VAP, or 5+ days of hospitalization preceding VAP

ARDS, acute respiratory distress syndrome; CAP, community-acquired pneumonia; COPD, chronic obstructive pulmonary disease; HAP, hospital-acquired pneumonia; ICP, intracranial pressure; MDR, multidrug-resistant; MRSA, methicillin-resistant *S. aureus*; VAP, ventilator-associated pneumonia.

- Viral pathogens (RSV and human rhinovirus) predominate in CAP among pediatric patients with a prevalence of up to 80% in those less than 2 years of age.
- HAP is predominantly caused by gram-negative aerobic bacilli and *S. aureus* and is much more likely to be caused by a multidrug-resistant isolate. *P. aeruginosa* and *Acinetobacter* spp. are the most common cause of HAP (about 25%–45%) while *K. pneumoniae* and *E. coli* are also common. HAP can be subclassified as VAP, which is pneumonia occurring after 48 or more hours of endotracheal intubation. The risk for developing pneumonia in the hospital increases by 6–21 times after a patient is intubated.
- The risk of HAP is exacerbated by the wide use of acid-suppressing drugs (eg, H2-receptor blocking agents and proton pump inhibitors) in the intensive care unit, which increases the pH of gastric secretions and may promote the proliferation of microorganisms in the upper GI tract.
- Aspiration pneumonia has a bacteriology similar to CAP or HAP and anaerobic pathogens are less common and typically seen in patients with specific risk factors such as periodontal disease or alcoholism.

CLINICAL PRESENTATION

GRAM-POSITIVE AND GRAM-NEGATIVE BACTERIAL PNEUMONIA

- The common signs, symptoms, physical exam findings, and diagnostic features of patients with pneumonia are both constitutional (fever, chills, malaise) and respiratory (cough, increased sputum production, dyspnea). These signs and symptoms coupled with physical exam findings suggestive of a pulmonary infiltrate, with or without abnormal WBC count or oxygen saturation, can form the basis of a presumed clinical diagnosis of pneumonia.

- The chest radiograph and sputum examination and culture are the most useful diagnostic tests for gram-positive and gram-negative bacterial pneumonia.
- Signs and symptoms: Abrupt onset of fever, chills, dyspnea, and productive cough; rust-colored sputum or hemoptysis; pleuritic chest pain; and dyspnea.
- Physical examination findings: Tachypnea and tachycardia; dullness to percussion; increased tactile fremitus, whispered pectoriloquy, and egophony; chest-wall retractions and grunting respirations; diminished breath sounds over affected area; and Inspiratory crackles during lung expansion.
- Chest radiograph findings: Dense lobar or segmental infiltrate.
- Laboratory tests: Leukocytosis with predominance of polymorphonuclear cells. Low oxygen saturation on arterial blood gas or pulse oximetry.
- Blood cultures and noninvasive sputum cultures (ie, expectorated sputum, sputum induction, or nasotracheal suctioning) are recommended for all adult patients with suspected HAP or VAP.

ATYPICAL PNEUMONIA (*M. PNEUMONIAE* AND *C. PNEUMONIAE*)

- Pneumonia caused by atypical pathogens, such as *M. pneumoniae* and *C. pneumoniae*, often has a more gradual onset and overall lower severity compared with other bacterial causes. Patients with atypical pneumonia also commonly have extrapulmonary, constitutional symptoms.

TREATMENT

- Goals of Treatment: The primary goal is the eradication of the offending organism and complete clinical cure. The secondary goals include minimization of the unintended consequences of therapy, including toxicities and selection for secondary infections such as *Clostridioides difficile* or antibiotic-resistant pathogens, and minimizing costs through outpatient and oral therapy when the patient's severity of illness and clinical considerations permit.
- The supportive care of the patient with pneumonia includes the use of humidified oxygen for hypoxemia, fluid resuscitation, administration of bronchodilators (**albuterol**) when bronchospasm is present, and chest physiotherapy with postural drainage if there is evidence of retained secretions.
- Important therapeutic adjuncts include adequate hydration (by IV route if necessary), optimal nutritional support, and fever control.
- Severity scoring systems such as pneumonia severity index (PSI) are used with age, comorbidities, physical exam findings, diagnostic test results, and laboratory test results to compute a patient's mortality risk and to guide treatment. Another scoring system is CURB-65, where patients receive 1 point for each criterion present: **C**onfusion, **U**remia (BUN >20 mg/dL [7.1 mmol/L]), **R**espiratory rate ≥30 breaths/min, **B**lood pressure (systolic <90 mm Hg, diastolic ≤60 mm Hg), age ≥65 years. Patients with CURB-65 score <2 are generally candidates for outpatient treatment. Patients with a score of 2 are typically admitted to the general ward of the hospital with ICU admission considered for patients with scores ≥3.
- The treatment of bacterial pneumonia initially involves the empiric use of a relatively broad-spectrum antibiotic therapy effective against probable pathogens after appropriate cultures and specimens for laboratory evaluation have been obtained. Therapy should be narrowed to cover specific pathogens once the results of cultures are known. The minimum duration of therapy for CAP is 5 days although CAP is commonly treated for 7–10 days.
- Appropriate empiric choices for the treatment of bacterial pneumonias relative to a patient's underlying disease are shown in **Table 44-4** for adults and **Table 44-5** for children. Dosages for antibiotics to treat pneumonia are provided in **Table 44-6**. Pathogen-directed antimicrobial therapy for common pneumonia pathogens in adult patients is given in **Table 44-7**.
- Antibiotic concentrations in respiratory secretions in excess of the pathogen minimum inhibitory concentration (MIC) are necessary for successful treatment of pulmonary infections.

TABLE 44-4 Evidence-Based Empirical Antimicrobial Therapy for Pneumonia in Adults[a]

Clinical Setting and/or Patient Characteristics	Usual Pathogens	Empirical Therapy
Outpatient/Community-Acquired		
No at-risk comorbidity (diabetes, heart/lung/liver/renal disease, alcoholism, malignancy, asplenia)	S. pneumoniae, M. pneumoniae, H. influenzae, C. pneumoniae, M. catarrhalis	Amoxicillin (preferred) OR Doxycycline (second preferred) OR Macrolide[b] (nonpreferred)
At-risk comorbidity (diabetes, heart/lung/liver/renal disease, alcoholism, malignancy, asplenia) OR immunosuppressive condition/drugs	S. pneumoniae (including drug-resistant), M. pneumoniae, H. influenzae, C. pneumoniae, M. catarrhalis	Antipneumococcal fluoroquinolone[c] OR β-lactam[d] + EITHER macrolide[b] OR doxycycline
Inpatient/Community-Acquired		
Nonsevere CAP	S. pneumoniae, H. influenzae, M. pneumoniae, C. pneumoniae, Legionella sp.	β-Lactam[e] + EITHER macrolide[b] OR doxycycline OR
	If prior respiratory MRSA (1 year)	Antipneumococcal fluoroquinolone[c]
	If prior respiratory P. aeruginosa (1 year)	ADD vancomycin OR linezolid AND obtain cultures, de-escalate in 48 hour if MRSA negative and clinically improving
	If prior hospitalization AND IV antibiotic (90 days) OR	ADD[f] cefepime, piperacillin-tazobactam, ceftazidime, imipenem, meropenem, OR aztreonam AND obtain cultures, de-escalate in 48 hour if P. aeruginosa negative and clinically improving
	Locally validated risk factor	Obtain cultures, escalate if needed based on results
Severe CAP	S. pneumoniae, H. influenzae, M. pneumoniae, C. pneumoniae, Legionella sp.	β-Lactam[e] + EITHER macrolide[b] OR antipneumococcal fluoroquinolone[c]
	If prior respiratory MRSA (1 year)	ADD vancomycin OR linezolid AND obtain cultures, de-escalate in 48 hour if MRSA negative and clinically improving

(Continued)

TABLE 44-4	Evidence-Based Empirical Antimicrobial Therapy for Pneumonia in Adults[a] (Continued)

Clinical Setting and/or Patient Characteristics	Usual Pathogens	Empirical Therapy
	If prior respiratory P. aeruginosa (1 year)	ADD[f] cefepime, piperacillin-tazobactam, ceftazidime, imipenem, meropenem, OR aztreonam AND obtain cultures, de-escalate in 48 hour if P. aeruginosa negative and clinically improving
	If prior hospitalization AND IV antibiotic (90 days)	ADD vancomycin OR Linezolid AND ADD[e] cefepime, ceftazidime, imipenem, meropenem, piperacillin-tazobactam, OR aztreonam AND obtain cultures, de-escalate if MRSA/P. aeruginosa-negative and clinically improving
Hospital-Acquired Pneumonia		
Low mortality risk[g] AND No MDR HAP[h] risk factors AND Local MRSA prevalence <20%	Nonfermenting gram-negative bacilli,[i] enteric gram-negative bacilli, MSSA	Piperacillin-tazobactam, cefepime, levofloxacin, imipenem, OR meropenem
Low mortality[g] risk AND No MDR HAP[h] risk factors AND Local MRSA ≥20% OR unknown	Nonfermenting gram-negative bacilli,[i] enteric gram-negative bacilli, MRSA	Piperacillin-tazobactam, cefepime, levofloxacin, ciprofloxacin, imipenem, meropenem, OR aztreonam + vancomycin OR linezolid
High mortality risk[g] OR MDR risk factor(s)[h]	Nonfermenting gram-negative bacilli,[i] enteric gram-negative bacilli, MRSA	Double cover P. aeruginosa with two of the following, avoiding two from the same class: piperacillin-tazobactam, cefepime, levofloxacin, ciprofloxacin, imipenem, meropenem, aztreonam, gentamicin, tobramycin, amikacin + vancomycin OR linezolid
Ventilator-Associated Pneumonia		
No MDR VAP risk factors[i] AND Local MRSA and gram-negative bacilli-resistance both <10%[j]	Nonfermenting gram-negative bacilli, enteric gram-negative bacilli, MSSA	Piperacillin-tazobactam, cefepime, levofloxacin, imipenem OR meropenem
No MDR VAP risk factors[i] AND Local MRSA ≥10% or unknown AND gram-negative bacilli-resistance <10%[j]	Nonfermenting gram-negative bacilli, enteric gram-negative bacilli, MRSA	Piperacillin-tazobactam, cefepime, levofloxacin, ciprofloxacin, imipenem, meropenem, OR aztreonam + vancomycin OR linezolid

(Continued)

455

TABLE 44-4	Evidence-Based Empirical Antimicrobial Therapy for Pneumonia in Adults[a] (Continued)	
Clinical Setting and/or Patient Characteristics	**Usual Pathogens**	**Empirical Therapy**
MDR VAP risk factor(s)[i] OR local MRSA and gram-negative bacilli-resistance >10%[j] or unknown	MDR nonfermenting gram-negative bacilli, MDR enteric gram-negative bacilli, MRSA	Double cover *P. aeruginosa* with two of the following, avoiding two from the same class: piperacillin-tazobactam, cefepime, levofloxacin, ciprofloxacin, imipenem, meropenem, aztreonam, gentamicin, tobramycin, amikacin, colistin, polymyxin B + vancomycin OR linezolid
Aspiration Pneumonia		
Community-acquired	*S. pneumoniae, M. pneumoniae, H. influenzae, C. pneumoniae*	Treat as above for CAP
Hospital-acquired	*S. aureus, P. aeruginosa* enteric gram-negative bacilli	Treat as above for HAP
	If anaerobes suspected	Treat as above for CAP/HAP using antibiotic with anaerobic coverage OR add clindamycin OR metronidazole

CAP, community-acquired pneumonia; HAP, hospital-acquired pneumonia; MDR, multidrug resistant; MRSA, methicillin-resistant Staphylococcus aureus; MSSA, methicillin-sensitive Staphylococcus aureus; VAP, Ventilator-acquired pneumonia.

[a]See the section "Selection of Antimicrobial Agents," Chapter 35, *Dipiro's Pharmacotherapy: A Pathophysiologic Approach,* 12 edition.

[b]Macrolide: erythromycin, clarithromycin, and azithromycin.

[c]Antipneumococcal fluoroquinolone: levofloxacin and moxifloxacin.

[d]Infectious Diseases Society of America recommended outpatient β-lactams: high-dose amoxicillin or amoxicillin/clavulanate preferred, cefpodoxime, cefuroxime, ceftriaxone (intramuscular) alternatives.

[e]Infectious Diseases Society of America recommended inpatient β-lactams: ceftriaxone (intravenous), cefotaxime, ampicillin, ampicillin-sulbactam, ceftaroline.

[f]If β-lactam-based CAP regimen selected, substitute antipseudomonal β-lactam for standard CAP β-lactam, unless ceftazidime or aztreonam chosen.

[g]Indicators of high HAP mortality risk: need for ventilator support due to pneumonia; septic shock.

[h]MDR HAP risk factors: receipt of IV antibiotics in previous 90 days; structural lung disease (bronchiectasis or cystic fibrosis).

[i]MDR VAP risk factors: receipt of IV antibiotics in previous 90 days; septic shock; acute respiratory distress syndrome preceding VAP; ≥5 days hospitalization preceding VAP; acute renal replacement therapy preceding VAP.

[j]Resistance to antibiotic being considered for empiric gram-negative monotherapy.

EVALUATION OF THERAPEUTIC OUTCOMES

- For patients with pneumonia of mild-to-moderate clinical severity, the time to resolution of cough, decreasing sputum production, and fever, as well as other constitutional symptoms of malaise, nausea, vomiting, and lethargy, should be noted. Progress should be observed in the first 2 days, with complete resolution in 5–7 days.
- When discontinuing therapy, patients should be afebrile for 48–72 hours and have no more than one CAP-related sign of clinical instability (ie, tachycardia, tachypnea, hypotension, hypoxia, altered mental status).

TABLE 44-5 Empirical Antimicrobial Therapy for Pneumonia in Pediatric Patients[a]

Clinical Setting and/or Patient Characteristics	Usual Pathogen(s)	Empirical Therapy
Outpatient/Community-Acquired		
<1 month	Group B *Streptococcus*, *H. influenzae* (nontypeable), *E. coli*, *S. aureus*, *Listeria* CMV, RSV, adenovirus	Ampicillin–sulbactam, cephalosporin,[b] carbapenem[c] Ribavirin for RSV[d]
1–3 months	*C. pneumoniae*, possibly *Ureaplasma*, CMV, *Pneumocystis carinii* (afebrile pneumonia syndrome) *S. pneumoniae*, *S. aureus*	Macrolide/azalide,[e] trimethoprim–sulfamethoxazole Semisynthetic penicillin[f] OR cephalosporin[g]
Preschool-aged children	Viral (rhinovirus, RSV, influenza A and B, parainfluenzae, adenovirus, human metapneumovirus, coronavirus)	Antimicrobial therapy not routinely required
Previously healthy, fully immunized infants and preschool children with suspected mild–moderate bacterial CAP	*S. pneumonia* *M. pneumoniae*, other atypical	Amoxicillin, cephalosporin[b,g] Macrolide/Azalide or fluoroquinolone
Previously healthy, fully immunized school-aged children and adolescents with mild–moderate CAP	*S. pneumonia* *M. pneumoniae*, other atypical	Amoxicillin, cephalosporin,[b,g] or fluoroquinolone Macrolide/Azalide, fluoroquinolone, or tetracycline
Moderate–severe CAP during influenza virus outbreak	Influenza A and B, other viruses	Oseltamivir or zanamivir
Inpatient/Community-Acquired		
Fully immunized infants and school-aged children	*S. pneumonia* CA-MRSA *M. pneumoniae*, *C. pneumoniae*	Ampicillin, penicillin G, cephalosporin[b] β-Lactam + vancomycin/clindamycin β-Lactam + macrolide/fluoroquinolone/doxycycline

(Continued)

TABLE 44-5	Empirical Antimicrobial Therapy for Pneumonia in Pediatric Patients[a] (Continued)	
Clinical Setting and/or Patient Characteristics	**Usual Pathogen(s)**	**Empirical Therapy**
Not fully immunized infants and children; regions with invasive penicillin-resistant pneumococcal strains; patients with life-threatening infections	S. pneumoniae, PCN-resistant	Cephalosporin[b]
	MRSA	Add vancomycin/ clindamycin
	M. pneumoniae, other atypical pathogens	Macrolide/azalide[e] + β-lactam/ doxycycline/ fluoroquinolone

CAP, community-acquired pneumonia; CMV, cytomegalovirus; MRSA, methicillin-resistant
Staphylococcus aureus; RSV, respiratory syncytial virus.
[a]See the section "Selection of Antimicrobial Agents," Chapter 35, Dipiro's Pharmacotherapy: A
Pathophysiologic Approach, 12 edition.
[b]Third-generation cephalosporin: ceftriaxone and cefotaxime. Note that cephalosporins are not active
against Listeria.
[c]Carbapenem: imipenem–cilastatin and meropenem.
[d]See Pharmacotherapy: A Pathophysiologic Approach, 12th edition, for details regarding possible
ribavirin treatment for RSV infection.
[e]Macrolide/Azalide: erythromycin and clarithromycin/azithromycin.
[f]Semisynthetic penicillin: nafcillin and oxacillin.
[g]Second-generation cephalosporin: cefuroxime and cefprozil.

TABLE 44-6	Antibiotic Doses for Treatment of Bacterial Pneumonia		
		Antibiotic Dose[a]	
Antibiotic Class	**Antibiotic**	**Pediatric**	**Usual Adult Dose**
Penicillin	Ampicillin ± sulbactam	150–200 mg/kg/ day IV	2 g IV every 4–6 hour (6 hours if ampicillin/ sulbactam)
	Amoxicillin ± clavulanate[b]	45–100 mg/kg/day orally	875–2000 mg orally twice daily
	Piperacillin–tazobactam	200–300 mg/kg/day IV	3.375–4.5 g IV every 6–8 hours
	Penicillin	100,000–250,000 units/kg/day IV	12–24 million units/day in divided doses IV every 4–6 hours
Extended-spectrum cephalosporins	Ceftriaxone	50–75 mg/kg/day IV	1–2 g IV daily
	Cefotaxime	150 mg/kg/day IV	1–2 g IV every 8 hours
	Ceftazidime	90–150 mg/kg/day IV	1–2 g IV every 8 hours
	Cefepime	100–150 mg/kg/ day IV	1–2 g IV every 6–8 hours
	Ceftolozane–tazobactam	–	3 g IV every 8 hours
	Ceftazidime–avibactam	–	2.5 g IV every 8 hours
Monobactam	Aztreonam	90–120 mg/kg/day IV	1–2 g IV every 8 hours
			(Continued)

TABLE 44-6 Antibiotic Doses for Treatment of Bacterial Pneumonia (*Continued*)

Antibiotic Class	Antibiotic	Antibiotic Dose[a] Pediatric	Usual Adult Dose
Macrolide/Azalide	Clarithromycin	15 orally mg/kg/day orally	0.5–1 g orally once or twice daily
	Erythromycin	30–50 IV or orally mg/kg/day orally	500 mg IV or orally every 6–8 hours
	Azithromycin	10 mg/kg × 1 day (×2 days if parenteral), and then 5 mg/kg days 2–5 IV or orally	500 mg × 1 day (×2 days if parenteral), and then 250 mg days 2–5 IV or orally
Fluoroquinolones[c]	Moxifloxacin	–	400 mg IV or orally daily
	Levofloxacin	8–20 mg/kg/day IV or orally	750 mg IV or orally daily
	Ciprofloxacin	30 mg/kg/day IV or orally	400 mg IV every 8 hours / 750 mg orally twice daily
Tetracycline[d]	Doxycycline	2–5 mg/kg/day IV or orally	100 mg IV or orally twice daily
	Tetracycline HCl	25–50 mg/kg/day orally	–
Aminoglycosides	Gentamicin	7.5–10 mg/kg/day IV	7.5 mg/kg IV daily
	Tobramycin	7.5–10 mg/kg/day IV	7.5 mg/kg IV daily
	Amikacin	15–20 mg/kg/day IV	15–20 mg/kg IV daily
	Plazomicin		15 mg/kg IV daily
Carbapenems	Imipenem	60–100 mg/kg/day IV	500–1000 mg IV every 6–8 hours
	Meropenem	30–60 mg/kg/day IV	500–2000 mg IV every 6–8 hours
	Meropenem–vaborbactam		2 g/2 g IV every 8 hours
	Imipenem-relabactam		1.25 g every 8 hours IV
Polymyxins	Colistin	2.5–5 mg/kg/day IV	IV: 300 mg × 1, then 150 mg daily/Neb: 150 mg every 8 hours
	Polymyxin B	15,000–30,000 units/kg/day IV	IV: 2–2.5 mg/kg × 1, then 1.25–1.5 mg/kg every 12 hours

(*Continued*)

TABLE 44-6 Antibiotic Doses for Treatment of Bacterial Pneumonia *(Continued)*

Antibiotic Class	Antibiotic	Antibiotic Dose[a]	
		Pediatric	Usual Adult Dose
Other	Vancomycin	45–60 mg/kg/day IV	15–20 mg/kg IV every 8–12 hours
	Linezolid	20–30 mg/kg/day IV or orally	600 mg IV or orally every 12 hours
	Clindamycin	30–40 mg/kg/day IV or orally	600 mg IV or orally every 8 hours or 450 mg orally every 6 hours

[a]Doses can be increased for more severe disease and may require modification for patients with organ dysfunction.
[b]Higher-dose amoxicillin and amoxicillin/clavulanate (eg, 90 mg/kg/day) are used for penicillin-resistant *S. pneumoniae*.
[c]Fluoroquinolones have been avoided for pediatric patients because of the potential for cartilage damage; however, they have been used for MDR bacterial infection safely and effectively in infants and children (see Chapter 35, *Dipiro's Pharmacotherapy: A Pathophysiologic Approach*, 12 edition).
[d]Tetracyclines are rarely used in pediatric patients, particularly in those younger than 8 years because of tetracycline-induced permanent tooth discoloration.

TABLE 44-7 Directed Antimicrobial Therapy for Common Pneumonia Pathogens in Adult Patients

Pathogen	Preferred Antibiotic Therapy	Alternative Antibiotic Therapy
Penicillin-susceptible *S. pneumoniae* (MIC ≤2 mg/L)	Ampicillin, amoxicillin, penicillin G	Ceftriaxone, cefotaxime, macrolide, levofloxacin, moxifloxacin, doxycycline, clindamycin, vancomycin
Penicillin-resistant *S. pneumoniae* (MIC >2 mg/L)	Ceftriaxone, cefotaxime, levofloxacin, moxifloxacin	High-dose amoxicillin (3 g/day), linezolid, clindamycin, vancomycin
Non-β-lactamase-producing *H. influenzae*	Ampicillin (IV), amoxicillin	Fluoroquinolone, doxycycline, azithromycin, clarithromycin
β-Lactamase-producing *H. influenzae*	Ceftriaxone, cefotaxime, ampicillin–sulbactam, amoxicillin–clavulanate	Fluoroquinolone, doxycycline, azithromycin, clarithromycin
Mycoplasma pneumoniae	Macrolide, doxycycline	Fluoroquinolone, doxycycline, azithromycin, clarithromycin
Chlamydophila pneumoniae	Macrolide, doxycycline	Fluoroquinolone
Legionella pneumophila	Fluoroquinolone or azithromycin	Doxycycline
MSSA	Cefazolin, antistaphylococcal penicillin	Clindamycin, vancomycin

(Continued)

TABLE 44-7	Directed Antimicrobial Therapy for Common Pneumonia Pathogens in Adult Patients (*Continued*)	
Pathogen	**Preferred Antibiotic Therapy**	**Alternative Antibiotic Therapy**
MRSA	Vancomycin, linezolid	Telavancin, ceftaroline, quinupristin/dalfopristin, clindamycin, sulfamethoxazole/ trimethoprim
P. aeruginosa	Antipseudomonal β-lactam[a] or fluoroquinolone[b] based on antimicrobial susceptibility testing results. Can consider adding aminoglycoside if patient in septic shock or at high mortality risk	IV colistin or polymyxin B + inhaled colistin for isolates resistant to all preferred therapies
Acinetobacter spp.	Carbapenem OR ampicillin–sulbactam based on antimicrobial susceptibility testing results	IV colistin or polymyxin B + inhaled colistin for isolates resistant to all preferred therapies
Extended-spectrum β-lactamase-producing gram-negative bacilli	Carbapenem	Piperacillin–tazobactam or cefepime potential options depending on susceptibility/adequate dosing
Carbapenem-resistant organisms	New β-lactam/β-lactamase inhibitors[c] based on antimicrobial susceptibility testing OR IV colistin or polymyxin B + inhaled colistin	

MIC, minimum inhibitory concentration; MRSA, methicillin-resistant *Staphylococcus aureus*; MSSA, methicillin-sensitive *Staphylococcus aureus*; PCN, penicillin.
[a]Antipseudomonal β-lactam: piperacillin/tazobactam, cefepime, ceftazidime, meropenem, imipenem/cilastatin, doripenem, aztreonam.
[b]Antipseudomonal fluoroquinolone: ciprofloxacin and levofloxacin
[c]New β-lactam/β-lactamase inhibitors: ceftazidime/avibactam, meropenem/vaborbactam, ceftolozane/tazobactam.

- With HAP some resolution of symptoms should be observed within 2 days of instituting antibiotic therapy. If no resolution of symptoms is observed within 2 days of starting seemingly appropriate antibiotic therapy or if the patient's clinical status is deteriorating, the appropriateness of initial antibiotic therapy should be critically reassessed. The clinician should consider the possibility of changing the initial antibiotic therapy to expand antimicrobial coverage not included in the original regimen if the patient's clinical status is worsening or failing to improve after 48–72 hours of therapy.
- De-escalation of antibiotic therapy to be more narrow spectrum in patients with HAP/VAP is strongly recommended. Evidence suggests this approach does not affect clinical outcomes while reducing excess antibiotic use. The recommended duration of therapy for HAP/VAP is 7 days, as the clinical benefit of longer durations of therapy (≥10 days) is not clear based on available clinical evidence.

See Chapter 129, Lower Respiratory Tract Infections, authored by Evan J. Zasowski and Martha G. Blackford, for a more detailed discussion of this topic.

45

CHAPTER

Respiratory Tract Infections, Upper

ACUTE OTITIS MEDIA

- *Otitis media* is an inflammation of the middle ear that is most common in infants and children. There are three subtypes of otitis media: acute otitis media, otitis media with effusion, and chronic otitis media. The three are differentiated by: (a) acute signs of infection, (b) evidence of middle ear inflammation, and (c) presence of fluid in the middle ear.

PATHOPHYSIOLOGY

- Bacteria have been found in more than 80% of cases of otitis media. Common bacterial pathogens include *Streptococcus pneumoniae*, nontypeable *Haemophilus influenzae*, and *Moraxella catarrhalis*.
- Acute otitis media usually follows a viral upper respiratory tract infection that impairs the mucociliary apparatus and causes eustachian tube dysfunction in the middle ear.
- *S. pneumoniae, H. influenzae,* and *M. catarrhalis* can all possess resistance to β-lactams. *S. pneumoniae* develops resistance through alteration of penicillin-binding proteins, whereas *H. influenzae* and *M. catarrhalis* produce β-lactamases.

CLINICAL PRESENTATION

- Acute otitis media is characterized as acute onset of otalgia (ear pain). Irritability and tugging on the ear are often the first clues that a child has acute otitis media.
- Children should be diagnosed with acute otitis media if they have middle ear effusion and either (1) moderate-to-severe bulging of the tympanic membrane or new onset otorrhea not due to acute otitis externa or (2) mild bulging of the tympanic membrane and onset of ear pain within the last 48 hours or intense erythema of the tympanic membrane.
- Nonverbal children with ear pain might hold, rub, or tug their ear. Very young children might cry, be irritable, and have difficulty sleeping. Signs and symptoms include bulging of the tympanic membrane, otorrhea, otalgia (considered to be moderate or severe if pain lasts at least 48 hours), and fever (considered to be severe if temperature is 39°C [102.2°F] or higher).

TREATMENT

- Goals of Treatment: Pain management and prudent antibiotic use. Acute otitis media should first be differentiated from otitis media with effusion or chronic otitis media.
- Primary prevention of acute otitis media with pneumococcal conjugate vaccine and annual influenza vaccine are recommended for all children.
- Pain of otitis media should be addressed with oral analgesics. **Acetaminophen** or a nonsteroidal anti-inflammatory agent, such as **ibuprofen**, should be offered early to relieve pain of acute otitis media.
- Antibiotic therapy should be initiated for children 6 months and older with acute otitis media showing severe symptoms (ie, toxic-appearing, persistent ear pain lasting more than 48 hours, or temperature of 39°C [102.2°F] or higher), for children 6 months and older with acute otitis media with otorrhea, and for children 6–23 months of age, with bilateral acute otitis media.
- Observation without initial antibiotic treatment can be considered for children 6 months and older with nonsevere unilateral acute otitis media without otorrhea, and children 24 months and older with bilateral acute otitis media without otorrhea.
- The central principle is to administer antibiotics quickly when the diagnosis is certain, but to withhold antibiotics, at least initially, when the diagnosis is uncertain.
- High-dose **amoxicillin** (80–90 mg/kg/day in two divided doses) is recommended for most children. Children who have received amoxicillin in the last 30 days, have

concurrent purulent conjunctivitis, or have a history of recurrent infection unresponsive to amoxicillin should receive high-dose **amoxicillin–clavulanate** (90 mg/kg/day of amoxicillin, with 6.4 mg/kg/day of clavulanate, in two divided doses) instead of amoxicillin.

- Antibiotic treatment recommendations for acute otitis media are given in Table 45-1.
- Patients with a penicillin allergy can be treated with several alternative antibiotics, including a cephalosporin in patients without history of severe or type 1 penicillin allergy.
- If treatment failure occurs with amoxicillin, an agent should be chosen with activity against β-lactamase-producing *H. influenzae* and *M. catarrhalis*, as well as drug-resistant *S. pneumoniae*, such as high-dose amoxicillin–clavulanate (recommended) or **cefuroxime, cefdinir, cefpodoxime**, or intramuscular or intravenous **ceftriaxone**.
- In children at least 6 years old who have mild-to-moderate acute otitis media, a 5- to 7-day course of antibiotics may be used. Short-course treatment is not recommended in children younger than 2 years of age.
- Patients with acute otitis media should be reassessed after 48–72 hours. A switch in regimen is recommended if there is no clinical improvement by the third day of therapy.

TABLE 45-1	Antibiotics and Doses for Acute Otitis Media		
Antibiotic	**Brand Name**	**Dose**	**Comments[a]**
Initial diagnosis			
Amoxicillin	Amoxil®	80–90 mg/kg/day orally divided twice daily	First line
Amoxicillin–clavulanate	Augmentin®	90 mg/kg/day orally of amoxicillin plus 6.4 mg/kg/day orally of clavulanate, divided twice daily	First line if certain criteria are present[b]
Cefdinir, cefuroxime, cefpodoxime	Omnicef®, Ceftin®, Vantin®	Cefdinir (14 mg/kg/day orally in 1–2 doses), cefuroxime (30 mg/kg/day orally in two divided doses), cefpodoxime (10 mg/kg/day orally in two divided doses)	Second line or nonsevere penicillin allergy
Ceftriaxone (1–3 days)	Rocephin®	50 mg/kg/day IM or IV for 3 days	Second line or nonsevere penicillin allergy
Failure at 48–72 hours			
Amoxicillin–clavulanate[b]	Augmentin®	90 mg/kg/day orally of amoxicillin plus 6.4 mg/kg/day orally of clavulanate, divided twice daily	First line
Ceftriaxone (1–3 days)	Rocephin®	50 mg/kg/day IM or IV for 3 days	First line or nonsevere penicillin allergy

IM, intramuscular; IV, intravenous.

[a]Amoxicillin–clavulanate 90:6.4 or 14:1 ratio is available in the United States; 7:1 ratio is available in Canada (use amoxicillin 45 mg/kg for one dose, amoxicillin 45 mg/kg with clavulanate 6.4 mg/kg for second dose).

[b]If a patient has received amoxicillin in the last 30 days, has concurrent purulent conjunctivitis, or has a history of recurrent infection unresponsive to amoxicillin.

PHARYNGITIS

- *Pharyngitis* is an acute infection of the oropharynx or nasopharynx that is responsible for 6% of visits by children to their primary care provider annually. Although viral causes are most common, group A β-hemolytic *Streptococcus* (GAS, also known as *S. pyogenes* is the primary bacterial cause.
- Viruses (eg, rhinovirus, coronavirus, adenovirus, and herpes suimplex virus) cause most of the cases of acute pharyngitis. A bacterial etiology for acute pharyngitis is far less likely. Of all the bacterial causes, GAS is the most common (10%–30% of cases in pediatric patients and 5%–15% in adults).
- Suppurative and nonsuppurative complications include acute rheumatic fever, acute glomerulonephritis, reactive arthritis, peritonsillar abscess, retropharyngeal abscess, cervical lymphadenitis, mastoiditis, otitis media, rhinosinusitis, and necrotizing fasciitis.

CLINICAL PRESENTATION

- The most common symptom of pharyngitis is sore throat of sudden onset that is mostly self-limited.
- Fever and constitutional symptoms resolve in about 3–5 days.
- Signs and symptoms of GAS pharyngitis include sore throat; pain on swallowing; fever; headache; nausea; vomiting; and abdominal pain (especially in children); erythema/inflammation of the tonsils and pharynx with or without patchy exudates; enlarged; tender lymph nodes; red swollen uvula; petechiae on the soft palate; and a scarlatiniform rash.
- Signs suggestive of viral origin for pharyngitis include conjunctivitis, coryza, and cough.
- Diagnosis can be confirmed by throat swab and culture and a rapid antigen-detection test (RADT).

TREATMENT

- <u>Goals of Treatment</u>: Improve clinical signs and symptoms, minimize adverse drug reactions, prevent transmission to close contacts, and prevent acute rheumatic fever and suppurative complications such as peritonsillar abscess, cervical lymphadenitis, and mastoiditis.
- Antimicrobial therapy should be limited to those who have clinical and epidemiologic features of GABHS pharyngitis, preferably with a positive laboratory test.
- Because pain is often the primary reason for visiting a physician, emphasis on analgesics such as **acetaminophen** and nonsteroidal anti-inflammatory drugs (NSAIDs) to aid in pain relief is strongly recommended.
- **Penicillin** and **amoxicillin** are the treatments of choice; however, amoxicillin suspension is more palatable. Antimicrobial treatment should be limited to those who have clinical and epidemiologic features of GAS pharyngitis with a positive laboratory test (**Table 45-2**). Table 45-3 presents antibiotics and doses for eradication of GAS in chronic carriers. The duration of therapy for GAS pharyngitis is 10 days, except for **benzathine penicillin** and **azithromycin**.
- **Amoxicillin–clavulanate, clindamycin, penicillin/rifampin** combination, and **benzathine penicillin G/rifampin** combination may be considered for recurrent episodes of pharyngitis to maximize bacterial eradication in potential carriers and to counter copathogens that produce β-lactamases.
- Most cases of pharyngitis are self-limited; however, antimicrobial therapy will hasten resolution when given early to proven cases of GAS. Symptoms generally resolve by 3 or 4 days even without antibiotics; however, symptoms will improve 0.5–2.5 days earlier with antibiotic therapy. Follow-up testing is generally not necessary for index cases or in asymptomatic contacts of the index patient; however, throat cultures 2–7 days after completion of antibiotics are warranted for patients who remain symptomatic or when symptoms recur despite completion of treatment.

TABLE 45-2 Antibiotics and Doses for Group A β-Hemolytic Streptococcal Pharyngitis

Antibiotic	Brand Name	Dose	Route/Duration	Rating
Preferred antibiotics if no penicillin allergy				
Penicillin V	Pen-V	Children: 250 mg twice daily or three times daily orally; adult: 250 mg four times daily or 500 mg twice daily orally	Orally 10 days	IB
Penicillin G benzathine	Bicillin L-A	<27 kg: 0.6 million units; 27 kg or greater: 1.2 million units IM	IM One dose	IB
Amoxicillin[a]	Amoxil	50 mg/kg once daily (maximum 1000 mg); 25 mg/kg (maximum 500 mg) twice daily	Orally 10 days	IB
Penicillin allergy				
Cephalexin	Keflex	20 mg/kg/dose orally twice daily (maximum 500 mg/dose)	Orally 10 days	IB
Cefadroxil	Duricef	30 mg/kg orally once daily (maximum 1 g)	Orally 10 days	IB
Clindamycin	Cleocin	7 mg/kg/dose orally thrice daily (maximum 300 mg/dose)	Orally 10 days	IIaB
Azithromycin[b]	Zithromax	12 mg/kg orally once daily (maximum 500 mg) for 1 day, then 6 mg/kg orally once daily (maximum 250 mg) for 4 days	Orally 5 days	IIaB
Clarithromycin[b]	Biaxin	15 mg/kg orally per day divided in two doses (maximum 250 mg twice daily)	Orally 10 days	IIaB

IM, intramuscularly.

[a]Standard formulation, not extended release.

[b]Resistance of group A β-hemolytic *Streptococcus* (GAS) to these agents may vary and local susceptibilities should be considered with these agents.

These guidelines provide a systematic weighting of the strength of the recommendation (Class I, conditions for which there is evidence and/or general agreement that a given procedure or treatment is beneficial, useful, and effective; Class II, conditions for which there is conflicting evidence and/or a divergence of opinion about the usefulness/efficacy of a procedure or treatment; Class IIa, weight of evidence/opinion is in favor of usefulness/efficacy; Class IIb, usefulness/efficacy is less well established by evidence/opinion; Class III, conditions for which there is evidence and/or general agreement that a procedure/treatment is not useful/effective and in some cases may be harmful) and quality of evidence (A, data derived from multiple randomized clinical trials or meta-analyses; B, data derived from a single-randomized trial or nonrandomized studies; C, only consensus opinion of experts, case studies, or standard of care).

TABLE 45-3	Antibiotics and Doses for Eradication of Group A β-Hemolytic Streptococcal Pharyngitis in Chronic Carriers	
Antibiotic	**Brand Name**	**Dose**
Clindamycin	Cleocin	20–30 mg/kg/day orally in three divided doses (maximum 300 mg/dose) for 10 days
Amoxicillin–clavulanate	Augmentin	40 mg/kg/day orally in three divided doses (maximum 2000 mg/day of amoxicillin) for 10 days
Penicillin V and rifampin	Pen-V, Rifadin	Penicillin V: 50 mg/kg/day orally in four doses for 10 days (maximum 2000 mg/day); *and* rifampin: 20 mg/kg/day orally in one dose for the last 4 days of treatment (maximum 600 mg/day)
Penicillin G benzathine and rifampin	Bicillin L-A, Rifadin	Penicillin G benzathine: <27 kg–0.6 million units IM once; 27 kg or greater: 1.2 million units IM; *and* rifampin: 20 mg/kg/day orally in two doses during last 4 days of treatment with penicillin (maximum 600 mg/day)

IM, intramuscularly.

ACUTE BACTERIAL RHINOSINUSITIS

- *Sinusitis* is an inflammation and/or infection of the paranasal sinuses, or membrane-lined air spaces, around the nose. The term *rhinosinusitis* is preferred, because sinusitis typically also involves the nasal mucosa. The majority of these infections are viral in origin. It is important to differentiate between viral and bacterial sinusitis to aid in optimizing treatment decisions.
- Acute bacterial sinusitis is most often caused by the same bacteria implicated in acute otitis media: *S. pneumoniae* and *H. influenzae*. These organisms are responsible for ~50%–70% of bacterial causes of acute sinusitis in both adults and children.

CLINICAL PRESENTATION

- There are three clinical presentations that are most consistent with acute bacterial versus viral rhinosinusitis: (1) onset with *persistent* signs or symptoms compatible with acute rhinosinusitis, lasting for ≥10 days without any evidence of clinical improvement; (2) onset with severe signs or symptoms of high fever (≥39°C [102.2°F]) and purulent nasal discharge or facial pain lasting for at least 3–4 consecutive days at the beginning of illness; (3) onset with *worsening* signs or symptoms characterized by new-onset fever, headache, or increase in nasal discharge following a typical viral URI that lasted 5–6 days and were initially improving ("double sickening").
- Signs and symptoms of bacterial rhinosinusitis include purulent anterior nasal discharge, purulent or discolored posterior nasal discharge, nasal congestion or obstruction, facial congestion or fullness, facial pain or pressure, fever, headache, ear pain/pressure/fullness, halitosis, dental pain, cough, and fatigue.
- Viral rhinosinusitis typically improves in 7–10 days. In contrast, acute bacterial rhinosinusitis symptoms persist for 10 days or greater without improvement or with worsening symptoms after 10 days, or can manifest worsening after initial improvement ("double-sickness" pattern).

TREATMENT

- <u>Goals of Treatment</u>: Reducing signs and symptoms, achieving and maintaining patency of the ostia, limiting antimicrobial treatment to those who may benefit, eradicating bacterial infection with appropriate antimicrobial therapy, minimizing the duration of illness, preventing complications, and preventing progression from acute disease to chronic disease.

- Symptomatic management for acute rhinosinusitis aims to relieve symptoms due to nasal drainage and obstruction such as pain with use of analgesics. Intranasal saline irrigation with either physiologic or hypertonic saline or intranasal corticosteroids are recommended as adjunct to antibiotics therapy in patients with acute bacterial rhinosinusitis, primarily in patients with a history of allergic rhinitis.
- Topical or oral decongestants or antihistamines are generally not recommended as adjunctive treatment for acute bacterial rhinosinusitis. These agents can dry mucosa and disturb clearance of mucosal secretions.
- **Amoxicillin–clavulanate** is first-line treatment in children and adults for acute bacterial rhinosinusitis. See **Tables 45-4** and **45-5**.
- High-dose amoxicillin–clavulanate is preferred in the following situations: (1) geographic regions with high endemic rates (10% or greater) of invasive penicillin-nonsusceptible *S. pneumoniae*, (2) severe infection, (3) attendance at daycare, (4) age less than 2 or greater than 65 years, (5) recent hospitalization, (6) antibiotic use within the last month, and (7) immunocompromised persons. Doxycycline is also second line for adults but should be avoided in children.

TABLE 45-4	Antibiotics and Doses for Acute Bacterial Rhinosinusitis in Children		
Antibiotic	**Brand Name**	**Dose**	**Comments**
Initial empirical therapy			
Amoxicillin–clavulanate	Augmentin	45 mg/kg/day orally twice daily	First line
Amoxicillin–clavulanate	Augmentin	90 mg/kg/day orally twice daily	Second line
β-Lactam allergy			
Clindamycin plus cefixime or cefpodoxime	Cleocin Suprax, Vantin	Clindamycin (30–40 mg/kg/day orally three times daily) plus cefixime (8 mg/kg/day orally twice daily) or cefpodoxime (10 mg/kg/day orally twice daily)	Nontype 1 allergy
Levofloxacin	Levaquin	10–20 mg/kg/day orally every 12–24 hours	Type 1 allergy
Risk for antibiotic resistance or failed initial therapy			
Amoxicillin–clavulanate	Augmentin	90 mg/kg/day orally twice daily	
Clindamycin plus cefixime or cefpodoxime	Cleocin, Suprax, Vantin	Clindamycin (30–40 mg/kg/day orally three times daily) plus cefixime (8 mg/kg/day orally twice daily) or cefpodoxime (10 mg/kg/day orally twice daily)	
Levofloxacin	Levaquin	10–20 mg/kg/day orally every 12–24 hours	
Severe infection requiring hospitalization			
Ampicillin–sulbactam	Unasyn	200–400 mg/kg/day IV every 6 hours	
Ceftriaxone	Rocephin	50 mg/kg/day IV every 12 hours	
Cefotaxime	Claforan	100–200 mg/kg/day IV every 6 hours	
Levofloxacin	Levaquin	10–20 mg/kg/day IV every 12–24 hours	

TABLE 45-5		Antibiotics and Doses for Acute Bacterial Rhinosinusitis in Adults	
Antibiotic	**Brand Name**	**Dose**	**Comments**
Initial empirical therapy			
Amoxicillin–clavulanate	Augmentin®	500 mg/125 mg orally three times daily, or 875 mg/125 mg orally twice daily	First line
Amoxicillin–clavulanate	Augmentin®	2000 mg/125 mg orally twice daily	Second line
Doxycycline		100 mg orally twice daily or 200 mg orally once daily	Second line
β-Lactam allergy			
Doxycycline		100 mg orally twice daily or 200 mg orally once daily	
Levofloxacin	Levaquin®	500 mg orally once daily	
Moxifloxacin	Avelox®	400 mg orally once daily	
Risk for antibiotic resistance or failed initial therapy			
Amoxicillin–clavulanate	Augmentin®	2000 mg/125 mg orally twice daily	
Levofloxacin	Levaquin®	500 mg orally once daily	
Moxifloxacin	Avelox®	400 mg orally once daily	
Severe infection requiring hospitalization			
Ampicillin–sulbactam	Unasyn®	1.5–3 g IV every 6 hours	
Levofloxacin	Levaquin®	500 mg orally once daily	
Moxifloxacin	Avelox®	400 mg orally once daily	
Ceftriaxone	Rocephin®	1–2 g IV every 12–24 hours	
Cefotaxime	Claforan®	2 g IV every 4–6 hours	

- The duration of therapy for the treatment of uncomplicated acute bacterial rhinosinusitis is 5–7 days for most adults. A longer duration of 10–14 days is still recommended for children.
- If symptoms persist or worsen after 48–72 hours of appropriate antibiotic therapy, then the patient should be reevaluated and alternative antibiotics should be considered.

See Chapter 130, Upper Respiratory Tract Infections, authored by Grace C. Lee, Christopher Frei and Bradi Frei, for a more detailed discussion of this topic.

- Sepsis-3 redefined sepsis by combining sepsis and severe sepsis from the Sepsis-2 guideline. The older and more recent definitions of terms related to *sepsis* are given in **Table 46-1**.

ETIOLOGY AND PATHOPHYSIOLOGY

- Patients at risk for infection who are predisposed to sepsis include advanced or very young age; preexisting conditions including heart failure, diabetes, chronic obstructive pulmonary disease, cirrhosis, alcohol dependence, and end-stage renal disease; and other immunosuppressive diseases such as neoplasm and human immunodeficiency virus (HIV) disease.
- The most common anatomic source of infection that leads to sepsis is the lung (40%–42%), followed by intra-abdominal space (31%–34%) and genitourinary tract (11%–15%). The microorganisms isolated from blood cultures of patients with sepsis or septic shock include gram-negative organisms in 44%–59% of patients, gram-positive bacteria in 37%–52%, anaerobic organisms in 5%, and fungi in 4%–10%.
- *Escherichia coli* is by far the most commonly isolated gram-negative microorganism in sepsis (55%–60%), followed by *Klebsiella* species, *Proteus* species, *Enterobacter* species, and *Pseudomonas aeruginosa*. Mortality increases significantly with increasing severity of sepsis (3.5% for sepsis, 9.9% in severe sepsis, and 29% in septic shock), especially in presence of *P. aeruginosa*. The most common gram-positive organisms are *Staphylococcus aureus*, followed by coagulase-negative *Staphylococci*, *Enterococcus* species, and *Streptococcus pneumoniae*.
- *Candida* species (particularly *Candida albicans*) are common fungal etiologic agents of bloodstream infections. The 30-day mortality rate for septic shock due to candidemia is 54%.
- The pathophysiologic focus of gram-negative sepsis has been on the lipopolysaccharide (endotoxin) component of the gram-negative cell wall membrane. Lipid A is a part of the endotoxin molecule from the gram-negative bacterial cell wall that is highly immunoreactive and is responsible for most of the toxic effects. In gram-positive sepsis, the exotoxin peptidoglycan on the cell wall surface appears to exhibit proinflammatory activity.

TABLE 46-1 Comparison of Definitions from Sepsis-2 and Sepsis-3 Guidelines	
Sepsis-2 Guideline (2012)	**Sepsis-3 Guideline (2016)**
Systemic inflammatory response syndrome (SIRS) to infectious or noninfectious insults: Two or more of the following: • Temperature >38°C or <36°C • Heart rate >90 beats/minute • Respiratory rate >20 breaths/minute • WBC >12,000/mm³ (12 × 10⁹/L) or <4000 cells/ mm³ (4 × 10⁹/L) or >10% (0.10) immature bands	**Sepsis:** Life-threatening organ dysfunction caused by a dysregulated host response to infection • Acute change in total SOFA score ≥2 points
Sepsis: SIRS + probable or documented infection	**Septic shock:** Sepsis + persistent hypotension requiring vasopressor use and serum lactate >2 mmol/L despite adequate fluid resuscitation
Severe sepsis: Sepsis + one or more organ dysfunction or hypoperfusion	
Septic shock: Sepsis + refractory hypotension despite fluid resuscitation (30 mL/kg) or serum lactate >1 mmol/L	

SOFA, sequential organ failure assessment; WBC, white blood cell.

- Sepsis involves a complex interaction of proinflammatory (eg, tumor necrosis factor-α [TNF-α]; interleukin [IL]-1, IL-6, IL-12) and anti-inflammatory mediators (eg, IL-1 receptor antagonist, IL-4, and IL-10).
- TNF-α concentrations are elevated early in the inflammatory response during sepsis. TNF-α also stimulates release of cyclooxygenase-derived arachidonic acid metabolites (thromboxane A2 and prostaglandins) that contribute to vascular endothelial damage.
- A primary mechanism of injury with sepsis is through endothelial cells. With inflammation, endothelial cells allow circulating cells (eg, granulocytes) and plasma constituents to enter inflamed tissues, which may result in organ damage.
- A key endogenous substance involved in inflammation of sepsis is activated protein C, which enhances fibrinolysis and inhibits inflammation. Levels of protein C are reduced in patients with sepsis.
- Septic shock is the most ominous complication associated with gram-negative sepsis. Another complication is disseminated intravascular coagulation (DIC). Simultaneous widespread microvascular thrombosis and profuse bleeding from various sites characterize DIC. DIC can produce acute renal failure, hemorrhagic necrosis of the gastrointestinal (GI) mucosa, liver failure, acute pancreatitis, acute respiratory distress syndrome (ARDS), and pulmonary failure.
- ARDS and acute kidney injury are other common complications of sepsis. ARDS can result in loss of functional alveolar volume, impaired pulmonary compliance, and profound hypoxemia.
- The hallmark of the hemodynamic effect of sepsis is the hyperdynamic state characterized by low systemic vascular resistance (SVR) and high cardiac output with tachycardia and arterial hypotension.

CLINICAL PRESENTATION

- The clinical presentation of sepsis varies significantly depending on the site of the infection (ie, pulmonary versus urinary tract), host response to the infection based on the patient's underlying health status and risk factors, and organ dysfunction. The initial presentations may include general malaise or myalgia and nonspecific signs such as fever (or hypothermia), chills, tachycardia, tachypnea, or change in mental status.
- Progression of uncontrolled sepsis leads to evidence of organ dysfunction, which may include oliguria, hemodynamic instability with hypotension or shock, lactic acidosis, hyperglycemia or hypoglycemia, possibly leukopenia, DIC, thrombocytopenia, ARDS, GI hemorrhage, or coma.
- Sepsis-3 redefined sepsis to "life-threatening organ dysfunction caused by a dysregulated host response to infection." Early recognition using a formal screening tool is critical, such as the SOFA scoring system. SOFA encompasses various organ systems such as pulmonary, hepatic, cardiovascular, renal, and neurological and gives a score ranging from 0 to 4 for each system. A SOFA score of 2 or more is associated with an increased risk of mortality by 10% in hospitalized patients with presumed infection.

TREATMENT

- <u>Goals of Treatment</u>: The primary goals include timely diagnosis and identification of the pathogen, prompt hemodynamic support, rapid identification of the pathogen and source control either medically and/or surgically, early initiation of appropriate broad-spectrum antimicrobial therapy, and avoidance complications such as organ failure and septic shock.
- Evidence-based treatment recommendations for sepsis and septic shock from the *Surviving Sepsis* campaign are presented in **Table 46-2**.

TABLE 46-2 Evidence-Based Treatment Recommendations and Best Practice Statements

Recommendations	Recommendation Grades
Fluid therapy	
Initial resuscitation from sepsis-associated hypotension with at least 30 mL/kg of IV crystalloid fluid within 1 hour	Strong recommendation, low evidence
Either balanced crystalloids or saline for additional fluids guided by frequent assessment of dynamic measures	Weak recommendation, low evidence
Antimicrobial therapy	
IV broad-spectrum antibiotic within 1 hour of diagnosis of sepsis and septic shock against likely bacterial/fungal pathogens	Strong recommendation, moderate evidence
Reassess antibiotic therapy daily with microbiology and clinical data to narrow coverage (de-escalation)	BPS
Combination therapy for patients at high risk for multidrug-resistant bacterial pathogens	Weak recommendation, low-quality evidence
Optimize dosing strategies based on pharmacokinetics/pharmacodynamics parameters in patients with sepsis or septic shock	BPS
Empiric antifungal therapy for patients at high risk of fungal infection	Weak recommendation, low evidence
Shorter duration of treatment duration using clinical evaluation and procalcitonin	Weak recommendation, low evidence
Vasopressors	
Initiate vasopressor therapy to maintain MAP ≥65 mm Hg	Strong recommendation, moderate evidence
Norepinephrine as the first-choice vasopressor	Strong recommendation, moderate evidence
Add vasopressin to norepinephrine instead of increasing norepinephrine dose to achieve adequate MAP	Weak recommendation, moderate evidence
Corticosteroids	
IV hydrocortisone for septic shock with ongoing requirement for vasopressor	Weak recommendation, low evidence
Hydrocortisone should be tapered when vasopressors are no longer required	Weak recommendation, low evidence
Glucose control	
Use insulin dosing protocol when two consecutive blood glucose levels are >180 mg/dL (10 mmol/L), targeting an upper blood glucose <180 mg/dL (10 mmol/L)	Strong recommendation, high-level evidence

(Continued)

TABLE 46-2	Evidence-Based Treatment Recommendations and Best Practice Statements (*Continued*)
Recommendations	**Recommendation Grades**
Venous thromboembolism prophylaxis	
Use daily low-molecular-weight heparin (LMWH) over unfractionated heparin	Strong recommendation, moderate evidence
Stress ulcer prophylaxis	
Stress ulcer prophylaxis should be given to patients who have bleeding risk factors	Strong recommendation, low evidence
Either proton pump inhibitors or H2 receptor blockers	Weak recommendation, low evidence

BPS, best practice statement; MAP, mean arterial pressure.

ANTIMICROBIAL THERAPY

- Once the source of infection is identified, prompt efforts to eradicate that source should be made as progression of sepsis can occur despite rapid initial resuscitation including fluid and appropriate antimicrobials in the absence of adequate source control.
- The Sepsis-3 guidelines recommend administration of empiric broad-spectrum therapy with one or more IV antimicrobials within 1 hour of recognition of sepsis or septic shock to treat most likely pathogens. Rapid identification of candidemia is critical in prompt initiation of appropriate therapy.
- The selection of an optimal empiric regimen requires assessment of patient factors including age, concomitant underlying diseases, chronic organ dysfunction (ie, liver or renal failure), presence of immunosuppression (ie, active cancer, neutropenia, or uncontrolled HIV infection), or presence of indwelling devices (ie, central venous lines or urinary catheter).
- The antibiotics that may be used for empiric treatment of sepsis based on site of infection based on the most likely pathogens are listed in **Table 46-3**.
- Patients with nosocomial infections are at risk for sepsis with MRSA, and an anti-MRSA agent such as vancomycin should be initiated empirically in most cases.
- If *P. aeruginosa* is suspected, or with sepsis from hospital-acquired infections, an antipseudomonal cephalosporin (**ceftazidime** or **cefepime**), antipseudomonal fluoroquinolone (**ciprofloxacin** or **levofloxacin**), or an aminoglycoside should be included in the regimen.
- The average duration of antimicrobial therapy in a patient with sepsis is 7–10 days in the absence of source control issues, and fungal infections can require 10–14 days. The Surgical Infection Society recommends no more than 4 full days of antimicrobial therapy for patients with adequate source control and no more than 5–7 days in patients in whom a definitive source control was not performed.
- Preferred empiric therapy for suspected invasive candidiasis in nonneutropenic patients in the intensive care unit (ICU) is an echinocandin (**anidulafungin, micafungin**, or **caspofungin**).
- Triazoles (**fluconazole, voriconazole**) are recommended in hemodynamically stable patients who have not had previous triazole exposure and not known to be colonized with azole-resistant *Candida* species.
- Empiric antimicrobial agents should be initiated immediately after the diagnosis of sepsis and septic shock is suspected due to the serious nature of the disease, but the antimicrobial regimen should be reassessed daily based on the microbiological and clinical data.

FLUID AND HEMODYNAMIC SUPPORT

- Early effective fluid resuscitation is crucial for preventing further sepsis-induced tissue hypoperfusion or septic shock. The Sepsis-3 guidelines recommend treating and resuscitating from sepsis-induced hypoperfusion immediately with at least 30 mL/kg

TABLE 46-3 Empiric Antimicrobial Regimens in Sepsis

Infection (Site or Type)	Antimicrobial Regimen		
	Community-Acquired	Hospital-Acquired	
Urinary tract	Ceftriaxone or ciprofloxacin/ levofloxacin	Ceftriaxone/ceftazidime or ciprofloxacin/levofloxacin	
Respiratory tract	Levofloxacin[a]/ moxifloxacin or ceftriaxone + clarithromycin/ azithromycin	Piperacillin/tazobactam or ceftazidime or cefepime or carbapenem[b] + levofloxacin/ciprofloxacin or aminoglycoside	±Vancomycin or linezolid
Intra-abdominal	Ertapenem or ciprofloxacin/ levofloxacin + metronidazole or ceftriaxone + metronidazole	Carbapenem[b] or piperacillin/ tazobactam or ceftazidime/cefepime + metronidazole	
Skin/Soft tissue	Vancomycin or linezolid or daptomycin	Vancomycin + piperacillin/ tazobactam	
Catheter-related		Vancomycin	
Unknown	Piperacillin/ Tazobactam or carbapenem[b]	Carbapenem[b]	

[a]750 mg once daily.
[b]Imipenem, meropenem, and doripenem.

of IV crystalloid fluid given judiciously within the first 3 hours. Target MAP is 65 mm Hg (8.6 kPa) to assess the need for vasopressors. Lactate should be normalized in patients with elevated lactate levels as a marker of tissue hypoperfusion.

- Fluid therapy guided by dynamic assessment of fluid responsiveness by examining cardiac output was associated with decreased mortality compared to standard care.
- The Sepsis-3 guidelines recommend a crystalloid product (balanced solution such as lactated Ringers and Plasma-Lyte or normal saline) based on accessibility and cost. Colloid (ie, albumin) can be used in patients who have already received considerable amount of crystalloids and continue to require fluid.
- Hetastarch products should be avoided at all times because they increased the risk of renal failure, need for renal replacement therapy, and death in multiple studies.
- Fluid therapy is based on the four phases of septic shock: ROSE—resuscitation, optimization, stabilization, and evacuation. **R**esuscitation phase occurs within minutes, and the patient will most likely have a positive fluid balance especially after the 30 mL/kg bolus. During the **O**ptimization phase, within hours, the goal is to keep a neutral fluid balance between intake and output. During the **S**tabilization phase, which usually occurs in days, the focus should be on organ support and keeping fluid balance neutral to net negative with maintenance doses (30 mL/kg/day) of fluid only. Lastly, the **E**vacuation phase occurs in days to weeks, and it is suggested to keep fluid balance negative.

INOTROPE AND VASOACTIVE DRUG SUPPORT

- Vasopressors should be used to achieve and maintain MAP goal of 65 mmHg in fluid-resuscitation refractory shock, and they are titrated up carefully to an end point of adequate organ perfusion. Selection and dosage are based on the pharmacologic properties of various catecholamines and how they influence hemodynamic parameters (**Table 46-4**).

TABLE 46-4 Mechanism of Action and Hemodynamic Effects of Vasopressors in Septic Shock

Drug	Receptor Affinity				Physiologic Outcome			
	Dopamine	Alpha-1	Beta-1	Beta-2	HR	SV	SVR	CO
Dopamine (0.5–2)[a]	+++	–	+	–	↔↑	↑	↔ or ↑	↑
Dopamine (5–10)[a]	++	+	+++	+	↑	↑	↔ or ↑	↑↑
Dopamine (10–20)[a]	++	+++	++	–	↑	↑	↑↑	↑
Epinephrine	–	++++	++++	+++	↑	↑	↑↑	↑↑
Norepinephrine	–	++++	++	+	↔ or ↑	↕	↑↑	↑
Phenylephrine	–	+++	–	–	↔ or ↓	–	↑↑	↔
Vasopressin	V1 receptor				↔ or ↓	–	↑↑	↔ or ↓
Angiotensin II	AT receptor				↓	–	↑	↑

CO, cardiac output; HR, heart rate; SV, stroke volume; SVR, systemic vascular resistance; V1, vasopressin receptor 1; V2, vasopressin receptor 2.
[a]mcg/kg/min.

TABLE 46-5	Sepsis-3 (2016) Performance Improvement Checklist for Bundle-Care Compliance

One-hour bundle
- Measure initial lactate
- Repeat in 2 hours if initial lactate $\geq$18 mg/dL ($\geq$2 mmol/L)
- Obtain cultures (blood, urine, sputum, etc.) prior to administration of antibiotics
- Administer broad-spectrum IV antibiotics within 1 hour
- Initial fluid resuscitation of 30 mL/kg crystalloid for hypotension or lactate $\geq$36 mg/dL ($\geq$4 mmol/L)
- Vasopressors if MAP <65 mm Hg during or after completion of fluid resuscitation

Outcome measurements
- Length of stay in ICU and hospital
- Rate of organ dysfunction
- Mortality rate

CVP, central venous pressure; ICU, intensive care unit; MAP, mean arterial pressure; ScvO$_2$, central venous oxygen saturation.

- For septic patients with clinical signs of shock and significant hypotension unresponsive to aggressive fluid therapy, norepinephrine is the first-line agent for patients with septic shock. In comparison to dopamine, it is less arrhythmogenic and was associated with lower risk of mortality.

PERFORMANCE IMPROVEMENT BUNDLE

- The Sepsis-3 guidelines recommend the 3-hour bundle with the use of a 1-hour care, putting the importance of beginning the initial treatment immediately (Table 46-5).

ADJUNCTIVE THERAPY

- Initiate insulin therapy at a glucose level of greater than 180 mg/dL (10 mmol/L) with a target range between 144 and 180 mg/dL (8–10 mmol/L).
- Add low dose **hydrocortisone** 200 mg/day for patients with septic shock who require ongoing norepinephrine dose of >0.25 mcg/kg/min at least 4 hours to maintain the target MAP. Hydrocortisone should be tapered when vasopressors are no longer required because hemodynamic and immunologic rebound effects have been reported with abrupt cessation of corticosteroids.
- Venous thromboembolism (VTE) prophylaxis with daily subcutaneous low-molecular-weight heparin should be initiated in all patients admitted to the ICU with sepsis and septic shock If pharmacologic prophylaxis is contraindicated, mechanical prophylactic measures should be considered.
- Stress ulcer prophylaxis should be initiated in all patients with sepsis and septic shock who have risk factors for GI bleeding.

See Chapter 142, Severe Sepsis and Septic Shock, authored by S. Lena Kang-Birken and Sul R. Jung, for a more detailed discussion of this topic.

Sexually Transmitted Infections

- The spectrum of sexually transmitted infections (STIs) includes the classic venereal diseases—gonorrhea, syphilis, chancroid, lymphogranuloma venereum, and granuloma inguinale—as well as a variety of other pathogens known to be spread by sexual contact (**Table 47-1**). Selected clinical syndromes associated with STIs are listed in **Table 47-2**. The most current information on epidemiology, diagnosis, and treatment of STIs provided by the Centers for Disease Control and Prevention (CDC) can be found at www.cdc.gov.

TABLE 47-1	Sexually Transmitted Infections
Disease	**Associated Pathogens**
Bacterial	
Gonorrhea	*Neisseria gonorrhoeae*
Syphilis	*Treponema pallidum*
Chancroid	*Haemophilus ducreyi*
Granuloma inguinale	*Calymmatobacterium granulomatis*
Enteric disease	*Salmonella* spp., *Shigella* spp., *Campylobacter* fetus
Campylobacter infection	*Campylobacter jejuni*
Bacterial vaginosis	*Gardnerella vaginalis, Mycoplasma hominis, Bacteroides* spp., *Mobiluncus* spp.
Chlamydial	
Nongonococcal urethritis	*Chlamydia trachomatis*
Lymphogranuloma venereum	*C. trachomatis*, type L
Viral	
Acquired immunodeficiency syndrome	Human immunodeficiency virus
Herpes genitalis	Herpes simplex virus, types I and II
Viral hepatitis	Hepatitis A, B, C, and D viruses
Condylomata acuminata	Human papillomavirus
Molluscum contagiosum	Poxvirus
Mycoplasmal	
Nongonococcal urethritis	*Mycoplasma genitalium*
Protozoal	
Trichomoniasis	*Trichomonas vaginalis*
Fungal	
Vaginal candidiasis	*Candida albicans*
Parasitic	
Scabies	*Sarcoptes scabiei*
Pediculosis pubis	*Phthirus pubis*
Enterobiasis	*Enterobius vermicularis*

TABLE 47-2	Selected Syndromes Associated with Common Sexually Transmitted Pathogens	
Syndrome	**Commonly Implicated Pathogens**	**Common Clinical Manifestations[a]**
Urethritis	C. trachomatis, herpes simplex virus, N. gonorrhoeae, Trichomonas vaginalis, Ureaplasma urealyticum, Mycoplasma genitalium	Urethral discharge, dysuria
Epididymitis	C. trachomatis, N. gonorrhoeae, Enterobacterales	Scrotal pain, inguinal pain, flank pain, urethral discharge
Cervicitis/Vulvovaginitis	C. trachomatis, Gardnerella vaginalis, herpes simplex virus, human papillomavirus, N. gonorrhoeae, T. vaginalis	Abnormal vaginal discharge, vulvar itching/irritation, dysuria, dyspareunia
Genital ulcers (painful)	Haemophilus ducreyi, herpes simplex virus	Usually multiple vesicular/pustular (herpes) or papular/pustular (H. ducreyi) lesions that can coalesce; painful, tender lymphadenopathy[b]
Genital ulcers (painless)	Treponema pallidum	Usually single papular lesion
Genital/Anal warts	Human papillomavirus	Multiple lesions ranging in size from small papular warts to large exophytic condylomas
Pharyngitis	C. trachomatis, herpes simplex virus, N. gonorrhoeae	Symptoms of acute pharyngitis, cervical lymphadenopathy, fever[c]
Proctitis	C. trachomatis, herpes simplex virus, N. gonorrhoeae, T. pallidum	Constipation, anorectal discomfort, tenesmus, mucopurulent rectal discharge
Salpingitis	C. trachomatis, N. gonorrhoeae	Lower abdominal pain, purulent cervical or vaginal discharge, adnexal swelling, fever[d]

[a]For some syndromes, clinical manifestations can be minimal or absent.
[b]Recurrent herpes infection can manifest as a single lesion.
[c]Most cases of pharyngeal gonococcal infection are asymptomatic.
[d]Salpingitis increases the risk of subsequent ectopic pregnancy and infertility.

Gonorrhea

- *Neisseria gonorrhoeae* is a gram-negative diplococcus causing 16,392 new infections in 2019 in the United States. Humans are the only known host of this intracellular parasite.
- The CDC identified drug-resistant *N. gonorrhoeae* as a top three pathogen presenting an urgent level threat, posing an immediate health threat requiring urgent and aggressive action.

CLINICAL PRESENTATION

- Infected individuals may be symptomatic or asymptomatic, have complicated or uncomplicated infections, and have infections involving several anatomical sites. The majority of women diagnosed with gonorrhea are asymptomatic.
- The most common clinical features of gonococcal infections are presented below.
- Incubation period: 1–14 days, symptom onset in 2–8 days (males) and 10 days (females).
- Most common site of infection: Urethra (males), endocervical canal (females); other sites: rectum (usually caused by rectal intercourse in MSM), oropharynx, eye (males) and urethra, rectum (usually caused by perineal contamination), oropharynx, eye (females).
- Symptoms
  ✓ Males: Commonly symptomatic, may be asymptomatic; urethral infection: dysuria and urinary frequency; anorectal infection: asymptomatic to severe rectal pain; pharyngeal infection: asymptomatic to mild pharyngitis.
  ✓ Females: Can be asymptomatic or minimally symptomatic; endocervical infection: usually asymptomatic or mildly symptomatic; urethral infection: dysuria, urinary frequency; anorectal and pharyngeal infection; symptoms same as for men.

- Signs: Purulent urethral or rectal discharge can be scant to profuse; anorectal: pruritus, mucopurulent discharge, bleeding (males) and abnormal vaginal discharge or uterine bleeding; purulent urethral or rectal discharge can be scant to profuse (females).
- Complications: Rare (epididymitis, prostatitis, inguinal lymphadenopathy, urethral stricture) in males; pelvic inflammatory disease (PID) and associated complications (ie, ectopic pregnancy, infertility) in females.
- Ninety percent of males experience symptoms within 2–6 days following exposure, most commonly mucopurulent penile discharge and dysuria. Approximately 10%–20% of women with gonorrhea develop PID. Left untreated, PID can be an indirect cause of infertility and ectopic pregnancies.
- In 0.5%–3% of patients with gonorrhea, the gonococci invade the bloodstream and produce disseminated disease. The usual clinical manifestations of disseminated gonococcal infection are tender necrotic skin lesions, tenosynovitis, and monoarticular arthritis.
- Diagnosis of gonococcal infections can be made by gram-stained smears, culture or detection of cellular components (eg, enzymes, antigens, or DNA).
- Nucleic acid amplification techniques (NAATs) have replaced culture in most settings as the primary diagnostic or screening test.
- Bacterial cultures are highly sensitive and specific, provide opportunity for susceptibility testing, and can be performed on a variety of specimens.
- The CDC and US Preventative Services Task Force recommend routine annual screening for gonococcal infection for all sexually active women younger than 25.

TREATMENT

- Goals of Treatment: Resolution of infection without complications or reinfection or recurrence.
- A single 500-mg ceftriaxone dose is recommended for treatment of uncomplicated gonococcal infections (Table 47-3). Patients weighing 150 kg or more should receive ceftriaxone 1 g. An 800-mg oral dose of **cefixime** may be substituted if ceftriaxone is unavailable.
- Because coexisting chlamydial infections are common, chlamydia treatment should be added with doxycycline 100 mg orally twice daily for 7 days.
- Ceftriaxone is the recommended therapy for disseminated gonococcal infection (DGI) including meningitis and endocarditis, and any type of gonococcal infection in children.
- Pregnant females infected with N. gonorrhoeae should be treated with a single intramuscular dose of ceftriaxone 500 mg, with the addition of 1 g of oral azithromycin if chlamydia has not been ruled out.

TABLE 47-3	Treatment of Gonorrhea	
Type of Infection	**Recommended Regimens[a]**	**Alternative Regimens[a]**
Uncomplicated infections of the cervix, urethra, and rectum in adults	Ceftriaxone 500 mg IM once[b,c]	Gentamicin 240 mg IM[d] *plus* Azithromycin 2 g orally once *or* When ceftriaxone administration is not feasible, cefixime 800 mg orally once[c]
Uncomplicated infections of the pharynx	Ceftriaxone 500 mg IM once[b,c]	Consult with infectious disease expert
DGI in adults (>45 kg)	Ceftriaxone 1–2 g IM or IV every 12–24 hours[c,e]	Cefotaxime 1 g IV every 8 hours[c,e] or ceftizoxime 1 g IV every 8 hours[c,e]
Gonococcal conjunctivitis in adults	Ceftriaxone 1 g IM once[f]	
Ophthalmia neonatorum	Ceftriaxone 25–50 mg/kg IV or IM once (not to exceed 250 mg)	
Infants born to mothers with gonococcal infection (prophylaxis)	Erythromycin (0.5%) ophthalmic ointment in a single application[g"] Ceftriaxone 25–50 mg/kg IM or IV once (not to exceed 125 mg)	

[a]Recommendations are those of the CDC.
[b]For patients weighing >150 kg, a 1 g dose of ceftriaxone is recommended.
[c]If chlamydial infection cannot be ruled out, treatment for chlamydia should be administered. Preferred therapy is doxycycline 100 mg orally twice daily × 7 days. Azithromycin 1 g orally once may be used as an alternative. Tetracyclines are contraindicated during pregnancy. Pregnant women should be treated with recommended cephalosporin-based combination therapy. In severe cephalosporin allergy, consultation with an infectious diseases expert is recommended.
[d]For patients with severe cephalosporin allergy.
[e]Parenteral treatment duration should be determined in consultation with an infectious diseases expert. Gonococcal meningitis should be treated with ceftriaxone 2 g IV every 12 hours. Parenteral therapy for meningitis should be continued for at least 10 to 14 days and at least 4 weeks in endocarditis.
[f]A single lavage of the infected eye with normal saline should be considered; empiric therapy for *C. trachomatis* is recommended.
[g]Efficacy in preventing chlamydial ophthalmia is unclear.

- Treatment of gonorrhea during pregnancy is essential to prevent ophthalmia neonatorum. The CDC recommends that **erythromycin (0.5%) ophthalmic ointment** be instilled in each conjunctival sac immediately postpartum to prevent ophthalmia neonatorum.
- The CDC recommends all treatment failures receive culture and sensitivity testing.

Syphilis

- The causative organism of syphilis is *Treponema pallidum*, a spirochete.
- Syphilis is usually acquired by sexual contact with infected mucous membranes or cutaneous lesions, although on rare occasions it can be acquired by nonsexual personal contact, accidental inoculation, or blood transfusion. Rates of coinfection with HIV have remained high, particularly among MSM.

CLINICAL PRESENTATION AND DIAGNOSIS

- The clinical presentation of syphilis is varied, with progression through multiple stages possible in untreated or inadequately treated patients.

PRIMARY SYPHILIS

- Primary syphilis is characterized by the appearance of a chancre on cutaneous or mucocutaneous tissue exposed to the organism and is highly infectious. Chancres heal within 4–6 weeks, although lymphadenopathy may persist longer.
- Incubation period: 10–90 days (mean, 21 days).
- Site of infection: External genitalia, perianal region, mouth, and throat.
- Signs and symptoms: Single, painless, indurated lesion (chancre) that erodes, ulcerates, and eventually heals (typical); regional lymphadenopathy is common; multiple, painful, purulent lesions possible but uncommon.

SECONDARY SYPHILIS

- The secondary stage of syphilis is characterized by a variety of mucocutaneous eruptions, resulting from widespread hematogenous and lymphatic spread of *T. pallidum*. There is multisystem involvement secondary to hematogenous and lymphatic spread.
- Skin lesions are often maculopapular and are usually nonpruritic, developing first on trunk and proximal arms and disseminating bilaterally. Secondary syphilis lesions typically involve the palms and soles, can present as mucous patches, and/or can have a wart-like appearance (condylomata lata). Patchy alopecia is another finding periodically seen.
- If untreated, secondary syphilis disappears spontaneously within 1–6 months.

LATENT SYPHILIS

- Persons with a positive serologic test for syphilis but with no other evidence of disease have latent syphilis.
- If left untreated, syphilis can slowly produce an inflammatory reaction in virtually any organ in the body. Most patients with late syphilis will have no further sequelae. However, approximately 28% will develop further disease years after the initial infection.

TERTIARY SYPHILIS AND NEUROSYPHILIS

- Neurologic manifestations, including ocular and otic, may present at any stage of syphilis.
- Non-neurologic manifestations of late syphilis include benign gumma formation and cardiovascular syphilis. Gummas, nonspecific granulomatous lesions, are the classic lesions of late syphilis and can infiltrate any organ or tissue.
- Because *T. pallidum* is difficult to culture in vitro, diagnosis is based primarily on dark-field or direct fluorescent antibody microscopic examination of serous material from a suspected syphilitic lesion or on results from serologic testing.
- Serologic tests are the mainstay in the diagnosis of syphilis and are categorized as nontreponemal or treponemal. Common nontreponemal tests include the venereal disease research laboratory (VDRL) slide test, rapid plasma reagin (RPR) card test, unheated serum reagin (USR) test, and the toluidine red unheated serum test (TRUST).
- Treponemal tests are more sensitive than nontreponemal tests and are used to confirm the diagnosis (ie, the fluorescent treponemal antibody absorption).

TREATMENT

- Goals of Treatment: Resolution of infection and prevention of medical complications. Also, to prevent spread of infection including to the newborn. Treatment recommendations from the CDC for syphilis are presented in Table 47-4. Parenteral penicillin G is the treatment of choice for all stages of syphilis. **Benzathine penicillin G** is the only penicillin effective for single-dose therapy. The recommended treatment for syphilis of less than 1 year's duration is benzathine penicillin G 2.4 million units as a single IM dose.

TABLE 47-4 Drug Therapy and Follow-up of Syphilis

Stage/Type of Syphilis	Recommended Regimens[a,b]	Follow-up Serology
Primary, secondary, or early latent syphilis (<1 year's duration)	Adults: benzathine penicillin G 2.4 million units IM in a single dose Children: Benzathine penicillin G 50,000 units/kg IM in a single dose, up to 2.4 million units	Quantitative nontreponemal tests at 6 and 12 months with failure if titer does not decrease at least fourfold in 12 months[c]
Late latent syphilis (>1 year's duration) or latent syphilis of unknown duration or tertiary syphilis or retreatment after failure	Adults: benzathine penicillin G 2.4 million units IM once a week for 3 successive weeks (7.2 million units total) Children: benzathine penicillin G 50,000 units/kg IM once a week for 3 successive weeks, up to 7.2 million units total	Quantitative nontreponemal tests at 6, 12, and 24 months with failure if titer does not increase at least fourfold in 24 months[c]
Neurosyphilis, including ocular or otic involvement	Aqueous crystalline penicillin G 18–24 million units IV (3–4 million units every 4 hours or by continuous infusion) for 10–14 days[d,e] *or* Aqueous procaine penicillin G 2.4 million units IM daily plus probenecid 500 mg orally four times daily, both for 10–14 days	Repeat CSF examination is no longer required at 6 months if adequate RPR response (decrease by fourfold or greater)
Congenital syphilis (infants with proven or highly probable disease)	Aqueous crystalline penicillin G 50,000 units/kg/dose IV every 12 hours during the first 7 days of life and every 8 hours thereafter for a total of 10 days *or* Procaine penicillin G 50,000 units/kg IM daily for 10 days[d]	Serologic follow-up only recommended if antimicrobials other than penicillin are used
Penicillin-allergic patients[e,f]		
Primary, secondary, or early latent syphilis	Doxycycline 100 mg orally two times daily for 14 days *or* Tetracycline 500 mg orally four times daily for 14 days *or* Ceftriaxone 1–2 g IM or IV daily for 10–14 days	Same as for non–penicillin-allergic patients

(Continued)

TABLE 47-4	Drug Therapy and Follow-up of Syphilis (*Continued*)	
Stage/Type of Syphilis	**Recommended Regimens[a,b]**	**Follow-up Serology**
Late latent syphilis (>1 year's duration) or syphilis of unknown duration	Doxycycline 100 mg orally twice a day for 28 days *or* Tetracycline 500 mg orally four times daily for 28 days	Same as for non–penicillin-allergic patients

CDC, Centers for Disease Control and Prevention; CSF, cerebrospinal fluid; HIV, human immunodeficiency virus; RPR, rapid plasma reagin.

[a]Recommendations are those of the CDC.
[b]The CDC recommends that all patients diagnosed with syphilis be tested for HIV infection.
[c] No specific recommendations exist for tertiary syphilis because of the lack of available data.
[d] Some experts administer benzathine penicillin G 2.4 million units IM once per week for up to 3 weeks after completion of the neurosyphilis regimens to provide a total duration of therapy comparable to that used for late syphilis in the absence of neurosyphilis.
[e] Growing data support ceftriaxone efficacy, although the optimal dosage and treatment duration are unclear; in neurosyphilis, 2 g IV daily for at least 10 days found to be as effective as intravenous penicillin G.
[f] For nonpregnant patients; pregnant patients should be treated with penicillin after desensitization.

- Alternative regimens recommended for penicillin-allergic patients are **doxycycline** 100 mg orally twice daily or **tetracycline** 500 mg orally four times daily for 2–4 weeks depending on the duration of syphilis infection.
- For pregnant patients, penicillin is the treatment of choice at the dosage recommended for that particular stage of syphilis. To ensure treatment success and prevent transmission to the fetus, some experts advocate an additional IM dose of benzathine penicillin G, 2.4 million units, 1 week after completion of the recommended regimen.
- Patients treated for primary and secondary syphilis experience the Jarisch–Herxheimer reaction after treatment, characterized by flu-like symptoms such as transient headache, fever, chills, malaise, arthralgia, myalgia, tachypnea, peripheral vasodilation, and aggravation of syphilitic lesions. The Jarisch–Herxheimer reaction should not be confused with penicillin allergy. Most reactions can be managed symptomatically with analgesics, antipyretics, and rest.
- The CDC recommendations for serologic follow-up of patients treated for syphilis are given in **Table 47-4**. Quantitative nontreponemal tests should be performed at 6 and 12 months in all patients treated for primary and secondary syphilis and at 6, 12, and 24 months for early and late latent disease.
- For women treated during pregnancy, monthly, quantitative, nontreponemal tests are recommended in those at high risk of reinfection.

Chlamydia

- Infections caused by *Chlamydia trachomatis* are believed to be the most common STI in the United States. *C. trachomatis* is an obligate intracellular parasite that has some similarities to viruses and bacteria.

CLINICAL PRESENTATION

- In comparison with gonorrhea, chlamydial genital infections are more frequently asymptomatic, and when present, symptoms tend to be less noticeable. The usual clinical presentation of chlamydial infections is as follows.
- Incubation period: 35 days (males), 7–35 days (females).
- Symptom onset: 7–21 days (males and females).
- Most site of infection: Urethra (males), endocervical canal (females); other sites: rectum (receptive anal intercourse), oropharynx, eye (males), urethra, rectum (usually caused by perineal contamination), oropharynx, eye (females).

- Symptoms:
  - ✓ Males: More than 50% of urethral and rectal infections are asymptomatic; urethral infection: mild dysuria, discharge; pharyngeal infection: asymptomatic to mild pharyngitis.
  - ✓ Females: More than 66% of cervical infections are asymptomatic; urethral infection: usually subclinical; dysuria and frequency uncommon; rectal and pharyngeal infection: symptoms same as for men.
- Signs:
  - ✓ Males: Scant to profuse, mucoid to purulent urethral or rectal discharge; rectal infection: pain, discharge, bleeding.
  - ✓ Females: Abnormal vaginal discharge or uterine bleeding, purulent urethral or rectal discharge can be scant to profuse.
- Complications include epididymitis, Reiter's syndrome (rare) in males, PID and associated complications (ie, ectopic pregnancy, infertility), Reiter's syndrome (rare) in females.
- Similar to gonorrhea, chlamydia may be transmitted to an infant during contact with infected cervicovaginal secretions. Nearly two-thirds of infants acquire chlamydial infection after endocervical exposure, with the primary morbidity associated with seeding of the infant's eyes, nasopharynx, rectum, or vagina.
- Culture of endocervical or urethral epithelial cell scrapings is the most specific method (close to 100%) for detection of chlamydia, but sensitivity is as low as 70%. Between 3 and 7 days are required for results.
- Tests that allow rapid identification of chlamydial antigens and nucleic acid provide more rapid results are technically less demanding to perform, less costly, and in some situations have greater sensitivity than culture. NAATs are the most sensitive tests for first-catch urine, endocervix and vaginal swab specimens in women, and urethral swab specimens in men, and are therefore the recommended tests for detecting chlamydia infection.

TREATMENT

- Goal of Treatment: Resolution of infection without reinfection.
- **Azithromycin** 1000 mg orally as a single-dose and **doxycycline** 100 mg orally twice daily for 7 days are the regimens of choice for the treatment of uncomplicated urogenital chlamydia infections (**Table 47-5**).

TABLE 47-5	Treatment of Chlamydia Infections	
Infection	**Recommended Regimens[a]**	**Alternative Regimens[a]**
Uncomplicated urethral, endocervical, or rectal infection in adults	Doxycycline 100 mg orally twice daily for 7 days	Azithromycin 1 g orally once[b], *or* levofloxacin 500 mg orally once daily for 7 days
Urogenital infections during pregnancy	Azithromycin 1 g orally as a single dose	Amoxicillin 500 mg orally three times daily for 7 days
Conjunctivitis of the newborn or pneumonia in infants	Erythromycin base or ethylsuccinate 50 mg/kg/day orally in four divided doses for 14 days[c,d]	Azithromycin suspension 20 mg/kg/day orally once daily for 3 days[c]

[a]Recommendations are those of the CDC.
[b]Azithromycin may be used if there are concerns for nonadherence. Test after treatment is recommended due to reduced efficacy in rectal chlamydia.
[c]An association between oral erythromycin and azithromycin and infantile hypertrophic pyloric stenosis (IHPS) has been reported in infants aged <6 weeks. Infants treated with either of these antimicrobials should be followed for signs and symptoms of IHPS.
[d]Topical therapy alone is inadequate for ophthalmia neonatorum and is unnecessary when systemic therapy is administered. Effectiveness of erythromycin treatment is approximately 80%; therefore, a second course of therapy may be required.

- Treatment of chlamydial infections with the recommended regimens is highly effective; therefore, posttreatment cultures are not routinely recommended.
- Infants with pneumonitis should receive follow-up testing because **erythromycin** is only 80% effective.
- For infected pregnant females azithromycin is the recommended treatment.

Genital Herpes

- The term *herpes* is used to describe two distinct but antigenically related serotypes of herpes simplex virus (HSV). HSV type 1 (HSV-1) is most commonly associated with oropharyngeal disease; type 2 (HSV-2) is most closely associated with genital disease.
- First-episode primary infection is when initial genital infection occurs in individuals lacking antibody to either HSV-1 or HSV-2.
- First-episode nonprimary infection is when initial genital infection occurs in individuals with clinical or serologic evidence of prior HSV (usually HSV-1) infection.
- Recurrent infection occurs when appearance of genital lesions occurs at some time following healing of first-episode infection.

CLINICAL PRESENTATION

- A summary of the clinical presentation of genital herpes is provided below.
- Incubation period: 2–14 days (mean, 4 days).
- Signs and symptoms:
  - ✓ First-episode infections:
    - Most primary infections are asymptomatic or minimally symptomatic.
    - Multiple painful pustular or ulcerative lesions on external genitalia developing over a period of 7–10 days; lesions heal in 2–4 weeks (mean, 21 days).
    - Flu-like symptoms (eg, fever, headache, malaise) during first few days after appearance of lesions.
    - Others—local itching, pain, or discomfort; vaginal or urethral discharge, tender inguinal adenopathy, paresthesias, urinary retention.
    - Severity of symptoms greater in females than in males.
    - Symptoms are less severe (eg, fewer lesions, more rapid lesion healing, fewer or milder systemic symptoms) with nonprimary infections.
    - Symptoms more severe and prolonged in immunocompromised patients.
    - On average viral shedding lasts approximately 11–12 days for primary infections and 7 days for nonprimary infections.
  - ✓ Recurrent:
    - Prodrome seen in approximately 50% of patients prior to appearance of recurrent lesions; mild burning, itching, or tingling are typical prodromal symptoms.
    - Compared to primary infections, recurrent infections are associated with (1) fewer lesions that are more localized, (2) shorter duration of active infection (lesions heal within 7 days), and (3) milder symptoms.
    - Severity of symptoms greater in females than in males.
    - Symptoms more severe and prolonged in immunocompromised patients.
    - On average viral shedding lasts approximately 4 days.
    - Asymptomatic viral shedding is more frequent during the first year after infection with HSV.

- Primary infections caused by HSV-1 and HSV-2 are virtually indistinguishable. Recurrent infections and subclinical viral shedding are less frequent with HSV-1 and recurrent infections with HSV-2 tend to be more severe.
- Complications from genital herpes infections result from both genital spread and autoinoculation of the virus and occur most commonly with primary first episodes. Lesions at extragenital sites, such as the eye, rectum, pharynx, and fingers, are not uncommon. Central nervous system involvement is seen occasionally and can take several forms, including encephalitis, aseptic meningitis, and transverse myelitis. A major concern is the effect of genital herpes on neonates exposed during pregnancy.

• Viral culture and HSV DNA detection with PCR assays (preferred) are primary modalities used to confirm the diagnosis of first-episode genital herpes.

TREATMENT

• <u>Goals of Treatment:</u> To relieve symptoms and to shorten the clinical course, prevent complications and recurrences, and to decrease disease transmission.
• Specific treatment recommendations are given in **Table 47-6**.
• Oral **acyclovir, valacyclovir**, and **famciclovir** are the treatments of choice for outpatients with first-episode genital herpes. All patients with first episodes genital herpes should receive systemic antiviral therapy to prevent severe or prolonged symptoms associated with newly acquired infections.
• Suppressive with oral antiviral agents reduces the frequency and the severity of clinical episodes and asymptomatic shedding in 70%–80% of patients experiencing frequent recurrences.

TABLE 47-6	Treatment of Genital Herpes	
Type of Infection	**Recommended Regimens[a,b]**	**Alternative Regimen**
First clinical episode of genital herpes[c]	Acyclovir 400 mg orally three times daily for 7–10 days[d] *or* Famciclovir 250 mg orally three times daily for 7–10 days[d] *or* Valacyclovir 1 g orally twice daily for 7–10 days[d]	Acyclovir 5–10 mg/ kg IV every 8 hours for 2–7 days or until clinical improvement occurs, followed by oral therapy to complete at least 10 days of total therapy[e]
Recurrent infection		
Episodic therapy	Acyclovir 800 mg orally twice daily for 5 days[f] *or* Acyclovir 800 mg orally three times daily for 2 days[f] *or* Famciclovir 125 mg orally twice daily for 5 days[f] *or* Famciclovir 1 g orally twice daily for 1 day[f] *or* Famciclovir 500 mg orally once, followed by 250 mg orally twice daily for 2 days[f] *or* Valacyclovir 500 mg orally twice daily for 3 days[f] *or* Valacyclovir 1 g orally once daily for 5 days[f]	

(Continued)

TABLE 47-6	Treatment of Genital Herpes (Continued)	
Type of Infection	**Recommended Regimens[a,b]**	**Alternative Regimen**
Suppressive therapy[g]	Acyclovir 400 mg orally twice daily	
	or	
	Famciclovir 250 mg orally twice daily[h]	
	or	
	Valacyclovir 500 mg or 1000 mg orally once daily[i]	

CDC, Centers for Disease Control and Prevention; HIV, human immunodeficiency virus; IV, intravenous.
[a]Recommendations are those of the CDC.
[b]HIV-infected patients can require more aggressive therapy.
[c]Primary or nonprimary first episode.
[d]Treatment duration can be extended if healing is incomplete after 10 days.
[e]Only for patients with severe symptoms or complications that necessitate hospitalization. HSV encephalitis requires 21 days of IV therapy.
[f]Requires initiation of therapy within 24 hours of lesion onset or during the prodrome that precedes some outbreaks.
[g]Consider discontinuation of treatment after 1 year to assess frequency of recurrence.
[h]Famciclovir appears less effective for suppression of viral shedding.
[i]Valacyclovir 500 mg appears less effective than other valacyclovir and acyclovir regimens in patients with 10 or more recurrences per year.

- Acyclovir, valacyclovir, and famciclovir have been used to prevent reactivation of infection in patients seropositive for HSV who undergo transplantation procedures or induction chemotherapy.
- The safety of famciclovir and valacyclovir therapy during pregnancy is not well established, although experience with both agents in animal studies suggests a low risk of fetal harm. Acyclovir has been used in pregnant patients and has produced no evidence of teratogenicity.

Trichomoniasis

- Trichomoniasis is caused by *Trichomonas vaginalis,* a flagellated, motile protozoan that was responsible for 6.9 million cases in the United States in 2018. *T. vaginalis* is primarily transmitted through sexual contact.
- Coinfection with other STIs (eg, gonorrhea) is not unusual, and the inflammatory response produced by trichomoniasis increases the risk of acquiring HIV.

CLINICAL PRESENTATION

- The typical presentation of trichomoniasis in men and women is presented below.
- Incubation period: 3–28 days. The organism can be detectable within 48 hours after exposure to infected partner.
- Most common sites of infection are the urethra (males) and endocervical canal (females); other sites of infection: rectum (usually caused by rectal intercourse in MSM), oropharynx, eye in males and urethra, rectum (usually caused by perineal contamination), oropharynx, eye in females.
- Symptoms:
  ✓ Males: Can be asymptomatic (more common in males than females) or minimally symptomatic; urethral discharge (clear to mucopurulent); dysuria, pruritus.
  ✓ Females: Can be asymptomatic or minimally symptomatic; scant to copious, typically malodorous vaginal discharge (50%–75%) and pruritus (worse during menses); dysuria, dyspareunia.
- Signs: Urethral discharge (males), Vaginal discharge, vaginal pH 4.5–6, inflammation/erythema of vulva, vagina, and/or cervix, urethritis (females).

- Complications:
  - ✓ Males: Epididymitis and chronic prostatitis (uncommon); male infertility (decreased sperm motility and viability).
  - ✓ Females: PID and associated complications (ie, ectopic pregnancy, infertility); premature labor, premature rupture of membranes, and low-birth-weight infants (risk of neonatal infections is low); cervical neoplasia.
- *T. vaginalis* produces nonspecific symptoms also consistent with bacterial vaginosis; thus, laboratory diagnosis is required.
- The simplest and most reliable means of diagnosis is a wet-mount examination of the vaginal discharge. Trichomoniasis is confirmed if characteristic pear-shaped, flagellating organisms are observed. Newer diagnostic tests, such as NAATs are highly sensitive and specific. Rapid point of care tests are also readily available, allowing for office-based testing.

TREATMENT

- Goal of Treatment: To achieve cure of the infection, relief of symptoms, and prevent reinfection and transmission.
- Recommended and alternative treatment regimens for *T. vaginalis* include either **metronidazole** or **tinidazole**, both of which produce high cure rates.
- Treatment recommendations for *Trichomonas* infections are given in **Table 47-7**.
- To achieve maximal cure rates and prevent relapse with the single 2-g dose of metronidazole, simultaneous treatment of infected sexual partners is recommended.
- In patients who fail to respond to an initial course of metronidazole therapy, a second course of therapy with metronidazole 500 mg twice daily for 7 days is recommended.
- The CDC guidelines do not link metronidazole use with the potential for a disulfiram-like reaction in those that consume alcohol concurrently.
- Because metronidazole is secreted in breast milk, it is recommended that breast-feeding be interrupted for 12–24 hours after maternal ingestion of a single 2-g dose. Some clinicians prefer to delay treatment in women in the first trimester; however, metronidazole is pregnancy category B and may be used for treatment in any trimester. Tinidazole is pregnancy category C and should be avoided. However, the CDC now recommends that all symptomatic pregnant women, regardless of pregnancy stage, be tested and considered for treatment with metronidazole.

TABLE 47-7	Treatment of Trichomoniasis	
Type	**Recommended Regimens[a]**	**Alternative Regimen**
Symptomatic and asymptomatic infections	Women: Metronidazole 500 mg orally two times daily for 7 days[a,b,c]	Tinidazole 2 g orally in single dose
	Men: Metronidazole 2 g orally in a single dose[b,d]	
Persistent or recurrent infections	Metronidazole 500 mg orally two times daily for 7 days	Tinidazole 2 g orally daily for 7 days
Treatment in pregnancy	Metronidazole 500 mg orally twice daily for 7 days	

[a]Recommendations are those of the CDC.
[b]Metronidazole labeling approved by the FDA does not include this regimen. Dosage regimens for treatment of trichomoniasis included in the product labeling are the single 2 g dose; 250 mg three times daily for 7 days; and 375 mg twice daily for 7 days. The 250-mg and 375-mg dosage regimens are currently not included in the CDC recommendations.
[c]For men, data is lacking for alternative treatment regimens and regimens for persistent infection. Consult an infectious diseases specialist.
[d]Randomized controlled trial comparing metronidazole 500 mg twice daily for 7 days and a single 2-g dose in women found fewer treatment failures in the 7-day regimen.

- Retesting for *T. vaginalis* is recommended for all sexually active women within 3 months following initial treatment due to the high rates of reinfection. Concurrent treatment of all sex partners is critical to ensure relief of symptoms and prevent reinfection and transmission.
- When patients remain symptomatic, it is important to ensure patient adherence and to determine if reinfection has occurred. In these cases, a repeat course of therapy, including sexual partner(s) is indicated.

Other Sexually Transmitted Infections

- Several STIs other than those previously discussed occur with varying frequency in the United States and throughout the world. Although an in-depth discussion of these diseases is beyond the scope of this chapter, recommended treatment regimens are given in **Table 47-8**.

TABLE 47-8	Treatment Regimens for Miscellaneous STIs	
Infection	**Recommended Regimens[a]**	**Alternative Regimens**
Cervicitis[b]	Doxycycline 100 mg orally twice daily for 7 days	Azithromycin 1 g orally in a single dose
Epididymitis		
Acute infection most likely caused by *C. trachomatis* or *N. gonorrhoeae*	Ceftriaxone 500 mg IM in a single dose PLUS doxycycline 100 mg orally twice daily for 7 days	
Acute infection most likely caused by *C. trachomatis*, *N. gonorrhoeae*, or enteric organisms (men who practice insertive anal sex)	Ceftriaxone 500 mg IM in a single dose PLUS levofloxacin 500 mg orally daily for 10 days	
Acute infection most likely caused by enteric organisms only	Levofloxacin 500 mg orally daily for 10 days	
Lymphogranuloma venereum	Doxycycline 100 mg orally twice daily for 21 days[c]	Azithromycin 1 g weekly for 3 weeks or erythromycin base 500 mg orally four times daily for 21 days[c,d]
Nongonococcal urethritis (NGU)	Doxycycline 100 mg orally twice daily for 7 days	Azithromycin 1 g orally in a single dose or 500 mg orally in a single dose followed by 250 mg daily for 4 days
NGU (persistent or recurrent or due to *M. genitalium*)	Doxycycline 100 mg orally twice daily for 7 days followed by moxifloxacin 400 mg orally daily for 7 days	If azithromycin resistance can be ruled out, moxifloxacin may be substituted with oral azithromycin 1 g and then 500 mg daily for 3 days
		(Continued)

TABLE 47-8	Treatment Regimens for Miscellaneous STIs (Continued)	
Infection	**Recommended Regimens[a]**	**Alternative Regimens**
HPV infection		
External genital/perianal warts	*Provider-Administered Therapies:* Cryotherapy (eg, liquid nitrogen or cryoprobe); repeat weekly as necessary, *or* TCA 80%–90% *or* BCA 80%-90% applied to warts; repeat weekly as necessary, *or* Surgical removal (tangential scissor excision, tangential shave excision, curettage, or electrosurgery) *Patient-Applied Therapies:* Podofilox 0.5% solution or gel applied twice daily for 3 days, followed by 4 days of no therapy; cycle is repeated as necessary for up to four cycles. Imiquimod 3.75% or 5% cream applied at bedtime three times weekly for up to 16 weeks,[e,f] *or* Sinecatechins 15% ointment applied three times daily for up to 16 weeks	
Vaginal and anal warts	Cryotherapy with liquid nitrogen, or TCA or BCA 80%–90% as for external HPV warts; repeat weekly as necessary Surgical removal (not for vaginal or urethral meatus warts)	
Urethral meatus warts	Cryotherapy with liquid nitrogen, or surgical removal	
Prevention (ages 9–14 years)[f]	Gardasil9® (HPV 9-valent [types 6, 11, 16, 18, 31, 33, 45, 52, 58]) recombinant vaccine 0.5 mL IM on day 1; a second dose administered 6–12 months following the first dose	

(Continued)

TABLE 47-8	Treatment Regimens for Miscellaneous STIs (*Continued*)	
Infection	**Recommended Regimens**[a]	**Alternative Regimens**
Prevention (age ≥15–26 years)[f]	Gardasil (HPV 9-valent [types 6, 11, 16, 18, 31, 33, 45, 52, 58]) recombinant vaccine 0.5 mL IM on day 1; a second and third dose are administered 1 and 6 months following the first dose	

BCA, bichloracetic acid; HPV, human papillomavirus; TCA, trichloroacetic acid.

[a]Recommendations are those of the CDC.
[b]Consider concurrent treatment for gonorrhea infection if the patient is at risk for gonorrhea.
[c]Pregnant patients should be treated with erythromycin.
[d]If NGU is due to *C. trachomatis*, refer to treatment in Table 140-6, Chapter 140, *Dipiro's Pharmacotherapy: A Pathophysiologic Approach*, 12 ed. If NGU not due to *C. trachomatis*, consider HSV, trichomoniasis, *M. genitalium*, or HPV as potential causes of NGU and perform testing when appropriate.
[e]Safety during pregnancy is not established.
[f]CDC recommendations: vaccination is recommended in adolescents 11–12 years of age, and can be given as early as age 9. Catch up vaccination is recommended through age 26 years for those who either were not previously vaccinated, or who did not complete the vaccination series. Vaccination for adults ages 27–45 can be considered.

See Chapter 140, Sexually Transmitted Infections, authored by Yvonne Burnett and Humberto Jimenez for a more detailed discussion of this topic.

CHAPTER 48

Skin and Soft-Tissue Infections

- Bacterial infections of the skin can be classified as primary or secondary (Table 48-1). Primary bacterial infections are usually caused by a single bacterial species and involve areas of generally healthy skin (eg, impetigo and erysipelas). Secondary infections develop in areas of previously damaged skin and are frequently polymicrobic.
- The conditions that may predispose a patient to the development of skin and soft-tissue infections (SSTIs) include: (1) a high concentration of bacteria; (2) excessive moisture of the skin; (3) inadequate blood supply; (4) availability of bacterial nutrients; and (5) damage to the corneal layer, allowing for bacterial penetration.
- The majority of SSTIs are caused by gram-positive organisms on the skin surface. *Staphylococcus aureus* and *Streptococcus pyogenes* account for the majority of SSTIs. Other common nosocomial pathogens include *Pseudomonas aeruginosa* (11%), enterococci (9%), and *Escherichia coli* (7%). The emergence of community-associated methicillin-resistant *S. aureus* (MRSA) is particularly problematic.

Erysipelas

- *Erysipelas* (Saint Anthony's fire) is a distinct form of cellulitis involving the superficial layers of the skin and cutaneous lymphatics. The infection is almost always caused by β-hemolytic streptococci, with *S. pyogenes* responsible for most infections.
- The lower extremities are the most common sites for erysipelas. Patients often experience flu-like symptoms (fever, chills, and malaise) prior to the appearance of the lesions. The infected area is painful, often a burning pain. The lesion is intensely erythematous and edematous, often with lymphatic streaking. It has a raised border, which is sharply demarcated from uninfected skin. Leukocytosis is common, and C-reactive protein is generally elevated.
- Mild-to-moderate cases of erysipelas in adults are treated with intramuscular **procaine penicillin G** or **penicillin VK** for 7–10 days. For more serious infections, the patient should be hospitalized and **aqueous penicillin G** administered IV. Penicillin-allergic patients can be treated with **clindamycin**.
- Evidence-based recommendations for treatment of SSTIs are given in Table 48-2, and recommended drugs and dosing regimens for outpatient treatment of mild-to-moderate SSTIs are given in Tables 48-3 and 48-4.

Impetigo

- *Impetigo* is a superficial skin infection that is seen most commonly in children. It is highly communicable and spreads through close contact especially among siblings and children in daycare centers and schools. Most cases are caused by *S. pyogenes*, but *S. aureus* either alone or in combination with *S. pyogenes* has emerged as a principal cause of impetigo. The bullous form is caused by strains of *S. aureus* capable of producing exfoliative toxins.

CLINICAL PRESENTATION

- Exposed skin, especially the face, is the most common site for impetigo.
- Pruritus is common, and scratching of the lesions may further spread infection through excoriation of the skin. Other systemic signs of infection are minimal.
- Weakness, fever, and diarrhea are sometimes seen with bullous impetigo.

TABLE 48-1	Bacterial Classification of Important Skin and Soft-Tissue Infections
Primary infections	
Erysipelas	Group A streptococci (*Streptococcus pyogenes*)
Impetigo	*Staphylococcus aureus* (including methicillin-resistant strains), group A streptococci
Lymphangitis	Group A streptococci; occasionally *S. aureus*
Cellulitis	Group A streptococci, *S. aureus* (potentially including methicillin-resistant strains); occasionally other gram-positive cocci, gram-negative bacilli, and/or anaerobes
Necrotizing fasciitis	
Type I	Anaerobes (*Bacteroides* spp., *Peptostreptococcus* spp.) and facultative bacteria (streptococci, Enterobacteriaceae)
Type II	Group A streptococci
Type III	*Clostridioides perfringens*
Secondary infections	
Diabetic foot infections	*S. aureus*, streptococci, Enterobacteriaceae, *Bacteroides* spp., *Peptostreptococcus* spp., *Pseudomonas aeruginosa*
Pressure sores	*S. aureus* including methicillin-resistant strains, streptococci, Enterobacteriaceae, *Bacteroides* spp., *Peptostreptococcus* spp., *P. aeruginosa*
Bite wounds	
Animal	*Pasteurella* spp., *S. aureus*, streptococci, *Bacteroides* spp.
Human	*Eikenella corrodens*, *S. aureus*, streptococci, *Corynebacterium* spp., *Bacteroides* spp., *Peptostreptococcus* spp.
Burn wounds	*P. aeruginosa*, Enterobacteriaceae, *S. aureus*, streptococci

- Nonbullous impetigo manifests initially as small, fluid-filled vesicles. These lesions rapidly develop into pus-filled blisters that readily rupture. Purulent discharge from the lesions dries to form golden yellow crusts that are characteristic of impetigo.
- In the bullous form of impetigo, the lesions begin as vesicles and turn into bullae containing clear yellow fluid. Bullae soon rupture, forming thin, light brown crusts.
- Regional lymph nodes may be enlarged.

TREATMENT

- Although impetigo may resolve spontaneously, antimicrobial treatment is indicated to relieve symptoms, prevent formation of new lesions, and prevent complications such as cellulitis. Preventing transmission to others is also important.
- Topical **mupirocin** ointment or **retapamulin** ointment for 5 days is recommended as first-line treatment of mild cases of impetigo not involving multiple lesions or the face.
- Penicillinase-resistant penicillins (eg, **dicloxacillin**) are the systemic agents of choice because of the increased isolation of *S. aureus*. First-generation cephalosporins (eg, **cephalexin**) are also used (see Table 48-3). **Penicillin** may be used for impetigo caused by *S. pyogenes*. Penicillin-allergic patients can be treated with oral **clindamycin, doxycycline, or trimethoprim–sulfamethoxazole**. Recommended doses for antimicrobials are given in **Table 48-4**. The duration of treatment is 7 days.

TABLE 48-2 Evidence-Based Recommendations for Treatment of SSTIs

Recommendations	Recommendation Grade[a]
Folliculitis, furuncles, carbuncles	
Gram stain and culture of pus from carbuncles and abscesses are recommended, but treatment without cultures is reasonable in most patients	Strong, moderate
Carbuncles, abscesses, and large furuncles of mild severity should be treated with incision and drainage	Strong, high
Administration of antibiotics with activity against *Staphylococcus aureus* as an adjunct to incision and drainage should be based on presence or absence of systemic signs of infection	Strong, low
Antibiotics with activity against MRSA are recommended for patients with carbuncles or abscesses of higher severity who have failed initial antibiotic therapy, have severe systemic signs of infection, or are immunocompromised	Strong, low
Erysipelas	
Most infections are caused by *Streptococcus pyogenes*. Penicillin (oral or IV depending on clinical severity) is the drug of choice	A-I
If *S. aureus* is suspected, a penicillinase-resistant penicillin or first-generation cephalosporin should be used	A-I
Impetigo	
Gram stain and culture of pus or exudates should be obtained to help identify causative pathogens	Strong, moderate
Bullous and nonbullous impetigo should be treated with either mupirocin or retapamulin for 5 days	Strong, high
Impetigo should be treated with oral antibiotics active against *S. aureus* unless cultures show streptococci alone; dicloxacillin or cephalexin is recommended for 7 days; doxycycline, clindamycin, or sulfamethoxazole–trimethoprim should be used when MRSA is suspected or confirmed	Strong, moderate
Cellulitis	
Cultures of blood or cutaneous aspirates, biopsies, or swabs are not routinely recommended	Strong, moderate
Blood cultures are recommended, and cultures of cutaneous aspirates, biopsies, or swabs should be considered, in patients receiving chemotherapy for malignancies, neutropenia, severe cell-mediated immunodeficiency, immersion injuries, or animal bites	Strong, moderate (blood)
	Weak, moderate (other cultures)

(Continued)

TABLE 48-2 Evidence-Based Recommendations for Treatment of SSTIs (*Continued*)

Recommendations	Recommendation Grade[a]
Typical cases of mild nonpurulent cellulitis should be treated with antibiotics active against streptococci	Strong, moderate
Systemic antibiotics are recommended for moderate nonpurulent cellulitis with systemic signs of infection; use of antibiotics active against methicillin-susceptible *S. aureus* could be considered	Weak, low
Patients with severe nonpurulent cellulitis associated with penetrating trauma, MRSA infection in another location, MRSA nasal colonization, injection drug use, or systemic signs of infection should be treated with vancomycin or other antibiotics active against both MRSA and streptococci	Strong, moderate
Broad-spectrum antibiotic therapy with vancomycin plus either piperacillin–tazobactam, imipenem, or meropenem may be considered for empiric treatment of severe nonpurulent cellulitis in severely immunocompromised patients	Weak, moderate (need for broad-spectrum therapy); strong, moderate (recommended broad-spectrum antibiotic regimen if used)
A treatment duration of 5 days is recommended for cellulitis, but may be extended if lack of clinical response within that time	Strong, high
Elevation of the affected area and treatment of predisposing factors are recommended for cellulitis	Strong, moderate
Systemic corticosteroids for 7 days can be considered for adjunctive treatment of cellulitis in nondiabetic patients	Weak, moderate
Patients with mild nonpurulent cellulitis who do not have systemic signs of infection, altered mental status, or hemodynamic instability should be treated as outpatients	Strong, moderate
Hospitalization is recommended for patients with moderate-to-severe nonpurulent cellulitis who have failed outpatient therapy, have poor adherence to therapy, are immunocompromised, or in whom there is a concern for deeper or necrotizing infection	Strong, moderate
Empiric antibiotics for outpatients with purulent cellulitis should provide activity against community-associated MRSA; coverage of β-hemolytic streptococci is likely not required. Mild-to-moderate infections can generally be treated with oral agents (dicloxacillin, cephalexin, clindamycin) unless resistance is high in the community	A-II
Recommended antibiotics for empiric coverage of MRSA in outpatients include orally administered trimethoprim–sulfamethoxazole, doxycycline, minocycline, clindamycin, and linezolid	A-II for all listed options

If coverage of both β-hemolytic streptococci and community-associated MRSA is desired, empiric antibiotic regimens for outpatient therapy include orally administered clindamycin alone; linezolid alone; or trimethoprim–sulfamethoxazole, doxycycline, or minocycline in combination with amoxicillin	A-II for all listed options
Hospitalized patients with complicated or purulent cellulitis should receive IV antibiotics with activity against MRSA pending culture data; antibiotic options include vancomycin, linezolid, daptomycin, telavancin, and clindamycin	A-I for all except clindamycin; clindamycin A-III
In the treatment of S. aureus infections, trough serum vancomycin concentrations should always be maintained >10 mg/L (7 μmol/L) to avoid development of resistance	B-III

Necrotizing fasciitis

Patients with severe nonpurulent cellulitis characterized by aggressive infection and associated with signs of systemic toxicity, necrotizing fasciitis, or gas gangrene should have prompt surgical consultation	Strong, low
Early and aggressive surgical debridement of all necrotic tissue is essential	A-III
Necrotizing fasciitis should be empirically treated with broad-spectrum antibiotics such as vancomycin or linezolid plus piperacillin–tazobactam or a carbapenem, or vancomycin or linezolid plus ceftriaxone and metronidazole	Strong, low
Necrotizing fasciitis caused by S. pyogenes should be treated with the combination of clindamycin and penicillin	Strong, low
In the treatment of necrotizing fasciitis caused by methicillin-resistant S. aureus infections, trough serum vancomycin concentrations of 15–20 mg/L (10–14 μmol/L) are recommended	B-II
Clostridial gas gangrene (myonecrosis) should be treated with clindamycin and penicillin	B-III

Diabetic foot infections

Clinically uninfected wounds should not be treated with antibiotics	A-III
Empiric antibiotic regimens should be selected based on severity of infection and likely pathogens	A-III
Antibiotic therapy should target only aerobic gram-positive cocci in patients with mild-to-moderate infection who have not received antibiotics within the previous month	C-III
Broad-spectrum empiric antibiotic therapy should be initiated in most patients with severe infections, until culture and susceptibility data are available	A-III

(Continued)

TABLE 48-2   Evidence-Based Recommendations for Treatment of SSTIs (Continued)

Recommendations	Recommendation Grade[a]
Empiric antibiotics directed against *Pseudomonas aeruginosa* are usually unnecessary except in patients with specific risk factors for infection with this pathogen: patient has been soaking feet, patient has failed previous antibiotic therapy with nonpseudomonal agents, or clinically severe infection	A-III
Empiric antibiotics directed against MRSA should be considered in patients with specific risk factors, including prior history of infection or colonization with MRSA, high local prevalence of MRSA (eg, ≥50% for mild infections, ≥30% for severe infection), or clinically severe infection	C-III
Oral agents with high bioavailability may be used in the treatment of most mild, and many moderate, infections	A-II
Parenteral therapy is initially preferred for all severe, and some moderate, infections; after initial response, step-down therapy to oral agents can be considered	C-III
Definitive therapy should be based on results of appropriately collected cultures and sensitivities, as well as clinical response to empiric antimicrobial agents	A-III
Appropriate wound care, in addition to appropriate antimicrobial therapy, is often necessary for healing of infected wounds	A-III
Antibiotic therapy should only be continued until resolution of signs/symptoms of infection, but not necessarily until the wound is fully healed; the duration of therapy should initially be 1–2 weeks for mild infections and 2–3 weeks for moderate-to-severe infection	C-III
Pressure ulcers	
Optimize the host response by evaluating nutritional status and addressing deficits; stabilizing glycemic control; improving arterial blood flow; and/or reducing immunosuppressant therapy if possible	A-III
Consider the use of topical antiseptics for pressure ulcers that are not expected to heal and are critically colonized/topically infected	B-III
Consider use of silver sulfadiazine in heavily contaminated or infected pressure ulcers until definitive debridement is accomplished	B-III
Consider the use of medical-grade honey in heavily contaminated or infected pressure ulcers until definitive debridement is accomplished	C-III
Limit the use of topical antibiotics on infected pressure ulcers, except in special situations where the benefit to the patient outweighs the risk of antibiotic side effects and resistance	B-III

Use systemic antibiotics for individuals with clinical evidence of systemic infection, such as positive blood cultures, cellulitis, fasciitis, osteomyelitis, systemic inflammatory response syndrome (SIRS), or sepsis	B-III

Animal bites

Preemptive early antibiotics should be administered for 3–5 days in patients with any of the following: immunocompromised; asplenic; advanced liver disease; preexisting or resultant edema of the bitten area; moderate-to-severe bite-related injuries, especially to the hands or face; or bite injuries that have penetrated the periosteum or joint capsule	Strong, low
Amoxicillin–clavulanic acid or other antibiotics active against both aerobic and anaerobic bacteria should be used for treatment of infected animal bites	Strong, moderate
Serious infections requiring IV antimicrobial therapy can be treated with a β-lactam/β-lactamase inhibitor combination or second-generation cephalosporin with activity against anaerobes (eg, cefoxitin)	B-II
Penicillinase-resistant penicillins, first-generation cephalosporins, macrolides, and clindamycin should not be used for treatment of infected wounds because of their poor activity against *Pasteurella multocida*	D-III

Human bites

Antimicrobial therapy should provide coverage against *Eikenella corrodens*, *S. aureus*, and β-lactamase–producing anaerobes	B-III

^a Cited evidence-based guidelines utilize different systems for grading the strengths of recommendation and quality of the associated evidence. Qualitative (descriptive) recommendations are from: Stevens DL, Bisno AL, Chambers HF, et al. Practice guidelines for the diagnosis and management of skin and soft-tissue infections: 2014 update by the Infectious Diseases Society of America. Clin Infect Dis. 2014;59:e10–e52.

Strength of recommendation: A, good evidence for use; B, moderate evidence for use; C, poor evidence for use, optional; D, moderate evidence to support not using; E, good evidence to support not using. *Quality of evidence:* I, evidence from ≥1 properly randomized controlled trials; II, evidence from ≥1 well-designed clinical trials without randomization, case–control analytic studies, multiple time series, or dramatic results from uncontrolled experiments; III, evidence from expert opinion, clinical experience, descriptive studies, or reports of expert committees.

Qualitative (descriptive) recommendations: *strong, high:* strong recommendation, high-quality evidence from well-performed randomized controlled trials (RCTs) or exceptionally strong evidence from unbiased observational studies; *strong, moderate:* strong recommendation, moderate quality evidence from RCTs with important limitations or exceptionally strong evidence from unbiased observational studies; *strong, low:* strong recommendation, low-quality evidence for at least one critical outcome from observational studies, RCTs with serious flaws, or indirect evidence; *weak, moderate:* weak recommendation, moderate quality evidence from RCTs with important limitations or exceptionally strong evidence from unbiased observational studies; *weak, low:* weak recommendation, low-quality evidence for at least one critical outcome from observational studies, RCTs with serious flaws, or indirect evidence.

TABLE 48-3	Recommended Oral Drugs for Outpatient Treatment of Mild-to-Moderate SSTIs	
Infection	**Adults**	**Children**
Folliculitis	None; warm saline compresses usually sufficient	
Furuncles and carbuncles	Trimethoprim–sulfamethoxazole[a,b] Doxycycline[a,b] Minocycline[a,b]	Trimethoprim–sulfamethoxazole[a,b] Clindamycin[a,b]
Erysipelas	Procaine penicillin G Penicillin VK Clindamycin[a] Erythromycin[a]	Penicillin VK Clindamycin[a] Erythromycin[a]
Impetigo	Mupirocin ointment[a] Retapamulin ointment[a] Dicloxacillin Cephalexin Trimethoprim–sulfamethoxazole[a,b] Clindamycin[a,b] Doxycycline[a,b]	Mupirocin ointment[a] Retapamulin ointment[a] Dicloxacillin Cephalexin Trimethoprim–sulfamethoxazole[a] Clindamycin[a]
Lymphangitis	Initial IV therapy, followed by penicillin VK Clindamycin[a]	Initial IV therapy, followed by penicillin VK Clindamycin[a]
Cellulitis	Penicillin VK[c] Cephalexin[c] Dicloxacillin[c] Clindamycin[b,c] Trimethoprim–sulfamethoxazole[b,d] Doxycycline[b,d] Minocycline[b,d] Linezolid[b]	Penicillin VK[c] Cephalexin[c] Dicloxacillin[c] Clindamycin[b,c] Trimethoprim–sulfamethoxazole[b,d] Linezolid[b]
Diabetic foot infections	Dicloxacillin Clindamycin Cephalexin Amoxicillin–clavulanate Levofloxacin ± metronidazole or clindamycin[a,e] Ciprofloxacin ± metronidazole or clindamycin[a,e] Moxifloxacin	

(Continued)

TABLE 48-3	Recommended Oral Drugs for Outpatient Treatment of Mild-to-Moderate SSTIs (*Continued*)	
Infection	**Adults**	**Children**
Bite wounds (animal or human)	Amoxicillin–clavulanate	Amoxicillin–clavulanate
	Doxycycline[a]	Trimethoprim–sulfamethoxazole + metronidazole or clindamycin[a]
	Moxifloxacin[a]	
	Trimethoprim–sulfamethoxazole + metronidazole or clindamycin[a]	Cefuroxime axetil + metronidazole or clindamycin
	Levofloxacin or ciprofloxacin + metronidazole or clindamycin[a]	Dicloxacillin + penicillin VK
	Cefuroxime axetil + metronidazole or clindamycin	
	Dicloxacillin + penicillin VK	

[a]May be used in patients with penicillin allergy.
[b]Recommended if CA-MRSA is suspected.
[c]For nonpurulent cellulitis when CA-MRSA is not suspected, or purulent cellulitis when CA-MRSA not documented (not penicillin VK).
[d]May be combined with amoxicillin if additional coverage for streptococci is desired.
[e]Fluoroquinolone alone may be suitable for mild infections, while addition of drugs with antianaerobic activity may be recommended for more severe infections.

Cellulitis

- Cellulitis is an acute, spreading infectious process that initially affects the epidermis and dermis and may subsequently spread within the superficial fascia. Cellulitis is considered a serious disease because of the propensity of the infection to spread through lymphatic tissue and to the bloodstream. This process is characterized by inflammation but with little or no necrosis or suppuration of soft tissue.
- Cellulitis is most often caused by *S. pyogenes* or *S. aureus* (see **Table 48-1**).
- Acute cellulitis with mixed aerobic and anaerobic pathogens may occur in diabetics, following traumatic injuries, at sites of surgical incisions to the abdomen or perineum, or where host defenses have been otherwise compromised (vascular insufficiency).

CLINICAL PRESENTATION

- Cellulitis is characterized by erythema and edema of the skin. The lesions are nonelevated and have poorly defined margins. Tender lymphadenopathy associated with lymphatic involvement is common. Malaise, fever, and chills are also commonly present. There is usually a history of an antecedent wound from minor trauma, an ulcer, or surgery.
- A Gram stain of a smear obtained by injection and aspiration of 0.5 mL of saline (using a small-gauge needle) into the advancing edge of the erythematous lesion may help in making the microbiologic diagnosis but often yields negative results.

TREATMENT

- <u>Goals of Treatment</u>: The primary goal is the rapid eradication of the infection and prevention of further complications. Antimicrobial therapy of bacterial cellulitis is directed toward the type of bacteria either documented to be present or suspected. Local care of cellulitis includes elevation and immobilization of the involved area to decrease local swelling. Surgical intervention (incision and drainage) is rarely indicated in the treatment of uncomplicated cellulitis, but may play an important role in

TABLE 48-4 Drug Dosing Table[a]

Drug	Brand Name	Usual Dosing Range	Special Population Dose	Other
Oral agents				
Amoxicillin–clavulanate	Augmentin	875/125 mg orally every 12 hours	Pediatric: 40 mg/kg (of the amoxicillin component) orally in two divided doses	
Cefaclor	Ceclor	500 mg orally every 8 hours	Pediatric: 20–40 mg/kg/day (not to exceed 1 g) orally in three divided doses	
Cefadroxil	Duricef	250–500 mg orally every 12 hours	Pediatric: 30 mg/kg orally in two divided doses	
Cefuroxime axetil	Ceftin	250–500 mg orally every 12 hours	Pediatric: 20–30 mg/kg orally in two divided doses	
Cephalexin	Keflex	250–500 mg orally every 6 hours	Pediatric: 25–50 mg/kg orally in four divided doses	
Ciprofloxacin	Cipro	500–750 mg orally every 12 hours		
Clindamycin	Cleocin	300–600 mg orally every 6–8 hours	Pediatric: 10–30 mg/kg/day orally in three to four divided doses	May be used for oral treatment of MRSA infection
Delafloxacin	Baxdela	450 mg orally every 12 hours		May be used for oral treatment of MRSA infection
Dicloxacillin	Dynapen	250–500 mg orally every 6 hours	Pediatric: 25–50 mg/kg orally in four divided doses	
Doxycycline	Vibramycin	100–200 mg orally every 12 hours		May be used for oral treatment of MRSA infection
Erythromycin	E-Mycin Erythrocin	250–500 mg orally every 6 hours	Pediatric: 30–50 mg/kg orally in four divided doses[a]	
Levofloxacin	Levaquin	500–750 mg orally once daily		
Linezolid	Zyvox	600 mg orally every 12 hours	Pediatric: 20–30 mg/kg/day orally in two to three divided doses	For oral treatment of MRSA infection
Metronidazole	Flagyl	250–500 mg orally every 8 hours	Pediatric: 30 mg/kg orally in three to four divided doses	

Generic	Brand	Adult dose	Pediatric dose	Comments
Moxifloxacin	Avelox	400 mg orally once daily		
Mupirocin ointment	Bactroban	Apply to affected areas every 8 hours	Pediatric: apply to affected areas every 8 hours	
Penicillin VK	Veetids, Pen-V	250–500 mg orally every 6 hours	Pediatric: 25,000–90,000 units/kg orally in four divided doses	
Retapamulin ointment	Altabax	Apply to affected area every 12 hours	Pediatric: apply to affected area every 12 hours	
Tedizolid	Sivextro	200 mg orally once daily		For oral treatment of MRSA infection
Trimethoprim–sulfamethoxazole	Bactrim, Septra, Cotrimoxazole	160/800 mg orally every 12 hours	Pediatric: 4–6 mg/kg (of the trimethoprim component) orally every 12 hours	Up to double the usual dose may be considered for oral treatment of MRSA infection
Parenteral agents				
Ampicillin	Omnipen, Polycillin, Principen	1–2 g IV every 6 hours	Pediatric: 200–300 mg/kg/day IV in four to six divided doses	
Aztreonam	Azactam	1 g IV every 6 hours	Pediatric: 100–150 mg/kg/day IV in four divided doses	
Cefazolin	Ancef, Kefzol	1 g IV every 6–8 hours	Pediatric: 75 mg/kg/day IV in three divided doses	
Cefepime	Maxipime	1–2 g IV every 12 hours	Pediatric: 100 mg/kg/day IV in two divided doses	
Cefotaxime	Claforan	1–2 g IV every 6 hours	150–200 mg/kg/day in three to four divided doses	
Cefoxitin	Mefoxin	1–2 g IV every 6 hours	Pediatric: 30–40 mg/kg/day IV in four divided doses	
Ceftazidime	Fortaz	1–2 g IV every 8 hours	Pediatric: 150 mg/kg/day IV in three divided doses	

(Continued)

TABLE 48-4 Drug Dosing Table[a] (Continued)

Drug	Brand Name	Usual Dosing Range	Special Population Dose	Other
Ceftaroline	Teflaro	600 mg IV every 12 hours		For MRSA infection
Ceftriaxone	Rocephin	1 g IV once daily		
Cefuroxime	Zinacef	0.75–1.5 g IV every 8 hours	Pediatric: 150 mg/kg/day IV in three divided doses	
Ciprofloxacin	Cipro	400 mg IV every 8–12 hours		
Clindamycin	Cleocin	300–600 mg IV every 6–8 hours; 600–900 mg IV every 6–8 hours for necrotizing fasciitis	Pediatric: 30–50 mg/kg/day IV in three to four divided doses	
Dalbavancin	Dalvance	1000 mg IV once on day 1 of therapy, followed by 500 mg IV once on day 8 of therapy; OR 1500 mg IV once with no additional doses		For MRSA infection
Daptomycin	Cubicin	4 mg/kg IV once daily		For MRSA infection
Delafloxacin	Baxdela	300 mg IV every 12 hours		For MRSA infection
Doripenem	Doribax	500 mg IV every 8 hours		
Ertapenem	Invanz	1 g IV once daily	Pediatric: 30 mg/kg/day IV in one to two divided doses	
Gentamicin	Garamycin	Traditional: 2 mg/kg loading dose, followed by 1.5 mg/kg IV every 8 hours and guided by measured serum concentrations. Alternative: 5–7 mg/kg IV once daily	Pediatric: 5–7 mg/kg/day IV in three divided doses; doses guided by serum concentrations	
Imipenem–cilastatin	Primaxin	250–500 mg IV every 6–8 hours	Pediatric: 40–80 mg/kg/day IV in four divided doses	
Levofloxacin	Levaquin	500–750 mg IV once daily		

Drug	Brand	Dose	Pediatric Dose	Notes
Linezolid	Zyvox	600 mg IV every 12 hours	Pediatric: 20–30 mg/kg/day IV in two to three divided doses	For MRSA infection
Meropenem	Merrem	1 g IV every 8 hours	Pediatric: 60 mg/kg/day IV in three divided doses	
Metronidazole	Flagyl	500 mg IV every 8 hours	Pediatric: 30–50 mg/kg/day IV in three divided doses	
Moxifloxacin	Avelox	400 mg IV once daily		
Nafcillin	Nafcil	1–2 g IV every 4–6 hours	Pediatric: 100–200 mg/kg/day IV in four to six equally divided doses	
Oritavancin	Orbactiv	1200 mg IV once with no additional doses		For MRSA infection
Penicillin G	Pfizerpen Bicillin Wycillin	1–2 million units IV every 4–6 hours	Pediatric: 100,000–200,000 units/kg/day IV in four divided doses[a]	
Piperacillin–tazobactam	Zosyn	3.375–4.5 g IV every 6 hours	Pediatric: 250–350 mg/kg/day IV in three to four divided doses	
Procaine penicillin G	Bicillin C-R	0.6–1.2 million units IM every 12 hours	Pediatric: 25,000–50,000 units/kg (maximum 1.2 million units) IM once daily	
Tedizolid	Sivextro	200 mg IV once daily		For MRSA infection
Telavancin	Vibativ	10 mg/kg IV once daily		For MRSA infection
Tigecycline	Tigacil	100 mg IV once, and then 50 mg IV every 12 hours		For MRSA infection

(Continued)

TABLE 48-4 Drug Dosing Table[a] (Continued)

Drug	Brand Name	Usual Dosing Range	Special Population Dose	Other
Tobramycin	Nebcin	Traditional: 2 mg/kg loading dose, followed by 1.5 mg/kg IV every 8 hours and guided by measured serum concentrations. Alternative: 5–7 mg/kg IV once daily	Pediatric: 5–7 mg/kg/day IV in three divided doses; doses guided by serum concentrations	
Vancomycin	Vancocin	30–40 mg/kg/day IV in two divided doses; dosing guided by serum concentrations to achieve 24-hour AUC/MIC ratios of 400–600 for serious MRSA infections	Pediatric: 40–60 mg/kg/day IV in three to four divided doses; doses guided by serum concentrations	For MRSA infection

IM, intramuscularly; IV, intravenously; MRSA, methicillin-resistant *S. aureus*.
[a]Dosing guidelines in patients with normal renal function.

management of more severe or complicated cases. Systemic antibiotic therapy is often unnecessary in such cases.

- Antibiotic therapy is recommended along with incision and drainage in patients with more complicated abscesses associated with the following: severe or extensive disease involving multiple sites of infection; rapidly progressive infection in the presence of associated cellulitis; signs and symptoms of systemic illness; complicating factors such as extremes of age, comorbidities, or immunosuppression; abscesses in areas that are difficult to drain, such as hands, face, and genitalia; or lack of response to previous drainage alone.

- Oral agents recommended for moderate purulent cellulitis include **trimethoprim-sulfamethoxazole** and **doxycycline** (Fig. 48-1). Oral **linezolid** or **tedizolid** is also recommended in such cases but is significantly more expensive and apparently no more efficacious than other treatment options.

- Patients with severe purulent cellulitis should be hospitalized for empiric treatment with parenteral antibiotics having activity against MRSA. **Vancomycin, daptomycin, linezolid,** and **tedizolid** are all acceptable treatment options with comparable efficacy in adults (Fig. 48-1). In children, **vancomycin, linezolid,** or **clindamycin** are the preferred treatment options.

- Empiric therapy of nonpurulent cellulitis is directed primarily against group A β-hemolytic streptococci. Recommended empiric therapy of mild nonpurulent cellulitis (ie, no focus of purulence or systemic signs of infection) consists of an orally administered β-lactam such as **penicillin VK, cephalexin,** or **dicloxacillin**.

- Hospitalization and treatment with parenteral antibiotics are also recommended for patients with severe nonpurulent cellulitis as indicated by the presence of systemic findings of infection, failure of previous oral antibiotic therapy, immunocompromised states, or presence of clinical signs of deeper infection such as bullae, skin sloughing, hypotension, or organ dysfunction. Recommended regimens include vancomycin plus **piperacillin–tazobactam**, and **vancomycin** plus **imipenem–cilastatin** or **meropenem**.

- Empiric treatment of MRSA should be considered for patients with either moderate or severe nonpurulent cellulitis that is associated with penetrating trauma, evidence of MRSA infection at another site or nasal colonization with MRSA, injection drug use, or in patients meeting SIRS criteria (fever, tachycardia, tachypnea, or leukocytosis or leukopenia as previously defined). Recommended drugs for the coverage of MRSA in this setting are the same as those for purulent cellulitis.

Diabetic Foot Infections

- Three key factors are involved in the causation of diabetic foot problems: neuropathy, angipathy, and ischemia, and immunologic defects. Any of these disorders can occur in isolation; however, they frequently occur together.

- There are three major types of diabetic foot infections (DFIs): deep abscesses, cellulitis of the dorsum, and mal perforans ulcers of the sole of the foot. Osteomyelitis may occur in 30%–40% of infections.

- Mild cases of DFIs are often monomicrobial. However, more severe infections are typically polymicrobic; up to 60% of hospitalized patients have polymicrobial infections. Staphylococci and streptococci are the most common pathogens, although gram-negative bacilli and anaerobes occur in 50% of cases.

- Patients with peripheral neuropathy often do not experience pain but seek medical attention for swelling or erythema. Lesions vary in size and clinical features (eg, erythema, edema, warmth, presence of pus, draining sinuses, pain, and tenderness). A foul-smelling odor suggests anaerobic organisms. Temperature may be mildly elevated or normal.

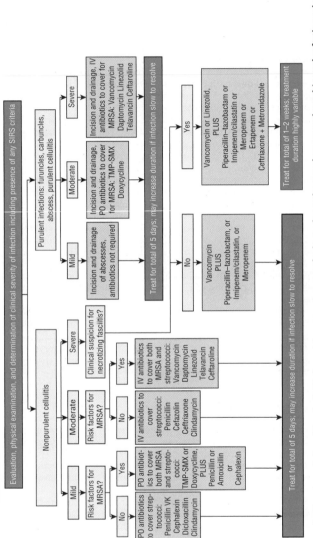

FIGURE 48-1. **Recommended treatment algorithm for initial empiric management of selected purulent and nonpurulent skin and soft-tissue infections.** GNR, aerobic gram-negative rods; GPC, aerobic gram-positive cocci; IV, intravenous; MRSA, methicillin-resistant *S. aureus*; PO, oral; SIRS, systemic inflammatory response syndrome; TMP-SMX, trimethoprim–sulfamethoxazole.

TREATMENT

- <u>Goals of Treatment</u>: The primary goals are to: (1) Successfully treat infected wounds by using effective nondrug and antibiotic therapy; (2) prevent additional infectious complications; (3) preserve as much normal limb function as possible; (4) avoid unnecessary use of antimicrobials that contribute to increased resistance; and (5) minimize toxicities and cost while increasing patient quality of life.
- Up to 90% of infections can be treated successfully with a comprehensive treatment approach that includes both wound care and antimicrobial therapy. After carefully assessing the extent of the lesion and obtaining necessary cultures, necrotic tissue must be thoroughly debrided, with wound drainage and amputation as required.
- Diabetic glycemic control should be maximized to ensure optimal healing.
- The patient should initially be restricted to bed rest, leg elevation, and control of edema, if present.
- Suggested antibiotic regimens for empiric treatment of DFIs are given in Table 48-5. Treatment algorithms for initial management of mild-to-moderate DFIs and severe DFIs are shown in Figs. 48-2 and 48-3.

Infected Pressure Injuries

- A pressure injury or "sore" is also called a "decubitus ulcer" or "bed sore." A classification system for pressure sores is presented in Table 48-6. Many factors are thought to predispose patients to the formation of pressure injuries: paralysis, paresis, immobilization, malnutrition, anemia, infection, and advanced age. Factors thought to be most critical to their formation are pressure, shearing forces, friction, and moisture; however, there is still debate as to the exact pathophysiology of pressure sore formation. The areas of highest pressure are generated over the bony prominences.
- Most pressure injuries are heavily colonized by microorganisms. A large variety of aerobic gram-positive and gram-negative bacteria, as well as anaerobes, are frequently isolated from wound cultures.

CLINICAL PRESENTATION

- Most pressure injuries are in the pelvic region and lower extremities. The most common sites are the sacral and coccygeal areas, ischial tuberosities, and greater trochanter.
- A dark red color on the surface of a pressure-injury related ulcer may indicate local infection. Surrounding erythema, swelling, and heat are commonly present with infection. Purulent discharge, foul odor, and systemic signs (fever and leukocytosis) may be present.
- Pressure injuries vary greatly in their severity, ranging from an abrasion to large lesions that can penetrate into the deep fascia involving both bone and muscle.

PREVENTION AND TREATMENT

- <u>Goals of Treatment</u>: The primary goal for pressure injuries is prevention. Once a pressure sore has developed, the goals of therapy are prevention of complications (ie, infections), preventing injuries from growing larger, and preventing the development of injuries in other locations.
- Prevention is the single most important aspect in managing pressure injuries. Friction and shearing forces can be minimized by proper positioning. Skin care and prevention of soilage are important, with the intent being to keep the surface relatively free from moisture. Relief for a period of only 5 minutes once every 2 hours gives protection against pressure injury formation.
- The goal of therapy is to clean and decontaminate the ulcer in order to permit formation of healthy granulation tissue that promotes wound healing or prepares the

TABLE 48-5 Suggested Antibiotic Regimens for Empiric Treatment of DFIs

Severity of Infection	Probable Pathogens	Drug(s)[a]	Duration of Therapy
Mild	*Staphylococcus aureus* (MSSA) *Streptococcus* spp. *S. aureus* (MRSA) • Patients with history of MRSA infection or colonization in past year • Prevalence of MRSA ≥50% in local geographic area • Recent hospitalization	Amoxicillin–clavulanate Cephalexin Dicloxacillin Clindamycin Levofloxacin Moxifloxacin[b]	1–2 weeks; may increase up to 4 weeks if infection slow to resolve
Moderate-to-severe (initially oral or IV antibiotics for moderately severe infections, IV antibiotics for severe infections)	MSSA *Streptococcus* spp. Enterobacteriaceae Obligate anaerobes MRSA • Patients with history of MRSA infection or colonization in past year • Prevalence of MRSA ≥30% in local geographic area • Recent hospitalization • Infection severe enough that not empirically covering MRSA poses unacceptable risk of treatment failure	Ampicillin/Sulbactam Cefoxitin Ceftriaxone Imipenem/Cilastatin Ertapenem Levofloxacin Moxifloxacin Tigecycline Levofloxacin or ciprofloxacin + clindamycin Add to one of the above regimens: • Vancomycin • Daptomycin	Moderately severe infection: 1–3 weeks; severe infection: 2–4 weeks

Pseudomonas aeruginosa • Patient has been soaking feet • Patient has previously failed therapy with nonpseudo-monal antibiotic regimen • Severe infection	Piperacillin/Tazobactam
Mixed infections potentially including all of the above	Cefepime, ceftazidime, or aztreonam + metronidazole or clindamycin + vancomycin[c] *or* Piperacillin–tazobactam or imipenem–cilastatin or meropenem[b] + vancomycin[c]

MRSA, methicillin-resistant *S. aureus*; MSSA, methicillin-susceptible *S. aureus*.

[a]Agents not shown in any particular order of preference.
[b]Not specifically recommended in IDSA guidelines but may be appropriate treatment option.
[c]Linezolid or daptomycin may be used in place of vancomycin.

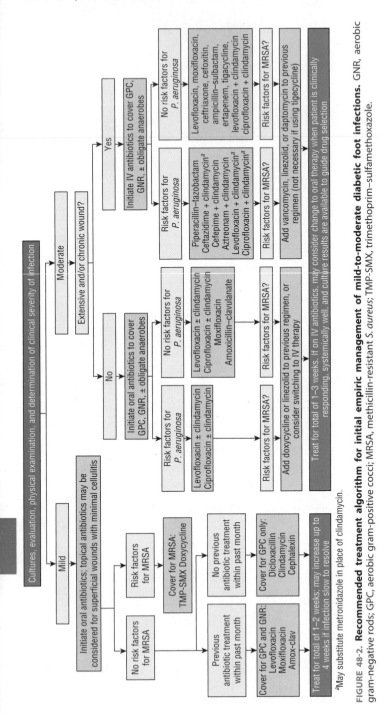

FIGURE 48-2. Recommended treatment algorithm for initial empiric management of mild-to-moderate diabetic foot infections. GNR, aerobic gram-negative rods; GPC, aerobic gram-positive cocci; MRSA, methicillin-resistant *S. aureus*; TMP-SMX, trimethoprim-sulfamethoxazole.

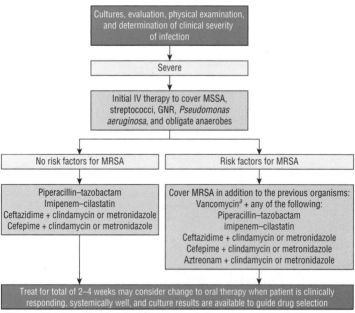

*a*May substitute linezolid or daptomycin for vancomycin.

FIGURE 48-3. Recommended treatment algorithm for initial empiric management of severe diabetic foot infections. GNR, aerobic gram-negative rods; MRSA, methicillin-resistant *S. aureus*; MSSA, methicillin-susceptible *S. aureus*.

wound for an operative procedure. The main factors to be considered for successful wound care are: (1) relief of pressure; (2) debridement of necrotic tissue; (3) wound cleansing; (4) dressing selection; and (5) prevention, diagnosis, and treatment of infection.

- Medical management is generally indicated for lesions that are of moderate size and of relatively shallow depth (stage 1 or 2 lesions) and are not located over a bony prominence. Surgical intervention is almost always necessary for ulcers that extend through superficial layers or into bone (stage 3, stage 4, and unstageable lesions).
- Debridement can be accomplished by surgical, mechanical (wet-to-dry dressing changes), or chemical means. Other effective therapies are hydrotherapy, wound irrigation, and dextranomers. Pressure injury wounds should be cleaned with normal saline.
- A short, 2-week trial of topical antibiotic (**silver sulfadiazine** or **triple antibiotic**) is recommended for a clean ulcer that is not healing or is producing a moderate amount of exudate despite appropriate care.
- Empiric therapy for infected pressure sores or associated infectious complications should cover MRSA, anaerobes, enterococci, and more resistant gram-negative bacteria such as Pseudomonas (see Table 48-5).

Infected Bite Wounds

- Patients at risk of acquiring an infection after a bite have had a puncture wound, have not sought medical attention within 8 hours of injury, or are older than 50 years.

TABLE 48-6	Pressure Injury Classification
Stage 1	Intact skin with a localized area of nonblanchable erythema. Presence of blanchable erythema or changes in sensation, temperature, or firmness may precede visual changes. Color changes do not include purple or maroon discoloration; these may indicate deep tissue pressure injury.
Stage 2	Partial-thickness loss of skin with exposed dermis. Wound bed is viable, pink or red, moist, and may also present as an intact or ruptured serum-filled blister. Adipose tissue is not visible and deeper tissues are not visible. Granulation tissue, slough, and eschar are not present.
Stage 3[a]	Full-thickness loss of skin, in which adipose tissue is visible in the ulcer and granulation tissue and epibole (rolled wound edges) are often present. Slough and/or eschar may be visible. Depth of tissue damage varies by anatomical location; areas of significant adiposity can develop deep wounds. Undermining and tunneling may occur. Fascia, muscle, tendon, ligament, cartilage, and/or bone are not exposed.
Stage 4[a]	Full-thickness skin and tissue loss with exposed or directly palpable fascia, muscle, tendon, ligament, cartilage, or bone in the ulcer. Slough and/or eschar may be visible. Epibole (rolled edges), undermining, and/or tunneling often occur. Depth varies by anatomical location.
Unstageable[a]	Full-thickness skin and tissue loss in which the extent of tissue damage within the ulcer cannot be confirmed because it is obscured by slough or eschar. If slough or eschar is removed, a stage 3 or stage 4 pressure injury will be revealed.
Deep-tissue pressure injury	Intact or nonintact skin with localized area of persistent nonblanchable deep red, maroon, purple discoloration or epidermal separation revealing a dark wound bed or blood-filled blister. Pain and temperature change often precede skin color changes. This injury results from intense and/or prolonged pressure and shear forces at the bone-muscle interface. The wound may evolve rapidly to reveal the actual extent of tissue injury, or may resolve without tissue loss.

[a]Stage 3, stage 4, and unstageable lesions are unlikely to resolve on their own and often require surgical intervention.

- Infections in bite wounds are caused predominantly by mouth flora from the animal or human biter, and from the victim's own skin flora.
- Most infections from dog and cat bites are polymicrobial. *Pasteurella* is the most frequent isolate.
- Bite wounds should be irrigated thoroughly with a copious volume of sterile water or saline, and the wound washed vigorously with soap or povidone–iodine in order to reduce the bacterial count in the wound. Surgical debridement and immobilization of the affected area are often required in dog and human bites associated with more extensive tissue injury.
- The role of antimicrobials for non-infected dog bite wounds remains controversial. A 3–5 day antibiotic prophylaxis regimen is recommended in patients with the following factors associated with increased risk for infection: immunocompromised; asplenic; advanced liver disease; preexisting or resultant edema of the affected area; moderate-to-severe bite-related injuries, especially to the hands or face; or bite injuries that have penetrated the periosteum or joint capsule.

- Empiric antibiotics for the treatment of established infection of dog and cat bite wounds should be directed at a variety of aerobic and anaerobic flora. **Amoxicillin–clavulanic** acid is commonly recommended for oral outpatient therapy. Alternative oral agents include **moxifloxacin** or **doxycycline** alone, or **trimethoprim–sulfamethoxazole, levofloxacin, ciprofloxacin**, or a second- or third-generation cephalosporin in combination with **metronidazole** or **clindamycin** to provide activity against oropharyngeal anaerobes.
- Treatment options for patients requiring IV therapy include β-lactam–β-lactamase inhibitors (**ampicillin–sulbactam** and **piperacillin–tazobactam**), second-generation cephalosporins with antianaerobic activity (**cefoxitin**), and **ertapenem**. Therapy should generally be continued from 7 to 14 days.
- If the immunization history of a patient with anything other than a clean minor wound is not known, or if the last known vaccination was longer than 10 years ago, tetanus/diphtheria toxoids (TD) should be administered. Both TD and tetanus immunoglobulin should be administered to patients who have never been immunized.
- If a patient has been exposed to rabies, postexposure procedures should be initiated and current treatment guidelines should be consulted for appropriate management recommendations.

Human Bites

- Human bite wounds are notable for potential involvement of *Eikenella corrodens* in approximately 30% of infections.
- Management of bite wounds consists of aggressive irrigation and topical wound dressing, surgical debridement, and immobilization of the affected area. Primary closure for human bites is not generally recommended. Tetanus toxoid and antitoxin may be indicated.
- Because transmission of viruses (HIV, herpes, hepatitis B and C) is a possibility with human bites, information about the biter is important. Bite victims exposed to blood-tainted saliva may be offered antiretroviral chemoprophylaxis, but each case should be individually assessed based on the potential for significant exposure and potential risks and benefits of antiretroviral therapy.
- All patients with human bite injuries should receive prophylactic antibiotic therapy ("early preemptive therapy") for 3–5 days due to high infection risk.
- **Amoxicillin–clavulanic** acid (500 mg every 8 hours) is commonly recommended.
- Patients with serious injuries or clenched-fist injuries should be started on IV antibiotics. Treatment options for patients requiring IV therapy include β-lactam–β-lactamase inhibitor combinations (**ampicillin–sulbactam, piperacillin–tazobactam**), second-generation cephalosporins with antianaerobic activity (eg, **cefoxitin**), and **ertapenem**.

See Chapter 133, Skin and Soft-Tissue Infections, authored by Douglas N. Fish, for a more detailed discussion of this topic.

Surgical Prophylaxis

49 CHAPTER

- Antibiotics administered prior to the contamination of previously sterile tissues or fluids are considered prophylactic. The goal of prophylactic antibiotics is to prevent an infection from developing.
- Presumptive antibiotic therapy is administered when an infection is suspected but not yet proven. Therapeutic antibiotics are required for established infection.
- *Surgical-site infections* (SSIs) are classified as either incisional (eg, cellulitis of the incision site) or involving an organ or space (eg, with meningitis). Incisional SSIs may be superficial (skin or subcutaneous tissue) or deep (fascial and muscle layers). Both types, by definition, occur by postoperative day 30. This period extends to 1 year from the date of surgery in the case of prosthesis implantation involvement with a deep incisional or organ/space infection.

RISK FACTORS FOR SURGICAL WOUND INFECTION

- The traditional classification system developed by the National Research Council (NRC) stratifying surgical procedures by infection risk is reproduced in Table 49-1. The NRC wound classification for a specific procedure is determined intraoperatively and is the primary determinant of whether antibiotic prophylaxis is warranted.
- The NRC classification system proposes that the risk of an SSI depends on the microbiology of the surgical site, the presence of a preexisting infection, the likelihood of contaminating previously sterile tissue during surgery, and the events during and after surgery. Abdominal operations, operations lasting more than 2 hours, contaminated or dirty procedures, and presence of more than three underlying medical diagnoses are factors associated with an increased incidence of SSI. When the NRC classification described in Table 49-1 was stratified by the number of SENIC risk factors present, the infection rates varied by as much as a factor of 15 within the same operative category.
- The SENIC risk assessment technique has been modified to include the American Society of Anesthesiologists preoperative assessment score (Table 49-2). An American Society of Anesthesiologists score greater than or equal to three was a strong predictor for the development of an SSI.

BACTERIOLOGY

- Bacteria involved in SSIs are acquired either from the patient's normal flora (endogenous) or from contamination during the surgical procedure (exogenous).
- The loss of normal flora through the use of broad-spectrum antibiotics can destabilize homeostasis, allowing pathogenic bacteria to proliferate and infection to occur.
- Normal flora can become pathogenic when translocated to a normally sterile tissue site or fluid during surgical procedures.
- The five most common pathogens encountered in surgical wounds are *Staphylococcus aureus*, coagulase-negative staphylococci, Enterococci, *Escherichia coli*, and *Pseudomonas aeruginosa*.
- Impaired host defenses, vascular occlusive states, traumatized tissues, and the presence of a foreign body greatly decrease the number of bacteria required to cause an SSI.

	SSI Rate (%)			
Classification	**Preoperative Antibiotics**	**No Preoperative Antibiotics**	**Criteria**	**Antibiotics**
Clean	0.8	5.1	No acute inflammation or transection of GI, oropharyngeal, genitourinary, biliary, or respiratory tracts; elective case, no technique break	Not indicated unless high-risk procedure[a]
Clean–contaminated	1.3	10.1	Controlled opening of aforementioned tracts with minimal spillage/minor technique break; clean procedures performed emergently or with major technique breaks	Prophylactic antibiotics indicated
Contaminated	10.2	21.9	Acute, nonpurulent inflammation present; major spillage/technique break during clean–contaminated procedure	Prophylactic antibiotics indicated
Dirty	N/A	N/A	Obvious preexisting infection present (abscess, pus, or necrotic tissue present)	Therapeutic antibiotics required

TABLE 49-1 National Research Council Wound Classification, Risk of Surgical Site Infection, and Indication for Antibiotics

GI, gastrointestinal; N/A, not applicable; SSI, surgical site infection.
[a]High-risk procedures include implantation of prosthetic materials and other procedures where surgical site infection is associated with high morbidity (see Chapter 146, *Dipiro's Pharmacotherapy: A Pathophysiologic Approach*, 12 ed.).

ANTIBIOTIC ISSUES

SCHEDULING ANTIBIOTIC ADMINISTRATION

- The following principles must be considered when providing antimicrobial surgical prophylaxis:
  - ✓ Antimicrobials should be delivered to the surgical site prior to the initial incision. They should be administered within 60 minutes prior to the initial incision, preferably at the time of anesthetic induction. Antibiotics should not be prescribed to be given "on-call to the OR (operating room)."
  - ✓ Bactericidal antibiotic tissue concentrations should be maintained throughout the surgical procedure.

TABLE 49-2	Surgical Site Infection Incidence (%) Stratified by NRC Wound Classification and SENIC Risk Factors[a]			
Number of SENIC Risk Factors	Clean	Clean–Contaminated	Contaminated	Dirty
0	1.1	0.6	N/A	N/A
1	3.9	2.8	4.5	6.7
2	8.4	8.4	8.3	10.9
3	15.8	17.7	11.0	18.8
4	N/A	N/A	23.9	27.4

N/A, not applicable; NRC, National Research Council; SENIC, Study on the Efficacy of Nosocomial Infection Control.

[a]Study on the Efficacy of Nosocomial Infection Control (SENIC) risk factors include abdominal operation, operations lasting >2 hours, contaminated or dirty procedures by National Research Council (NRC) classification, and more than three underlying medical diagnoses.

Data from Wilson AP, Hodgson B, Liu M, et al. Reduction in wound infection rates by wound surveillance with postdischarge follow-up and feedback. Br J Surg. 2006;93:630-638.

- Strategies to ensure appropriate antimicrobial prophylaxis use are described in Table 49-3.

ANTIMICROBIAL CHOICE

- The choice of the prophylactic antimicrobial depends on the type of surgical procedure, most likely pathogenic organisms, safety and efficacy of the antimicrobial, current literature evidence supporting its use, and cost.
- Typically, gram-positive coverage is included in the choice of surgical prophylaxis because organisms such as *S. aureus* and *S. epidermidis* are common skin flora.
- Parenteral antibiotic administration is favored because of its reliability in achieving suitable tissue concentrations.
- First-generation cephalosporins (particularly **cefazolin**) are the preferred choice, particularly for clean surgical procedures. Antianaerobic cephalosporins (eg, **cefoxitin** or **cefotetan**) are appropriate choices when broad-spectrum anaerobic and gram-negative coverage are desired.
- Although third-generation cephalosporins (eg, **ceftriaxone**) have been advocated for prophylaxis because of their increased gram-negative coverage and prolonged

TABLE 49-3	Strategies for Implementing an Institutional Program to Ensure Appropriate Use of Antimicrobial Prophylaxis in Surgery

1. **Educate:** Develop an educational program that enforces the importance and rationale of timely antimicrobial prophylaxis. Make this educational program available to all healthcare practitioners involved in the patient's care.

2. **Standardize the ordering process:** Establish a protocol (eg, a preprinted order sheet) that standardizes antibiotic choice according to current published evidence, formulary availability, institutional resistance patterns, and cost.

3. **Standardize the delivery and administration process:** Use system that ensures antibiotics are prepared and delivered to the holding area in a timely fashion. Standardize the administration time to <1 hour preoperatively. Designate responsibility and accountability for antibiotic administration. Provide visible reminders to prescribe/administer prophylactic antibiotics (eg, checklists). Develop a system to remind surgeons/nurses to readminister antibiotics intraoperatively during long procedures.

4. **Provide feedback:** Follow up with regular reports of compliance and infection rates.

half-lives, their inferior gram-positive and anaerobic activity and high cost have discouraged the widespread use of these agents.

- **Vancomycin** may be considered for prophylactic therapy in surgical procedures involving implantation of a prosthetic device in which the rate of methicillin-resistant *S. aureus* (MRSA) is high. If the risk of MRSA is low and a β-lactam hypersensitivity exists, **clindamycin** can be used instead of cefazolin in order to limit vancomycin use.

RECOMMENDATIONS FOR SPECIFIC TYPES OF SURGERIES

- Specific recommendations are summarized in Table 49-4.

GASTRODUODENAL SURGERY

- The risk of infection rises with conditions that increase gastric pH and subsequent bacterial overgrowth, such as obstruction, hemorrhage, malignancy, and acid-suppression therapy (clean-contaminated).
- A single dose of intravenous (IV) **cefazolin** given 30 minutes preoperatively will provide adequate prophylaxis for most cases.
- Postoperative therapeutic antibiotics may be indicated if perforation is detected during surgery, depending on whether an established infection is present.

HEPATOBILIARY SURGERY

- Antibiotic prophylaxis has been proven beneficial for surgery involving the biliary tract.
- Most frequently encountered organisms include *E. coli, Klebsiella*, and Enterococci. Single-dose prophylaxis with **cefazolin** is currently recommended. **Ciprofloxacin** and **levofloxacin** are alternatives for patients with β-lactam hypersensitivity undergoing open cholecystectomy.
- For patients undergoing elective laparoscopic cholecystectomy, antibiotic prophylaxis has traditionally not been recommended but newer trials and systematic reviews are conflicting and assessments of current practice are reflective of this.
- Detection of an active infection during surgery (gangrenous gallbladder or suppurative cholangitis) is an indication for therapeutic postoperative antibiotics.

COLORECTAL SURGERY

- Anaerobes and gram-negative aerobes predominate in SSIs (see Table 49-4), although gram-positive aerobes are also important. Therefore, the risk of an SSI in the absence of an adequate prophylactic regimen is substantial.
- Risk factors for SSIs include age over 60 years, hypoalbuminemia, poor preoperative bowel preparation, corticosteroid therapy, malignancy, and operations lasting longer than 3.5 hours.
- Reducing bacteria load with a thorough bowel preparation regimen (4 L of polyethylene glycol solution or 90 mL of sodium phosphate solution administered orally the day before surgery) is controversial, even though it is used by most surgeons.
- While oral or parenteral antimicrobials have been used, combination therapy (oral and IV) was superior to oral regimens alone and IV regimens alone. The combination of 1 g of **neomycin** and 1 g of **erythromycin base** given orally 19, 18, and 9 hours preoperatively is the most commonly used oral regimen in the United States. **Cefoxitin** and **cefotetan** are the IV agents used most commonly, but other second- and some third-generation cephalosporins also are effective.
- Postoperative antibiotics are unnecessary in the absence of any untoward events or findings during surgery.

APPENDECTOMY

- Preoperative antimicrobials are effective at reducing the risk of infection after appendectomy and should be administered in all cases.

TABLE 49-4 Most Likely Pathogens and Specific Recommendations for Surgical Prophylaxis

Type of Operation	Likely Pathogens	Recommended Prophylaxis Regimen[a]	Comments	Grade of Recommendation[b]
GI surgery				
Gastroduodenal	Enteric gram-negative bacilli, gram-positive cocci, oral anaerobes	Cefazolin 1 g × 1	High-risk patients only (obstruction, hemorrhage, malignancy, acid suppression therapy, morbid obesity)	IA
Bariatric Surgery	Enteric gram-negative bacilli, gram-positive cocci, oral anaerobes	Cefazolin 2 g × 1	Intraoperative redosing required for procedures longer than 4 hours	IB
Cholecystectomy	Enteric gram-negative bacilli, anaerobes	Cefazolin 1 g × 1 for high-risk patients; laparoscopic: controversial	High-risk patients only (open biliary tract procedures, acute cholecystitis, common duct stones, previous biliary surgery, jaundice, age >60 years, obesity, diabetes mellitus)	IA
Transjugular intrahepatic portosystemic shunt (TIPS)	Enteric gram-negative bacilli, anaerobes	Ceftriaxone 1 g × 1	Longer-acting cephalosporins preferred	IA
Appendectomy	Enteric gram-negative bacilli, anaerobes	Cefoxitin or cefotetan 1 g × 1 or cefazolin 1 g plus metronidazole 1 g × 1	Second intraoperative dose of cefoxitin may be required if procedure lasts longer than 3 hours	IA
Colorectal	Enteric gram-negative bacilli, anaerobes	Orally: neomycin 1 g + erythromycin base 1 g at 1, 2, and 11 pm 1 day preoperatively plus mechanical bowel preparation IV: cefoxitin or cefotetan 1 g × 1	Role of mechanical bowel preparation is controversial. It is widely used despite evidence suggesting it may have no effect on SSI or other clinical outcomes	IA

(Continued)

Procedure	Organisms	Antibiotic/Dose	Comments	Strength
GI endoscopy	Variable, depending on procedure, but typically enteric gram-negative bacilli, gram-positive cocci, oral anaerobes	Orally: amoxicillin 2 g × 1 IV: ampicillin 2 g × 1 or cefazolin 1 g × 1	Recommended only for high-risk patients undergoing high-risk procedures (see Chapter 146, *Dipiro's Pharmacotherapy: A Pathophysiologic Approach*, 12 ed.)	IA
Urologic surgery				
Prostate resection, shock-wave lithotripsy, ureteroscopy	*E. coli*	Ciprofloxacin 500 mg orally *or* Trimethoprim–sulfamethoxazole 1 DS tablet	All patients with positive preoperative urine cultures should receive a course of antibiotic treatment	IA–IB
Removal of external urinary catheters, cystography, urodynamic studies, simple cystourethroscopy	*E. coli*	Ciprofloxacin 500 mg orally *or* Trimethoprim–sulfamethoxazole 1 DS tablet	Should be considered only in patients with risk factors (see Chapter 146, *DiPiro's Pharmacotherapy: A Pathophysiologic Approach*, 12 ed.)	IB
Gynecological surgery				
Cesarean section	Enteric gram-negative bacilli, anaerobes, group B streptococci, enterococci	Cefazolin 1 g × 1 (<80 kg); Cefazolin 2 g × 1 (>80 kg); add azithromycin 500 mg IV × 1 if nonelective procedure	Antimicrobial administration should be prior to the initial incision as opposed to after umbilical cord clamping	IA
Hysterectomy	Enteric gram-negative bacilli, anaerobes, group B streptococci, enterococci	Vaginal: cefazolin 2 g × 1 (3 g if >120 kg); Abdominal: cefotetan 1 g × 1 or cefazolin 2 g × 1	Metronidazole 1 g IV × 1 is recommended alternative for penicillin allergy	IA
Head and neck surgery				
Maxillofacial surgery	*Staphylococcus aureus*, streptococci spp., oral anerobes	Cefazolin 2 g or clindamycin 600 mg	Repeat intraoperative dose for operations longer than 4 hours	IA

TABLE 49-4 Most Likely Pathogens and Specific Recommendations for Surgical Prophylaxis *(Continued)*

Type of Operation	Likely Pathogens	Recommended Prophylaxis Regimen[a]	Comments	Grade of Recommendation[b]
Head and neck cancer resection	S. aureus, streptococci spp., oral anerobes	Clindamycin 600 mg at induction and every 8 hours × 2 more doses	Add gentamicin for clean–contaminated procedures	IA
Cardiothoracic surgery				
Cardiac surgery	S. aureus, S. epidermidis, Corynebacterium	Cefazolin 1 g every 8 hours × 48 hours Intranasal mupirocin twice daily for 5 days preoperatively for patients colonized with S. aureus	Patients >80 kg (>176 lb) should receive 2 g of cefazolin instead; in areas with high prevalence of S. aureus resistance, vancomycin should be considered	IA
Thoracic surgery	S. aureus, S. epidermidis, Corynebacterium, enteric gram-negative bacilli	Cefuroxime 750 mg IV every 8 hours × 48 hours	First-generation cephalosporins are deemed inadequate, and shorter durations of prophylaxis have not been adequately studied	IA
Vascular surgery				
Abdominal aorta and lower extremity vascular surgery	S. aureus, S. epidermidis, enteric gram-negative bacilli	Cefazolin 1 g at induction and every 8 hours × 2 more doses	Although complications from infections may be infrequent, graft infections are associated with significant morbidity	IB
Orthopedic surgery				
Joint replacement	S. aureus, S. epidermidis	Cefazolin 1 g × 1 preoperatively, then every 8 hours × 2 more doses Intranasal mupirocin twice daily for 5 days preoperatively for patients colonized with S. aureus	Vancomycin reserved for penicillin-allergic patients or where institutional prevalence of methicillin-resistant S. aureus warrants use	IA
Hip fracture repair	S. aureus, S. epidermidis	Cefazolin 1 g × 1 preoperatively, then every 8 hours for 48 hours	Compound fractures are treated as if infection is presumed	IA

Open/Compound fractures	S. aureus, S. epidermidis, gram-negative bacilli, polymicrobial	Cefazolin 1 g × 1 preoperatively, then every 8 hours for a course of presumed infection	Gram-negative coverage (ie, gentamicin) often indicated for severe open fractures	IA
Neurosurgery				
CSF shunt procedures	S. aureus, S. epidermidis	Cefazolin 1 g every 8 hours × 3 doses or ceftriaxone 2 g × 1	No agents have been shown to be better than cefazolin in randomized comparative trials	IA
Spinal surgery	S. aureus, S. epidermidis	Cefazolin 1 g × 1	Limited number of clinical trials comparing different treatment regimens	IB
CSF shunt procedures	S. aureus, S. epidermidis	Cefazolin 1 g every 8 hours × 3 doses or ceftriaxone 2 g × 1	No agents have been shown to be better than cefazolin in randomized comparative trials	IA
Craniotomy	S. aureus, S. epidermidis	Cefazolin 1 g × 1 or cefotaxime 1 g × 1	Vancomycin 1 g IV × 1 can be substituted for patients with penicillin allergy	IA

CSF, cerebrospinal fluid; DS, double strength.

[a]One-time doses are optimally infused at induction of anesthesia except as noted. Repeat doses may be required for long procedures. See Chapter 146, *Dipiro's Pharmacotherapy: A Pathophysiologic Approach*, 12 ed., for references.

[b]Strength of recommendations: Category IA: Strongly recommended and supported by well-designed experimental, clinical, or epidemiologic studies. Category IB: Strongly recommended and supported by some experimental, clinical, or epidemiologic studies and strong theoretical rationale. Category II: Suggested and supported by suggestive clinical or epidemiologic studies or theoretical rationale.

- A cephalosporin with antianaerobic activity, such as **cefoxitin** or **cefotetan**, is recommended as first-line therapy; however, cefotetan may be superior for longer operations because of its longer duration of action.
- Single-dose therapy with cefotetan is adequate. Intraoperative dosing of cefoxitin may be required if the procedure extends beyond 3 hours.

UROLOGIC PROCEDURES

- As long as the urine is sterile preoperatively, the risk of SSI after urologic procedures is low, and the benefit of prophylactic antibiotics in this setting is controversial. *E. coli* is the most frequently encountered organism.
- Antibiotic prophylaxis is warranted for all patients undergoing transurethral resection of the prostate or bladder tumors, shock wave lithotripsy, percutaneous renal surgery, or ureteroscopy.
- Specific recommendations are listed in Table 49-4.
- Urologic procedures requiring an abdominal approach such as a nephrectomy or cystectomy require prophylaxis appropriate for a clean-contaminated abdominal procedure.

CESAREAN SECTION

- Antibiotics are efficacious to prevent SSIs for all women undergoing cesarean section regardless of underlying risk factors.
- **Cefazolin** remains the drug of choice and a single 2-g IV dose for patients weighing 80 kg or more and a single 1-g dose for patients weighing less than 80 kg is recommended. For patients with a β-lactam allergy, preoperative **metronidazole** is an acceptable alternative. Azithromycin should be administered in addition to the standard cephalosporin regimen for patients undergoing nonelective cesarean section.
- Antimicrobial administration should occur at the time of the initial incision instead of at the time of umbilical cord clamping.

HYSTERECTOMY

- Vaginal hysterectomies are associated with a high rate of postoperative infection when performed without the benefit of prophylactic antibiotics.
- A single preoperative dose of **cefazolin** or **cefoxitin** is recommended for vaginal hysterectomy. For patients with β-lactam hypersensitivity, a single preoperative dose of **metronidazole** or **doxycycline** is effective.
- Abdominal hysterectomy SSI rates are correspondingly lower than vaginal hysterectomy rates. However, prophylactic antibiotics are still recommended regardless of underlying risk factors.
- First- (cefazolin), second- (cefotetan), or third-generation cephalosporins can be used for prophylaxis.

HEAD AND NECK SURGERY

- Use of prophylactic antibiotics during head and neck surgery depends on the procedure type. Clean procedures, such as thyroidectomy or a simple tooth extraction, are associated with low rates of SSI and antimicrobial prophylaxis is not recommended. Head and neck procedures involving an incision through a mucosal layer carry a high risk of SSI.
- Specific recommendations for prophylaxis are listed in Table 49-4.
- Although typical doses of **cefazolin** are ineffective for anaerobic infections, the recommended 2-g dose produces concentrations high enough to be inhibitory to these organisms. A 24-hour duration has been used in most studies, but single-dose therapy may also be effective.
- A single dose of **clindamycin** is adequate for prophylaxis in maxillofacial surgery unless the procedure lasts longer than 4 hours, when a second dose should be administered intraoperatively. For most head and neck cancer resection surgeries, including free-flap reconstruction, 24 hours of clindamycin is appropriate.

CARDIAC SURGERY

- Although most cardiac surgeries are technically clean procedures, prophylactic antibiotics have been shown to lower rates of SSI.
- The usual pathogens are skin flora (see Table 49-4) and, rarely, gram-negative enteric organisms.
- Risk factors for developing an SSI after cardiac surgery include obesity, renal insufficiency, connective tissue disease, reexploration for bleeding, and poorly timed administration of antibiotics.
- **Cefazolin** has been extensively studied and is currently considered the drug of choice. Patients weighing more than 80 kg should receive 2 g cefazolin rather than 1 g. Doses should be administered no earlier than 60 minutes before the first incision and no later than the beginning of induction of anesthesia.
- Extending antibiotic administration beyond 48 hours does not lower SSI rates.
- **Vancomycin** use may be justified in hospitals with a high incidence of SSI with MRSA or when sternal wounds are to be explored for possible mediastinitis.

NONCARDIAC VASCULAR SURGERY

- Prophylactic antibiotics are beneficial, especially in procedures involving the abdominal aorta and the lower extremities.
- Twenty-four hours of prophylaxis with IV **cefazolin** is adequate. For patients with β-lactam allergy, 24 hours of oral **ciprofloxacin** is effective.

ORTHOPEDIC SURGERY

- Prophylactic antibiotics are beneficial in cases involving implantation of prosthetic material (pins, plates, and artificial joints).
- The most likely pathogens mirror those of other clean procedures and include staphylococci and, infrequently, gram-negative aerobes.
- **Cefazolin** is the drug of choice. For hip fracture repairs and joint replacements, it should be administered for 24 hours. **Vancomycin** is not recommended unless a patient has a history of β-lactam hypersensitivity or the propensity for MRSA infection at the institution necessitates its use.

NEUROSURGERY

- The use of prophylactic antibiotics in neurosurgery is controversial.
- Single doses of **cefazolin** appear to lower SSI risk after craniotomy.

See Chapter 146, Antimicrobial Prophylaxis in Surgery, authored by Salmaan Kanji, for a more detailed discussion of this topic.

Tuberculosis

- *Tuberculosis* (TB) is a communicable infectious disease caused by *Mycobacterium tuberculosis*. It can produce silent, latent infection, as well as progressive, active disease. In 2019, there were about 10 million new cases and 1.2 million deaths from TB reported.

PATHOPHYSIOLOGY AND ETIOLOGY

- *M. tuberculosis* is transmitted from person to person by coughing or other activities that cause the organism to be aerosolized. Close contacts of TB patients are most likely to become infected.
- Human immunodeficiency virus (HIV) is the most important risk factor for progressing to active TB, especially among people 25–44 years of age. An HIV-infected individual with TB infection is over 100-fold more likely to develop active disease than an HIV-seronegative persons.
- Approximately 90% of patients who experience primary disease have no further clinical manifestations other than a positive skin or blood test for immune response (70%), whereas some also have radiographic evidence of stable granulomas. The radiodense area is referred to as a *Ghon complex*.
- Approximately 10% of patients develop reactivation disease, nearly half of these cases occur within 2 years of infection. In the United States, most cases of TB are believed to result from reactivation.
- Occasionally, a massive inoculum of organisms may be introduced into the bloodstream, causing widely disseminated disease and granuloma formation known as *miliary TB*.

CLINICAL PRESENTATION AND DIAGNOSIS

- Patients with TB typically present with weight loss, fatigue, a productive cough, fever, and night sweats. Symptom onset may be gradual.
- Frank hemoptysis usually occurs late in the course of disease but may present earlier.
- On physical examination, the patient is usually thin with evidence or recent weight loss. Dullness to chest percussion, rales, and increased vocal fremitus are often present, but a normal lung examination is common compared to the degree of radiological lung involvement.
- The white blood cell (WBC) count is usually moderately elevated with lymphocyte predominance. A high platelet count (thrombocytosis) and mild-to-moderate anemia are common.
- Sputum smear is done to detect mycobacteria. A fiber-optic bronchoscopy is performed if sputum tests are inconclusive and suspicion is high.
- Chest radiograph shows patchy or nodular infiltrates in the apical areas of the upper lobes or the superior segment of the lower lobes. There may be cavitation that shows air–fluid levels as the infection progresses.
- Clinical features associated with extrapulmonary TB vary depending on the organ system(s) involved but typically consist of slowly progressive decline of organ function with low-grade fever and other constitutional symptoms.
- Patients with HIV may have atypical presentation. HIV-positive patients are less likely to have positive skin tests, cavitary lesions, or fever. They have a higher incidence of extrapulmonary TB and are more likely to present with progressive primary disease.
- TB in older persons is easily confused with other respiratory diseases. It is far less likely to present with positive skin tests, fevers, night sweats, sputum production, or hemoptysis. TB in children may present as typical bacterial pneumonia and is called *progressive primary TB*.

TABLE 50-1 Criteria for Tuberculosis Positivity

Reaction ≥5 mm of Induration	Reaction ≥10 mm of Induration	Reaction ≥15 mm of Induration
HIV-infected persons A recent contact of a person with TB disease Fibrotic changes on chest radiograph consistent with prior TB	Recent immigrants (ie, within the last 5 years) from high-prevalence countries Injection drug users Residents and employees[a] of the following high-risk congregate settings: prisons and jails, nursing homes and other long-term facilities for the elderly, hospitals and other healthcare facilities, residential facilities for patients with AIDS, and homeless shelters	Persons with no risk factors for TB
Patients with organ transplants and other immunosuppressed patients (receiving the equivalent of 15 mg/day or more of prednisone for 1 month or longer, taking TNF-α antagonists)[a]	Mycobacteriology laboratory personnel, persons with the following clinical conditions that place them at high risk: silicosis, diabetes mellitus, chronic renal failure, some hematologic disorders, other specific malignancies, gastrectomy, and jejunoileal bypass Children younger than 5 years of age or infants, children, and adolescents exposed to adults at high risk	

Interpretation of Interferon Gamma Release Assay (IGRA) Results

The interpretation of IGRAs is based on the amount of IFN-γ, in T-SPOT®.TB. An IGRA is recommended over a tuberculin skin test (TST) in persons at least 5 years of age who are likely to have *M. tuberculosis* infection; who are at low or moderate risk of the disease progressing; in whom it has been determined that latent tuberculosis infection (LTBI) testing is necessary; and who have been vaccinated against Calmette-Guerin or are not likely to return for follow up after a TST. The TST is a viable second option in certain circumstances, such as if an IGRA is unavailable. Laboratories should provide both the qualitative and quantitative results.

Qualitative results are reported positive, negative, indeterminate, or borderline.

Quantitative results are reported as numerical values that include a response to the TB antigen and two controls, nil and mitogen.

Quantitative results may be useful for clinical decision making in individual cases, in combination with risk factors.

AIDS, acquired immunodeficiency syndrome; HIV, human immunodeficiency virus; TB, tuberculosis.
[a]Risk of TB for patients treated with corticosteroids increases with higher dose and longer duration.
Data from Centers for Disease Control and Prevention. Screening for tuberculosis and tuberculosis infection in high-risk populations: recommendations of the Advisory Council for the Elimination of Tuberculosis. M.M.W.R. 1995;44(No. RR-11):19–34.

- The most widely used screening method for TB infection is the tuberculin skin test, which uses purified protein derivative (PPD). Populations most likely to benefit from skin testing are listed in **Table 50-1**. Testing for latent TB is summarized in **Fig. 50-1**.
- The Mantoux method of PPD administration consists of the intracutaneous injection of PPD containing five tuberculin units. The test is read 48–72 hours after injection by measuring the diameter of the zone of induration.
- Some patients may exhibit a positive test when retested 1 week after an initial negative test; this is referred to as a *booster effect*.

Group	Testing Strategy	Considerations
Likely to Be Infected **High** Risk of Progression (TST ≥5 mM)	**Adults** **Acceptable:** IGRA OR TST Consider dual testing where a positive result from either result would be considered **positive** **Children ≤5 years of age** **Acceptable:** TST **Acceptable:** IGRA OR TST Consider dual testing where a positive result from either result would be considered **positive**[a]	
Likely to Be Infected **Low** to **Intermediate** Risk of Progression (TST ≥10 mM)	**Preferred:** IGRA where available **Acceptable:** IGRA or TST	Prevalence of BCG vaccination Expertise of staff and/or laboratory Test availability Patient perceptions Staff perceptions Programmatic concerns

Unlikely to Be Infected
(TST >15 mM)
	Testing for LTBI is not recommended
	If necessary:
	    Preferred: IGRA where available
	    Acceptable: Either IGRA OR TST
	For serial testing:
	    Acceptable: Either IGRA OR TST
	
	Consider repeat or dual testing where a negative result from either would be considered **negative**[b]	

[a]Performing a second diagnostic test when the initial test is a negative is a strategy to increase sensitivity. This may reduce specificity, but the panel decided that this is an acceptable trade off in situations in which the consequences of missing LTBI exceed the consequences of inappropriate therapy. [b]Performing a confirmatory test following an initial positive result is based upon both the evidence that false-positive results are common among individuals who are unlikely to be infected with *M. tuberculosis* and the committee's presumption that performing a second test on those patients whose initial test was positive will help identify initial false-positive results. (Reprinted with permission from Lewinsohn D, Leonard M. Official American Thoracic Society/Infectious Diseases Society of America/Centers for Disease Control and Prevention Clinical Practice Guidelines: Diagnosis of Tuberculosis in Adults and Children. 2017;64:e1–e33.)

FIGURE 50-1. Summary of recommendations for testing for latent tuberculosis infection (LTBI).

- Interferon-γ release assays (IGRA) measure the release of INF-γ in blood in response to the TB antigens. IGRA may provide quick and specific results for identifying *M. tuberculosis*.
- Confirmatory diagnosis of a clinical suspicion of TB must be made via chest radiograph and microbiologic examination of sputum or other infected material to rule out active disease.
- When active TB is suspected, attempts should be made to isolate *M. tuberculosis* from the infected site. Daily sputum collection over 3 consecutive days is recommended.

TREATMENT

- <u>Goals of Treatment</u>: The goals are: (1) rapid identification of a new TB case; (2) initiation of specific anti-TB treatment; (3) eradicating *M. tuberculosis* infection; (4) achievement of a noninfectious state in the patient, thus ending isolation; (5) preventing the development of resistance; (6) adherence to the treatment regimen by the patient; and (7) cure of the patient as quickly as possible (generally at least 6 months of treatment).
- Patients with active disease should be isolated to prevent spread of the disease.
- Patients with active disease should receive four drugs.
- Drug treatment is the cornerstone of TB management. A minimum of two drugs, and generally three or four drugs, must be used simultaneously. Directly observed therapy (DOT) by a healthcare worker is a cost-effective way to ensure completion of treatment and is considered the standard of care.
- Drug treatment is continued for at least 6 months, and 18–24 months for cases of multidrug-resistant TB (MDR-TB).
- Debilitated patients may require therapy for other medical conditions, including substance abuse and HIV infection, and some may need nutritional support.
- Surgery may be needed to remove destroyed lung tissue, space-occupying lesions, and some extrapulmonary lesions.

PHARMACOLOGIC THERAPY

LATENT INFECTION

- As described in Table 50-2, chemoprophylaxis should be initiated in patients to reduce the risk of progression to active disease. There are three recommended treatment regimens for latent tuberculosis infection (LTBI): 3 months of once-weekly **isoniazid** plus **rifapentine**, 4 months of daily rifampin, or 3 months of daily isoniazid plus rifampin.
- The CDC recommends the 12-week **isoniazid/rifapentine** regimen as an equal alternative to 9 months of daily isoniazid for treating LTBI in otherwise healthy patients aged 12 years or older who have a predictive factor for greater likelihood of developing active TB, which included recent exposure to contagious TB, conversion from negative to positive on an indirect test for infection (ie, interferon-gamma release assays [IGRA] or tuberculin skin test), and radiographic findings of healed pulmonary TB.
- Pregnant females, persons who misuse alcohol, and those with poor diets who are treated with isoniazid should receive pyridoxine, 10–50 mg daily, to reduce the incidence of central nervous system (CNS) effects or peripheral neuropathies.

TREATING ACTIVE DISEASE

- Table 50-3 lists options for treatment of culture-positive pulmonary TB caused by drug-susceptible organisms. Doses of antituberculosis drugs are given in Table 50-4. Other sources should be consulted for treatment recommendations when TB is concurrent with HIV infection. The standard TB treatment regimen is **isoniazid, rifampin, pyrazinamide**, and **ethambutol** for 2 months, followed by isoniazid and rifampin for 4 months. Ethambutol can be stopped if susceptibility to isoniazid, rifampin, and pyrazinamide is shown.

TABLE 50-2	Doses Recommended for Latent Tuberculosis Treatment Regimens	
Drug	**Duration**	**Dose**
Isoniazid and rifapentine	Once weekly for 3 months	Adults and children ≥12 years:
		Isoniazid: 15 mg/kg
		Rifapentine:
		10–14 kg: 300 mg
		14.1–25 kg: 450 mg
		25.1–32 kg: 600 mg
		32.1–49.9 kg: 750 mg
		≥50 kg: 900 mg
		Children 2–11 years:
		Isoniazid: 25 mg/kg
		Rifapentine: see above
Isoniazid and rifampin	Daily for 3 months	Adult:
		Isoniazid: 5 mg/kg
		Rifampin: 10 mg/kg
		Children:
		Isoniazid: 10–20 mg/kg
		Rifampin: 15–20 mg/kg
Rifampin	Daily for 4 months	Adults: 10 mg/kg
		Children: 15–20 mg/kg

Data from Sterling TR, Njie G, Zenner D, et al. Guidelines for the Treatment of Latent Tuberculosis Infection: Recommendations from the National Tuberculosis Controllers Association and CDC, 2020. MMWR Recomm Rep. 2020;69:1.

- Appropriate samples should be sent for culture and susceptibility testing prior to initiating therapy for all patients with active TB. The data should guide the initial drug selection for the new patient. If susceptibility data are not available, the drug resistance pattern in the area where the patient likely acquired TB should be used.
- If the patient is being evaluated for the retreatment of TB, it is imperative to know what drugs were used previously and for how long.
- The standard TB treatment regimen is isoniazid, rifampin, pyrazinamide, and ethambutol for 2 months, followed by isoniazid and rifampin for 4 months, a total of 6 months of treatment.
- Patients who are slow to respond, those who remain culture positive at 2 months of treatment, those with cavitary lesions on chest radiograph, and HIV-positive patients should be treated for 9 months and for at least 6 months from the time they convert to smear and culture negativity.

DRUG RESISTANCE

- If the organism is drug resistant, the aim is to introduce two or more active agents that the patient has not received previously. With MDR-TB, no standard regimen can be proposed. It is critical to avoid monotherapy or adding only a single drug to a failing regimen.
- Drug resistance should be suspected in the following situations:
  - ✓ Patients who have received prior therapy for TB.
  - ✓ Patients from geographic areas with a high prevalence of resistance (South Africa, Mexico, Southeast Asia, the Baltic countries, and the former Soviet states).

TABLE 50-3 Drug Regimens for Microbiologically Confirmed Pulmonary Tuberculosis Caused by Drug Susceptible Organisms

		Initial Phase		Continuation Phase	
Regimen	Drugs[a]	Interval and Doses (Minimal Duration)[b]	Drugs	Interval and Doses[a]	Comments[b,c]
1	Isoniazid Rifampin Pyrazinamide Ethambutol	Daily for 8 weeks, 7 days/week for 56 doses or 5 days/week for 40 doses[d]	Isoniazid/ Rifampin	7 days/week for 126 doses (18 weeks) or 5 days/week for 90 doses (18 weeks)[c]	This is preferred regimen for patient with newly diagnosed pulmonary TB.
2	Isoniazid Rifampin Pyrazinamide Ethambutol	Daily for 8 weeks, 7 days/week for 56 doses or 5 days/week for 40 doses[d]	Isoniazid/ Rifampin	Three times weekly for 54 doses (18 weeks)[e]	Preferred alternative regimen in situations in which more frequent DOT during continuation phase is difficult to achieve.
3	Isoniazid Rifampin Pyrazinamide Ethambutol	3 times weekly for 8 weeks (24 doses)	Isoniazid/ Rifampin	Three times weekly for 54 doses (18 weeks)	Use regimen with caution in patients with HIV and/or cavitary disease. Missed doses can lead to treatment failure, relapse, and acquired drug resistance.

(Continued)

TABLE 50-3	Drug Regimens for Microbiologically Confirmed Pulmonary Tuberculosis Caused by Drug Susceptible Organisms *(Continued)*				
	Initial Phase		**Continuation Phase**		
Regimen	Drugs[a]	Interval and Doses (Minimal Duration)[b]	Drugs	Interval and Doses[a]	Comments[b,c]
4	Isoniazid Rifampin Ethambutol Pyrazinamide	Daily for 2 weeks, then twice weekly for 6 weeks. 7 days/week for 14 doses, then twice weekly for 12 doses[e]	Isoniazid/ Rifampin	Twice weekly for 36 doses (18 weeks)	Do not use twice weekly regimens in HIV-infected patients or patients with smear positive and/ or cavitary disease. If doses are missed, then therapy is equivalent to once weekly, which is inferior.

DOT, directly observed therapy; EMB, ethambutol; HIV, human immunodeficiency virus; INH, isoniazid; PZA, pyrazinamide; RIF, rifampin.

[a]When DOT is used, drugs may be given 5 days/week and the necessary number of doses adjusted accordingly. Although there are no studies that compare 5 with 7 daily doses, extensive experience indicates this would be an effective practice. DOT should be used when drugs are administered <7 days/week.

[b]Based on expert opinion, patients with cavitation on initial chest radiograph and positive cultures at completion of 2 months of therapy should receive a 7-month (31-week) continuation phase.

[c]Pyridoxine (vitamin B₆), 25–50 mg/day, is given with INH to all persons at risk of neuropathy (eg, pregnant women; breastfeeding infants; persons with HIV; patients with diabetes, alcoholism, malnutrition, or chronic renal failure; or patients with advanced age). For patients with peripheral neuropathy, experts recommend increasing pyridoxine dose to 100 mg/day.

[d]Five-day-a-week administration is always given by DOT.

[e]Alternatively, some US TB control programs have administered intensive-phase regimens 5 days/week for 15 doses (3 weeks), then twice weekly for 12 doses.

Reprinted, with permission, from Nahid P, et al. Executive Summary: Official American Thoracic Society/Centers for Disease Control and Prevention/Infectious Diseases Society of America Clinical Practice Guidelines: Treatment of Drug-Susceptible Tuberculosis, Clinical Infectious Diseases, Volume 63, Issue 7, 1 October 2016, pp. 853–867.

TABLE 50-4 Suggested Starting Doses[a] of First-Line Antituberculosis Drugs for Adults and Children[b,c]

Drug	Preparation	Adults/ Children	Typical Doses			
			Daily	1 × Per Week	2 × Per Week	3 × Per Week
First-Line Drugs						
Isoniazid	Tablets (50, 100, 300 mg); elixir (50 mg/5 mL); aqueous solution (100 mg/mL) for IV or intramuscular injection	Adults[c]	5 mg/kg	15 mg/kg	15 mg/kg	15 mg/kg
		Children[c]	10–15 mg/kg	—	20–30 mg/kg	—
Rifampin	Capsule (150, 300 mg); powder may be suspended for oral administration; aqueous solution for IV injection	Adults[d,e]	10 mg/kg	—	10 mg/kg	10 mg/kg
		Children[c]	10–20 mg/kg	—	10–20 mg/kg	—
Rifabutin	Capsule (150 mg)	Adult[d,e]	5 mg/kg	—	—	—
		Children	Appropriate dosing for children is unknown	Appropriate dosing for children is unknown	Appropriate dosing for children is unknown	Appropriate dosing for children is unknown
Rifapentine	Tablet (150 mg, film coated)	Adults[c]	20 mg per kg daily is now being used for active TB	—	—	—
		Children	The drug is not approved for use in children	The drug is not approved for use in children	The drug is not approved for use in children	The drug is not approved for use in children
Pyrazinamide	Tablet (500 mg, scored)	Adults[c]	Weight 40–55 kg: 1000 mg; Weight 56–75 kg: 1500 mg	—	Weight 40–55 kg: 2000 mg; Weight 56–75 kg: 3000 mg	Weight 40–55 kg: 1500 mg; Weight 56–75 kg: 2500 mg

(Continued)

531

TABLE 50-4 Suggested Starting Doses[a] of First-Line Antituberculosis Drugs for Adults and Children[b,c] (*Continued*)

Drug	Preparation	Adults/ Children	Typical Doses			
			Daily	1× Per Week	2× Per Week	3× Per Week
			Weight 76–90 kg: 2000 mg	—	Weight 76–90 kg: 4000 mg	Weight 76–90 kg: 3000 mg
		Children[c]	15–30 mg/kg	—	50 mg/kg	—
Ethambutol	Tablet (100, 400 mg)	Adults[c]	Weight 40–55 kg: 800 mg	—	Weight 40–55 kg: 2000 mg	Weight 40–55 kg: 1200 mg
			Weight 56–75 kg: 1200 mg	—	Weight 56–75 kg: 2800 mg	Weight 56–75 kg: 2000 mg
			Weight 76–90 kg: 1600 mg	—	Weight 76–90 kg: 4000 mg	Weight 76–90 kg: 2400 mg
		Children[d,e]	15–20 mg/kg daily	—	50 mg/kg	—

Higher doses of rifampin and rifapentine are being studied. Rifabutin dose may need to be adjusted when there is concomitant use of protease inhibitors or non-nucleoside reverse transcriptase inhibitors.

[a]Dose per weight is based on ideal body weight. Children weighing more than 40 kg should be dosed as adults.

[b]For purposes of this document, adult dosing begins at age 15 years.

[c]The authors of this chapter do not agree with the use of maximum doses, since this arbitrarily caps doses for patients who otherwise might need larger doses. These maximum doses were not based on prospective studies in large or overweight individuals, and do not consider patients with documented malabsorption of their medications. Clinical judgment should be used in such circumstances.

[d]The drug can likely be used safely in older children but should be used with caution in children younger than 5 years, in whom visual acuity cannot be monitored. In younger children, ethambutol at the dose of 15 mg/kg/day can be used if there is suspected or proven resistance to isoniazid or rifampin.

[e]It should be noted that, although this is the dose recommended generally, most clinicians with experience using cycloserine indicate that it is unusual for patients to be able to tolerate this amount. Serum concentration measurements are often useful in determining the optimal dose for a given patient.

✓ Patients who are homeless, institutionalized, IV drug abusers, and/or infected with HIV.

✓ Patients who still have acid-fast bacilli–positive sputum smears after 2 months of therapy.

✓ Patients who still have positive cultures after 2–4 months of therapy.

✓ Patients who fail therapy or relapse after retreatment.

✓ Patients known to be exposed to MDR-TB cases.

SPECIAL POPULATIONS

Tuberculous Meningitis and Extrapulmonary Disease

- In general, **isoniazid, pyrazinamide, ethionamide**, cycloserine and linezolid penetrate the cerebrospinal fluid readily. Patients with CNS TB are often treated for longer periods (9–12 months). Extrapulmonary TB of the soft tissues can be treated with conventional regimens. TB of the bone is typically treated for 9 months, occasionally with surgical debridement.

Children

- TB in children may be treated with regimens similar to those used in adults, although some physicians still prefer to extend treatment to 9 months. Pediatric doses of drugs should be used.

Pregnant Females

- The usual treatment of pregnant females is **isoniazid, rifampin, and ethambutol** for 9 months.

- Females with TB should be cautioned against becoming pregnant, as the disease poses a risk to the fetus as well as to the mother. Isoniazid or ethambutol is relatively safe when used during pregnancy. Supplementation with B vitamins is particularly important during pregnancy. **Rifampin** has been rarely associated with birth defects, but those seen are occasionally severe, including limb reduction and CNS lesions. **Pyrazinamide** has not been studied in a large number of pregnant females, but anecdotal information suggests that it may be safe. **Ethionamide** may be associated with premature delivery, congenital deformities, and Down syndrome when used during pregnancy, so it cannot be recommended in pregnancy. **Cycloserine** is not recommended during pregnancy. Fluoroquinolones should be avoided in pregnancy and during nursing.

Renal Failure

- In nearly all patients, isoniazid and rifampin do not require dose modifications in renal failure. Pyrazinamide and ethambutol typically require a reduction in dosing frequency from daily to three times weekly (Table 50-5).

EVALUATION OF THERAPEUTIC OUTCOMES AND PATIENT MONITORIG

- The most serious problem with TB therapy is nonadherence to the prescribed regimen. The most effective way to ensure adherence is with DOT.

- Patients who are AFB smear positive should have sputum samples sent for acid-fast bacilli stains every 1–2 weeks until two consecutive smears are negative. Once on maintenance therapy, patients should have sputum cultures performed monthly until negative, which generally occurs over 2–3 months. If sputum cultures continue to be positive after 2 months, drug susceptibility testing should be repeated, and serum drug concentrations should be checked.

- Patients should have blood urea nitrogen, serum creatinine, aspartate transaminase or alanine transaminase, and a complete blood count determined at baseline and

TABLE 50-5	Dosing Recommendations for Adults with Reduced Renal Function and for Adults Receiving Hemodialysis	
Drug	**Change in Frequency?**	**Recommended Dose and Frequency for Patients with Creatinine Clearance <30 mL/min (0.50 mL/sec) or for Patients Receiving Hemodialysis[a,b,c,d]**
Isoniazid	No change	300 mg once daily, or 900 mg three times per week
Rifampin	No change	600 mg once daily, or 600 mg three times per week
Pyrazinamide	Yes	25–35 mg/kg per dose three times per week (not daily)
Ethambutol	Yes	15–25 mg/kg per dose three times per week (not daily)
Levofloxacin	Yes	750–1000 mg per dose three times per week (not daily)
Cycloserine	Yes	250 mg once daily, or 500 mg/dose three times per week[e]
Ethionamide	No change	250–500 mg/dose daily
p-Aminosalicylic acid	No change	4 g/dose, twice daily
Streptomycin	Yes	12–15 mg/kg per dose two or three times per week (not daily)
Capreomycin	Yes	12–15 mg/kg per dose two or three times per week (not daily)
Kanamycin	Yes	12–15 mg/kg per dose two or three times per week (not daily)
Amikacin	Yes	12–15 mg/kg per dose two or three times per week (not daily)

[a]Standard doses are given unless there is intolerance.
[b]The medications should be given after hemodialysis on the day of hemodialysis.
[c]Monitoring of serum drug concentrations should be considered to ensure adequate drug absorption, without excessive accumulation, and to assist in avoiding toxicity.
[d]Data currently are not available for patients receiving peritoneal dialysis. Until data become available, begin with doses recommended for patients receiving hemodialysis and verify adequacy of dosing, using serum concentration monitoring.
[e]The appropriateness of 250-mg daily doses has not been established. There should be careful monitoring for evidence of neurotoxicity.

Reprinted, with permission, from Nahid P, et al. Executive Summary: Official American Thoracic Society/Centers for Disease Control and Prevention/Infectious Diseases Society of America Clinical Practice Guidelines: Treatment of Drug-Susceptible Tuberculosis, Clinical Infectious Diseases, Volume 63, Issue 7, 1 October 2016, pp. 853–867.

periodically, depending on the presence of other factors that may increase the likelihood of toxicity (advanced age, alcohol abuse, and possibly pregnancy). Hepatotoxicity should be suspected in patients whose transaminases exceed five times the upper limit of normal or whose total bilirubin exceeds 3 mg/dL (51.3 μmol/L). At this point, the offending agent(s) should be discontinued and alternatives selected.

• See Table 50-6 for drug monitoring recommendations.

See Chapter 135, Tuberculosis, authored by Rocsanna Namdar and Charles A. Peloquin, for a more detailed discussion of this topic.

TABLE 50-6 Recommended Regimens for the Concomitant Treatment of TB and HIV Infection in Adults

Combined Regimen for Treatment of HIV and TB	Pharmacokinetic Effect of the Rifamycin	Tolerability/ Toxicity	Antiviral Activity when Used with Rifamycin	Recommendations (Comments)
Efavirenz-based antiretroviral therapy[a] with rifampin-based TB treatment	Well-characterized, modest decrease in concentrations in some patients	Low rates of discontinuation	Excellent	Preferred (efavirenz should not be used during the first trimester of pregnancy)
PI-based antiretroviral therapy[a] with rifabutin-based TB treatment	Little effect of rifabutin on PI concentrations, but marked increases in rifabutin concentrations	Low rates of discontinuation (if rifabutin is appropriately dose-reduced)	Favorable, although published clinical experience is not extensive	Preferred for patients unable to take efavirenz[b] (caution to ensure patients who discontinue PI not to continue to receive reduced rifabutin dose)
Nevirapine-based antiretroviral therapy with rifampin-based TB treatment	Moderate decrease in concentrations	Concern about hepatotoxicity when used with isoniazid, rifampin, and pyrazinamide	Suboptimal when nevirapine is initiated using once-daily dosing largely favorable when nevirapine is given twice daily throughout cotreatment	Alternative for patients who cannot take efavirenz, though efavirenz is preferred (nevirapine should not be initiated among women with CD4 >250 [0.25 × 10^9/L] or men with CD4 >400 cells/μL [0.40 × 10^9/L])
Raltegravir-based antiretroviral therapy with rifampin-based TB treatment	Significant decrease in concentrations with standard dosing	Limited experience	Limited published clinical experience	Alternative at higher doses for patients who cannot take efavirenz and who have baseline viral load <100,000 copies/mL (100 × 10^6/L)
Dolutegravir-based antiretroviral therapy with rifampin-based TB-treatment	Coadministration with rifampicin results in decreases in dolutegravir plasma exposure requiring increased dose of dolutegravir	Limited experience	Limited published clinical experience	Alternative for patients who cannot take efavirenz

(Continued)

TABLE 50-6 Recommended Regimens for the Concomitant Treatment of TB and HIV Infection in Adults (Continued)

Combined Regimen for Treatment of HIV and TB	Pharmacokinetic Effect of the Rifamycin	Tolerability/ Toxicity	Antiviral Activity when Used with Rifamycin	Recommendations (Comments)
Zidovudine/Lamivudine/ Abacavir/Tenofovir with rifampin-based TB treatment	50% decrease in zidovudine, possible effect on abacavir not evaluated	Anemia	No published clinical experience, but this regimen is less effective than efavirenz- or atazanavir-based regimens in person not taking rifampin	Alternative for patients who cannot take efavirenz or nevirapine and if rifabutin not available
Zidovudine/Lamivudine/ Tenofovir with rifampin-based TB treatment	50% decrease in zidovudine, no other effects predicted	Anemia	Favorable, but not evaluated in a randomized trial	Alternative for patients who cannot take efavirenz and abacavir and if rifabutin not available
Zidovudine/Lamivudine/Abacavir with rifampin-based TB treatment	50% decrease in zidovudine, possible effect on abacavir not evaluated	Anemia	Early favorable experience, but this combination is less effective than efavirenz- or nevirapine-based regimens in persons not taking rifampin	Alternative for patients who cannot take efavirenz and tenofovir and if rifabutin not available
Superboosted[c] lopinavir-based antiretroviral therapy or double dose lopinavir/ ritonavir-based therapy with rifampin-based TB treatment	Moderate decrease in concentrations	Hepatitis	Early favorable experience of superboosting among young children and double dose among adults already on antiretroviral drugs at the time of rifampin initiation	Alternative if rifabutin not available; double dose an option among adults already taking lopinavir-based antiretroviral therapy and virologically suppressed at the time of tuberculosis treatment initiation; superboosting has not been adequately tested in adults but may be effective

ART, antiretroviral therapy; HIV, human immunodeficiency virus; TB, tuberculosis.

[a]With two nucleoside analogues.

[b]Includes patients with NNRTI-resistant HIV, those unable to tolerate efavirenz, and women during the first one to two trimesters of pregnancy.

[c]Superboosting of lopinavir is achieved by giving lopinavir 400 mg together with 400 mg ritonavir twice daily. Double dose lopinavir/ritonavir is lopinavir 800 mg plus ritonavir 200 mg twice daily.

Data from CDC. Managing Drug Interactions in the Treatment of HIV-Related Tuberculosis [online]. 2013. Available at: http://www.cdc.gov/tb/TB_HIV_Drugs/default.htm.

Urinary Tract Infections and Prostatitis

- Infections of the urinary tract include a wide variety of clinical syndromes including urethritis, cystitis, prostatitis, and pyelonephritis.
- A *urinary tract infection* (UTI) is defined as the presence of microorganisms in the urine that cannot be accounted for by contamination. The organisms have the potential to invade the tissues of the urinary tract and adjacent structures.
- Lower tract infections include cystitis (bladder), urethritis (urethra), prostatitis (prostate gland), and epididymitis. Upper tract infections involve the kidney and are referred to as *pyelonephritis.*
- *Uncomplicated* UTIs are not associated with structural or functional abnormalities that may interfere with the normal flow of urine or the voiding mechanism. *Complicated* UTIs are the result of a predisposing lesion of the urinary tract, such as a congenital abnormality or distortion of the urinary tract, stone, indwelling catheter, prostatic hypertrophy, obstruction, or neurologic deficit that interferes with the normal flow of urine and urinary tract defenses.
- *Recurrent* UTIs, two or more UTIs occurring within 6 months or three or more within 1 year, are characterized by multiple symptomatic episodes with asymptomatic periods occurring between these episodes. These infections are due to reinfection or relapse. Reinfections are caused by a different organism and account for the majority of recurrent UTIs. Relapse represents the development of repeated infections caused by the same initial organism.

PATHOPHYSIOLOGY

- The bacteria causing UTIs usually originate from bowel flora of the host. Organisms typically gain entry into the urinary tract via three routes: the ascending, hematogenous (descending), and lymphatic pathways.
- The most common cause of uncomplicated UTIs is *Escherichia coli*, accounting for more than 80%–90% of community-acquired infections. Additional causative organisms are *Staphylococcus saprophyticus, Klebsiella pneumoniae, Proteus* spp., *Pseudomonas aeruginosa*, and *Enterococcus* spp.
- The urinary pathogens in complicated or nosocomial infections may include *E. coli*, which accounts for less than 50% of these infections, *Proteus* spp., *K. pneumoniae, Enterobacter* spp., *P. aeruginosa*, staphylococci, and enterococci. Enterococci represent the second most frequently isolated organisms in hospitalized patients.
- Most UTIs are caused by a single organism; however, in patients with stones, indwelling urinary catheters, or chronic renal abscesses, multiple organisms may be isolated.
- Vancomycin-resistant *E. faecalis* and *E. faecium* (vancomycin-resistant enterococci) have become more widespread, especially in patients with long-term hospitalizations or underlying malignancies.

CLINICAL PRESENTATION

- The typical signs and symptoms of urinary tract infections are:
  - ✓ Lower UTI: Dysuria, urgency, frequency, nocturia, and suprapubic heaviness, gross hematuria, and costovertebral tenderness.
  - ✓ Upper UTI: Flank pain, fever, nausea, vomiting, and malaise.
- Symptoms alone are unreliable for the diagnosis of bacterial UTIs. The key to the diagnosis of a UTI is the ability to demonstrate significant numbers of microorganisms present in an appropriate urine specimen to distinguish contamination from infection.
- Older patients frequently do not experience specific urinary symptoms, but they will present with altered mental status, change in eating habits, or gastrointestinal (GI) symptoms.

- A standard urinalysis should be obtained in the initial assessment of a patient. Microscopic examination of the urine should be performed by preparation of a Gram stain of unspun or centrifuged urine. The presence of at least one organism per oil-immersion field in a properly collected uncentrifuged specimen correlates with greater than 100,000 colony-forming units (CFU)/mL (10^5 CFU/mL [$>10^8$ CFU/L]) of urine.
- A quantitative count of 10^5 CFU/mL (10^8 CFU/L) or more is considered indicative of a UTI; however, up to 50% of females will present with clinical symptoms of a UTI with lower counts (10^3 CFU/mL [10^6CFU/L]).
- The presence of pyuria (>10 white blood cells [WBC]/mm^3 [10×10^6/L]) in a symptomatic patient correlates with significant bacteriuria. A count of 5–10 WBC/mm^3 (5×10^6–10×10^6/L) is accepted as the upper limit of normal.
- The nitrite test can be used to detect the presence of nitrate-reducing bacteria in the urine (eg, *E. coli*). The leukocyte esterase test is a rapid dipstick test to detect pyuria.
- The most reliable method of diagnosing UTIs is by quantitative urine culture. Patients with infection usually have more than 10^5 bacteria/mL (10^8/L) of urine, although as many as one-third of females with symptomatic infection have less than 10^5 bacteria/mL (10^8/L).

TREATMENT

- <u>Goals of Treatment</u>: Eradicate the invading organisms, prevent or treat systemic consequences of infection, prevent recurrence of infection, and decrease the potential for collateral damage with excessively broad antimicrobial therapy.
- The management of a patient with a UTI includes initial evaluation, selection of an antibacterial agent and duration of therapy, and follow-up evaluation.
- The initial selection of an antimicrobial agent for the treatment of UTI is primarily based on the severity of the presenting signs and symptoms, the site of infection, and whether the infection is determined to be complicated or uncomplicated. Other considerations include antibiotic susceptibility, side-effect potential, cost, current antimicrobial exposure, and the comparative inconvenience of different therapies.

PHARMACOLOGIC TREATMENT

- Eradication of bacteria from the urinary tract is directly related to the sensitivity of the organism and the achievable concentration of the antimicrobial agent in the urine.
- Management of UTIs is best accomplished by first categorizing the type of infection: acute uncomplicated cystitis, symptomatic abacteriuria, asymptomatic bacteriuria, complicated UTIs, recurrent infections, or prostatitis.
- Most *E. coli* remain susceptible to **trimethoprim–sulfamethoxazole**, although resistance is increasing and has been reported as high as 27%. In light of rising resistance and in order to decrease the overuse of broad-spectrum antimicrobials, agents such as **nitrofurantoin** and **fosfomycin** are considered first-line treatments along with trimethoprim–sulfamethoxazole in acute uncomplicated cystitis.
- Table 51-1 lists the most common agents used to treat lower UTIs in adults, along with comments concerning their general use.
- Table 51-2 presents an overview of various therapeutic options for outpatient therapy for UTI.
- Table 51-3 describes empiric treatment regimens for specific clinical situations.

Acute Uncomplicated Cystitis

- These infections are predominantly caused by *E. coli,* and antimicrobial therapy should be directed against this organism initially. Because the causative organisms and their susceptibilities are generally known, a cost-effective approach to management is

TABLE 51-1	Commonly Used Antimicrobial Agents in the Treatment of UTIs		
Drug	**Adverse Drug Reactions**	**Monitoring Parameters**	**Comments**
Oral therapy			
Trimethoprim–sulfamethoxazole	Rash, Stevens–Johnson syndrome, renal failure, photosensitivity, hematologic (neutropenia, anemia, etc.)	Serum creatinine, BUN, electrolytes, signs of rash, and CBC	Highly effective against most aerobic enteric bacteria except *P. aeruginosa*. High urinary tract tissue concentrations and urine concentrations are achieved, which may be important in complicated infection treatment. Also effective as prophylaxis for recurrent infections.
Nitrofurantoin	GI intolerance, neuropathies, and pulmonary reactions	Baseline serum creatinine and BUN	Effective as both a therapeutic and prophylactic agent in patients with recurrent UTIs. Main advantage is the lack of resistance even after long courses of therapy.
Fosfomycin trometamol	Diarrhea, headache, and angioedema	No routine tests recommended	Single-dose therapy for uncomplicated infections, low levels of resistance, use with caution in patients with hepatic dysfunction.
Fluoroquinolones			
Ciprofloxacin Levofloxacin	Hypersensitivity, photosensitivity, GI symptoms, dizziness, confusion, and tendonitis (black box warning)	CBC, baseline serum creatinine, and BUN	Greater spectrum of activity, including *P. aeruginosa*. Effective for pyelonephritis and prostatitis. Avoid in pregnancy and children. Moxifloxacin should not be used owing to inadequate urinary concentrations.
Amoxicillin–clavulanate	Hypersensitivity (rash, anaphylaxis), diarrhea, superinfections, and seizures	CBC, signs of rash, or hypersensitivity	Due to increasing *E. coli* resistance, amoxicillin–clavulanate is the preferred penicillin for uncomplicated cystitis.

(Continued)

TABLE 51-1	Commonly Used Antimicrobial Agents in the Treatment of UTIs (*Continued*)		
Drug	**Adverse Drug Reactions**	**Monitoring Parameters**	**Comments**
Cephalosporins			
Cefaclor Cefpodoxime- proxetil	Hypersensitivity (rash, anaphylaxis), diarrhea, superinfections, and seizures	CBC, signs of rash, or hypersensitivity	No major advantages over other agents for treating UTIs, and they are more expensive. Not active against enterococci.
Parenteral therapy			
Aminoglycosides			
Gentamicin Tobramycin Amikacin	Ototoxicity, nephrotoxicity	Serum creatinine and BUN, serum drug concentrations, and individual pharmacokinetic monitoring	Renally excreted and achieve good concentrations in the urine. Amikacin generally is reserved for multidrug-resistant bacteria.
Penicillins			
Ampicillin–sulbactam Piperacillin–tazobactam	Hypersensitivity (rash, anaphylaxis), diarrhea, superinfections, and seizures	CBC, signs of rash, or hypersensitivity	Generally are equally effective for susceptible bacteria. The extended-spectrum penicillins are more active against *P. aeruginosa* and enterococci and often are preferred over cephalosporins. They are very useful in renally impaired patients or when an aminoglycoside is to be avoided.
Cephalosporins			
Ceftriaxone Ceftazidime Cefepime Ceftozolane/Tazobactam Ceftazidime/Avabactam	Hypersensitivity (rash, anaphylaxis), diarrhea, superinfections, and seizures	CBC, signs of rash, or hypersensitivity	Second- and third-generation cephalosporins have a broad spectrum of activity against gram-negative bacteria, but are not active against enterococci and have limited activity against *P. aeruginosa*. Ceftazidime and cefepime are active against *P. aeruginosa*. They are useful for nosocomial infections and urosepsis due to susceptible pathogens.

(Continued)

Drug	Adverse Drug Reactions	Monitoring Parameters	Comments
TABLE 51-1	Commonly Used Antimicrobial Agents in the Treatment of UTIs *(Continued)*		
Carbapenems/ Monobactams			
Imipenem–cilistatin Meropenem Meropenem/ Vaborbactam Doripenem Ertapenem Aztreonam	Hypersensitivity (rash, anaphylaxis), diarrhea, superinfections, and seizures	CBC, signs of rash, or hypersensitivity	Carbapenems have a broad spectrum of activity, including gram-positive, gram-negative, and anaerobic bacteria. Imipenem, meropenem, and doripenem are active against *P. aeruginosa* and enterococci, but ertapenem is not. Aztreonam is a monobactam that is only active against gram-negative bacteria, including some strains of *P. aeruginosa*. Generally useful for nosocomial infections when aminoglycosides are to be avoided and in penicillin-sensitive patients.
Fluoroquinolones			
Ciprofloxacin Levofloxacin	Hypersensitivity, photosensitivity, GI symptoms, dizziness, confusion, and tendonitis (black box warning)	CBC, baseline serum creatinine, and BUN	Broad-spectrum activity against both gram-negative and gram-positive bacteria. They provide urine and high-tissue concentrations and are actively secreted in reduced renal function.

BUN, blood urea nitrogen; CBC, complete blood count; GI, gastrointestinal; UTIs, urinary tract infections.

recommended that includes a urinalysis and initiation of empiric therapy without a urine culture (Fig. 51-1).

- Short-course therapy (3-day therapy) with **trimethoprim–sulfamethoxazole** or a **fluoroquinolone** (eg, **ciprofloxacin** or **levofloxacin**, but not moxifloxacin) is superior to single-dose therapy for uncomplicated infection. Fluoroquinolones should be reserved for patients with suspected or possible pyelonephritis due to the collateral damage risk. Instead, a 3-day course of trimethoprim–sulfamethoxazole, a 5-day course of nitrofurantoin, or a one-time dose of **fosfomycin** should be considered

TABLE 51-2	Overview of Outpatient Antimicrobial Therapy for Lower Tract Infections in Adults			
Indications	**Antibiotic**	**Oral Dose**	**Interval**[a]	**Duration**
Lower tract infections				
Uncomplicated	Trimethoprim–sulfamethoxazole	1 DS tablet	Twice a day	3 days
	Nitrofurantoin monohydrate	100 mg	Twice a day	5 days
	Fosfomycin trometamol	3 g	Single dose	1 day
	Ciprofloxacin	250 mg	Twice a day	3 days
	Levofloxacin	250 mg	Once a day	3 days
	Amoxicillin–clavulanate	500 mg	Every 8 hours	5–7 days
	Pivmecillinam	400 mg	Twice a day	3 days
Complicated	Trimethoprim–sulfamethoxazole	1 DS tablet	Twice a day	7–10 days
	Ciprofloxacin	250–500 mg	Twice a day	7–10 days
	Levofloxacin	250 mg	Once a day	10 days
		750 mg	Once a day	5 days
	Amoxicillin–clavulanate	500 mg	Every 8 hours	7–10 days
Recurrent infections	Nitrofurantoin	50 mg	Once a day	6 months
	Trimethoprim–sulfamethoxazole	1/2 SS tablet	Once a day	6 months
Acute pyelonephritis	Trimethoprim–sulfamethoxazole	1 DS tablet	Twice a day	14 days
	Ciprofloxacin	500 mg	Twice a day	14 days
		1000 mg ER	Once a day	7 days
	Levofloxacin	250 mg	Once a day	10 days
		750 mg	Once a day	5 days
	Amoxicillin–clavulanate	500 mg	Every 8 hours	14 days

DS, double strength; SS, single strength.
[a]Dosing intervals for normal renal function.

as first-line therapy. In areas where there is more than 20% resistance of *E. coli* to trimethoprim–sulfamethoxazole, nitrofurantoin or fosfomycin should be utilized.

Complicated Urinary Tract Infections

Acute Pyelonephritis

- The presentation of high-grade fever (>38.3°C [100.9°F]) and severe flank pain should be treated as acute pyelonephritis, and aggressive management is warranted. Severely ill patients with pyelonephritis should be hospitalized and IV drugs administered initially. Milder cases may be managed with oral antibiotics in an outpatient setting.
- At the time of presentation, a Gram stain of the urine should be performed, along with urinalysis, culture, and sensitivity tests.
- In the mild to moderately symptomatic patient for whom oral therapy is considered, an effective agent should be administered for 7–14 days, depending on the

TABLE 51-3 Evidence-Based Empirical Treatment of UTIs and Prostatitis

Diagnosis	Pathogens	Treatment Recommendation	Comments
Acute uncomplicated cystitis	*Escherichia coli, Staphylococcus saprophyticus*	1. Nitrofurantoin × 5 days (A,I)[a]	Short-course therapy more effective than single dose
		2. Trimethoprim–sulfamethoxazole × 3 days (A,I)[a]	Reserve fluoroquinolones as alternatives to development of resistance (A-III)[a]
		3. Fosfomycin trometamol × 1 dose (A,I)[a]	β-Lactams as a group are not as effective in acute cystitis than trimethoprim–sulfamethoxazole or the fluoroquinolones, do not use amoxicillin or ampicillin[a]
		4. Fluoroquinolone × 3 days (A,I)[a]	
		5. β-Lactams × 3–7 days (B,I)[a]	
		6. Pivmecillinam × 3–7 days (A,I)	Pivmecillinam not available in the United States
Pregnancy	As above	1. Amoxicillin–clavulanate × 7 days	Avoid trimethoprim–sulfamethoxazole during the third trimester
		2. Cephalosporin × 7 days	
		3. Trimethoprim–sulfamethoxazole × 7 days	
Acute pyelonephritis			
Uncomplicated	*E. coli*	1. Fluoroquinolone × 7 days (A,I)[a]	Can be managed as outpatient
		2. Trimethoprim–sulfamethoxazole (if susceptible) × 14 days (A,I)[a]	
	Gram-positive bacteria	1. Amoxicillin or amoxicillin–clavulanic acid × 14 days	
Complicated	*E. coli*	1. Quinolone × 14 days	Severity of illness will determine duration of IV therapy; culture results should direct therapy
	P. mirabilis	2. Extended-spectrum penicillin plus aminoglycoside	
	K. pneumoniae		
	P. aeruginosa		Oral therapy may complete 14 days of therapy
	Enterococcus faecalis		
Prostatitis	*E. coli*	1. Trimethoprim–sulfamethoxazole × 4–6 weeks	Acute prostatitis may require IV therapy initially
	K. pneumoniae		
	Proteus spp.	2. Fluoroquinolone 4–6 weeks	Chronic prostatitis may require longer treatment periods or surgery
	P. aeruginosa		

UTI, urinary tract infection.

[a]Strength of recommendations: A, good evidence for; B, moderate evidence for; C, poor evidence for and against; D, moderate against; E, good evidence against. Quality of evidence: I, at least one proper randomized, controlled study; II, one well-designed clinical trial; III, evidence from opinions, clinical experience, and expert committees.

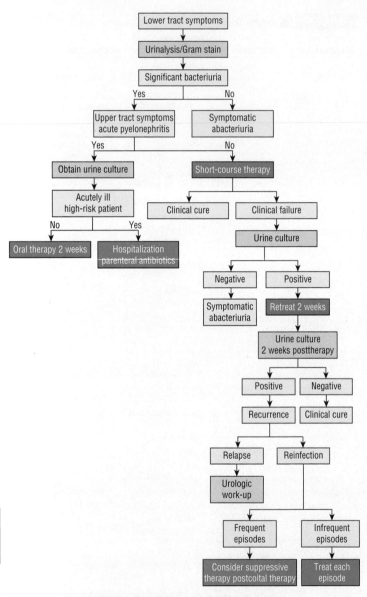

FIGURE 51-1. **Management of urinary tract infections in women.**

agent used. Fluoroquinolones (**ciprofloxacin** or **levofloxacin**) orally for 7–10 days are the first-line choice in mild-to-moderate pyelonephritis. Other options include **trimethoprim–sulfamethoxazole** for 14 days. If a Gram stain reveals gram-positive cocci, *Enterococcus faecalis* should be considered and treatment must be directed against this pathogen (**ampicillin**).

- In the seriously ill patient, the traditional initial therapy is an IV fluoroquinolone, an aminoglycoside with or without ampicillin, or an extended-spectrum cephalosporin with or without an aminoglycoside.
- If the patient has been hospitalized in the last 6 months, has a urinary catheter, or is in a nursing home, the possibility of *P. aeruginosa* and enterococci infection, as well as multiple-resistant organisms, should be considered. In this setting, broad-spectrum coverage, such as an extended spectrum beta-lactam/beta-lactamase inhibitor or carbapenem, is recommended.
- Follow-up urine cultures should be obtained 2 weeks after the completion of therapy to ensure a satisfactory response and to detect possible relapse.

Urinary Tract Infections in Men

- Therapy in men requires prolonged treatment (Fig. 51-2).
- A urine culture should be obtained before treatment, because the cause of infection in men is not as predictable as in females.
- If gram-negative bacteria are presumed, trimethoprim–sulfamethoxazole or a fluoroquinolone should be considered. Initial therapy is for 10–14 days. For recurrent infections in men, cure rates are much higher with a 6-week regimen of trimethoprim–sulfamethoxazole.

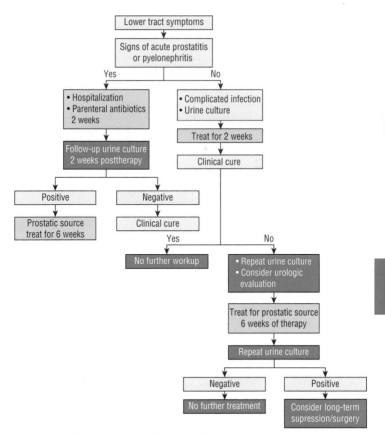

FIGURE 51-2. Management of urinary tract infections in men.

Recurrent Infections

- Recurrent episodes of UTI (reinfections and relapses) account for a significant portion of all UTIs. These patients are most commonly female and can be divided into two groups: those with fewer than two or three episodes per year and those who develop more frequent infections.
- In patients with infrequent infections (ie, fewer than three infections per year), each episode should be treated as a separately occurring infection. Short-course therapy should be used in symptomatic female patients with lower tract infection.
- In patients who have frequent symptomatic infections and no apparent precipitating event, long-term prophylactic antimicrobial therapy may be instituted (see Table 51-2). Therapy is generally given for 6 months, with urine cultures followed monthly.
- In females who experience symptomatic reinfections in association with sexual activity, voiding after intercourse may help prevent infection. Also, self-administered, single-dose prophylactic therapy with **trimethoprim–sulfamethoxazole** taken after intercourse significantly reduces the incidence of recurrent infection in these patients.
- Females who relapse after short-course therapy should receive a 2-week course of therapy. In patients who relapse after 2 weeks, therapy should be continued for another 2–4 weeks. If relapse occurs after 6 weeks of treatment, urologic examination should be performed, and therapy for 6 months or even longer may be considered.

SPECIAL CONDITIONS

URINARY TRACT INFECTION IN PREGNANCY

- In females with significant bacteriuria, symptomatic or asymptomatic treatment is recommended to avoid possible complications during the pregnancy. Therapy should consist of an agent with a relatively low adverse-effect potential (**cephalexin, amoxicillin**, or **amoxicillin/clavulanate**) administered for 7 days.
- Tetracyclines should be avoided because of teratogenic effects and sulfonamides should not be administered during the third trimester because of the possible development of kernicterus and hyperbilirubinemia. Also, the fluoroquinolones should not be given because of their potential to inhibit cartilage and bone development in the newborn.

CATHETERIZED PATIENTS

- When bacteriuria occurs in asymptomatic, short-term catheterized patients (<30 days), the use of systemic antibiotic therapy should be withheld and the catheter removed as soon as possible. If the patient becomes symptomatic, the catheter should again be removed, and treatment as described for complicated infections should be started.
- In long-term catheterized patients, however, antibiotics only postpone the development of bacteriuria and lead to emergence of resistant organisms.

See Chapter 139, Urinary Tract Infections and Prostatitis, authored by Julianna M. Fernandez and Elizabeth A. Coyle, for a more detailed discussion of this topic.

CHAPTER 52

Vaccines, Toxoids, and Other Immunobiologics

- *Vaccines* are substances administered to generate a protective immune response. They can be live attenuated or inactivated.
- *Adjuvants* are chemicals that stimulate a strong, but short-lived inflammatory response which strengthens the immune response to the antigen.
- *Immunoglobulins (Igs)* are sterile solutions containing antibody derived from human (immunoglobulin [Ig]) sources.

VACCINE RECOMMENDATIONS

- The latest vaccine schedules can be found at https://www.cdc.gov/vaccines/schedules/hcp/index.html.
- The childhood, adolescent, and adult immunization schedules are updated frequently and published annually. Recommendations for the use of influenza vaccine are issued annually. Healthcare providers involved in primary care and immunization delivery must keep themselves abreast of these changes in a systematic way. Electronic newsletters and browsing reliable websites are efficient methods for obtaining information (Table 52-1).
- In general, inactivated and live-attenuated vaccines can be administered simultaneously at separate sites. If two or more inactivated vaccines cannot be administered simultaneously, they can be administered without regard to spacing between doses. Inactivated and live vaccines can be administered simultaneously or, if they cannot be administered simultaneously, at any interval between doses. If live vaccines are not administered simultaneously, their administration should be separated by at least 4 weeks.

TABLE 52-1	Web Resources for Vaccine Information
Recommended Internet Sites for Vaccine Information	
http://www.cdc.gov/vaccines/	Vaccines and Immunizations
	Centers for Disease Control and Prevention
www.immunize.org	Immunization Action Coalition
www.nfid.org/	National Foundation for Infectious Diseases
www.cdc.gov/mmwr/	Morbidity and Mortality Weekly Report
http://www.nationalacademies.org/hmd/	The National Academies of Sciences, Engineering, and Medicine. Health and Medicine Division
http://www.hrsa.gov/vaccinecompensation/	Vaccine Injury Compensation Program
http://www.chop.edu/centers-programs/vaccine-education-center/	Vaccine Education Center
	Children's Hospital of Philadelphia
https://vaers.hhs.gov/index.html	Vaccine Adverse Event Reporting System
Recommended Electronic Newsletters	
www.immunize.org/express	The Immunization Action Coalition's newsletter
www.cdc.gov/mmwr/	Morbidity and Mortality Weekly Report

- Administration of live vaccines, such as rubella or varicella, is deferred until pregnancy is completed and are routinely recommended for those who do not have evidence of immunity prior to hospital discharge. These live vaccines can be administered without regard to administration of Rho(D) Ig (RDIg) in the postpartum period. Additionally, Tdap is recommended for all new mothers who have not received a Tdap before because household contacts are frequently implicated as the source of pertussis infection in a young infant.
- Severely immunocompromised individuals should not receive live vaccines.
- Patients with chronic pulmonary, renal, hepatic, or metabolic disease and who are not receiving immunosuppressants may receive live-attenuated and killed vaccines, as well as toxoids.
- Patients with active malignant disease may receive killed vaccines or toxoids but should not be given live vaccines. Live virus vaccines may be administered to persons with leukemia who have not received chemotherapy for at least 3 months.
- If a person has been receiving high-dose corticosteroids or has had a course lasting longer than 2 weeks, then at least 1 month should pass before immunization with live virus vaccines.
- Patients with HIV infection may have suboptimal immune responses to live and inactivated vaccines.
- Whenever possible, transplant patients should be immunized before transplantation. Live vaccines generally are not given after transplantation.

DIPHTHERIA TOXOID ADSORBED AND DIPHTHERIA ANTITOXIN

- Two strengths of diphtheria toxoid are available: pediatric strength (D) and adult strength (d), which contain less antigen. Primary immunization with D is indicated for children older than 6 weeks. Generally, D is given along with tetanus and acellular pertussis (DTaP) vaccines at 2, 4, and 6 months of age, and then at 15–18 months and 4–6 years of age.
- For nonimmunized adults, a complete three-dose series of diphtheria toxoid should be administered, with the first two doses given at least 4 weeks apart and the third dose 6–12 months after the second. One dose in the series should be Tdap. The combined preparation, tetanus–diphtheria (Td), is recommended in adults because it contains less diphtheria toxoid than DTaP, with fewer reactions seen from the diphtheria preparation. Booster doses of Td or Tdap are given every 10 years.
- Adverse effects to diphtheria toxoid include mild to moderate tenderness, erythema, and induration at the injection site.

TETANUS TOXOID, TETANUS TOXOID ADSORBED, AND TETANUS IMMUNOGLOBULIN

- In children, primary immunization against tetanus is usually done in conjunction with diphtheria and pertussis vaccination using DTaP or a combination vaccine that includes other antigens. A 0.5-mL dose is recommended at 2, 4, 6, and 15–18 months of age.
- In children 7 years and older and in adults who have not been previously immunized, a series of three 0.5-mL doses of Td is administered intramuscularly (IM) initially. The first two doses are given 1–2 months after the second dose and the third dose 6–12 months after the second dose. Boosters are recommended every 10 years.
- Tetanus Ig (TIg) is used to provide passive tetanus immunization after the occurrence of traumatic wounds in nonimmunized or suboptimally immunized persons (Table 52-2). A dose of 250–500 units is administered IM. When administered with tetanus toxoid, separate sites for administration should be used.
- TIg is also used for the treatment of tetanus. In this setting, a single dose of 3000–6000 units is administered IM.

TABLE 52-2	Tetanus Prophylaxis			
Vaccination History	**Clean, Minor Wounds**		**All Other Wounds**	
	Td[a]	TIg	Td or Tdap[a]	TIg
Unknown or fewer than three doses	Yes	No	Yes	Yes
Three or more doses	No[a,b]	No	No[a,c]	No

[a]A single dose of Tdap should be used for the next dose of tetanus–diphtheria toxoid for individuals aged >10 years.
[b]Yes, if more than 10 years since last dose.
[c]Yes, if more than 5 years since last dose.

SARS CORONAVIRUS-19 VACCINES

- See Chapter 37, for Coronavirus-19 vaccines.

HAEMOPHILUS INFLUENZAE TYPE B VACCINES

- Hib conjugate vaccines are indicated for routine use in all infants and children younger than 5 years.
- The primary series of Hib vaccination consists of 0.5-mL IM doses at 2, 4, and 6 months of age. A booster dose is recommended at age 12–15 months.
- For infants 7–11 months of age who have not been vaccinated, three doses of Hib vaccine should be given: two doses spaced 4 weeks apart and then a booster dose at age 12–15 months (but at least 8 weeks since the second dose). For unvaccinated children ages 12–14 months, two doses should be given, with an interval of 2 months between doses. In a child older than 15 months, a single dose of any of the four conjugate vaccines is indicated.

HEPATITIS VACCINES

- Information on hepatitis vaccines can be found in Chapter 25.

HUMAN PAPILLOMAVIRUS VACCINE

- The Advisory Committee on Immunization Practices (ACIP) recommends human papillomavirus (HPV) vaccine for the prevention of HPV-related disease in individuals aged 9–26 years. Individuals who start the HPV series between the ages of 9 and 14 years should receive two doses separated by 6 months. This vaccine is administered as a three-dose series using a schedule of 0, 1–2, and 6 months for individuals who start the series at age 15 years or older. The vaccines are recommended for adolescents aged 11–12 years and catch-up immunization for individuals aged 13–26 years.
- The ACIP recommended shared clinical decision-making for HPV vaccine for individuals aged 27–45 years. The vaccine is administered as a three-dose series (0, 1–2, and 6 months).
- The vaccine is well tolerated, with injection site reactions and headache and fatigue occurring as commonly as in placebo groups.

INFLUENZA VIRUS VACCINE

- See Chapter 43 for information regarding influenza vaccination.

MEASLES VACCINE

- Measles vaccine is a live-attenuated vaccine that is administered for primary immunization to persons 12–15 months of age or older, usually as a combination of measles, mumps, and rubella (MMR). A second dose is recommended at 4–6 years of age.

- Measles-containing vaccine should not be given to pregnant females or immunosuppressed individuals. An exception is HIV-infected patients, who are at very high risk for severe complications if they develop measles.
- The vaccine should not be given within 1 month of any other live vaccine unless the vaccine is given on the same day (as with the MMR vaccine).
- Measles vaccine is indicated in all persons born after 1956 or in those who lack documentation of wild virus infection by either history or antibody titers.

MENINGOCOCCAL VACCINES

- There are two meningococcal (MenACWY) conjugate vaccines: Menactra is licensed for individuals 9 months–55 years old and Menveo for those 2 months–55 years old. They are recommended for all children 11–12 years old with a second dose at 16 years of age.
- Reimmunization at 5-year intervals is recommended for individuals who are at high risk.
- Also, there are two meningococcal serogroup B (MenB) vaccines (Trumenba and Bexsero), and are licensed for individuals at high risk for invasive meningococcal disease.

MUMPS VACCINE

- The live attenuated vaccine (usually given in conjunction with measles and rubella, MMR) is given beginning at age 12–15 months, with a second dose prior to entry into elementary school.
- Two doses of mumps vaccine are recommended for school-age children, international travelers, students in post-high school educational institutions, and healthcare workers born after 1956.
- Postexposure vaccination is of no benefit.
- Mumps vaccine should not be given to pregnant women or immunosuppressed patients.

PERTUSSIS VACCINE

- Acellular pertussis vaccine is usually administered in combination with diphtheria and tetanus toxoids (as DTaP).
- The primary immunization series for pertussis vaccine consists of four doses given at ages 2, 4, 6, and 15–18 months. A booster dose is recommended at age 4–6 years. Administration of an acellular pertussis-containing vaccine is also recommended for adolescents once between ages 11 and 18 years and a single dose of Tdap should be administered to all adults.
- Tdap should be administered to persons in their late second or third trimester of pregnancy. Tdap should also be administered to all close contacts, including household contacts and out of home care providers.
- Systemic reactions, such as moderate fever, occur in 3%–5% of those receiving vaccines. Rarely, high fever, febrile seizures, persistent crying spells, and hypotonic hyporesponsive episodes occur after vaccination.

PNEUMOCOCCAL VACCINES

- Four pneumococcal vaccine preparations, PCV13, PCV15, PCV20, and 23-valent pneumococcal polysaccharide vaccine (PPSV23), are available. The vaccines have different indications and are not interchangeable.
- Pneumococcal polysaccharide vaccine (Pneumovax 23) is a mixture of highly purified capsular polysaccharides from 23 of the most prevalent or invasive types of *S. pneumoniae* seen in the United States. The vaccine is administered IM or subcutaneously as a single 0.5-mL dose.
- PCV20 or PCV15 followed by PPSV23 in 8 weeks is recommended for adults with immunocompromising conditions listed below. Either PCV15 or PCV20 should be administered with at least a year interval in those adults for whom it has been

recommended and have already received one or more doses of PPSV23. For PCV13-immunized adults conjugate vaccine should not be repeated.

- Indications for PCV20 or PCV15 followed by PPSV23 for adults 19 years and older are:
  - ✓ Functional or anatomic aspleniia.
  - ✓ Sickle cell disease or other hemaglobinopathies.
  - ✓ Congenital or acquired immunodeficiencies.
  - ✓ HIV infection.
  - ✓ Chronic renal failure or nephrotic syndrome.
  - ✓ Leukemias, lymphomas, Hodgkin's lymphoma.
  - ✓ Generalized malignancy.
  - ✓ Diseases requiring treatment with immunosuppressive drugs, including long-term systemic corticosteroids or radiation therapy.
  - ✓ Solid organ transplantation.
  - ✓ Multiple myeloma.
  - ✓ High-risk medical conditions: chronic heart disease, chronic liver disease, chronic lung disease, diabetes mellitus, alcoholism, cigarette smoking.
- PCV13 or PCV15 valent is administered as a 0.5-mL IM injection at 2, 4, and 6 months of age and between 12 and 15 months of age. A single dose of PCV13 or PCV15 should be administered to children aged 6–18 years with sickle cell disease or splenic dysfunction, HIV infection, immunocompromising conditions, cochlear implant, or cerebral spinal fluid leak.

POLIOVIRUS VACCINES

- Two types of trivalent poliovirus vaccines are currently licensed for distribution in the United States: an enhanced inactivated poliovirus vaccine (IPV) and a live-attenuated, oral poliovirus vaccine (OPV). IPV is the recommended vaccine for the primary series and booster dose for children in the United States, whereas OPV is recommended in areas of the world that have circulating poliovirus.
- IPV is given to children ages 2, 4, and 6–18 months and 4–6 years. Primary poliomyelitis immunization is recommended for all children and young adults up to age 18 years. Allergies to any component of IPV, including streptomycin, polymyxin B, and neomycin, are contraindications to vaccine use.
- OPV will continue to be used in areas of the world that have circulating poliovirus.

RUBELLA VACCINE

- The vaccine is indicated for children older than 1 year of age. The vaccine is given with measles and mumps vaccines (MMR) at 12–15 months of age, then at 4–6 years.
- The vaccine should not be given to immunosuppressed individuals, although MMR vaccine should be administered to young children with HIV without evidence of immunity.
- All females of childbearing potential should have documentation of receiving at least one dose of a rubella-containing vaccine or laboratory evidence of immunity. Although the vaccine has not been associated with congenital rubella syndrome, its use in pregnancy is contraindicated. Women should be counseled not to become pregnant for 4 weeks after vaccination.

VARICELLA VACCINE

- Varicella virus vaccine is recommended for all children 12–15 months of age, with a second dose between 4 and 6 years of age. Two doses separated by 4–8 weeks should be administered to anyone who lacks immunity to varicella.
  - ✓ The vaccine is contraindicated in immunosuppressed or pregnant patients.
  - ✓ Children with humoral immune deficiencies may be immunized.

ZOSTER VACCINE

- A recombinant zoster vaccine (RZV) with an adjuvant is recommended by the ACIP for use in immunocompetent individuals aged 50 years and older as a two-dose series at 0 and 2–6 months. The recombinant zoster vaccine is 91% effective for preventing zoster.
- Almost 80% of those who receive the recombinant vaccine report injection site pain with 9% of those reporting injection site reactions that interfere with their normal activities.

IMMUNOGLOBULIN

- Ig is available as both IM (IGIM) and IV (IGIV) preparations.
- Table 52-3 lists the suggested dosages for IGIM in various disease states.
- The uses for IGIV are as follows:
  - ✓ Primary immunodeficiency states, including both antibody deficiencies and combined deficiencies.
  - ✓ Idiopathic thrombocytopenia.
  - ✓ Chronic lymphocytic leukemia in patients who have had a serious bacterial infection.
  - ✓ Kawasaki disease (mucocutaneous lymph node syndrome).
  - ✓ Pediatric HIV infection.
  - ✓ Allogeneic bone marrow transplant.
  - ✓ Chronic inflammatory demyelinating polyneuropathy and multifocal motor neuropathy.
  - ✓ Multifocal motor neuropathy.
  - ✓ Kidney transplantation involving a recipient with high antibody concentrations or an ABO incompatible donor.

RHO(D) IMMUNOGLOBULIN

- Rho(D) Ig (RDIg) suppresses the antibody response and formation of anti-Rho(D) in Rho(D)-negative, D^u-negative women exposed to Rho(D)-positive blood and prevents the future chance of erythroblastosis fetalis in subsequent pregnancies with a Rho(D)-positive fetus.
- RDIg, when administered IM within 72 hours of delivery of a full-term infant, reduces active antibody formation from 1% to 0.2%.

TABLE 52-3	Indications and Dosage of Intramuscular Immunoglobulin in Infectious Diseases
Primary immunodeficiency states	1.2 mL/kg IM then 0.6 mL/kg every 2–4 weeks
Hepatitis A exposure	0.02 mL/kg IM within 2 weeks if <1 year or >39 years of age
Hepatitis A prophylaxis	0.02 mL/kg IM for exposure <3 months' duration
	0.06 mL/kg IM for exposure up to 5 months' duration
Hepatitis B exposure	0.06 mL/kg (HBIG preferred in known exposures)
Measles exposure	0.5 mL/kg (maximum dose 15 mL) as soon as possible

- RDIg is also used in the case of a premenopausal woman who is Rho(D) negative and has inadvertently received Rho(D)-positive blood or blood products.
- RDIg may be used after abortion, miscarriage, amniocentesis, or abdominal trauma.

See Chapter 147, Vaccines and Immunoglobulins, authored by Mary S. Hayney, for a more detailed discussion of this topic.

CHAPTER

53 | Alzheimer Disease

- *Alzheimer disease* (AD) affects ~7.5 million Americans of all ages and is a progressive illness of unknown cause characterized by loss of cognitive and physical functioning, commonly with behavior symptoms.

PATHOPHYSIOLOGY

- Genetic susceptibility to late-onset AD is primarily linked to the apolipoprotein E (*APOE*) genotype, but a genetic × environmental interaction may be at play. AD occurrence at a young age is seen in less than 1% of cases. These dominantly inherited forms are attributed to chromosomal alterations that affect processing of the amyloid precursor protein.
- AD risk factors include age, decreased brain reserve capacity, head injury, Down syndrome, depression, mild cognitive impairment, and risk factors for vascular disease, including hypertension, elevated homocysteine, elevated low-density lipoprotein cholesterol, low high-density lipoprotein cholesterol, obesity, metabolic syndrome, and diabetes.
- Signature lesions include intracellular neurofibrillary tangles (NFTs), extracellular amyloid plaques in the cortex and medial temporal lobe, degeneration of neurons and synapses, and cortical atrophy. AD-affected individuals appear to have a higher burden of plaques and NFTs in their younger years compared to age-matched controls.
- Proposed mechanisms for these changes include: (1) β-amyloid protein aggregation, leading to formation of plaques; (2) hyperphosphorylation of tau protein, leading to NFTs; (3) synaptic failure and depletion of neurotrophin and neurotransmitters; (4) mitochondrial dysfunction; and (5) oxidative stress.
- The amyloid cascade hypothesis involves a β-amyloid production and clearance imbalance, with aggregation and accumulation leading to AD. It is unknown if this is the primary pathology in most forms of AD.
- Loss of cholinergic activity is the most prominent neurotransmitter deficit that correlates with AD severity. Cholinergic cell loss seems to be a consequence of AD pathology, not the cause of it.
- Other neurotransmitters involved include: (1) serotonergic neurons of the raphe nuclei and noradrenergic cells of the locus ceruleus are lost; (2) monoamine oxidase type B activity is increased; (3) glutamate pathways of the cortex and limbic structures are abnormal; and (4) excitatory neurotransmitters, including glutamate, may be neurotoxic.

CLINICAL PRESENTATION

- Early disease may be characterized by changes in learning and memory, planning, organization, and mood. As the disease progresses, further declines in these domains, as well as changes in personality, judgment, speech, and spatial orientation are seen. In the late stages, functional decline may result in gait, swallowing, incontinence symptoms, and behavioral changes. Patients become increasingly unable to care for themselves. **Table 53-1** shows the stages of AD.

TABLE 53-1	Stages of Alzheimer Disease
Mild (MMSE score 26–21)	Patient has difficulty remembering recent events. Ability to manage finances, prepare food, and carry out other household activities declines. May get lost while driving. Begins to withdraw from difficult tasks and to give up hobbies. May deny memory problems.
Moderate (MMSE score 20–10)	Patient requires assistance with activities of daily living. Frequently disoriented with regard to time (date, year, and season). Recent events recall is severely impaired. May forget some details of past life events and names of family and friends. Functioning may fluctuate from day to day. Patient generally denies problems. May become suspicious or tearful. Loses ability to drive safely. Agitation, paranoia, and delusions are common.
Severe (MMSE score 9–0)	Patient loses ability to speak, walk, and feed self. Incontinent of urine and feces. Requires care 24 hours a day, 7 days a week.

MMSE, Mini-Mental State Examination.

DIAGNOSIS

- AD is a spectrum beginning with an asymptomatic preclinical phase progressing to the symptomatic preclinical phase and then to the dementia phase. AD is a clinical diagnosis, based largely on identified symptoms and difficulty with activities of daily living revealed by patient and caregiver interviews.
- Patients with suspected AD should have a history and physical examination with appropriate laboratory tests (ie, serum B_{12}, folate, thyroid panel, blood cell counts, serum electrolytes, and liver function tests).
- Structural imaging (ie, noncontrast enhanced CT or MRI) may be performed to identify structural abnormalities consistent with AD or other pathology, such as brain atrophy, vascular damage, or tumors. To exclude other diagnoses, cerebrospinal fluid analysis or an electroencephalogram can occasionally be justified. *APOE* genetic testing is currently not recommended.
- Obtain information on medication and substance use; family medical history; and history of trauma, depression, or head injury. Rule out medications (eg, anticholinergics, sedatives, hypnotics, opioids, antipsychotics, and anticonvulsants) as contributors to dementia symptoms or contribute to delirium (eg, digoxin, nonsteroidal anti-inflammatory drugs [NSAIDs], histamine-2 [H_2] receptor antagonists, amiodarone, antihypertensives, and corticosteroids).
- The Folstein Mini-Mental State Examination (MMSE) can help establish a history of deficits in two or more areas of cognition at baseline against which to evaluate change in severity over time. The average expected decline in an untreated patient is 2–4 points per year (Table 53-1). The MMSE is copyrighted and therefore if used requires payment by the user. Other assessment scales are also available.
- In the future, improved brain imaging and validated biomarkers of disease will enable a more sophisticated diagnosis with identified cognitive strengths and weaknesses and neuroanatomic localization of deficits.

TREATMENT

- Goals of Treatment: To maintain cognitive functioning and activities of daily living as long as possible, with a secondary goal to treat the psychiatric and behavioral symptoms.

NONPHARMACOLOGIC THERAPY

- Identify the possible causative factors for cognitive and noncognitive symptoms, and adapt the caregiving environment to remedy the situation.
- Sleep disturbances, wandering, urinary incontinence, agitation, and aggression should be managed with behavioral and environmental interventions whenever possible, for example, redirecting the patient's attention and removing stressors and triggers.
- On initial diagnosis, the patient and caregiver should be educated on the course of illness, available treatments, legal decisions, lifestyle changes that will become necessary, and other quality-of-life issues.
- Primary prevention includes smoking cessation, increasing physical activity, and reducing midlife obesity, hypertension, and diabetes. Adherence to the Mediterranean Diet or Dietary Approaches to Stop Hypertension (DASH) Diet may reduce the risk of cognitive impairment or decline.

PHARMACOLOGIC THERAPY OF COGNITIVE SYMPTOMS

- Consider the anti-amyloid monoclonal antibody (mAb) **aducanumab** for mild cognitive impairment (MCI). Titrate to recommended maintenance dose as tolerated.
- In mild to moderate AD, consider a cholinesterase inhibitor (**donepezil, rivastigmine,** or **galantamine**) or aducanumab titrated to recommended maintenance dose as tolerated.
- In moderate to severe AD, consider adding the antiglutamatergic agent **memantine** titrated to recommended maintenance dose as tolerated; alternatively, consider memantine or cholinesterase inhibitor therapy alone.
- A reasonable response may be a slowed decline in abilities and delayed long-term care placement.
- Simplify dosing regimens, taking patient and caregiver preferences into consideration to improve medication adherence and persistence.
- Treatment gaps may be associated with a loss of benefits when medication is stopped but this is controversial.
- Behavioral symptoms may require additional pharmacologic approaches.

Cholinesterase Inhibitors

- Table 53-2 summarizes cholinesterase inhibitor dosing. **Donepezil, rivastigmine,** and **galantamine** are indicated in mild to moderate AD; donepezil is also indicated for severe AD. No trials have assessed the effectiveness of one agent over another.
- Successful treatment shows a MMSE score decline of less than 2 points per year with benefit lasting 3–24 months.
- If rivastigmine or galantamine are interrupted for several days or longer, retitrate starting at the lowest dose due to their short half-lives. Gradual dose titration over several months improves tolerability. When switching from one agent to another, a washout period is recommended.
- Table 53-3 lists common medication adverse reactions and monitoring parameters. Abrupt discontinuation can cause worsening of cognition and behavior in some patients.

N-Methyl-D-Aspartate (NMDA) Receptor Antagonist

- **Memantine** is used as monotherapy and in combination with a cholinesterase inhibitor and is indicated for moderate to severe AD, but not for mild AD. It is not metabolized but requires dosing adjustments in patients with renal impairment. It is usually well tolerated; adverse medication reactions are outlined in Table 53-3.
- Combination therapy with cholinesterase inhibitors and memantine, individually or as **Namzaric,** is generally used for moderate to severe AD. It slows cognitive and functional decline compared to cholinesterase inhibitor monotherapy or no treatment. Memantine may help mitigate some of the GI effects seen with cholinesterase inhibitors.

TABLE 53-2 Dosing of Medications Used for Cognitive Symptoms

Medication	Initial Dose	Usual Range	Dosage Adjustments	Comments
Cholinesterase inhibitors				
Donepezil	5 mg daily in the evening	5–10 mg daily in mild to moderate AD 10–23 mg daily in moderate to severe AD	No dosage adjustments recommended	Available as: tablet, ODT, oral solution Can be taken with or without food Incidence of GI adverse effects (including weight loss) are higher with 23-mg dose Therapy interruptions require retitration of dose
Rivastigmine	1.5 mg twice daily (capsule, oral solution) 4.6 mg/day (transdermal patch)	3–6 mg twice a day (capsule, oral solution) 9.5–13.3 mg/day (transdermal patch)	Capsule/oral solution: renal impairment, hepatic impairment, or low body weight (<50 kg [<110 lb]): patients may be able to only tolerate lower doses Transdermal patch: mild to moderate hepatic impairment or low body weight: consider maximum daily dose of 4.6 mg every 24 hours	Available as: capsule, oral solution, transdermal patch Therapy interruptions require retitration of dose Take with meals Also indicated for Parkinson disease dementia Use of multiple transdermal patches at same the time is associated with hospitalization and death
Galantamine	4 mg twice daily (tablet, oral solution) 8 mg daily in the morning (extended-release capsule)	8–12 mg twice a day (tablet, oral solution) 16–24 mg (extended-release capsule)	Moderate renal or hepatic impairment: maximum daily dose of 16 mg Severe renal or hepatic impairment: not recommended	Available as: tablet, oral solution, extended-release capsule Recommended to take with meals

N-methyl-D-aspartate (NMDA) receptor antagonist

Drug	Dose	Renal/Hepatic adjustment	Considerations
Memantine	5 mg daily (tablet, oral solution) 7 mg daily (extended-release capsule)	10 mg twice daily 28 mg daily (extended-release capsule)	Severe renal impairment: recommended maintenance dose of 5 mg twice daily (tablet, oral solution) or 14 mg daily (extended-release capsule) Severe hepatic impairment: administer with caution	Available as: tablet, oral solution, extended-release capsule Can be taken with or without food Can open capsule and sprinkle contents on applesauce for ease of administration Therapy interruptions require retitration of dose

Cholinesterase inhibitor + NMDA receptor antagonist

Memantine + donepezil	7 mg/10 mg (if patient is stabilized on donepezil and not currently on memantine) 28 mg/10 mg (if patient is stabilized on memantine and donepezil)	28 mg/10 mg daily	Severe renal impairment: 14 mg/10 mg daily	Available as: memantine extended-release and donepezil capsule Therapy interruptions require retitration of dose Can be taken with or without food Can open capsule and sprinkle contents on applesauce for ease of administration

Anti-amyloid Monoclonal Antibody

Aducanumab	1 mg/kg intravenous	Titrated up to 10 mg/kg intravenous once every 4 weeks	No dosage adjustments recommended	Available as 170 mg/1.7 mL and 300 mg/3 mL single-dose vials Must be diluted in 100 mL of 0.9% NaCl and administered over ~1 hour

GI, gastrointestinal; ODT, orally disintegrating tablet.

	TABLE 53-3	Adverse Medication Reaction Monitoring

Medication	Adverse Medication Reaction	Monitoring Parameters	Comments
Galantamine	Serious skin reactions (Stevens–Johnson syndrome and acute generalized exanthematous pustulosis)	Appearance of skin rash	Discontinue at first sign of skin rash, unless clearly not related If signs/symptoms are suggestive of a serious reaction, consider alternative treatment and do not rechallenge
Rivastigmine	Allergic dermatitis	Reaction spread beyond patch size, evidence of a more intense local reaction (increasing erythema, edema, papules, vesicles), and persistence of symptoms for more than 48 hours after patch removal	Discontinue if evidence of disseminated allergic dermatitis appears Patients sensitized by patch exposure may not be able to take rivastigmine by mouth; allergy testing and close medical supervision recommended
Cholinesterase inhibitors	Dizziness, syncope, bradycardia, atrial arrhythmias, sinoatrial and atrioventricular block, myocardial infarction	Report of dizziness or falls, pulse, blood pressure, and postural blood pressure change	Dizziness is usually mild, transient, and not related to cardiovascular problems Routine pulse checks at baseline, monthly during titration, and every 6 months thereafter
	Nausea, vomiting, diarrhea, anorexia, weight loss	Weight and GI complaints	Take with food to reduce GI upset Usually transient, dose-related GI adverse effects seen with initiation, dosage titration, or medication switch Frail patients or those with low body weight may experience more GI effects and significant weight loss, particularly when rivastigmine is prescribed or when titrating to donepezil 23 mg GI effects less prominent with transdermal versus oral rivastigmine

(Continued)

| | TABLE 53-3 | Adverse Medication Reaction Monitoring (*Continued*) |

Medication	Adverse Medication Reaction	Monitoring Parameters	Comments
	Peptic ulcer disease, GI bleeding	Signs or symptoms of active or occult GI bleeding	Increased concern for patients at increased risk of developing ulcers (eg, history of ulcer disease or concurrently taking NSAIDs)
	Insomnia, vivid/abnormal dreams, nightmares	Sleep disturbances, daytime drowsiness	Donepezil can be taken in the morning to decrease risk
Memantine	Headache, confusion, dizziness, hallucinations	Report of dizziness or falls, hallucinations	Confusion may be observed during dose titration and is usually transient
	Constipation	GI complaints	May mitigate GI effects associated with cholinesterase inhibitors
Aducanumab	ARIA	MRI at baseline, prior to 7th and 12th infusions, or if symptoms suggest ARIA, to identify brain edema, microhemorrhage, superficial siderosis	Vigilance for ARIA and focal neurologic changes recommended especially during dose titration and the first eight doses
		Symptoms of headache, confusion, dizziness, visual disturbances, and nausea	
	Hypersensitivity reactions	Angioedema and urticaria (rare)	

ARIA, Amyloid-related imaging abnormalities; GI, gastrointestinal; NSAIDs, nonsteroidal anti-inflammatory drugs.

Anti-amyloid Monoclonal Antibody

• Four humanized, immunoglobulin G1 mAbs have been designated as AD breakthrough therapies by the FDA (ie, aducanumab, lecanemab, donanemab, and gantenerumab). Aducanumab was controversially approved for use in MCI due to AD and mild AD.

• Dosing for aducanumab, outlined in Tables 53-2 and 53-3, discusses its adverse effect monitoring.

• The potential degree and duration of clinical benefit of anti-amyloid antibodies remains largely unclear.

Other Medications

- Use of estrogen, NSAIDS, prednisone, statins, or *Ginkgo biloba* is not recommended to prevent or treat dementia. Do not use *Ginkgo biloba* in individuals taking anticoagulants or antiplatelet medications, and use cautiously in those taking NSAIDs.
- Vitamin E is under investigation for AD prevention and is not recommended for treatment.
- There is currently insufficient evidence to recommend omega-3 fatty acids or medical foods such as Axona, Souvenaid, and Cerefolin NAC for treatment of AD.

PHARMACOLOGIC THERAPY OF NEUROPSYCHIATRIC SYMPTOMS

- No medication is FDA-approved for the treatment of AD behavioral and psychological symptoms of dementia (BPSD) that are: (1) psychotic; (2) hyperactive (eg, inappropriate or disruptive behavior); (3) affective (eg, depression); and (4) apathy.
- General guidelines include: (1) reserve for situations where nonpharmacologic therapies have failed; (2) starting with reduced doses and titrating slowly; (3) monitoring closely; (4) periodically attempting to taper and discontinue medication; and (5) careful documentation.
- Cholinesterase inhibitors and memantine may be beneficial in treating BPSD but they do not reduce acute agitation. Avoid anticholinergic medications as they may worsen cognition.

Antidepressants

- Antidepressants may help manage anxiety, apathy, as well as agitation and aggression.
- A selective serotonin reuptake inhibitor (SSRI) can be used to treat depression with the best evidence for **sertraline** and **citalopram**. Tricyclic antidepressants are usually avoided.

  ✓ Common SSRI adverse medication reactions can be found in Chapter 69.

Antipsychotics

- Antipsychotic medications have traditionally been used for psychotic and hyperactive symptoms, but the risks and benefits must be carefully weighed.
- Second-generation antipsychotics (ie, **aripiprazole, risperidone, olanzapine**, and **quetiapine**) are more effective compared to placebo; however, the higher risk of adverse effects and mortality offset this benefit. They should be restricted to patients with severe symptoms not responding to other measures. Taper treatment as early as possible and rarely used beyond 12 weeks.

  ✓ Common adverse medication reactions include somnolence, extrapyramidal symptoms, abnormal gait, worsening cognition, cerebrovascular events, and increased risk of death (black-box warning). See Chapter 72 for more information.

Miscellaneous Therapies

- Evidence for benzodiazepine use is lacking and is not advised due to significant adverse medication reactions.
- Use of antiseizure medications (also known as mood stabilizers), **carbamazepine**, **lamotrigine**, **pregabalin**, and **gabapentin,** may be alternatives for agitation, but evidence is conflicting.
- Use of **valproic acid** is no longer recommended due to severe adverse effects.

EVALUATION OF THERAPEUTIC OUTCOMES

- At baseline interview both patient and caregiver to identify target symptoms; define therapeutic goals; and document cognitive status, physical status, functional performance, mood, thought processes, and behavior.
- Use a validated scale to assess cognition, activities of daily living (eg, the Bristol Activities of Daily Living Scale), and behavioral disturbances (eg, Neuropsychiatric Inventory Questionnaire) to quantify symptom changes and functioning.

- Observe carefully for medication efficacy, need for dosage adjustments, adherence, potential adverse medication reactions, and document the method and frequency of monitoring.
- Medication changes and adjustments should occur at 2–4 and 8–12 weeks after initiation, with assessments being repeated every 3–6 months thereafter. Several months to 1 year of treatment may be required to determine whether medications for cognition are beneficial.
- Medication deprescribing for people with AD is aided by the availability of deprescribing guidelines. When to stop treatment due to lack of efficacy, if ever, is controversial.

See Chapter 73, Alzheimer Disease, authored by Ericka L Crouse, Kristin M. Zimmerman, Emily P. Peron, Lana J Sargent, and Sarah E. Hobgood, for a more detailed discussion of this topic.

Epilepsy

- *Epilepsy* is a common neurologic condition in which a person is prone to recurrent seizures. Epilepsies are characterized by different seizure types, ranging in severity and etiologies often with neurobiological, cognitive, psychological, and social consequences. *Status epilepticus* can occur when the length of the continuous seizure activity extends past 5 minutes or time of ongoing seizure activity extends past 30 minutes, after which there is a risk of long-term consequences. It is a neurologic emergency.

PATHOPHYSIOLOGY

- Seizures result from excessive excitation or disordered inhibition of neurons. Changes in electrical activity are measured by the electroencephalogram (EEG). Initially, a small number of neurons fire abnormally. Normal membrane conductances and inhibitory synaptic currents then break down, and excitability spreads locally (focal seizure) or more widely (generalized seizure). Epileptic seizures result only when there is also synchronization of excessive neuronal firing.
- Seizure initiation is likely caused by an imbalance between excitatory (eg, glutamate, calcium, sodium, substance P, and neurokinin B) and inhibitory (γ-aminobutyric acid [GABA], adenosine, potassium, neuropeptide Y, opioid peptides, and galanin) neurotransmission. Sustained depolarization can result in neuronal death.
- Epilepsy etiologies can be classified into six categories: (1) genetic; (2) structural; (3) infectious; (4) metabolic; (5) immune; and (6) unknown.

CLINICAL PRESENTATION

- **Figure 54-1** shows the International League Against Epilepsy (ILAE) framework for the classification of seizure types.
- Many patients, particularly those with focal onset seizures with dyscognitive features or generalized tonic–clonic (GTC) seizures, are amnestic to the actual seizure event.
- Symptoms depend on seizure type and where the abnormal firing occurs. Although seizures can vary between patients, they tend to be stereotyped within an individual.
- Focal seizures (ie, partial seizures) begin in one hemisphere of the brain, and unless they become secondarily generalized (ie, evolve to a bilateral convulsive seizure), result in an asymmetric seizure. Focal seizures manifest as alterations in motor functions (eg, twitching or shaking), sensory (eg, numbness or tingling) or somatosensory symptoms, aberrations in behavior, or automatisms. Focal seizures without dyscognitive features (formerly called simple partial seizures) are associated with no impairment of consciousness. In focal seizures with dyscognitive features (formerly called complex partial seizures), there is impairment of consciousness and awareness and no memory of the event.
- Absence seizures generally occur in young children or adolescents and exhibit a sudden onset, interruption of ongoing activities, a blank stare, and possibly a brief upward rotation of the eyes. There is only a very brief (seconds) period of altered consciousness. Absence seizures have a characteristic 2- to 4-cycles per second spike and slow-wave EEG pattern.
- GTC seizures are major convulsive episodes and are always associated with a loss of consciousness. Motor symptoms are bilateral. GTC seizures may be preceded by premonitory symptoms (ie, an aura). A tonic–clonic seizure that is preceded by an aura is likely a focal seizure that is secondarily generalized. Tonic–clonic seizures begin with a short tonic contraction of muscles followed by a period of rigidity and

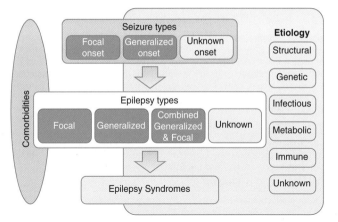

FIGURE 54-1. **ILAE framework for classification of seizure types—expanded version**.

clonic movements. The patient may lose sphincter control, bite the tongue, or become cyanotic. The episode is frequently followed by a deep sleep.

- Interictally (between seizure episodes), there are typically no objective, pathognomonic signs of epilepsy.
- Myoclonic seizures are brief shock-like muscular contractions (jerks) of the face, trunk, and extremities. They may be isolated events or rapidly repetitive. There is no alteration of consciousness.
- In atonic seizures (the hallmark of Lennox–Gastaut syndrome), there is a sudden loss of muscle tone that may be described as a head drop, dropping of a limb, or slumping to the ground.

DIAGNOSIS

- Ask the patient and family to characterize the seizure for signs/symptoms, triggers, frequency, duration, precipitating factors, time of occurrence, presence of an aura, impairment of consciousness, ictal activity, and postictal state.
- Physical, neurologic, and laboratory examinations may identify an etiology.
- A person is considered to have epilepsy if they have: (1) at least two unprovoked (or reflex) seizures occurring greater than 24 hours apart; (2) one unprovoked (or reflex) seizure and a probability of further seizures of at least 60% after two unprovoked seizures, occurring over the next 10 years; or (3) a diagnosis of an epilepsy syndrome.
- In some cases, particularly following GTC seizures, serum prolactin levels may be transiently elevated. A serum prolactin level obtained within 10–20 minutes of a tonic–clonic seizure can help differentiate seizure activity from pseudoseizure activity but not from syncope.
- Laboratory tests may rule out treatable causes of seizures (hypoglycemia, altered serum electrolyte concentrations, infections, etc.) that are not epilepsy.
- EEG is very useful in the diagnosis of various seizure disorders, but epileptiform activity is found in only about 50% of patients with epilepsy.
- Brain imaging with either a computerized tomography (CT) scan or magnetic resonance imaging (MRI) can detect structural lesions that can aid in the diagnosis of seizures and epilepsy types.

TREATMENT

- Goals of Treatment: Control or reduce the frequency and severity of seizures, minimize medication adverse effects, and ensure compliance, allowing the patient to live as normal a life as possible. Achieving complete suppression of seizures is often balanced with medication tolerability, with this decision involving the patient. Medication adverse effects, comorbidities (eg, anxiety and depression) and social factors (eg, driving, job security, relationships, and social stigma) have a significant impact on quality of life.

NONPHARMACOLOGIC THERAPY

- Nonpharmacologic therapies are available for patients in which the benefits of nonpharmacologic therapies outweigh its risk (ie, ketogenic diet, vagus nerve stimulation [VNS], and surgery among other modalities).

PHARMACOLOGIC THERAPY

- Medication selection depends on the seizure type and epilepsy classification as well as patient-specific characteristics including age, gender, susceptibility to medication adverse effects, comorbid medical conditions, medication interactions, ability for regimen adherence, and cost of therapy/insurance coverage. Figure 54-2 is a suggested algorithm for the treatment of epilepsy.
- Most antiseizure medications (ASMs) affect channel (sodium and Ca) kinetics, augment inhibitory neurotransmission (increasing central nervous system [CNS] GABA), and modulate excitatory neurotransmission (decreasing or antagonizing glutamate and aspartate). ASMs are effective against GTC and focal seizures and probably work by delaying recovery of sodium channels from activation. Medications that reduce corticothalamic T-type Ca currents are effective against generalized absence seizures.
- Begin with monotherapy, as ~65% of patients can be maintained on one ASM, although not necessarily seizure free.
- Up to 60% of patients with epilepsy have adherence issues, commonly leading to treatment failure.
- Patients who have had two or more seizures should generally be started on ASMs; however, some providers start after one seizure.
- Provide the patient with a seizure and medication adverse effect diary.
- ASM dosing is shown in Table 54-1.
- Many newer ASMs have approvals as only adjunctive therapy, but many providers will use them off-label as monotherapy.
- Evidence for comparable effectiveness is mostly available for older agents and for a few newer ones. In general, the newer ASMs appear to have comparable efficacy to the older medications, and some may be better tolerated.
- **Carbamazepine, ethosuximide, gabapentin, levetiracetam, oxcarbazepine, phenytoin valproic acid,** and **zonisamide** have strong enough evidence to be labeled efficacious or effective or as probably efficacious or effective as initial monotherapy in certain seizure types.
- Some ASMs may possibly precipitate or aggravate certain seizure types, and it is suggested that they be used with caution in those patients. Examples are **carbamazepine, gabapentin, oxcarbazepine, phenytoin, tiagabine,** and **vigabatrin** in children with absence or juvenile myoclonic epilepsy.
- Initiate ASMs with a low dose (ie, one-fourth to one-third of the anticipated maintenance dose), and titrated gradually over 3–4 weeks to a moderate dose. If seizures continue, titrate to a maximum dose. If the first ASM is ineffective or causes intolerable adverse effects, add a second ASM (preferably with a different mechanism of action), and then taper and discontinue the ineffective or intolerable ASM. If the second ASM is ineffective, then polytherapy may be indicated.
- Clinicians should determine the optimal serum concentration for each patient as seizure control may occur outside of the standard therapeutic serum range Table 54-1.

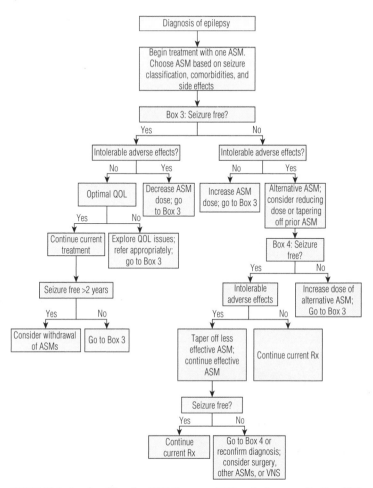

FIGURE 54-2. An algorithm for ASM therapy. ASM, antiseizure medication; VNS, vagal nerve stimulation; QOL, quality of life.

- The therapeutic range for ASMs may be different for different seizure types (eg, higher for focal seizures with dyscognitive features than for GTC seizures).
- Serum concentration determinations can be useful to document lack of or loss of efficacy, establish adherence issues, and guide therapy in patients with renal and/ or hepatic disease, those taking multiple medications, and in individuals who are pregnant or taking oral contraceptives.
- Lower doses of ASMs are often required in older individuals due to compromised renal or hepatic function and some patients have increased receptor sensitivity to CNS medications, making the accepted therapeutic range invalid. Older persons often take many medications, and thus are more prone to experience neurocognitive effects and medication interactions involving ASMs that affect the CPY450 system (eg, carbamazepine, phenytoin, valproic acid, and phenobarbital). Hypoalbumin-emia is common in older individuals, and highly bound ASMs (eg, valproic acid) can be problematic. They also experience body mass changes which can affect the

TABLE 54-1 Antiseizure Medication Dosing and Target Serum Concentration Ranges

Medication (Brand Name)	Initial Total Daily Dose (TTD)	Target Serum Concentration Range
First Generation		
Carbamazepine (Tegretol, Tegretol XR)	400 mg (>12 yrs)	4–12 mcg/mL (mg/L; 17–51 μmol/L)
	200 mg (6–12 yrs)	
	10–20 mg/kg (<6 yrs)	
Clonazepam (Klonopin)	Up to 1.5 mg (≥18 yrs)	20–70 ng/mL (mcg/L; 63–222 nmol/L)
	0.01–0.03 mg/kg (<10 yrs or <30 kg)	
Ethosuximide (Zarontin)	500 mg (≥6 yrs)	40–100 mcg/mL (mg/L; 283–708 μmol/L)
	250 mg (3–6 yrs)	
Phenobarbital (Various)	300 mg (≥18 yrs)	10–40 mcg/mL (mg/L; 43–172 μmol/L)
	5 mg/kg (<18 yrs)	
	(15–20 mg/kg LD)	
Phenytoin (Dilantin)	300 mg (≥18 yrs)	Total: 10–20 mcg/mL (mg/L; 40–79 μmol/L)
	5 mg/kg (<18 yrs)	Unbound: 0.5–3 mcg/mL (mg/L; 2–12 μmol/L)
	(15–20 mg/kg LD)	
Primidone (Mysoline)	100–125 mg (≥8 yrs)	5–10 mcg/mL (mg/L; 23–46 μmol/L)
Valproic acid, Divalproex, Valproate (Depakene, Depakote DR, Depakote ER, Depacon)	10–15 mg/kg (≥10 yrs)	50–100 mcg/mL (mg/L; 347–693 μmol/L)
Second Generation		
Felbamate (Felbatol)	1200 mg (≥14 yrs)	30–60 mcg/mL (mg/L; 126–252 μmol/L)
	15 mg/kg (2–14 yrs)	
Gabapentin (Neurontin)	300–900 mg (≥12 yrs)	2–20 mcg/mL (mg/L; 12–117 μmol/L)
	10–15 mg/kg (3–11 yrs)	

Lamotrigine (Lamictal, Lamictal XR)	25 mg (>12 years)	4–20 mcg/mL (mg/L; 16–78 µmol/L)
	0.3 mg/kg (2–12 yrs)	
Levetiracetam (Keppra, Keppra XR)	1000 mg (≥16 yrs)	12–46 mcg/mL (mg/L; 70–270 µmol/L)
	20 mg/kg (6–15 yrs)	
	Varies by age (<6 yrs)	
Oxcarbazepine (Trileptal, Oxtellar XR)	600 mg (>17 yrs)	3–35 mcg/mL (MHD) (mg/L; 12–138 µmol/L)
	8–10 mg/kg-max 600 mg (2–16 yrs)	
Tiagabine (Gabitril)	4 mg if on other ASMs that are inducers and <4 mg if not on inducers (≥12 yrs)	0.02–0.2 mcg/mL (mg/L; 0.05–0.5 µmol/L)
Topiramate (Topamax, Trokendi XR)	25–50 mg (≥10 yrs)	5–20 mcg/mL (mg/L; 15–59 µmol/L)
	25 mg (2–9 yrs)	
Zonisamide (Zonegran)	100 mg (>16 yrs)	10–40 mcg/mL (mg/L; 47–188 µmol/L)
Third Generation		
Brivaracetam (Briviact)	100 mg (≥16 yrs)	Not defined
	50–100 mg if >50 kg or 1–3 mg/kg if <50 kg (1 mo – 15 yrs)	
Cenobamate (Xcopri)	12.5 mg (≥18 yrs)	Not defined
Eslicarbazepine (Aptiom)	400 mg (≥18 yrs)	Not defined
Lacosamide (Vimpat)	200–400 mg (4–17 yrs)	Not defined
	100–200 mg (>17 yrs)	
Perampanel (Fycompa)	100 mg if >50 kg and 2 mg/kg if <50 kg (4–17 yrs)	Not defined
	2 mg	

(Continued)

TABLE 54-1 Antiseizure Medication Dosing and Target Serum Concentration Ranges *(Continued)*

Medication (Brand Name)	Initial Total Daily Dose (TTD)	Target Serum Concentration Range
Pregabalin (Lyrica)	150 mg (≥17 yrs)	Not defined
	2.5 mg/kg if >30 kg and 3.5 mg/kg between 11–29 kg (4–17 yrs)	
Third Generation with Indications for Specific Epilepsy Syndromes		
Cannabadiol (Epidiolex)	5 mg/kg (≥2 yrs)	Not defined
Clobazam (Onfi)	5 mg if ≤30 kg and 10 mg if >30 kg (≥2 yrs)	0.03–0.3 ng/mL (mcg/L; 0.1–1.0 nmol/L)
Fenfluramine (Fintepla)	0.2 mg/kg if not on STP and 0.1 mg/kg if on STP and CLB (≥2 yrs)	Not defined
Rufinamide (Banzel)	400–800 mg (≥17 yrs)	Not defined
	10 mg/kg (1–16 yrs)	
Stiripentol (Diacomit)	50 mg/kg (≥2 yrs)	4–22 mg/L (mcg/mL; 17–94 μmol/L)
Vigabatrin (Sabril)	1000 mg (≥17 yrs)	0.8–36 mcg/mL (mg/L; 6–279 μmol/L)
	350–500 mg depending on weight (2–16 yrs)	
	50 mg/kg (Infants)	

CLB, clobazam; CBZ, carbamazepine; DR, delayed-release; FDA, Food and Drug Administration; ER, extended-release; LD, loading dose; LGS, Lennox–Gastaut Syndrome; MHD, 10-monohydroxycarbazepine derivative; PB, phenobarbital; PHT, phenytoin; PI, prescribing information; PRM, primidone; STP, stiripentol; TDD, total daily dose; yrs, years; VPA, valproate; XR, extended-release.

elimination half-life and volume of distribution. **Lamotrigine** is often considered a medication of choice for older patients with focal onset seizures because of effectiveness and tolerability.

- After 12 months of treatment, the percentage who are seizure free is highest for those with only GTC seizures (48%–55%), lowest for those who have only focal seizures (23%–26%), and intermediate for those with mixed seizure types (25%–32%).

- ASM withdrawal can be considered if the patient is seizure free for 2–5 years, has a history of a single type of focal seizure or primary generalized seizures with a normal neurologic exam and normal IQ, and an EEG that has normalized with treatment. Factors favoring an unsuccessful ASM withdrawal include a high seizure frequency history, repeated episodes of status epilepticus, combination seizure types, and abnormal cognition. Always withdraw ASMs gradually.

- Medication resistance occurs if there is inadequate seizure control after two trials of tolerated and appropriately chosen and scheduled ASMs (whether as monotherapies or in combination).

- Measure free rather than total serum concentrations of highly protein-bound ASMs if suspected altered protein binding. Example situations include chronic renal failure, liver disease, hypoalbuminemia, burns, pregnancy, malnutrition, displacing medications, and in neonates and older persons. Unbound concentration monitoring is especially useful for phenytoin.

- Neonates and infants display decreased efficiency in renal elimination and may metabolize medications more slowly, but by age 2 or 3 years they may metabolize medications more rapidly than adults. Thus, neonates and infants require lower ASM doses, but children may require higher doses than adults.

- ASM monitoring is shown in Table 54-2. Concentration-dependent effects can often be alleviated by decreasing the dose or avoided by slow dose titration.

- CNS adverse medication effects are frequent and include sedation, dizziness, blurred vision, poor concentration, and ataxia.

- Barbiturates can cause more cognitive impairment than other ASMs, but in children can cause paradoxical excitement. The newer agents have less effect on cognition in general, except topiramate.

  ✓ The most widely recognized idiosyncratic reactions are ASM-induced rashes, which can progress to Stevens–Johnson syndrome/toxic epidermal necrolysis. The HLA-B*1502 variant has been associated with increased risk of developing Stevens–Johnson syndrome as well as toxic epidermal necrolysis with carbamazepine (and possibly phenytoin, lamotrigine, and oxcarbazepine) and occurs in ~15% of individuals of Asian, southeast Asian, and south Asian origin. Patients with this variant should not use these ASMs. The HLA genotype HLA-A*3101 is associated with carbamazepine-induced skin reactions in individuals of Chinese, Japanese, and European populations and this ASM should also be avoided in those with this variant.

  ✓ Others reactions include hepatitis and blood dyscrasias. Acute organ failure usually happens within the first 6 months of ASM therapy. Any patient taking an ASM who complains of lethargy, vomiting, fever, or rash should have a laboratory assessment, including white blood cell counts and liver function tests.

  ✓ An adverse effect of long-term use of ASMs is osteomalacia or osteoporosis as phenytoin, phenobarbital, carbamazepine, oxcarbazepine, felbamate, and valproic acid may interfere with vitamin D metabolism. Patients taking these medications should receive vitamin D supplementation and calcium and bone mineral density testing if other risk factors for osteoporosis are present. Laboratory tests may reveal elevated bone-specific alkaline phosphatase and decreased serum Ca and 25-OH vitamin D, as well as intact parathyroid hormone.

- Table 54-3 shows ASM elimination pathways and major effects on hepatic enzymes. Use caution when ASMs are added to or discontinued from a regimen. Pharmacokinetic interactions are a common complicating factor in ASN selection.

- Phenobarbital, phenytoin, primidone, and carbamazepine are potent inducers of cytochrome P450 (CYP450), epoxide hydrolase, and uridine diphosphate

TABLE 54-2 Antiseizure Medications (ASMs)	
ASM and Available Formulations	**Advantages/Disadvantages**
First-Generation ASM	
Carbamazepine (CBZ) Chewable tablet, ER tablet, liquid suspension	**Advantages**: Useful in comorbid bipolar disorder and trigeminal neuralgia **Disadvantages**: Worsens other seizure types in patients with absence epilepsy; HLA-B*1502 and HLA-A*3101 may be a risk factor for the development of SJS/TEN in patients of Asian ancestry; avoid if prior rash with other ASMs due to possible cross-reaction auto-inducer; active metabolite carbamazepine-10,11 epoxide contributes to idiosyncratic adverse reactions; avoid if history of bone marrow depression or sensitivity to tricyclic compounds; cannot use within 14 days of MAO inhibitor; can cause fetal harm
Clonazepam (Schedule IV) Tablet, ODT	**Advantages**: Useful when there is a need for a benzodiazepine with long half-life **Disadvantages**: May increase TC seizures when used in mixed seizure types; tolerance and dependence may occur; risk of respiratory depression which is increased when used with other CNS depressants including opioids; contraindicated in acute narrow angle glaucoma and severe hepatic impairment; metabolites may accumulate with impaired renal function and may require dose adjustment; some loss of effect may occur after 3 months; withdrawal symptoms including status epilepticus may occur after discontinuation; may increase hypersalivation; no adequate data in pregnancy—may cause fetal harm
Ethosuximide (ETX) Capsule, liquid solution	**Advantages**: Medication of choice for absence seizures **Disadvantages**: May worsen generalized TC seizures and other seizure types when used alone in mixed types of epilepsy; contraindicated in those with allergies to succinimides; may cause fetal harm; use with caution in hepatic/renal dysfunction

Interactions	Adverse Medication Reactions
Effect of CBZ on ASMs: Potent inducer of CYP3A4, CYP1A2, CYP2B6, CYP2C9/19; CBZ decreases or possibly decreases levels of brivaracetam, clonazepam, eslicarbazepine, ethosuximide, felbamate, lacosamide, lamotrigine, oxcarbazepine, perampanel, phenytoin, rufinamide, stiripentol tiagabine, topiramate, valproate, zonisamide	**BOXED WARNING**: Increased risk of SJS/TEN with HLA-B*1502 allele; aplastic anemia and agranulocytosis
	Common: CNS effects including diplopia, dizziness, drowsiness; unsteadiness, lethargy; hyponatremia from SIADH
Effect of ASMs on CBZ: Cenobamate, eslicarbazepine, felbamate, phenobarbital, phenytoin, primidone, rufinamide may decrease CBZ levels; brivaracetam, felbamate, valproate may increase carbamazepine-10,11 epoxide levels; vigabatrin may increase CBZ levels	**Serious but rare**: Other blood dyscrasias including thrombocytopenia, leukopenia; DRESS; increased intraocular pressure; cardiovascular effects including second and third degree AV heart block; hepatotoxicity
Others (partial list): CYP3A4 inhibitors/inducers may increase/decrease CBZ levels; CBZ may decrease levels of hormonal contraceptives; do not administer with other liquid agents due to possibility of precipitate occurrence	**Long term**: Hyponatremia from SIADH; metabolic bone disease including osteoporosis, osteopenia, osteomalacia
Effect of clonazepam on ASMs: Clonazepam may affect levels of phenytoin	**BOXED WARNING**: Concomitant use with opioids may result in profound sedation, respiratory depression, coma, and death
Effect of ASMs on clonazepam: Carbamazepine, lamotrigine, phenobarbital, phenytoin may decrease clonazepam levels; vigabatrin increases clonazepam, clonazepam may be affected by other enzyme inducing or enzyme-inhibiting ASMs	**Common**: CNS effects including impairment of cognitive and motor performance due to sedation and ataxia; behavior problems; paradoxical reactions such as agitation, irritability, aggression, anxiety, anger, nightmares, hallucinations and psychoses
Other (partial list): Use with opioids increases risk of respiratory depression	**Serious but rare**: Respiratory depression; hepatomegaly; muscle weakness
	Long term: Physiologic dependence; hair loss; hirsutism; ankle and facial edema
Effect of ETX on ASMs: ETX may affect levels of carbamazepine, phenobarbital, phenytoin, primidone, valproate	**Common**: GI distress including nausea/vomiting, cramps diarrhea; epigastric and abdominal pain; anorexia and weight loss; CNS effects including lethargy, fatigue, drowsiness, dizziness, ataxia
Effect of ASMs on ETX: Valproate may increase or decrease ETX levels	
	Serious but rare: Blood dyscrasias including leukopenia, agranulocytosis, pancytopenia, eosinophilia; rash including SJS; DRESS; hepatic/renal dysfunction; lupus erythematosus; psychiatric abnormalities including night terrors and paranoid psychosis
	Long-term: Behavioral changes

(Continued)

TABLE 54-2	Antiseizure Medications (ASMs) (*Continued*)
ASM and Available Formulations	**Advantages/Disadvantages**
Phenobarbital (PB) (Schedule III) Tablet, elixir, injectable solution	**Advantages**: Easily available world-wide; extensive knowledge and experience with PHB use; not FDA-approved as PHB developed in early 1900s prior to establishment of FDA and current regulatory practices **Disadvantages**: Tolerance and dependence may occur; slow taper needed when discontinuing after prolonged use; use with other CNS depressants may produce additive CNS effects; may cause respiratory depression; can cause fetal harm
Phenytoin (PHT) ER capsule; liquid suspension; injectable; chewable tablet (Fosphenytoin, a prodrug desterified by esterases in the blood to phenytoin, also available as injectable solution only)	**Advantages**: May be orally or intravenously loaded in patients who require rapid steady-state serum levels; ER formulation useful in nonadherence as dosed once daily **Disadvantages**: May aggravate seizures in patients with absence seizures; can increase blood sugar levels in diabetes; HLA-B*1502 may be a risk factor for the development of SJS/TEN in patients of Asian ancestry; CYP2C9*3 carriers may increase development of SCARS; monitoring of free phenytoin levels required in renal, hepatic impairment, hypoalbuminemia, and pregnancy; compromised absorption with concomitant tube feeds; dose adjustments required to switch between free acid and sodium salt formulations; phenytoin dose adjustments needed in older adults due to decreased clearance; may exacerbate porphyria

Interactions	Adverse Medication Reactions
Effect of PB on ASMs: PB is inducer of CYP1A2, CYP2C9, CYP2C19, CYP3A4; PB may decrease levels of carbamazepine, eslicarbazepine, ethosuximide, felbamate, lacosamide, lamotrigine, oxcarbazepine, perampanel, phenytoin, rufinamide, stiripentol, tiagabine, topiramate, valproate, zonisamide **Effect of ASMs on PB**: Cenobamate, felbamate, rufinamide, valproate may increase PB levels; phenytoin may increase or decrease PB levels **Other (partial list)**: PB may decrease levels of oral contraceptives	**Common**: CNS effects including residual sedation or "hangover," impaired cognition, drowsiness, dizziness, vertigo, ataxia, headache, sleep disturbance; paroxysmal effects including excitement, irritability and hyperactivity in older adults and children; GI effects including epigastric pain, nausea, vomiting, diarrhea, and constipation **Serious but rare**: Respiratory depression and apnea; rash (SJS, TEN); cardiac effects including bradycardia, hypotension with IV administration, syncope; hepatotoxicity; megaloblastic anemia; apnea and hypoventilation **Long term**: Behavioral changes; connective tissue disorder; intellectual blunting; metabolic bone disease (Rickets, osteopenia, osteoporosis, osteomalacia); folate deficiency (with megaloblastic anemia)
Effect of PHT on ASMs: PHT may decreases levels of brivaracetam, carbamazepine, cenobamate, clonazepam, eslicarbazepine, felbamate, ethosuximide, felbamate, lacosamide, lamotrigine, oxcarbazepine, perampanel, rufinamide, stiripentol, tiagabine, topiramate, valproate, zonisamide **Effect of ASMs on PHT**: Carbamazepine, eslicarbazepine, vigabatrin may decrease PHT levels; brivaracetam, cenobamate, ethosuximide, felbamate, methsuximide, oxcarbazepine, rufinamide, topiramate may increase PHT levels; phenobarbital, valproate may increase or decrease PHT levels **Other (partial list)**: PHT can substantially reduce delavirdine concentrations and cause loss of virologic response and resistance; may decrease contraceptive levels, may increase/decrease PT/INR when given with warfarin	**Common**: CNS effects including ataxia, nystagmus, slurred speech, decreased coordination, mental confusion, dizziness, insomnia, transient nervousness, headaches **Serious but rare**: Blood dyscrasias including thrombocytopenia, leukopenia, granulocytopenia, agranulocytosis, pancytopenia; lymphadenopathy; rash (SJS/TEN/SCARS); DRESS; hepatotoxicity; angioedema; bradycardia/cardiac arrest; purple glove syndrome with IV administration **Long term**: Connective tissue changes including skin thickening, gingival hyperplasia, coarsening of facial features, enlargement of lips; hirsutism; metabolic bone disease (osteoporosis, osteopenia, osteomalacia); peripheral neuropathy; cerebellar atrophy; folate deficiency (with megaloblastic anemia)

(Continued)

TABLE 54-2	Antiseizure Medications (ASMs) (*Continued*)
ASM and Available Formulations	**Advantages/Disadvantages**
Primidone (PRM) Tablet	**Advantages**: Useful in patients with essential tremor **Disadvantages**: Contraindicated in porphyria
Valproate (VPA) Divalproex DR sprinkle capsule and tablet, Divalproex ER 24-hour tablet, valproic acid IR capsule, valproate sodium injectable solution	**Advantages**: Useful in comorbid bipolar disorder and migraine; commonly used in all age groups including ages <10 years **Disadvantages**: Contraindicated in significant hepatic dysfunction, mitochondrial disorders caused by DNA polymerase γ (POLG) mutations, urea cycle disorders; use with caution in pancreatitis, bleeding and other hematopoietic disorders; risk of hyperammonemia with and without encephalopathy associated with concomitant topiramate use; pregnancy category D—contraindicated in females of childbearing potential and pregnancy category X for pregnant patients treated for migraine prophylaxis

Interactions	Adverse Medication Reactions
Effect of PRM on ASMs: PRM may decrease levels of carbamazepine, eslicarbazepine, ethosuximide, felbamate, lacosamide, lamotrigine, oxcarbazepine, perampanel, phenytoin, rufinamide, stiripentol, tiagabine, topiramate, valproate, zonisamide	**Common**: CNS effects including ataxia, vertigo, nystagmus, diplopia, drowsiness, fatigue; GI effects including nausea/vomiting, anorexia, fatigue; emotional disturbances including hyperirritability
Effect of ASMs on PRM: Valproate may increase PRM levels; phenytoin may increase or decrease PRM levels; carbamazepine, eslicarbazepine may affect levels	**Serious but rare**: Blood dyscrasias including granulocytopenia, agranulocytosis; rash (SJS, TEN); liver dysfunction
	Long term: Behavioral changes; intellectual blunting; connective tissue disorder; metabolic bone disease (rickets, osteomalacia); folate deficiency (with megaloblastic anemia)
Effect of VPA on ASMs: VPA may increase levels of eslicarbazepine, ethosuximide, felbamate, lamotrigine, oxcarbazepine, phenytoin, phenobarbital, rufinamide, tiagabine, topiramate, zonisamide	**BOXED WARNING**: Hepatotoxicity especially for children <2 years of age and with mitochondrial disorders; fetal risk including neural tube defects, other major malformations, and decreased IQ; pancreatitis including fatal hemorrhagic pancreatitis
Effect of ASMs on VPA: Carbamazepine, phenobarbital, phenytoin, primidone may decrease VPA levels; felbamate may increase VPA levels	**Common**: GI effects including abdominal pain/GI upset (worse with valproic acid IR), constipation, diarrhea, anorexia, increased appetite, weight gain, nausea/vomiting; CNS effects including blurred vision, ataxia, dizziness, headache, insomnia, nystagmus, somnolence, thinking abnormal, tremor; dose-dependent thrombocytopenia (>100 mg/mL)
Other (partial list): Estrogen OCP may affect VPA levels	**Serious but rare**: Hyperammonemia with and without encephalopathy; hypothermia with and without hyperammonemia; DRESS; bleeding and other hematopoietic disorders
	Long-term: Hair and nail changes including alopecia, hirsutism, hair texture and color changes, nail and nail bed disorders; irregular menses and polycystic ovary-like syndrome; weight gain; cerebral pseudoatrophy; osteoporosis and osteopenia

(Continued)

TABLE 54-2 Antiseizure Medications (ASMs) (*Continued*)

ASM and Available Formulations	Advantages/Disadvantages
Second-Generation ASMs	
Gabapentin (GBP) Tablet, capsule, oral solution	**Advantages**: Useful in post-herpetic neuralgia, chronic pain, and neuropathy; few interactions **Disadvantages**: Considered weakly efficacious; potential abuse when taken with opioids; withdrawal reaction characterized by anxiety, insomnia, nausea, sweating, and increased pain; absorption may be impaired for single oral doses >1200 mg; no adequate data in pregnancy—may cause fetal harm
Lamotrigine (LTG) Tablet, chewable tablet,[a] ODT,[a] XR tablet[a]	**Advantages**: Useful in bipolar disease; XR useful in nonadherence as dosed once daily **Disadvantages**: Slow titration required to avoid rash including SJS; rash more likely to occur if patient with prior rash to other ASM and concomitant use of valproic acid; rash incidence higher in children; may exacerbate myoclonus; dosage adjustment required in patients with moderate and severe liver impairment; no adequate data in pregnancy—may cause fetal harm
Levetiracetam (LEV) Tablet, XR tablet,[a] injectable solution	**Advantages**: Minimal interactions; XR useful in nonadherence as dosed once daily **Disadvantages**: May worsen depression, PTSD, anxiety, thought disorders; must dose adjust in dialysis/renal failure; pregnancy category C
Oxcarbazepine (OXC) Tablet, tablet ER,[a] liquid suspension[a]	**Advantages**: Useful in bipolar disorder; ER useful in nonadherence as dosed once daily **Disadvantages**: Higher incidence of hyponatremia, (as high as 25%); HLA-B*1502 in Asians may increase SJS or TEN risk; may require slower titration in renal impairment; active MHD metabolite may decrease in pregnancy; no adequate data in pregnant patients—may cause fetal harm

Interactions	Adverse Medication Reactions
Effect of GBP on ASMs: No significant effects **Effect of ASMs on GBP**: No significant effects	**Common**: CNS effects including somnolence, dizziness, ataxia, fatigue, nystagmus; peripheral edema and weight gain; GI effects including nausea/vomiting **Serious but rare**: Anaphylaxis, angioedema, DRESS; neuropsychiatric symptoms in children 3–12 years of age **Long-term**: Weight gain, peripheral edema
Effect of LTG on ASMs: No significant effects **Effect of ASMs on LTG**: Carbamazepine, cenobamate, oxcarbazepine, phenytoin, phenobarbital, primidone, rufinamide may decrease LTG levels; Cannabidiol increases LTG and valproate increases LTG levels by 2-fold **Other (partial list)**: Estrogen OCPs may decrease LTG by 50%	**BOXED WARNING**: Rash including SJS, TEN with increased risk if given with valproate, exceeding recommended initial dose or dose escalation **Common**: CNS effects including dizziness, headache, diplopia, ataxia, blurred vision, somnolence, tremor; GI effects including nausea/vomiting, abdominal pain, diarrhea; other effects including rhinitis, pharyngitis, infection, fever; rash **Serious but rare**: DRESS; blood dyscrasias; hemophagocytic lymphohistiocytosis (HLH). Rash usually appears after 3–4 weeks of therapy and is typically generalized, erythematous, and morbilliform but can progress to SJS
Effect of LEV on ASMs: No significant effects **Effect of ASMs on LEV**: No significant effects	**Common**: CNS effects including somnolence, fatigue; behavior effects including aggression, agitation, anger, anxiety, apathy, depersonalization, depression, emotional liability, hostility, irritability **Serious but rare**: Psychosis, hallucinations
Effects of OXC on ASMs: OXC is inhibitor of CYP2C19 and inducer of CYP3A4/5; OXC may decrease lamotrigine levels through UGT induction and decrease perampane levels; OXC may increase phenytoin levels **Effect of ASMs on OXC**: Carbamazepine, phenobarbital, phenytoin, primidone may decrease levels of OXC active metabolites; valproate may increase levels of OXC **Other (partial list)**: OXC may decrease estrogen OCP levels	**Common**: CNS effects including dizziness, somnolence, diplopia, fatigue, ataxia, abnormal vision, headache, nystagmus, tremor; GI effects including nausea, vomiting; hyponatremia due to SIADH; rash **Serious but rare**: SJS, TEN; DRESS; blood dyscrasias

(Continued)

TABLE 54-2	Antiseizure Medications (ASMs) (*Continued*)
ASM and Available Formulations	**Advantages/Disadvantages**
Tiagabine (TGB) Tablet	**Advantages**: None noted **Disadvantages**: Has been associated with new onset seizure, status epilepticus, and exacerbation of EEG abnormalities in those with existing epilepsy; dosage reduction may be necessary in patients with liver disease; pregnancy category C
Topiramate (TPM) Sprinkle capsule, tablet, ER capsule	**Advantages**: Useful in comorbid migraine and obesity; ER useful in nonadherence as dosed once daily **Disadvantages**: Avoid in patients with preexisting cognitive issues; renally dose adjust with CrCl <70 mL/min (1.17 mL/s); can cause fetal harm
Zonisamide (ZON) Capsule	**Advantages**: Useful in tremor; useful in nonadherence as dosed once daily **Disadvantages**: Contraindicated in those with sulfa allergy; dose efficacy may plateau at 400 mg; should not be used in renal failure due to increases in SCr and BUN and possible effects on GFR; pregnancy category C

Interactions	Adverse Medication Reactions
Effect of TGB on ASMs: TGB may decrease VPA levels by 10% **Effects of ASMs on TGB**: Carbamazepine, phenobarbital, phenytoin, primidone increases TGB clearance by 60% and may decrease TGB levels; valproate may increase TGB levels by 40%	**Common**: CNS effects including dizziness, lightheadedness, somnolence, thinking abnormal; behavior effects including asthenia, lack of energy, nervousness, irritability, difficulty with concentration or attention; GI effects including abdominal pain, nausea, and vomiting **Serious but rare**: Increase in generalized seizures and non-convulsive SE in patients with refractory epilepsy; occurrence of seizures and SE in patients without epilepsy; moderately severe to incapacitating generalized weakness; exacerbation of EEG abnormalities; rash including SJS **Long-term**: Possibility of long-term ophthalmologic effects
Effect of TPM on ASMs: TPM is weak inhibitor of CYP2C19 and inducer of CYP3A4; TPM may increase or decrease ASMs metabolized by CYP2C19 and 3A4 including felbamate and topiramate **Effect of ASMs on TPM**: Carbamazepine, phenobarbital, phenytoin, primidone may decrease TPM levels; valproate may increase TPM levels **Other (partial list)**: TPM at higher doses may decrease estrogen OCP levels	**Common**: CNS effects including fatigue, difficulty concentrating, confusion, language problems, tremor, paresthesias; behavioral effects including nervousness, anxiety **Serious but rare**: Renal stones, glaucoma, hypo/hyperthermia, oligohidrosis, metabolic acidosis, SJS, TEN, and hyperammonemia with and without encephalopathy when used with valproate **Long term**: Weight loss; renal stones; metabolic acidosis
Effect of ZON on ASMs: No significant DDIs **Effect of ASMs on ZON**: CYP3A4 inhibitors or inducers may alter ZON levels; carbamazepine, phenobarbital, phenytoin, valproate may decrease ZON levels	**Common**: CNS effects including sedation, ataxia, confusion, depression, difficulty concentrating, word-finding difficulties **Serious but rare**: Oligohidrosis and hyperthermia; renal stones; metabolic acidosis; rash (SJS, TEN); DRESS; fulminant hepatic necrosis; blood dyscrasias **Long term**: Weight loss; renal stones; metabolic acidosis

(Continued)

TABLE 54-2 Antiseizure Medications (ASMs) (*Continued*)	
ASM and Available Formulations	**Advantages/Disadvantages**
Third-Generation ASMs	
Brivaracetam (BRV, Schedule V) Tablet, oral solution, injectable solution	**Advantages**: Can consider converting well-controlled patients from levetiracetam if intolerable psychiatric adverse reactions **Disadvantages**: Dosage adjustments required in hepatic impairment; no adequate data in pregnancy—may cause fetal harm
Cenobamate (CBM, Schedule V) Tablet	**Advantages**: None **Disadvantages**: Must be slowly titrated every 2 weeks to avoid DRESS; contraindicated in familial short QT syndrome; caution when administering with other medications that shorten QT interval; use with caution and dose reduce in hepatic and renal impairment; use not recommended in end-stage hepatic or renal disease; no adequate data in pregnancy—may cause fetal harm
Eslicarbazepine (ESL) Tablet	**Advantages**: Useful in nonadherence as dosed once daily **Disadvantages**: Avoid in severe hepatic impairment; dose adjustment in renal failure; avoid concomitant use with carbamazepine and oxcarbazepine; no adequate data in pregnancy—may cause fetal harm

Interactions	Adverse Medication Reactions
Effect of BRV on ASMs: BRV may increase carbamazepine metabolite; BRV may increase phenytoin levels; no added therapeutic benefit when given with levetiracetam **Effect of ASMs on BRV**: CYP2C19 inhibitors may alter BRV levels **Other (partial list)**: rifampin will reduce BRV levels	**Common**: CNS effects including sedation, fatigue, ataxia, nystagmus; behavioral effects including irritability, aggressive behavior, anxiety, agitation, restlessness, tearfulness, apathy, altered mood, mood swings, hyperactivity, adjustment disorder; GI effects including nausea, vomiting **Serious but rare**: Angioedema; bronchospasm; decreased neutrophils; psychosis and depression; hematologic abnormalities including leukopenia and neutropenia
Effect of CBM on ASMs: CBM is a CYP2C19, CYP2B6, CYP3A inhibitor and may increase substrate levels; CBM is a CY2B6, CYPC8, CYP3A4 inducer and may decrease substrate levels; CBM may increase phenytoin, phenobarbital, clobazam concentrations; CBM may decrease lamotrigine, carbamazepine concentrations; CBM does not affect valproic acid, levetiracetam, or lacosamide **Effect of ASMs on CBM**: Phenytoin may decrease CBM; valproate, phenobarbital, carbamazepine do not significantly impact CBM **Other (partial list)**: CBM may decrease estrogen OCP levels; additive risk with other medications that shorten the QT interval; use with CNS depressants increases CNS toxicity	**Common**: CNS effects including somnolence, dizziness, fatigue, diplopia, headache; dizziness and disturbance in gait and coordination; cognitive dysfunction including memory impairment, disturbance in attention, confusional state, slowness of thought; vision changes including diplopia, blurred vision, and impaired vision; laboratory abnormalities including hepatic transaminases, potassium elevation **Serious but rare**: DRESS with fast titration (weekly intervals); QT interval shortening; appendicitis
Effect of ESL on ASMs: Inhibitor of CYP2C19; ESL may affect carbamazepine, perampanel, phenytoin, phenobarbital, primidone levels **Effect of ASMs on ESL**: Carbamazepine, phenobarbital, primidone, and phenytoin may decrease ESL levels **Other (partial list)**: ESL decreases estrogen OCP levels	**Common**: CNS effects include dizziness, somnolence, nausea, headache, diplopia, fatigue, vertigo, ataxia, blurred vision, tremor; hyponatremia due to SIADH; rash **Serious but rare**: SJS; anaphylaxis, angioedema, DRESS; cardiac effects including prolonged PR interval, AV block; hepatotoxicity; blood dyscrasias **Long-term**: Hyponatremia

(Continued)

TABLE 54-2 Antiseizure Medications (ASMs) *(Continued)*	
ASM and Available Formulations	**Advantages/Disadvantages**
Lacosamide (LCM) (Schedule V) Tablet, oral solution, injectable solution	**Advantages**: Minimal interactions **Disadvantages**: Avoid in third degree heart block; must obtain ECG prior to intravenous infusion; use with caution in patients with underlying proarrhythmic conditions or on concomitant medications that affect cardiac conduction; not recommended in severe hepatic impairment; requires dose adjustment in renal impairment; oral solution contains phenylalanine and is a risk in patients with phenylketonuria no adequate data in pregnancy—may cause fetal harm
Perampanel (PER) (Schedule III) Tablet, oral suspension	**Advantages**: Useful in mixed seizure types; useful in nonadherence as dosed once daily **Disadvantages**: Avoid in active psychosis or unstable recurrent affective disorders with significant hostility or aggressive behavior; avoid in severe hepatic/renal impairment or hemodialysis; no adequate data in pregnancy—may cause fetal harm
Pregabalin (PGB) (Schedule V) Capsule, tablet CR, oral solution	**Advantages**: Useful in patients with diabetic peripheral neuropathy, postherpetic neuralgia, fibromyalgia, neuropathic pain with spinal cord injury; minimal DDIs due to renal excretion **Disadvantages**: Caution in preexisting cognitive disorders; no adequate data in pregnancy—may cause fetal harm
Third-Generation ASMs with FDA Approval for Specific Epilepsy Syndrome Indications	
Cannabidiol (CBD, Schedule V) Oral solution	**Advantages**: Useful for refractory seizures in LGS and Dravet Syndrome **Disadvantages**: Avoid in patients with hypersensitivity reactions to cannabis, THC; liver function and bilirubin monitoring before and at 1, 3, and 6 months of treatment specially if given with valproate; no adequate data in pregnant woman—may cause fetal harm

Interactions	Adverse Medication Reactions
Effect of LCM on ASMs: LCM is a potential CYP2C19 inhibitor but no clinically significant effects of LCM on other ASMs have been observed **Effect of ASMs on LCM**: LCM is a substrate of CYP3A4, CYP2C9, and CYP2C19; carbamazepine, phenytoin, phenobarbital, primidone may decrease LCM levels by 15%–20%	**Common**: CNS effects including diplopia, headache, nausea, somnolence, dizziness, ataxia; GI effects including constipation, diarrhea, nausea, vomiting, dyspepsia, dry mouth, oral hypoesthesia/paresthesia; laboratory abnormalities including LFT elevations
Other (partial list): LCM may increase levels of strong CYP3A4 or CYP2C9 inhibitors in renal or hepatically impaired patients; risk of cardiac abnormalities increased with concomitant medications that affect cardiac conduction	**Serious but rare**: Cardiac effects including AV conduction abnormalities, prolonged PR interval, atrial arrhythmias, syncope (especially in patients with diabetes); DRESS and hypersensitivity reactions; blood abnormalities including neutropenia and anemia
Effect of PER on ASMs: PER is a modest enzyme inducer at high doses	**BOXED WARNING**: Aggression, hostility, irritability, anger, and homicidal ideation
Effect of ASMs on PER: Carbamazepine, eslicarbazepine, oxcarbazepine, phenobarbital, phenytoin, primidone, topiramate decrease PER levels; valproate has no effect on PER levels	**Common**: CNS effects including dizziness, somnolence, fatigue, falls, vertigo, ataxia, headache, confusion; GI effects including nausea, weight gain, vomiting, abdominal pain; behavioral effects including irritability anxiety; weight gain; falls sometimes leading to serious head injuries
Other (partial list): PER decreases estrogen OCP levels	**Serious but rare**: DRESS
Effect of PGB on ASMs: No significant effects **Effect of ASMs on PGB**: No significant effects	**Common**: CNS effects including dizziness, somnolence, blurred vision, difficulty with concentration and attention; dry mouth; edema and weight gain
	Serious: Potential for misuse when taken with opiates
	Long term: Weight gain
Effect of CBD on ASMs: CBD increases lamotrigine levels; CBD increase levels of clobazam's active metabolite 3-fold	**Common**: CNS effects including somnolence, fatigue, malaise, asthenia; sleep disorders including insomnia, poor quality sleep; GI effects including decreased appetite; diarrhea; transaminase elevations
Effect of ASMs on CBD: CYP3A4 and CYP2C19 inhibitors will increase CBD levels; CYP3A4 and CYP2C19 inducers will decrease CBD levels	**Serious but rare**: Hepatotoxicity; hypoxia; respiratory failure

(Continued)

TABLE 54-2	Antiseizure Medications (ASMs) (Continued)
ASM and Available Formulations	**Advantages/Disadvantages**
Clobazam (CLB, Schedule IV) Tablet, oral suspension	**Advantages**: Despite FDA approval for LGS only, may be useful in all types of epilepsy; less sedating benzodiazepine
	Disadvantages: Monitor patients with history of substance use; use with other CNS depressant may produce additive CNS effects; may cause respiratory depression, coma, and death; no adequate data in pregnant patients—may cause fetal harm
Fenfluramine (FEN, Schedule IV) Oral solution	**Advantages**: Useful for refractory seizures in Dravet Syndrome
	Disadvantages: Contraindicated within 13 days of MAO inhibitors due to risk of serotonin syndrome; may increase blood pressure; not recommended in severe hepatic or renal impairment; available only through FINETPLA REMS; no adequate data in pregnancy—may cause fetal harm
Rufinamide (RFN) Tablet, oral suspension	**Advantages**: Useful for refractory seizures in LGS
	Disadvantages: Contraindicated in severe liver impairment or in familial short QT syndrome; use caution with other drugs that shorten QT interval; no adequate data in pregnancy—may cause fetal harm

Interactions	Adverse Medication Reactions
Effect of CLB on ASMs: CLB is inhibitor of CYP2C9 and inducer of CYP3A4; CLB may affect levels of CYP2C9, CYP3A4 substrates	**BOXED WARNING**: Concomitant use with opioids increases risk of death
Effect of ASMs on CLB: Carbamazepine, felbamate, phenobarbital, phenytoin, primidone may decrease CLB levels; cannabidiol, cenobamate, stiripentol increase CLB levels	**Common**: CNS effects including somnolence, sedation, lethargy; pyrexia; constipation; drooling
Other (partial list): CLB decreases estrogen OCP levels	**Rare but serious**: Rash (SJS, TEN); anemia; liver enzyme elevations; respiratory depression
Effect of FEN on ASMs: No significant effects	**BOXED WARNING**: Risk of valvular heart disease and pulmonary arterial hypertension; echocardiograms required before, during, and after treatment
Effect of ASMs on FEN: CYP1A2, 2B6 inducers will decrease FEN; stiripentol + clobazam will increase FEN concentrations (max daily dose of FEN is reduced to 17 mg); cyproheptadine and potent 5-HT serotonin receptor binding agents may decrease efficacy of FEN	**Common**: GI effects like decreased appetite/weight, vomiting, diarrhea, constipation; CNS effects like somnolence, sedation, lethargy; fatigue, malaise, asthenia; ataxia, balance disorder, gait disturbance; blood pressure increase; salivary effects like drooling, hypersecretion; pyrexia; falls; status epilepticus; abnormal echocardiogram
Other (partial list): Rifampin will decrease FEN, strong CYP1A2 and CYP2B6 inducers will decrease FEN	**Rare but serious**: increased blood pressure including hypertensive crisis; risk of valvular disease and pulmonary arterial hypertension; mydriasis precipitating acute angle closure glaucoma
Effect of RFN on ASMs: RFN is a weak inhibitor of CYP2E1 and weak inducer of CYP3A4; RFN modestly decreases levels of carbamazepine, lamotrigine; RFN increases levels of phenobarbital, phenytoin	**Common**: CNS effects including somnolence, fatigue, coordination abnormalities, dizziness, gait disturbances, ataxia; GI effects including nausea
Effect of ASMs on RFN: Carbamazepine, phenobarbital, phenytoin decrease RFN levels by 19%-46%; valproate increases RFN levels up to 70%	**Rare but serious**: DRESS; rash (SJS); status epilepticus; leukopenia; QT interval shortening
	Other (partial list): RFN decreases estrogen OCP levels

(Continued)

TABLE 54-2	Antiseizure Medications (ASMs) (Continued)
ASM and Available Formulations	**Advantages/Disadvantages**
Stiripentol (STP) Capsule	**Advantages**: Useful for refractory seizures in Dravet Syndrome
	Disadvantages: Must be used as adjunctive therapy with clobazam; hematologic testing is required prior to first dose and q6months after due to risk of neutropenia and thrombocytopenia; powder formulation contains phenylalanine and is a risk in patients with phenylketonuria; not recommended in moderate or severe hepatic or renal impairment; no adequate data in pregnancy—may cause fetal harm
Vigabatrin (VGB) Tablet, powder packet	**Advantages**: Useful in infantile spasms for whom potential benefit outweighs risk of vision loss; renally cleared and has less DDIs than other ASMs
	Disadvantages: Permanent vision loss in most patients after a certain duration of exposure requiring eye exams Q3 months; requires REMS program registration; no adequate data in pregnancy—may cause fetal harm

Interactions	Adverse Medication Reactions
Effect of STP on ASMs: STP is inhibitor and inducer of CYP1A2, 2B6, 3A4 and possible inhibitor of CYP2C8, 2C19, P-gp transporter, BCRP transporter; STP increases clobazam concentration 2-fold and clobazam active metabolite 5-fold (must decrease clobazam dosage when used together)	**Common**: Somnolence, decreased appetite/weight, agitation, ataxia, hypotonia, nausea, tremor, dysarthria, insomnia
Effect of ASMs on STP: STP is substrate of CYP1A2, CYP2C19, CYP3A4 and phenytoin, phenobarbital, carbamazepine may decrease stiripentol levels	**Rare but serious**: Neutropenia and thrombocytopenia; monitor
Effect of VGB on ASMs: VGB is inducer of CYP2C9; VGB decreases levels of phenytoin by 20%; VGB possibly increases levels of carbamazepine by 10%; VGB increases C_{max} of clonazepam	**BOXED WARNING**: Progressive and permanent bilateral peripheral visual loss including tunnel vision and decrease in visual acuity
Effect of ASMs on VGB: Carbamazepine, primidone, valproate have no effect on VGB	**Common**: CNS effects including fatigue, somnolence, nystagmus, tremor, blurred vision, memory impairment, abnormal coordination, confusion; weight gain; edema; peripheral neuropathy; laboratory abnormalities including decreases in ALT/AST in pediatric patients; aggression; infection including upper respiratory tract infection, bronchitis, ear infection, and acute otitis media constriction; vision loss
Other (partial list): Unlikely to affect estrogen OCP levels	
	Serious but rare: Seizure exacerbation, particularly absence and myoclonic seizures in patients with generalized epilepsies; anemia; onset of vision loss is unpredictable and can occur after weeks, months, or years with risk increasing in a dose-related and life exposure–related manner; abnormal MRI signal changes in infants treated for infantile spasms strongly suggestive of intramyelinic edema in select brain areas

AMPA, A-Amino-3-Hydroxy-5-Methyl-4-Isoxazolepropionic Acid; ASM, antiseizure medication; AV, atrioventricular; BUN, blood urea nitrogen; C_{max}, maximum concentration; CNS, central nervous system; CR, controlled-release; CrCl, creatinine clearance; CYP, cytochrome p450 isoenzyme system; DDI, drug-drug interaction; DR, delayed-release; DRESS, drug rash with eosinophilia and systemic symptoms; EEG, electroencephalogram; FDA, Food and Drug Administration; ER, extended-release; GABA, gamma-aminobutyric acid; GAT1, GABA transporter type 1; GI, gastrointestinal; GFR, glomerular filtration rate; HLA, human leukocyte antigen; IQ, intelligence quotient; IR, immediate release; IV, intravenous; LGS, Lennox–Gastaut syndrome; OCP, oral contraceptives; ODT, orally dissolving tablet; PTSD, posttraumatic stress disorder; SJS, Steven–Johnson syndrome; TEN, toxic epidermal necrolysis; TBI, traumatic brain injury; TC, tonic–clonic; UGT, UDP-glucuronosyltransferase; XR, extended-release.

[a]All ASMs may increase the risk of suicidal thoughts or behavior and patients treated with an ASM should be monitored for the emergence or worsening of depression, suicidal thoughts or behavior, or any unusual changes in mood or behavior.

TABLE 54-3 Antiseizure Medication Elimination Pathways and Major Effects on Hepatic Enzymes

Antiepileptic Medications	Major Hepatic Enzymes	Induces	Inhibits
First Generation			
Carbamazepine	CYP3A4	CYP1A2; CYP2B6; CYP2C9/19; CYP3A; GT	None
Clonazepam	CYP3A	None	None
Ethosuximide	CYP3A4; CYP2E1	None	None
Phenobarbital	CYP2C9; CYP2C19	CYP 3A4/2C9/2C19/1A2; GT	None
Phenytoin	CYP2C9; CYP2C19	CYP3A; CYP2C; GT	None
Primidone			
Valproate	GT; β-oxidation	None	CYP2C9; GT epoxide hydrolase
Second Generation			
Felbamate	CYP3A4; CYP2E1; other	CYP3A4	CYP2C19; β-oxidation
Gabapentin	None	None	None
Lamotrigine	GT	GT	None
Levetiracetam	None (undergoes nonhepatic hydrolysis)	None	None
Oxcarbazepine (MHD is the active metabolite.)	Cytosolic system	CYP3A4; CYP3A5; GT	CYP2C19
Tiagabine	CYP3A4; CYP1A2; CYP2D6; CYP2C19	None	None
Topiramate	Not known	CYP3A (dose dependent)	CYP2C19
Zonisamide	CYP3A4	None	None
Third Generation			
Brivaracetam	CYP2C19	None	CYP2C19 (weak), GT epoxide hydrolase
Cenobamate	UGT2B7/B4; CYP2E1; CYP2A6; CYP2B6; CYP2C19; CYP3A4/5	CYP2B6; CYP2C8; CYP3A4	CYP 2B6; CYP2C19; CYP3A

Eslicarbazepine	Undergoes hydrolysis	GT (mild)	CYP2C19
Lacosamide	CYP2C9/19; CYP3A4	None	CYP2C19
Perampanel	CYP3A4/5; CYP1A2; CYP2B6	CYP3A4/5; CYP2B6; GT	CYP3A4/5; CYP2C8; GT
Pregabalin	None	None	None
Third Generation with Indications for Specific Epilepsy Syndromes			
Cannabadiol	CYP2C19; CYP3A4; GT	CYP1A2; CYP2B6; GT	CYP2C8/9/19
Clobazam	CYP3A4; CYP2C19; CYP2B6	CYP3A4 (weak)	CYP2C9
Fenfluramine	CYP1A2; CYP2B6; CYP2D6	None	None
Rufinamide	Hydrolysis	CYP3A4 (weak)	CYP2E1 (weak)
Stiripentol	CYP1A2; CYP2C19; CYP3A4	CYP1A2; CYP2B6; CYP3A4	CYP1A2; CYP2B6; CYP3A4; CYP 2C8/19
Vigabatrin	None	CYP2C9	None

CYP, cytochrome P450 isoenzyme system; GT, glucuronyltransferase; MHD, monohydroxy derivative, 10-OH-carbazepine.

glucuronosyltransferase enzyme systems. Valproic acid inhibits many hepatic enzyme systems and displaces some medications from plasma albumin.

- Felbamate and topiramate can act as inducers with some isoforms and inhibitors with others.

First-Generation ASMs

Carbamazepine

- Food, especially fat, may enhance the bioavailability of carbamazepine.
- Controlled- and sustained-release preparations dosed every 12 hours are bioequivalent to immediate-release preparations dosed every 6 hours. The sustained-release capsule can be opened and sprinkled on food.
- Carbamazepine may be continued unless the white blood cell count drops to less than 2500/mm^3 (2.5×10^9/L) and the absolute neutrophil count drops to less than 1000/mm^3 (1×10^9/L).
- Carbamazepine may interact with other medications by inducing their metabolism. The interaction of erythromycin and clarithromycin (CYP3A4 inhibition) with carbamazepine is particularly significant. Autoinduction of its own metabolism starts 3–5 days after initiating and is complete in 21–28 days. Reversal of autoinduction is rapid after discontinuation.

Ethosuximide

- Titration over 1–2 weeks to maintenance doses of 20 mg/kg/day usually produces therapeutic serum concentrations. It is usually given in two equal doses daily.
- There is some evidence for nonlinear metabolism at higher serum concentrations.

Phenobarbital

- Phenobarbital, a potent enzyme inducer, interacts with many medications.

Phenytoin

- Phenytoin is a first-line ASM for many seizure types (see Table 54-2).
- Absorption may be saturable at higher doses (above 400 mg). Do not change brands without careful monitoring. The intramuscular (IM) route is best avoided, as absorption is erratic. Fosphenytoin can safely be administered IV and IM. Equations are available to normalize the phenytoin concentration in patients with hypoalbuminemia or renal failure.
- Zero-order kinetics occurs within the usual therapeutic range, so any change in dose may produce disproportional changes in serum concentrations.
- Most adult patients can be maintained on a single-daily dose, but children often require more frequent administration. Only extended-release preparations should be used for single-daily dosing.
- For phenytoin serum concentration less than 7 mcg/mL (28 μmol/L), the daily dose should be increased by 100 mg; if the concentration is 7–12 mcg/mL (28–48 μmol/L), the daily dose can be increased by 50 mg; and if the concentration is greater than 12 mcg/mL (48 μmol/L), the daily dose can be increased by 30 mg or less. At concentrations greater than 50 mcg/mL (200 μmol/L), phenytoin can exacerbate seizures.
- If protein-binding interactions are suspected, free rather than total phenytoin serum concentrations are a better therapeutic guide.
- Folic acid replacement enhances phenytoin clearance and can result in loss of efficacy. Phenytoin tablets and suspension contain phenytoin acid, whereas the capsules and parenteral solution are phenytoin sodium. Ninety-two milligrams of phenytoin acid is approximately equal to 100 mg of phenytoin sodium.

Valproic acid and Divalproex Sodium

- The free fraction may increase as the total serum concentration increases, and monitoring free concentrations may be more useful than total concentrations, especially at higher serum concentrations and in patients with hypoalbuminemia.

- At least 10 metabolites have been identified, and some may be active.
- It is first-line therapy for primary generalized seizures, such as absence, myoclonic, and atonic seizures, and is approved for adjunctive and monotherapy treatment of focal onset seizures. It can also be useful in mixed seizure disorders.
- GI complaints may be minimized with the enteric-coated formulation or by giving food.
- Although carnitine supplementation may partially ameliorate hyperammonemia, it is expensive and is not generally supported.
- Valproic acid is an enzyme inhibitor. Carbapenems and combination oral contraceptives may lower serum levels of valproic acid.
- Once-daily dosing is possible with the extended-release divalproex, but more frequent dosing is the norm due to reports of breakthrough seizures.
- The enteric-coated tablet divalproex sodium causes fewer GI adverse effects. It is metabolized in the gut to valproic acid. When switching from Depakote to Depakote-ER, the dose should be increased by 14%–20%.

Second-Generation ASMs

Felbamate

- Felbamate is approved as an adjunctive treatment for seizures of Lennox–Gastaut syndrome and is effective as monotherapy or adjunctive therapy for focal onset seizures as well. Felbamate is recommended only for patients refractory to other ASMs given the risk of aplastic anemia and hepatitis. Risk factors for aplastic anemia may include a history of cytopenia, ASM allergy or toxicity, viral infection, and/or immunologic problems.

Gabapentin

- Gabapentin is a second-line agent for patients with focal onset seizures.
- Binding is saturable, causing dose-dependent bioavailability. It is eliminated exclusively renally, and dosage adjustment is necessary in patients with impaired renal function.
- Dosing is initiated at 300 mg at bedtime and increased to 300 mg twice daily on the second day and 300 mg three times daily on the third day. Further titrations are then made. When the total daily dose is 3600 mg/day or greater, divide the daily dose into at least four doses.

Lamotrigine

- Lamotrigine is useful as both adjunctive therapy and monotherapy for partial seizures and can be considered first- or second-line therapy. It is also approved for primary GTC seizures, and for primary generalized seizure of Lennox–Gastaut syndrome.

Levetiracetam

- Renal elimination of unchanged medication accounts for 66% of levetiracetam clearance, and the dose should be adjusted for impaired renal function. It is metabolized in blood by nonhepatic enzymatic hydrolysis.
- It is effective in the adjunctive treatment of focal onset seizures in patients 1 month of age and older, myoclonic seizures in patients 12 years and older, and primary GTC seizures in patients 6 years and older.
- The recommended initial adult dose is 500 mg orally twice daily. In some intractable seizure patients, the oral dose has been titrated rapidly over 3 days up to 3000 mg/day (1500 mg twice daily). It can be loaded orally or intravenously.

Oxcarbazepine

- The relationship between dose and serum concentration is linear. It does not autoinduce its own metabolism.
- It is indicated for use as adjunctive therapy for partial seizures in patients 6 years and older.

- Concurrent use of oxcarbazepine with ethinyl estradiol and levonorgestrel-containing contraceptives may render these agents less effective.
- In patients converted from carbamazepine, the typical maintenance doses of oxcarbazepine are 1.5 times the carbamazepine dose or less if patients are on larger carbamazepine doses. See manufacturer's recommendations for dosing by weight.

Tiagabine

- Tiagabine is adjunctive therapy for patients 12 years and older with focal onset seizures who have failed initial therapy.
- Tiagabine is displaced from protein by naproxen, salicylates, and valproate.

Topiramate

- Topiramate is a first-line ASM for patients with partial seizures as an adjunct or for monotherapy. It is also approved for tonic–clonic seizures in primary generalized epilepsy and for generalized seizures in Lennox–Gastaut syndrome.
- The dose should be adjusted in renally impaired patients.
- It increases the clearance of ethinyl estradiol.
- Dose increments may occur every 1 or 2 weeks. For patients on other ASMs, doses greater than 400 mg/day do not appear to lead to improved efficacy and may increase medication adverse effects.

Zonisamide

- Zonisamide, a broad-spectrum sulfonamide ASD, is approved as adjunctive therapy for partial seizures in adults.
- Start dosing in adults at 100 mg/day and increase by 100 mg/day every 2 weeks. It is suitable for once- or twice-daily dosing, but once-daily dosing may cause more adverse effects.

Third-Generation ASMs

Brivaracetam

- Dosage adjustment is required in all stages of hepatic impairment.

Cenobamate

- Cenobamate mostly has CNS adverse effects but there is a risk of DRESS (drug reaction with eosinophilia and systemic symptoms) with fast titration more rapid than every 2 weeks. It has also associated with QT interval shortening and a rate of appendicitis which is higher than in the general population.

Eslicarbazepine

- Eslicarbazepine acetate is a prodrug that undergoes hydrolysis to S-licarbazepine, the major active metabolite of oxcarbazepine. It is FDA-approved for monotherapy or adjunctive therapy of focal onset seizures.
- It is mostly renally excreted, and dosage adjustment is needed when creatinine clearance is less than 50 mL/min (0.8 mL/sec). It may increase the PR interval on the ECG. It causes less hyponatremia than oxcarbazepine

Lacosamide

- Lacosamide is approved as adjunctive therapy in patients 17 years old or greater with focal onset seizures.
- There is a linear relationship between daily doses and serum concentrations up to 800 mg/day. Moderate hepatic and renal impairment both increase systemic drug exposure by up to 40%.
- The starting dose is 100 mg/day in two divided doses, with dose increase by 100 mg/day every week until a daily dose of 200–400 mg has been reached.

Perampanel

- Perampanel has a half-life of approximately 100 hours, and its clearance is increased two- to threefold by enzyme-inducing ASMs.
- It is FDA-approved for adjunctive therapy of focal onset seizures in patients 12 years and older and as adjunctive therapy for primary GTC in patients 12 years and older.

Pregabalin

- Pregabalin is FDA-approved as adjunctive therapy for adults with focal onset seizures. It is considered a second-line agent for those who have failed initial treatment.
- It is eliminated unchanged primarily by renal excretion; dosage adjustment is required in patients with significant renal dysfunction.

Third Generation ASMs Approved for Specific Epilepsy Syndromes

Cannabadiol

- Cannabadiol is a purified drug derived from cannabis whose exact antiseizure mechanism is unknown.
- It is FDA-approved for Dravet syndrome and LGS.

Clobazam

- Abrupt discontinuation can cause a withdrawal syndrome (eg, behavioral disorder, tremor, anxiety, dysphoria, insomnia, convulsions, and psychosis).
- As an inducer of CYP3A4, clobazam may lower serum levels of some oral contraceptives. It is an inhibitor of CYP2D6. In older persons and poor metabolizers of CYP2C19, initiate dosing as in patients weighing less than 30 kg.
- It is more effective than clonazepam for LGS but less effective than clonazepam for myoclonic jerks and absence seizures. It is an adjunctive treatment for seizures of LGS.

Fenfluramine

- Fenfluramine is approved for Dravet syndrome and LGS.
- Fenfluramine goes through hepatic metabolism by CYP1A2, CYP2B6, and CYP2D6 with minor involvement of a few other CYP enzymes to an active metabolite norfenfluramine which is inactivated.
- Stiripentol and clobazam combination act upon fenfluramine to increase its levels and other potent serotonin receptor binding agents may decrease its efficacy.
- Fenfluramine does not generally act upon other ASMs and therefore has less medication interactions.
- Fenfluramine was previously used as a weight-loss drug has known cardiac effects at higher doses and has a boxed warning regarding risk of valvular heart disease and pulmonary arterial hypertension, which requires echocardiograms before, during and after treatment.

Rufinamide

- Rufinamide is an adjunctive agent used for seizures of LGS in patients 1 year and older and in adults. Reserve rufinamide for patients who have failed other ASMs.
- Children may have a higher clearance of rufinamide than adults.
- It is dosed twice daily because of slow absorption and a short half-life. Drug interactions are common.
- Multiorgan hypersensitivity has occurred within 4 weeks of dose initiation in children younger than 12 years.

Stiripentol

- Stiripentol is approved for Dravet syndrome.

- It is metabolized by CYP1A2, CYP2C19, and CYP3A4. It also induces and inhibits multiple CYP enzymes and may also possibly be an inhibitor of the P-glycoprotein and breast cancer resistance protein transporters.
- Stiripentol may cause neutropenia and thrombocytopenia which necessitates frequent monitoring of blood counts including prior to the first dose and every 6 months during and 6 months after discontinuing.

Vigabatrin

- Vigabatrin is monotherapy for infantile spasms in infants 1 month–2 years of age, and a third-line adjunctive agent for refractory complex partial seizures in patients 10 years and older.
- It is excreted unchanged in the urine. Dosage adjustment is necessary in pediatric and renally impaired patients.
- Access to vigabatrin is restricted as all providers must be certified in the Vigabatrin Risk Evaluation and Mitigation Strategy (REMS) Program.

Special Considerations in Patients of Reproductive Age

- Estrogen has a seizure-activating effect, and progesterone has a seizure-protective effect. Enzyme-inducing ASMs (eg, phenobarbital, phenytoin, carbamazepine, topiramate, oxcarbazepine, and perhaps rufinamide, lamotrigine, clobazam, and felbamate) may cause oral contraceptive failures; supplemental birth control is advised if breakthrough bleeding occurs. Individuals taking these ASMs should take twice the usual dose of emergency contraception.
- For catamenial epilepsy (seizures just before or during menses) or seizures that occur during ovulation, conventional ASMs should be tried first, but intermittent supplementation with higher-dose ASMs or benzodiazepines should be considered. Acetazolamide has been used with limited success. Progestational agents may also be effective.
- Seizures often improve in frequency at menopause.
- Individuals with epilepsy who are seizure free for 9–12 months before becoming pregnant, have an 84%–92% chance of being seizure free during pregnancy. Fluctuations in ASM serum concentrations during pregnancy may be due to reduced gastric motility, nausea and vomiting, increased medication distribution, increased renal elimination, altered hepatic enzyme activity, or changes in protein binding.
- ASM monotherapy is preferred in pregnancy. Clearance of phenytoin, carbamazepine, lamotrigine, oxcarbazepine, and levetiracetam increases during pregnancy, and protein binding may be reduced. Serum concentrations of phenobarbital, primidone, ethosuximide, and valproic acid may also fluctuate during pregnancy. Serum concentrations of ASMs should be monitored closely during pregnancy. There is a higher incidence of adverse pregnancy outcomes in individuals taking ASDs, including an increased risk of major congenital malformation (MCMs).
- Although data are insufficient to show that folate is effective in preventing MCM in pregnant individuals with epilepsy, there is no evidence of harm. Therefore, the American Association of Neurology recommends that all females of childbearing potential, take at least 0.4 mg of folic acid prior to conception and during pregnancy. Higher folate doses should be used for those who have previously delivered a child with a neural tube defect and who are taking valproic acid.
- Valproic acid is associated with a risk of MCMs 3.5–4 times that of offspring of non-epileptic individuals. There is also an increased risk of neurodevelopmental effects including effects on cognition in children. **Valproic** acid should not be used in pregnancy, but when it is used, doses should not exceed 500–600 mg/day.
- Topiramate use during pregnancy has been associated with cleft palate and possibly low birth weight and hypospadias.
- ASMs with low protein binding will accumulate in human milk.
- Other adverse outcomes of maternal seizures are growth, psychomotor, and intellectual delays. Vitamin K, 10 mg/day orally, given during the last month of pregnancy

may prevent neonatal hemorrhagic disorder. Alternatively, parenteral vitamin K can be given to the newborn at delivery.

- Data suggest that males with epilepsy have reduced fertility, and that carbamazepine, oxcarbazepine, and valproic acid are associated with sperm abnormalities. Valproic acid seems to cause testicular atrophy resulting in reduced testosterone volume, whereas levetiracetam appears to slightly increase serum testosterone.

EVALUATION OF THERAPEUTIC OUTCOMES

- The goal of therapeutic outcome for all ASMs is seizure freedom or reduction in seizure frequency, while minimizing medication adverse effects.
- Monitor long term for seizure control, adverse effects, social adjustment including quality of life, medication interactions, and adherence. Clinical response is more important than serum drug concentrations.
- Screen periodically for mental health disorders (eg, anxiety and depression).
- Ask patients and caregivers to record severity and frequency of seizures. Medication adherence should be assessed continually.

See Chapter 75, Epilepsy, authored by Viet-Huong V. Nguyen, Sunita Dergalust, and Edward Chang for a more detailed discussion of this topic.

Headache: Migraine and Tension-Type

Migraine Headache

- *Migraine*, a common, recurrent, primary headache of moderate-to-severe intensity, interferes with normal functioning and is associated with gastrointestinal (GI), neurologic, and autonomic symptoms. In migraine with aura, focal neurologic symptoms precede or accompany the attack.

PATHOPHYSIOLOGY

- Activation of trigeminal sensory nerves triggers the release of vasoactive neuropeptides, including calcitonin gene-related peptide (CGRP), neurokinin A, and substance P from perivascular axons. Vasodilation of dural blood vessels may occur with extravasation of dural plasma resulting in inflammation.
- Genetics may play a role in the occurrence of migraines as well as response to various triggers.
- Specific populations of serotonin (5-HT) receptors appear to be involved in the pathophysiology and treatment of migraine headache.

CLINICAL PRESENTATION

- Migraine headache is characterized by recurring episodes of throbbing head pain, frequently unilateral.
- About 77% of patients with migraines have premonitory symptoms (not to be confused with aura) in the hours or days before headache onset. Neurologic symptoms (phonophobia, photophobia, hyperosmia, and difficulty concentrating) are most common, but psychological (anxiety, depression, euphoria, irritability, drowsiness, hyperactivity, and restlessness), autonomic (eg, polyuria, diarrhea, and constipation), and constitutional (eg, stiff neck, yawning, thirst, food cravings, and anorexia) symptoms may also occur.
- A migraine aura is experienced by approximately 25% of patients with migraines. Aura evolves over 5–20 minutes and lasts less than 60 minutes. Visual auras can include both positive features (eg, scintillations, photopsia, teichopsia, and fortification spectrum) and negative features (eg, scotoma and hemianopsia). Sensory symptoms such as paresthesias or numbness of the arms and face, dysphasia or aphasia, weakness, and hemiparesis may also occur.
- Migraine headache pain is usually gradual in onset, peaking in intensity over minutes to hours and lasting 4–72 hours. Pain is typically in the frontotemporal region and is moderate to severe. Headache is usually unilateral and throbbing with GI symptoms (eg, nausea and vomiting) almost invariably accompanying the headache. Other systemic symptoms include anorexia, constipation, diarrhea, abdominal cramps, nasal stuffiness, blurred vision, diaphoresis, facial pallor, and localized facial, scalp, or periorbital edema. Sensory hyperacuity (photophobia, phonophobia, or osmophobia) is frequent. Many patients seek a dark, quiet place.
- Once the headache pain wanes, a resolution phase characterized by exhaustion, malaise, and irritability ensues.

DIAGNOSIS

- Diagnosis can be refined based on the frequency of monthly migraine days (MMDs) and monthly headache days (MHDs). Patients with fewer than 15 MMDs or MHDs have episodic migraine, whereas chronic migraine is diagnosed in those with at least 15 MHDs for at least three months, of which at least eight are MMDs.

- A comprehensive headache history is essential and includes age at onset; frequency, timing, and duration of attacks; possible triggers; ameliorating factors; description and characteristics of symptoms; associated signs and symptoms; treatment history; and family and social history.
- Neuroimaging should be considered in patients with unexplained abnormal neurologic examination or atypical headache history.
- Onset of migraine headaches after age 50 suggests an organic etiology, such as a mass lesion, cerebrovascular disease, or temporal arteritis.

TREATMENT

- Goals of Treatment: The goal is to prevent headaches and achieve consistent, rapid headache relief with minimal adverse effects. Additionally goals include minimizing disability and emotional distress, and enabling resumption of normal activities. Headache management without emergency department or physician office visits is also a goal.

NONPHARMACOLOGIC TREATMENT

- Apply ice to the head and recommend periods of rest or sleep, usually in a dark, quiet environment.
- Identify and avoid triggers of migraine attacks (Table 55-1).
- Behavioral interventions (relaxation therapy, biofeedback, and cognitive therapy) may help those preferring nonpharmacologic approaches or when medications are ineffective or not tolerated.

PHARMACOLOGIC TREATMENT

- Administer acute migraine therapies at the onset of migraine (Table 55-2 and Fig. 55-1).

Antiemetic Pretreatment

- Pretreatment with an antiemetic (eg, **metoclopramide**, **chlorpromazine**, or **prochlorperazine**) 15–30 minutes before oral or nonoral migraine treatments (rectal suppositories, nasal spray, or injections) may be advisable when nausea and vomiting are severe. In addition to its antiemetic effects, metoclopramide helps reverse gastroparesis and enhances absorption of oral medications.

TABLE 55-1	Commonly Reported Triggers of Migraine
Food triggers	
Alcohol	Monosodium glutamate (eg, in Chinese food, seasoned salt, and instant foods)
Caffeine/Caffeine withdrawal	Nitrate-containing foods (eg, processed meats)
Chocolate	Saccharin/Aspartame (eg, diet foods or diet sodas)
Fermented and pickled foods	Tyramine-containing foods
Environmental triggers	**Behavioral–physiologic triggers**
Glare or flickering lights	Excess or insufficient sleep
High altitude	Fatigue
Loud noises	Menstruation, menopause
Strong smells and fumes	Sexual activity
Tobacco smoke	Skipped meals/fasting
Weather changes	Strenuous physical activity (eg, prolonged overexertion)
	Stress or poststress

TABLE 55-2	Dosing of Self-Administered Acute Migraine Therapies[a]	
Medication	**Dose**	**Maximum Dose/Comments**
Analgesics		
Acetaminophen[a] (Tylenol)	500–1000 mg every 4–6 hours as needed	Maximum daily dose is 4 g
Acetaminophen 250 mg/ aspirin 250 mg/ caffeine 65 mg[a] (Excedrin Migraine)	Two tablets every 6 hours as needed	Available over-the-counter as Excedrin Migraine
Nonsteroidal anti-inflammatory drugs		
Aspirin[a]	500–1000 mg every 4–6 hours as needed	Maximum daily dose is 4 g
Ibuprofen[a] (Advil, Motrin)	400–800 mg every 4–6 hours as needed	Maximum daily dose is 3.2 g
Naproxen sodium[a] (Aleve, Anaprox)	220–550 mg every 8–12 hours as needed	Avoid doses greater than 1.375 g/day
Diclofenac potassium[a] (Cataflam, Cambia)	50–100 mg every 8 hours as needed	Avoid doses greater than 150 mg/day
Ketorolac nasal (Sprix)	31.5 mg (one spray each nostril) every 6–8 hours as needed	Maximum daily dose is 126 mg/ day × 5 days
Ketorolac IM[b]	30–60 mg every 6 hours as needed	Maximum daily dose is 120 mg/ day × 5 days
Ergotamine tartrate		
Oral tablet (1 mg) with caffeine 100 mg[b] (Cafergot)	2 mg at onset; can repeat 1–2 mg every 30 minutes as needed	Maximum dose is 6 mg/day or 10 mg/week; consider pretreatment with an antiemetic
Sublingual tablet (2 mg) (Ergomar)	2 mg at onset; can repeat 2 mg every 30 minutes as needed	Maximum dose is 4 mg/day or 10 mg/week; consider pretreatment with an antiemetic
Rectal suppository (2 mg) with caffeine 100 mg[b] (Cafergot, Migergot)	Insert half to one suppository at onset; can repeat after 1 hour if needed	Maximum dose is 4 mg/day or 10 mg/week; consider pretreatment with an antiemetic
Dihydroergotamine		
Injection 1 mg/mL (DHE 45)[b]	0.25–1 mg (IM, IV, or subcutaneous) at onset; can repeat every hour as needed	Maximum dose is 3 mg/day or 6 mg/week
Nasal spray 4 mg/mL[a] (Migranal, Trudhesa)	One spray (0.5 mg) in each nostril at onset; can repeat sequence 15 minutes later (total dose is 2 mg or four sprays) (Migranal)	Maximum dose is 3 mg/day or 6 mg/week; prime sprayer four times before using; do not tilt head back or inhale through nose while spraying; discard open ampules after 8 hours (Migranal)
	0.725 mg (one spray) in each nostril, may repeat once in 1 hour (Trudhesa)	Two (four sprays)/day or three (six sprays)/week (Trudhesa)

(Continued)

TABLE 55-2 Dosing of Self-Administered Acute Migraine Therapies[a] (*Continued*)

Medication	Dose	Maximum Dose/Comments
Triptans		
Sumatriptan[a]		
Injection (Imitrex, Zembrace Symtouch)	1–6 mg subcutaneous at onset; can repeat after 1 hour if needed	Maximum daily dose is 12 mg
Oral tablets (Imitrex)	25, 50, 85, or 100 mg at onset; can repeat after 2 hours if needed	Maximum daily dose is 200 mg; combination product with naproxen, 85/500 mg
Nasal spray (Imitrex)	5 or 20 mg at onset; can repeat after 2 hours if needed	Maximum daily dose is 40 mg
Nasal spray (Tosymra)	10 mg intranasally at onset; can repeat after 1 hour if needed	Maximum daily dose is 30 mg
Nasal powder (Onzetra Xsail)	22 mg (one 11-mg nosepiece in each nostril) at onset; can repeat after 2 hours if needed	Maximum daily dose is 44 mg (four nosepieces, 11 mg each)
Transdermal (Zecuity)	Apply 6.5 mg patch to upper arm or thigh over 4 hours; can apply second patch after 2 hours	Maximum daily dose is two patches
Zolmitriptan[a]		
Oral tablets/ODT (Zomig, Zomig-ZMT)	1.25, 2.5, or 5 mg at onset; can repeat after 2 hours if needed	Maximum daily dose is 10 mg; do not divide ODT dosage form
Nasal spray (Zomig)	2.5 or 5 mg intranasally at onset; can repeat after 2 hours if needed	Maximum daily dose is 10 mg
Naratriptan[a] (Amerge)	1 or 2.5 mg at onset; can repeat after 4 hours if needed	Maximum daily dose is 5 mg
Rizatriptan[a] oral tablets/ ODT (Maxalt, Maxalt-MLT)	5 or 10 mg at onset; can repeat after 2 hours if needed	Maximum daily dose is 30 mg; use 5 mg dose (15 mg/day maximum) in individuals on propranolol
Almotriptan[a] (Axert)	6.25 or 12.5 mg at onset; can repeat after 2 hours if needed	Maximum daily dose is 25 mg
Frovatriptan[a] (Frova)	2.5 or 5 mg at onset; can repeat in 2 hours if needed	Maximum daily dose is 7.5 mg
Eletriptan[a] (Relpax)	20 or 40 mg at onset; can repeat after 2 hours if needed	Maximum daily dose is 80 mg
Ditans		
Lasmiditan (Reyvow)	50, 100, or 200 mg at onset	Maximum of one dose per 24 hours; safety of treating more than four migraine attacks in a 30-day period has not been established

(Continued)

TABLE 55-2	Dosing of Self-Administered Acute Migraine Therapies[a] (Continued)	
Medication	**Dose**	**Maximum Dose/Comments**
CGRP antagonists		
Ubrogepant (Ubrelvy)	50 or 100 mg at onset; can repeat after 2 hours if needed	Maximum daily dose is 200 mg; safety of treating more than eight migraine attacks in a 30-day period has not been established
Rimegepant (Nurtec ODT)	75 mg at onset	Maximum of one dose per 24 hours; take on an empty stomach
Anti-emetics/Miscellaneous		
Acetaminophen, Isometheptene, and Dichloralphenazone (generic Midrin)	Two capsules to start followed by one capsule every hour until relief is obtained	Maximum five capsules/12 hours
Metoclopramide[b] (Reglan)	10 mg every 4–6 mg hours as needed	Maximum daily dose is 40 mg (also available as ODT)
Metoclopramide[a] and Aspirin[a]	10 mg (metoclopramide) and 1000 mg (aspirin) every 4–6 hours as needed	Maximum daily dose is 40 mg (metoclopramide) + 4 g (aspirin)
Prochlorperazine[b] (Compazine)	5–10 mg orally 3–4 times daily as needed or 25 mg via rectal suppository up to twice daily as needed	Maximum daily dose is 40 mg for oral and 50 mg for suppository
Promethazine (Phenergan)	25 mg oral or via rectal suppository every 4–6 hours as needed	Maximum daily dose is 100 mg

DHE, dihydroergotamine; IM, intramuscular; IV, intravenous; ODT, orally disintegrating tablet.
[a]Level A—established efficacy (≥2 Class I studies).
[b]Level B—probably effective (1 Class I or 2 Class II studies).

- **Prochlorperazine** (IM, IV, or rectal), **metoclopramide** (IV), as well as parenteral chlorpromazine and **droperidol** provide more effective pain relief than placebo.
- Frequent or excessive use of acute migraine medications can result in increasing headache frequency known as medication-overuse headache. This occurs commonly with simple or combination analgesics, **opioids ergotamine tartrate**, and **triptans**. Limit use of acute migraine therapies to 15 days or less per month.

Analgesics and Nonsteroidal Anti-Inflammatory Drugs

- Simple analgesics and nonsteroidal anti-inflammatory drugs (NSAIDs) are first-line treatments for mild to moderate migraine attacks; some severe attacks are also responsive. **Aspirin, diclofenac, ibuprofen, naproxen sodium**, and the combination of **acetaminophen plus aspirin and caffeine** are effective.
- NSAIDs appear to prevent neurogenically mediated inflammation in the trigemino-vascular system by inhibiting prostaglandin synthesis.
- Rectal analgesic preparations are options for patients with severe nausea and vomiting.
- The combination of acetaminophen, aspirin, and caffeine is approved in the United States for relieving migraine pain.
- Aspirin and acetaminophen are also available by prescription in combination with a short-acting barbiturate (**butalbital**). Use of these analgesics or narcotics should

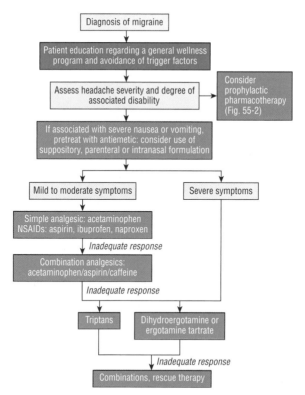

FIGURE 55-1. Treatment algorithm for migraine headaches.

be limited because of concerns about overuse, medication-overuse headache, and withdrawal.

• Metoclopramide combined with aspirin has similar efficacy to sumatriptan and may be used when triptans are contraindicated.

Ergot Alkaloids and Derivatives

• Ergot alkaloids are useful for moderate-to-severe migraine attacks. They are nonselective 5-HT$_1$ receptor agonists that constrict intracranial blood vessels and inhibit the development of neurogenic inflammation in the trigeminovascular system. Venous and arterial constriction occurs.

• **Ergotamine tartrate** is available for oral, sublingual, and rectal administration. Oral and rectal preparations contain caffeine to enhance absorption and potentiate analgesia.

• **Dihydroergotamine (DHE)** can be self-administered IM or SC, while IV administration should occur in in the hospital. The nasal spray formulation is also effective.

  ✓ Nausea and vomiting are common ergotamine derivative adverse effects, so consider antiemetic pretreatment and titrate to a dose that is not nauseating. Others include abdominal pain, weakness, fatigue, paresthesias, muscle pain, diarrhea, and chest tightness. Symptoms of severe peripheral ischemia (ergotism) include cold, numb, painful extremities; continuous paresthesias; diminished peripheral pulses; and claudication. Gangrenous extremities, myocardial infarction (MI), hepatic necrosis, and bowel and brain ischemia have occurred rarely with ergotamine. Do not use ergotamine derivatives and triptans within 24 hours of each other.

✓ Contraindications to ergot derivatives include renal and hepatic failure; coronary, cerebral, or peripheral vascular disease; uncontrolled hypertension; sepsis; and individuals who are pregnant or nursing.

✓ DHE does not appear to cause rebound headache, but dosage restrictions for ergotamine tartrate should be strictly observed to prevent this complication.

Serotonin Receptor Agonists (Triptans)

• The triptans are appropriate first-line therapies for patients with mild-to-severe migraine or as rescue therapy when nonspecific medications are ineffective.

• They are selective agonists of the 5-HT_{1B} and 5-HT_{1D} receptors. Relief of migraine headache results from: (1) normalization of dilated intracranial arteries, (2) inhibition of vasoactive peptide release, and (3) inhibition of transmission through second-order neurons ascending to the thalamus.

• **Sumatriptan** SC injection is packaged as an autoinjector device for self-administration. It also offers enhanced efficacy and more rapid onset of action. Intranasal sumatriptan also has a faster onset of effect and produces similar rates of response to the oral.

• Second-generation triptans (all except sumatriptan) have higher oral bioavailability and longer half-lives than oral sumatriptan, which could theoretically increase efficacy. However, comparative clinical trials are necessary to determine their relative efficacy. **Frovatriptan** and **naratriptan** have the longest half-lives, slowest onset of action, and less headache recurrence. Pharmacokinetic characteristics of the triptans are shown in Table 55-3.

• Lack of response to one triptan does not preclude effective therapy with another triptan.

✓ Triptan adverse effects include paresthesias, fatigue, dizziness, flushing, warm sensations, and somnolence. Minor injection site reactions are reported with SC use, and taste perversion and nasal discomfort may occur with intranasal administration.

✓ Up to 25% of patients report chest tightness, pressure, heaviness, or pain in the chest, neck, or throat due to an unknown mechanism. A cardiac source is unlikely, although isolated MI and coronary vasospasm with ischemia have been reported. Use triptans cautiously in patients at risk for unrecognized coronary artery disease. Assess cardiovascular risk before giving triptans to menopausal individuals, males over 40 years of age, and patients with uncontrolled risk factors. Administer the first dose under medical supervision. Ischemic heart disease, uncontrolled hypertension, cerebrovascular disease, hemiplegic and basilar migraine, and pregnancy are contraindications to their use.

✓ Do not give triptans within 24 hours of ergotamine derivative administration or within 2 weeks of therapy with monoamine oxidase inhibitors. Concomitant use of triptans with serotonin antidepressants has been reported to cause serotonin syndrome.

Ditans

• **Lamiditan** is in a new class of abortive migraine medications known as "ditans" that acts by blocking both neurogenic inflammation in dura and simulation of the trigeminal nucleus caudalis.

✓ Common adverse effects include dizziness, parethesia, sedation and nausea/vomiting. It has a specific warning in its labeling regarding not driving a motor vehicle or operating heavy machinery for at least 8 hours following each dose due to drowsiness.

Calcitonin Gene-Related Peptide (CGRP) Antagonists

• **Ubrogepant** and **rimegepant** are also known as "gepants" work by blocking CGRP receptors, resulting in vasoconstriction and a reduction in neurogenic inflammation.

TABLE 55-3 Pharmacokinetic Characteristics of Triptans

Medication	Half-Life (Hours)	Time to Maximal Concentration (t_{max})	Bioavailability (%)	Elimination
Almotriptan	3–4	1.4–3.8 hours	80	MAO-A, CYP3A4, CYP2D6
Eletriptan	4–5	1–2 hours	50	CYP3A4
Frovatriptan	25	2–4 hours	24–30	Mostly unchanged, CYP1A2
Naratriptan	5–6	2–3 hours	63–74	Largely unchanged, CYP450 (various isoenzymes)
Rizatriptan	2–3		45	MAO-A
Oral tablets		1–1.2 hours		
Disintegrating		1.6–2.5 hours		
Sumatriptan	2			MAO-A
SC injection		12–15 minutes	97	
Oral tablets		2.5 hours	14	
Nasal spray		10 minutes	17	
Nasal powder		45 minutes		
Patch		1.1 hours	45	
Zolmitriptan	3		40–48	CYP1A2, MAO-A
Oral		2 hours		
Disintegrating		3.3 hours		
Nasal		4 hours		

CYP, cytochrome P450; MAO-A, monoamine oxidase type A.

- Their efficacy is similar to the triptans and lasmiditan, however they tend to be better tolerated. A history of cardiovascular disease is not a contraindication and medication overuse headache may not occur with their use.
  - ✓ Adverse medication effects include nausea for rimegepant and nausea, xerostomia, and somnolence for ubrogepant.
  - ✓ Rimegepant has a half-life of 11 hours and is not recommended for repeat dosing within 24 hours, while ubrogepant's half-life is 5–7 hours and the dose can repeated 2 hours after the initial administration.
  - ✓ There are significant medication interactions and concomitant use with strong CYP3A4 inhibitors, P-glycoprotein (P-gp) inhibitors, and Breast Cancer Resistance Protein (BCRP) inhibitors should be avoided. Use of "gepants" should also be avoided in severe renal or hepatic impairment.

Opioids

- There is inadequate evidence for opioids and derivatives (eg, **meperidine**, **butorphanol**, **oxycodone**, and **hydromorphone**) for the treatment of migraines. Combinations of either oral **codeine** or **tramadol** and acetaminophen are probably effective, and **butorphanol** nasal spray has established efficacy.
- Reserve these for patients with moderate-to-severe infrequent headaches in whom conventional therapies are contraindicated or as rescue medication after failure to respond to conventional therapies. Closely supervise therapy.

Prophylactic Therapy

- Prophylactic therapies (Table 55-4 and Fig. 55-2) are administered daily to reduce the frequency, severity, and duration of attacks, and to increase responsiveness to acute therapies.

TABLE 55-4	Dosing of Prophylactic Migraine Therapies		
Medication	**Initial Dose**	**Usual Range**	**Comments**
β-Adrenergic antagonists			
Atenolol[a] (Tenormin)	25–50 mg/day	50–200 mg/day	
Metoprolol[b] (Toprol, Toprol XL)	25–100 mg/day in divided doses	100–200 mg/day in divided doses	Dose short-acting two to four times a day and extended-release one to two times a day
Nadolol[a] (Corgard)	40–80 mg/day	80–240 mg/day	
Propranolol[b] (Inderal, Inderal LA)	40 mg/day in divided doses	40–160 mg/day in divided doses	Dose short-acting two to three times a day and extended-release one to two times a day
Timolol[b] (Blocadren)	20 mg/day in divided doses	20–60 mg/day in divided doses	
Antidepressants			
Amitriptyline[a] (Elavil)	10 mg at bedtime	20–50 mg at bedtime	
Venlafaxine[a] (Effexor, Effexor-XR)	37.5 mg/day	75–150 mg/day	Dose short-acting two times a day and extended-release once daily
Antiseizure medications			
Topiramate[b] (Topamax)	12.5–25 mg/day	50–200 mg/day in divided doses or only at bedtime	Increase by 12.5–25 mg/week
Valproic acid/ divalproex sodium[b] (Depakene, Depakote, Depakote ER)	250–500 mg/day in divided doses, or daily for extended-release	500–1500 mg/day	Dose short-acting two times a day and extended-release once daily; monitor levels if compliance is an issue
CGRP antagonists (Anti-CGRP antibodies)			
Erenumab-aooe (Aimovig)	70 mg subcutaneously monthly	70–140 mg subcutaneously every month	
Fremanezumab-vfrm (Ajovy)	225 mg subcutaneously monthly or 675 mg subcutaneously every 3 months	225 mg subcutaneously monthly or 675 mg subcutaneously every 3 months	

(Continued)

TABLE 55-4	Dosing of Prophylactic Migraine Therapies (*Continued*)		
Medication	**Initial Dose**	**Usual Range**	**Comments**
Galcanezumab-gnlm (Emgality)	240 mg subcutaneous loading dose, followed by 120 mg subcutaneously monthly	120 mg subcutaneously every month	
Eptinezumab-jjmr (Vyepti)	100 mg via IV infusion over 30 minutes every 3 months	100–300 mg IV infusion over 30 minutes every 3 months	
CGRP antagonists ("gepants")			
Atogepant (Quilpta)	10 mg/day	60 mg/day	Taken with or without food
Rimegepant (Nurtec ODT)	75 mg every other day	75 mg/day	No titration required and taken on an empty stomach
Nonsteroidal anti-inflammatory drugs—*For prevention of menstrual migraine only*			
Ibuprofen[a] (Motrin)	200 mg/day in three to four divided doses	200–800 mg/day in three to four divided doses (maximum daily dose is 3200 mg)	Use intermittently only; daily or prolonged use may lead to medication-overuse headaches
Ketoprofen[a] (Orudis)	150 mg/day in divided doses	150 mg/day in divided doses	Use intermittently only; daily or prolonged use may lead to medication-overuse headaches
Naproxen sodium[a] (Aleve, Anaprox)	550 mg/day in divided doses	550–1100 mg/day in divided doses	Use intermittently only; daily or prolonged use may lead to medication-overuse headaches
Triptans—*For prevention of menstrual migraine only*			
Frovatriptan[b] (Frova)	2.5 mg/day or 5 mg/day in divided doses; start 6 days prior to anticipated start of menstruation	5 mg/day in divided doses	Use intermittently only; daily or prolonged use may lead to medication-overuse headaches
Naratriptan[a] (Amerge)	2 mg/day in divided doses; start 6 days prior to anticipated start of menstruation	2 mg/day in divided doses	Use intermittently only; daily or prolonged use may lead to medication-overuse headaches

(*Continued*)

TABLE 55-4	Dosing of Prophylactic Migraine Therapies (*Continued*)		
Medication	**Initial Dose**	**Usual Range**	**Comments**
Zolmitriptan[a] (Zomig)	5–7.5 mg/day in divided doses; start 6 days prior to anticipated start of menstruation	5–7.5 mg/day in divided doses	Use intermittently only; daily or prolonged use may lead to medication-overuse headaches
Miscellaneous			
Histamine[a] (Histatrol)	1–10 ng two times/ week	Same as initial dose	May cause transient itching and burning at injection site
Magnesium[a]	400 mg/day	800 mg/day in divided doses	May be more helpful in migraine with aura and menstrual migraine
MIG-99[a] (feverfew)	10–100 mg/day in divided doses	Same as initial dose	Withdrawal may be associated with increased headaches
Petasites[b]	100–150 mg/day in divided doses	150 mg/day in divided doses	Use only commercial preparations, plant is carcinogenic
Riboflavin[a]	400 mg/day in divided doses	400 mg/day in divided doses	Benefit only after 3 months

[a]Level B—probably effective (1 Class I or 2 Class II studies).
[b]Level A—established efficacy (≥2 Class I studies).

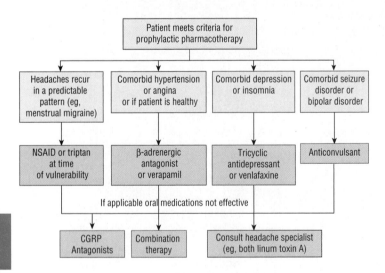

FIGURE 55-2. Treatment algorithm for prophylactic management of migraine headaches. (NSAID, nonsteroidal anti-inflammatory drug.)

- Consider prophylaxis in the setting of recurring migraines producing significant disability; frequent attacks requiring symptomatic medication more than twice per week; symptomatic therapies that are ineffective, contraindicated, or produce serious adverse effects; profound disruption or risk of neurologic injury; and patient preference to limit the number of attacks.
- Preventive therapy may also be given intermittently when headaches recur in a predictable pattern (eg, exercise-induced or menstrual migraine).
- Because efficacy appears to be similar, medication selection is based on adverse effect profiles and comorbid conditions. Response to an agent is unpredictable, and a 2- to 3-month trial is necessary to achieve clinical benefit.
- Only **propranolol**, **timolol**, **divalproex sodium**, **topiramate**, **erenumab-aooe**, **fremanezumab-vfrm**, and **galcanezumab-gnlm** are Food and Drug Administration (FDA) approved for migraine prevention. Other established agents also have probable efficacy.
- Initiate prophylaxis with low doses, and advance slowly until a therapeutic effect is achieved or adverse effects become intolerable. Continue prophylaxis for at least 6–12 months after headache frequency and severity have diminished, and then gradual tapering or discontinuation may be reasonable.

B-Adrenergic Antagonists

- **Propranolol**, **timolol**, and **metoprolol** reduce the frequency of migraine attacks by half in >50% of patients. **Atenolol** and **nadolol** are probably also effective.
  ✓ Adverse effects include drowsiness, fatigue, sleep disturbances, vivid dreams, memory disturbance, depression, sexual dysfunction, bradycardia, and hypotension.
  ✓ Use with caution in patients with heart failure, peripheral vascular disease, atrioventricular conduction disturbances, asthma, depression, and diabetes.

Antidepressants

- The tricyclic antidepressants (TCAs) **amitriptyline** and **venlafaxine** are probably effective for migraine prophylaxis. Data regarding other antidepressants is insufficient.
- Their beneficial effects in migraine prophylaxis are independent of antidepressant activity and may be related to downregulation of central 5-HT$_2$ receptors, increased synaptic norepinephrine, and enhanced opioid receptor actions.
  ✓ TCAs are usually well tolerated at the doses used for migraine prophylaxis, but anticholinergic effects may limit use, especially in older patients or those with benign prostatic hyperplasia or glaucoma. Evening doses are due to sedation. Increased appetite and weight gain can occur. Orthostatic hypotension and slowed atrioventricular conduction are occasionally reported.

Antiseizure Medications

- **Valproic acid**, **divalproex sodium**, and **topiramate** can reduce the frequency, severity, and duration of headaches. **Carbamazepine** is possibly effective and **lamotrigine** is probably ineffective.
  ✓ Adverse effects of valproic acid and divalproex sodium include nausea, tremor, somnolence, weight gain, hair loss, and hepatotoxicity. Obtain baseline liver function tests. The extended-release formulation of divalproex sodium is administered once daily and is better tolerated than the enteric-coated formulation. Valproate is contraindicated in pregnancy and patients with a history of pancreatitis or chronic liver disease.
  ✓ Paresthesias (~50% of patients) and weight loss (9%–12% of patients) are common adverse effects of topiramate. Others include fatigue, anorexia, diarrhea, difficulty with memory, language problems, taste perversions, and nausea. Use topiramate cautiously or avoid in those with a history of kidney stones or cognitive impairment.

Nonsteroidal Anti-Inflammatory Drugs

- NSAIDs are modestly effective for reducing the frequency, severity, and duration of migraine attacks. For migraine prevention, evidence for efficacy is strongest for naproxen and weakest for aspirin.
- They may be used intermittently to prevent headaches that recur in a predictable pattern (eg, menstrual migraine). Initiate up to 1 week before the time of headache vulnerability, and continue until vulnerability is passed.
  ✓ Potential GI and renal toxicity limit daily or prolonged use.

Triptans

- Frovatriptan has established prophylactic efficacy, while naratriptan and zolmitriptan are probably effective. They are usually started one or two days before the expected headache onset and continued during the period of vulnerability.

Calcitonin Gene-Related Peptide Antagonists

- Several anti-CGRP receptor monoclonal antibodies (**erenumab-aooe, fremanezumab-vfrm,** and **eptinezumab-jjmr,** and **galcanezumab-gnlm**) have demonstrated efficacy in the prevention of episodic and chronic migraines (with or without aura). Data regarding long-term safety and efficacy are still needed. Cost and access may limit their use.
  ✓ Injection site reactions are the most common adverse event for all of the subcutaneous agents. Other adverse effects include constipation, nasopharyngitis, and hypersensitivity. There are no known medication interactions.

Miscellaneous Prophylactic Agents

- The angiotensin-converting enzyme inhibitor **lisinopril** and the angiotensin II receptor blocker **candesartan** have been found to be effective. The calcium channel blocker **verapamil** has been used clinically fairly extensively. **Clonidine** and **guanfacine** have also demonstrated possible efficacy, although adverse effects limit their use.
- Localized injections of **botulinum toxin type A** is FDA-approved for individuals who have 15 or more headache days per month lasting four or more hours daily. A six-week trial is as effective as other second line therapies.

EVALUATION OF THERAPEUTIC OUTCOMES

- Monitor patients taking abortive therapy for frequency of use of prescription and nonprescription medications and for adverse effects.
- Document patterns of abortive medication used to establish the need for prophylactic therapy. Monitor prophylactic therapies closely for adverse effects, abortive therapy needs, adequate dosing, and compliance.

Tension-Type Headache

- *Tension-type headache*, the most common type of primary headaches, is more common in females than males. Pain is usually mild to moderate and nonpulsatile. These headaches are classified as either episodic (infrequent or frequent) or chronic based on the frequency and duration of the attacks.

PATHOPHYSIOLOGY

- Pain is thought to originate from myofascial factors and peripheral sensitization of nociceptors. Central mechanisms are also involved. Mental distress, nonphysiologic motor stress, a local myofascial release of irritants, or a combination of these may be the initiating stimulus.

CLINICAL PRESENTATION

- Premonitory symptoms and aura are absent, and pain is usually mild to moderate, bilateral (having a hatband pattern), and nonpulsatile.
- Mild photophobia or phonophobia may occur. Pericranial or cervical muscles may have tender spots or localized nodules in some patients.

DIAGNOSIS

- A comprehensive headache history is essential and includes age at onset; frequency, timing, and duration of attacks; possible triggers; ameliorating factors; description and characteristics of symptoms; associated signs and symptoms; treatment history; and family and social history.

TREATMENT

- <u>Goals of Treatment</u>: Pain relief and prevention of further headaches are the main desired outcomes of treatment.

NONPHARMACOLOGIC THERAPY

- Nonpharmacologic therapies include reassurance and counseling, stress management, relaxation training, and biofeedback. Evidence supporting physical therapeutic options (eg, heat or cold packs, ultrasound, electrical nerve stimulation, massage, acupuncture, trigger point injections, and occipital nerve blocks) has been inconsistent.

PHARMACOLOGIC THERAPY

Acute Treatment

- Simple analgesics (alone or in combination with caffeine) and NSAIDs are the mainstay of acute therapy. **Acetaminophen**, **aspirin**, **diclofenac**, **ibuprofen**, **naproxen**, **ketoprofen**, and **ketorolac** are effective.
- The combination of aspirin or acetaminophen with **butalbital** is an effective option. **Codeine** can by effective in select patients, but butalbital and codeine combinations should be avoided when possible due to the risk of overuse and unhealthy use. There is no evidence to support the efficacy of muscle relaxants.
- Give acute medication for episodic headache no more often than 10 days a month for butalbital-containing or combination analgesics, or 15 days a month for NSAIDs to prevent the development of chronic tension-type headache.

Prophylactic Therapy

- Preventive treatment is used if headache frequency is more than two per week, have a duration longer than 3–4 hours, or cause substantial disability.
- The TCAs are used most often for prophylaxis of tension headache, but **venlafaxine**, **mirtazapine**, **gabapentin**, **topiramate**, and **tizanidine** may also be effective. Limited data suggest that trigger point injections of lidocaine may reduce headache frequency and data regarding botulinum toxin injections is inconsistent.

EVALUATION OF THERAPEUTIC OUTCOMES

- Monitor for frequency, intensity, and duration of headaches and for any change in the headache pattern. Encourage patients to keep a headache diary to document frequency, duration, and severity of headaches, headache response, and potential triggers of migraine headaches.

See Chapter 80, Headache Disorders, authored by Kimberly B. Tallian and Natalie T. Heinrich , for a more detailed discussion of this topic.

Multiple Sclerosis

- *Multiple Sclerosis* (MS) is an autoimmune illness characterized by central nervous system (CNS) demyelination and axonal damage. It is classified into several categories, differentiated by disease progression over time, clinical presentation, and response to therapy.

PATHOPHYSIOLOGY

- The true etiology of MS is unknown; however, substantial evidence suggests an autoimmune process directed against myelin and oligodendrocytes, the cells that make myelin.
- The actual mediator of myelin and axonal destruction has not been established but may reflect a combination of macrophages, antibodies, destructive cytokines, and reactive oxygen intermediates.
- MS lesions are heterogeneous, possibly due to differences in lesion evolution over time, underlying immunopathogenesis, or a combination.

CLINICAL PRESENTATION

- MS clinical presentation is highly variable among patients and over time.
- The clinical course is classified into relapsing-remitting MS (RRMS), progressive MS (PPMS), and secondary-progressive MS (SPMS).
- Patients with RRMS have relapses/exacerbations with new symptoms lasting at least 24 hours. Most patients with RRMS enter a progressive phase (SPMS) where attacks and remissions are challenging to identify. Patients with PPMS have progressive disease at the outset of diagnosis.
- Signs and symptoms of MS are divided into three categories: primary symptoms, secondary symptoms, and tertiary symptoms.

PRIMARY SYMPTOMS

- Direct consequence of demyelination.
- These include: visual complaints/optic neuritis, gait problems and falls, paresthesias, pain, spasticity, weakness, ataxia, speech difficulty, psychological changes, cognitive changes, fatigue, bowel/bladder dysfunction, sexual dysfunction, tremor.

SECONDARY SYMPTOMS

- Complications resulting from primary symptoms.
- May include recurrent urinary tract infections, urinary calculi, decubiti and osteomyelitis, osteoporosis, respiratory infections, poor nutrition, and depression.

TERTIARY SYMPTOMS

- These reflect the effect of the disease on the patient's everyday life.
- These include financial, personal/social, vocational, and emotional problems.

DIAGNOSIS

- MS is a diagnosis of exclusion as symptoms can frequently be attributed to other neurologic diseases, just as many syndromes can mimic MS.
- The three diagnostic criteria are: (1) MS [either RRMS or PPMS], (2) possible MS, and (3) not MS. There should be at least two episodes of neurologic disturbance, which reflect specific CNS damage not explained by other mechanisms. **Figure 56-1** outlines diagnostic decision-making.

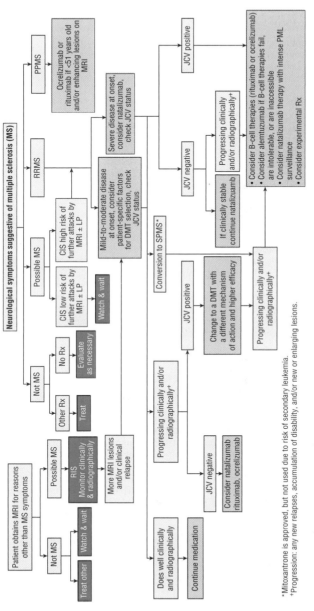

FIGURE 56-1. **Algorithm for management of clinically definite multiple sclerosis.** (MRI, magnetic resonance imaging; LP, lumbar puncture; MS, multiple sclerosis; CIS, clinically isolated syndrome; JCV, John Cunningham virus; PML, progressive multifocal leukoencephalopathy; RRMS, relapsing-remitting multiple sclerosis; PPMS, primary progressive multiple sclerosis; RIS, radiologically isolated syndrome; SPMS, secondary progressive multiple sclerosis; Rx, prescription medication; DMT, disease modifying therapy.)

*Mitoxantrone is approved, but not used due to risk of secondary leukemia.
+Progression: any new relapses, accumulation of disability, and/or new or enlarging lesions.

- There are no tests specific for MS. Evidence is gathered through (1) MRI of the brain and spine, (2) CSF evaluation examining for increased oligoclonal bands and increased IgG, (3) evoked potentials, and (4) optic coherence tomography.

TREATMENT

- <u>Goals of Treatment</u>: To improve the overall quality of life, maintain employment, and minimize long-term disability for MS patients.
- Treatment falls into three broad categories: (1) treatment of exacerbations, (2) disease-modifying therapies (DMTs), and (3) symptomatic therapies.

NONPHARMACOLOGIC THERAPY

- Occupational therapy may improve daily living activities by helping learn new techniques or tools to accomplish these tasks and remain active.
- Physical therapy may improve muscle strength, gait, and balance, and stretching exercises reduce muscle spasms. Mobility may improve with aids such as canes or walkers active.

PHARMACOLOGIC THERAPY

- Symptom severity at the initial presentation will determine whether an induction or escalation algorithm is assigned to an individual.
- An algorithm for the management of MS is shown in **Fig. 56-1**. **Table 56-1** summarizes available disease-modifying treatments (DMTs) and dosing, and **Table 56-2** shows medication adverse event monitoring.
- Treating exacerbations will shorten the duration and possibly decrease attack severity. Treat relapses that are (1) mono- or polysymptomatic presentations; (2) localized to the optic nerve, spinal cord, or brainstem; (3) those with functional limitations that affect activities of daily living; and (4) symptoms that worsen over a 2-week period.
- DMTs can alter the course of the illness and diminish progressive disability over time; however, symptomatic disease management is required to maintain quality of life.
- Treatment guidelines exist, but decisions are frequently based on the patient's wishes and goals.

Glucocorticoids

- An IV injection of high-dose corticosteroids is recommended when the patient's functional ability is affected by a relapse.
- **Adrenocorticotropic hormone** (ACTH) is the only FDA-approved agent for MS exacerbation treatment; it is rarely used due to cost and availability.
- **Methylprednisolone** doses range from 500 to 1000 mg/day, given IV for three to (rarely) 10 days. If initiated within 2 weeks of symptom onset, functional recovery after an exacerbation is more rapid, with improvement beginning after 3–5 days.
- Equipotent doses of oral **prednisone** or **dexamethasone** can be substituted for IV methylprednisolone, although dexamethasone use is not well supported in the literature.
  ✓ Common adverse medication reactions include sleep disturbance, a metallic taste in the mouth, and rarely gastrointestinal (GI) upset (See Table 56-2).

Disease-Modifying Therapy (DMT)

- DMTs are either immunomodulatory (ie, alter the immune signals without cytotoxic effect or bone marrow suppression) or immunosuppressive (ie, alter the immune system through a direct cytotoxic activity or bone marrow suppression).
- Four **interferon** (IFN) formulations and **glatiramer acetate** (a non-IFN) make up first-generation DMTs.
- The FDA has also approved several second-generation DMTs, **ocrelizumab, natalizumab, mitoxantrone, fingolimod, siponimod, ozanimod, ponesimod, teriflunomide, dimethyl fumarate, diroximel fumarate, monomethyl fumarate, cladribine, ofatumumab**, and **alemtuzumab** for the treatment of relapsing forms of MS.

TABLE 56-1	Disease-Modifying Therapy				
Medication	Brand Name	Indication	Initial Dose	Usual Dose	Comment
First-generation agents					
Self-injectables					
Interferon-β$_{1a}$	Avonex	Relapsing forms of MS	30 mcg (6 million IU) IM once weekly	30 mcg IM once weekly	Considered low-potency interferon
	Rebif	Relapsing forms of MS	22 mcg SQ three times a week	22 or 44 mcg SQ three times a week	Considered a high-potency interferon
Interferon-β$_{1b}$	Betaseron, Extavia	Relapsing forms of MS	250 mcg (8 million IU) SQ every other day	250 mcg SQ every other day	Betaseron/Extavia is considered a high-potency interferon. Pregnancy category C
Pegylated Interferon-β$_{1a}$	Plegridy	RRMS	6.3 mcg SQ day 1, then 94 mcg SQ on day 15, then 125 mcg SQ on day 29, then 125 mcg SQ every 14 days	125 mg SQ every 14 days	Can premedicate or concurrently use an antipyretic/analgesic for flu-like symptoms. Pregnancy category C
Glatiramer acetate	Copaxone, Glatopa	CIS, RRMS	20 mg SQ once daily or 40 mg SQ three times a week	20 mg SQ once daily or 40 mg SQ three times a week	Glatopa is the generic version of Copaxone. Pregnancy category B
IV infusion					
Mitoxantrone	Novantrone	SPMS and worsening RRMS	12 mg/m² IV every 3 months	12 mg/m² IV every 3 months	Lifetime dose should not exceed 140 mg/m². Pregnancy category D
Second-generation agents					
Oral					
Fingolimod	Gilenya	Relapsing forms of MS, in patients 10 years and older	Adult: 0.5 mg orally once daily. Pediatric: <40 kg 0.25 mg orally once daily, >40 kg 0.5 mg orally once daily	Adult: 0.5 mg orally once daily. Pediatric: <40 kg 0.25 mg orally once daily, >40 kg 0.5 mg orally once daily	Medication guide required. Pregnancy category C

(Continued)

TABLE 56-1 Disease-Modifying Therapy (*Continued*)

Medication	Brand Name	Indication	Initial Dose	Usual Dose	Comment
Siponimod	Mayzent	Relapsing forms of MS	CYP2C9 *1/*1, *1/*2, *2/*2: 0.25 mg once daily on days 1 and 2, then 0.5 mg once daily on day 3, then 0.75 mg once daily on day 4, then 1.25 mg once daily on day 5. CYP2C9 *1/*3, *2/*3: 0.25 mg once daily on days 1 and 2, then 0.5 mg once daily on day 3, then 0.75 mg once daily on day 4	CYP2C9 *1/*1, *1/*2, *2/*2: 2 mg once daily beginning on day 6. CYP2C9 *1/*3, *2/*3: 1 mg once daily beginning on day 5	Medication guide required. May cause fetal harm. CYP2C9 genotype testing required prior to initiating dose
Ozanimod	Zeposia	Relapsing forms of MS	0.23 mg once daily on days 1–4, then 0.46 mg once daily on days 5–7	0.92 mg once daily beginning on day 8	Medication guide required. May cause fetal harm
Ponesimod	Ponvory	Relapsing forms of MS	2 mg on days 1 and 2, 3 mg on days 3 and 4, 4 mg on days 5 and 6, 5 mg on day 7, 6 mg on day 8, 7 mg on day 9, 8 mg on day 10, 9 mg on day 11, 10 mg on days 12–14	20 mg on day 15 and thereafter	Medication guide required. May cause fetal harm
Dimethyl fumarate	Tecfidera	Relapsing forms of MS	120 mg delayed release twice daily for 7 days	240 mg delayed release twice daily	Pregnancy category C
Diroximel fumarate	Vumerity	Relapsing forms of MS	231 mg twice daily for 7 days	462 mg twice daily	May cause fetal harm based on animal data
Monomethyl fumarate	Bafiertam	Relapsing forms of MS	95 mg twice daily for 7 days	190 mg twice daily	May cause fetal harm based on animal data
Teriflunomide	Aubagio	Relapsing forms of MS	7 mg orally once daily	7 or 14 mg orally once daily	Cholestyramine and charcoal accelerate teriflunomide elimination. Pregnancy category X

Cladribine	Mavenclad	RRMS and active SPMS	3.5 mg/kg over 2-year treatment course, administered as 1.75 mg/kg in each year. Divide the 1.75 mg/kg dose over 2 cycles, each cycle lasting 4 to 5 consecutive days; do not administer more than 20 mg/day. In the first-year treatment course, initiate the first cycle at any time; administer the second cycle 23–27 days after the last dose of the first cycle	Second-year treatment course: Initiate the first cycle ≥43 weeks after the last dose of the first year's second cycle. Administer the second cycle 23–27 days after the last dose of the second year's first cycle. Following 2 years of treatment, do not administer oral cladribine during the next 2 years	Medication guide required Contraindicated for use in females and males of reproductive potential. Lymphocytes must be within normal limits before initiating first treatment course and >800 cells/mm³ (0.8 × 10⁹/L) before the second treatment course
IV infusion					
Natalizumab	Tysabri	Relapsing forms of MS	300 mg IV every 4 weeks	300 mg IV every 4 weeks	REMS program required. Pregnancy category C
Alemtuzumab	Lemtrada	RRMS	First treatment course: 12 mg/day IV for 5 consecutive days (60 mg total dose)	Second treatment course: 12 mg/day IV for 3 consecutive days (36 mg total dose) administered 12 months after first treatment course	REMS program required. Pregnancy category C. May premedicate with 1,000 mg methylprednisolone (or equivalent) immediately prior to infusion for first 3 days. Also, administer herpes viral prophylaxis starting on first day of treatment and continued for at least 2 months after completion of treatment or until CD4⁺ count is at least 200 cells/mm³ (0.2 × 10⁹/L), whichever occurs last *(Continued)*

TABLE 56-1	Disease-Modifying Therapy (Continued)				
Medication	Brand Name	Indication	Initial Dose	Usual Dose	Comment
Ocrelizumab	Ocrevus	Relapsing forms of MS and PPMS	First treatment course: 300 mg IV followed by 300 mg IV 2 weeks later. Start infusion at 30 mL/h, then increase by 30 mL/h every 30 minutes as tolerated to a maximum of 180 mL/h for a duration of 2.5 hours or longer	Maintenance treatment (given 6 months after the end of first treatment, and every 6 months thereafter): 600 mg IV starting at 40 mL/h and increased by 40 mL/h every 30 minutes as tolerated to a maximum rate of 200 mL/h for a duration of 3.5 hours or longer	REMS program required. Fetal risk cannot be ruled out. Premedication: antihistamine 30–60 minutes prior to infusion and 100-mg methylprednisolone or equivalent corticosteroid 30 minutes prior to infusion. Can also consider an antipyretic. Observe patient for at least 1 hour post infusion
Self-injectable					
Ofatumumab	Kesimpta	Relapsing forms of MS	20 mg once weekly for 3 doses (weeks 0, 1, 2)	20 mg once monthly starting at week 4	Medication guide required. Single-dose prefilled syringe pen. Based on animal data, may cause fetal harm

CIS, clinically isolated syndrome; IM, intramuscular; IU, international units; PRMS, primary relapsing multiple sclerosis; REMS, Risk Evaluation and Mitigation Strategy; RRMS, relapsing-remitting multiple sclerosis; SPMS, secondary progressive multiple sclerosis; SQ, subcutaneous.

TABLE 56-2 Adverse Medication Reactions and Monitoring Parameters

Medication	Adverse Medication Reaction	Monitoring Parameter	Comments
Interferon-β_{1a}	Depression, flu-like symptoms, leukopenia, injection site reactions	Electrolytes, CBC, LFTs, thyroid function, LVEF, depression LFTs at baseline, 1 month, and every 3 months for a year, and every 6 months thereafter	Avoid use in untreated severe depression
Interferon-β_{1b}	Depression, injection site reactions, leukopenia, flu-like symptoms	Electrolytes, CBC, LFTs, thyroid function, depression	Avoid use in untreated severe depression. More frequent injection site reactions reported
Glatiramer acetate	Injection site reactions, infection, hypersensitivity, chest tightness, urticaria	MRI, tissue necrosis, postinjection reaction	Chest tightness, urticaria can occur at any dose
Mitoxantrone	Bone marrow suppression, neutropenia, cardiotoxicity, AML, nausea, vomiting, diarrhea, alopecia	CBC, ECG, LVEF, LFTs	Secondary leukemia. Lifetime maximum dose due to cardiac toxicity
Fingolimod	Lymphocytopenia, macular retinal edema, AV block, infection, headache	CBC, ECG, varicella zoster antibody, blood pressure, ophthalmic examination, LFTs	Requires first-dose observation. Contraindicated in patients receiving Class I and III antiarrhythmic medications and those with recent cardiac diseases,[a] second- and third-degree AV block. Ketoconazole increases serum concentrations (3A4 inhibition). Vaccine efficacy may be decreased
Siponimod	Infections, macular edema, bradyarrhythmia and atrioventricular conduction delays, decreased pulmonary function, liver injury, increased blood pressure	CBC, ECG, varicella zoster antibody, blood pressure, ophthalmic examination, LFTs	Requires CYP2C9 genomic testing. Contraindicated in *3/*3 genotype. Medication interactions with 2C9 and 3A4 inhibitors and inducers

(Continued)

TABLE 56-2	Adverse Medication Reactions and Monitoring Parameters (Continued)		
Medication	**Adverse Medication Reaction**	**Monitoring Parameter**	**Comments**
Ozanimod	Infections (URTI), AV block, bradycardia, hepatotoxicity, increased blood pressure, lymphopenia, macular edema, neurotoxicity, PML, decreased pulmonary function, varicella zoster infections	CBC, ECG, varicella zoster antibody, blood pressure, ophthalmic examination, LFTs	Medication interactions with strong CYP2C8 inhibitors and inducers and BCRP inhibitors. Avoid use of live attenuated vaccines during and for up to 3 months after treatment
Ponesimod	Infections, bradyarrhythmia and atrioventricular conduction delays, pulmonary function, liver injury, increased blood pressure, cutaneous malignancies, macular edema	CBC, ECG, LFTs, ophthalmic examination, varicella zoster antibody	Contraindicated in patients with recent cardiac diseases,[a] second- and third-degree AV block, sick sinus syndrome, or sinoatrial block unless patient has functioning pacemaker. Four-hour observation monitoring for patients with certain preexisting cardiac conditions
Dimethyl fumarate	Flushing, rash, pruritus, GI discomfort, lymphocytopenia, increased LFTs, albuminuria, PML	CBC, LFTs, MRI	Taking with food decreases incidence of flushing
Diroximel fumarate	Flushing, GI upset, hepatotoxicity, infections, lymphopenia, PML	CBC, LFTs, MRI	Less GI adverse events compared to dimethyl fumarate and may be better tolerated
Monomethyl fumarate	Flushing, GI upset, hepatotoxicity, infections, lymphopenia, PML	CBC, LFTs, MRI	Less GI adverse events compared to dimethyl fumarate and may be better tolerated
Teriflunomide	Steven-Johnson syndrome, liver failure, neutropenia, respiratory infection, activation of TB, alopecia, neuropathy	CBD, LFTs, blood pressure, pregnancy, TB test	Contraindicated in severe hepatic impairment. Possibility of TB reactivation. Active metabolite of leflunomide
Cladribine	Bone marrow suppression, cardiotoxicity, hepatotoxicity, infection, malignancy, neurotoxicity, PML, renal toxicity, hypersensitivity, headache	CBC before starting, 2 and 6 months after the first course of each cycle and periodically. HIV, HBV, HCV, TB screening, VZV antibody, pregnancy test, LFTs, MRI, PML infection	Contraindicated with current malignancy, HIV infection or active chronic infections, pregnancy, and lactation

Drug	Adverse Effects	Monitoring	Comments
Natalizumab	PML, depression, fatigue, respiratory infection, arthralgia, hepatotoxicity	JCV antibody, infection, MRI, LFTs, hypersensitivity reactions	Risk of PML. Risk of IRIS when discontinued due to PML
Alemtuzumab	Infusion reactions, infections (nasopharyngitis, UTI, URI, herpes viral infections), autoimmune disorders; thyroid disorders, immune-mediated thrombocytopenic purpura, goodpasture syndrome	CBC, thyroid function, antibodies to varicella zoster virus, HPV screening, serum creatinine, TB prior to treatment, infusion reactions, skin exams, urinalysis	Contraindicated with HIV infection. Birth control should be used during treatment and for 4 months after each treatment course. Nursing is not recommended during treatment and for 4 months following each treatment course
Ocrelizumab	Infusion reactions, nasopharyngitis, upper respiratory tract infection, headache, urinary tract infection, herpes virus–related infections, neoplasms	MRI, active infection before infusion, infusion reactions during and after infusion, skin infections	Live vaccines are not recommended during treatment and after treatment until B-cell repletion; administer all live vaccines 6 weeks before treatment. Evaluate for hepatitis B infection before first dose. Avoid pregnancy during treatment and for 6 months after stopping treatment
Ofatumumab	Infections, injection site reactions, reduction in immunoglobulins, headache	HBV screen, serum immunoglobulins, CBC, PML, MRI	Contraindicated in active HBV infection. Immunize at least 4 weeks prior to initiation for live or live-attenuated vaccines and 2 weeks prior for inactivated vaccines

AML, acute myeloid leukemia; CBC, complete blood count; ECG, electrocardiogram; LVEF, left ventricular ejection fraction; IRIS, immune reconstitution inflammatory syndrome; PML, progressive multifocal leukoencephalopathy; LFT, liver function test.
[a]Cardiac disease including myocardial infarction, unstable angina, stroke, transient ischemic attack, and heart failure NYHA Class III/IV.

- Ocrelizumab is also FDA-approved for PPMS, and mitoxantrone has an additional FDA indication for progressive or worsening MS.
- These therapies are considered specialty medications, are only available through specialty pharmacies, and have a yearly cost of $100,000 or greater.
- DMT efficacy varies considerably between individual patients and for any given patient at different time points.
- Several DMTs have a black box warning regarding progressive multifocal leukoencephalopathy (PML), with required enrollment in a Risk Evaluation and Mitigation Strategy (REMS) program.
- Evidenced-based recommendations for DMT of MS are included in Table 56-3.
- Questions related to MS treatment include (1) when to begin therapy, (2) which agent to initiate, and (3) when to switch and stop therapies. Key recommendations regarding initiating, switching, and stopping DMTs are summarized in Table 56-3.
- These medications slow the course of the illness but do not suppress it completely. In some individuals, there is no apparent benefit; however, very early therapy is effective.
- The majority of untreated patients will have progressive disease over time, and even in acute lesions, there is significant axonal damage that is essentially irreversible.

Symptomatic Management

- Pharmacologic management of the primary symptoms of MS is outlined in Table 56-4.

TABLE 56-3	Key Recommendations on Treatment and Access Considerations

- Initiate therapy with an FDA-approved DMT as soon as possible following a definite diagnosis of RRMS. It can also be considered for selected patients with a first clinical attack consistent with MS where other potential causes have been excluded, as well as for patients with PPMS with clinical relapses and/or inflammatory activity.
- Choice of initial or alternative DMT is complex and should be collaboratively done by the treating clinician and the patient.
- Clinicians should evaluate barriers to treatment adherence and counsel patients on its importance.
- Continue therapy indefinitely unless there is a clear lack of benefit, intolerable adverse medication reactions, inadequate patient adherence, new data that reveal other reasons for cessation, or a better therapy becomes available.
- The absence of relapses while on treatment should not justify treatment discontinuation. When switching DMTs due to suboptimal response, choose an agent with an alternative mechanism of action.
- For patients with highly active MS, use alemtuzumab, fingolimod, or natalizumab.
- Natalizumab can be used in patients with MS and positive anti-JCV antibody indexes above 0.9 only when the benefit outweighs the severe but low risk of PML.
- Ocrelizumab can be offered to patients with PPMS when the risks of treatment do not outweigh the benefits.
- Clinicians should counsel female patients to stop their DMT before conception for planned pregnancies. If accidental exposure occurs, discontinue DMTs during pregnancy and do not initiate during pregnancy unless the risk of MS activity outweighs the DMT risk.
- Due to the significant variability in therapeutic response, contraindications, risk tolerance, and treatment adherence seen in the MS population, patient and clinician access to all available therapies is necessary as this may influence decisions regarding the route of administration and/or adverse medication effect tolerance.
- Patient access to medication should not be limited by the frequency of relapses, age or other personal characteristics, or level of disability. Therapy should not be withheld to allow for determination of coverage by payers, as this puts the patient at increased risk for recurrent disease activity.

TABLE 56-4	Treatment of Select Primary MS Symptoms
Spasticity	Baclofen, Dantrolene, Diazepam, Clonazepam, Tizanidine, Tiagabine, Gabapentin, Pregabalin, Botulinum toxin type A, Dalfampridine
Bladder symptoms	Propantheline, Oxybutynin, Dicyclomine, DDAVP, Imipramine, Amitriptyline, Prazosin, Terazosin, Botulinum toxin type A, Solifenacin, Darifenacin, Trospium, Hyoscyamine, Mirabegron, Tamsulosin, Tolerodine, Self-catheterization
Sensory symptoms	Carbamazepine, Phenytoin, Amitriptyline; other TCAs, Gabapentin, Lamotrigine, Pregabalin, Duloxetine
Fatigue	Amantadine, Antidepressants, Modafinil, Methylphenidate, Dextroamphetamine, Armodafinil, Fluoxetine

DDAVP, desmopressin acetate; TCA, tricyclic antidepressant.

Complementary and Alternative Therapies for MS

- Antioxidant supplements vitamin A, C, E, α-lipoic acid, coenzyme Q10, grape seed, pine bark extracts, mangosteen, and acai have suggestive benefits in MS, but the use of antioxidant supplements may hold risk due to possible immune system activation.

Vaccine Recommendations

- Avoid live vaccine administration in patients receiving DMTs due to immunosuppression and the potential for increased MS activity. Those considered safe include the human papillomavirus, tetanus, rabies, COVID-19, and inactivated polio.
- A yearly flu shot is recommended for all patients, while the live-attenuated intranasal vaccine is not.
- Patients taking fingolimod, and alemtuzumab, who are negative for varicella-zoster antibodies should receive the non-live virus immunization at least 2 months before starting treatment.
- Unvaccinated patients at high risk for Hepatitis B exposure should be vaccinated prior to starting ocrelizumab.

EVALUATION OF THERAPEUTIC OUTCOMES

- Therapeutic outcome evaluation is conducted over months to years by monitoring MS exacerbations, hospitalizations, disease progression, and disability measured using scales such as the Expanded Disability Status Scale (EDSS).
- Patients should be given realistic treatment goals and expectations, including adverse medication reactions, to maximize adherence. They should also be encouraged to participate in the evaluation of therapeutic responses.
- Each DMTs has specific safety monitoring recommendations and patients should receive regular laboratory monitoring and close observation, including regular neurologic examinations, frequent evaluation for adverse medication reactions, and/or changes in disability.
- Several DMTs have REMS or medication guides to monitor safety.

See Chapter 74, Multiple Sclerosis, authored by Jacquelyn L Bainbridge, Augusto Miravelle, Pei Shieen Won, Matthew J. Makelky Sr., and Sarah Rajkovic, for a more detailed discussion of this topic.

CHAPTER 57

Pain Management

- *Pain* is a subjective, unpleasant, sensory, and emotional experience associated with actual or potential tissue damage or abnormal functioning of nerves. It may be classified as acute, chronic, or cancer pain.

PATHOPHYSIOLOGY

ADAPTIVE (PHYSIOLOGIC) PAIN

- Nociceptive (eg, from touching something too hot, too cold, or sharp) and inflammatory pain (eg, trauma or surgery) are both adaptive and protective.
- The steps in processing pain are:
  - ✓ Transduction—Stimulation of nociceptors.
    - o Nociceptors, found in both somatic and visceral structures, are activated by mechanical, thermal, and chemical stimuli. Noxious stimuli may cause release of cytokines and chemokines that sensitize and/or activate nociceptors.
  - ✓ Conduction—Receptor activation leads to action potentials that continue along afferent fibers to the spinal cord. Stimulation of large-diameter, sparsely myelinated fibers evokes sharp, well-localized pain. Stimulation of small-diameter, unmyelinated fibers produces aching, poorly localized pain.
  - ✓ Transmission—Afferent nociceptive fibers synapse in the spinal cord's dorsal horn, releasing excitatory neurotransmitters (eg, glutamate and substance P). The neo- and paleospinothalamic tract and other pathways bring the signal to the brain's higher cortical structures.
  - ✓ Modulation—Possible modulating factors include glutamate, substance P, endogenous opioids, γ-aminobutyric acid (GABA), norepinephrine, and serotonin.
  - ✓ Perception—The experience of pain occurs when signals reach higher cortical structures. Cognitive and behavioral functions can modify pain, thus relaxation, meditation, and distraction can lessen pain, and anxiety and depression can worsen pain.
- The interface between neurons and immune cells in the central nervous system (CNS) may facilitate maintenance of chronic pain.

MALADAPTIVE (PATHOLOGIC) PAIN

- Pathophysiologic pain (eg, postherpetic neuralgia, diabetic neuropathy, fibromyalgia, irritable bowel syndrome, chronic headaches) is often described as chronic pain. It results from damage or abnormal functioning of nerves in the CNS or peripheral nervous system (PNS). Pain circuits sometimes rewire themselves anatomically and biochemically, resulting in chronic pain, hyperalgesia, or allodynia.

CLINICAL PRESENTATION

ACUTE PAIN

Symptoms

- Pain can be sharp or dull, burning, shock-like, tingling, shooting, radiating, fluctuating in intensity, varying in location, and occurring in a temporal relationship with an obvious noxious stimulus. Infants and older individuals may present differently.

Signs

- Hypertension, tachycardia, diaphoresis, mydriasis, and pallor. In some cases there are not obvious physical signs. There are no laboratory tests for pain.

CHRONIC PAIN

Symptoms

• Very similar to acute pain, and may change over time (ie, sharp to dull). Attention must also be given to emotional factors that alter the pain threshold.

Signs

• In most cases there are no obvious signs. Depression, sleep disturbances, and anxiety are often present. No laboratory tests are diagnostic, but may identify etiology.

DIAGNOSIS

• Pain is always subjective and best diagnosed using a patient-centered approach with assessment measures used in other medical conditions. This includes a baseline description of pain using a symptom assessment mnemonic (ie, OLDCARTS, SOCRATES, SCHOLAR-MAC, PQRST). Ongoing assessment should include a consistent and validated method.

• Adult cancer pain can be categorized by level of pain intensity (0-no pain, 10-worst pain; mild [1–3], moderate [4–], and severe [8–10]) which can be used to help guide treatment decisions.

TREATMENT

• <u>Goals of Treatment:</u> The goals of pain management are to optimize patient treatment outcomes in five dimensions, also known as the 5As of pain management outcomes: **A**nalgesia (optimize, analgesia); **A**ctivities (optimize activities of daily living); **A**dverse effects (minimize ADRs); **A**berrant medication use (avoid misuse "aberrant" use); **A**ffect (relationship between pain and mood).

• **Figures 57-1** and **57-2** are algorithms for management of acute pain and cancer pain crisis, respectively.

• **Table 57-1** outlines recommendations for treating cancer pain of different intensities. A three-step ladder approach using the nonopioids as initial treatment and escalating treatment to either "weak" or "strong" opioids based on pain intensity ratings is recommended.

GENERAL APPROACH

• Multimodal therapy, with concomitant use of different nonpharmacologic and pharmacologic therapies can optimize treatment.

• In patients with cancer, determine if pain is related to a life-threatening oncologic emergency or indirectly related to a patient's cancer or anticancer treatment.

• Use of pharmacogenomic testing results may be beneficial in making therapeutic decisions among agents.

NONPHARMACOLOGIC THERAPY

• Nonpharmacologic therapies should always be considered first-line therapy, either alone or in combination with appropriate analgesics.

• These include physical therapy, exercise programs, weight loss, and electroanalgesia as well as complementary and integrative approaches (ie, acupuncture, Tai chi, yoga, mindfulness, meditation, relaxation, and biofeedback).

• Electroanalgesia includes application of electrical stimulation to various locations ranging from noninvasive (eg, transcutaneous or percutaneous electrical nerve stimulation) to highly invasive (implanted spinal cord stimulation).

• For patients with severe pain, pain crisis, or uncontrolled pain, hospital or inpatient hospice may be required.

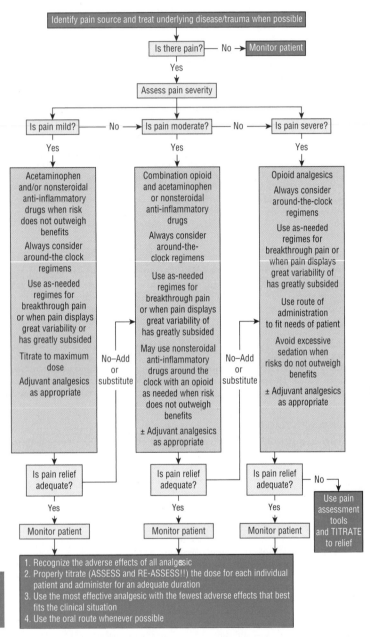

FIGURE 57-1. Algorithm for acute pain. Patients should first be assessed regarding severity of pain and then managed accordingly. Pain assessment tools should be used to monitor response and dose titration for pain relief.

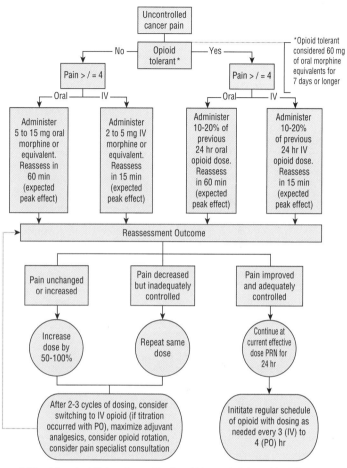

FIGURE 57-2. Treatment algorithm for cancer pain crisis. Patients should first be assessed for opioid tolerance and then managed according to their pain score on the 0–10 numeric rating scale. Patients in pain crisis require frequent monitoring and reassessment of their pain score to determine if redosing of opioids are needed to achieve adequate pain control.

PHARMACOLOGIC THERAPY

Nonopioid Agents

Acetaminophen and Nonsteroidal Anti-Inflammatory Drugs

- Initiate treatment with the most effective analgesic with the fewest adverse effects. See Table 57-2 for adult dosages of nonopioid analgesics.
- **Acetaminophen** and **nonsteroidal anti-inflammatory drugs** (NSAIDs) are often preferred over opioids for mild to moderate pain. The NSAIDs reduce prostaglandins, decreasing the number of pain impulses received by the CNS.

TABLE 57-1	Cancer-Related Pain Treatment Recommendations	
Pain Intensity (Numerical Rating Score)	**Opioid-Naïve**	**Opioid-Tolerant**
Mild (1–3)	Nonopioid analgesics + adjuvant analgesics	Nonopioid analgesics + adjuvant analgesics
		Re-evaluate need for opioid analgesics and initiate gradual dose reductions if indicated
Moderate (4–6)	Nonopioid analgesics + adjuvant analgesics + shortacting opioids as needed Titrate every 3–4 hours If ≥ 4 doses are needed/day consider addition of long-acting opioid based on TDD	Nonopioid analgesics + adjuvant analgesics + short-acting opioids as needed
		Titrate short-acting opioids with goal of increasing total daily dose by 30%–50% until pain relief is achieved
		If ≥4 doses are needed/day consider addition or increase in dose of long-acting opioid based on total daily dose
Severe (7–10)	Consider hospital or inpatient hospice admission IV or oral short-acting opioids	

- An adequate NSAID trial is about 1 month in duration. Chronic use may cause gastrointestinal (GI), cardiac, and renal toxicities.
- NSAIDs may be useful for chronic low back pain and used in combination with opioids for cancer-related nonemergency bone pain.
- Topical NSAIDs may have similar efficacy as oral NSAIDs with improved safety when treating small or superficial joint arthritis.
- Regular alcohol use and of acetaminophen may result in liver toxicity. Use combination products cautiously to avoid overdoses.
- Underlying renal impairment, hypovolemia, and CHF may predispose to nephrotoxicity.

Antiseizure medications

- The antiseizure medications (ASMs) **carbamazepine** and **oxcarbazepine** preferred for trigeminal neuralgia (Table 57-3).
  - ✓ Common adverse effects include dizziness, drowsiness, unsteadiness, nausea, and vomiting which can be avoided with low starting doses.
  - ✓ Serious dermatologic reactions can occur, including toxic epidermal necrolysis and Stevens–Johnson syndrome (SJS). The risk of dermatological adverse effects is higher in patients with Asian ethnicity with specific HLA variants. Testing for these should be done prior to treatment.
  - ✓ Cardiovascular effects include hyper/hypotension, congestive heart failure, edema, arrhythmias, atrioventricular block. Elevation in hepatic enzymes should be monitored periodically during treatment.
  - ✓ The primary metabolic pathway for carbamazepine is CYP3A4. Additionally, carbamazepine autoinduces its own metabolism, making titration difficult also resulting in many interactions through induction of CYP3A4, CYP1A2, CYP2B6, CYP2C9, and CYP2C19.
- Gabapentinoids, including **gabapentin** and **pregabalin**, are considered first line for neuropathic pain and may be part of enhanced recovery after surgery protocols.
  - ✓ Dizziness and sedation can be mitigated with slow dose titration.
  - ✓ All ASMs have an increased risk for suicidal thoughts and behavior. They are controlled substances due to the risk of misuse.

TABLE 57-2 Nonopioid Analgesics

Class and Generic Name (Brand Name)	Usual Dosage Range (mg)	Maximal Dose (mg/day)
Salicylates		
Acetylsalicylic acid[a]—aspirin (various)	325–1000 every 4–6 hours	4000
Choline and magnesium trisalicylate (various)	1000–1500 every 12 hours 750 every 8 hours (older patients)	3000
Diflunisal (Dolobid, various)	500–1000 initial then 250–500 every 8–12 hours	1500
Salsalate (various)	1000 every 12 hours or 500 every 6 hours	3000
Para-aminophenol		
Acetaminophen[a] (oral: Tylenol, various; parenteral: Ofirmev)	325–1000 every 4–6 hour	4000[b] Dosing for peds lower based on weight
Fenamates		
Meclofenamate (various)	50–100 every 4–6 hours	400
Mefenamic acid (Ponstel)	Initial 500 then 250 every 6 hours (max. 7 days)	1000[c]
Pyranocarboxylic acid		
Etodolac (various) (immediate release)	200–400 every 6–8 hours	1000 (1200 with extended-release product)
Acetic acid		
Diclofenac potassium (Cataflam, various, Flector [patch] Voltaren Gel, Pennsaid [solution])	Initial 100 then 50 three times per day Patch available: to be applied twice daily to painful area (intact skin only), gel and solution dosing joint specific	150[d]
Propionic acids		
Ibuprofen[a] (Motrin, Caldolor, various)	200–400 every 4–6 hours injectable, 400–800 every 6 hours (infused over 30 minutes)	3200[e], 2400[e], 1200[f]
Fenoprofen (Nalfon, various)	200 every 4–6 hours	3200
Ketoprofen (various)	25–50 every 6–8 hours	300 (200 with extended-release product)
Naproxen (Naprosyn, Anaprox, various)	500 every 12 hours or 250 mg every 6–8 hours	1000[c]
Naproxen sodium[a] (Aleve, various, combined with esomeprazole [Vimovo])	Initial 440 mg then 220 mg every 8–12 hours[f]	660[f]

(Continued)

TABLE 57-2 Nonopioid Analgesics *(Continued)*		
Class and Generic Name (Brand Name)	**Usual Dosage Range (mg)**	**Maximal Dose (mg/day)**
Pyrrolizine carboxylic acid		
Ketorolac–parenteral (Toradol, various)	30[g]–60 (single IM dose only)	30[g]–60
	15[g]–30 (single IV dose only)	15[g]–30
	10[g]–30 every 6 hours (IV dose) (max. 5 days)	60[g]–120
Ketorolac—oral, indicated for continuation with parenteral only (various)	10 every 4–6 hours (max. 5 days, which includes parenteral doses)	40
	In non-older patients, initial oral dose of 20	126
Ketorolac—nasal spray, indicated for acute, moderate to moderately severe pain	1 spray (15.75 mg) in each nostril every 6–8 hours in adults <65 years and weight ≥50 kg	
Pyrazols		
Celecoxib (Celebrex)	Initial 400 followed by another 200 on first day, then 200 twice daily (note some recommend maintenance doses of 200 mg/day due to cardiovascular concerns)	400

FDA, Food and Drug Administration; IM, intramuscular; IV, intravenous; ND, no data.
[a]Available both as an over-the-counter preparation and as a prescription medication.
[b]Food and Drug Administration maximum dose. OTC maximum dose 3000 mg daily. Lower with weight-based dosing in pediatric patients.
[c]Up to 1250 mg on the first day.
[d]Up to 200 mg on the first day.
[e]Some individuals may respond better to 3200 mg as opposed to 2400 mg, although well-controlled trials show no better response; consider risk versus benefits when using 3200 mg/day.
[f]Over-the-counter dose.
[g]Dose for older individuals and those under 50 kg (110 lb).

- **Lamotrigine** is a fourth-line agent for use in a specialist setting due to risk of life-threatening rash requiring increased monitoring and careful dose titration (Table 57-3).
  - ✓ Other adverse effects include dizziness, nausea, headache, insomnia, somnolence, fatigue, rhinitis, abdominal pain diplopia, ataxia, and blurred vision.
- **Topirmate** is also listed as a fourth-line agent for migraines and low back pain.

Antidepressants

- **Tricyclic antidepressants** (TCAs) are often used for neuropathic pain (Table 57-4) and some guidelines list them as first line.
- **Duloxetine, venlafaxine,** and **milnacipran** are serotonin norepinephrine reuptake inhibitors (SNRIs) that have evidence to support their use in various chronic pain syndromes.
- Pharmacogenomic testing may be helpful to reduce medication adverse effects.

Skeletal Muscle Relaxants

- Skeletal muscle relaxants (SMRs) include antispasmodic (**baclofen, diazepam,** and **tizanidine**) and antispasticity medications (**carisoprodol, chlorzoxazone, cyclobenzaprine, diazepam, metaxalone, methocarbamol, orphenadrine,** and **tizanidine**) (Table 57-5).

TABLE 57-3	Co-analgesics: Oral Antiseizure Medications	
Medication	**Dosing**	**Notes**
Carbamazepine and carbamazepine XR	Initial dose: 100 mg twice daily Titrate dose by 100 mg twice daily Target dose: 300–900 mg/day Maximum dose: 1200 mg/day	Significant medication interactions Monitor CBC, LFTs, sodium level Recommended HLA testing in patients with Asian ancestry Therapeutic levels only indicated for high-dose therapy to avoid toxicity. No correlation between analgesia and serum concentration
Gabapentin	100–300 mg steps Increase every 3–5 days as tolerated by 100–300 mg increments	Median dose for response 1600–2400 mg/day Risk of misuse Requires renal dose adjustment
Gabapentin (Gralise)	Take once daily with evening meal Day 1: 300 mg Day 2: 600 mg Day 3–6: 900 mg Days 7–10: 1200 mg Days 11–14: 1500 mg Day 15: 1800 mg Maximum dose: 1800 mg/day	Refer to gabapentin
Gabapentin enacarbil	Initial dose: 600 mg every morning × 3 days Titrate dose: 600 mg twice daily Maximum dose: 1200 mg/day	Refer to gabapentin
Lamotrigine	Initial 25 mg daily Titrate every 2 weeks to 50 mg/day, 100 mg/day, and 200 mg/day Maximum dose: 400 mg/day	Stevens–Johnson syndrome
Oxcarbazepine	Initial: 150 mg BID Titrate by 300 mg every 3 days Target dose: 300–600 mg twice daily Max dose: 1800 mg/day	Improved tolerability and less medication interactions compared to CBZ
Oxcarbamazepine XR	Initial dose: 600 mg daily Titrate by 600 mg/day weekly Maximum: 2400 mg/day	Refer to oxcarbazepine
Pregabalin	Initial dose: 150 mg/day in 2 or 3 divided doses Titrate dose by 300 mg/day at 1 week Maximum dose: varies by indication. Overall 600 mg/day	Refer to gabapentin

(Continued)

TABLE 57-3	Co-analgesics: Oral Antiseizure Medications (*Continued*)	
Medication	**Dosing**	**Notes**
Pregabalin CR	Initial dose: 165 mg daily	Refer to gabapentin
	Maximum dose: 330 mg/day (DPN) or 330–660 mg/day (PHN)	
Topiramate and Topiramate XR	Initial dose: 25 mg daily × 1 week	Monitor serum bicarbonate and renal function
	Titrate by 25–50 mg week	Increase risk for kidney stones
	Target dose: 50 mg twice daily (migraine) or 200–400 mg/day neuropathic pain	Weight loss
		Decreased sweating/ hyperthermia
		Hyperammonemia

BID, twice daily dosing; CBC, complete blood count; CBZ, carbamazepine; DPN, diabetic peripheral neuropathy; HLA, human leukocyte antigens; LFT, liver function tests; PHN, postherpetic neuralgia. All anticonvulsants associated with increased risk for suicidal thoughts and behaviors.

TABLE 57-4	Co-analgesics: Antidepressants		
Medication	**Uses**	**Dosing**	**Notes**
Tricyclic antidepressants (TCAs)			
Amitriptyline	Fibromyalgia	Initial: 10–25 mg at bedtime	Secondary amines (desipramine, nortriptyline) less anticholinergic activity = less adverse effects
Desipramine	Low back pain		
Imipramine	Migraine prophylaxis	Titrate by 10–25 mg every 3–7 days	
Nortriptyline	Neuropathic pain	Maximum: 150 mg	
			Cardiac adverse effects (QTc prolongation, orthostatic hypotension, arrhythmias, tachycardia)
			Doses >100 mg/day associated with sudden cardiac death
			Lowers seizure threshold
Serotonin norepinephrine reuptake inhibitors (SNRIs)			
Duloxetine	Chronic musculoskeletal pain (low back pain [LBP], osteoarthritis)[a]	Initial: 30 mg daily × 1 week (2 weeks if older patient)	Avoid eGFR <30 mL/min (0.50 mL/sec)
	Diabetic peripheral neuropathy (DPN)[a]	Target dose: 60 mg daily	Avoid chronic liver disease or cirrhosis
	Fibromyalgia[a]	Maximum dose: 120 mg/day though limited evidence for doses >60 mg providing additional benefit in pain	Hypertension
	Chemotherapy-induced neuropathic pain (CINP)		Hyponatremia
			Increased risk of bleeding (GI and CNS)

(*Continued*)

TABLE 57-4	Co-analgesics: Antidepressants *(Continued)*		
Medication	**Uses**	**Dosing**	**Notes**
Serotonin norepinephrine reuptake inhibitors (SNRIs) *(Continued)*			
Milnacipran	Fibromyalgia[a]	Day 1: 12.5 mg daily	Avoid eGFR <30 mL/min (0.50 mL/sec)
		Days 2–3: 12.5 mg BID	
		Days 4–7: 25 mg BID	Caution with severe hepatic impairment
		Then increase to 50 mg BID	Increase risk for bleeding
		Target dose: 100 mg/day	
		Maximum dose: 200 mg/day	
Venlafaxine	CINP	Initial: venlafaxine SA 37.5 mg daily	Higher doses needed to achieve SNRI effect
	DPN		
	Fibromyalgia	Titrate: by no more than 75 mg/day every 4 days	Dose adjustments with renal/hepatic impairment
	LBP		
	Migraine prophylaxis	Maximum dose: 225 mg/day	Hypertension
	Painful polyneuropathy		Hyponatremia
	Tension-type headache		QTc prolongation
			Increased bleeding risk

eGFR, estimated glomerular filtration rate; GI, gastrointestinal; CNS central nervous system.
[a]FDA-approved indication(s).

TABLE 57-5	Skeletal Muscle Relaxants	
Medication	**Dosing**	**Notes**
Baclofen	Initial: 5 mg 3 times daily	Withdrawal syndrome (hallucinations, seizures)
	Titrate: every 3 days to effect	
	Maximum: 80 mg/day	Respiratory depression
		Requires renal dose adjustment
Carisoprodol	250–300 mg 4 times daily	Meprobamate (a barbiturate) is primary metabolite and has misuse potential (Schedule IV).
		Respiratory depression with opioids, benzodiazepines, or barbiturates
		Metabolized by CYP2C19 which has genetic variabilities
Chlorzoxazone	Initial: 250–500 mg 3–4 times daily	Rare hepatotoxicity
		Urine discoloration
	Maximum dose: 750 mg 3–4 times daily	Respiratory depression when combined with opioids, benzodiazepines, or barbiturates

(Continued)

TABLE 57-5	Skeletal Muscle Relaxants *(Continued)*	
Medication	**Dosing**	**Notes**
Cyclobenzaprine	Initial: 5 mg 3 times daily	Anticholinergic effects
	Titrate: increase to 7.5–10 mg 3 times daily × 2–3 weeks	Avoid in older paints and caution in those with cardiac conduction/arrhythmias
	Older patients: 5 mg dose with less frequent doses	Avoid closed angle glaucoma
	Doses for fibromyalgia 10mg QAM, 20mg QHS	Hepatic dose adjustments
Diazepam	Adults: 2–10 mg 3–4 times daily	Long half-life
		Avoid in older patients and those with renal/hepatic impairment
		Withdrawal with abrupt discontinuation
Methocarbamol	Initial: 1500 mg 4 times daily × 2–3 days	Urine discoloration
	Then: 750–1000 mg 4 times daily	Respiratory depression with opioids, benzodiazepines, or barbiturates
Metaxalone	800 mg 3–4 times daily	Respiratory depression when used with opioids, benzodiazepines, or barbiturates
		Contraindicated in severe liver/renal impairment
Orphenadrine	100 mg twice daily	Anticholinergic effects
		Rare aplastic anemia
Tizanidine	Initial: 4 mg	Hypotension
	Titrate by 2–4 mg every 6–8 hours	Hepatotoxicity
	Maximum: 36 mg/day	Tablets and capsules not bioequivalent
		Withdrawal syndrome with abrupt discontinuation

Topicals

- Topicals address local symptoms while minimizing systemic exposure and adverse effects (Table 57-6). Guidelines suggest use of topical NSAIDs before oral treatment for knee or hand osteoarthritis.
- **Capsaicin** is recommended for peripheral neuropathic pain. It is more effective used on a schedule basis. The burning that may occur with initial application decreases over time with repeated, scheduled use.
- Topical **lidocaine** may be the treatment of choice when CNS adverse effects are a concern.

Emerging Agents

- **Cannabis** has been primarily studied in the treatment of neuropathic pain; however, the route of administration, dose, and monitoring recommendations are still unclear.
- The non-psychoactive cannabinoid, cannabidiol (CBD) may have a role in the treatment of chronic pain, although its utility in the absence of delta-9-tetrahydrocannabinol (THC) is unclear.

TABLE 57-6 Topical Analgesics

Medication	Uses	Dosing	Notes
Capsaicin cream (various)	Temporary relief of minor aches and pains of muscles and joints Localized neuropathic pain	Apply 3–4 times daily	Continue scheduled use for 2–4 weeks for best results
Capsaicin 8% patch (Qutenza)	PHN	Apply 1–4 patches to affected area for 60 minutes (PHN) or 30 minutes (DPN) Cleansing gel must be used on application site after patch removal Repeat no more frequently than every 3 months Max: Four patches	Specific administration directions in packaging information Apply topical anesthetic before applying Monitor blood pressure due to transient increase in blood pressure during application
Diclofenac 1% gel (Voltaren)	Pain of osteoarthritis of joints amenable to topical treatment (knees, hands)	Lower extremities: 4 g four times daily, max. 16 g/day Upper extremities: 2 g four times daily, max. 8 g/day Total dose maximum: 32 g/day	Same black box warnings as PO NSAIDs despite low systemic bioavailability (6% of systemic exposure from oral diclofenac) Use dosing card to measure amount
Diclofenac epolamine 1.3% patch (Flector)	Topical treatment of acute pain due to minor strains, sprains, and contusions	1 patch to most painful area twice daily	Systemic effects were <1% after 4 days of repeated dosing
Diclofenac topical solution (Pennsaid)	Pain from osteoarthritis of the knee	1.5%: 40 drops to each affected knee 4 times daily. Apply 10 drops at a time 2%: 2 pumps (40 mg) on each painful knee twice daily	Same black box warnings as PO NSAIDs

(Continued)

TABLE 57-6 Topical Analgesics (*Continued*)

Medication	Uses	Dosing	Notes
Lidocaine gel/Ointment/Patch (various)	Neuropathic pain	Cream/Ointment: Apply to affected area 3 times daily Patch: apply 1 patch to affected area up to 12 hours	Apply to intact skin only
Lidocaine 5% patch (Lidoderm, also available over the counter at 4%)	PHN	Apply 1–3 patches to site of pain for 12 hours Maximum: 3 patches	May cut lidocaine patches Apply to intact skin only Severe hepatic impairment increases risk of adverse effects
Menthol/Methyl salicylate (various)	Minor aches and pains of muscles and joints (simple backache, arthritis, strains, bruises, sprains)	Apply topically 3–4 times a day to affected area	Do not apply to damaged skin
Trolamine salicylate cream 10% (various)	Aches and pains of muscles and joints (arthritis, simple backache, bruises, sprains, strains)	Apply topically 3–4 times a day to affected area	Do not apply to damaged skin

DPN, diabetic peripheral neuropathy; NSAIDs, nonsteroidal anti-inflammatory drugs; PHN, postherpetic neuralgia.

- Guidelines for the use of **ketamine** for treating maladaptive pain syndrome are available, but appropriate dose, duration, and patient selection for chronic pain are still unclear.

Opioid Agents

- Opioids are often the next step in the management of acute pain and cancer-related chronic pain.
- Equianalgesic doses, dosing guidelines, and major adverse effects are shown in Tables 57-7 and 57-8. Equianalgesic doses are only a guide, and doses must be individualized based on response and adverse effects.
- Combining opioid analgesics with alcohol or other CNS depressants amplifies CNS depression and risk of death.
- Partial agonists and antagonists (eg, **nalbuphine**) compete with agonists for opioid receptor sites and exhibit mixed agonist–antagonist activity. They may produce analgesia with fewer adverse effects.
- Initially give analgesics around-the-clock for acute pain. As pain subsides, as-needed schedules can be used. Around-the-clock administration is also useful for management of chronic pain.
- Patients with severe pain may receive high doses of opioids with no unwanted adverse effects, but as pain subsides, may not tolerate low doses.
- Most opioid-related itching or rash is due to histamine release from cutaneous mast cells, and is not a true allergic response. When opioid allergies occur, an opioid from a different structural class may be cautiously tried. For these purposes, the mixed agonist–antagonist class behaves most like the morphine-like agonists.
- With patient-controlled analgesia (PCA), patients self-administer preset amounts of IV opioids via a syringe pump electronically interfaced with a timing device. PCA provides better pain control, improved patient satisfaction, and relatively few differences in adverse effects compared to traditional as needed administration.
- Administration of opioids directly into the CNS (see Table 57-9) (eg, epidural and intrathecal/subarachnoid routes) can be used for acute pain, chronic noncancer pain, and cancer pain. This requires preservative free formulations and careful monitoring for marked sedation, respiratory depression, pruritus, vomiting, urinary retention, and hypotension.

Morphine and Congeners (Phenanthrenes)

- **Morphine** is a first-line agent for moderate-to-severe pain. It may be used for pain associated with myocardial infarction, as it decreases myocardial oxygen demand, but this is controversial.
  - ✓ Tidal exchange and minute volume can be affected by opioids. Patients with underlying pulmonary dysfunction are at increased risk for respiratory depression, which can be reversed by **naloxone**.
  - ✓ Morphine-induced respiratory depression can increase intracranial pressure and cloud the neurologic examination results.
  - ✓ Hypovolemic patients are at risk for morphine-induced orthostatic hypotension.
  - ✓ Most clinicians avoid morphine in patients with creatinine clearance less than or equal to 30 mL/min [0.5 mL/sec] due to accumulation of active metabolites.
- **Hydromorphone** may have fewer adverse effects, especially pruritus, compared with other opioids and **levorphanol** has an extended half-life and purported NMDA glutamate receptor activity.
- **Codeine**, alone or combined with other analgesics (eg, acetaminophen), is commonly used for mild-to-moderate pain. **Oxycodone** is useful for moderate-to-severe pain, especially when combined with nonopioids.
- **Oliceridine** is approved IV for moderate-severe pain and is classified as a biased opioid agonist. It is structurally dissimilar from other opioid analgesics and is associated with fewer tolerability concerns.

TABLE 57-7 Opioid Dosing Guidelines

Agent(s)	Standard Dose Ranges	Equianalgesic Dose in Adults (mg)	Notes
Morphine	PO 5–30 mg every 4 hours[a]	25	Medication of choice in severe pain
	IM 5–20 mg every 4 hours[a]	10	Use immediate-release product with SR product to control breakthrough pain in cancer patients
	IV 5–15 mg every 4 hours[a]	10	Typical patient controlled analgesia IV dose is 1 mg with a 10-minutes lock-out interval
	SR 15–30 mg every 12 hours (may need to be every 8 hours in some patients)		Every 24-hour products available
	Rectal 10–20 mg every 4 hours[a]		
Hydromorphone	PO 2–4 mg every 4–6 hours[a]	7.5	Use in severe pain
	XR 8 mg to 64 mg every 24 hours		More potent than morphine; otherwise, no advantages
	IM 1–2 mg every 4–6 hours[a]	1.5	
	IV 0.5–2 mg every 4 hours[a]	1.5	Typical patient-controlled analgesia IV dose is 0.2 mg with a 10-minute lock-out interval
	Rectal 3 mg every 6–8 hours[a]		Every 24-hour product (Exalgo) available
Oxymorphone	IM 1–1.5 mg every 4–6 hours[a]	1	Use in severe pain
	IV 0.5 mg every 4–6 hours[a]	1	No advantages over morphine
	PO immediate-release 5–10 mg every 4–6 hours[a]	10	Use immediate-release product with controlled-release product to control breakthrough pain in cancer or chronic pain patients
	PO extended-release 5–10 mg every 12 hours[a]		Manufacturer recommends 5 mg every 12 hours in opioid-naive patients
			Take ER on empty stomach

Levorphanol	PO 2–3 mg every 6–8 hours[a] (Levo-Dromoran)	Variable	Use in severe pain
	PO 2 mg every 3–6 hours[a] (Levorphanol Tartrate)		Extended half-life useful in cancer patients
	IM 1–2 mg every 6–8 hours[a]		In chronic pain, wait 3 days between dosage adjustments
	IV 1 mg every 3–6 hours[a]		
Codeine	PO 15–60 mg every 4–6 hours[a]		Use in mild-to-moderate pain
	IM 15–60 mg every 4–6 hours[a]		Weak analgesic; analgesic prodrug
Hydrocodone	PO 5–10 mg every 4–6 hours[a]		Use in moderate/severe pain
Oxycodone	PO 5–15 mg every 4–6 hours[a]	15–30	Use in moderate/severe pain
	Controlled release 10–20 mg every 12 hours		Use immediate-release product with controlled-release product to control breakthrough pain in cancer or chronic pain patients
			CR reformulated to deter misuse
Meperidine	IM 50–150 mg every 3–4 hours[a]	75	Use in severe pain
	IV 5–10 mg every 5 minutes prn[a]	75	Oral not recommended
			Do not use in renal failure
			May precipitate tremors, myoclonus, and seizures
			Monoamine oxidase inhibitors can induce hyperpyrexia and/or seizures or opioid overdose symptoms

(Continued)

TABLE 57-7 Opioid Dosing Guidelines (Continued)

Agent(s)	Standard Dose Ranges	Equianalgesic Dose in Adults (mg)	Notes
Fentanyl	IV 25–50 mcg/h	0.125	Used in severe pain
	IM 50–100 mcg every 1–2 hours[a]	0.125	**Do not use transdermal in acute pain**
	Transdermal 25 mcg/h every 72 hours	Variable	Transmucosal for breakthrough cancer pain in patients already receiving or tolerant to opioids
	Transmucosal (Actiq/OTFC Lozenge and Onsolis buccal film) 200 mcg may repeat × 1, 30 minutes after first dose is started, then titrate	Variable	**Always start with lowest dose despite daily opioid intake; product-specific titration recommendations exist**
	Transmucosal (Fentora Buccal Tablet) 100 mcg, may repeat × 1, 30 minutes after first dose is started, then titrate	Variable	
	Intranasal (Lazanda Spray) 100 mcg (one spray) in one nostril; wait 2 hours prior to redosing	Variable	
	Sublingual (Subsys Spray) 100 mcg (1 spray); wait 4 hours prior to redosing	Variable	
	Sublingual (Abstral Tablet) 100 mcg tablets placed sublingually. Must wait 2 hours prior to redosing	Variable	
Methadone[g]	PO 2.5–10 mg every 8–12 hours[a]	Variable	Effective in severe chronic pain
	IM 2.5–10 mg every 8–12 hours[a]	Variable	Some chronic pain patients can be dosed every 12 hours

Drug	Dose		Comments
Pentazocine	PO 50–100 mg every 3–4 hours[b] (max. 600 mg daily, for those 50-mg tablet containing 0.5 mg of naloxone)		Equianalgesic dose of methadone when compared with other opioids will decrease progressively the higher the previous opioid dose. Avoid dose titrations more frequently than weekly in chronic pain maintenance
	PO 25 mg every 4 hours[b] (max. 150 mg daily, for those 25 mg tablet containing 325 mg of acetaminophen)		Second-line agent for moderate-to-severe pain; may precipitate withdrawal in opiate-dependent patients; parenteral doses not recommended
Butorphanol	IM 1–4 mg every 3–4 hours[b]	2	Second-line agent for moderate-to-severe pain
	IV 0.5–2 mg every 3–4 hours[b]	2	May precipitate withdrawal in opiate-dependent patients
	Intranasal 1 mg (1 spray) every 3–4 hours[b]		
	If inadequate relief after initial spray, may repeat in other nostril × 1 in 60–90 minutes		
	Max. 2 sprays (one per nostril) every 3–4 hours[b]		
Nalbuphine	IM/IV 10 mg every 3–6 hours[b] (max. 20 mg dose, 160 mg daily)	10	Second-line agent for moderate-to-severe pain; may precipitate withdrawal in opiate-dependent patients
			Used frequently in low doses to treat/prevent opioid-induced pruritus

(Continued)

TABLE 57-7 Opioid Dosing Guidelines (*Continued*)

Agent(s)	Standard Dose Ranges	Equianalgesic Dose in Adults (mg)	Notes
Buprenorphine	IM 0.3 mg every 6 hours[b]	0.3	Second-line agent for moderate-to-severe pain
	Slow IV 0.3 mg every 6 hours[b]	0.3	May precipitate withdrawal in opiate-dependent patients
			Transdermal delivery systems (5, 7.5, 10, 15, 20 mcg/h) available for every 7 day administration; detailed manufacturer dosing conversion recommendations exist
Naloxone	May repeat × 1, 30–60 minutes after initial dose		Naloxone may not be effective in reversing respiratory depression
	IV/IM 0.4–2 mg		When reversing opiate adverse effects in patients needing analgesia, dilute and titrate (0.1–0.2 mg every 2–3 minutes) so as not to reverse analgesia
Tramadol	PO 50–100 mg every 4–6 hours[a]		Maximum dose for nonextended-release, 400 mg/24 h maximum for extended release, 300 mg/24 h
	If rapid onset not required, start 25 mg/day and titrate over several days		Decrease dose in older patients and those renal impairment
	Extended release PO 100 mg every 24 hours		
Tapentadol	PO 50–100 mg every 4–6 hours[a]		First day of therapy may administer second dose after the first within 1 hour, maximum dose first day 700 mg, max. dose thereafter 600 mg (maximum dose for CR 500 mg)

CR, controlled release; HCL, hydrochloride; IM, intramuscular; IV, intravenous; ; mcg, microgram; mg, milligram; NSAID, nonsteroidal anti-inflammatory drug; OTFC, Oral transmucosal fentanyl citrate; PO, oral; prn, as needed; SR, sustained release; XR, extended release.
[a]May start with an around-the-clock regimen and switch to prn if/when the painful signal subsides or is episodic.
[b]May reach a ceiling analgesic effect.

TABLE 57-8	Major Adverse Medication Effects of the Opioid Analgesics
Effect	**Manifestation**
Mood changes	Dysphoria, euphoria
Somnolence	Sedation, inability to concentrate
Chemoreceptor trigger zone stimulation	Nausea, vomiting
Respiratory depression	Decreased respiratory rate, periodic breathing, oxygen desaturation
Decreased gastrointestinal motility	Constipation
Increase in sphincter tone	Biliary spasm, urinary retention (varies among agents)
Histamine release	Urticaria, pruritus, rarely exacerbation of asthma due to bronchospasm (varies among agents)
Tolerance	Larger doses for same effect
Physical Dependence	Withdrawal symptoms upon abrupt discontinuation
Hypogonadism	Fatigue, depression, loss of analgesia, sexual dysfunction, amenorrhea (females)
Sleep	Disrupts sleep–wake cycle, causes dose-dependent rapid eye movement (REM) suppression

TABLE 57-9	Intraspinal Opioids			
Medication	**Single Dose (mg)**	**Onset of Pain Relief (minutes)**	**Duration of Pain Relief (hour)**	**Continual Infusion Dose (mg/h)**
Epidural route				
Morphine	1–6	30	6–24	0.1–1
Hydromorphone	0.8–1.5	5–8	4–8	0.1–0.3
Fentanyl	0.025–0.1	5	2–8	0.025–0.1
Sufentanil	0.01–0.06	5	2–4	0.01–0.05
Subarachnoid route				
Morphine	0.1–0.3	15	8–34	–
Fentanyl	0.005–0.025	5	3–6	–

Doses above should not be interpreted as equianalgesic doses for conversion to or from the specific opioid or route of administration.

Meperidine and Congeners (Phenylpiperidines)

• **Meperidine** is less potent and has a shorter duration of action than morphine.
  ✓ With high doses or in patients with renal failure, the metabolite normeperidine accumulates, causing tremor, muscle twitching, and possibly seizures. In most settings, meperidine offers no advantages over morphine.
  ✓ Do not combine meperidine with monoamine oxidase inhibitors because severe respiratory depression or serotonin syndrome may occur.

- **Fentanyl**, often used as an adjunct to general anesthesia, is more potent and faster acting than meperidine. It can be administered parenterally, transmucosally, sublingually, intranasally, and transdermally.
- Numerous fentanyl-like agents exist including **remifentanil**, **alfentanil**, and **sufentanil**.

Methadone and Congeners (Diphenylheptanes)

- **Methadone** has an extended duration of action. High doses cause cardiac arrhythmias and there are specific echocardiogram recommendations for monitoring. Although effective for acute pain, it is used for chronic cancer pain.
- The equianalgesic dose of methadone may decrease with higher doses of the previous opioid. Doses should not be titrated more frequently than every 5–7 days.

Mixed Opioid Agonist–Antagonists

- This analgesic class may cause less respiratory depression and may have lower misuse potential. However, psychotomimetic responses (eg, hallucinations and dysphoria), a limited analgesic effect, and the propensity to initiate withdrawal in opioid-dependent patients have limited their use.
- Buprenorphine is a pharmacologically complex opioid. When used with or without naloxone, for opioid use disorder, a special DEA license is required by the prescriber.

Centrally Acting Opioids

- **Tramadol** and **tapentadol** are indicated for relief of moderate to moderately severe pain.
  ✓ Their adverse effects are similar to other opioids, although the seizure risk with tramadol may be higher.

Opioid Antagonists

- **Naloxone**, a pure opioid antagonist that binds competitively to opioid receptors, does not produce analgesia or opioid adverse effects. It reverses respiratory depression, but may need repeated or continuous dosing. Monitor respiratory function for at least 24 hours after a single dose of intrathecal or epidural morphine with standing orders for naloxone if needed. See Chapter 71 on other naloxone formulations. Many states have standing orders for naloxone so individuals can purchase without a prescription.
- Opioid antagonists may act centrally (eg, naloxone or **naltrexone**) or be limited to peripheral action only (eg, **naloxegol, methylnaltrexone, or naldemedine**).
- Table 57-10 lists dosing for central and peripheral opioid antagonists.

REGIONAL ANALGESIA

- Regional analgesia with local anesthetics (Table 57-11) is useful for both acute and chronic pain. Anesthetics can be positioned by injection (eg, in the joints, epidural or intrathecal space, nerve plexus, or along nerve roots), or applied topically.
- High plasma concentrations of local anesthetics can cause dizziness, tinnitus, drowsiness, seizures, and respiratory arrest. Cardiovascular effects include myocardial depression, heart block, hypotension, bradycardia, and cardiac arrest. Skillful application, frequent administration, and specialized follow-up are required.

SPECIAL POPULATIONS

- Older and younger patients are at higher risk of undertreatment. In these populations, it is important to monitor signs (eg, heart rate) and to talk with parents or caregivers.
- Those with chronic, debilitating, and life-threatening illnesses need specialized pain control and palliative care.

TABLE 57-10 Central and Peripheral Opioid Antagonists

Generic Name (Brand Name)	Activity	Role	Route	Dose in Adults (mg)	Special Considerations
Naldemedine (Symproic)	Peripheral	CNMP[a], OIC[b]	PO	0.2 mg qday	Avoid with severe hepatic impairment
Naloxone (Narcan, various)	Central	Opioid reversal	IV, IM, IN	0.4–2 mg[c]	Onset 1–2 (IV) minutes; 2–5 (IM) minutes Half-life 0.5–1.3 hours
Methylnaltrexone (Relistor)	Peripheral	Cancer and CNMP[a] OIC[b]	SC (both), PO (CNMP)	Variable	Renal dose adjustments
Naltrexone (ReVia, Vivitrol)	Central	AUD[d], OUD[e]	PO, IM	12 mg QD-Q12 (PO) 380 mg q4weeks (IM)	Opioid free for 7–10 days before initiation
Alvimopan (Entereg)	Peripheral	Postoperative ileus	PO	12 mg PO 30 minutes to 5 hours before surgery then 12 mg PO BID starting day after surgery for maximum of 7 days	Limited to 15 doses
Naloxegol (Movantik)	Peripheral	CNMP[a], OIC[b]	PO	12.5–25 mg qday 1 hour before, 2 hours after a meal	Renal dose adjustments Avoid with moderate 3A4 inhibitors

[a]Chronic nonmalignant pain.
[b]Opioid-induced constipation.
[c]Starting doses to be used in cases of opioid overdose.
[d]Alcohol use disorder.
[e]Opioid use disorder.
Data from individual package inserts.

TABLE 57-11 Local Anesthetics[a]

Generic Name (Brand Name)	Onset (minutes)	Duration (hours)
Esters		
Procaine (Novocain, various)	2–5	0.25–1
Chloroprocaine (Nesacaine, various)	6–12	0.5
Tetracaine (Pontocaine)	≤15	2–3
Amides		
Mepivacaine (Polocaine, various)	3–5	0.75–1.5
Bupivacaine (Marcaine, various)	5	2–4
Bupivacaine liposomal	Variable	24 local
(Exparel—wound infiltration only)		96 systemic
Lidocaine (Xylocaine, various)	<2	0.5–1
Prilocaine (Citanest)	<2	1–2
Ropivacaine[b] (Naropin)	10–30	0.5–6

[a]Unless otherwise indicated, values are for infiltrative anesthesia.
[b]Epidural administration.

EVALUATION OF THERAPEUTIC OUTCOMES

- Pain intensity, pain relief, and medication adverse effects must be assessed regularly. The frequency of assessment depends on the type of pain, analgesic used, route of administration, and concomitant medications. Postoperative pain and acute exacerbations of cancer pain may require hourly assessment. Chronic nonmalignant pain may need only daily (or less frequent) monitoring. Quality of life must be assessed regularly.
- Use the five As to assess pain and response to treatment for patients with chronic pain.
- Patients taking opioids should be counseled on proper intake of fluids and fiber, and a stimulant laxative should be added with chronic opioid use. Peripherally acting mu-opioid receptor antagonists (PAMORAs) are available for treating opioid-induced constipation.
- Concomitant use of CNS depressants should be avoided with opioid analgesics.

See Chapter 79, Pain Management, authored by Chris M. Herndon, Courtney M. Kominek, and Amanda M. Mullins and Chapter 150, Supportive Care in Cancer, authored by Amber B. Clemmons, and Ashley E. Glode for a more detailed discussion of this topic.

58 Parkinson Disease

- *Parkinson disease* (PD) has highly characteristic neuropathologic findings and a clinical presentation, including motor deficits and, in some cases, mental deterioration.

PATHOPHYSIOLOGY

- Its true etiology is unknown. Reduced activation of dopamine$_1$ and dopamine$_2$ receptors results in greater inhibition of the thalamus and reduced activation of the motor cortex. Clinical improvement may be tied to restoring activity more at the dopamine$_2$ receptor than at the dopamine$_1$ receptor. Antagonism of adenosine A$_{2A}$ receptors located in GABAergic neurons can prolong dopaminergic action.
- Two hallmark features in the substantia nigra pars compacta are loss of neurons and presence of Lewy bodies. The degree of nigrostriatal dopamine loss correlates positively with severity of motor symptoms.

CLINICAL PRESENTATION

- PD develops insidiously and progresses slowly over many years.

GENERAL FEATURES

- Bradykinesia (slowness of movements) and at least one of the following: resting tremor, rigidity, or postural instability.

MOTOR SYMPTOMS

- Only two-thirds of patients with PD have tremor on diagnosis, and some never develop this sign. Tremor in PD is present most commonly in the hands, sometimes with a characteristic pill-rolling motion. Motor features may be asymmetric.
- Hypokinetic movements, decreased manual dexterity, difficulty arising from a seated position, diminished arm swing during ambulation, dysarthria (slurred speech), dysphagia (difficulty with swallowing), festinating gait (tendency to pass from a slow to a quickened pace), flexed posture, "freezing" at the initiation of movement, hypomimia (reduced facial animation), hypophonia (reduced voice volume), and micrographia.

AUTONOMIC AND SENSORY SYMPTOMS

- Bladder dysfunction, constipation, diaphoresis, fatigue, olfactory impairment, orthostatic intolerance, pain, paresthesia, paroxysmal vascular flushing, seborrhea, sexual dysfunction, and sialorrhea (drooling).

MENTAL STATUS CHANGES

- Anxiety, apathy, bradyphrenia (slowness of thought processes), cognitive impairment, depression, and hallucinosis/psychosis.

SLEEP DISTURBANCES

- Excessive daytime sleepiness, insomnia, obstructive sleep apnea, and rapid eye movement (REM) sleep behavior disorder.

DIAGNOSIS

- The clinical diagnosis of PD is outlined in Table 58-1.
- Laboratory or genetic testing, cannot diagnose PD. Neuroimaging may be useful for excluding other diagnoses.
- Obtain a medication history to rule out medication-induced parkinsonism.

| **TABLE 58-1** | Diagnostic Criteria and Differential Diagnosis for Parkinson Disease |

Parkinson disease
- Step 1: Presence of bradykinesia and at least one of the following: resting tremor, rigidity, or postural instability
- Step 2: Exclude other types of parkinsonism or tremor disorders (see "Differential Diagnosis")
- Step 3: Presence of at least three supportive positive criteria:
  - Asymmetry of motor signs/symptoms
  - Unilateral onset
  - Progressive disorder
  - Resting tremor
  - Excellent response to carbidopa/levodopa
  - levodopa response for 5 years or longer
  - Presence of levodopa dyskinesias

Differential diagnosis
- Essential tremor
- Pharmacotoxicity (medication-induced)
  - Antiemetics (eg, metoclopramide, prochlorperazine)
  - Antipsychotics (eg, chlorpromazine, fluphenazine, haloperidol, olanzapine, risperidone, thioridazine)
  - Other medications (α-methyldopa, cinnarizine, flunarizine, tetrabenazine)
- Environmental toxicity (eg, manganese, organophosphates)
- Infections (eg, human immunodeficiency virus, subacute sclerosing panencephalitis)
- Metabolic disorder (eg, hypothyroidism, parathyroid abnormalities)
- Neoplasms, strokes, traumatic lesions involving the nigrostriatal pathways
- Normal-pressure hydrocephalus
- Parkinsonism with other neuronal system degenerations
  - Corticobasal ganglionic degeneration
- Multiple-system atrophies
- Progressive supranuclear palsy
- Familial (hereditary) parkinsonism
  - Autosomal dominant
    - α-Synuclein gene mutation (*PARK1* and *PARK4*)
    - L-responsive dystonia
    - Leucine-rich repeat kinase 2 (LRRK2) mutation
    - Rapid-onset dystonia-parkinsonism (DYT12)
    - Spinocerebellar ataxias (SCA2, SCA3)
  - Autosomal recessive
    - Wilson disease
    - Young-onset parkinsonism (DJ-1, parkin, PINK1)
  - X-linked recessive
    - Fragile X tremor/ataxia syndrome (FXTAS)
    - Lubag (DYT3 or Filipino dystonia-parkinsonism)

TREATMENT

- <u>Goals of Treatment</u>: The goals of treatment are to minimize symptoms, disability, and medication adverse effects while maintaining quality of life. Education of patients and caregivers, exercise, and proper nutrition are essential.
- To date, no treatments have been shown to effectively change the course of PD by slowing or halting its progression (disease modification).

NONPHARMACOLOGIC THERAPY

- Exercise, physiotherapy, yoga, Tai Chi, and dance can improve PD symptoms. The Lee Silvermann Voice Treatment-BIG Therapy may be of particular benefit.

- Surgery should be considered an adjunct to pharmacotherapy for patients experiencing frequent motor fluctuations or disabling dyskinesia or tremor despite an optimized medical regimen. Bilateral, chronic, high-frequency electrical stimulation, also known as deep-brain stimulation (DBS), is the preferred surgical modality.

PHARMACOLOGIC THERAPY

General Approach

- An algorithm for management of early to advanced PD is shown in Fig. 58-1. Table 58-2 is a summary of available antiparkinson medications and their dosing, and Table 58-3 shows adverse effect monitoring.

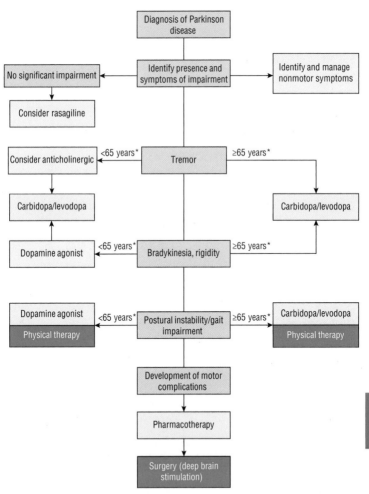

FIGURE 58-1. **General approach to the management of early to advanced Parkinson disease.**

TABLE 58-2	Dosing of Medications Used in Parkinson Disease[a]	
Medication (Brand Name)	**Starting Dose[b] (mg/day)**	**Maintenance Dose[b] (mg/day)**
Adenosine-Receptor Antagonist		
Istradefylline	20	20–40
Anticholinergic Medications		
Benztropine	0.5–1	1–6
Trihexyphenidyl	1–2	6–15
Carbidopa/Levodopa products		
Carbidopa/levodopa	300[c]	300–2000[c]
Carbidopa/levodopa ODT	300[c]	300–2000[c]
Carbidopa/levodopa CR	400[c]	400–2000[c]
Carbidopa/levodopa IR/ER	435[c]	435–2450[c]
Carbidopa/levodopa enteral suspension	1000[c]	1000–2000[c]
Carbidopa/levodopa/entacapone	600[d]	600–1600[d]
Carbidopa	25	25–75
Levodopa	84	84–420
Dopamine agonists		
Apomorphine (Apokyn)	1–3	3–12
Apomorphine (Kynmobi)	10	10-150
Bromocriptine	2.5–5	15–40
Pramipexole	0.125	1.5–4.5
Pramipexole ER	0.375	1.5–4.5
Ropinirole	0.75	9–24
Ropinirole XL	2	8–24
Rotigotine	2	2–8
COMT inhibitors		
Entacapone	200–600	200–1600
Ocicapone	25-50	50
Tolcapone	300	300–600
MAO-B inhibitors		
Rasagiline	0.5–1	0.5–1
Safinamide	50	50–100
Selegiline	5–10	5–10
Selegiline ODT	1.25	1.25–2.5

(Continued)

TABLE 58-2	Dosing of Medications Used in Parkinson Disease[a] (Continued)		
Medication (Brand Name)	**Starting Dose[b] (mg/day)**	**Maintenance Dose[b] (mg/day)**	
Miscellaneous			
Amantadine	100	200–300	
Amantadine ER (Gocovri)	137	274	
Amantadine ER (Osmolex)	129	129–258	

COMT, catechol-*O*-methyltransferase; CR, controlled-release; IR, immediate-release; ER, extended-release; MAO, monoamine oxidase; ODT, orally disintegrating tablet.
[a]Marketed in the United States for Parkinson disease.
[b]Dosages may vary.
[c]Dosages expressed as levodopa component.
[d]Dosages expressed as entacapone component.

TABLE 58-3	Monitoring of Potential Adverse Effects for Parkinson Disease		
Medication	**Adverse Medication Effect**	**Monitoring Parameter**	**Comments**
Amantadine	Confusion	Mental status; renal function	Reduce dosage; adjust dose for renal impairment
	Livedo reticularis	Lower extremity examination; ankle edema	Reversible upon medication discontinuation
Benztropine and Trihexyphenidyl	Anticholinergic effects, confusion, drowsiness	Dry mouth, mental status, constipation, urinary retention, vision	Reduce dosage; avoid in older persons and in those with a history of constipation, memory impairment, urinary retention
Carbidopa/ levodopa	Drowsiness, dyskinesias, nausea	Mental status, abnormal involuntary movements, nausea	Reduce dose, add amantadine, take with food (eg, nonprotein snack)
Istradefylline	Insomniam dizziness, nausea, constipation	Sleep, nausea, bowel movements	Take in the morning with food
COMT inhibitors			
Entacapone	Augmentation of levodopa adverse effects; also diarrhea	See carbidopa/ levodopa; also bowel movements	Reduce dose of levodopa; antidiarrheal agents
Opicapone	Augmentation of L-dopa adverse effects, constipation	Mental status, abnormal involuntary movements, bowel movements	Reduce dose of L-dopa

(Continued)

TABLE 58-3	Monitoring of Potential Adverse Effects for Parkinson Disease (*Continued*)		
Medication	**Adverse Medication Effect**	**Monitoring Parameter**	**Comments**
Tolcapone	See entacapone; also liver toxicity	See carbidopa/levodopa; also ALT/AST	See carbidopa/levodopa, ALT and AST levels at baseline and every 2–4 weeks for the first 6 months of therapy; afterward monitor based on clinical judgment.
Dopamine agonists			
Apomorphine	Drowsiness, nausea, orthostatic hypotension	Mental status, nausea, blood pressure, dizziness upon standing	Reduce dose, premedicate with trimethobenzamide
Bromocriptine	See pramipexole; also pulmonary fibrosis	Mental status; also chest radiograph	Reduce dose; chest radiograph at baseline and once yearly
Pramipexole and Ropinirole	Confusion, drowsiness, edema, hallucinations/ delusions, impulsivity, nausea, orthostatic hypotension	Mental status, lower extremity swelling, nausea, blood pressure, dizziness upon standing	Reduce dose or discontinue medication, titrate dose upward slowly, take with food
Rotigotine	See pramipexole; also skin irritation at site of patch application	See pramipexole; also skin examination	See pramipexole; rotate patch application site
MAO-B inhibitors			
Rasagiline	Nausea	Nausea	Take with food
Safinamide	Nausea Elevation in blood pressure Insomnia	Nausea Blood pressure Sleep	Take with food Monitor blood pressure if have a history of uncontrolled hypertension Take in the morning
Selegiline	Agitation/Confusion, insomnia, hallucinations, orthostatic hypotension	Mental status, sleep, blood pressure, dizziness upon standing	Reduce dose or administer earlier in the day

ALT, alanine aminotransferase; AST, aspartate aminotransferase; COMT, catechol-*O*-methyltransferase; MAO, monoamine oxidase.

- For mild functional impairment, initial monotherapy usually begins with a monoamine oxidase-B (MAO-B) inhibitor.
- Ultimately, all patients will require the use of **carbidopa/levodopa** either as monotherapy or in combination with other agents.

- With the development of motor fluctuations, administer carbidopa/levodopa more frequently or add a COMT inhibitor, MAO-B inhibitor, adenosine receptor antagonist, or dopamine agonist to the carbidopa/levodopa regimen.
- To manage carbidopa/levodopa–induced peak-dose dyskinesias, reduce the levodopa dose and/or add amantadine.

Anticholinergic Medications

- **Anticholinergic** medication can improve tremor and sometimes dystonic features, but they rarely substantially improve bradykinesia or other disabilities. They can be used as monotherapy but are most often used adjunctively.
  ✓ Adverse effects include dry mouth, blurred vision, constipation, and urinary retention. More serious reactions include forgetfulness, confusion, sedation, depression, and anxiety (see Table 58-3). Patients with preexisting cognitive deficits and advanced age are at greater risk for central anticholinergic adverse effects.

Amantadine

- **Amantadine** often provides modest benefit for tremor, rigidity, and bradykinesia and is often used for levodopa-induced dyskinesia.
- There are three different formulations available for use (one immediate-release and two extended-release products) (See Table 58-2).
- Doses should be reduced in renal dysfunction (100 mg/day with creatinine clearances of 30–50 mL/min [0.50–0.84 mL/sec]; 100 mg every other day for creatinine clearances of 15–29 mL/min [0.25–0.49 mL/sec], and 200 mg every 7 days for creatinine clearances less than 15 mL/min [0.25 mL/sec]) and those on hemodialysis.
  ✓ Adverse effects (See Table 58-3) include livedo reticularis (a diffuse mottling of the skin in the upper or lower extremities) which is common but reversible.

Levodopa and Carbidopa/Levodopa

- **Levodopa** is the immediate precursor of dopamine and, in combination with a peripherally acting L-amino acid decarboxylase (L-AAD) inhibitor (**carbidopa** or **benserazide**), remains the most effective medication for the symptomatic treatment of PD.
- In the central nervous system (CNS) and peripherally, levodopa is converted by L-AAD to dopamine. In the periphery, carbidopa or benserazide can block L-AAD, which increases levodopa CNS penetration and decreases dopamine adverse effects (eg, nausea, cardiac arrhythmias, postural hypotension, and vivid dreams). Benserazide is unavailable in the United States.
- The usual maximal levodopa dose tolerated is approximately 1000 to 1500 mg/day.
- About 75 mg of carbidopa is required to effectively block peripheral L-AAD, but some patients need more. Controlled-release preparations of carbidopa/levodopa are also available (Table 58-2). For patients with difficulty swallowing, an orally disintegrating tablet is available, and a capsule containing beads is available which can be sprinkled on food (Rytary).
- After oral levodopa administration, time to peak plasma concentrations varies intra- and intersubject. Meals delay gastric emptying, but antacids promote gastric emptying. Levodopa is absorbed primarily in the proximal duodenum via a saturable large neutral amino acid transport system, thus high-protein meals can interfere with bioavailability.
- Levodopa is not bound to plasma proteins, and the elimination half-life is approximately 1 hour. Adding carbidopa or benserazide can extend the half-life to 1.5 hours, and adding a COMT inhibitor (eg, **entacapone**) can extend it to approximately 2–2.5 hours.
- Sinemet CR and Rytary are 70% and 75% bioavailable compared to the standard immediate-release carbidopa/levodopa formulation.
  ✓ Long-term, levodopa-associated motor complications can be disabling but are manageable (Table 58-4). The risk of developing these is approximately 10% per year; however, they can occur 5–6 months after starting levodopa. Risk factors associated with their occurrence are higher levodopa doses and younger age of PD onset.

TABLE 58-4	Common Motor Complications and Possible Initial Treatments
Complication and Management	
End-of-dose "wearing off" (motor fluctuation): Relates to the increasing loss of neuronal dopamine storage capability and the short half-life of levodopa.	Management includes bedtime administration of a dopamine agonist or a formulation that provides sustained medication levels overnight (eg, carbidopa/levodopa CR or IR/ER, ropinirole XL, pramipexole ER, rotigotine transdermal patch); Increase frequency of carbidopa/levodopa doses; add either COMT inhibitor or MAO-B inhibitor or dopamine agonist; add or switch to extended-release carbidopa/levodopa (ie, Rytary); use levodopa inhalation or apomorphine subcutaneous or sublingual.
"Delayed on" or "no on" response: can result from delayed gastric emptying or decreased absorption in the duodenum.	Give carbidopa/levodopa on empty stomach; use carbidopa/levodopa ODT or crush or chew regular tablets and take on an empty stomach; avoid carbidopa/levodopa SR; use apomorphine subcutaneous or sublingual or levodopa inhalation.
Start hesitation ("freezing"): an episodic inhibition of lower extremity motor function, may be worsened by anxiety and may increase falls.	To manage increase the carbidopa/levodopa dose; add a dopamine agonist or MAO-B inhibitor; utilize physical therapy along with assistive walking devices or sensory cues (eg, rhythmic commands, stepping over objects)
Peak-dose dyskinesia: involuntary choreiform movements usually involving the neck, trunk, and extremities, are usually associated with peak striatal dopamine levels.	Provide smaller doses of carbidopa/levodopa at the same or increased dosing frequency; reduce dose of adjunctive dopamine agonist; add amantadine
"Off-period" dystonia: muscle contractions occur most commonly in distal lower extremities (eg, feet or toes), often in the early morning	Consider bedtime administration of sustained-release products, use of baclofen, or selective denervation with botulinum toxin.

COMT, catechol-*O*-methyltransferase; MAO, monoamine oxidase; ODT, orally disintegrating tablet; SR, sustained release.

Adenosine Receptor Antagonist

- **Istradefylline** is used adjunctively to levodopa for "off" episodes (See Table 58-2). For patients who smoke >20 cigarettes a day use the 40-mg dose.
  - ✓ Common adverse effects include insomnia, hallucination, nausea, and constipation.
  - ✓ It is metabolized by CYP1A1 and CYP3A4 and has an elimination half-life of approximately 80 hours. Avoid use with CYP3A4 strong inducers and reduce the dose with strong inhibitors.

Monoamine Oxidase B Inhibitors

- Three selective MAO-B inhibitors (**rasagiline, safinamide, selegiline**) are available for PD (See Table 58-2).
- Rasagiline and selegiline contain a propargylamine moiety, which is essential for conferring irreversible inhibition of MAO-B, in contrast to safinamide, which is reversible. At therapeutic doses, all three agents preferentially inhibit MAO-B over MAO-A.
- Concomitant use of MAO-B inhibitors with meperidine and other selected opioid analgesics is contraindicated due to serotonin syndrome but serotonergic antidepressants can be used concomitantly when clinically warranted.
- As monotherapy in early PD, both selegiline and rasagiline provide modest improvements in motor function.

- All can provide up to 1 hour of extra "on" time for patients, when used adjunctively.
- Selegiline increases levodopa peak effects and can worsen preexisting dyskinesias or psychiatric symptoms, such as delusions. Metabolites of selegiline are L-methamphetamine and L-amphetamine. The oral disintegrating tablet may provide improved response and fewer adverse effects.

  ✓ Adverse effects of selegiline include agitation, insomnia (especially if administered at bedtime), hallucinations, and orthostatic hypotension. Both rasagiline and safinamide are well tolerated with minimal GI or neuropsychiatric adverse effects.

Catechol-*O*-Methyltransferase Inhibitors

- **Tolcapone**, **entacapone,** and **opicapone** are used adjunctively with carbidopa/levodopa to prevent the peripheral conversion of levodopa to dopamine which increases levodopa's area under the curve ~35%), increases "on" time by ~1–2 hours (longer with opicapone), and reduces levodopa dosage requirements. Avoid concomitant nonselective MAO inhibitors to prevent inhibition of normal catecholamine metabolism pathways.
- Table 58-2 outlines dosing. Opicapone can be dosed once daily but entacapone is given with each dose of carbidopa/levodopa up to eight times a day.

  ✓ Tolcapone's use is limited due to the potential for fatal liver toxicity, requiring strict monitoring.
  ✓ Dopaminergic adverse effects may occur and are managed by reducing the carbidopa/levodopa dose. Brownish orange urine discoloration may occur (as with tolcapone), but hepatotoxicity is not reported with entacapone.

Dopamine Agonists

- The ergot derivative **bromocriptine** and the nonergots **pramipexole**, **rotigotine,** and **ropinirole** are beneficial adjuncts in patients experiencing fluctuation in levodopa response as they decrease the frequency of "off" periods and provide a levodopa-sparing effect.
- Titrate the dose slowly to enhance tolerability, and find the optimal dose (See Table 58-2).
- The nonergots are effective as monotherapy in mild-to-moderate PD and adjunctively to levodopa in patients with motor fluctuations and are safer.
- **Pramipexole** is primarily renally excreted, and the dose must be adjusted in renal insufficiency.
- **Ropinirole** is metabolized by cytochrome P4501A2; fluoroquinolones and cigarette smoking may alter clearance.
- **Rotigotine** patch provides continuous release over 24 hours, and disposition is not affected by hepatic or renal impairment.
- **Apomorphine** is a nonergot dopamine agonist given as a subcutaneous "rescue" injection. For patients with advanced PD with intermittent "off" episodes despite optimized therapy, subcutaneous apomorphine triggers an "on" response within 20 minutes, and duration of effect is up to 100 minutes. Most patients require 0.06 mg/kg. Prior to injection, patients should be premedicated with the antiemetic **trimethobenzamide**. It is contraindicated with the serotonin-3-receptor blockers (eg, ondansetron).

  ✓ Common adverse effects are in Table 58-3. Additional effects include vivid dreams and sleep attacks. Adding levodopa may worsen dyskinesias. Hallucinations or delusions should be managed by dosage reduction or discontinuation and if needed addition of **clozapine**, **quetiapine**, or **pimavanserin** (FDA approved for psychosis in PD).
  ✓ **Bromocriptine** is not commonly used given its safety profile, which includes a risk of pulmonary fibrosis.
  ✓ Motor complication risk is less with dopamine agonist monotherapy than levodopa. They are preferred in younger patients due to the increased risk of motor fluctuations. Carbidopa/levodopa may be the best in older patients due to the risk of psychosis and orthostatic hypotension from dopamine agonists. For patients with cognitive problems or dementia, avoid dopamine agonists.

EVALUATION OF THERAPEUTIC OUTCOMES

- Comprehensive monitoring is essential to achieve desired outcomes (Table 58-5). Educate patients and caregivers about recording medication doses and administration times and duration of "on" and "off" periods.
- Concomitant medications that may worsen motor symptoms, memory, falls, or behavioral symptoms should be discontinued if possible.

TABLE 58-5	Monitoring and Education for Parkinson Disease Therapy

1. Monitor medication administration times. Educate the patient that immediate-release carbidopa/levodopa is absorbed best on an empty stomach but is commonly taken with food (preferably a non-protein snack) to minimize nausea. Avoid conventional selegiline in the late afternoon or evening to minimize insomnia.

2. Monitor to ensure that the patient and/or caregivers understand the medication regimen. For example, they should understand that catechol-*O*-methyltransferase inhibitors work by enhancing levodopa's effect and medication should not be discontinued without notifying the clinician.

3. Monitor and inquire specifically about dose-by-dose effects, including response and the presence of common motor symptoms (**Table 58-4**) and adverse effects (**Table 58-3**). Offer suggestions to help alleviate these, encourage the patient to discuss them with the clinician, and monitor caregiver involvement in their early detection.

4. Monitor adherence and if there are problems inquire for possible reasons (eg, dosing convenience, financial issues, and adverse effects) and offer suggestions.

5. Monitor for presence of medications that can exacerbate idiopathic Parkinson disease motor features (eg, D_2-receptor blockers).

6. Monitor for presence of medications that can exacerbate nonmotor symptoms. Evaluate if an anticholinergic agent is causing confusion or cognitive impairment.

See Chapter 78, Parkinson Disease, authored by Jessa M. Koch, Khashayar Dashtipour, and Jack J. Chen, for a more detailed discussion of this topic.

CHAPTER 59

Obesity

- *Obesity* occurs when there is an imbalance between energy intake and energy expenditure over time, resulting in increased energy storage.

PATHOPHYSIOLOGY

- The etiology of obesity is usually unknown, but it is likely multifactorial and related to varying contributions from genetic, environmental, and physiologic factors.
- Genetic factors appear to be the primary determinants of obesity in some individuals, determining both obesity and distribution of fat, whereas environmental factors are more important in others. The total number and identity of contributing genes are still being determined.
- Environmental factors include reduced physical activity or work, abundant food supply, relatively sedentary lifestyles, increased availability of high-fat foods, and cultural factors and religious beliefs.
- Medical conditions including Cushing syndrome, growth hormone deficiency, insulinoma, leptin deficiency, and psychiatric disorders such as depression, binge-eating disorder, and schizophrenia and genetic syndromes such as Prader–Willi syndrome can be associated with weight gain.
- Medications associated with unintended weight gain include insulin, corticosteroids, some antidepressants, atypical and conventional antipsychotics, and several anticonvulsants.
- Many neurotransmitters and neuropeptides stimulate or depress the brain's appetite network, impacting total calorie intake.
- The degree of obesity is determined by the net balance of energy ingested relative to energy expended over time. The single largest determinant of energy expenditure is metabolic rate, which is expressed as *resting energy expenditure* or *basal metabolic rate*. Physical activity is the other major factor that affects total energy expenditure and is the most variable component.
- Major types of adipose tissue are: (1) white adipose tissue, which stores energy; and (2) brown adipose tissue, which uncouples oxidative phosphorylation to produce heat and maintain body temperature. Adrenergic stimulation activates lipolysis in fat cells and increases energy expenditure in adipose tissue and skeletal muscle.

CLINICAL PRESENTATION

- Obesity is associated with serious health risks and increased risk of all-cause mortality. Central obesity reflects high levels of intra-abdominal or visceral fat that is associated with the development of hypertension, dyslipidemia, type 2 diabetes, and cardiovascular disease (sometimes referred to as the "metabolic syndrome").
- Body mass index (BMI) and waist circumference (WC) are recognized, acceptable markers of excess body fat that independently predict disease risk (Table 59-1). Both measurements should be assessed and monitored during therapy for obesity.
- BMI is calculated as weight (kg) divided by the square of the height (m^2).
- WC, the most practical method of characterizing central adiposity, is the narrowest circumference between the last rib and the top of the iliac crest.

TABLE 59-1 Classification of Overweight and Obesity by Body Mass Index, Comorbidity Risk, Waist Circumference, and Associated Disease Risk

	BMI (kg/m^2)	Obesity Class	Comorbidity Risk	Disease Risk[a] (Relative to Normal Weight and Waist Circumference) Men ≤40 in (102 cm) / Women ≤35 in (89 cm)	Men >40 in (102 cm) / Women >35 in (89 cm)
Underweight	<18.5		Low but other problems	—	—
Normal weight[b]	18.5–24.9		Average	—	High
Overweight	25.0–29.9		Increased	Increased	High
Obesity	30.0–34.9	I	Moderate	High	Very high
	35.0–39.9	II	Severe	Very high	Very high
Extreme obesity	≥40	III	Very severe	Extremely high	Extremely high

BMI, body mass index.
[a]Disease risk for type 2 diabetes, hypertension, and cardiovascular disease.
[b]Increased waist circumference can also be a marker for increased risk even in persons of normal weight.
Data from WHO Consultation on Obesity (1999: Geneva, Switzerland) & World Health Organization. (2000). Obesity: preventing and managing the global epidemic: report of a WHO consultation. World Health Organization. Available at: https://apps.who.int/iris/handle/10665/42330.

TREATMENT

- <u>Goals of Treatment</u>: Current clinical practice guidelines recommend a "complication-centric approach" to assess the presence and severity of weight-related complications to determine appropriate treatment and intensity of weight loss therapy in individuals with overweight and obesity. The primary goal is to ameliorate weight-related complications and ultimately improve health and quality of life rather than a preset decrease in body weight.

GENERAL APPROACH

- Successful obesity treatment plans include comprehensive lifestyle interventions such as healthy diet, adequate physical activity, and behavior modifications as the cornerstone of weight management. Establish specific weight goals consistent with medical needs, weight-related complications, and patient's personal desire.
- Current adult practice guidelines recommend reduced caloric intake through adherence to a low-calorie diet. Adherence to this type of diet with increased exercise, and in-person behavioral counseling sessions result in an average weight loss of 8 kg (17.6 lb) over 6 months.
- Bariatric surgery, which reduces the stomach volume or absorptive surface of the alimentary tract, remains the most effective intervention for obesity. Surgery should be reserved for those with extreme obesity (BMI ≥40 kg/m^2) or BMI >35 kg/m^2 with significant comorbidities such as hypertension, type 2 diabetes, or obstructive sleep apnea.

- Implantable medical devices are an option for individuals who do not qualify for bariatric surgery or choose to not undergo the procedure. These devices are designed to work in conjunction with prescribed diet and exercise programs.

PHARMACOLOGIC THERAPY

- Pharmacotherapy is an adjunct to comprehensive lifestyle intervention in adults who are motivated to lose weight, have failed to achieve or sustain weight loss with lifestyle change alone, and have a BMI $\geq$30 kg/m^2 or BMI $\geq$27 kg/m^2 with at least one weight-related comorbidity (Table 59-2).
- Long-term pharmacotherapy may have a role for patients who have no contraindications to approved drug therapy (Table 59-3). Guidelines recommend discontinuation of medication therapy after 3 months if insufficient body weight is lost or significant adverse reactions are experienced.
- **Orlistat** (180 or 360 mg in three divided doses/day) is a lipase inhibitor that induces weight loss by lowering dietary fat absorption; it also improves lipid profiles, glucose control, and other metabolic markers. Soft stools, abdominal pain or colic, flatulence, fecal urgency, and/or incontinence occur in 80% of individuals using prescription strength, are mild to moderate in severity, and improve after 1–2 months of therapy. Orlistat is approved for long-term use. It interferes with the absorption of fat-soluble vitamins, **cyclosporine**, **levothyroxine**, and **antiretrovirals**. A nonprescription formulation is also available.
- **Phentermine** in combination with **topiramate extended-release** is indicated for chronic weight management. Doses are gradually titrated from phentermine 3.75 to 15 mg and topiramate 23 to 92 mg over 4 months, but the drug should be stopped after 12 weeks if 5% weight loss is not achieved. Common adverse effects include constipation, dry mouth, paraesthesia, dysgeusia, and insomnia.
- **Naltrexone** in combination with **bupropion extended-release** is indicated for chronic weight management. Doses are gradually increased over 4 weeks, starting with one tablet daily (8 mg naltrexone/90 mg bupropion) to a maintenance dose of two tablets twice daily. Patients should avoid taking their dose with a high-fat meal. Common adverse effects include nausea, constipation, headache, vomiting, dizziness, insomnia, dry mouth, and diarrhea. Discontinue treatment if 5% weight loss is not achieved after 12 weeks.
- **Liraglutide** and **semaglutide** are glucagon-like peptide-1 receptor agonists indicated for chronic weight management. See **Table 59-2** for dose escalation schedules to improve tolerability of gastrointestinal adverse effects. Both are administered subcutaneously and available in prefilled, multidose pens. Common adverse effects include nausea, diarrhea, constipation, vomiting, dyspepsia, hypoglycemia, and abdominal pain. Discontinue liraglutide if weight loss of at least 4% is not achieved after 16 weeks.

- **Setmelanotide** is a peptide analog of endogenous alpha-melanocyte stimulating hormone indicated for chronic weight management in patients with genetically confirmed or suspected proopiomelanocortin (POMC), proprotein convertase subtilisin/kexin type 1 (PCSK1) or leptin receptor (LEPR) deficiency. It is administered once daily as a subcutaneous injection with a starting dose of 2 mg daily for those 12 years and older and 1 mg daily for children aged 6 to less than 12 years. Common adverse effects include injection site reactions, skin hyperpigmentation, nausea, headache, diarrhea, abdominal pain, and spontaneous penile erections. Discontinue setmelanotide if weight loss of 5% is not achieved after 12–16 weeks.
- Many complementary and alternative therapy products are promoted for weight loss. Regulation of dietary supplements is less rigorous than that of prescription and over-the-counter drug products; manufacturers do not have to prove safety and effectiveness prior to marketing.

TABLE 59-2	FDA-Approved Pharmacotherapeutic Agents for Weight Loss				
Medication	Brand Name	Initial Dose	Usual Range	Special Population Dose	Comments
Gastrointestinal Lipase Inhibitor					
Orlistat	Xenical®	120 mg three times daily with each main meal containing fat	120 mg three times daily with each main meal containing fat	120 mg three times daily is approved for adolescents ages 12 or greater with BMI for age equivalent to 30 kg/m² in adults	Approved for long-term use Take during or up to 1 hour after the meal Omit dose if meal is occasionally missed or contains no fat
Orlistat	Alli®ᵃ	60 mg three times daily with each main meal containing fat	60 mg three times daily with each main meal containing fat		Same as Xenical®
Phentermine–Topiramate Combination					
Phentermine and topiramate extended-release	Qsymia®	3.75 mg of phentermine and 23 mg of topiramate once daily for 14 days; then increase to 7.5 mg of phentermine and 46 mg of topiramate once daily	7.5 mg of phentermine and 46 mg of topiramate once daily to a maximum dose of phentermine 15 mg and topiramate 92 mg once daily	Maximum dose for patients with moderate or severe kidney impairment or patients with moderate hepatic impairment is 7.5 mg of phentermine and 46 mg of topiramate	Approved for long-term use Take dose in the morning to avoid insomnia Controlled substance: C–IV

Naltrexone-Bupropion Combination

| Bupropion and naltrexone extended-release | Contrave® | 8 mg naltrexone/90 mg bupropion (one tablet) once daily in the morning for 1 week; then 8 mg naltrexone/90 mg bupropion twice daily (morning and evening) for 1 week; then 16 mg naltrexone/180 mg bupropion in the morning and 8 mg naltrexone/90 mg bupropion in the evening for 1 week; then 16 mg naltrexone/180 mg bupropion twice daily (morning and evening) | 16 mg naltrexone and 180 mg bupropion (two tablets) twice daily | Maximum dose for patients with moderate or severe kidney impairment is 8 mg naltrexone/90 mg bupropion (one tablet) twice daily

Maximum dose for patients with hepatic impairment is 8 mg naltrexone/90 mg bupropion (one tablet) once daily in the morning | Approved for long-term use
Do not take dose with high-fat meal |

Glucagon-Like Peptide-1 Agonists

| Liraglutide | Saxenda® | 0.6 mg once daily for 1 week
1.2 mg once daily for 1 week
1.8 mg once daily for 1 week
2.4 mg once daily for 1 week
3.0 mg once daily for 1 week | 3 mg once daily | Use with caution in mild, moderate, and severe kidney and hepatic impairment Dose escalation to 3.0 mg once daily is approved for adolescents ages 12 or greater with weight 60 kg (132 lb) or greater and BMI for age equivalent to 30 kg/m^2 in adults | Approved for long-term use
Inject subcutaneously in the abdomen, thigh, or upper arm |

(Continued)

TABLE 59-2 FDA-Approved Pharmacotherapeutic Agents for Weight Loss (*Continued*)

Medication	Brand Name	Initial Dose	Usual Range	Special Population Dose	Comments
		Administered by subcutaneous injection			Administer at any time of day without regard to the timing of meals
Semaglutide	Wegovy™	0.25 mg once weekly for 4 weeks 0.5 mg once weekly for 4 weeks 1 mg once weekly for 4 weeks 1.7 mg once weekly for 4 weeks 2.4 mg once weekly Administered by subcutaneous injection	2.4 mg once weekly		Approved for long-term use Inject subcutaneously in the abdomen, thigh, or upper arm Administer at any time of day without regard to the timing of meals
Melanocortin 4 (MC4) Receptor Agonist					
Setmelanotide	Imcivree™	Adults and adolescents >12 years: 2 mg once daily for 2 weeks, then increase to 3 mg once daily if tolerated and additional weight loss is desired (or decrease to 1 mg once daily based on tolerability) Children aged 6 to <12 years: 1 mg once daily for 2 weeks, then increase to 2 mg once daily if tolerated (or decrease to 0.5 mg once daily based on tolerability), then increase to 3 mg once daily if tolerated and additional weight loss is desired Administered by subcutaneous injection	2–3 mg once daily	Not recommended for patients with moderate to severe kidney impairment	Approved for long-term use in patients aged 6 years and above with genetically confirmed or suspected deficiency of POMC, PCSK1, or LEPR Inject subcutaneously in the abdomen, thigh, or upper arm rotating sites each day Administer at the beginning of the day without regard to timing of meals

Noradrenergic Agents

Phendimetrazine	Bontril® PDM; Bontril® Slow-Release	Conventional tablet: start at 17.5 mg two or three times daily, given 1 hour before meals Extended-release capsule: 105 mg once daily 30–60 minutes before morning meal	70–105 mg/day	Use caution in patients with kidney impairment	Approved for short-term monotherapy Controlled substance: C–III Prescriptions should be written for the smallest quantity to minimize possibility of overdose
Phentermine	Lomaira™, Adipex-P®	8 mg three times daily, given ½ hour before meal Orally disintegrating tablet: 15 or 30 mg once every morning Phentermine hydrochloride: 15–37.5 mg/day given in one or two divided doses; administer before breakfast or 1–2 hours after breakfast	8 mg three times daily, given ½ hour before meal Orally disintegrating tablet: 15 or 30 mg once every morning Phentermine hydrochloride: 15–37.5 mg/day given in one or two divided doses; administer before breakfast or 1–2 hours after breakfast	Use with caution in patients with kidney impairment	Approved for short-term monotherapy Controlled substance: C–IV Prescriptions should be written for the smallest quantity to minimize possibility of overdose Individualize to achieve adequate response with lowest effective dose

(Continued)

TABLE 59-2 FDA-Approved Pharmacotherapeutic Agents for Weight Loss *(Continued)*

Medication	Brand Name	Initial Dose	Usual Range	Special Population Dose	Comments
Diethylpropion	Tenuate®, Tenuate Dospan	Immediate release: 25 mg three times daily administered 1 hour before meals Controlled release: 75 mg once daily administered at midmorning	75 mg/day	Use with caution in patients with kidney impairment	Approved for short-term monotherapy Dose should not be administered in the evening or at bedtime Controlled substance: C–IV

^aAvailable without a prescription.

TABLE 59-3 Clinical and Economic Considerations for Long-Term Pharmacotherapy Options

Medication	Brand Name	Weight Loss Above Diet and Exercise Alone (1 year)	Cost for 30 Days of Therapy[a]	Comments
Orlistat	Xenical®	2.9–3.4 kg (6.5–7.5 lb)	$685.81	Use may be limited by GI intolerance
Phentermine and topiramate extended-release	Qsymia®	6.6–8.6 kg (14.5–18.9 lb)	$186.00, 7.5–46 mg $199.50, 15–92 mg	Limited distribution under FDA Risk Evaluation Mitigation Strategy (REMS)
Bupropion and naltrexone extended-release	Contrave®	4.9 kg (10.8 lb)	$303.60	Lowers seizure threshold (bupropion) Rare reports of hepatotoxicity (naltrexone) Drug interactions with opioids, CYP2B6 inducers, and CYP2D6 substrates
Liraglutide	Saxenda®	5.2 kg (11.4 lb)	$1349.00	Injectable (daily dosing) Available as pre-filled dosing pen Reduces HbA1c and fasting glucose Risk of medullary thyroid carcinoma and multiple endocrine neoplasia syndrome type 2 Rare reports of pancreatitis, gallbladder disease, and suicidal ideation
Semaglutide	Wegovy™	15.5 kg (34.1 lb)[b]	$1349.00	Injectable (weekly dosing) Available as pre-filled dosing pen Reduces HbA1c and fasting glucose Risk of medullary thyroid carcinoma and multiple endocrine neoplasia syndrome type 2 Rare reports of pancreatitis, gallbladder disease, and suicidal ideation

(Continued)

| | | **Weight Loss Above Diet** | **Cost for** | |
Medication	**Brand Name**	**and Exercise Alone (1 year)**	**30 Days of Therapy[a]**	**Comments**
Setmelanotide	Imcivree™	23.1% (patients with POMC or PCSK1 deficiency) 9.7% (patients with LEPR deficiency)	$19,800	Injectable (daily dosing) Available as multiple-dose vial (10 mg/mL) Indicated for genetically confirmed or suspected deficiency POMC, PCSK1, or LEPR

TABLE 59-3 Clinical and Economic Considerations for Long-Term Pharmacotherapy Options (*Continued*)

[a]Cost of therapy based on maintenance dose using wholesaler acquisition cost (WAC) as of September 29, 2021.
[b]Data from 68-week trial.

EVALUATION OF THERAPEUTIC OUTCOMES

- Assess progress monthly for the first 3 months, then every 3 months. Each encounter should document weight, WC, BMI, blood pressure, medical history, and patient assessment of tolerability of drug therapy.
- Discontinue medication therapy after 3 months if the patient has failed to demonstrate weight loss or maintenance of prior weight.
- Diabetic patients require more intense medical monitoring and self-monitoring of blood glucose. Weekly healthcare visits for 1–2 months may be necessary until the effects of diet, exercise, and weight loss medication become more predictable.
- Monitor patients with hyperlipidemia or hypertension to assess effects of weight loss on appropriate end points.

See Chapter 167, Obesity, authored by Amy H. Sheehan, Judy T. Chen, and Jack A. Yanovski, for a more detailed discussion of this topic.

CHAPTER 60

Nutrition Assessment and Support

- Malnutrition encompasses both undernutrition and overnutrition (obesity) and is a consequence of nutrient imbalance. Starvation-associated malnutrition, marasmus, results from inadequate intake, absorption, or utilization of protein and energy. Patients with severe acute disease or injury (major infections, burns, trauma) or with chronic inflammatory diseases (Crohn's disease), organ failure, or cancer can develop disease-related malnutrition because of increased metabolic demands. Undernutrition and overnutrition can result in changes in subcellular, cellular, or organ function that increase morbidity and mortality.
- For information on overnutrition or obesity, see Chapter 59.
- Nutrition screening provides a systematic way to identify individuals in any care environment with preexisting malnutrition or those at risk for malnutrition for whom a detailed nutrition assessment is warranted.
- Nutrition assessment is the first step in developing a nutrition care plan. This assessment should include a comprehensive medical, surgical, and dietary history and a nutrition-focused physical exam (NFPE) including anthropometrics and laboratory measurements. The NFPE uses a system-based approach to assess for abnormal nutrition-related clinical and physical findings in each region of the body.
- Goals of nutrition assessment are to identify the presence of risk factors associated with malnutrition and increased risk of developing undernutrition and complications, estimate nutrition needs, and establish baseline parameters for assessing the outcome of therapy.

NUTRITION ASSESSMENT

ANTHROPOMETRIC MEASUREMENTS

- Anthropometric measurements are physical measurements of the size, weight, and proportions of the human body used to compare an individual with normative population standards. Common measurements are weight, stature, head circumference (for children younger than 3 years of age), and waist circumference. Measurements of limb size (eg, skinfold thickness and mid-arm muscle and wrist circumferences), along with bioelectrical impedance analysis (BIA), may be useful in selected individuals.
- Interpretation of actual body weight (ABW) should consider ideal body weight (IBW) for height, usual body weight (UBW), fluid status, and age. Change over time can be calculated as the percentage of UBW. Unintentional weight loss, especially rapid weight loss (5% of UBW in 1 month or 10% of UBW in 6 months), increases the risk of nutrition-related poor clinical outcomes in adults.
- The best indicator of adequate nutrition in children is appropriate growth. Weight, stature, head circumference (until 3 years), and body mass index (BMI) (after 2 years) should be plotted on the appropriate growth curve. Average weight gain for newborns is 10–20 g/kg/day (24–35 g/day for term infants and 10–25 g/day for preterm infants depending on gestational age).
- BMI is another index of weight-for-height. Interpretation of BMI should include consideration of sex, frame size, race/ethnicity, and age. BMI values greater than 25 kg/m^2 are indicative of overweight, and values less than 18.5 kg/m^2 are indicative of undernutrition. BMI is calculated as follows:

Body weight (kg)/[height (m)]^2 **or** [Body weight (lb) × 703]/[height (in)]^2

- Measurements of skinfold thickness estimate subcutaneous fat, mid-arm muscle circumference estimates skeletal muscle mass, and waist circumference estimates abdominal (visceral) fat content.

- BIA is a simple, noninvasive, and relatively inexpensive way to assess LBM, total body water (TBW), and water distribution. It is based on differences between fat tissue and lean tissue's resistance to conductivity. Hydration status should be considered in interpretation of BIA results. Current guidelines do not provide recommendations regarding the use of BIA in clinical practice.

BIOCHEMICAL AND IMMUNE FUNCTION STUDIES

- Interpret visceral protein concentrations (Table 60-1) relative to the individual's overall clinical condition and inflammatory state. Factors other than nutrition can affect the serum protein concentrations including age; abnormal kidney (nephrotic syndrome), gastrointestinal (GI) tract (protein-losing enteropathy) or skin (burns) losses; hydration (dehydration results in hemoconcentration, overhydration in hemo-dilution); liver function (synthesis); and metabolic stress and inflammation (chronic disease, sepsis, trauma, surgery, infection).
- Nutrition status affects immune function either directly or indirectly. Total lympho-cyte count and delayed cutaneous hypersensitivity reactions are immune function tests useful in nutrition assessment, but their lack of specificity limits their usefulness as nutrition status markers.
  ✓ Delayed cutaneous hypersensitivity is commonly assessed using antigens to which the patient was likely previously sensitized. The recall antigens used most frequently are mumps and *Candida albicans*. Anergy is associated with severe malnutrition; immune response can be restored with nutrition repletion.

TABLE 60-1	Serum Proteins Associated with Nutrition Risk			
Serum Protein	Half-Life (Days)	Function	Factors Resulting in Increased Values	Factors Resulting in Decreased Values
Albumin	18–20	Maintains plasma oncotic pressure; transports small molecules	Dehydration, anabolic steroids, insulin, infection	Fluid overload; edema; kidney dysfunction; nephrotic syndrome; poor dietary intake; impaired digestion; burns; heart failure; cirrhosis; thyroid, adrenal, or pituitary hormones; trauma; sepsis
Transferrin	8–9	Binds Fe in plasma; transports Fe to bone	Fe deficiency, pregnancy, hypoxia, chronic blood loss, estrogens	Chronic infection, cirrhosis, burns, enteropathies, nephrotic syndrome, cortisone, testosterone
Prealbumin (transthyretin)	2–3	Binds T_3 and, to a lesser extent, T_4; retinol-binding protein carrier	Impaired kidney function	Cirrhosis, hepatitis, stress, surgery, inflammation, hyperthyroidism, cystic fibrosis, burns, zinc deficiency

Fe, iron; T_3, triiodothyronine; T_4, thyroxine.

SPECIFIC NUTRIENT DEFICIENCIES

- Biochemical assessment of trace element, vitamin, and essential fatty acid deficiencies should be based on the nutrient's function, but few practical methods are available. Therefore, most assays measure serum concentrations of the individual nutrient.
- Clinical syndromes are associated with deficiencies of the following trace elements: zinc, copper, manganese, selenium, chromium, iodine, molybdenum, and iron.
- Single vitamin deficiencies are uncommon; multiple vitamin deficiencies more commonly occur with malnutrition. For information on iron deficiency and other anemias, see Chapter 33.
- Essential fatty acid deficiency is rare but can occur with prolonged lipid-free parenteral nutrition (PN), very low-fat enteral formulations or diets, high medium chain triglyceride–containing diets, severe fat malabsorption, or severe malnutrition. The body can synthesize all fatty acids except for linoleic and α-linolenic acid.
- Carnitine can be synthesized from lysine and methionine, but hepatic synthesis is decreased in premature infants. Low carnitine levels can occur in premature infants receiving PN or carnitine-free diets.

ASSESSMENT OF NUTRIENT REQUIREMENTS

- Assessment of nutrient requirements must be made in the context of patient-specific factors (eg, age, sex, size, clinical condition, nutrition status, and physical activity).
- Adults should consume 45%–65% of total calories from carbohydrates, 20%–35% from fat, and 10%–35% from protein. Recommendations are similar for children, except that infants should consume 40%–50% of total calories from fat.

Energy Requirements

- Energy requirements of individuals can be estimated using validated predictive equations or directly measured, depending on factors including severity of illness and resources available. The simplest method is to use population estimates of calories required per kilogram of body weight.
- Healthy adults with normal nutrition status and minimal illness severity require an estimated 20–25 kcal ABW/kg/day (84–105 kJ ABW/kg/day). Daily energy requirements for children are approximately 130%–150% of basal metabolic rate with additional calories to support activity and growth. Consult references for equations used to estimate energy expenditure in adults and children.
- Energy requirements for all ages increase with fever, sepsis, major surgery, trauma, burns, long-term growth failure, and with chronic conditions (eg, bronchopulmonary dysplasia, congenital heart disease, and cystic fibrosis).

Protein, Fluid, and Micronutrient Requirements

Protein

- Protein requirements are based on age, sex, nutrition status, disease state, and clinical condition. The usual recommended daily protein allowances are 0.8 g/kg for adults, 1.5 g/kg for adults over 60 years of age, 1.5–2 g/kg for patients with metabolic stress (eg, infection, trauma, and surgery), and 2.5–3 g/kg for patients with burns.

Fluid

- Daily adult fluid requirements are approximately 30–40 mL/kg.
- Fluid requirements for children and preterm infants who weigh less than 10 kg are at least 100 mL/kg/day. An additional 50 mL/kg should be provided for each kilogram of body weight between 11 and 20 kg, and 20 mL/kg for each kilogram greater than 20 kg.
- Factors that may result in increased fluid requirements include but are not limited to GI losses, fever, sweating, and increased metabolism, whereas kidney or heart failure and hypoalbuminemia with starvation are examples of factors that may result in decreased fluid requirements.

- Assess fluid status by monitoring urine output and specific gravity, serum electrolytes, and weight changes. An hourly urine output of at least 1 mL/kg for children and 40–50 mL for adults is needed to ensure tissue perfusion.

Micronutrients

- Requirements for micronutrients (ie, electrolytes, minerals, trace elements, and vitamins) vary with age, sex, route of ingestion, and underlying clinical conditions.
- Sodium, potassium, magnesium, and phosphorus requirements are typically decreased in patients with kidney failure, whereas calcium requirements are increased (see Chapters 75 and 76).

Drug–Nutrient Interactions

- Concomitant drug therapy can alter serum concentrations of vitamins (Table 60-2), minerals, and electrolytes.
- Some drug delivery vehicles contain nutrients. For example, the vehicle for propofol is 10% lipid emulsion, and most IV therapies include dextrose or sodium.

NUTRITION SUPPORT

- The primary objective of nutrition support therapy is to promote positive clinical outcomes of an illness and improve quality of life.

ENTERAL NUTRITION

- Enteral nutrition (EN) delivers nutrients by tube or mouth into the GI tract; we will focus on delivery through a feeding tube. The goal of EN is to provide calories, macronutrients, and micronutrients to those who are unable to achieve these requirements from an oral diet.
- EN is indicated for the patient who cannot or will not eat enough to meet nutritional requirements and who has a functioning GI tract and a method of enteral access. Potential indications include neoplastic disease, organ dysfunction, hypermetabolic states, GI disease, and neurologic impairment.
- Distal mechanical intestinal obstruction, bowel ischemia, and necrotizing enterocolitis are contraindications to EN. Contraindications to tube placement include active peritonitis and uncorrectable coagulopathy. Conditions that challenge the success of EN include severe diarrhea, protracted vomiting, enteric fistulas, severe GI hemorrhage, hemodynamic instability, and intestinal dysmotility.
- EN has replaced PN as the preferred method for the feeding of critically ill patients requiring specialized nutrition support. Advantages of EN over PN include maintaining GI tract structure and function; fewer metabolic, infectious, and technical complications; and lower costs.
- The timing of initiation of EN in critically ill patients is of clinical significance. Initiation within 24–48 hours of admission to an intensive care unit is associated with decreased disease severity and infectious complications when compared with the initiation of feedings after 48 hours. If patients are only mildly to moderately stressed and well nourished, EN initiation can be delayed until oral intake is inadequate for 5–7 days.

Access

- EN can be administered through four routes, which have different indications, tube placement options, advantages, and disadvantages (Table 60-3). The choice depends on the anticipated duration of use and the feeding site (ie, stomach vs. small bowel).
- The stomach is generally the least expensive and least labor-intensive access site; however, patients who have impaired gastric emptying are at risk for aspiration and pneumonia.
- Long-term access with gastrostomy and jejunostomy tubes should be considered when EN is anticipated for more than 4–6 weeks.

TABLE 60-2	Drug and Nutrient Interactions
Drug	**Effect**
Angiotensin-converting enzyme inhibitors	Increased urinary zinc losses
Angiotensin receptor blockers	Increased urinary zinc losses
Antacids	Thiamine deficiency
Antibiotics	Vitamin K deficiency
Aspirin	Folic acid deficiency; increased vitamin C excretion
Cathartics	Increased requirements for vitamins D, C, and B_6
Cholestyramine	Vitamins A, D, E, and K and β-carotene malabsorption
Colestipol	Vitamins A, D, E, and K and β-carotene malabsorption
Corticosteroids	Decreased vitamins A, D, and C
Diuretics (loop)	Thiamine deficiency
Diuretics (thiazides)	Increased urinary zinc losses
Efavirenz	Vitamin D deficiency caused by increased metabolism of $25(OH)D$ and $1,25(OH)_2D$
Histamine$_2$ antagonists	Vitamin B_{12} malabsorption (reduced acid results in an impaired release of B_{12} from food)
Isoniazid	Vitamin B_6 and niacin deficiency
Isotretinoin	Vitamin A increases toxicity
Mercaptopurine	Niacin deficiency
Methotrexate	Folic acid inhibits effect
Orlistat	Vitamins A, D, E, and K malabsorption caused by fat malabsorption
Pentamidine	Folic acid deficiency
Phenobarbital	Increased vitamin D metabolism
Phenytoin	Increased vitamin D metabolism; decreased folic acid concentrations
Primidone	Folic acid deficiency
Protease inhibitors	Vitamin D deficiency (impaired renal hydroxylation)
Proton pump inhibitors	Decreased iron and vitamin B_{12} absorption (reduced acid results in an impaired release of B_{12} from food)
Sulfasalazine	Folic acid malabsorption
Trimethoprim	Folic acid depletion
Warfarin	Vitamin K inhibits effect; vitamins A, C, and E may affect prothrombin time
Valproic acid	Zinc
Zidovudine	Folic acid and B_{12} deficiencies increase myelosuppression

Administration Methods

- EN can be administered by continuous, cyclic, bolus, and intermittent methods. The choice depends on the location of the feeding tube tip, patient's clinical condition, intestinal function, and tolerance to tube feeding.
- Continuous EN is preferred for initiating therapy and has the advantage of being well tolerated. Disadvantages include cost and inconvenience associated with pump and administration sets.

TABLE 60-3	Options and Considerations in the Selection of Enteral Access			
Access	**EN Duration/Patient Characteristics**	**Tube Placement Options**	**Advantages**	**Disadvantages**
Nasogastric or orogastric	Short term Intact gag reflex Normal gastric emptying	Manually at bedside	Ease of placement Allows for all methods of administration Inexpensive Multiple commercially available tubes and sizes	Potential tube displacement Potential increased aspiration risk
Nasojejunal	Short term Impaired gastric motility or emptying High risk of GER or aspiration	Manually at bedside Fluoroscopically Endoscopically	Potential reduced aspiration risk Allows for early postinjury or postoperative feeding Multiple commercially available tubes and sizes	Manual transpyloric passage requires greater skill Potential tube displacement or clogging Bolus or intermittent feeding not tolerated
Gastrostomy	Long term Normal gastric emptying	Surgically Endoscopically Radiologically Laparoscopically	Allows for all methods of administration Low-profile buttons available Large-bore tubes less likely to clog Multiple commercially available tubes and sizes	Attendant risks associated with each type of procedure Potential increased aspiration risk Risk of stoma site complications
Jejunostomy	Long term Impaired gastric motility or gastric emptying High risk of GER or aspiration	Surgically Endoscopically Radiologically Laparoscopically	Allows for early postinjury or postoperative feeding Potential reduced aspiration risk Multiple commercially available tubes and sizes Low-profile buttons available	Attendant risks associated with each type of procedure Bolus or intermittent feeding not tolerated Risk of stoma site complications

EN, enteral nutrition; GER, gastroesophageal reflux.

- Cyclic EN has the advantage of allowing breaks from the infusion system, thereby increasing mobility, especially if EN is administered nocturnally.
- Bolus EN is most commonly used in patients in the home or long-term care setting who have a gastrostomy. Advantages include short administration time (eg, 5–10 minutes) and minimal equipment (eg, a syringe). Bolus EN has the potential disadvantages of causing cramping, nausea, vomiting, aspiration, and diarrhea.
- Intermittent EN is similar to bolus EN except that the feeding is administered over 20–60 minutes, which improves tolerability but requires more equipment (eg, reservoir bag and infusion pump). Like bolus EN, intermittent EN mimics normal eating patterns.
- Protocols outlining initiation and advancement criteria are a useful strategy to optimize achievement of nutrient goals based on GI tolerance. Clinical signs of intolerance include abdominal distention or cramping, high gastric residual volumes, aspiration, and diarrhea.

Formulations

- Historically, EN formulations were created to provide essential nutrients, including macronutrients (eg, carbohydrates, fats, and proteins) and micronutrients (eg, electrolytes, trace elements, vitamins, and water).
- Over time, formulations have been enhanced to improve tolerance and meet specific patient needs. For example, immunonutrients or pharmaconutrients are added to modify the disease process or improve clinical outcome; however, these health claims are not regulated by the FDA.
- The molecular form of the protein source determines the amount of digestion required for absorption within the small bowel. The carbohydrate component usually provides the major source of calories; polymeric entities are preferred over elemental sugars. Vegetable oils rich in polyunsaturated fatty acids are the most common sources of fat in EN formulations.
- Soluble and insoluble fiber has been added to several EN formulations. Potential benefits of soluble fiber include trophic effects on colonic mucosa, promotion of sodium and water absorption, and regulation of bowel function.
- Osmolality is a function of the size and quantity of ionic and molecular particles primarily related to protein, carbohydrate, electrolyte, and mineral content. The osmolality of EN formulations for adults ranges from 280 to 875 mOsm/kg (mmol/kg). Osmolality is commonly thought to affect GI tolerability, but there is a lack of supporting evidence.

Classification of Enteral Feeding Formulations

- EN formulations are classified by their composition and intended patient population (Table 60-4). The development of an evidence-based, enteral formulary should focus on clinically significant characteristics of available formulations and avoid duplication.

Complications and Monitoring

- Monitor patients for metabolic, GI, and mechanical complications of EN (Table 60-5).
- Metabolic complications associated with EN are similar to those of PN, but the incidence is lower.
- GI complications include nausea, vomiting, abdominal distention, cramping, aspiration, diarrhea, and constipation. Diarrhea may be caused by a number of factors, and management should be directed at identifying and correcting the most likely cause(s).
- Mechanical complications include tube occlusion or malposition and inadvertent nasopulmonary intubation. Techniques for clearing occluded tubes include pancreatic enzymes in sodium bicarbonate and using a declogging device. Techniques for maintaining patency include flushing with at least 15–30 mL of water before and after medication administration and intermittent feedings and at least every 8 hours during continuous feeding.

TABLE 60-4	Adult Enteral Feeding Formulation Classification System	
Category	**Features**	**Indications**
Standard polymeric	Isotonic	Designed to meet the needs of the majority of patients
	1–1.2 kcal/mL (4.2–5 kJ/mL)	
	NPC:N 125:1–150:1	Patients with functional GI tract
	May contain fiber	Not suitable for oral use
High protein	NPC:N <125:1	Patients with protein requirements >1.5 g/kg/day, such as trauma patients and those with burns, pressure sores, or wounds
	May contain fiber	
		Patients receiving propofol
High caloric density	1.5–2 kcal/mL (6.3–8.4 kJ/mL)	Patients requiring fluid and/or electrolyte restriction, such as kidney insufficiency
	Lower electrolyte content per calorie	
	Hypertonic	
Elemental	High proportion of free amino acids	Patients who require low fat
	Low in fat	Use has generally been replaced by peptide-based formulations
Peptide-based	Contains dipeptides and tripeptides	Indications/benefits not clearly established
	Contains MCTs	Trial may be warranted in patients who do not tolerate intact protein due to malabsorption
Disease specific		
Kidney	Caloric dense	Alternative to high-caloric density formulations, but generally more expensive
	Protein content varies	
	Low-electrolyte content	
Liver	Increased branched-chain and decreased aromatic amino acids	Patients with hepatic encephalopathy
Lung	High fat, low carbohydrate	Patients with ARDS and severe ALI
	Anti-inflammatory lipid profile and antioxidants	
Diabetes mellitus	High fat, low carbohydrate	Alternative to standard, fiber-containing formulation in patients with uncontrolled hyperglycemia
Immune-modulating	Supplemented with glutamine, arginine, nucleotides, and/or omega-3 fatty acids	Patients undergoing major elective GI surgery, trauma, burns, head and neck cancer, and critically ill patients on mechanical ventilation
		Use with caution in patients with sepsis
		Select nutrients may be beneficial or harmful in subgroups of critically ill patients
Oral supplement	Sweetened for taste	Patients who require supplementation to an oral diet
	Hypertonic	

ALI, acute lung injury; ARDS, acute respiratory distress syndrome; MCT, medium-chain triglyceride; NPC:N, nonprotein calorie-to-nitrogen ratio.

	During Initiation	
Parameter	**of EN Therapy**	**During Stable EN Therapy**
Vital signs	Every 4–6 hours	As needed with suspected change (ie, fever)
Clinical assessment		
Weight	Daily	Weekly
Total intake/Output	Daily	As needed with suspected change in intake/output
Tube-feeding intake	Daily	Daily
Enterostomy tube site assessment	Daily	Daily
GI tolerance		
Stool frequency/Volume	Daily	Daily
Abdomen assessment	Daily	Daily
Nausea or vomiting	Daily	Daily
Tube placement	Prior to starting, then ongoing	Ongoing
Laboratory		
Electrolytes, blood urea nitrogen/serum creatinine, glucose	Daily until stable, then 2–3 times/week	Every 1–3 months
Calcium, magnesium, phosphorus	Daily until stable, then 2–3 times/week	Every 1–3 months
Liver function tests	Weekly	Every 1–3 months
Trace elements, vitamins	If deficiency/toxicity suspected	If deficiency/toxicity suspected

TABLE 60-5 Suggested Monitoring for Adult Patients on Enteral Nutrition

EN, enteral nutrition.

Medication Delivery Via Feeding Tube

- Administering medications via tube feeding is a common practice. If the medication is a solid that can be crushed (eg, *not* a sublingual, sustained-release, or enteric-coated formulation) or is a capsule, mix with 15–30 mL of water or other appropriate solvent and administer. Otherwise, a liquid dosage preparation should be used. Administer multiple medications separately, each followed by flushing the tube with 5–15 mL of water.
- Mixing of liquid medications with EN formulations can cause physical incompatibilities that inhibit drug absorption and clog small-bore feeding tubes. Incompatibility is more common with formulations containing intact (vs. hydrolyzed) protein and medications formulated as acidic syrups. Mixing of liquid medications and EN formulations should be avoided whenever possible.
- The most significant drug–nutrient interactions result in reduced bioavailability and suboptimal pharmacologic effect (Table 60-6). Continuous feeding requires interruption for drug administration, and medications should be spaced between bolus feedings.

PARENTERAL NUTRITION

- PN provides macro- and micronutrients by central or peripheral venous access to meet specific nutritional requirements of the patient.
- PN should be considered when a patient cannot meet nutritional requirements enterally for an extended time period.

TABLE 60-6	Select Medications with Special Considerations for Enteral Feeding Tube Administration	
Drug	**Interaction**	**Comments**
Phenytoin	Reduced bioavailability in the presence of tube feedings	To minimize interaction, holding tube feedings 1–2 hours before and after phenytoin has been suggested
	Possible phenytoin binding to calcium caseinates or protein hydrolysates in enteral feeding	Adjust tube-feeding rate to account for time held for phenytoin administration
		Monitor phenytoin serum concentration and clinical response closely
		Consider switching to IV phenytoin or an alternative-treatment option if unable to reach therapeutic serum concentration
Fluoroquinolones Tetracyclines	Potential for reduced bioavailability because of complexation of drug with divalent and trivalent cations found in enteral feeding	Consider holding tube feeding 1 hour before and after administration
		Avoid jejunal administration of ciprofloxacin
		Monitor clinical response
Warfarin	Decreased absorption of warfarin because of enteral feeding; therapeutic effect antagonized by vitamin K in enteral formulations	Adjust warfarin dose based on INR
		Anticipate need to increase warfarin dose when enteral feedings are started and decrease dose when enteral feedings are stopped
		Consider holding tube feeding 1 hour before and after administration
Omeprazole Lansoprazole	Administration via feeding tube complicated by acid-labile medication within delayed-release, base-labile granules	Granules become sticky when moistened with water and may occlude small-bore tubes
		Granules should be mixed with acidic liquid when given via a gastric feeding tube
		An oral liquid suspension can be extemporaneously prepared for administration via a feeding tube

INR, International normalized ratio.

Components of Parenteral Nutrition

- Macronutrients (ie, water, protein, dextrose, and lipid) are used for energy (dextrose and lipid) and as structural substrates (protein and lipid).
- Protein is provided as crystalline amino acids (CAAs). When oxidized, 1 g of protein yields 4 calories (∼17 J). Including the caloric contribution from protein in calorie calculations is controversial; therefore, PN calories can be calculated as either total or nonprotein calories.
- Standard CAA products contain a balanced profile of essential, semi-essential, and nonessential L-amino acids and are designed for patients with "normal" organ function and nutritional requirements. Standard CAA products differ in protein concentration, total nitrogen, and electrolyte content but have similar effects on protein markers.

- The primary energy source in PN solutions is carbohydrate, usually as dextrose monohydrate, which is available in concentrations ranging from 5% to 70%. When oxidized, 1 g of hydrated dextrose provides 3.4 kcal (14.2 kJ).
- Commercially available lipid injectable emulsions (ILE) provide calories and essential fatty acids. These products differ in triglyceride source, fatty acid content, and essential fatty acid concentration.
- When oxidized, 1 g of fat yields 9 kcal (38 kJ). Because of the caloric contribution from egg phospholipid and glycerol, caloric content of ILE is 1.1 kcal/mL (4.6 kJ/mL) for the 10%, 2 kcal/mL (8.4 kJ/mL) for the 20%, and 3 kcal/mL (12.6 kJ/mL) for the 30% emulsions.
- Essential fatty acid deficiency can be prevented by giving soybean oil ILE, 0.5–1 g/kg/day for neonates and infants and 100 g/wk for adults.
- ILE 10% and 20% products can be administered by a central or peripheral vein, added directly to PN solution as a total nutrient admixture (TNA) or three-in-one system (lipids, protein, glucose, and additives), or co-infused with a CAA and dextrose solution, commonly referred to as a two-in-one solution. ILE 30% is approved only for TNA preparation.
- Micronutrients (ie, vitamins, trace elements, and electrolytes) support metabolic activities for cellular homeostasis such as enzyme reactions, fluid balance, and regulation of electrophysiologic processes.
- Multivitamin products have been formulated to comply with guidelines for adults, children, and infants. These products contain 13 essential vitamins, including vitamin K.
- Requirements for trace elements depend on the patient's age and clinical condition.
- Copper, manganese, selenium, and zinc are considered essential and available as single- or multiple-entity products for addition to adult, neonate, and pediatric PN solutions.
- Sodium, potassium, calcium, magnesium, phosphorus, chloride, and acetate are necessary components of PN for maintenance of numerous cellular functions.
- Electrolyte requirements depend on the patient's age, disease state, organ function, previous and current medication therapy, nutrition status, and extrarenal losses.

Specifics of Parenteral Nutrition

- The patient's clinical condition determines whether PN is administered through a peripheral or central vein.
- Peripheral parenteral nutrition (PPN) candidates do not have large nutritional requirements, are not fluid restricted, and are expected to regain GI tract function within 10–14 days. Solutions for PPN have lower final concentrations of amino acid (3%–5%), dextrose (5%–10%), and micronutrients as compared with central parenteral nutrition (CPN).
- Primary advantages of PPN include a lower risk of infectious and technical complications.
- CPN is useful in patients who require PN for more than 7–14 days and who have large nutrient requirements, poor peripheral venous access, or fluctuating fluid requirements.
- CPN solutions are highly concentrated hypertonic solutions that must be administered through a large central vein. The choice of venous access site depends on factors including patient age and anatomy. Peripherally inserted central catheters (PICCs) are often used for both short- and long-term central venous access in acute or home care settings.
- Disadvantages of CPN include risks associated with catheter insertion, use, and care. Central venous access has a greater potential for infection.
- PN regimens for adults can be ordered on traditional paper order forms or by using standardized electronic order forms. Standardized order forms are popular because they help educate practitioners and foster cost-efficient nutrition support by minimizing errors in ordering, compounding, and administering.
- Pediatric PN regimens typically require an individualized approach because practice guidelines often recommend nutrient intake based on weight. Labeling should reflect the "amount per kilogram per day."

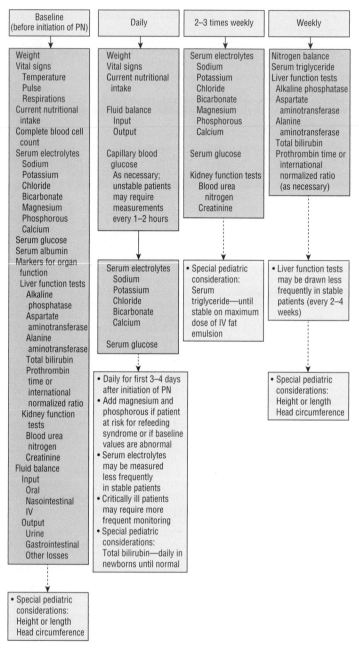

FIGURE 60-1. Monitoring strategy for patients receiving parenteral nutrition (PN). ALT, alanine aminotransferase; AST, aspartate aminotransferase; BUN, blood urea nitrogen; CBC, complete blood cell count; INR, international normalized ratio; PN, parenteral nutrition; PT, prothrombin time; SCr, serum creatinine.

EVALUATION OF THERAPEUTIC OUTCOMES

• Assessing the outcome of EN includes monitoring objective measures of body composition, protein and energy balance, and subjective outcome for physiologic muscle function and wound healing.

• Measures of disease-related morbidity include length of hospital stay, infectious complications, and patient's sense of well-being. Ultimately, the successful use of EN avoids the need for PN.

• Outcomes with PN are determined through routine assessment of the clinical condition of the patient, with a focus on the nutritional and metabolic effects of the PN regimen.

• Biochemical and clinical parameters should be monitored routinely in patients receiving PN (**Fig. 60-1**).

See Chapter 164, Assessment of Nutrition Status and Nutrition Requirements, authored by Katherine Hammond Chessman and Angela L. Bingham; Chapter 165, Parenteral Nutrition, authored by Todd W. Mattox and Catherine M. Crill; and Chapter 166, Enteral Nutrition, authored by Diana W. Mulherin, for a more detailed discussion of this topic.

CHAPTER

61 Breast Cancer

- *Breast cancer* is a malignancy originating from breast tissue. Disease confined to a localized breast lesion is referred to as *early, primary, localized*, or *curable*. Disease detected clinically or radiologically in sites distant from the breast is referred to as *advanced* or *metastatic breast cancer* (MBC), which is incurable.

EPIDEMIOLOGY

- Two variables most strongly associated with the occurrence of breast cancer are biological sex and age. Additional risk factors include endocrine factors (eg, menarche before age 11, age 55, or later for natural menopause, nulliparity, late age at first birth, and hormone replacement therapy), genetic factors (eg, personal and family history, mutations of tumor suppressor genes [*BRCA1* and *BRCA2*]), and environmental and lifestyle factors (eg, radiation exposure, tobacco use, and alcohol consumption).
- Breast cancer cells often spread undetected by contiguity, lymph channels, and through the blood early in the course of the disease, resulting in metastatic disease after local therapy. The most common metastatic sites are lymph nodes, skin, bone, liver, lungs, and brain.

PREVENTION OF BREAST CANCER

- Risk reduction strategies include prophylactic mastectomy, oophorectomy, and pharmacologic agents.
- Agents available for pharmacologic risk reduction include selective estrogen receptor modulators (SERMs) and aromatase inhibitors (AIs). The SERMs, **tamoxifen** and **raloxifene** taken for 5 years, reduce the risk of invasive and noninvasive breast cancer by about 50% in women at high risk for developing the disease. Tamoxifen increased the incidence of endometrial cancer and both agents increased thromboembolic events.
- A similar reduction in the risk of contralateral primary breast cancers in high-risk, postmenopausal individuals was demonstrated with the AIs, **exemestane** and **anastrozole**.
- Clinical guidelines recommend the use of SERMs or AIs for risk reduction in postmenopausal women at high risk.

CLINICAL PRESENTATION

- A painless, palpable lump is the initial sign of breast cancer in most women. The typical malignant mass is solitary, unilateral, solid, hard, irregular, and nonmobile. Nipple changes are less commonly seen. More advanced cases present with prominent skin edema, redness, warmth, and induration.
- Symptoms of MBC depend on the site of metastases but may include bone pain, difficulty breathing, abdominal enlargement, jaundice, and mental status changes.
- Many women first detect some breast abnormalities themselves, but it is increasingly common for breast cancer to be detected during routine screening mammography in asymptomatic women.

DIAGNOSIS

- Initial workup should include a careful history, physical examination of the breast, three-dimensional mammography, and, possibly, other breast imaging techniques, such as ultrasound, magnetic resonance imaging (MRI), digital mammography, and tomosynthesis.
- Breast biopsy is indicated for a mammographic abnormality that suggests malignancy or for a palpable mass on physical examination.

PATHOLOGIC EVALUATION

- Development of malignancy is a multistep process involving preinvasive (or noninvasive) and invasive phases. The goal of treatment for noninvasive carcinomas is to prevent the development of invasive disease.
- Pathologic evaluation of breast lesions establishes the histologic diagnosis and confirms the presence or absence of prognostic factors.
- Most breast carcinomas are adenocarcinomas and are classified as ductal or lobular.

PROGNOSTIC FACTORS

- The ability to predict prognosis is used to design personalized treatment recommendations.
- Age at diagnosis and ethnicity can affect prognosis.
- Alcohol use, dietary factors, weight, and exercise are potentially modifiable prognostic factors.
- Tumor size and presence and the number of involved axillary lymph nodes are independent factors that influence the risk for breast cancer recurrence and subsequent metastatic disease. Other disease characteristics that provide prognostic information are histologic subtype, nuclear or histologic grade, lymphovascular invasion, and proliferation indices.
- Hormone receptors (estrogen [ER] and progesterone [PR]) are not strong prognostic markers but are used clinically to predict response to endocrine therapy.
- *HER2* overexpression occurs in about 15%–20% of breast cancers and is associated with increased tumor aggressiveness, increased rates of recurrence, and increased rates of mortality.
- Genetic profiling tools provide additional prognostic information to aid in treatment decisions for subgroups of patients with otherwise favorable prognostic features.

STAGING

- Stage (anatomical extent of disease) is based on primary tumor extent and size (T_{1-4}), presence and extent of lymph node involvement (N_{1-3}), and presence or absence of distant metastases (M_{0-1}). The staging system determines prognosis and assists with treatment decisions. Simplistically stated, these stages may be represented as follows:
  ✓ *Early breast cancer*
    - Stage 0: Carcinoma in situ or disease that has not invaded the basement membrane.
    - Stage I: Small primary invasive tumor without lymph node involvement or with micrometastatic nodal involvement.
    - Stage II: Involvement of regional lymph nodes.
  ✓ *Locally advanced breast cancer*
    - Stage III: Usually a large tumor with extensive nodal involvement in which the node or tumor is fixed to the chest wall.
  ✓ *Advanced or metastatic breast cancer*
    - Stage IV: Metastases in organs distant from the primary tumor.
- Staging for breast cancer is separated into clinical and pathologic staging. Clinical stage is assigned before surgery and is based on physical examination (assessment of

tumor size and presence of axillary lymph nodes), imaging (eg, mammography, ultrasonography), and pathologic examination of tissues (eg, biopsy results). Pathologic staging occurs after surgery and adds data from surgical exploration and resection.

TREATMENT

- Goals of Treatment: The intent of adjuvant systemic therapy for Stage I–III is to eradicate micrometastatic disease with cure as the desired outcome.   Neoadjuvant systemic therapy may be administered for Stage III to decrease tumor size prior to surgery and/or to allow for breast conserving surgery if desired by the patient. Palliation is the desired therapeutic outcome in the treatment of MBC.
- Treatment is rapidly evolving. Specific information regarding the most promising interventions can be found only in the primary literature.
- Treatment can cause substantial toxicity, which differs depending on the individual agent, administration method, and combination regimen. A comprehensive review of toxicities is beyond the scope of this chapter; consult appropriate references.

CURATIVE BREAST CANCER (STAGES I-III)

Local-Regional Therapy

- Surgery alone can cure most patients with in situ cancers, 70%–80% of Stage I cancers, and approximately one-half of those with Stage II cancers.
- Breast-conserving therapy (BCT) maintains acceptable cosmetic results and rates of local and distant recurrence and mortality seen with mastectomy. BCT includes removal of part of the breast, surgical evaluation of axillary lymph nodes, and radiation therapy (RT) to prevent local recurrence.
- RT is administered to the entire breast over 3–5 weeks to eradicate residual disease after BCT. Reddening and erythema of the breast tissue with subsequent shrinkage of total breast mass are less common complications associated with short-term RT.
- Multiple sites of cancer within the breast and the inability to attain negative pathologic margins on the excised breast specimen are indications for mastectomy.
- Axillary lymph nodes should be sampled for staging and prognostic information. Lymphatic mapping with sentinel lymph node biopsy is a less invasive alternative to axillary dissection.

Systemic Therapy

- Chemotherapy, endocrine therapy, targeted therapy, or some combination of these agents improves disease-free and/or overall survival (OS) for high-risk patients in specific prognostic subgroups (eg, nodal involvement, menopausal status, hormone-receptor status, or *HER2* status) based on the results of several hundred randomized clinical trials.
- The National Comprehensive Cancer Network (NCCN) practice guidelines are updated at least every 2 years; treatment recommendations are complex and the reader is referred to the guidelines.
- Several multigene expression assays are commercially available as decision-support tools for adjuvant chemotherapy.

Cytotoxic Chemotherapy

- Systemic adjuvant therapy is the administration of systemic therapy following definitive local therapy (surgery, radiation, or both) when there is no evidence of metastatic disease but a high likelihood of disease recurrence. The goal of such therapy is cure. It is recommended in most women with lymph node metastases or with primary breast cancers larger than 1 cm in diameter (both node-negative and node-positive).
- Neoadjuvant (preoperative) systemic therapy is the standard of care for patients with locally advanced breast cancer; it consists of chemotherapy, either alone or combined with biologic or targeted therapy, but in special circumstances may also include endocrine therapy.

- The most common cytotoxic drugs that have been used alone and in combination as adjuvant therapy for breast cancer include **doxorubicin**, **epirubicin**, **cyclophosphamide**, **methotrexate**, **fluorouracil**, **carboplatin**, **paclitaxel**, and **docetaxel**. Combination regimens are more effective than single-agent chemotherapy; the most common combination regimens are listed in Table 61-1.
- Anthracyclines (doxorubicin or epirubicin) and taxanes (paclitaxel or docetaxel) are the cornerstones of modern chemotherapy for adjuvant treatment of breast cancer.
- Initiate chemotherapy within 12 weeks of surgical removal of the primary tumor. Optimal duration of adjuvant treatment is unknown but appears to be 12–24 weeks, depending on the regimen used.
- *Dose intensity* refers to the amount of drug administered per unit of time, which can be achieved by increasing dose, decreasing time between doses, or both. *Dose density* is one way of achieving dose intensity by decreasing time between treatment cycles.
- Dose increases in standard regimens appear to not be beneficial and may be harmful.
- Avoid dose reductions in standard regimens unless necessitated by severe toxicity.
- Short-term toxicities of adjuvant chemotherapy are generally well tolerated, especially with the availability of more effective antiemetics and myeloid growth factors with dose-dense regimens.

Biologic or Targeted Therapy

- Targeted therapies are directed at molecular targets through novel mechanisms; many are also biologic therapies because they are monoclonal antibodies (mAbs).
- **Trastuzumab** is an mAb targeted against the *HER2*-receptor protein used in combination with or sequentially after adjuvant chemotherapy in patients with early stage, *HER2*-positive breast cancer. The risk of recurrence was reduced up to 50% in clinical trials.

TABLE 61-1	Selected Neo/Adjuvant Chemotherapy Regimens for Breast Cancer
Dose-Dense AC → Paclitaxel[a]	**AC → Paclitaxel**
Doxorubicin 60 mg/m^2 IV bolus, day 1	Doxorubicin 60 mg/m^2 IV, day 1
Cyclophosphamide 600 mg/m^2 IV, day 1	Cyclophosphamide 600 mg/m^2 IV, day 1
Repeat cycles every 14 days for 4 cycles (must be given with growth factor support)	Repeat cycles every 21 days for 4 cycles
Followed by paclitaxel 80 mg/m^2 IV weekly	Followed by paclitaxel 80 mg/m^2 IV weekly
Repeat cycles every 7 days for 12 cycles	Repeat cycles every 7 days for 12 cycles
TC[a]	
Docetaxel 75 mg/m^2 IV, day 1	
Cyclophosphamide 600 mg/m^2 IV, day 1	
Repeat cycles every 21 days for 4 cycles	
Dose-Dense AC → Dose-Dense Paclitaxel[a]	
Doxorubicin 60 mg/m^2 IV bolus, day 1	
Cyclophosphamide 600 mg/m^2 IV, day 1	
Repeat cycles every 14 days for 4 cycles (must be given with growth factor support)	
Followed by paclitaxel 175 mg/m^2 IV over 3 hours	
Repeat cycles every 14 days for 4 cycles (must be given with growth factor support)	

AC, Adriamycin (doxorubicin), Cytoxan (cyclophosphamide); TC, Taxotere (docetaxel), cyclophosphamide.
[a]Designated as a preferred regimen in the NCCN Breast Cancer Guidelines.

- The benefit of adding trastuzumab is clear but the optimal regimen is less clear because the type of chemotherapy, sequence of administration, and duration of treatment differed among the trials.
- The risk of symptomatic heart failure with adjuvant trastuzumab regimens that contain an anthracycline ranges from 0.5% to 4%. Sequential administration of trastuzumab after chemotherapy and the use of non-anthracycline-based regimens are strategies to lower the incidence of cardiac toxicity.
- The addition of **pertuzumab** to trastuzumab and chemotherapy is another important treatment option for patients with *HER*2-positive breast cancer in the neoadjuvant setting (Table 61-2).
- **Neratinib** (240 mg by mouth daily for 1 year), an oral tyrosine kinase inhibitor of EGFR, *HER2*, and *HER4*, is indicated for extended adjuvant therapy after completion of trastuzumab. Common toxicities include diarrhea, nausea, fatigue, and vomiting.
- **Ado-trastuzumab emtansine** (also known as T-DM1) is used in the adjuvant setting following neoadjuvant therapy when residual disease is found at the time of surgery. Common toxicities include peripheral neuropathy, thrombocytopenia, and liver dysfunction.

Endocrine Therapy

- **Tamoxifen**, **toremifene**, oophorectomy, ovarian irradiation, luteinizing hormone–releasing hormone (LHRH) agonists, and AIs are endocrine therapies used in the treatment of primary or early-stage breast cancer. Menopausal status determines the

TABLE 61-2 Selected Regimens for HER2-Positive Early-Stage Breast Cancer

Neo/Adjuvant Regimen	Drugs	Doses	Frequency	Cycles
PH → H[a]	Paclitaxel	80 mg/m² IV over 1 hour	Every 7 days	12 weeks
	Trastuzumab	4 mg/kg IV → 2 mg/kg IV	Every 7 day	12 weeks
	Followed by			
	Trastuzumab	6 mg/kg IV	Every 21 days	Complete 1 year
TCH[a]	Docetaxel	75 mg/m² IV	Every 21 days	6
	Carboplatin	AUC 6 IV	Every 21 days	6
	Trastuzumab	4 mg/kg IV → 2 mg/kg IV	Every 7 days	18 weeks
	Followed by			
	Trastuzumab	6 mg/kg IV	Every 21 days	Complete 1 year
TCHP[a]	Docetaxel	75 mg/m² IV	Every 21 days	6
	Carboplatin	AUC 6 IV	Every 21 days	6
	Trastuzumab	8 mg/kg IV → 6 mg/kg IV	Every 21 days	6
	Pertuzumab	840 mg IV → 420 mg IV	Every 21 days	6
	Followed by			
	Trastuzumab	6 mg/kg IV	Every 21 days	Complete 1 year
	Pertuzumab	420 mg IV	Every 21 days	Complete 1 year

PH, paclitaxel, trastuzumab; TCH, docetaxel, carboplatin, trastuzumab; TCHP, docetaxel, carboplatin, trastuzumab, pertuzumab.
[a]Designated as a preferred regimen in the NCCN Breast Cancer Guidelines.

agent of choice. Tamoxifen is generally considered the adjuvant endocrine therapy of choice for premenopausal women; newer data also support the use of LHRH agonists or oophorectomy in combination with AIs.

- Tamoxifen 20 mg daily, beginning soon after completing chemotherapy and continuing for 5–10 years, reduces the risk of recurrence and mortality. It is usually well tolerated; hot flashes and vaginal discharge may occur. Tamoxifen reduces the risk of hip radius and spine fractures. It increases the risks of stroke, pulmonary embolism, deep vein thrombosis, and endometrial cancer, particularly in women aged 50 years or older.

- The combination of ovarian suppression with LHRH agonists (eg, **goserelin, triptorelin, and leuprolide**) and an AI is recommended in premenopausal women with hormone receptor-positive early-stage breast cancer. Tamoxifen is an option with low risk of recurrence and/or intolerance to ovarian suppression plus AI.

- Guidelines recommend incorporation of AIs (**anastrozole, letrozole**, and **exemestane**) into adjuvant endocrine therapy for postmenopausal, hormone-sensitive breast cancer. Guidelines consider AIs to similar antitumor efficacy and toxicity profiles; adverse effects include bone loss/osteoporosis, hot flashes, myalgia/arthralgia, vaginal dryness/atrophy, mild headaches, and diarrhea.

METASTATIC BREAST CANCER (STAGE IV)

- Treatment of MBC with cytotoxic, endocrine, or targeted therapy often results in regression of disease, improvements in quality of life, and improved OS with the addition of some biologic or targeted therapies.

- The choice of therapy for MBC is based on the extent of disease involvement and the presence or absence of certain tumor or patient characteristics. The most important predictive factors are the presence of *HER2*, ER, and PR receptors in the primary or metastatic tumor tissue.

- Consider adding bone-modifying agents (eg, **pamidronate, zoledronic acid**, or **denosumab**) to treat breast-cancer patients with metastases to the bone to decrease rates of skeletal-related events, such as fractures, spinal cord compression, and pain, and the need for radiation to the bones or surgery.

Biologic or Targeted Therapy

- Cyclin-dependent kinases (CDK) form complexes that control cell cycling; CDK-inhibitors, **abemaciclib, palbociclib**, and **ribociclib**, that selectively inhibit CDK-4 and -6, are approved for MBC; progression-free survival (PFS) has improved when used in combination with AIs (as first-line therapy) and fulvestrant (as first- and second-line therapy) (see Table 61-3). Addition of CDK-inhibitors to endocrine therapy increases toxicity of the regimen; neutropenia (all grades) is the dose-limiting toxicity of palbociclib and ribociclib, and diarrhea is the dose-limiting toxicity with abemaciclib.

- The mammalian target of rapamycin (mTOR) inhibitor **everolimus** improved PFS when used in combination with either exemestane, fulvestrant, or tamoxifen.

- The phosphatidylinositol 3-kinase (PI3k) inhibitor **apelisib** is approved in combination with fulvestrant for postmenopausal women and men, with hormone receptor–positive, *HER2*-negative, PIK3CA-mutated, advanced, or metastatic breast cancer as detected by an FDA-approved test following progression on or after an endocrine-based regimen. Monitor fasting glucose closely as hyperglycemia, including ketoacidosis, may occur. Other significant toxicities include rash and diarrhea.

- The poly (ADP-RIBOSE) polymerase (PARP) inhibitors **olaparib** and **talazoparib** improve PFS in appropriate patients.

- *HER2*-targeted agents available in the United States are trastuzumab, pertuzumab, ado-trastuzumab emtansine, **fam-trastuzumab deruxtecan, margetuximab, lapatinib**, neratinib, and **tucatinib**.

- First-line therapy with a pertuzumab-trastuzumab-taxane combination is the preferred option for *HER2*-overexpressing MBC in patients who have not received

TABLE 61-3 Therapies Used for Hormone Receptor–Positive Metastatic Breast Cancer

Drug	Initial Dose	Special Population Dose	Comments
Aromatase Inhibitors: Nonsteroidal			
Anastrozole	1 mg orally daily		
Letrozole	2.5 mg orally daily	Caution in severe liver impairment[a]	
Aromatase Inhibitor: Steroidal			
Exemestane	25 mg orally daily		Take after meals
Antiestrogens: SERMs			
Tamoxifen	20 mg orally daily	See Chapter 151, *Dipiro's Pharmacotherapy: A Pathophysiologic Approach*, 12 ed., regarding *CYP2D6*	
Toremifene	60 mg orally daily		
Antiestrogen: SERD			
Fulvestrant	500 mg IM every 28 days (after loading days 1, 15, 29)	Moderate liver impairment[a] administer 250 mg IM every 28 days (after loading days 1, 15, 29)	
LHRH Agonists			
Goserelin	3.6 mg SC every 28 days	Premenopausal women only	
Leuprolide	3.75 mg IM every 28 days	Premenopausal women only	Not FDA-approved for breast cancer; other formulations are administered differently
Triptorelin	3.75 mg IM every 28 days	Premenopausal women only	Not FDA-approved for breast cancer

(*Continued*)

TABLE 61-3 Therapies Used for Hormone Receptor–Positive Metastatic Breast Cancer (*Continued*)

Drug	Initial Dose	Special Population Dose	Comments
Biologic/Targeted Therapies			
Abemaciclib (+/– Letrozole or Fulvestrant)	Single-agent 200 mg orally twice a day continuously **OR** Combination 150 mg orally twice a day continuously	Adjust dose for diarrhea, myelosuppression, and/or severe hepatic impairment; monitor for hepatotoxicity and thromboembolism; avoid concomitant strong inhibitors of CYP3A4 and moderate/strong inducers of CYP3A4	Do not split tablets
Palbociclib (+ Letrozole or Fulvestrant)	125 mg orally daily × 21 days, followed by 7 days off, repeated every 28 days	Adjust dose for myelosuppression and severe hepatic impairment; monitor for nausea, diarrhea, and hepatotoxicity; avoid concomitant strong inhibitors of CYP3A4 and moderate/strong inducers of CYP3A4	Do not split tablets Take with meals (capsules only)
Ribociclib (+ Letrozole or Fulvestrant)	600 mg orally daily × 21 days, followed by 7 days off, repeated every 28 days	Adjust dose for myelosuppression and/or severe hepatic or renal impairment; monitor for hepatotoxicity and QT prolongation; avoid concomitant strong inhibitors of CYP3A4 and moderate/strong inducers of CYP3A4	Do not split tablets
Alpelisib (+ Fulvestrant)	300 mg orally daily	Adjust dose for dermatologic toxicity, hyperglycemia and diarrhea; monitor for hyperglycemia and dermatologic toxicity; avoid concomitant strong inducers of CYP3A4	Take after meals Do not split tablets
Everolimus (+ Exemestane or Fulvestrant or Tamoxifen)	10 mg orally daily	Adjust dose in mild, moderate and severe liver impairment; also monitor for myelosuppression, hyperglycemia, dyslipidemia, renal dysfunction. May need to adjust dose with concomitant CYP3A4 inhibitors/inducers	Do not split tablets

IM, intramuscular; SC, subcutaneous.

^aSevere liver impairment: Child–Pugh class C; moderate liver impairment: Child–Pugh class B; minor liver impairment: Child–Pugh class A.

pertuzumab in the neoadjuvant or adjuvant setting. Ado-trastuzumab emtansine is the recommended second-line *HER2*-targeted therapy after a patient progresses on or can no longer tolerate first-line therapy. Subsequent therapy (third-line) for *HER2*-positive MBC is controversial; choice of regimen may depend on the presence of brain metastases, organ function, and residual toxicities from previous regimens. All therapies in this class have some degree of cardiotoxicity. Other adverse drug reactions are drug-specific.

Endocrine Therapy

- Consider endocrine therapy in combination with a targeted agent as first-line therapy for patients with hormone-positive MBC, when feasible. These combinations address de novo or acquired resistance with endocrine therapy alone and have demonstrated efficacy over single agents in specific patient populations. The choice of endocrine therapy is based on the menopausal status of the patient, prior therapies and previous response, duration of response, or disease-free interval. Optimal subsequent therapy after progression on initial targeted-endocrine treatment is largely unknown and the subject of ongoing clinical trials. Most patients with hormone-positive MBC will receive several targeted-endocrine combination regimens or endocrine therapy alone sequentially before chemotherapy is considered.

- No one endocrine therapy has clearly superior survival benefit. The choice of agent is based primarily on mechanism of action, toxicity, and patient preference (Table 61-3). Based on these criteria, AIs, tamoxifen or toremifene, and **fulvestrant**, are the preferred initial agents in MBC except when the patient's cancer recurs during or within one year of adjuvant therapy with the same class of agent.

- AIs reduce circulating and target organ estrogens by blocking peripheral conversion from an androgenic precursor, the primary source of estrogens in postmenopausal women. The third-generation AIs, anastrozole, letrozole, and exemestane, are more selective and have an improved toxicity profile.

- SERMs (tamoxifen and toremifene) and selective estrogen receptor downregulators (SERDs; fulvestrant) are antiestrogens. In addition to the tamoxifen side effects described for adjuvant therapy, tumor flare or hypercalcemia occurs in approximately 5% of patients with MBC.

- Fulvestrant, an intramuscular agent, is approved for second-line therapy of postmenopausal patients with hormone receptor–positive tumors either alone or in combination with targeted therapy. Fulvestrant in combination with ovarian suppression or ablation is an appropriate therapy in premenopausal women. Common toxicities include injection-site reactions, hot flashes, asthenia, and headaches.

- Medical ovarian suppression with an LHRH analog (goserelin, leuprolide, or triptorelin) is a reversible alternative to oophorectomy in premenopausal women. Use of these agents is associated with amenorrhea, bone loss or osteoporosis, hot flashes, and occasional nausea. A 2- to 4-week flare response may also be seen.

Chemotherapy

- Chemotherapy is used as initial therapy for women with hormone receptor-negative tumors, with triple negative tumors, and after failure of endocrine/targeted therapy regimens. Combination chemotherapy results in an objective response in about 47%–55% of unselected, chemotherapy-naive patients.

- In the absence of predictive biomarkers, chemotherapy is chosen based on overall efficacy, the risk of toxicity, performance status and presence of comorbidities in the patient, aggressiveness of disease (eg, indolent vs visceral crisis), and patient preferences related to chemotherapy schedules, dosing route (eg, oral vs intravenous), and frequency (eg, weekly vs every 3 weeks).

- Response rates are high with combination chemotherapy, but sequential use of single agents is an effective strategy and may be preferred due to decreased rates of adverse events. In the palliative setting, when efficacy is similar, the least toxic approach is preferred (Table 61-4).

TABLE 61-4 Selected Regimens for *HER2*-Negative Metastatic Breast Cancer

Single Agent Chemotherapy

Paclitaxel[a]

Paclitaxel 175 mg/m^2 IV

Repeat cycle every 21 days

or

Paclitaxel 80 mg/m^2/week IV

Repeat dose every 7 days

Vinorelbine[a]

Vinorelbine 25 mg/m^2/week IV

Repeat dose every 7 days

Capecitabine[a]

Capecitabine 1000–1250 mg/m^2 orally twice daily for 14 days

Repeat cycle every 21 days

Gemcitabine[a]

Gemcitabine 800–1200 mg/m^2/week IV, days 1, 8, and 15

Repeat cycle every 28 days

Eribulin[a]

Eribulin 1.4 mg/m^2 IV, days 1 and 8

Repeat cycle every 21 days

Liposomal Doxorubicin[a]

Liposomal doxorubicin 50 mg/m^2 IV

Repeat cycle every 28 days

Combination Chemotherapy Regimens

Gemcitabine + Carboplatin

Gemcitabine 1000 mg/m^2 IV, days 1 and 8
Carboplatin AUC 2 IV, days 1 and 8

Repeat cycle every 21 days

Docetaxel + Capecitabine

Docetaxel 75 mg/m^2 IV, day 1

Capecitabine 950 mg/m^2 orally twice daily for 14 days

Repeat cycle every 21 days

Additional Targeted Therapies

Olaparib[a]

Olaparib tablet 300 mg orally twice daily

Repeat cycle every 28 days

Talazoparib[a]

Talazoparib tablet 1 mg orally daily

Repeat cycles every 28 days

Atezolizumab + albumin bound paclitaxel[a]

Atezolizumab 840 mg IV, days 1 and 15

Albumin-bound paclitaxel 100 mg/m^2 IV, days 1, 8, and 15

Repeat cycle every 28 days

Pembrolizumab + chemotherapy (albumin-bound paclitaxel, paclitaxel, or gemcitabine + carboplatin)[a]

Pembrolizumab 200 mg IV, day 1 (given every 21 days)

Albumin-bound paclitaxel 100 mg/m^2 IV, days 1, 8, and 15 (given every 28 days)

OR

Paclitaxel 90 mg/m^2 IV, days 1, 8, and 15 (given every 28 days)

OR

Pembrolizumab 200 mg IV, day 1

Gemcitabine 1000 mg/m^2 IV, days 1 and 8

Carboplatin AUC 2 IV, days 1 and 8

Repeat cycle every 21 days

[a]Designated as a preferred regimen in the NCCN Breast Cancer Guidelines.

- Treatment with sequential single agents is recommended over combination regimens unless the patient has rapidly progressive disease, life-threatening visceral disease, or the need for rapid symptom control.
- Most patients experience partial responses to chemotherapy. The median duration of response is highly variable, ranging from 3 to 15 months; the median OS is 10–33 months. A specific chemotherapy regimen is usually continued until progressive disease or intolerable side effects.
- **Anthracyclines** and **taxanes** produce response rates as high as 50% when used as first-line therapy for MBC. Single-agent **capecitabine**, **vinorelbine**, and **gemcitabine** have response rates of 20%–25% when used after an anthracycline and a taxane.
- **Ixabepilone**, a microtubule stabilizing agent, is indicated as monotherapy or in combination with capecitabine. **Eribulin** is another antimicrotubule agent approved as monotherapy in patients who have received at least two prior chemotherapy regimens for MBC.
- **Sacituzumab govitecan-hziy**, an antibody-drug conjugate (ADC), is approved for adult patients with metastatic triple negative breast cancer who received at least two prior therapies for metastatic disease.

Immunotherapy

- **Pembrolizumab** (mAb against programmed cell death protein 1 [PD-1]) is approved in combination with albumin-bound paclitaxel, paclitaxel, or the combination of carboplatin + gemcitabine. **Atezolizumab** (mAb against programmed death-ligand [PD-L1]) is approved in combination with albumin-bound paclitaxel (see Table 61-4). These agents have failed to demonstrate antitumor activity as single agents in MBC.

Radiation Therapy

- Commonly used to treat painful bone metastases or other localized sites of refractory disease, including brain, spinal cord, eye, or orbit lesions. Pain relief is seen in approximately 90% of patients who receive RT for painful bone metastases.

EVALUATION OF THERAPEUTIC OUTCOMES

- The goal of surgery, radiation, neoadjuvant/adjuvant therapy for early-stage breast cancer—chemotherapy, biologic or targeted therapy, and endocrine therapy—is cure which cannot be fully evaluated for years after initial diagnosis and treatment.
- Patients are recommended to have a history and physical every 3–6 months for the first 3 years after completion of primary therapy, every 6 months for the following 2 years, and then yearly thereafter.

METASTATIC BREAST CANCER

- Palliation is the therapeutic endpoint in the treatment of MBC. Optimizing benefits and minimizing toxicity are general therapeutic goals; careful consideration of quality of life is important in this setting and is an important therapeutic endpoint.
- Tumor response is measured by changes in laboratory tests, diagnostic imaging, or physical signs or symptoms.

See Chapter 151, Breast Cancer, authored by Bonnie Lin Boster, Neelam K. Patel, and Jaime Kaushik, for a more detailed discussion of this topic.

62

CHAPTER

- *Colorectal cancer* (CRC) is a malignant neoplasm involving the colon, rectum, and anal canal.

PATHOPHYSIOLOGY

- Development of a colorectal neoplasm is a multistep process of genetic and phenotypic alterations of normal bowel epithelium structure and function leading to dysregulated cell growth, proliferation, and tumor development.
- Features of colorectal tumorigenesis include genomic instability, activation of oncogene pathways, mutational inactivation or silencing of tumor-suppressor genes, DNA mismatch repairs, and activation of growth factor pathways.
- Adenocarcinomas account for about 92% of tumors of the large intestine.

PREVENTION AND SCREENING

- *Primary prevention* is aimed at preventing CRC in an at-risk population. Trials with celecoxib in people with familial adenomatous polyposis (FAP) showed reduction in size and number of polyps after 6–9 months of treatment, but there is a lack of long-term benefit. Daily low-dose aspirin for at least 10 years in adults aged 50–59 years with a ≥10% 10-year cardiovascular disease risk, a life expectancy of at least 10 years, and who are not at risk for bleeding, is endorsed for primary prevention of both cardiovascular disease and colorectal cancer.
- *Secondary prevention* is aimed at preventing malignancy in a population that has already manifested an initial disease process. Secondary prevention includes procedures ranging from colonoscopic removal of precancerous polyps detected during screening colonoscopy to total colectomy for high-risk individuals (eg, FAP).
- In recognition of the increasing incidence of CRC in adults younger than 50 years, national organizations recommend initiating CRC screening at age 45 for individuals at average risk for CRC.

CLINICAL MANIFESTATIONS

- Signs and symptoms of CRC can be extremely varied, subtle, and nonspecific. Early-stage CRC is often asymptomatic and detected by screening procedures.
- Blood in the stool is the most common sign; however, any change in bowel habits, abdominal discomfort, or abdominal distention may be a warning sign. Less common signs and symptoms include nausea, vomiting, and, if anemia is severe, fatigue.
- Twenty percent of patients present with metastatic disease most commonly in the liver, lungs, and bones.

DIAGNOSIS

- Perform a physical examination and obtain a careful personal and family history. Evaluate the entire large bowel by colonoscopy.
- Obtain baseline laboratory tests: complete blood cell count, international normalized ratio (INR), prothrombin time, activated partial thromboplastin time, liver and renal function tests, and serum carcinoembryonic antigen (CEA). Serum CEA serves as a marker for monitoring CRC response to treatment, but it is too insensitive and nonspecific to be used as a screening test for early-stage CRC.
- Radiographic imaging studies may include chest radiographs, bone scans, chest and abdominal computed tomography scans, positron emission tomography, ultrasonography, and magnetic resonance imaging.

- Determine CRC stage at diagnosis to predict prognosis and develop treatment options. Stage is based on size of the primary tumor (T_{1-4}), presence and extent of lymph node involvement (N_{0-2}), and presence or absence of distant metastases (M).
  - ✓ Stage I disease involves tumor invasion of the submucosa (T_1) or muscularis propria (T_2) and negative lymph nodes.
  - ✓ Stage II disease involves tumor invasion through the muscularis propria into pericolorectal tissues (T_3), or penetration to the surface of the visceral peritoneum (T_{4a}), or directly invades or is adherent to other organs or structures (T_{4b}), and negative lymph nodes.
  - ✓ Stage III disease includes T_{1-4} and positive regional lymph nodes.
  - ✓ Stage IV disease includes any T, any N, and distant metastasis.

PROGNOSIS

- Stage at diagnosis is the most important independent prognostic factor for survival and disease recurrence. Five-year relative survival is approximately 90% for those with localized tumor as compared with about 14% for those with metastatic disease at diagnosis.
- Poor prognostic clinical factors at diagnosis include bowel obstruction or perforation, high preoperative CEA level, distant metastases, and location of the primary tumor in the rectum or rectosigmoid area.
- Molecular markers, particularly MSI, 18q/*DCC* mutation or LOH, *BRAF V600E* mutation, and *RAS* mutations are also associated with CRC prognosis, although the pathologic stage of disease remains the primary prognostic assessment.

TREATMENT

- <u>Goals of Treatment</u>: The goals include cure for stages I, II, and III; the intent is to eradicate micrometastatic disease after surgical resection. Most stage IV disease is incurable; palliative treatment is given to reduce symptoms, avoid disease-related complications, and prolong survival. Twenty to 30% of patients with metastatic disease may be cured if their metastases are resectable.
- Treatment modalities are surgery, radiation therapy (RT), chemotherapy, and biomodulators.

OPERABLE DISEASE

Surgery

- Complete surgical resection of the primary tumor with regional lymphadenectomy is a curative approach for patients with operable CRC.
- The preferred surgical procedure for rectal cancer is total excision of the mesorectum that includes tissue containing perirectal fat and draining lymph nodes.
- Infection, anastomotic leakage, obstruction, adhesions, sexual dysfunction, and malabsorption syndromes.

Neoadjuvant Radiation Therapy

- RT has a limited role in colon cancer because most recurrences are extrapelvic and occur in the abdomen. A subset of patients with recurrent disease or with T_4 tumors that have penetrated fixed structures may benefit from neoadjuvant (preoperative) fluorouracil-based chemoradiation to improve resectability.

Adjuvant Chemotherapy for Colon Cancer

- Adjuvant therapy for 6 months is administered after complete tumor resection to eliminate residual micrometastatic disease. Adjuvant therapy is not indicated for stage I CRC because more than 90% of patients are cured by surgical resection alone.
- Offer adjuvant therapy to patients with stage II disease at higher risk for relapse, with a detailed discussion regarding the potential benefits versus treatment-related toxicities.

- Adjuvant chemotherapy significantly decreases risk of cancer recurrence and death and is standard of care for stage III colon cancer.
- Standard adjuvant regimens include a fluoropyrimidine (**fluorouracil** [with **leucovorin**] or **capecitabine**) as a single agent or in combination with **oxaliplatin**. Leucovorin enhances cytotoxic activity of fluorouracil.
- Administration method affects clinical activity and toxicity. In most common combination regimens, fluorouracil is administered by both IV bolus injection and by continuous IV infusion. No one treatment schedule is superior for overall patient survival.
- Continuous IV infusion of fluorouracil is generally well tolerated but is associated with palmar-plantar erythrodysesthesia (hand–foot syndrome) and stomatitis. IV bolus administration is associated with leukopenia, which is dose-limiting and can be life-threatening. Both administration methods are associated with a similar incidence of mucositis, diarrhea, nausea and vomiting, and alopecia.
- In rare cases, patients deficient in dihydropyrimidine dehydrogenase, responsible for the catabolism of fluorouracil, develop severe toxicity, including death, after fluorouracil administration.
- National guidelines recommend oxaliplatin-based regimens as the first-line option for patients with stage III colon cancer who can tolerate combination therapy. It is commonly administered with fluorouracil/leucovorin. Oxaliplatin is associated with both acute and persistent neuropathies, including rare, acute pharyngolaryngeal dysesthesia, neutropenia, and gastrointestinal (GI) toxicity.
- Selection of an adjuvant regimen (Table 62-1) is based on patient-specific factors, including performance status, comorbid conditions, and patient preference based on lifestyle factors. Age should also be considered as subset analysis of large clinical trials has shown that patients older than 70 years may not benefit from adjuvant oxaliplatin.
- Fluorouracil/leucovorin regimens currently have limited use but are acceptable options in patients who cannot receive oxaliplatin and are unable to tolerate oral capecitabine.

Adjuvant Therapy for Rectal Cancer

- Rectal cancer is more difficult to resect with wide margins, so local recurrences are more frequent than with colon cancer. Neoadjuvant chemoradiation followed by surgery and adjuvant chemotherapy or total neoadjuvant therapy (fluoropyrimidine-based chemotherapy followed by chemo RT (or vice versa) followed by surgery) is recommended for stages II and III rectal cancer. FOLFOX or CAPEOX are the preferred fluoropyrimidine-based chemotherapy regimens, but fluorouracil and leucovorin combination regimens and capecitabine can be used.
- Neoadjuvant chemoradiation significantly reduces local recurrence and has fewer toxicities, and improved sphincter-preserving surgeries as compared to postoperative chemoradiation. Offer preoperative RT alone to patients who can't tolerate chemoradiation.
- Patients should receive adjuvant (postoperative) chemotherapy to total 6 months of chemotherapy.

METASTATIC DISEASE

- Patients with metastatic colorectal cancer (MCRC) are considered to have resectable, potentially resectable, or unresectable metastatic disease. Surgery and RT are used to manage isolated sites of tumor. Chemotherapy is used for disseminated disease and is the primary treatment modality for unresectable MCRC.
- Tumor genotyping for *RAS* (*KRAS* and *NRAS*) and *BRAF* mutation status, *HER2* amplification, and determination of tumor methylation or mismatch repair (MMR) or microsatellite instability (MSI) status (if not previously done) are recommended to identify appropriate treatment options.

TABLE 62-1	Chemotherapy Regimens for the Adjuvant Treatment of Colorectal Cancer	
Regimen	**Agents**	**Comments**
FOLFOX	Oxaliplatin 85 mg/m² IV on day 1 Leucovorin 400 mg/m² IV on day 1 Fluorouracil 400 mg/m² IV bolus, after leucovorin on day 1, then 1200 mg/m²/day × 2 days CIV (total 2400 mg/m² over 46–48 hours) Repeat every 2 weeks × 24 weeks[a]	Preferred regimen for stage III colon and rectal cancers; common toxicities: sensory neuropathy, neutropenia.
CAPEOX	Oxaliplatin 130 mg/m² IV day 1 Capecitabine 1000 mg/m² twice daily orally days 1 through 14 Each cycle lasts 3 weeks × 24 weeks[b]	Improved DFS in patients with stage III colon cancer compared to capecitabine alone or Roswell Park Regimen; common dose-limiting toxicities: neuropathies and hand–foot syndrome. A preferred regimen for adjuvant rectal therapy.
Capecitabine	Capecitabine 1000 mg/m² to 1250 mg/m² PO twice daily on days 1 through 14 Each cycle lasts 14 days and is repeated every 3 weeks × 24 weeks	Equivalent DFS as compared with the Mayo Clinic regimen with improved tolerability; hand–foot syndrome common, useful for patients without vascular access or who have difficulties with travel to the– infusion center
Roswell Park Regimen	Leucovorin 500 mg/m² IV day 1 over 2 hours Fluorouracil 500 mg/m² IV bolus 1 hour after leucovorin Repeat weekly for 6 of 8 weeks × 4 cycles	Leukopenia common dose-limiting toxicity; diarrhea, and stomatitis common
Simplified Biweekly	Leucovorin 400 mg/m² per day IV Fluorouracil 400 mg IV bolus, after leucovorin, then 1200 mg/m²/day days 1 and 2 (total 2400 mg/m² over 46–48 hours) for 2 consecutive days Repeat every 2 weeks × 12 cycles	Hand–foot syndrome common

[a]Known as mFOLFOX6; survival benefit has not been demonstrated for patients 70 years and older.
[b]In patients with low-risk stage III (T1-3, any N), 3 months of CAPEOX is noninferior to 6 months of CAPEOX for DFS but this has not been proven for FOLFOX. In patients with high-risk stage III disease (T4, N1-2, or any T, N2), 3 months of FOLFOX is inferior to 6 months of FOLFOX for DFS, but this has not been proven with CAPEOX. Grade 3 neuropathy is lower with 3 months of CAPEOX or FOLFOX.
CIV, continuous intravenous infusion; DFS, disease-free survival; OS, overall survival; PO, by mouth.

Resectable or Potentially Resectable MCRC

- Surgical resection of metastases with curative intent is the primary goal.
- Neoadjuvant or conversional chemotherapy is administered to increase complete resection rates with resectable and potentially resectable liver or lung lesions (Table 62-2). The choice of neoadjuvant therapy depends on patient-specific factors and includes FOLFOX, CAPEOX, FOLFIRI (infusional fluorouracil, leucovorin, and irinotecan), or FOLFOXIRI (infusional fluorouracil, leucovorin, oxaliplatin, and irinotecan). It is typically administered for 2–3 months before surgery. Adjuvant

TABLE 62-2	Initial Chemotherapeutic Regimens for Metastatic Colorectal Cancer[a]		
Regimen	Agents	Major Dose-Limiting Toxicities	Comments
Patients Appropriate for Intensive Therapy with *RAS* Mutations			
FOLFOX +/− bevacizumab	Oxaliplatin 85 mg/m² IV day 1 Leucovorin 400 mg/m² IV day 1 Fluorouracil 400 mg/m² IV bolus, after leucovorin day 1, then 1200 mg/m²/day × 2 days CIV (total 2400 mg/m² over 46-48 hr) Repeat every 2 weeks +/− Bevacizumab 5 mg/kg IV day 1 before FOLFOX Repeat cycle every 2 weeks	FOLFOX: sensory neuropathy, neutropenia Bevacizumab: hypertension, thrombosis, proteinuria	Most commonly used first-line regimen
CAPEOX +/− bevacizumab	Oxaliplatin 130 mg/m² IV day 1 Capecitabine 1000 mg/m² orally twice a day, days 1-14 Repeat cycle every 3 weeks +/− Bevacizumab 7.5 mg/kg IV day 1 Repeat cycle every 3 weeks	CAPEOX: diarrhea, hand–foot syndrome, neuropathies Bevacizumab: hypertension, thrombosis, proteinuria	Reduced capecitabine dose better tolerated; patient must be able to be adherent and report adverse drug reactions in a timely fashion
FOLFIRI +/− bevacizumab	Irinotecan 180 mg/m² IV day 1 Leucovorin 400 mg/m² IV day 1 Fluorouracil 400 mg/m² IV bolus, after leucovorin day 1, then 1200 mg/m²/day × 2 days CIV (total 2400 mg/m² over 46-48 hr) +/− Bevacizumab 5 mg/kg IV day prior to FOLFIRI Repeat cycle every 2 weeks	FOLFIRI: diarrhea, mucositis, neutropenia Bevacizumab: hypertension, thrombosis, proteinuria	May be preferred in patients who have preexisting neuropathy or those in which neuropathy may be debilitating to their line of work (eg, musician)

Regimen	Details	Notes
FOLFOXIRI +/− bevacizumab	Irinotecan 165 mg/m² IV day 1 prior to oxaliplatin Oxaliplatin 85 mg/m² IV day 1 prior to leucovorin day 1 Leucovorin 400 mg/m² IV day 1 prior to fluorouracil Fluorouracil 1200 mg/m²/day × 2 days CIV (total 2400 mg/m² over 48 hr) Repeat cycle every 2 weeks +/− Bevacizumab 5 mg/kg IV day 1 before FOLFOXIRI Repeat cycle every 2 weeks	FOLFOXIRI: neutropenia, diarrhea, stomatitis, peripheral neurotoxicity, thrombocytopenia Bevacizumab: hypertension, thrombosis, proteinuria	[b]More neutropenia and peripheral neurotoxicity compared to FOLFIRI; often used in medically fit individuals with diffuse aggressive disease to palliate symptoms and as potential conversion therapy

Patients Appropriate for Intensive Therapy with *RAS* or *BRAF* Wild-Type and Left-Sided Colon Tumors

Regimen	Details	Toxicity	Notes
FOLFOX + cetuximab or panitumumab	FOLFOX regimen + cetuximab (400 mg/m² IV loading dose, then cetuximab 250 mg/m² IV weekly thereafter OR cetuximab 500 mg/m² IV every 2 weeks) before FOLFOX OR FOLFOX regimen + panitumumab 6 mg/kg IV day 1 before FOLFOX Repeat cycle every 2 weeks	FOLFOX: sensory neuropathy, neutropenia Cetuximab: Papulopustular and follicular rash, asthenia, constipation, diarrhea, allergic reactions, hypomagnesemia Panitumumab: rash, diarrhea, hypomagnesemia	Only *RAS* or *BRAF* wild-type and left-sided tumor
FOLFIRI + cetuximab or panitumumab	FOLFIRI + cetuximab (400 mg/m² IV loading dose, then cetuximab 250 mg/m² IV weekly thereafter OR cetuximab 500 mg/m² IV every 2 weeks) before FOLFIRI OR FOLFIRI + panitumumab 6 mg/kg IV day 1 before FOLFIRI Repeat cycle every 2 weeks	FOLFIRI: diarrhea, mucositis, neutropenia Cetuximab: papulopustular and follicular rash, asthenia, constipation, diarrhea, allergic reactions, hypomagnesemia Panitumumab: rash, diarrhea, hypomagnesemia	Only *RAS* or *BRAF* wild-type and left-sided tumor; preferred for patients with preexisting neuropathy or those in whom neuropathy may be debilitating to their line of work (eg, musician)

(Continued)

TABLE 62-2	Initial Chemotherapeutic Regimens for Metastatic Colorectal Cancer[a] (Continued)		
Regimen	Agents	Major Dose-Limiting Toxicities	Comments
Patients NOT Appropriate for Intensive Therapy with RAS Mutations			
Infusional fluorouracil + fluorouracil + leucovorin +/− bevacizumab	Fluorouracil 400 mg/m² IV bolus, after leucovorin on day 1, then 1200 mg/m²/day × 2 days CIV (total 2400 mg/m² over 46–48 h)	Infusional fluorouracil/leucovorin: neutropenia, diarrhea	Infusional fluorouracil/leucovorin regimen preferred to bolus fluorouracil regimen
	Repeat cycle every 2 weeks	Bevacizumab: hypertension, bleeding, proteinuria	
	+/− Bevacizumab 5 mg/kg IV day 1 prior to fluorouracil and leucovorin		
	Repeat cycle every 2 weeks		
Capecitabine +/− bevacizumab	Capecitabine 850–1250 mg/m² orally twice a day, days 1–14	Capecitabine: hand–foot syndrome, diarrhea, hyperbilirubinemia	
	+/− Bevacizumab 7.5 mg/kg IV day 1	Bevacizumab: hypertension, thrombosis, proteinuria	
	Repeat cycle every 3 weeks		
Patients NOT Appropriate for Intensive Therapy with RAS or BRAF Wild-Type and Left-Sided Tumors			
Cetuximab[c]	Cetuximab 400 mg/m² IV loading dose, then cetuximab 250 mg/m² IV weekly thereafter	Papulopustular and follicular rash, asthenia, constipation, diarrhea, allergic reactions, hypomagnesemia	Only RAS or BRAF wild-type and left-sided tumor
	Or		
	Cetuximab 500 mg/m² IV every 2 weeks		
Panitumumab[c]	6 mg/kg IV over 60 minutes every 2 weeks	Rash, diarrhea hypomagnesemia, rare allergic reactions	Only RAS or BRAF wild-type and left-sided tumor

Patients with dMMR or MSI-H

Pembrolizumab	2 mg/kg IV every 2 weeks or 200 mg IV every 3 weeks or 400 mg IV every 6 weeks[d]	Immune-mediated adverse drug reactions (most common: skin, liver, kidney, gastrointestinal tract, lung, and endocrine systems)	Only in MMR-d or MSI-H tumors. Patients should be closely monitored for adverse drug reactions and report any adverse drug reactions immediately as interruption of treatment or initiation of corticosteroids may be needed
Nivolumab +/- ipilimumab	Nivolumab 3 mg/kg IV over 30 minutes and ipilimumab 1 mg/kg IV over 30 minutes every 3 weeks × 4 doses, then nivolumab 3 mg/kg IV or nivolumab 240 mg IV every 2 weeks or 480 mg IV every 4 weeks[d]	Immune-mediated adverse drug reactions (most common: skin, liver, kidney, gastrointestinal tract, lung, and endocrine systems)	Only in MMR-d or MSI-H tumors. Patients should be closely monitored for adverse drug reactions and report any adverse drug reactions immediately as interruption of treatment or initiation of corticosteroids may be needed

Patients NOT Appropriate for Intensive Therapy with *HER*-Amplified and *RAS* and *BRAF* WT

Trastuzumab + (pertuzumab or lapatinib) or fam-trastuzumab deruxtecan-nxki	Trastuzumab 8 mg/kg IV day 1 of cycle 1 then 6 mg/kg IV every 21 days + pertuzumab 840 mg IV day 1 of cycle 1 then 420 mg IV every 21 days OR trastuzumab 4 mg/kg IV day of cycle 1 then 2 mg/kg IV weekly + lapatinib 1000 mg po daily OR fam-trastuzumab deruxtecan-nxki 6.4 mg/kg IV on day 1 every 21 days	Trastuzumab + pertuzumab: hypokalemia, abdominal pain, diarrhea, fatigue, nausea; trastuzumab + lapatinib: fatigue, elevated liver enzymes, diarrhea, and rash; fam-trastuzumab deruxtecan-nxki: interstitial pneumonitis	Only in *HER*-amplified and *RAS* and *BRAF* WT tumors. Evaluate all patients for left ventricular ejection fraction at baseline and monitor closely throughout therapy. Do not substitute conventional or biosimilar trastuzumab with ado-trastuzumab emtansine, fam-trastuzumab deruxtecan, or trastuzumab/hyaluronidase

[a]NCCN Guideline recommendations for initial therapy. All recommendations are category 2A unless otherwise noted. Category 2A: based on lower evidence, there is uniform NCCN consensus that intervention is appropriate.
[b]Original dosing was 1600 mg/m²/day but it is recommended that US patients use this dose as they do not tolerate fluorouracil as well.
[c]NCCN Category 2B: based upon lower-evidence, there is NCCN consensus that this intervention is appropriate.
[d]Flat dosing is preferred.

(postoperative) chemotherapy (preferably FOLFOX or CAPEOX) is administered to complete a total of 6 months of chemotherapy.

- The optimal sequencing of chemotherapy with initially resectable metastatic disease is controversial; as treatment options include surgery followed by chemotherapy or perioperative (pre- and postoperative) chemotherapy with surgery.
- Consider hepatic-directed therapy in addition to or as an alternative to surgical resection in patients with liver-only or liver-predominant MCRC. Hepatic artery infusion (HAI) delivers chemotherapy (eg, **floxuridine** and fluorouracil) through the hepatic artery directly into the liver. Tumor ablation uses radiofrequency ablation or microwave energy to generate heat to destroy tumor cells. Cryoablation is also used. These strategies are less successful than surgical interventions.

Unresectable MCRC

- Systemic chemotherapy palliates symptoms and improves survival in patients with unresectable disease. RT may control localized symptoms. Most MCRCs are incurable; however, randomized trials confirm that chemotherapy prolongs life and improves quality of life.
- Consider goals of therapy, history of prior chemotherapy, tumor *RAS* and MMR/MSI mutation status, performance status/comorbidities, and risk of drug-related toxicities to determine a management strategy. Regimens are the same for metastatic cancer of the colon and rectum.

  ✓ Most first-line chemotherapy regimens incorporate a fluoropyrimidine. Addition of **irinotecan** significantly improves response rates, progression-free survival (PFS), and overall survival (OS). Oxaliplatin in combination with infusional fluorouracil plus leucovorin is associated with higher response rates and prolonged PFS, with variable effects on OS (see Table 62-2).

- **Capecitabine** monotherapy is suitable for first-line therapy in patients not likely to tolerate IV chemotherapy. Available for oral administration, it is converted to fluorouracil and is a suitable replacement for infusional fluorouracil in combination with oxaliplatin (CAPEOX).
- **Bevacizumab** is a recombinant, humanized monoclonal antibody that inhibits vascular endothelial growth factor (VEGF). Addition of bevacizumab to fluorouracil-based regimens modestly increases PFS and OS as compared to chemotherapy alone.

  ✓ Hypertension is common with bevacizumab and easily managed with oral antihypertensive agents. Other safety concerns include bleeding, thrombocytopenia, and proteinuria. GI perforation is a rare but potentially fatal complication necessitating prompt evaluation of abdominal pain associated with vomiting or constipation. Bevacizumab can interfere with wound healing; schedule surgery at least 6–8 weeks after the last dose of bevacizumab and wait at least 6–8 weeks after surgery to restart.

- **Cetuximab** and **panitumumab** are epidermal growth factor receptor (EGFR) inhibitors used in patients with wild-type *RAS* and *BRAF* tumors in combination with FOLFOX or FOLFIRI or administered alone (Table 62-2). Patients with left-sided primary tumors have improved OS when treated with EGFR inhibitors while those with right-sided tumors (cecum to hepatic flexure) do not. Severe infusion reactions, including anaphylaxis, can occur with cetuximab (3%) and panitumumab (1%). Skin toxicity is also commonly seen and is not part of the infusion reaction. The presence of papulopustular skin rash correlates with response and survival and most commonly occurs within 2–4 weeks of therapy initiation.
- **Trastuzumab** and **pertuzumab** are monoclonal antibodies directed against HER2. The combination of trastuzumab + pertuzumab or **lapatinib**, or **fam-trastuzumab deruxtecan-nxki** alone is recommended as an option with HER2 amplification and wild-type *RAS* and *BRAF* tumors.
- Patients may receive multiple different regimens; the sequence of drugs appears less important than exposure to all active agents in the course of cancer treatments. Both

FOLFIRI and FOLFOX are considered the reference standards in metastatic colorectal cancer; their different toxicity profiles influence sequence of treatments.

METASTATIC DISEASE: SECOND-LINE AND SUBSEQUENT THERAPY

- The selection of second-line chemotherapy is primarily based on the type of and response to prior therapy received, site and extent of disease, and patient factors and treatment preferences. The optimal sequence of regimens has not been established (Table 62-3). **Trifluridine/tipiracil** is approved for treatment of MCRC patients who have been previously treated with an fluoropyrimidine-, oxaliplatin-, and irinotecan-containing regimens, an anti-VEGF targeted therapy, and an anti-EGFR monoclonal antibody if *RAS* wild-type.
- Patients with wild-type *RAS* and *BRAF* tumors who experience progression on therapies that do not contain an EGFR inhibitor may benefit from the combination of cetuximab or panitumumab and irinotecan, FOLFOX, or FOLFIRI.

TABLE 62-3	Second-Line and Salvage Chemotherapy Regimens for Metastatic Colorectal Cancer
Disease Progression with First-Line Regimen	**Comments**
Second-line options	
FOLFIRI or irinotecan	After previous oxaliplatin-based regimen (without irinotecan) (ie, FOLFOX, CAPEOX); use with caution in patients with elevated bilirubin
FOLFIRI + bevacizumab or ziv-aflibercept or ramucirumab	After previous oxaliplatin-based regimen (without irinotecan) (ie, FOLFOX, CAPEOX); use with caution in patients with elevated bilirubin; bevacizumab is preferred antiangiogenic agent based on toxicity and cost
FOLFOX or CAPEOX ± bevacizumab	After previous irinotecan-based regimen (without oxaliplatin) (ie, FOLFIRI); bevacizumab FDA-approved to continue with second-line options
FOLFOX + cetuximab or panitumumab	After previous irinotecan-based regimen (without oxaliplatin) (ie, FOLFIRI); only if *RAS* wild-type and *BRAF* wild-type
Irinotecan + bevacizumab or ziv-aflibercept or ramucirumab	After previous oxaliplatin-based regimen (without irinotecan) (ie, FOLFOX, CAPEOX); use with caution in patients with elevated bilirubin; bevacizumab is preferred antiangiogenic agent based on toxicity and cost
FOLFIRI + cetuximab or panitumumab	After previous oxaliplatin-based regimen (without irinotecan) (ie, FOLFOX, CAPEOX); only if *RAS* wild-type and *BRAF* wild-type; if neither previously given; use with caution in patients with elevated bilirubin
Irinotecan ± cetuximab or panitumumab	Only if *RAS* wild-type and *BRAF* wild-type; if neither previously given; use with caution in patients with elevated bilirubin
Encorafenib + (cetuximab or panitumumab)	Only if *BRAF V600E* mutation positive
Nivolumab ± ipilimumab	Only if dMMR/MSI-H
Dostarlimab	Only if dMMR/MSI-H
Pembrolizumab	Only if dMMR/MSI-H
Trastuzumab + (pertuzumab or lapatinib) or fam-trastuzumab deruxtecan-nxki	Only if *HER2*-amplified and *RAS* and *BRAF* wild-type

(Continued)

TABLE 62-3	Second-Line and Salvage Chemotherapy Regimens for Metastatic Colorectal Cancer (*Continued*)
Disease Progression with First-Line Regimen	**Comments**
Therapy After Second Progression or Third Progression (can use any of the previous recommendations)	
Regorafenib	Used after progressed through all available regimens
Trifluridine/tipiracil ± bevacizumab	Used after progressed through all available regimens
Clinical trial	If available and only if patient eligible
Best supportive care	Appropriate for patients who do not want to pursue treatment, or not eligible for cancer-directed therapy, or if quality of life is expected to decrease

CAPEOX, capecitabine plus oxaliplatin; dMMR, DNA mismatch repair deficiency; FOLFIRI, fluorouracil plus leucovorin plus irinotecan; FOLFOX, fluorouracil plus leucovorin plus oxaliplatin; MSI-H, high microsatellite instability.

- A two-drug regimen of **encorafenib** (a BRAF inhibitor) and an EGFR inhibitor (cetuximab or panitumumab) is recommended to improve overall outcomes in second- and subsequent-line therapies for patients with *BRAF V600E* mutations.
- Angiogenesis inhibitors including VEGF inhibitors bevacizumab, **ramucirumab**, and **ziv-aflibercept** and the oral multikinase inhibitor **regorafenib** may be used in patients with progressive disease on other therapies.
- *HER2*, a member of the same kinase family as EGFR, is rarely overexpressed in CRC; however, it is more common in those with *RAS* and *BRAF* wild-type tumors. *HER2* inhibitor therapy can be an option for those with *HER2* overexpression when other options have failed.
- **Pembrolizumab**, a humanized, IgG4 monoclonal antibody that binds to PD-L1 with high affinity, is effective in MCRC patients with dMMR who have progressed through 2–4 other regimens. **Nivolumab**, another humanized IgG4 monoclonal antibody PD-1 inhibitor, has also been evaluated with or without **ipilimumab** in patients with MCRC who have dMMR/MSI-H tumors.

EVALUATION OF THERAPEUTIC OUTCOMES

- Goals of monitoring are to evaluate benefit of treatment and detect recurrence.
- Patients who undergo curative surgical resection, with or without adjuvant therapy, require routine follow-up. Consult practice guidelines for specifics.
- Evaluate patients for anticipated side effects such as loose stools or diarrhea, nausea or vomiting, mouth sores, fatigue, and fever.
- Patients should be closely monitored for side effects that require prompt intervention, such as irinotecan-induced diarrhea, bevacizumab-induced GI perforation, hypertension and proteinuria, oxaliplatin-induced neuropathy, and cetuximab- and panitumumab-induced skin rash.
- Less than one-half of patients develop symptoms of recurrence, such as pain syndromes, changes in bowel habits, rectal or vaginal bleeding, pelvic masses, anorexia, and weight loss. Recurrences in asymptomatic patients can be detected because of increased serum CEA levels.
- Monitor quality-of-life indices, especially in patients with metastatic disease.

See Chapter 153, Colorectal Cancer, authored by Lisa M. Holle, Jessica M. Clement, and Lisa E. Davis, for a more detailed discussion of this topic.

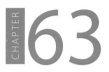

63 Lung Cancer

- *Lung cancer* is a solid tumor originating from the bronchial epithelial cells that have acquired multiple genetic lesions and express a variety of phenotypes. This chapter distinguishes between non-small cell lung cancer (NSCLC) and small cell lung cancer (SCLC) because they have different natural histories and responses to therapy.

PATHOPHYSIOLOGY

- Mutations cause activation of proto-oncogenes, inhibition of tumor suppressor genes, and production of autocrine (self-stimulatory) growth factors contributing to cellular proliferation and malignant transformation in lung tissue. Many molecular alterations are common to both SCLC and NSCLC, but certain mutations are found more frequently in specific subtypes of lung cancer and can be potentially treated with targeted interventions, such as overexpression of c-KIT in SCLC and numerous targetable mutations in NSCLC.
- Smoking is responsible for approximately 80% of lung cancer deaths. Other risk factors are exposure to environmental respiratory carcinogens (eg, asbestos, benzene, and arsenic), genetic risk factors, and history of other lung diseases (eg, chronic obstructive pulmonary disease [COPD] and asthma).
- The major cell types are SCLC (~15% of all lung cancers), adenocarcinoma (~50%), squamous cell carcinoma (<30%), and large cell carcinoma. The last three types are grouped together and referred to as NSCLC. Incorporation of genetics in NSCLC and the availability of targeted therapies have led to personalized treatment. Optimal therapy requires knowledge of histology, immunotherapy marker expression, and genetic mutational status.

CLINICAL PRESENTATION

- The most common initial signs and symptoms are cough, dyspnea, chest pain, or discomfort, with or without hemoptysis. Many patients also exhibit systemic symptoms such as anorexia, weight loss, and fatigue.
- Disseminated disease can cause neurologic deficits from CNS metastases, bone pain, or pathologic fractures secondary to bone metastases, or liver dysfunction from hepatic involvement.
- Paraneoplastic syndromes are signs and symptoms that occur at sites away from the tumor location(s) and are not associated with direct tumor involvement. They occur more frequently with lung cancer than any other tumor, and more frequently with SCLC than with NSCLC.

DIAGNOSIS

- Computed tomography (CT) scans of the chest and upper abdomen are the most common initial radiologic evaluations. The staging workup can include an endo-bronchial ultrasound, positron emission tomography (PET) scan, or other tests. Integrated CT–PET technology appears to improve diagnostic accuracy in staging NSCLC over CT or PET alone.
- Pathologic confirmation is established by examination of sputum cytology and/or tumor biopsy by bronchoscopy, mediastinoscopy, percutaneous needle biopsy, or open-lung biopsy. The tissue sample not only confirms malignancy, but it is also necessary to determine the specific tumor type and to provide tissue for molecular analysis.
- All patients must have a thorough history and physical examination to detect signs and symptoms of the primary tumor, regional spread, distant metastases, paraneo-plastic syndromes, and ability to withstand aggressive therapy.

STAGING

- Clinical staging of NSCLC with the TNM system incorporates tumor size (T), extent of nodal involvement (N), and presence or absence of distant metastases (M).
- A simpler system is commonly used to compare therapeutic modalities. Stage I includes tumors confined to the lung without lymphatic spread, stage II includes large tumors with ipsilateral peribronchial or hilar lymph node involvement, stage III includes other lymph nodes and regional involvement, and stage IV includes any tumor with distant metastases.
- A two-stage classification is widely used for SCLC. Limited disease is confined to one hemithorax and can be encompassed by a single radiation port. All other disease is classified as extensive.

TREATMENT

NON-SMALL CELL LUNG CANCER

- Goals of Treatment: Definitive cure is the desired outcome with early-stage disease. Prolongation of survival is desired in patients with advanced-stage disease. All therapies should improve quality of life.
- Surgery, radiation, and systemic therapies with cytotoxic chemotherapy, immunotherapy, or targeted therapies are used in the management of NSCLC. The applications of these treatment modalities are determined by stage- and patient-specific factors.
- Local disease (stages IA and IB) is associated with a favorable prognosis. Surgery is the primary treatment and may be used alone or in some situations with radiation therapy (RT) and/or systemic therapy.
- Stage IIA and IIB diseases are primarily treated with surgery followed by four cycles of adjuvant chemotherapy (Table 63-1). Platinum-based regimens are preferred and should be given concurrently rather than sequentially with RT. Chemoradiotherapy is recommended for medically inoperable patients who can tolerate combined modality therapy.
- Adjuvant targeted therapy in epidermal growth factor receptor (EGFR) positive disease with **osimertinib** improves 2-year disease-free survival (DFS). DFS at 2- and 3-year follow-up was improved with **atezolizumab** following complete resection and chemotherapy for the treatment of stage II–IIIA NSCLC disease positive for programmed death-ligand 1 (PD-L1).

Locally Advanced Disease (Stage III)

- Optimal outcomes for stage III disease are achieved with multimodality therapy. Patients with operable disease should be considered for surgery preceded or followed by systemic chemotherapy. Current recommendations for patients with resectable stage IIIA disease include chemotherapy (Table 63-1) followed by surgery or radiation, depending on individual patient and tumor features. Neoadjuvant chemotherapy should include **nivolumab**.
- Patients with stage IIIA disease who are not surgical candidates or have a tumor that cannot be resected are typically treated with both a platinum-containing regimen and concurrent RT. Stage IIIB and IIIC NSCLC are generally considered unresectable. Administer induction therapy with chemoradiation followed by consolidation therapy in those who respond with the PD-L1 inhibitor, **durvalumab**, for 1 year to improve PFS and overall survival (OS).

Advanced (Stage IV) and Relapsed Disease

- Patients with stage III disease who are not candidates for radiation are treated like those with stage IV disease. Chemotherapy is administered to palliate symptoms, improve quality of life, and increase duration of survival. Therapy depends on patient-specific factors (performance status is most important) and tumor characteristics.

		Frequency and
TABLE 63-1	**Common Chemotherapy Regimens Used in the Adjuvant Treatment of Non-Small Cell Lung Cancer**	

Regimen	Drugs and Doses	Frequency and Number of Cycles
Cisplatin/ Etoposide	Cisplatin 100 mg/m² IV day 1	Every 28 days for 4 cycles
	Etoposide 100 mg/m² IV daily on days 1, 2, and 3	
Cisplatin/ Vinorelbine	Cisplatin 50 mg/m² IV days 1 and 8	Every 28 days for 4 cycles
	Vinorelbine 25 mg/m² IV days 1, 8, 15, and 22	
	Cisplatin 100 mg/m² IV day 1	Every 28 days for 4 cycles
	Vinorelbine 30 mg/m² IV days 1, 8, 15, and 22	
Carboplatin/ Paclitaxel	Carboplatin AUC 6 IV day 1	Every 21 days for 4 cycles
	Paclitaxel 200 mg/m² IV day 1	
Cisplatin/ Pemetrexed	Cisplatin 75 mg/m² IV day 1	Every 21 days for 4 cycles (for nonsquamous histology only)
	Pemetrexed 500 mg/m² IV day 1	

- Three pathways have been identified for advanced NSCLC: (1) immune sensitive (PD-L1+), (2) targetable genetic mutation-driven, which is further divided based on the sensitizing mutation (EGFR), and (3) nonbiomarker-driven therapy treatment, which is further classified as squamous histology or nonsquamous histology due to drug toxicity and efficacy. Select regimens for first-line treatment of advanced NSCLC are outlined in Table 63-2; second-line treatment options are found in Table 63-3.

- Patients with advanced lung cancer positive for targetable genetic driver mutations have treatment options based on the specific mutation: EGFR, KRAS, ALK, ROS1, BRAF^V600E, METex14 skipping, NTRK, or RET-fusion.

- Treatment options for patients with advanced lung cancer and a targetable genetic driver mutation include the following (see Table 63-4) (consult practice guidelines for the most up-to-date recommendations):

  (1) Patients with a tumor that harbors a *mutation in the EGFR receptor* should receive a first-line EGFR kinase inhibitor. First- and second-generation EGFR kinase inhibitors include **afatinib**, **erlotinib**, or **gefitinib**. A meta-analysis suggests that these three agents have similar PFS results and response rates about two times higher than chemotherapy. **Dacomitinib** is another second-generation irreversible inhibitor. **Osimertinib**, a third-generation EGFR kinase inhibitor, shows the most impressive activity in EGFR-positive tumors and is considered first-line therapy. In addition to significantly longer PFS, osimertinib has improved CNS penetration resulting in improved CNS response rates and less CNS disease as the cause of progression. Subsequent therapy after progression during treatment with an EGFR inhibitor depends on initial treatment and further genetic evaluation. Most patients will proceed to a platinum doublet chemotherapy with or without an immunotherapy agent.

  (2) First-generation ALK inhibitors **crizotinib** and **ceritinib** established ALK inhibition as superior to chemotherapy. Patients with a tumor with an *ALK rearrangement* should receive initial treatment with a second (**alectinib** or **brigatinib**) or third (**lorlatinib**)–generation ALK inhibitor. Patients who relapse while receiving initial ALK-targeted therapy can receive an agent from the next generation.

  (3) Ceritinib, crizotinib, or **entrecitinib** are recommended first-line agents for tumors with a *mutation in ROS1*. Second-line therapy includes **lorlatinib** and entrecitinib.

  (4) Patients with a tumor with the *BRAF V600E mutation* should receive combination therapy with two kinase inhibitors, **trametinib** and **dabrafenib**. Entrectinib is also approved as a first-line treatment for patients with this mutation.

  (5) Patients with a tumor with *neurotrophic receptor kinases (NTRK) gene fusion* should receive **larotrectinib**.

TABLE 63-2 Selected Regimens for the First-Line Treatment of Advanced-Stage Non-Small Cell Lung Cancer

Place in Therapy	Nonsquamous		Squamous	
	PD-L1 ≥50%	PD-L1 1%-49%	PD-L1 ≥50%	PD-L1 1%-49%
First Line	Pembrolizumab 200 mg IV on day 1 every 21 days or 400 mg IV on day 1 every 42 days Repeat until disease progression or unacceptable toxicity for a maximum of 2 years Atezolizumab 840 mg IV on day 1 repeat every 14 days or 1200 mg IV on day 1 repeat every 21 days or 1680 mg IV on day 1 repeat every 28 days Continue until disease progression or unacceptable toxicity	Platinum + pemetrexed + pembrolizumab Cisplatin 75 mg/m² or Carboplatin AUC 5 IV on day 1 Pemetrexed 500 mg/m² IV on day 1 Pembrolizumab 200 mg IV on day 1 Repeat cycle every 3 weeks × 4 cycles—Pembrolizumab maintenance up to 31 additional doses or until progression Atezolizumab + carboplatin + paclitaxel + bevacizumab Atezolizumab 1200 mg IV on day 1 Carboplatin AUC 6 IV on day 1 Paclitaxel 200 mg/m² IV on day 1 Bevacizumab 15 mg/kg IV on day 1 Repeat cycle every 3 weeks × 6 cycles Atezolizumab and bevacizumab maintenance until progression	Pembrolizumab 200 mg IV on day 1 every 21 days or 400 mg IV on day 1 every 42 days Repeat until disease progression, or unacceptable toxicity for a maximum of 2 years Carboplatin + taxane + pembrolizumab Carboplatin AUC 6 IV on day 1 Paclitaxel 200 mg/m² IV on day 1 or nab-paclitaxel 100 mg/m² IV on day 1, 8, and 15 Pembrolizumab 200 mg IV on day 1 Repeat cycle every 3 weeks × 4 cycles Pembrolizumab maintenance up to 31 additional doses or until progression	Carboplatin + paclitaxel + pembrolizumab Carboplatin AUC 6 IV on day 1 Paclitaxel 200 mg/m² IV on day 1 or nab-paclitaxel 100 mg/m² IV on day 1, 8, and 15 Pembrolizumab 200 mg IV on day 1 Repeat cycle every 3 weeks × 4 cycles—Pembrolizumab maintenance up to 31 additional doses or until progression Nivolumab + ipilimumab + carboplatin + paclitaxel Nivolumab 360 mg IV on day 1 and 22 Ipilimumab 1 mg/kg IV on day 1 Paclitaxel 200 mg/m² on day 1 and 22 Carboplatin AUC 6 IV on day 1 and 22 Followed by nivolumab and ipilimumab maintenance every 42 days until disease progression or unacceptable toxicity for a maximum of 2 years

Cemiplimab
350 mg IV on day 1
Repeat every 21 days until disease
Continue until disease progression or unacceptable toxicity

Platinum + pemetrexed + pembrolizumab
Cisplatin 75 mg/m² or carboplatin AUC 5 IV on day 1
Pemetrexed 500 mg/m² IV on day 1
Pembrolizumab 200 mg IV on day 1
Repeat cycle every 3 weeks × 4 cycles
Pembrolizumab maintenance up to 31 additional doses or until progression

Nivolumab + ipilimumab + platinum + pemetrexed
Nivolumab 360 mg IV on days 1 and 22
Ipilimumab 1 mg/kg IV on day 1
Pemetrexed 500 mg/m² on days 1 and 22
Carboplatin AUC 6 IV or cisplatin 75 mg/m² on day 1 and 22
Followed by nivolumab and ipilimumab maintenance every 42 days until disease progression or unacceptable toxicity for a maximum of 2 years

Nivolumab + ipilimumab
Nivolumab 3 mg/kg IV on day 1, 15, and 29
Ipilimumab 1 mg/kg IV on day 1
Repeat every 42 days until disease progression or unacceptable toxicity for a maximum of 2 years

Atezolizumab
840 mg IV on day 1, repeat every 14 days or
1200 mg IV on day 1 repeat every 21 days or
1680 mg IV on day 1 repeat every 28 days
Continue until disease progression or unacceptable toxicity

Cemiplimab
350 mg IV on day 1
Repeat every 21 days until disease progression or unacceptable toxicity

Nivolumab + ipilimumab
Nivolumab 3 mg/kg IV on day 1, 15, and 29
Ipilimumab 1 mg/kg IV on day 1
Repeat every 42 days until disease progression or unacceptable toxicity for a maximum of 2 years

Pembrolizumab
200 mg IV on day 1 every 21 days or
400 mg IV on day 1 every 42 days
Repeat until disease progression, or unacceptable toxicity for a maximum of 2 years

(Continued)

TABLE 63-2 Selected Regimens for the First-Line Treatment of Advanced-Stage Non-Small Cell Lung Cancer (*Continued*)

Place in Therapy	Nonsquamous		Squamous	
	PD-L1 ≥50%	PD-L1 1%–49%	PD-L1 ≥50%	PD-L1 1%–49%
First-line: Contraindications to PD-1 or PD-L1 Inhibitors	Carboplatin + pemetrexed Carboplatin AUC 5 IV on day 1 Pemetrexed 500 mg/m² IV on day 1 Repeat cycle every 3 weeks × 4 or 6 cycles followed by pemetrexed maintenance		Gemcitabine + cisplatin Gemcitabine 1000 mg/m² IV on day 1, 8, and 15 Cisplatin 100 mg/m² IV on day 1 Repeat cycle every 28 days	

TABLE 63-3	Selected Regimens for the Second-Line Treatment of Advanced-Stage Nonsmall Cell Lung Cancer
Second Line: No previous checkpoint inhibitor	Nivolumab
	240 mg IV on day 1 repeat every 14 or
	480 mg IV on day 1 repeat every 28 days
	Continue until disease progression or unacceptable toxicity
	Atezolizumab
	840 mg IV on day 1, repeat every 14 days or
	1200 mg IV on day 1 repeat every 21 days or
	1680 mg IV on day 1 repeat every 28 days
	Continue until disease progression or unacceptable toxicity
	Pembrolizumab
	200 mg IV on day 1 every 21 days or
	400 mg IV on day 1 every 42 days
	Repeat until disease progression, or unacceptable toxicity
Second Line: Other recommend	Docetaxel + ramucirumab
	Docetaxel 75 mg/m^2 IV day 1
	Ramucirumab 10 mg/kg IV day 1
	Repeat every 21 days

- Combination chemotherapy is the standard of care for managing NSCLC without targetable genetic mutations. Platinum-based chemotherapy doublets consisting of **cisplatin** or **carboplatin** combined with **paclitaxel**, **gemcitabine**, or **pemetrexed** are considered standard care; in nonsquamous NSCLC, cisplatin and pemetrexed are the preferred chemotherapy regimen.
- Maintenance therapy is the ongoing use of one or more agents after a positive tumor response to four to six cycles of an initial chemotherapy regimen until disease progression. Several studies show that continuation or switch maintenance therapy improves survival of NSCLC patients with nonsquamous histology. In continuation maintenance therapy, patients receive ongoing treatment with at least one of the agents used in the initial chemotherapy regimen. Alternatively, switch maintenance therapy starts a new agent not included in the initial regimen. Pemetrexed is the most established maintenance chemotherapy option.
- Patients with PD-L1+ tumors and no sensitizing mutations are eligible for first-line immunotherapies with checkpoint inhibitors, including **pembrolizumab**, **atezolizumab**, **nivolumab**, and **cemiplimab**. These agents may be used alone, in combination with chemotherapy, or a CTLA-4 inhibitor, **ipilimumab**. The percentage of PDL1 expression on tumor cells is measured by tumor proportion score (TPS); this drives selection of treatment. Patients are divided into three distinct categories: PD-L1 ≥ 50%, PD-L1 1%–49%, and PD-L1 < 1% (see Table 63-2).
- Guidelines recommend adding **bevacizumab**, a recombinant, humanized monoclonal antibody that neutralizes vascular endothelial growth factor (VEGF) to chemotherapy for patients with advanced NSCLC of nonsquamous cell histology, no recent hemoptysis, no CNS metastasis, and not receiving therapeutic anticoagulation.
- The most recent treatment advance for metastatic NSCLC is chemoimmunotherapy with the addition of **atezolizumab**, a PD-L1 inhibitor, to first-line therapy with carboplatin, pemetrexed, and bevacizumab (ABCP) in patients with nonbiomarker-driven, nonsquamous NSCLC.

TABLE 63-4 Selected Oral Targeted Therapies for Advanced, Mutation-Driven NSCLC

Drug and Dosing	Adverse Reactions		Monitoring Parameters	Comments
	Common	Rare but Serious		
EGFR Exon 19 Deletion or EGFR I858R Mutation				
Osimertinib 80 mg (1 × 80 mg tablet) once daily	• Anorexia • Dermatologic reactions including dry skin and rash • Diarrhea • Fatigue • Myelosuppression • Paronychia • Stomatitis	• Cardiomyopathy • Interstitial lung disease • Keratitis • QTc interval prolongation	• Signs and symptoms of interstitial lung disease (dyspnea, cough, and fever) • Skin exam • CMP at baseline and periodically • Ophthalmic exam periodically and at the onset of any vision changes • CBC at baseline and periodically • ECG periodically in patients with congenital long QTc syndrome, heart failure, electrolyte abnormalities, or concomitantly receiving other QT prolonging agents • Ejection fraction at baseline and periodically in patients at risk for developing heart failure or if patients develop cardiac symptoms	• Can be taken without regard to meals • Increase dose by 50% if patient taking strong cytochrome P4503A4 inducer • Activity not effected by T790M mutation • Improved CNS activity compared to other EGFR-targeting agents • Can be used in patients who have progressed while receiving earlier-generation inhibitors (erlotinib, gefitinib, dacomitinib)
Erlotinib 150 mg (1 × 150 mg tablet) once daily	• Anorexia • Cough • Fatigue • Diarrhea • Dyspnea • Nausea and vomiting • Rash	• Cerebrovascular accident • Gastrointestinal perforation • Hemolytic anemia with thrombocytopenia • Hepatotoxicity including hepatorenal syndrome • Interstitial lung disease • Ocular disorders including corneal perforation, ulceration, or severe keratitis • Severe rash, including Stevens-Johnson syndrome and toxic epidermal necrolysis	• Signs and symptoms of interstitial lung disease • Skin exam • CMP at baseline and periodically • Ophthalmic examinations periodically and at the onset of any changes in vision • Signs and symptoms of hemorrhage if patients receiving warfarin	• Should be taken 1 hour before or 2 hours after meals • Best absorbed in acidic gastric environment • Cytochrome P450 3A4 substrate, use with caution with 3A4 inducers/inhibitors • Increased hemorrhage risk with warfarin • Resistance caused by T790M mutation • Has been studied in combination with bevacizumab or ramucirumab

Afatinib 40 mg (1 × 40 mg tablet) once daily	• Anorexia • Dermatologic reactions including dry skin and rash • Diarrhea • Nausea and vomiting • Paronychia • Pruritus • Stomatitis	• Hepatotoxicity • Interstitial lung disease • Keratitis • Renal impairment from dehydration due to diarrhea • Severe rash, including Stevens-Johnson syndrome and toxic epidermal necrolysis	• Signs and symptoms of interstitial lung disease • Skin exam • CMP at baseline and periodically • Ophthalmic examinations periodically and at onset of any changes in vision	• Should be taken 1 hour before or 2 hours after meals • Dose reduction recommended for severe renal impairment • Diarrhea can be severe and require dose reductions • Pharmacokinetics may be affected by P-glycoprotein inhibitors and inducers • Resistance caused by T790M mutation • Patients with reduced ejection fraction excluded from clinical trials

ALK Rearrangement

Alectinib 600 mg (4 × 150 mg capsules) twice daily	• Anemia • Constipation • Edema • Fatigue • Hepatotoxicity • Leukopenia • Myalgia • Photosensitivity	• Bradycardia • Endocarditis • Gastrointestinal perforation • Increased creatine kinase • Interstitial lung disease • Pulmonary embolism • Renal impairment	• Signs and symptoms of interstitial lung disease • CMP at baseline and periodically • CBC with differential monthly • Liver function tests every 2 weeks for the first 3 months of treatment then monthly • Heart rate and blood pressure should be monitored regularly • CPK every 2 weeks for the first month of treatment and with patient reports of unexplained muscle pain, tenderness, or weakness	• Should be taken with meals • Counsel regarding appropriate precautions to protect from UVA/UVB exposure

(Continued)

TABLE 63-4 Selected Oral Targeted Therapies for Advanced, Mutation-Driven NSCLC (*Continued*)

Drug and Dosing	Adverse Reactions		Monitoring Parameters	Comments
	Common	Rare but Serious		
Brigatinib 90 mg (1 × 90 mg tablet) orally once daily for 7 days then increase to 180 mg (1 × 180 mg tablet) daily if tolerated	• Cough • Diarrhea • Fatigue • Hyperglycemia • Increased creatine kinase • Increased serum lipase and amylase • Nausea	• Bradycardia • Hypertension • Interstitial lung disease • Pneumonitis, including pneumonia • Visual disturbances	• Signs and symptoms of interstitial lung disease • Ophthalmic examinations periodically and at the onset of any changes in vision • Blood pressure should be monitored after 2 weeks then monthly • Heart rate and blood pressure should be monitored regularly • CPK levels should be monitored regularly • Fasting serum glucose at baseline and regularly • Lipase and amylase levels be monitored regularly	• Can be taken without regard to meals • Dose reduction recommended for severe renal or hepatic impairment • Cytochrome P450 3A4 substrate, should not be used with moderate-to-strong inhibitors or inducers of 3A4
Lorlatinib 100 mg (1 × 100 mg tablet) once daily	• Arthralgia • Diarrhea • Dyslipidemia • Dyspnea • Edema • Fatigue • Peripheral neuropathy • Weight gain	• Atrioventricular block • CNS effects such as mood disorders or seizures • Hepatotoxicity • Hyperglycemia • Hypertension • Interstitial lung disease	• Signs and symptoms of interstitial lung disease • Blood pressure should be monitored after 2 weeks then monthly • Heart rate and blood pressure should be monitored regularly • Fasting serum glucose at baseline and regularly • Serum cholesterol and triglycerides at baseline, 1 month and 2 months after initiation then periodically • ECG at baseline and periodically	• Can be taken without regard to meals • Dose reduction recommended for severe renal impairment • Has demonstrated efficacy after the failure of previous ALK-targeted therapies • Patients with severe psychiatric illnesses excluded from clinical trials

ROS1 Rearrangement

| Crizotinib 250 mg (1 × 250 mg capsule) twice daily | • Anorexia
• Constipation
• Diarrhea
• Dizziness
• Edema
• Fatigue
• Hepatotoxicity
• Lymphopenia and neutropenia
• Nausea and vomiting
• Neuropathy
• Upper respiratory infection, including possible pneumonia
• Vision disorders | • Bradycardia
• Interstitial lung disease
• Pulmonary embolism
• QTc interval prolongation | • Signs and symptoms of interstitial lung disease
• CMP at baseline and periodically
• Ophthalmic evaluation in patients with new-onset vision changes
• CBC with differential monthly
• ECG should be monitored periodically in patients with heart failure, bradyarrhythmias, electrolyte abnormalities, or concomitantly receiving other QT prolonging agents
• Heart rate and blood pressure should be monitored regularly | • Can be taken without regard to meals
• Dose reduction recommended for severe renal or hepatic impairment
• Cytochrome P450 3A4 substrate, should not be used with strong inhibitors or inducers of 3A4
• Fatal hepatoxicity has occurred
• Ocular toxicity can lead to severe vision loss |
| Entrectinib 600 mg (3 × 200 mg capsules) once daily | • Arthralgia/myalgia
• Constipation
• Edema
• Fatigue
• Nausea/vomiting/diarrhea
• Vision disorders
• Weight gain | • Fractures
• Heart failure
• Hepatoxicity
• Hyperuricemia
• Mood disorder
• QT prolongation | • Liver function tests every 2 weeks for the first month of therapy then monthly
• Uric acid level at baseline and periodically
• CMP at baseline and periodically to anticipate risk of QT prolongation
• Ejection fraction at baseline and periodically | • Also indicated for *NTRK* mutation-positive NSCLC.
• Can be taken without regard to meals |

(Continued)

713

TABLE 63-4 Selected Oral Targeted Therapies for Advanced, Mutation-Driven NSCLC (*Continued*)

Drug and Dosing	Adverse Reactions		Monitoring Parameters	Comments
	Common	Rare but Serious		
BRAF V600E Mutation				
Trametinib 2 mg (1 × 2 mg tablet) once daily	• Edema • Fatigue • Fever • Nausea/vomiting/diarrhea • Rash	• Cutaneous or other malignancy • Hemorrhagic events • Cardiomyopathy • Colitis with or without perforation • Hyperglycemia • Interstitial lung disease • Ocular toxicity • Venous thromboembolism	• Signs and symptoms of interstitial lung disease • Fasting serum glucose at baseline and regularly • Dermatologic evaluations at baseline and every 2 months • Ejection fraction at baseline, 1 month after initiation of therapy then every 2–3 months • Ophthalmic evaluation at baseline and within 24 hours of any visual disturbances	• Should be used with dabrafenib • Can be taken without regard to meals • Permanently discontinue if symptomatic cardiomyopathy or decrease in ejection fraction by greater than 20% (0.20)
Dabrafenib 150 mg (2 × 75 mg capsules) twice daily	• Edema • Fatigue • Fever • Nausea/vomiting/diarrhea • Rash	• Cardiomyopathy • Cutaneous or other malignancy • Hemorrhagic events • Hyperglycemia • Uveitis	• Fasting serum glucose at baseline and regularly • Dermatologic evaluations at baseline and every 2 months • Ejection fraction at baseline, 1 month after initiation of therapy then every 2–3 months	• Should be used with trametinib • Should be taken 1 hour before or 2 hours after meals • Permanently discontinue if symptomatic cardiomyopathy or decrease in ejection fraction by greater than 20% (0.20) • Hemolytic anemia can occur if patient has glucose-6-phosphate dehydrogenase deficiency
MET exon 14 Mutation				
Capmatinib 400 mg (2 × 200 mg tablets) twice daily	• Edema • Decreased appetite • Dyspnea • Fatigue • Nausea/vomiting	• Hepatotoxicity • Interstitial lung disease • Photosensitivity	• Signs and symptoms of interstitial lung disease • Liver function tests at baseline then every 2 weeks for 3 months, then monthly	• Can be taken without regard to meals • Avoid coadministration of strong CYP3A inducers or inhibitors • Patients should be counseled regarding appropriate precautions to protect from ultraviolet light A/B exposure

Drug/Dose	Adverse Effects	Serious Adverse Effects	Monitoring Parameters	Comments
Tepotinib 450 mg (2 × 225 mg tablets) once daily	• Dyspnea • Edema • Fatigue • Myalgias • Nausea/diarrhea	• Hepatoxicity • Interstitial lung disease	• Signs and symptoms of interstitial lung disease (dyspnea, cough, and fever) • Liver function tests at baseline then every 2 weeks for 3 months, then monthly	• Should be taken with meals

RET Rearrangement

Drug/Dose	Adverse Effects	Serious Adverse Effects	Monitoring Parameters	Comments
Selpercatinib 160 mg (2 × 80 mg capsules) twice daily	• Diarrhea • Edema • Fatigue • Hepatotoxicity • Hyperglycemia • Hypertension • Hypocalcemia • Leukopenia • Rash • Thrombocytopenia • Xerostomia	• Hemorrhage • Hypersensitivity • Impaired wound healing QT prolongation • Tumor lysis syndrome	• Liver function tests at baseline then every 2 weeks for 3 months, then monthly • Electrolytes, including calcium, at baseline and periodically • Blood pressure at baseline, 1 week after therapy initiation, then monthly • ECG at baseline and periodically	• Can be taken without regard to meals • Dose reduce to 120 mg if patient is less than 50 kg • Dose reduction recommended for severe hepatic impairment • Patients should watch for signs/symptoms of hypersensitivity • Hold therapy for planned surgical procedures
Pralsetinib 400 mg (4 × 100 mg capsules) once daily	• Constipation • Edema • Fatigue • Hepatotoxicity • Hypertension • Musculoskeletal pain • Myelosuppression	• Hemorrhage • Impaired wound healing • Interstitial lung disease • Tumor lysis syndrome	• Signs and symptoms of interstitial lung disease • Liver function tests at baseline then every 2 weeks for 3 months, then monthly • Blood pressure at baseline, 1 week after therapy initiation, then monthly	• Should be taken 1 hour before or 2 hours after meals • Dosing modifications required if used concomitantly with strong P-glycoprotein inhibitors or strong CYP3A inhibitors or inducers • Hold therapy for planned surgical procedures

(Continued)

TABLE 63-4 Selected Oral Targeted Therapies for Advanced, Mutation-Driven NSCLC *(Continued)*

Drug and Dosing	Adverse Reactions		Monitoring Parameters	Comments
	Common	Rare but Serious		
NTRK Gene Fusion Positive				
Larotrectinib 100 mg (1 × 100 mg capsule) twice daily	• Constipation or diarrhea • Dizziness • Fatigue • Hepatotoxicity • Hypocalcemia • Musculoskeletal pain • Myelosuppression • Nausea/Vomiting	• CNS effects including cognitive impairment or mood disorders • Fractures	• Liver function tests at baseline then every 2 weeks for 1 month, then monthly	• Can be taken without regard to meals • Dosing modification required if used concomitantly with strong CYP3A4 inhibitors or inducers • Dose reduction recommended for patients with severe hepatic impairment • Inform patients to report signs/symptoms of possible fracture
KRAS G12C Mutation				
Sotorasib 960 mg (8 × 120 mg tablets) once daily	• Diarrhea • Fatigue • Hepatotoxicity • Musculoskeletal pain • Nausea	• Interstitial lung disease	• Signs and symptoms of interstitial lung disease • Liver function tests at baseline then every 3 weeks for 3 months, then monthly	• Can be taken without regard to meals • Avoid administration with drugs that decrease gastric acid • Has only been evaluated after progression on other therapies for advanced disease

- Monotherapy with nivolumab, pembrolizumab, atezolizumab, **docetaxel**, and peme-trexed is the most commonly considered option for second-line therapy in patients with a good performance status who progress during or after first-line chemotherapy. Nivolumab, pembrolizumab, and atezolizumab are options in the second-line setting for patients who have not previously received immunotherapy.
- For patients who have failed initial treatment with immunotherapy, second-line treat-ment with docetaxel, docetaxel-**ramucirumab**, or pemetrexed (if pemetrexed wasn't used as maintenance therapy) is recommended.

SMALL CELL LUNG CANCER

- <u>Goals of Treatment</u>: The goals include cure or prolonged survival, which requires aggressive combination chemotherapy. All therapies should improve quality of life.

Limited Disease

- Use of surgery in SCLC is limited to solitary nodules without evidence of metastasis to lymph nodes.
- SCLC is very radiosensitive; radiation is preferred for treatment of local disease over surgery. Radiation is given concurrently with chemotherapy, and the regimen of choice is **etoposide** and cisplatin (EP regimen; see Table 63-5).
- Radiotherapy is used to prevent and treat brain metastases, a frequent occurrence with SCLC. Prophylactic cranial irradiation (PCI) is used in patients with limited or extensive disease to reduce the risk of brain metastases.

Extensive Disease

- The EP regimen is the regimen of choice to treat extensive-stage SCLC. The addi-tion of the PD-L1 inhibitors atezolizumab or **durvalumab** to carboplatin/etoposide improves OS.
- Concurrent radiotherapy is not routinely used in extensive disease.

Relapsed Disease

- Relapsed SCLC is usually less sensitive to chemotherapy. **Topotecan** (IV and oral) is considered the second-line treatment of choice, but other agents should be con-sidered because of their modest efficacy. If relapse occurs more than 3 months after first-line chemotherapy, national guidelines recommend single-agent PD-L1 inhibi-tor, gemcitabine, **irinotecan**, paclitaxel, docetaxel, oral etoposide, **temozolomide**, and vinorelbine; CAV regimen (**cyclophosphamide, doxorubicin, and vincristine**); and participation in a clinical trial.
- SCLC that recurs within 3 months of first-line chemotherapy is considered refractory to chemotherapy and unlikely to respond to a second-line regimen. Patients should receive best supportive care or be enrolled in a clinical trial.

EVALUATION OF THERAPEUTIC OUTCOMES

- Evaluate tumor response to chemotherapy for NSCLC at the end of the second or third cycle and at the end of every second cycle thereafter. Patients with stable dis-ease, objective response, or measurable decrease in tumor size should continue treat-ment until four to six cycles have been administered. Consider maintenance therapy with pemetrexed in responding patients with nonsquamous histology.
- Immune checkpoint inhibitors can display a different response pattern than tradi-tional chemotherapy or targeted therapy. The median time-to-response for immune checkpoint inhibitors is 10–12 weeks and the initial tumor response can appear radiologically as progression.
- Evaluate efficacy of first-line therapy for SCLC after two or three cycles of chemo-therapy. If there is no response or progressive disease, therapy can be discontinued or changed to a non–cross-resistant regimen. If responsive to chemotherapy, the

TABLE 63-5	Chemotherapy Regimens Used in the Treatment of SCLC	
	Regimen	**Drugs and Doses**
First Line	Etoposide/ cisplatin (EP)	Cisplatin 75 mg/m² IV on day 1
		Etoposide 100 mg/m² IV on days 1-3; repeat cycle every 3 weeks for 4-6 cycles
		or
		Cisplatin 60 mg/m² IV on day 1
		Etoposide 120 mg/m² IV on days 1-3; repeat cycle every 3 weeks for 4-6 cycles
	Etoposide/ carboplatin (EC)	Carboplatin AUC 5-6 IV on day 1
		Etoposide 100 mg/m² IV on days 1-3; repeat cycle every 3 weeks for 4-6 cycles
	EC + atezolizumab[a]	Carboplatin AUC 5 IV on day 1
		Etoposide 100 mg/m² IV on days 1-3
		Atezolizumab 1,200 mg IV on day 1; repeat cycle every 3 weeks for 4 cycles
		followed by
		Atezolizumab 1,200 mg every 3 weeks or 1680 mg every 4 weeks as maintenance
	EP + durvalumab[a]	Carboplatin AUC 5-6 IV on day 1
		Etoposide 80-100 mg/m² IV on days 1-3
		Durvalumab 1,500 mg IV on day 1; repeat cycle every 3 weeks for 4 cycles
		followed by
		Durvalumab 1,500 mg every 4 weeks as maintenance
	EC + durvalumab[a]	Cisplatin 75-80 mg/m² IV on day 1
		Etoposide 80-100 mg/m² IV on days 1-3
		Durvalumab 1,500 mg IV on day 1; repeat cycle every 3 weeks for 4 cycles
		followed by
		Durvalumab 1,500 mg every 4 weeks as maintenance
Second Line	Topotecan	Topotecan 1.5 mg/m²/day IV days 1-5; repeat every 3 weeks
	Lurbinectedin	Lurbinectedin 3.2 mg/m²/day IV day 1; repeat every 3 weeks

[a]Extensive stage only.

induction regimen should be administered for four to six cycles. Responding patients benefit from the addition of PCI following initial therapy.

- Intensive therapeutic monitoring is required for all patients with lung cancer to avoid drug-related and radiotherapy-related toxicities. These patients frequently have numerous concurrent medical problems requiring close attention.
- References should be consulted for management of common toxicities associated with the aggressive chemotherapy regimens used for lung cancer.

See Chapter 152, Lung Cancer, authored by Keith A. Hecht and Eve M. Segal, for a more detailed discussion of this topic.

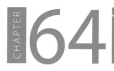
Lymphomas

- *Lymphomas* are a heterogeneous group of malignancies that arise from malignant transformation of immune cells residing predominantly in lymphoid tissues. Differences in histology have led to the classification of Hodgkin lymphoma (Reed-Sternberg cells) or non-Hodgkin lymphoma (NHL) (B- or T-cell lymphocyte markers).

Hodgkin Lymphoma: Pathophysiology

- B-cell transcriptional processes are disrupted during malignant transformation, preventing expression of B-cell surface markers and production of immunoglobulin messenger RNA. Alterations in the normal apoptotic pathways favor cell survival and proliferation.
- Malignant Reed–Sternberg cells overexpress nuclear factor-κB, which is associated with cell proliferation and antiapoptotic signals. Infections with viral and bacterial pathogens upregulate nuclear factor-κB. Epstein–Barr virus is found in many, but not all, HL tumors.

CLINICAL PRESENTATION

- Most patients with HL present with a painless, rubbery, enlarged lymph node in the supradiaphragmatic area and commonly have mediastinal nodal involvement. Asymptomatic adenopathy of the inguinal and axillary regions may also be present.
- Constitutional, or "B," symptoms (eg, fever, drenching night sweats, and weight loss) are present at diagnosis in approximately 25% of patients with HL.

DIAGNOSIS AND STAGING

- Diagnosis requires the presence of Reed–Sternberg cells in the lymph node biopsy.
- Staging is performed to provide prognostic information and to guide therapy. Clinical staging is based on noninvasive procedures such as history, physical examination, laboratory tests, and radiography, including positron emission tomography (PET). Pathologic staging is based on biopsy findings of strategic sites (eg, bone marrow, spleen, and abdominal nodes).
- At diagnosis, approximately half of patients have localized disease (stages I, II, and II$_E$) and the remainder have advanced disease (stage III or IV), of which 10%–15% is stage IV, metastatic disease.
- Prognosis predominantly depends on age and amount of disease; patients older than 65–70 years have a lower cure rate than younger patients. Patients with limited-stage disease (stages I and II) have a 90%–95% cure rate, whereas those with advanced disease (stages III and IV) have a 60%–80% cure rate.

TREATMENT

- <u>Goals of Treatment</u>: The goal is to maximize curability while minimizing short- and long-term treatment-related complications.
- Treatment options include radiation therapy (RT), chemotherapy, or both (combined-modality therapy). The therapeutic role of surgery is limited, regardless of stage.
- RT is an integral part of treatment and can be used alone for select patients with early-stage disease, although most patients will receive chemotherapy and radiation.
- Long-term complications of RT, chemotherapy, and chemoradiotherapy include gonadal dysfunction, secondary malignancies (eg, lung, breast, GI tract, and connective tissue), and cardiac disease.

INITIAL CHEMOTHERAPY

- Treat all stages and risk groups of HL with 8–12 weeks of chemotherapy and then obtain a restaging PET-CT (Table 64-1). Most patients with unfavorable disease will require RT.

SALVAGE CHEMOTHERAPY

- Response to salvage therapy depends on the extent and site of recurrence, previous therapy, and duration of first remission. Choice of salvage therapy should be guided by response to initial therapy and a patient's ability to tolerate therapy.
- Patients who relapse after an initial complete response can be treated with the same regimen, a non–cross-resistant regimen, or high-dose chemotherapy and autologous hematopoietic stem cell transplantation (HSCT).
- Lack of complete remission after initial therapy or relapse within 1 year after completing initial therapy is associated with a poor prognosis. Patients with these prognostic factors are candidates for high-dose chemotherapy and HSCT.
- **Brentuximab vedotin** is approved for the treatment of classical Hodgkin lymphoma after failure of autologous HSCT or after failure of at least two prior multi-agent chemotherapy regimens in patients who are not candidates for autologous HSCT, and also for patients with classical Hodgkin lymphoma at high risk of relapse or progression as consolidation therapy after autologous HSCT.
- Immune checkpoint inhibitors, specifically PD-1 (programmed death 1 pathway) inhibitors (eg, **nivolumab** and **pembrolizumab**), are approved for relapsed HL.

Non-Hodgkin Lymphoma: Pathophysiology

- NHLs are derived from monoclonal proliferation of malignant B or T lymphocytes and their precursors. Current classification schemes characterize NHLs according to cell of origin, clinical features, and morphologic features. Additional immunohistochemical markers, cytogenetic features, and genotypic characteristics may further classify NHL into subtypes.
- The World Health Organization (WHO) classification uses *grade* to refer to histologic parameters such as cell and nuclear size, density of chromatin, and proliferation fraction, and *aggressiveness* to denote clinical behavior of a tumor.

CLINICAL PRESENTATION

- Patients present with a variety of symptoms, which depend on site of involvement and whether it is nodal or extranodal.
- Adenopathy can be localized or generalized. Involved nodes are painless, rubbery, and discrete and usually located in the cervical and supraclavicular regions. Mesenteric or GI involvement can cause nausea, vomiting, obstruction, abdominal pain, palpable abdominal mass, or GI bleeding. Bone marrow involvement can cause symptoms related to anemia, neutropenia, or thrombocytopenia.
- Forty percent of patients with NHL present with B symptoms—fever, drenching night sweats, and weight loss.

DIAGNOSIS AND STAGING

- Diagnosis is established by biopsy of an involved lymph node. Diagnostic workup of NHL is generally similar to that of HL.
- NHL classification systems continue to evolve. Slow-growing or indolent lymphomas are favorable (untreated survival measured in years), whereas rapid-growing or aggressive lymphomas are unfavorable (untreated survival measured in weeks to months).
- Prognosis depends on histologic subtype and clinical risk factors (eg, age >60 years, performance status of two or more, abnormal lactate dehydrogenase, extranodal involvement, and stage III or IV disease). These risk factors are used to calculate the International Prognostic Index (IPI) which is most useful in patients with aggressive lymphomas.

TABLE 64-1 Combination Chemotherapy Regimens for Hodgkin Lymphoma

Drug	Dosage (mg/m²)	Route	Days
MOPP			
Mechlorethamine	6	IV	1, 8
Vincristine	1.4	IV	1, 8
Procarbazine	100	Oral	1–14
Prednisone	40	Oral	1–14
Repeat every 21 days			
ABVD			
Doxorubicin (Adriamycin)	25	IV	1, 15
Bleomycin	10	IV	1, 15
Vinblastine	6	IV	1, 15
Dacarbazine	375	IV	1, 15
Repeat every 28 days			
MOPP/ABVD			
Alternating months of MOPP and ABVD			
MOPP/ABV hybrid			
Mechlorethamine	6	IV	1
Vincristine	1.4	IV	1
Procarbazine	100	Oral	1–7
Prednisone	40	Oral	1–14
Doxorubicin	35	IV	8
Bleomycin	10	IV	8
Vinblastine	6	IV	8
Repeat every 28 days			
Stanford V			
Doxorubicin	25	IV	Weeks 1, 3, 5, 7, 9, 11
Vinblastine	6	IV	Weeks 1, 3, 5, 7, 9, 11
Mechlorethamine	6	IV	Weeks 1, 5, 9
Etoposide	60	IV	Weeks 3, 7, 11
Vincristine	1.4 add superscript a	IV	Weeks 2, 4, 6, 8, 10, 12
Bleomycin	5	IV	Weeks 2, 4, 6, 8
Prednisone	40	Oral	Every other day for 12 weeks; begin tapering at week 10
One course (12 weeks)			

(Continued)

	Dosage		
Drug	**(mg/m²)**	**Route**	**Days**
BEACOPP (standard dose)			
Bleomycin	10	IV	8
Etoposide	100	IV	1–3
Adriamycin (doxorubicin)	25	IV	1
Cyclophosphamide	650	IV	1
Oncovin (vincristine)	1.4[a]	IV	8
Procarbazine	100	Oral	1–7
Prednisone	40	Oral	1–14
Repeat every 21 days			
BEACOPP (escalated dose)			
Bleomycin	10	IV	8
Etoposide	200	IV	1–3
Adriamycin (doxorubicin)	35	IV	1
Cyclophosphamide	1250	IV	1
Oncovin (vincristine)	1.4[a]	IV	8
Procarbazine	100	Oral	1–7
Prednisone	40	Oral	1–14
Granulocyte colony-stimulating factor		Subcutaneously	8+
Repeat every 21 days			
A-AVD			
Brentuximab vedotin	1.2 mg/kg	IV	1, 15
Doxorubicin	25	IV	1, 15
Vinblastine	6	IV	1, 15
Dacarbazine	375	IV	1, 15

TABLE 64-1 Combination Chemotherapy Regimens for Hodgkin Lymphoma (*Continued*)

[a]Vincristine dose capped at 2 mg.

- A newer prognostic index for patients with indolent (follicular) lymphomas uses similar risk factors except that poor performance status is replaced with low hemoglobin (<12 g/dL [120 g/L; 7.45 mmol/L]). Current research is focused on prognostic importance of phenotypic and molecular characteristics of NHL, including molecular markers of apoptosis, cell-cycle regulation, cell lineage, and cell proliferation.

TREATMENT

- <u>Goals of Treatment</u>: The goals are to relieve symptoms and, whenever possible, cure the patient of disease while minimizing the risk of serious toxicity.

GENERAL PRINCIPLES

- Appropriate therapy for NHL depends on many factors, including patient age, histologic type, stage and site of disease, presence of adverse prognostic factors, and patient preference.

- Treatment options include RT, chemotherapy, and biological agents. RT is used for remission induction with early-stage, localized disease and, more commonly, as a palliative measure in advanced disease.
- Effective chemotherapy ranges from single-agent therapy for indolent (follicular) lymphomas to aggressive, complex combination regimens for aggressive disease.

FOLLICULAR LYMPHOMAS

- Follicular lymphomas occur in older adults, with a majority having advanced disease that includes the chromosomal translocation t(14;18). Clinical course is generally indolent, with median survival of 8–10 years. The natural history of follicular lymphoma is unpredictable, with spontaneous regression of objective disease seen in 20%–30% of patients.

Localized Follicular Lymphoma

- Options for stages I and II follicular lymphoma include locoregional RT and immunotherapy (ie, **rituximab**) with or without chemotherapy or RT.
- RT is the standard treatment and is usually curative. Chemotherapy is not recommended, unless the patient has high-risk, stage II disease.

Advanced Follicular Lymphoma

- Management of stages II bulky, III, and IV indolent lymphomas is controversial because standard approaches are not curative. Median time to relapse is only 18–36 months. After relapse, response can be reinduced; however, response rates and durations decrease with each retreatment.
- Therapeutic options are diverse and include watchful waiting, RT, single-agent chemotherapy, combination chemotherapy, biologic therapy, radioimmunotherapy, and combined-modality therapy. Immediate aggressive therapy does not improve survival compared with conservative therapy (ie, watchful waiting followed by single-agent chemotherapy, rituximab, or RT, when treatment is needed).
- Rituximab, a chimeric monoclonal antibody directed at the CD20 molecule on B cells, is one of the most widely used therapies for follicular lymphoma. It is approved for first-line therapy either alone or combined with chemotherapy and as maintenance therapy with stable disease or with partial or complete response following induction chemotherapy.
  - ✓ The most common chemotherapy regimen used with rituximab is the CHOP regimen (Table 64-2). Practice guidelines list rituximab maintenance for up to 2 years as an option in both first- and second-line therapy.
  - ✓ Rituximab adverse effects are usually infusion-related, especially after the first infusion, and consist of fever, chills, respiratory symptoms, fatigue, headache, pruritus, and angioedema. Pretreatment with oral acetaminophen, 650 mg, and diphenhydramine, 50 mg, 30 minutes before the infusion is recommended.
  - ✓ **Bendamustine** is an IV alkylating agent approved for relapsed or refractory indolent NHL that has been shown to be noninferior to R-CHOP when combined with rituximab.

TABLE 64-2	CHOP Regimen		
Drug	**Dose**	**Route**	**Treatment Days**
Cyclophosphamide	750 mg/m^2	IV	1
Doxorubicin[a]	50 mg/m^2	IV	1
Vincristine[b]	1.4 mg/m^2	IV	1
Prednisone	100 mg	Oral	1–5
One cycle is 21 days			

[a]Another name for doxorubicin is hydroxydaunorubicin.
[b]Vincristine dose is typically capped at 2 mg

- A second anti-CD20 monoclonal antibody, **obinutuzumab**, is approved in combination with chemotherapy, as first-line, second-line, and subsequent therapy options for treatment of follicular lymphoma.
- **Lenalidomide** is an immunomodulating agent approved in combination with rituximab for first- and second-line therapy of follicular lymphoma.
- ^{90}Y-ibritumomab tiuxetan is an anti-CD20 radioimmunoconjugate, linking mouse antibodies to radioisotopes. Radiation is selectively delivered to tumor cells expressing the CD20 antigen and to adjacent tumor cells that do not express it.
  - ✓ Radioimmunotherapy is generally well tolerated. Toxicities include infusion-related reactions, myelosuppression, and possibly myelodysplastic syndrome or acute myelogenous leukemia.
- Phosphatidylinositol-3-kinase (PI3K) inhibitors reduce a messenger that affects malignant B lymphocyte proliferation and survival. **Idelalisib, copanlisib,** and **duvelisib** are treatment options for second-line therapy, and **umbralisib** is listed as third-line therapy with relapsed or refractory follicular lymphoma. All of the PI3K inhibitors can cause severe neutropenia, diarrhea, infection, and pneumonia, as well as drug-specific toxicities.
- An activating mutation of the epigenetic regulator EZH2 is found in 20% to 25% of patients with follicular lymphoma. **Tazemetostat** is a first-generation EZH2 inhibitor currently approved for EZH2 mutation-positive relapsed or refractory disease after two prior therapies, or EZH2 wild-type or unknown relapsed/refractory disease with no satisfactory alternative treatment options.
- High-dose chemotherapy followed by autologous or allogeneic HSCT is an option for relapsed follicular lymphoma. The recurrence rate is lower after allogeneic than after autologous HSCT, but the benefit is offset by increased treatment-related mortality.

AGGRESSIVE LYMPHOMAS

- Diffuse large B-cell lymphomas (DLBCLs) are the most common lymphoma in patients of all ages but most commonly seen in the seventh decade. Extranodal disease is present at diagnosis in 30%–40% of patients. IPI score correlates with prognosis. Diffuse aggressive lymphomas are sensitive to chemotherapy, with cure achieved in some patients.

Treatment of Localized Disease

- Stage I and nonbulky stage II should be treated with three or four cycles of rituximab and CHOP (R-CHOP) followed by locoregional RT or six to eight cycles of R-CHOP with no RT.
- Consider six cycles of R-CHOP without radiation if disease presents at sites where radiotherapy may lead to significant morbidity.

Treatment of Advanced Disease

- Treat bulky stage II and stages III and IV lymphomas with R-CHOP or rituximab and CHOP-like chemotherapy until achieving complete response (usually 4–6 cycles). Maintenance therapy following a complete response does not improve survival.
- Consider high-dose chemotherapy with autologous HSCT in high-risk patients who respond to standard chemotherapy and meet HSCT criteria.
- Although historically elderly adults have lower complete response and survival rates than younger patients, full-dose R-CHOP is recommended as initial treatment for aggressive lymphoma in the elderly. **Lenalidomide** is an option if maintenance therapy is considered in older adults who have responded to treatment.

Treatment of Refractory or Relapsed Disease

- Approximately one-third of patients with aggressive lymphoma will require salvage therapy at some point. Salvage therapy is more likely to induce response if the response to initial chemotherapy was complete (chemosensitivity) than if it was primarily or partially resistant to chemotherapy.

- High-dose chemotherapy with autologous HSCT is the therapy of choice for younger patients with chemosensitive relapse.
- Salvage regimens incorporate drugs not used as initial therapy. Commonly used regimens include DHAP (**dexamethasone, cytarabine**, and **cisplatin**), ESHAP (**etoposide, methylprednisolone**, cytarabine, and cisplatin), ICE (**ifosfamide, carboplatin**, etoposide), and MINE (**mesna**, ifosfamide, **mitoxantrone**, and etoposide). None is clearly superior to the others.
- Rituximab is being evaluated in combination with many salvage regimens; exclude rituximab in second-line therapy if the disease is refractory or if the duration of remission is less than 6 months.
- Three chimeric antigen receptor (CAR) T-cell therapies, **tisagenlecleucel, axicabtagene ciloleucel**, and **lisocabtagene maraleucel** have been approved for relapsed and refractory disease after failure of two or more lines of systemic treatment. CAR T-cell therapies are associated with a high incidence of cytokine release syndrome, which is characterized by fever, hypoxia, and hypotension, and may require the use of vasopressors in severe cases. Severe neurological toxicities such as encephalopathy and seizures can also occur.

EVALUATION OF THERAPEUTIC OUTCOMES

- Evaluate therapeutic response based on physical examination, radiologic evidence, PET/computed tomography (CT) scanning, and other baseline findings.

See Chapter 155, Lymphomas, authored by Alexandre Chan, Chia Jie Tan, and Shawn Griffin, for a more detailed discussion of this topic.

CHAPTER 65

Prostate Cancer

- *Prostate cancer* is a malignant neoplasm that arises from the prosta surgery or radiation therapy, but advanced prostate cancer is not yet curable.

PATHOPHYSIOLOGY

- The normal prostate is composed of acinar secretory cells that are altered when invaded by cancer. The major pathologic cell type is adenocarcinoma (>95% of cases).
- Prostate cancer can be graded. Well-differentiated tumors grow slowly, whereas poorly differentiated tumors grow rapidly and have a poor prognosis.
- Metastatic spread can occur by local extension, lymphatic drainage, or hematogenous dissemination. Skeletal metastases from hematogenous spread are the most common sites of distant spread. The lung, liver, brain, and adrenal glands are the most common sites of visceral involvement, but these organs are not usually involved initially.
- Hormonal regulation of androgen synthesis is mediated through a series of biochemical interactions between the hypothalamus, pituitary, adrenal glands, and testes (Fig. 65-1).
- The testes and the adrenal glands are the major sources of androgens, specifically dihydrotestosterone (DHT).
- Luteinizing hormone–releasing hormone (LHRH) from the hypothalamus stimulates the release of luteinizing hormone (LH) and follicle-stimulating hormone (FSH) from the anterior pituitary gland.
- LH complexes with receptors on the Leydig cell testicular membrane, stimulating the production of testosterone and small amounts of estrogen.
- FSH acts on testicular Sertoli cells to promote maturation of LH receptors and produce an androgen-binding protein.
- Circulating testosterone and estradiol influence the synthesis of LHRH, LH, and FSH by a negative-feedback loop at the hypothalamic and pituitary level.

CHEMOPREVENTION

- The use of 5-α-reductase inhibitors, **finasteride** and **dutasteride**, to prevent prostate cancer has been debated for more than a decade. Based on the concern for the development of more aggressive tumors, lack of survival benefit, and increased risk of adverse drug reactions, these agents are not approved or recommended for preventing prostate cancer.

SCREENING

- Screening recommendations for prostate cancer have changed, and digital rectal examination (DRE) and prostate-specific antigen (PSA) are no longer recommended for patients without a discussion with their clinician about risks versus benefits. The American Urologic Association does not recommend routine screening in biologic males between the ages of 40 and 54 years of average risk but recommends that the risks and benefits of prostate cancer screening are discussed with individuals aged 55–69 years. Biologic males who elect to have screening should do so no more than every 2 years and screening every 5 years may be adequate.
- PSA is a glycoprotein produced and secreted by prostate epithelial cells. Acute urinary retention, acute prostatitis, prostatic ischemia or infarction, and benign prostatic hypertrophy (BPH) increase PSA, thereby limiting the usefulness of PSA alone for early detection, but it is a useful marker for monitoring response to therapy.

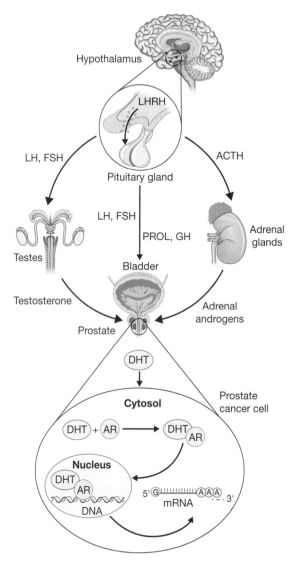

FIGURE 65-1. Hormonal regulation of the prostate gland. (ACTH, adrenocorticotropic hormone; DHT, dihydrotestosterone; DNA, deoxyribonucleic acid; FSH, follicle-stimulating hormone; GH, growth hormone; LH, luteinizing hormone; LHRH, luteinizing hormone–releasing hormone; mRNA, messenger RNA; PROL, prolactin.)

CLINICAL PRESENTATION

- Localized prostate cancer is usually asymptomatic.
- Locally invasive prostate cancer is associated with ureteral dysfunction or impingement, such as alterations in micturition (eg, urinary frequency, hesitancy, and dribbling), and impotence.

- Advanced disease commonly presents with back pain and stiffness due to osseous metastases. Untreated spinal cord lesions can lead to cord compression. Lower extremity edema can occur as a result of lymphatic obstruction. Anemia and weight loss are nonspecific signs of advanced disease.

TREATMENT

- <u>Goals of Treatment</u>: In early-stage prostate cancer, the goal is to minimize morbidity and mortality. Early-stage disease may be treated with surgery, radiation, or expectant management; surgery and radiation are curative but also associated with significant morbidity and mortality. In advanced prostate cancer, treatment focuses on providing symptom relief and maintaining quality of life.

GENERAL APPROACH

- Initial treatment depends on disease stage, Gleason score, presence of symptoms, and patient's life expectancy. See Table 65-1 for management recommendations based on risk of recurrence.
- Initial treatment modality for advanced prostate cancer is androgen ablation (eg, orchiectomy or LHRH agonists with or without antiandrogens). Patients with metastatic castration-resistant prostate cancer (CRPC) should receive best supportive care in addition to other treatments; genetic testing is recommended to help direct therapy.

NONPHARMACOLOGIC THERAPY

Observation

- Observation is utilized in biologic males with a shorter life expectancy and lower risk of disease. Observation involves monitoring the course of disease with laboratory testing and imaging, and starting palliative treatment if the cancer progresses.

TABLE 65-1	Initial Management of Prostate Cancer Based on Expected Survival and Recurrence Risk	
Recurrence Risk	**Expected Survival (Years)**	**Initial Therapy**
Very Low		
Has all of the following:	<10	Observation
• T_{1c}	10–20	Active surveillance
• Gleason group 1	20 or more	Active surveillance
• PSA less than 10 ng/mL (mcg/L)		or
• Fewer than 3 prostate biopsies positive, ≤50% cancer in each core		radical prostatectomy
• PSA density <0.15 ng/mL/g (mcg/L/g)		or
		radiation therapy
Low		
Has all of the following but does not qualify for very low risk:	10 or more	Active surveillance
• T_1–T_{2a}		or
• Gleason Group 1		radical prostatectomy
• PSA less than 10 ng/mL (mcg/L)		or
		radiation therapy
	<10	Observation
		(Continued)

| TABLE 65-1 | Initial Management of Prostate Cancer Based on Expected Survival and Recurrence Risk (*Continued*) |

Recurrence Risk		Expected Survival (Years)	Initial Therapy
Intermediate			
• Has no high-risk group features			
• Intermediate risk factors (IRFs):			
• T_{2b}–T_{2c}			
• Gleason Group 2-3			
• PSA10-20 ng/mL (mcg/L)			
Favorable Intermediate risk	Has all of following: • Only 1 intermediate risk factor • Gleason Grade Group 1–2 • <50% biopsy cores positive	10 or more	Active surveillance or radical prostatectomy +/– pelvic lymph node dissection or radiation therapy
		<10	Observation or Radiation therapy or Brachytherapy
Unfavorable intermediate risk	Has one or more of the following: • 2 or 3 intermediate risk factors • Gleason Grade Group 3 • ≥50% biopsy cores positive	10 or more	Radical prostatectomy +/– pelvic lymph node dissection or radiation therapy + ADT[a,b] or radiation therapy + brachytherapy +/– ADT
		<10	Observation or radiation therapy + ADT[a,b] or radiation therapy + brachytherapy +/– ADT
High			
Has no very-high risk features and has exactly ONE high-risk feature: • T_{3a} or • Gleason Grade Group 4–5 or 8 • PSA >20 ng/mL (mcg/L)		5 or more	Radiation therapy + ADT +/– docetaxel or radiation therapy + ADT + brachytherapy or radical prostatectomy and pelvic lymph node dissection

(*Continued*)

Recurrence Risk	Expected Survival (Years)	Initial Therapy
TABLE 65-1 Initial Management of Prostate Cancer Based on Expected Survival and Recurrence Risk (*Continued*)		
Very High		
Has at least one of the following: • T_{3b}–T_4 • Primary Gleason pattern 5 • 2 or 3 high-risk features • 4 cores with Gleason Grade Group 4 or 5	5 or more	Radiation therapy + ADT +/− docetaxel or radiation therapy + ADT + brachytherapy or radical prostatectomy and pelvic lymph node dissection
Locally Advanced/Metastatic disease		
Any T, N_1	5 or more	ADT +/− abiraterone and prednisone or radiation therapy + ADT +/− with or without abiraterone and prednisone)
Any T, Any N, M_1		ADT alone or in addition to: Apalutamide Abiraterone with prednisone Docetaxel Enzalutamide

[a]ADT therapy to achieve serum testosterone levels <50 ng/dL (1.7 nmol/L).
[b]LHRH agonists, LHRH/GnRH antagonists, or surgical castration are equivalent.

- Advantages include avoiding adverse effects of definitive therapies and minimizing risk of unnecessary therapies. The major disadvantage is the risk of cancer progression requiring more intense therapy.

Surgery and Radiation Therapy

- Bilateral orchiectomy rapidly reduces circulating androgens to castrate levels. Many patients are not surgical candidates due to advanced age, and other patients find this procedure psychologically unacceptable. Orchiectomy is the preferred initial treatment for patients with impending spinal cord compression or ureteral obstruction.
- Radical prostatectomy and radiation therapy are potentially curative therapies but are associated with complications that must be weighed against expected benefit. Consequently, many patients postpone therapy until symptoms develop.
- Complications of radical prostatectomy include blood loss, stricture formation, incontinence, lymphocele, fistula formation, anesthetic risk, and impotence. Nerve-sparing techniques facilitate return of sexual potency after prostatectomy.
- Acute complications of radiation therapy include cystitis, proctitis, hematuria, urinary retention, penoscrotal edema, and impotence.
- Chronic complications of radiation therapy include proctitis, diarrhea, cystitis, enteritis, impotence, urethral stricture, and incontinence.

PHARMACOLOGIC THERAPY

Drug Treatments of First Choice

Luteinizing Hormone–Releasing Hormone Agonists

- LHRH agonists are a reversible method of androgen ablation and are as effective as orchiectomy.
- There are no comparative trials of LHRH agonists, so the choice is usually based on cost and patient and physician preference for a dosing schedule (Table 65-2). **Leuprolide acetate, leuprolide depot, leuprolide implant, triptorelin depot, triptorelin implant,** and **goserelin acetate implant** are currently available. Dosing intervals range from once monthly to every 6 months. Leuprolide implant is a mini-osmotic pump that delivers daily doses for 1 year. Testosterone castration levels are achieved in 28 days with leuprolide.
- The most common adverse effects of LHRH agonists include disease flare-ups during the first week of therapy (eg, increased bone pain or urinary symptoms), hot flashes, erectile impotence, decreased libido, and injection-site reactions. Use of an antiandrogen (eg, **flutamide, bicalutamide,** or **nilutamide**) prior to initiation of LHRH therapy and continuing for 2–4 weeks is a strategy to minimize initial tumor flare.
- Decreases in bone mineral density complicate androgen deprivation therapy (ADT), resulting in increased risk of osteoporosis, osteopenia, and skeletal fractures. Calcium and vitamin D supplements and a baseline bone mineral density are recommended. Initiate an antiresorptive agent (eg, **alendronate**, **denosumab**, or **zoledronic acid**) to reduce the risk of skeletal-related events.
- Screen patients receiving ADT for cardiovascular disease and diabetes due to increased risk of metabolic effects.

Leutinizing Hormone–Releasing Hormone/Gonadotropin Releasing–Hormone Antagonists (GnRH Antagonists)

- GnRH antagonists **degarelix** and **relugolix** bind reversibly to GnRH receptors in the pituitary gland, reducing the production of testosterone to castrate levels in 7 days or less. A major advantage of GnRH antagonists over LHRH agonists is the lack of tumor flare.
- Degarelix is administered as a subcutaneous injection every 28 days. Injection site reactions and hot flashes are the most frequently reported adverse effects. Osteoporosis may develop, and calcium and vitamin D supplementation should be considered.
- Relugolix is an oral agent taken daily; adherence is critical for maintenance of testosterone suppression. Cardiovascular risk is not increased with relugolix in contrast to the other FDA-approved LHRH agonists and GnRH antagonists. Hot flashes, hyperglycemia, hypertriglyceridemia, musculoskeletal pain, and fatigue were common toxicities, and providers should use with caution the medications that increase QTC interval, or are inhibitors of cytochrome P450 (CYP) 3A4 or the p-glycoprotein(P-gp) efflux transporter.

Antiandrogens

- Monotherapy with first-generation antiandrogens flutamide, bicalutamide, and nilutamide is no longer recommended due to decreased efficacy as compared with patients treated with LHRH agonist therapy. Antiandrogens are indicated for advanced prostate cancer only when combined with an LHRH agonist (flutamide and bicalutamide]) or orchiectomy (nilutamide). In combination, antiandrogens can reduce the LHRH agonist–induced flare in patients with metastatic disease.
- Adverse reactions with first-generation antiandrogens include but are not limited to gynecomastia, hot flashes, GI disturbances, decreased libido, LFT abnormalities, and breast tenderness.
- **Apalutamide**, **enzalutamide**, and **darolutamide** are second-generation antiandrogens. Apalalutamide is approved for the treatment of nonmetastatic CRPC and

TABLE 65-2	Hormonal Therapies for Prostate Cancer			
Drug	Usual Dose	Hepatic/Renal Adjustments	Monitoring Parameters	Administration
First-Generation Antiandrogens				
Bicalutamide	50 mg/day PO (up to 150 mg/day unlabeled use)	Discontinue if ALT >2 times upper limit of normal or patient develops jaundice	Serum transaminases should be monitored prior to start of therapy and monthly for the first 4 months, then periodically thereafter Periodic monitoring of CBC, EKG, echocardiograms, serum testosterone, luteinizing hormone, and PSA	May be taken with or without food
Flutamide	750 mg/day PO	Contraindicated in patients with hepatic impairment No dosage adjustment necessary in chronic renal impairment	Serum transaminases should be monitored prior to start of therapy and monthly for the first 4 months, then periodically thereafter Monitor for tumor reduction, PSA, testosterone/estrogen, and phosphatase serum levels	Administered orally in three divided doses; capsule may be opened into applesauce, pudding, or other soft foods
Nilutamide	300 mg/day PO for first month then 150 mg/day	Contraindicated in patients with hepatic impairment Discontinue if ALT >2 times upper limit of normal or patient develops jaundice	Serum transaminases should be monitored prior to start of therapy and monthly for the first 4 months, then periodically thereafter Chest x-ray at baseline and consideration of pulmonary function testing (at baseline), PSA periodically	May be taken with or without food
Second-Generation Antiandrogens				
Apalutamide	240 mg/day PO	No adjustment necessary for renal or hepatic impairment	Complete blood counts baseline and periodically LFTs baseline and periodically TSH at baseline and every 4 months, PSA periodically	May be taken with or without food

Drug	Dosing	Renal/Hepatic Adjustment	Monitoring	Administration
Darolutamide	1200 mg/day PO	For moderate hepatic impairment or severe renal impairment (not on dialysis); dose should be reduced to 600 mg/day	Complete blood counts baseline and periodically LFTs baseline and periodically, PSA periodically	Take with food
Enzalutamide	160 mg/day PO	No adjustment necessary for renal or hepatic impairment	Complete blood counts baseline and periodically LFTs baseline and periodically, PSA periodically	May be taken with or without food
Androgen Synthesis Inhibitor				
Abiraterone acetate	Abiraterone acetate: 1000 mg/day PO + prednisone 5 mg daily PO (castration-naïve) or BID PO (CRPC). Micronized abiraterone: 500 mg daily PO + methylprednisolone 4 mg BID PO (CRPC)	250 mg daily for Child-Pugh Class B; avoid use in Child-Pugh Class C Withhold treatment if LFTs >5 times the ULN or bilirubin >3 ULN	Serum transaminases should be monitored prior to start of therapy, every 2 weeks for 3 months, then monthly thereafter Monitor for signs and symptoms of adrenocorticoid insufficiency; monthly for hypertension, hypokalemia, and fluid retention, PSA periodically	For standard abiraterone, administer on an empty stomach, at least 1 hour before and 2 hours after food (micronized abiraterone can be given regardless of food)
Luteinizing-Hormone Releasing Hormone Agonists				
Goserelin	3.6 mg SQ implant every month 10.8 mg SQ implant every 3 months	No adjustment necessary for renal or hepatic impairment	Monitor bone mineral density, serum calcium, and cholesterol/lipids, PSA periodically	Vary injection site
Leuprolide	7.5 mg IM every month 22.5 mg IM every 3 months 30 mg IM every 4 months 45 mg IM every 6 months	No adjustment necessary for renal or hepatic impairment	Serum testosterone ~4 weeks after initiation, PSA, blood glucose, and HgbA$_{1c}$ prior to initiation and periodically thereafter, PSA periodically	Vary injection site
Triptorelin	3.75 mg IM every month 11.25 mg IM every 3 months 22.5 mg IM every 6 months	No adjustment necessary for renal or hepatic impairment	Monitor serum testosterone levels and PSA periodically	Vary injection site

(Continued)

TABLE 65-2 Hormonal Therapies for Prostate Cancer (*Continued*)

Drug	Usual Dose	Hepatic/Renal Adjustments	Monitoring Parameters	Administration
Luteinizing-Hormone Releasing Hormone/Gonadotropin-Releasing Hormone Receptor Antagonists				
Degarelix	240 mg SQ loading dose 80 mg SQ every 28 days (following 28 days after loading dose)	Use with caution with CL$_{cr}$ <50 mL/min (0.83 mL/s) Do not use in patients with severe hepatic impairment	PSA periodically, serum testosterone monthly until castration achieved then every other month, LFTs at baseline in addition to serum electrolytes and bone mineral density	Vary injection site
Relugolix	360 mg PO followed by 120 mg PO daily	No adjustment necessary for renal or hepatic impairment	PSA periodically, LFTs and serum electrolytes at baseline and periodically; bone mineral density periodically	May be taken with or without food

ALT, alanine aminotransferase; BID, twice daily; CBC, complete blood count; CL$_{cr}$, creatinine clearance; CNS, central nervous system; CYP, cytochrome P450; CRPC, castrate-resistant prostate cancer; EKG, electrocardiogram; GI, gastrointestinal; HgbA1$_c$, hemoglobin A1$_c$; IM, intramuscular injection; INR, international normalized ratio; LFT, liver function test; PO, oral administration; PSA, prostate-specific antigen; SQ, subcutaneous injection; TSH, thyroid stimulating hormone; ULN, upper limit of normal.

metastatic castration-naïve prostate cancer. Enzalutamide may be used in the first-line setting to delay the initiation of chemotherapy in nonmetastatic CRPC, as well as metastatic castration-naïve and metastatic CRPC. Darolutamide is approved for nonmetastatic CRPC.

- Adverse effects of second-generation antiandrogens include, but are not limited to, fatigue, GI disturbances, musculoskeletal disorders, and seizures.

Combined Androgen Blockade

- Up to 80% of patients with advanced prostate cancer will respond to initial hormonal manipulation with disease progression seen within 2–4 years. The rationale for combined androgen blockade (CAB) is to interfere with multiple hormonal pathways to completely eliminate androgen action. Antiandrogen therapy should precede, or be co-administered with LHRH agonists; studies of short-term or long-term CAB have shown that any survival advantage for patients treated with CAB, if present, is small.

Alternative Drug Treatments

- Selection of salvage therapy depends on what was used as initial therapy. Radiotherapy can be used after failed radical prostatectomy. ADT can be used after progression of disease following radiation therapy or radical prostatectomy.
- **Abiraterone** is an androgen synthesis inhibitor that targets CYP17A1, resulting in decreased circulating levels of testosterone. It is indicated in patients with metastatic castration-naïve prostate cancer or metastatic CRPC. Prednisone is prescribed concurrently to mitigate potential adverse reactions due to abiraterone-induced hypoadrenalism (eg, hypertension, hypokalemia, and edema). Review medication profiles for potential drug interactions because abiraterone is an inhibitor of CYP2D6.

Chemotherapy

- **Docetaxel,** 75 mg/m^2 every 3 weeks, combined with **prednisone**, 5 mg twice daily, improves survival in CRPC. The most common adverse events include nausea, alopecia, and myelosuppression (Table 65-3).
- **Cabazitaxel** 25 mg/m^2 every 3 weeks with prednisone 10 mg daily significantly improves progression-free and overall survival in patients previously treated with docetaxel and prednisone. Neutropenia, febrile neutropenia, neuropathy, and diarrhea are the most significant toxicities.

Immunotherapy

- **Sipuleucel-T** is a novel autologous cellular immunotherapy approved for asymptomatic or minimally symptomatic metastatic CRPC. No clinical trials have compared sipuleucel-T to secondary hormonal therapies. Hypersensitivity, chills, fatigue, and fever are common toxicities.
- The immune checkpoint inhibitor **pembrolizumab** inhibits signals that lead to T-cell senescence which increases the immune response to cancer. Approximately 5%–12% of metastatic CRPC patients have documented MSI-H or dMMR by molecular testing which makes pembrolizumab a viable treatment option. Fatigue and immune-mediated adverse reactions are most commonly seen.

Targeted Therapy

- Poly (ADP ribose) polymerase (PARP) inhibitors, including **olaparib** and **rucaparib**, can be considered in men with metastatic CRPC who have specific somatic or germline alterations in genes involved in homologous recombination, such as *BRCA1* and *BRCA2*.
- Fatigue (including asthenia), nausea, anemia, and decreased appetite are the most common toxicities for these two PARP inhibitors.

TABLE 65-3	Chemotherapy, Immunotherapy, and Targeted Therapy for Prostate Cancer			
Drug	Usual Dose	Hepatic/Renal Adjustments	Monitoring Parameters	Administration
Antimicrotubule Agents				
Cabazitaxel	25 mg/m^2 IV every 3 weeks	Discontinue if ALT >2 times upper limit of normal or patient develops jaundice	CBC weekly during the first cycle, then prior to each treatment, PSA periodically Monitor for hypersensitivity	Administer IV infusion over 1 hour
Docetaxel	75 mg/m^2 IV every 3 weeks	AST/ALT >1.5 times the upper limit of normal and alkaline phosphatase >2.5 times the upper limit of normal do not administer	CBC with differential, LFTs, bilirubin, alkaline phosphatase, renal function, PSA periodically Monitor for hypersensitivity reactions	Administer IV infusion over 1 hour Premedication with corticosteroids for 3 days beginning the day before
Immunotherapy				
Pembrolizumab	200 mg IV every 3 weeks or 400 mg IV every 6 weeks	No adjustment needed for baseline renal/hepatic impairment; treat as immune-mediated toxicity if occurs during treatment	CBC, LFTs, renal function, thyroid function, glucose at baseline and during therapy, PSA periodically	Administer over 30 minutes
Sipuleucel-T	Each injection contains >50 million autologous CD54+ cells (obtained through leukapheresis) activated with PAP-GM-CSF Dose is given every 2 weeks for 3 total doses	No dosage adjustment necessary for renal or hepatic dysfunction	No specific laboratory monitoring recommended, PSA periodically	Administer IV infusion over 1 hour Observe the patient for 30 minutes after the completion of the infusion Premedicate with acetaminophen and an antihistamine 30 minutes prior to administration

Targeted Therapy

Olaparib	300 mg PO BID	Reduce dose for moderate renal impairment	CBC at baseline and monthly, renal function periodically, PSA periodically	Administer with or without food
Rucaparib	600 mg PO BID	None	CBC at baseline and monthly, PSA periodically	Administer with or without food

Nuclear Medicine

Radium-223	50 kBq/kg (1.35 µCi) administered every 4 weeks for 6 injections	None	CBC should be monitored prior to every injection, PSA periodically	Administer radium-223 by slow IV injection over 1 minute

ALT, alanine aminotransferase; AST, asparate aminotransferase; BID, twice daily; CBC, complete blood count; CYP, cytochrome P450; IV, intravenous administration; LFT, liver function test; PAP-GM-CSF, prostatic acid phosphatase granulocyte-macrophage colony-stimulating factor; PO, oral administration; PSA, prostate surface antigen.

Nuclear Medicine

- Radium-223, an alpha emitter, can be used in first-, second-, or third-line therapy in patients with metastatic CRPC with symptomatic primary bone metastases. It has not been approved for use with concomitant abiraterone, second-generation antiandrogens, chemotherapy, immunotherapy, or targeted therapy.
- Radium-223 improved survival, pain-related outcomes, quality of life, and decreased opioid needs. The most common adverse effects include nausea, diarrhea, vomiting, peripheral edema, and bone marrow suppression.

EVALUATION OF THERAPEUTIC OUTCOMES

- Monitor primary tumor size, involved lymph nodes, and tumor marker response such as PSA with definitive, curative therapy. PSA level is checked every 6–12 months for the first 5 years, then annually.
- Monitor medication adherence for orally administered treatments.

See Chapter 154, Prostate Cancer, authored by Daniel J. Crona and Amber B. Cipriani, for a more detailed discussion of this topic.

66

Glaucoma

- *Glaucomas* are ocular disorders that lead to an optic neuropathy characterized by changes in the optic nerve head (optic disc) that is associated with loss of visual sensitivity and field.

PATHOPHYSIOLOGY

- There are two major types of glaucoma: *primary open-angle glaucoma* (POAG) or ocular hypertension, which accounts for most cases and is therefore the focus of this chapter, and *primary angle closure glaucoma* (PACG). Either type can be a primary inherited disorder, congenital, or secondary to disease, trauma, or drugs.
- In POAG, the specific cause of optic nerve damage is unknown. Increased intraocular pressure (IOP) was historically considered to be the sole cause. Additional contributing factors include increased susceptibility of the optic nerve to ischemia, excitotoxicity, autoimmune reactions, and other abnormal physiologic processes.
- Although IOP is a poor predictor of which patients will have visual field loss, the risk of visual field loss increases with increasing IOP. IOP is not constant; it changes with pulse, blood pressure, forced expiration or coughing, neck compression, and posture. IOP demonstrates diurnal variation with a minimum pressure around 6 PM and a maximum pressure upon awakening.
- The balance between the inflow and outflow of aqueous humor determines IOP. Pharmacologic studies suggest that α_2-adrenergic agonists, β-adrenergic blockers, dopamine blockers, carbonic anhydrase inhibitors (CAIs), melatonin-1 agonists, and adenylate cyclase stimulators decrease aqueous inflow by reducing aqueous humor production. Outflow is increased by cholinergic agents (eg, pilocarpine), which contract the ciliary muscle and open the trabecular meshwork, and by prostaglandin analogs and α_2-adrenergic agonists, which increase uveoscleral outflow.
- Secondary OAG has many causes, including exfoliation syndrome, pigmentary glaucoma, systemic diseases, trauma, surgery, ocular inflammatory diseases, and medications. Secondary glaucoma can be classified as pretrabecular (normal meshwork is covered and prevents outflow of aqueous humor), trabecular (meshwork is altered or material accumulates in the intertrabecular spaces), or posttrabecular (episcleral venous blood pressure is increased).
- Many medications can increase IOP (Table 66-1). The potential to induce or worsen glaucoma depends on the type of glaucoma and on whether it is adequately controlled.
- PACG occurs when there is a physical blockage of the trabecular meshwork, resulting in increased IOP.

CLINICAL PRESENTATION

- POAG is a bilateral, often asymmetric, genetically determined disorder constituting 60%–70% of all glaucomas and 90%–95% of primary glaucomas in the United States. progresses slowly, and is usually asymptomatic until the onset of substantial visual field loss. Central visual acuity is maintained, even in the late stages.
- Patients with PACG typically experience intermittent prodromal symptoms (eg, blurred or hazy vision with halos around lights and, occasionally, headache). Acute episodes produce symptoms associated with a cloudy, edematous cornea; ocular pain; nausea, vomiting, and abdominal pain; and diaphoresis.

TABLE 66-1	Drugs That May Induce or Potentiate Increased Intraocular Pressure

Open-angle glaucoma
Ophthalmic corticosteroids (high risk)
Systemic corticosteroids
Nasal/Inhaled corticosteroids
Fenoldopam
Ophthalmic anticholinergics
Succinylcholine
Vasodilators (low risk)
Cimetidine (low risk)

Closed-angle glaucoma
Topical anticholinergics
Topical sympathomimetics
Systemic anticholinergics
Heterocyclic antidepressants
Low-potency phenothiazines
Antihistamines
Ipratropium
Benzodiazepines (low risk)
Theophylline (low risk)
Vasodilators (low risk)
Systemic sympathomimetics (low risk)
CNS stimulants (low risk)
Serotonin-selective reuptake inhibitors
Imipramine
Venlafaxine
Topiramate
Tetracyclines (low risk)
Carbonic anhydrase inhibitors (low risk)
Monoamine oxidase inhibitors (low risk)
Topical cholinergics (low risk)

DIAGNOSIS

- POAG is confirmed by the presence of characteristic optic disc changes and visual field loss, with or without increased IOP. *Normal tension glaucoma* refers to disc changes, visual field loss, and IOP less than 21 mm Hg (2.8 kPa). *Ocular hypertension* refers to IOP greater than 21 mm Hg (2.8 kPa) without disc changes or visual field loss.
- IOP is generally markedly elevated (eg, 40–90 mm Hg [5.3–12 kPa]) in PACG when symptoms are present. Additional signs include hyperemic conjunctiva, cloudy cornea, shallow anterior chamber, and occasionally edematous and hyperemic optic disc.

TREATMENT OF OCULAR HYPERTENSION AND OPEN-ANGLE GLAUCOMA

- Goal of Treatment: The goal is to lower the IOP to a level associated with a decreased risk of optic nerve damage, usually at least a 20%, if not a 25%–30% decrease from baseline to decrease the risk of optic nerve damage.
- Treat ocular hypertension if the patient has a significant risk factor such as IOP greater than 25 mm Hg (3.3 kPa), vertical cup-to-disc ratio greater than 0.5, and central corneal thickness less than 555 μm. Additional risk factors to be considered include family history of glaucoma, black, Latino/Hispanic ethnicity, severe myopia, and presence of only one eye.
- Initiate drug therapy in a stepwise manner (Fig. 66-1), starting with lower concentrations of a single well-tolerated topical agent (Table 66-2). Therapy can be started in one eye (except for patients with very high IOP or advanced visual field loss) to evaluate drug efficacy and tolerance.
- Topical β-blockers (eg, **timolol, levobunolol, metipranolol, carteolol,** and **betaxolol** are first-line agents with a long history of successful use, providing a combination of clinical efficacy and general tolerability. Prostaglandin analogs (eg, **latanoprost, bimatoprost, travoprost,** and **tafluprost**) are also used as first-line therapy; they offer once-daily dosing, better IOP reduction, good tolerance, and availability of lower-cost generics. **Latanoprostene bunod** is a prodrug of latanoprost and is also metabolized to a nitric-oxide-donating moiety, thus providing dual mechanisms for increasing aqueous outflow. **Brimonidine** and topical CAIs are well-tolerated and effective agents for second-line therapy.
- If more than one agent is needed, fixed combination products reduce the number of daily doses, which might improve adherence and prevent washout effect seen when a second medication is administered too soon after the initial medication. They also reduce exposure to ophthalmic preservatives.
- **Pilocarpine** is used as third-line therapy because of adverse events or reduced efficacy as compared with newer agents.
- **Carbachol, dipivefrin,** topical cholinesterase inhibitors, and oral CAIs (eg, **acetazolamide**) are used as last-resort options after the failure of less toxic combinations.
- **Netarsudil** is the first approved Rho kinase inhibitor with efficacy similar to that of β-blockers. It may be used in combination therapy.
- Surgical procedures such as laser trabeculoplasty or surgical trabeculectomy can be considered when drug therapy fails, is not tolerated, or is excessively complicated. Antiproliferative agents such as **fluorouracil** and **mitomycin C** are used for patients undergoing glaucoma-filtering surgery to improve success rates by reducing fibroblast proliferation and consequent scarring.

TREATMENT OF CLOSED-ANGLE GLAUCOMA

- Acute angle-closure crisis (AACC) with high IOP requires rapid reduction in IOP. Iridectomy is the definitive treatment producing a hole in the iris that permits aqueous humor flow to move directly from the posterior to the anterior chamber.
- Drug therapy of an acute attack typically consists of a miotic (eg, pilocarpine), secretory inhibitor (eg, β-blocker, α_2-agonist, or CAI), or prostaglandin agonist.
- Osmotic agents are used to rapidly decrease IOP. Examples include oral **glycerin,** 1–2 g/kg, and **mannitol,** 1–2 g/kg IV.
- Topical corticosteroids can be used to reduce ocular inflammation and synechiae.

EVALUATION OF THERAPEUTIC OUTCOMES

- Successful outcomes require identifying an effective, well-tolerated regimen; closely monitoring therapy; and patient adherence. Many drugs or combinations may need to be tried before the optimal regimen is identified.

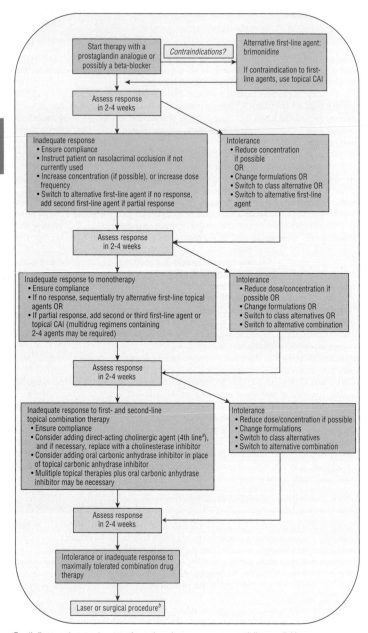

Start therapy with a prostaglandin analogue or possibly a beta-blocker → *Contraindications?* → Alternative first-line agent: brimonidine. If contraindication to first-line agents, use topical CAI

Assess response in 2-4 weeks

Inadequate response
• Ensure compliance
• Instruct patient on nasolacrimal occlusion if not currently used
• Increase concentration (if possible), or increase dose frequency
• Switch to alternative first-line agent if no response, add second first-line agent if partial response

Intolerance
• Reduce concentration if possible OR
• Change formulations OR
• Switch to class alternative OR
• Switch to alternative first-line agent

Assess response in 2-4 weeks

Inadequate response to monotherapy
• Ensure compliance
• If no response, sequentially try alternative first-line topical agents OR
• If partial response, add second or third first-line agent or topical CAI (multidrug regimens containing 2-4 agents may be required)

Intolerance
• Reduce dose/concentration if possible OR
• Change formulations OR
• Switch to class alternatives OR
• Switch to alternative combination

Assess response in 2-4 weeks

Inadequate response to first- and second-line topical combination therapy
• Ensure compliance
• Consider adding direct-acting cholinergic agent (4th lineᵃ), and if necessary, replace with a cholinesterase inhibitor
• Consider adding oral carbonic anhydrase inhibitor in place of topical carbonic anhydrase inhibitor
• Multiple topical therapies plus oral carbonic anhydrase inhibitor may be necessary

Intolerance
• Reduce dose/concentration if possible
• Change formulations
• Switch to class alternatives
• Switch to alternative combination

Assess response in 2-4 weeks

Intolerance or inadequate response to maximally tolerated combination drug therapy

Laser or surgical procedureᵇ

ᵃFourth-line agents are not commonly used any longer or are commercially unavailable.
ᵇMost clinicians believe the laser procedure should be performed earlier (eg, after three-drug maximum, poorly adherent patient).

FIGURE 66-1. Algorithm for the pharmacotherapy of open-angle glaucoma. (CAI, carbonic anhydrase inhibitor.)

TABLE 66-2 Topical Drugs Used in the Treatment of Open-Angle Glaucoma

Drug	Pharmacologic Properties	Dose Form	Strength (%)	Usual Dose[a]	Mechanism of Action
β-Adrenergic blocking agents					
Betaxolol	Relative β_1 selective	Solution	0.5	One drop twice a day	All reduce aqueous production of ciliary body
		Suspension	0.25	One drop twice a day	
Carteolol	Nonselective, intrinsic sympathomimetic activity	Solution	1	One drop twice a day	
Levobunolol	Nonselective	Solution	0.25, 0.5	One drop twice a day	
Metipranolol	Nonselective	Solution	0.3	One drop twice a day	
Timolol	Nonselective	Solution	0.25, 0.5	One drop every day—one to two times a day	
		Gelling solution	0.25, 0.5	One drop every day[a]	
Adrenergic agonists					
α_2-Adrenergic agonists					
Apraclonidine	Specific α_2-agonists	Solution	0.5, 1	One drop two to three times a day	Both reduce aqueous humor production; brimonidine is known to also increase uveoscleral outflow; only brimonidine has primary indication
Brimonidine		Solution	0.2, 0.15, 0.1	One drop two to three times a day	

(Continued)

TABLE 66-2 Topical Drugs Used in the Treatment of Open-Angle Glaucoma (*Continued*)

Drug	Pharmacologic Properties	Dose Form	Strength (%)	Usual Dose[a]	Mechanism of Action
Cholinergic agonists direct acting					
Carbachol	Direct and indirect acting	Solution	1.5, 3	One drop two to three times a day[a]	All increase aqueous humor outflow through trabecular meshwork
Pilocarpine	Direct acting	Solution	1, 2, 4	One drop two to three times a day[a]	One drop four times a day
Cholinesterase inhibitor					
Echothiophate	Indirect-acting cholinesterase inhibitor	Solution	0.125	Once or twice a day	
Carbonic anhydrase inhibitors					
Topical					
Brinzolamide	Carbonic anhydrase type II inhibition	Suspension	1	Two to three times a day	All reduce aqueous humor production of ciliary body
Dorzolamide		Solution	2	Two to three times a day	
Systemic					
Acetazolamide		Tablet	125 mg, 250 mg	125–250 mg two to four times a day	
		Injection	250–500 mg		
		Capsule	500 mg	500 mg twice a day	
Methazolamide		Tablet	25 mg, 50 mg	25–50 mg two to three times a day	

Prostaglandin analogs

Latanoprost	Prostanoid agonist	Solution	0.005	One drop every night	Increases aqueous uveoscleral outflow and to a lesser extent trabecular outflow
Latanoprostene Bunod	Prostanoid agonist	Solution	0.024	One drop every night	
Bimatoprost	Prostamide agonist	Solution	0.01, 0.03	One drop every night	
Travoprost	Prostanoid agonist	Solution	0.004	One drop every night	
Tafluprost	Prostanoid agonist	Preservative free solution	0.0015	One drop every night	
Rho kinase inhibitor					
Netarsudil	Rho kinase inhibitor	Solution	0.02	One drop every night	
Combinations					
Timolol—dorzolamide		Solution	Timolol 0.5/Dorzolamide 2	One drop twice daily	
Timolol—brimonidine		Solution	Timolol 0.5/Brimonidine 0.2	One drop twice daily	
Brinzolamide—brimonidine		Suspension	Brinzolamide 1/Brimonidine 0.2	One drop three times daily	
Netarsudil-latanoprost		Solution	Netarsudil 0.02/Latanoprost 0.005	One drop every night	

[a]Use of nasolacrimal occlusion will increase the number of patients successfully treated with longer dosage intervals.

- Monitoring therapy for POAG should be individualized. Assess IOP response every 4–6 weeks initially, every 3–4 months after IOPs become acceptable, and more frequently if therapy is changed. Visual field and disc changes are monitored every 6–12 months, unless glaucoma is unstable or worsening.
- There is no specific target IOP because the correlation between IOP and optic nerve damage is poor. Typically, a reduction of 25%–30% is desired.
- The target IOP also depends on disease severity and is generally less than 21 mm Hg (2.8 kPa). Targets as low as less than 10 mm Hg (1.3 kPa) are desired for very advanced disease, continued damage at higher IOPs, normal-tension glaucoma, and pretreatment pressures in the low to middle teens.
- Monitor medication adherence because it is commonly inadequate and a cause of therapy failure.

See Chapter 114, Glaucoma, authored by Richard G. Fiscella, Ohoud A. Owaidhah, and Deepak P. Edward, for a more detailed discussion of this topic.

Edited by Vicki L. Ellingrod

CHAPTER

67 | Anxiety Disorders

- *Anxiety disorders* (eg, generalized anxiety disorder [GAD] and panic disorder [PD]) have prominent features of anxiety and avoidance that are irrational or that impair functioning. In posttraumatic stress disorder (PTSD), there is previous exposure to trauma and the occurrence of intrusive, avoidant, and hyperarousal symptoms.

ETIOLOGY

- Evaluation of anxiety requires a physical and mental status examination; complete psychiatric diagnostic exam; appropriate laboratory tests.
- Anxiety symptoms may be associated with medical illnesses (Table 67-1) or medications (Table 67-2), and may be comorbid with other mental illnesses (eg, mood disorders, schizophrenia, and substance withdrawal).

PATHOPHYSIOLOGY

- The *noradrenergic model* suggests the autonomic nervous system is hypersensitive and overreacts to stimuli. The locus ceruleus (LC) activates norepinephrine release and stimulates the sympathetic and parasympathetic nervous systems. This down-regulates α_2-adrenoreceptors in patients with GAD and PTSD, while this receptor is hypersensitive in PD. Medications with anxiolytic or antipanic effects (eg, benzodiazepines and antidepressants) inhibit LC firing and decrease noradrenergic activity.
- *γ-Aminobutyric acid (GABA) receptor model.* GABA is the major inhibitory neurotransmitter in the central nervous system (CNS). Benzodiazepines enhance GABA's inhibitory effects, which regulates or inhibits serotonin (5-hydroxytryptamine; 5-HT), norepinephrine, and dopamine activity. The number of $GABA_A$ receptors can change with environmental alterations, and hormones can alter subunit expression. Abnormal functioning of norepinephrine, GABA, glutamate, dopamine, and 5-HT may affect manifestations of anxiety disorders.
- *5-HT model* suggests that greater 5-HT function facilitates avoidance behavior and that reducing 5-HT increases aggression. GAD symptoms may reflect excessive 5-HT

TABLE 67-1	Common Medical Illnesses Associated with Anxiety Symptoms

Cardiovascular: Angina, arrhythmias, cardiomyopathy, congestive heart failure, hypertension, ischemic heart disease, mitral valve prolapse, myocardial infarction

Endocrine and metabolic: Cushing disease, diabetes, hyperparathyroidism, hyperthyroidism, hypothyroidism, hypoglycemia, hyponatremia, hyperkalemia, pheochromocytoma, vitamin B_{12} or folate deficiencies

Gastrointestinal: Crohn's disease, irritable bowel syndrome, ulcerative colitis, peptic ulcer disease

Neurologic: Migraine, seizures, stroke, neoplasms, poor pain control

Respiratory system: Asthma, chronic obstructive pulmonary disease, pulmonary embolism, pneumonia

Others: Anemias, cancer, systemic lupus erythematosus, vestibular dysfunction

TABLE 67-2	Medications and Substances Associated with Anxiety Symptoms

Antiseizure medications: carbamazepine, phenytoin

Antidepressants: bupropion, selective serotonin reuptake inhibitors, serotonin-norepinephrine reuptake inhibitors

Antihypertensives: clonidine, felodipine

Antibiotics: quinolones, isoniazid

Bronchodilators: albuterol, theophylline

Corticosteroids: prednisone

Dopamine agonists: amantadine, levodopa

Herbals: ma huang, ginseng, ephedra

Unhealthy substance use: ecstasy, cannabis

Nonsteroidal anti-inflammatory drugs: ibuprofen, indomethacin

Stimulants: amphetamines, caffeine, cocaine, methylphenidate, nicotine

Sympathomimetics: pseudoephedrine, phenylephrine

Thyroid hormones: levothyroxine

Toxicity: anticholinergics, antihistamines, digoxin

---

transmission or overactivity of the stimulatory 5-HT pathways. The selective serotonin reuptake inhibitors (SSRIs) increase synaptic 5-HT and are effective in blocking manifestations of panic and anxiety.

- Cortisol reduces the stress response by tempering the sympathetic reaction. Patients with PTSD hypersecrete corticotropin-releasing factor but have subnormal levels of cortisol at the time of trauma and chronically. Dysregulation of the hypothalamic–pituitary–adrenal axis may be a risk factor for eventual development of PTSD.
- Neuroimaging studies support the role of the amygdala, anterior cingulate cortex, and insula in the pathophysiology of anxiety. In GAD, there is an abnormal increase in the brain's fear circuitry and activity in the prefrontal cortex. Patients with PD have midbrain structural abnormalities. In PTSD, the amygdala plays a role in the persistence of traumatic memory. Hypofunctioning in the ventromedial prefrontal cortex is theorized to prevent extinction in patients with PTSD and is inversely correlated with severity of symptoms.
- Glutamate signaling abnormalities may distort amygdala-dependent emotional processing under stress, which may contribute to the dissociative and hypervigilant symptoms in PTSD.

GENERALIZED ANXIETY DISORDER: CLINICAL PRESENTATION AND DIAGNOSIS

- Psychological and cognitive symptoms of GAD include excessive anxiety, worries that are difficult to control, feeling keyed up or on edge, and trouble concentrating or mind going blank.
- Physical symptoms include restlessness, fatigue, muscle tension, sleep disturbance, and irritability.
- The diagnosis of GAD requires excessive anxiety and worry most days for at least 6 months with at least three physical symptoms present. Significant distress or impairment in functioning is present, and the disturbance is not caused by a substance or another medical condition.
- Females are twice as likely as males to have GAD. The illness has a gradual onset at an average age of 21 years. The course is chronic, with multiple exacerbations and remissions.

TREATMENT

- <u>Goals of Treatment</u>: The goals are to reduce severity, duration, and frequency of symptoms and improve functioning. The long-term goal is minimal or no anxiety symptoms, no functional impairment, prevention of recurrence, and improved quality of life.

NONPHARMACOLOGIC THERAPY

- Nonpharmacologic modalities include psychotherapy, short-term counseling, stress management, psychoeducation, meditation, and exercise. Ideally, patients with GAD should have psychological therapy, alone or in combination with antianxiety medications. Cognitive behavioral therapy (CBT), though not widely available, is the most effective psychological therapy. Patients should avoid caffeine, nicotine, stimulants, excessive alcohol, and diet pills.
- A treatment algorithm from the International Psychopharmacology Algorithm Project (IMAP) is shown in Fig. 67-1.

PHARMACOLOGIC THERAPY

- Pharmacologic choices for GAD and PD are shown in Table 67-3, and non-benzodiazepine antianxiety agents for GAD and their dosing are shown in Table 67-4.

Antidepressants

- Antidepressants are effective for acute and long-term management of GAD (Table 67-4) and are the treatment of choice, especially in the presence of depressive symptoms. An 8–12 week trial with an SSRIs (eg, escitalopram, paroxetine, sertraline), or the serotonin-norepinephrine reuptake inhibitors (SNRIs) (eg, venlafaxine extended-release and duloxetine), results in response rates between 60% and 68%, and remission rates of ~30%. **Venlafaxine, escitalopram, paroxetine, duloxetine,** and **quetiapine** are more likely to achieve remission of GAD symptoms; however, **sertraline** may be the best tolerated. See Chapter 68 for additional information on antidepressants.
- Common adverse medication reactions and monitoring parameters are shown in Table 67-5.
- Patients may require small initial doses for the first week to limit the development of transient increased anxiety, also known as jitteriness syndrome.
- All antidepressants carry a black box warning regarding suicidal thinking and behaviors in children, adolescents, and young adults less than 25 years and recommend specific monitoring parameters (consult the FDA-approved labeling or the FDA website).
- Clinical practice guidelines recommend **fluoxetine,** sertraline, or **citalopram** for pregnant persons; however, jitteriness, myoclonus, and irritability in the neonate and premature infant have been reported and paroxetine should be avoided due to cardiovascular malformation risk.

Benzodiazepines

- All benzodiazepines possess anxiolytic properties, although only seven are FDA-approved for the treatment of GAD.
- Benzodiazepines are the most effective and frequently prescribed treatment for acute anxiety (Table 67-6). About 65%–75% of patients with GAD have a marked to moderate response, with most improvement in the first 2 weeks. They are more effective for somatic and autonomic symptoms of GAD, whereas antidepressants are more effective for the psychic symptoms (eg, apprehension and worry).
- The dose must be individualized. Older patients are more sensitive to benzodiazepines and may experience falls when taking them.
- Their most common adverse effect is CNS depression but tolerance usually develops. Others include disorientation, psychomotor impairment, confusion, aggression, excitement, ataxia, and anterograde amnesia (see Table 67-5).

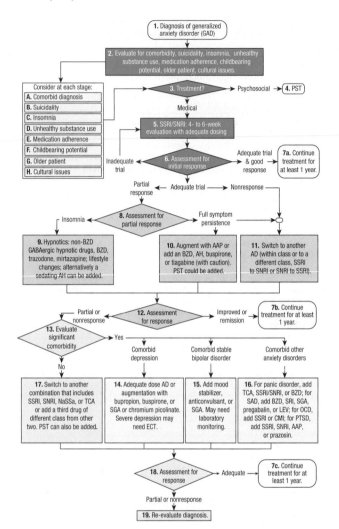

FIGURE 67-1. International Psychopharmacology Algorithm Project (IPAP) generalized anxiety disorder (GAD) algorithm flowchart. First-line treatment (nodes 2, 3, 5, 6); second-line treatment (nodes 8-12); third-line treatment, no comorbidity (nodes 13, 17, 18, 19); third-line treatment, with comorbidity (nodes 14-16); assessment and evaluation. Levels of evidence used in development of the flowchart were: 1, more than one placebo-controlled trial with sample sizes over 30; 2, one placebo-controlled trial (or active vs active medication comparison) with sample size of 30 or greater; 3, one or small ($n < 30$) placebocontrolled trial; 4, case reports or open-label trials; and 5, expert consensus without published evidence. AD, antidepressant; AH, antihistamine; BZD, benzodiazepine; CMI, clomipramine; ECT, electroconvulsive therapy; GAD, generalized anxiety disorder; LEV, levetiracetam; NaSSa, noradrenergic and selective serotonergic antidepressant; PST, psychosocial treatment; SAD, social anxiety disorder; SGA, second-generation antipsychotic; SNRI, serotonin-norepinephrine reuptake inhibitor; SRI, serotonin reuptake inhibitor; SSRI, selective serotonin reuptake inhibitor; TCA, tricyclic antidepressant.

TABLE 67-3 Medications of Choice for Anxiety Disorders

Anxiety Disorder	First-Line Medications	Second-Line Medications	Alternatives
Generalized anxiety disorder	Duloxetine	Benzodiazepines	Hydroxyzine
	Escitalopram	Buspirone	Quetiapine
	Paroxetine	Imipramine	
	Sertraline	Pregabalin	
	Venlafaxine XR		
Panic disorder	SSRIs	Alprazolam	Phenelzine
	Venlafaxine XR	Citalopram	
		Clomipramine	
		Clonazepam	
		Imipramine	

SSRI, selective serotonin reuptake inhibitor; XR, extended-release.

TABLE 67-4 Nonbenzodiazepine Antianxiety Agents for Generalized Anxiety Disorder

Medications	Initial Dose (mg/day)	Usual Range (mg/day)[a]
Duloxetine	30 or 60	60–120
Escitalopram	10	10–20
Imipramine	50	75–200
Paroxetine	20	20–50[c]
Sertraline	50	50–200
Venlafaxine XR	37.5 or 75	75–225
Vilazodone	10	20–40[d]
Vortioxetine	5	5–20
Buspirone	15	15–60[b]
Hydroxyzine	100-200	200–400[e]
Pregabalin	150	150–600[f]
Quetiapine XR	50	150–300

XR, extended-release.
[a]Older patients are usually treated with approximately one-half of the dose listed.
[b]No dosage adjustment is required in older patients.
[c]avoid in pregnancy
[d]During concomitant use of a strong CYP3A4 inhibitor (eg, itraconazole, clarithromycin, voriconazole), dose should not exceed 20 mg daily
[e]FDA approved for children with anxiety and tension
[f]Dosage adjustment required in renal impairment.

- Start with low doses, and adjust weekly (see Table 67-6). Benzodiazepines should be used with a regular dosing regimen and not on an as-needed basis when used for the treatment of an anxiety disorder.
- Treatment of acute anxiety generally should be 2–4 weeks. Manage persistent symptoms with antidepressants.
- Long half-life benzodiazepines may be dosed once daily at bedtime, providing nighttime hypnotic and next-day anxiolytic effects.
- Use low doses of short-elimination half-life agents in older patients.

TABLE 67-5 Monitoring of Adverse Medication Reactions for Anxiety Disorders

Medication Class/ Medication	Adverse Medication Reaction	Monitoring Parameter	Comments
SSRIs			
	Jitteriness syndrome	Patient interview	
	Suicidality	Patient interview	Monitor weekly in first few weeks in patients with comorbid depression and patients under age 25
	Nausea, diarrhea	Patient interview	Typically transient
	Headache	Patient interview	Typically transient
	Weight gain	Body weight, BMI, waist circumference	Paroxetine may be more likely to cause weight gain
	Sexual dysfunction	Patient interview	Significant reason for nonadherence
	Hyponatremia	Basic metabolic panel	Monitor at baseline and periodically thereafter. More frequent monitoring required in high-risk groups, especially older adults (>65 years)
	Thrombocytopenia	Complete blood count	Reported with citalopram
	Teratogenicity	Pregnancy test at baseline	Avoid paroxetine in pregnancy
	QT prolongation	ECG	Before starting citalopram, consider ECG and measurement of QT interval in patients with cardiac disease
	Discontinuation syndrome	Patient interview	Avoid abrupt discontinuation in all but fluoxetine
SNRIs			
	Jitteriness syndrome	Patient interview	
	Suicidality	Patient interview	Monitor weekly in first few weeks in patients with comorbid depression and patients under age 25

	Nausea, diarrhea	Patient interview	Typically transient
	Headache	Patient interview	Typically transient
	Elevated blood pressure	Blood pressure	Monitor blood pressure on initiation and regularly during treatment
	Sexual dysfunction	Patient interview	Significant reason for nonadherence
	Discontinuation syndrome	Patient interview	Avoid abrupt discontinuation
TCAs			
	Jitteriness syndrome	Patient interview	
	Suicidality	Patient interview	Monitor weekly in first few weeks in patients with comorbid depression and patients under age 25
	Anticholinergic effects	Patient interview	Contraindicated with narrow-angle glaucoma, prostatic hypertrophy, and urinary retention
	Weight gain	Body weight, BMI, waist circumference	
	Sexual dysfunction	Patient interview	Significant reason for nonadherence
	Sedation	Patient interview	Administer dosage at bedtime when feasible
	Arrhythmia	ECG	At baseline and periodically in children and patients >40 years of age
	Orthostatic hypotension	Blood pressure with position changes	
	Cholinergic rebound	Patient interview	Avoid abrupt discontinuation; taper doses

(Continued)

TABLE 67-5 Monitoring of Adverse Medication Reactions for Anxiety Disorders (*Continued*)

Medication Class/ Medication	Adverse Medication Reaction	Monitoring Parameter	Comments
Benzodiazepines			
	Drowsiness, fatigue	Patient interview	Avoid operating large machinery; tolerance to sedation develops after repeated dosing
	Anterograde amnesia and memory impairment	Patient interview	Risk of anterograde amnesia is worsened with concomitant intake of alcohol
	Use disorder	Patient interview; prescription monitoring program	Monitor for early refills or escalation of dosage
	Withdrawal symptoms	Physical examination; patient interview	Taper doses on discontinuation
	Respiratory depression	Respiratory rate	Avoid administering with other CNS depressants (ie, opioids, alcohol)
	Psychomotor impairment	Physical examination	Increased risk of falls
	Paradoxical disinhibition	Physical examination; family report	Increase in anxiety, irritability, or agitation may be seen in older adults or children
Other Medications			
Buspirone	Nausea, abdominal pain	Patient interview	Typically transient
	Drowsiness, dizziness	Patient interview	Typically transient

BMI, body mass index; ECG, electrocardiogram; SNRI, serotonin–norepinephrine reuptake inhibitor; SSRIs, selective serotonin reuptake inhibitors; TCAs, tricyclic antidepressants.

TABLE 67-6	Benzodiazepine Antianxiety Medications		
Medication	Approved Dosage Range (mg/day)	Maximum Dosage for Older Patients (mg/day)	Approximate Equivalent Dose (mg)
Alprazolam[a]	0.75–4	2	0.5
	1–10 (XR form)[b]		
Chlordiazepoxide	25–400	40	10
Clonazepam	1–4[b]	3	0.25–0.5
Clorazepate	7.5–60	30	7.5
Diazepam	2–40	20	5
Lorazepam[c]	0.5–10	3	1
Oxazepam[c]	30–120	60	30

XR, extended-release.
[a]Associated with interdose rebound anxiety
[b]Dose for Panic disorder.
[c]Preferred in older adults

- **Diazepam** and **clorazepate** have high lipophilicity and are rapidly absorbed and distributed into the CNS. They have rapid antianxiety effects, but a shorter duration of effect after a single dose than would be predicted based on half-life, as they are rapidly distributed to the periphery.
- **Lorazepam** and **oxazepam** are less lipophilic, have a slower onset, but a longer duration of action. They are not recommended for immediate relief of anxiety.
- **Avoid intramuscular (IM) diazepam** and **IM chlordiazepoxide** because of variability in rate and extent of absorption. **IM lorazepam** provides rapid and complete absorption.
- Several benzodiazepines are converted to desmethyldiazepam, which has a long half-life and can accumulate. Intermediate- or short-acting benzodiazepines are preferred for chronic use in older patients and those with liver disorders because of minimal accumulation and achievement of steady state within 1–3 days.
- Combining benzodiazepines with alcohol or other CNS depressants may be fatal.
- Addition of nefazodone, ritonavir, or ketoconazole (CYP3A4 inhibitors) can increase the blood levels of alprazolam and diazepam. Medications that induce cytochrome CYP3A4 (eg, carbamazepine, St. John's wort) can reduce benzodiazepine levels. Medications that inhibit or induce CYP2C19 (eg, fluoxetine, fluvoxamine, omeprazole) or N-acetyltransferase 2 activity can alter diazepam and clonazepam metabolism, respectively.
- Consult the medication interaction literature for more information on benzodiazepine interactions.
- Benzodiazepine use in pregnant persons has been associated with teratogenic effects (ie, cleft lip and palate, "floppy baby syndrome," and neonatal withdrawal). Antidepressants are preferred. If a benzodiazepine must be used, diazepam and chlordiazepoxide may be preferred. In infants receiving human milk from an individual receiving a benzodiazepine, sedation, lethargy, and weight loss may be seen.

Benzodiazepine Discontinuation

- After benzodiazepines are abruptly discontinued, three events can occur: (1) rebound symptoms are an immediate but transient return of original symptoms with an increased intensity compared with baseline; (2) recurrence or relapse is the return of original symptoms at the same intensity as before treatment; or (3) withdrawal is the emergence of new symptoms and a worsening of preexisting symptoms.
- The onset of withdrawal symptoms is within 24–48 hours after discontinuation of short-elimination half-life benzodiazepines and 3–8 days after discontinuation of a long-elimination half-life medication.

- Discontinuation strategies include:
  - ✓ A 25% per week reduction in dosage until 50% of the dose is reached, and then reduce by one-eighth every 4–7 days. If therapy duration exceeds 8 weeks, a taper over 2–3 weeks is recommended, but if duration of treatment is 6 months, a taper over 4–8 weeks is reasonable. Longer durations of treatment may require a 2- to 4-month taper.
- Adjunctive use of **pregabalin** can help to reduce withdrawal symptoms during the benzodiazepine taper.

Physical Dependence, Withdrawal, and Tolerance

- Benzodiazepine physical dependence is defined by appearance of a withdrawal syndrome (ie, anxiety, insomnia, agitation, muscle tension, irritability, nausea, diaphoresis, nightmares, depression, hyperreflexia, tinnitus, delusions, hallucinations, and seizures) upon abrupt discontinuation.
- Those with a history of a substance use disorder should not receive benzodiazepines, if possible. Those with GAD and PD are at high risk for unhealthy use and possibly physical dependence because of illness chronicity.

Buspirone

- **Buspirone** is a 5-HT$_{1A}$ partial agonist that lacks antiseizure, muscle relaxant, sedative-hypnotic, motor impairment, and dependence-producing properties.
- It is a second-line agent for GAD because of inconsistent long-term efficacy, and delayed onset of effect. It is an option for patients who fail other anxiolytic therapies or patients with a history of unhealthy alcohol or substance use. It does not provide rapid or "as-needed" antianxiety effects.
- Buspirone can be titrated in increments of 5 mg/day every 2 or 3 days as needed.
- The onset of anxiolytic effects requires 2 weeks or more; maximum benefit may require 4–6 weeks. Improvement in psychic symptoms precedes improvement in somatic symptoms.
- It may be less effective in patients who have previously taken benzodiazepines.
- It has a mean t$_{1/2}$ of 2.5 hours, and it is dosed two to three times daily (see Table 67-4).
- Buspirone may elevate blood pressure in patients taking a monoamine oxidase inhibitor (MAOI).
- Verapamil, itraconazole, and fluvoxamine can increase buspirone levels through CYP3A4 inhibition, and rifampin reduces buspirone blood levels 10-fold.

Alternative Pharmacotherapy

- **Hydroxyzine** is considered a second-line agent.
- **Pregabalin** produced anxiolytic effects similar to lorazepam, alprazolam, and venlafaxine in acute trials. Sedation and dizziness are common adverse medication effects.
- **Quetiapine** extended- release, 150 mg/day, was superior to placebo and as effective as **paroxetine** 20 mg/day and **escitalopram** 10 mg/day, but with earlier onset of action. Quetiapine is not FDA-approved for GAD and the long-term risks are unknown.

EVALUATION OF THERAPEUTIC OUTCOMES

- Initially, monitor every 2 weeks for symptom reduction, improvement in functioning, and medication adverse effects. The Hamilton Rating Scale for Anxiety (HAM-A) or the Sheehan Disability Scale can help measure response.
- Treatment resistance may be diagnosed after poor, partial, or lack of response is seen with at least two antidepressants from different classes. For those not achieving an appropriate response with a first-line agent, the dose may be increased. Other options include augmentation, or changing to a different agent. If treatment fails, assess for (a) symptoms (eg, psychotic symptoms) that need additional medications or (b) treatment nonadherence. Patients should also be assessed for concurrent substance use disorder, concurrent illnesses, and suicidal thoughts.

PANIC DISORDER: CLINICAL PRESENTATION AND DIAGNOSIS

- Psychological symptoms include depersonalization (feeling detached from oneself); derealization (feelings of being detached from one's environment); and fear of losing control or dying.
- Physical symptoms include abdominal distress, chest pain or discomfort, chills, dizziness or lightheadedness, feeling of choking, heart sensations, nausea, palpitations, paresthesias, sensation of shortness of breath or smothering, sweating, tachycardia, and trembling or shaking.
- Recurrent unexpected panic attacks. At least one attack has been followed by at least 1 month of either or both (1) persistent worry about having another panic attack or their consequences or (2) maladaptive change in behavior related to the attacks.
- During an attack, there must be at least four symptoms in addition to intense fear or discomfort. Symptoms reach a peak within 10 minutes and usually last no more than 20 or 30 minutes.
- Up to 50% of patients with panic disorder (PD) develop agoraphobia, which is marked fear or anxiety about being in at least two situations where escape could be difficult or help unavailable (eg, being in crowded places or crossing bridges). Patients may become homebound.

TREATMENT

- <u>Goals of Treatment</u>: Complete resolution of panic attacks, marked reduction in anticipatory anxiety, elimination of phobic avoidance, and no functional impairment.

NONPHARMACOLOGIC THERAPY

- Cognitive Behavioral Therapy (CBT) is associated with short-term improvement in 80%–90% of patients and 6-month improvement in 75% of patients. Adding psychosocial treatment to pharmacotherapy may reduce the likelihood of relapse when medications are stopped.
- Educate patients to avoid caffeine, nicotine, alcohol, stimulants, and misused substances and medications. Aerobic exercise may benefit patients with PD.

PHARMACOLOGIC THERAPY

- SSRIs or **venlafaxine XR** are first-line agents for PD (Table 67-7), but benzodiazepines (second-line agents) are used most commonly. **Imipramine** is considered second line. An algorithm for pharmacologic therapy of PD is shown in Fig. 67-2.
- If pharmacotherapy is used, antidepressants, especially the SSRIs, are preferred in older patients and youth, asbenzodiazepines are second line in these patients due to potential problems with disinhibition.
- The acute phase of treatment usually lasts 1–3 months with SSRIs. Therapy should be altered if there is no response after 6–8 weeks of an adequate dose. With benzodiazepines, the acute phase lasts approximately 1 month.
- Usually, patients are treated for 12–24 months before discontinuation is attempted over 4–6 months. Many patients require long-term therapy.

Antidepressants

- **Citalopram** use is limited by QT prolongation.
- Stimulatory effects (eg, anxiety, insomnia, and jitteriness) that can occur in patients treated with tricyclic antidepressants (TCA) and SSRIs may hinder adherence and dose escalation. Low initial doses and gradual dose titration may eliminate these effects (see Table 67-7).
- Imipramine blocks panic attacks within 4 weeks in 75% of patients, but reducing anticipatory anxiety and phobic avoidance requires 8–12 weeks.
- One-quarter of PD patients discontinue TCAs because of adverse medication reactions.

TABLE 67-7	Medications Used in the Treatment of Panic Disorder	
Class/Medication	**Starting Dose (mg/day)**	**Antipanic Dosage Range (mg)**
SSRIs		
Citalopram	10	20–40
Escitalopram	5	10–20
Fluoxetine	5	10–30
Fluvoxamine	25	100–300
Paroxetine	10	20–60
	12.5	25–75
Sertraline	25	50–200
SNRI		
Venlafaxine XR	37.5	75–225
Benzodiazepines		
Alprazolam	0.5 TID	4–10
	0.5–1	3–10
Clonazepam	0.25 QD or BID	1–4
Diazepam	2–5 mg TID	5–20
Lorazepam	0.5–1 TID	2–8
TCA		
Imipramine	10	75–250
MAOI		
Phenelzine	15	45–90

BID, twice daily; CR, controlled release; MAOI, monoamine oxidase inhibitor; QD, once daily; SNRI, serotonin-norepinephrine reuptake inhibitor; SSRIs, selective serotonin reuptake inhibitors; TCA, tricyclic antidepressant; TID, three times daily; XR, extended release.

- SSRIs eliminate panic attacks in 60%–80% of patients within about 4 weeks, but some patients require 8–12 weeks.
- Venlafaxine extended-release is superior to placebo and similar in efficacy to **paroxetine** in relieving panic attacks, anticipatory anxiety, fear, and avoidance.

Benzodiazepines

- Benzodiazepines are second-line PD agents except when rapid response is essential. Avoid benzodiazepine monotherapy in patients who are depressed, have a history of depression, or a history of alcohol or substance use disorders. They are often used concomitantly with antidepressants in the first 4–6 weeks to achieve a more rapid antipanic response.
- Relapse rates of 50% or higher are common despite slow tapering.
- **Alprazolam** and **clonazepam** are the preferred benzodiazepines for PD. Therapeutic response typically occurs within 1–2 weeks. The use of extended-release alprazolam or clonazepam avoids breakthrough symptoms between doses.
  - ✓ A regular dosing schedule helps prevent panic attacks rather than reduce symptoms once an attack has already occurred.
  - ✓ The starting dose of clonazepam is 0.25 mg once or twice daily, with a dose increase of 0.25–0.5 mg every 3 days to 4 mg/day if needed.
  - ✓ The starting dose of alprazolam is 0.25 three times daily (or 0.5 mg once daily of extended-release alprazolam), slowly increasing over several weeks as needed. Most patients require 3–6 mg/day.

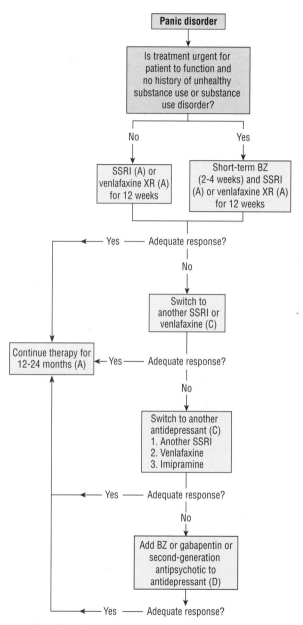

FIGURE 67-2. Algorithm for the pharmacotherapy of panic disorder. Strength of recommendations: A, directly based on category I evidence (ie, meta-analysis of randomized controlled trials [RCT] or at least one RCT); C, directly based on category III evidence (ie, nonexperimental descriptive studies); D, directly based on category IV evidence (ie, expert committee reports or opinions and/or clinical experience of respected authorities). BZ, benzodiazepine; SSRI, selective serotonin reuptake inhibitor.

759

EVALUATION OF THERAPEUTIC OUTCOMES

- Evaluate patients with PD every 1–2 weeks to begin with to fine-tune dosing and monitor adverse medication reactions. Once stabilized, they can be seen every 2 months. The Panic Disorder Severity Scale (with a remission goal of three or less with no or mild agoraphobic avoidance, anxiety, disability, or depressive symptoms) and the Sheehan Disability Scale (with a goal of less than or equal to one on each item) can be used to measure disability. During mediation discontinuation, the frequency of appointments should be increased.

POSTTRAUMATIC STRESS DISORDER: CLINICAL PRESENTATION AND DIAGNOSIS

- In adults and children older than 6, there is exposure to actual or threatened death, serious injury, or sexual violence, either directly, or by witnessing the event(s) happening to others, learning about the event(s) happening to someone close, or experiencing repeated or extreme exposure to details of the event(s).
- Duration of intrusive, avoidance, alterations in thinking and mood, and hyperarousal symptoms (Table 67-8) must be present longer than 1 month and cause significant distress or impairment. There must be at least one intrusive symptom, one symptom of avoidance of stimuli associated with the trauma, at least two symptoms of negative alterations in thinking and mood, and at least two symptoms of increased arousal.
- PTSD co-occurs with mood, anxiety, and substance use disorders and has been shown to increase the risk of lifetime suicide attempts.

TABLE 67-8	Clinical Presentation of Posttraumatic Stress Disorder
Intrusion symptoms	Recurrent, intrusive distressing memories of the trauma
	Recurrent, disturbing dreams of the event
	Feeling that the traumatic event is recurring (eg, dissociative flashbacks)
	Physiologic reaction to or psychological distress from reminders of the trauma
Avoidance symptoms	Avoidance of conversations, thoughts, or feelings about the trauma
	Avoidance of people, places, or activities that are reminders of the event
Persistent negative alterations in thinking and mood	Inability to recall an important aspect of the trauma
	Anhedonia and restricted
	Estrangement from others
	Restricted affect
	Negative beliefs about oneself
	Distorted beliefs causing one to blame others or themselves for the trauma
	Negative mood state
Hyperarousal symptoms	Decreased concentration and easily startled
	Easily startled
	Self-destructive behavior
	Hypervigilance
	Insomnia
	Irritability or anger outbursts
Specifiers	Dissociative symptoms: depersonalization or derealization
	With delayed expression: full criteria are not met until at least 6 months posttrauma

TREATMENT

- <u>Goals of Treatment</u>: Reduction in core symptoms, disability, comorbidity, and improved quality of life.
- Brief courses of trauma-focused cognitive behavioral therapy (TF-CBT) in close proximity to the trauma can help prevent PTSD.
- If symptoms persist for 3–4 weeks, and there is social or occupational impairment, treatment should start. Treatment regimens usually combine psychoeducation, psychosocial support and/or treatment, and pharmacotherapy; however, newer guidelines specifically emphasize the utility of individual trauma-focused psychotherapies.

NONPHARMACOLOGIC THERAPY

- Psychotherapies include stress management, TF-CBT, cognitive processing therapy (CPT), eye movement desensitization and reprocessing (EMDR), and psychoeducation. TF-CBT and EMDR are more effective than stress management or group therapy to reduce PTSD symptoms. Veterans Health Administration clinical practice guidelines emphasize the role of trauma-focused psychotherapy as the preferred treatment approach.

PHARMACOLOGIC THERAPY

- **Figure 67-3** shows an algorithm for the pharmacotherapy of PTSD.
- The SSRIs and venlafaxine are first-line pharmacotherapy for PTSD (**Table 67-9**). The TCAs and MAOIs also can be effective, but adverse effects can be problematic and limit their use.
- **Sertraline** and **paroxetine** are approved for acute treatment of PTSD, and sertraline is approved for long-term management.
- Long-term use of SSRIs (9–12 months) is effective in preventing relapse.
- In a 12-week trial comparing **venlafaxine XR** and sertraline, venlafaxine XR was effective in reducing the avoidance/numbing and hyperarousal cluster, whereas sertraline improved all PTSD symptom clusters.

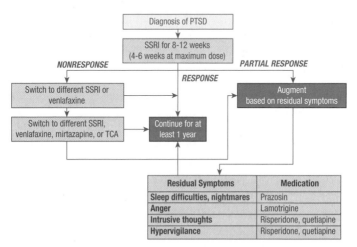

FIGURE 67-3. Algorithm for the pharmacotherapy of social anxiety disorder. Strength of recommendations: A, directly based on category I evidence (ie, meta-analysis of randomized controlled trials [RCT] or at least one RCT); C, directly based on category III evidence (ie, nonexperimental descriptive studies); D, directly based on category IV evidence (ie, expert committee reports or opinions and/or clinical experience of respected authorities). SSRI, selective serotonin reuptake inhibitor.

TABLE 67-9	Dosing of Antidepressants in the Treatment of PTSD	
Medication	**Initial Dose (mg/day)**	**Usual Range (mg/day)**
SSRIs		
Fluoxetine[a]	10	10–40[b]
Paroxetine[a]	10–20	20–40; max 50 mg/day[c]
Sertraline[a]	25	50–100; max 200 mg/day[c]
Other agents		
Amitriptyline[a]	25 or 50	75–200[b]
Imipramine[a]	25 or 50	75–200[b]
Mirtazapine[a]	15[d]	30–60[b]
Phenelzine[a]	15 or 30[d]	45–90[b]
Venlafaxine extended-release[a]	37.5	75–225[b]

[a]Available generically.
[b]Dosage used in clinical trials but not FDA-approved.
[c]Dosage is FDA-approved.
[d]Given at night.
PTSD, posttraumatic stress disorder; SSRIs, selective serotonin reuptake inhibitors.

- **Mirtazapine,** amitriptyline, and imipramine are second-line therapies and **phenelzine** and **nefazodone** are considered third-line agents. **Bupropion** is not recommended.
- SSRIs should be started in a low dose with slow titration upward toward antidepressant doses. Eight to 12 weeks is an adequate duration for the acute phase of treatment.
- During the continuation phase, medication dosages may vary and symptoms continue to improve.
- Patients who respond should continue treatment for at least 12 months. When discontinued, the medications should be tapered slowly over 1 month or more to reduce the likelihood of relapse.
- **Prazosin,** in daily doses of 1–25 mg, can be useful in some patients with PTSD. It may be particularly helpful for nightmares and insomnia; however, recent Veteran's Administration guidelines do not recommend its use.
- **Risperidone, quetiapine, α_1-adrenergic antagonists, mood stabilizers,** and **anti-seizure medications** may be used as augmenting agents in partial responders. The second-generation antipsychtoics may be useful in targeting intrusive symptoms but their use should be weighed against their metabolic effects.

EVALUATION OF THERAPEUTIC OUTCOMES

- See patients frequently for the first 3 months, then monthly for 3 months. In months 6–12, patients can be seen every 2 months. Those who respond to pharmacotherapy should continue treatment for at least 12 months.
- Monitor for symptom response, suicidal ideation, disability, adverse medication reactions, and treatment adherence. The Clinician-Administered PTSD Scale (CAPS) can be useful to assess symptom severity.

See Chapter 90, Generalized Anxiety Disorder, Panic Disorder, and Social Anxiety Disorder, authored by Sarah T. Melton and Cynthia K. Kirkwood, and Chapter 91, Posttraumatic Stress Disorder and Obsessive-Compulsive Disorder, authored by Kristen N. Gardner, Jolene R. Bostwick, and Ericka L. Crouse, for a more detailed discussion of these topics.

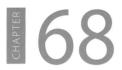

68 Bipolar Disorder

- *Bipolar disorder* is a common, lifelong, often severe cyclic mood disorder characterized by recurrent fluctuations in mood, energy, and behavior. The mania or hypomania is not substance-related or caused by other medical or psychiatric disorders.

PATHOPHYSIOLOGY

- Table 68-1 lists medical conditions, medications, and substances that may induce mania.
- Bipolar disorder is influenced by developmental, genetic, neurobiological, and psychological factors. Multiple gene loci are likely involved in the heredity of mood disorders.

CLINICAL PRESENTATION

- Different types of episodes may occur sequentially with or without a period of normal mood (euthymia) between them. There can be mood fluctuations that continue for months or after one episode, and there can be years without recurrence of any type of mood episode.

DIAGNOSIS

- The *Diagnostic and Statistical Manual of Mental Disorders*, 5th edition classifies bipolar disorders into five subtypes:
  (1) Bipolar I disorder: At least one mania episode, which may have been preceded by and may be followed by hypomania or major depressive episode(s).
  (2) Bipolar II disorder: At least one hypomania episode and a current or past major depressive episode.
  (3) Cyclothymic disorder: Chronic fluctuations between subsyndromal depressive and hypomania episodes.
  (4) Other specified bipolar and related disorder.
  (5) Unspecified bipolar and related disorder.
- See Table 68-2 for diagnostic criteria for a major depressive episode, mania episode, and hypomania episode.
- A medical, psychiatric, and medication history; physical examination; and laboratory testing are necessary to rule out organic causes of mania or depression.
- Delusions, hallucinations, and suicide attempts are more common in bipolar depression than in unipolar depression.
- Acute mania usually begins abruptly, and symptoms increase over several days. Bizarre behavior, hallucinations, and paranoid or grandiose delusions may occur. There is marked impairment in functioning. Mania episodes may be precipitated by stressors, sleep deprivation, antidepressants, central nervous system (CNS) stimulants, or bright light.
- In hypomania episodes, there is no marked impairment in social or occupational functioning, no delusions, and no hallucinations. Some patients may be more productive than usual, but 5%–15% of patients may rapidly switch to a mania episode.

COURSE OF ILLNESS

- Childhood onset is associated with more mood episodes, rapid cycling, and comorbid psychiatric conditions.

TABLE 68-1   Secondary Causes of Mania

Medical conditions that induce mania
- CNS disorders (brain tumor, strokes, head injuries, subdural hematoma, multiple sclerosis, systemic lupus erythematosus, temporal lobe seizures, Huntington disease)
- Infections (encephalitis, neurosyphilis, sepsis, human immunodeficiency virus)
- Electrolyte or metabolic abnormalities (calcium or sodium fluctuations, hyperglycemia or hypoglycemia)
- Endocrine or hormonal dysregulation (Addison disease, Cushing disease, hyperthyroidism or hypothyroidism, menstrual-related or pregnancy-related or perimenopausal mood disorders)

Medications or substances that induce mania
- Alcohol intoxication, hallucinogens (LSD, PCP) and cannabis intoxication precipitates psychosis, paranoid thoughts, anxiety, and restlessness
- Medication withdrawal (alcohol, α_2-adrenergic agonists, antidepressants, barbiturates, benzodiazepines, opiates)
- Antidepressants (MAOIs, TCAs, 5-HT and/or NE and/or DA reuptake inhibitors, 5-HT antagonists)
- DA-augmenting agents (CNS stimulants: amphetamines, cocaine, sympathomimetics; DA agonists, releasers, and reuptake inhibitors)
- NE-augmenting agents (α_2-adrenergic antagonists, β-agonists, NE reuptake inhibitors)
- Steroids (anabolic, adrenocorticotropic hormone, corticosteroids)
- Thyroid preparations and Xanthines (caffeine, theophylline)
- Nonprescription weight loss agents and decongestants (ephedra, pseudoephedrine)
- Herbal products (St. John's wort)

Somatic therapies that induce mania
- Bright light therapy, deep brain stimulation, sleep deprivation

CNS, central nervous system; DA, dopamine; 5-HT, serotonin; LSD, lysergic acid diethylamide; MAOI, monoamine oxidase inhibitor; NE, norepinephrine; PCP, phencyclidine; TCA, tricyclic antidepressant.

- Rapid cycling (have four or more episodes per year [major depressive, mania, or hypomania]) affects up to 43% of patients and is associated with frequent and severe episodes of depression and a poorer long-term prognosis.
- Females are more likely to have depressive symptoms, older age of onset, better adherence, and thyroid abnormalities. Males may have more mania episodes and substance use.
- Suicide attempts occur in up to 50% of patients with bipolar disorder, and ~7% of individuals with bipolar I disorder die by suicide. Patients with bipolar II disorder may have a higher rate of suicide attempts than bipolar I patients.

TREATMENT

- <u>Goals of Treatment</u>: The goals are to: (1) eliminate mood episode with complete remission of symptoms (ie, acute treatment); (2) prevent recurrences or relapses of mood episodes (ie, continuation phase treatment); (3) return to baseline psychosocial functioning; (4) maximize adherence with therapy; (5) minimize adverse medication effects; (6) use medications with the best tolerability and fewest interactions; (7) minimize polypharmacy when possible; (8) treat comorbid substance use disorders; (9) minimize nicotine use and stop caffeine intake at least 8 hours prior to bedtime; and (10) avoid stressors or substances that precipitate an acute episode.

TABLE 68-2	Evaluation and Diagnosis of Mood Episodes
Diagnosis Episode[a]	**DSM-5 Criteria**[b]
Major depressive	At least 2-week period of either depressed mood or loss of interest or pleasure in normal activities, associated with at least five of the following symptoms: • Depressed, sad mood (adults); can be irritable mood in children • Decreased interest and pleasure in normal activities • Decreased or increased appetite, weight loss or weight gain • Insomnia or hypersomnia • Psychomotor retardation or agitation • Decreased energy or fatigue • Feelings of excessive guilt or worthlessness • Impaired concentration or indecisiveness • Recurrent thoughts of death, suicidal thoughts or attempts
Mania	At least 1-week period of abnormally and persistently elevated mood (expansive or irritable) and energy, associated with at least three of the following symptoms (four if the mood is only irritable): • Inflated self-esteem (grandiosity) • Decreased need for sleep • Increased talking (pressure of speech) • Racing thoughts (flight of ideas) • Distractibility (poor attention) • Increased goal-directed activity (socially, at work, or sexually) or psychomotor agitation • Excessive involvement in activities that are pleasurable but have a high risk for serious consequences (buying sprees, sexual indiscretions, poor judgment in business ventures)
Hypomania	At least 4 days of abnormally and persistently elevated mood (expansive or irritable) and energy, associated with at least three of the symptoms listed under "Mania" above (four if the mood is only irritable)

[a]Impairment in social or occupational functioning; may include need for hospitalization because of potential self-harm, harm to others, or psychotic symptoms.
[b]The disorder is not caused by a medical condition (eg, hypothyroidism) or substance-induced (eg, antidepressants or other medications). Numerous specifiers are available to further characterize episodes (eg, with mixed features, with anxious distress, with rapid cycling, with melancholic features).

GENERAL APPROACH

• Table 68-3 shows an algorithmic approach to treating acute episodes including refractory episodes in adults. Treatment should be individualized. Treatment adherence is the most important factor in achieving goals.
• During acute episodes, medications can be added but then tapered once the patient is stabilized and euthymic.
• Patients with bipolar disorder should remain on a mood stabilizer (eg, **lithium, valproate, or a second-generation antipsychotic** [SGA]) lifelong.

NONPHARMACOLOGIC THERAPY

• Patients and family members should be educated about bipolar disorder (eg, symptoms, causes, and course) and treatment options.
• Nonpharmacologic approaches should address nutrition, sleep, exercise, and stress reduction.

TABLE 68-3	Algorithm and Guidelines for the Acute Treatment of Mood Episodes in Patients with Bipolar I Disorder

Acute Manic or Mixed Episode	Acute Depressive Episode		
• Assess for secondary causes of mania or mixed states (eg, alcohol or drug use) • Discontinue antidepressants • Taper off stimulants and caffeine if possible • Treat substance use/misuse • Encourage good nutrition with regular protein and essential fatty acid intake, exercise, adequate sleep, stress reduction, and psychosocial therapy	• Assess for secondary causes of depression (eg, alcohol or drug use) • Taper off antipsychotics, benzodiazepines, or sedative–hypnotic agents if possible • Treat substance use/misuse • Encourage good nutrition with regular protein and essential fatty acid intake, exercise, adequate sleep, stress reduction, and psychosocial therapy		
Hypomania	**Mania**	**Mild-to-Moderate Depressive Episode**	**Severe Depressive Episode**
• **First**, optimize current mood stabilizer if nonadherence is suspected or initiate mood-stabilizing medication: lithium,[a] valproate,[a] carbamazepine,[a] or SGAs • Consider adding a benzodiazepine (eg, lorazepam or clonazepam) for short-term adjunctive treatment of agitation or insomnia if needed • Oxcarbazepine is an alternative medication treatment option • **Second**, if response is inadequate, consider a two-drug combination: • Lithium[a] **plus** an antiseizure medication (ASM) or an SGA, or • ASM **plus** an ASM or SGA	• **First**, optimize the previously prescribed mood stabilizer or medication regimen if nonadherence suspected or initiate new mood-stabilizing two- or three-drug combinations (lithium,[a] valproate,[a] or SGA) **plus** a benzodiazepine (eg, lorazepam or clonazepam) and/or antipsychotic for short-term adjunctive treatment of agitation or insomnia; lorazepam is recommended for catatonia • Do not combine antipsychotics • Alternative options: carbamazepine[a]; if patient does not respond or tolerate, consider oxcarbazepine • **Second**, if response is inadequate, consider a three-drug combination: • Lithium[a] **plus** an ASM **plus** an antipsychotic, or • ASM **plus** an ASM **plus** an antipsychotic	• **First**, initiate and/or optimize mood-stabilizing medication: lithium,[a] quetiapine, lurasidone • Alternative ASMs: lamotrigine,[c] valproate[a] • Alternative antipsychotics: fluoxetine/olanzapine combination, cariprazine, lumateperone	• **First**, optimize current mood stabilizer if nonadherence is suspected or initiate a new mood-stabilizing medication: lithium,[a] quetiapine, or lurasidone • Fluoxetine/olanzapine combination • If psychosis is present, optimize current antipsychotic or initiate in combination with above • Alternative antipsychotics: cariprazine, lumateperone • Do not combine antipsychotics • Alternative ASM: lamotrigine,[c] valproate[a] • **Second**, if response is inadequate, consider carbamazepine[a] or adding antidepressant[d]

(Continued)

TABLE 68-3	Algorithm and Guidelines for the Acute Treatment of Mood Episodes in Patients with Bipolar I Disorder (*Continued*)

Acute Manic or Mixed Episode		Acute Depressive Episode	
Hypomania	**Mania**	**Mild-to-Moderate Depressive Episode**	**Severe Depressive Episode**
	• **Third**, if response is inadequate, consider ECT for mania with psychosis or catatonia[b] or add clozapine for treatment-refractory illness		• **Third**, if response is inadequate, consider a three-drug combination: • Lithium **plus** lamotrigine[c] **plus** an antidepressant[d] • Lithium **plus** quetiapine **plus** antidepressant[d] • **Fourth**, if response is inadequate, consider ECT for treatment-refractory illness and depression with psychosis or catatonia[b]

ASM, antiseizure medication; ECT, electroconvulsive therapy; SGA, second-generation antipsychotic.

[a]Use standard therapeutic serum concentration ranges if clinically indicated; if partial response or breakthrough episode, adjust dose to achieve higher serum concentrations without causing intolerable adverse effects; lithium, SGAs, and/or lamotrigine are preferred over valproate and carbamazepine for bipolar depression.

[b]ECT is used for severe mania or depression during pregnancy and for mixed episodes; prior to treatment, ASM, lithium, and benzodiazepines should be tapered off to maximize therapy and minimize adverse effects.

[c]Lamotrigine is not approved for the acute treatment of depression, and the dose must be started low and slowly titrated up to decrease adverse effects if used for maintenance therapy. Lamotrigine may be initiated during acute treatment with plans to transition to this medication for long-term maintenance. A medication interaction and a severe dermatologic rash can occur when lamotrigine is combined with valproate (ie, lamotrigine doses must be halved from standard dosing titration).

[d]Controversy exists concerning the use of antidepressants, and they are often considered third line in treating acute bipolar depression, except in patients with no recent history of severe acute mania or potentially in bipolar II patients.

- Current evidence suggests adjunctive psychosocial interventions are useful for acute depressive episodes and in maintenance and relapse prevention. These include cognitive behavioral therapy (CBT), interpersonal and social rhythm therapy, group psychoeducation, family-focused therapy, and enhanced relapse prevention/individual psychoeducation.

PHARMACOLOGIC THERAPY

- See Table 68-4 for product and dosing information on medications for bipolar disorder.
- Differing therapies are approved by the U.S. Food and Drug Administration (FDA) for treatment of acute mania, acute bipolar depression, and/or maintenance treatment (see Table 68-4).
- Combination therapies (see Table 68-3) can provide better acute response and long-term prevention of relapse and recurrence than monotherapy in some bipolar patients.
- Sources of useful guidelines include the Canadian Network for Mood and Anxiety Treatments (CANMAT), International Society for Bipolar Disorders (ISBD), and International Task Force of the World Federation of Societies of Biological Psychiatry (WFSBP).

TABLE 68-4 Agents Used in the Treatment of Bipolar Disorder

Drug (Brand Name)	Initial Dosing	Usual Dosing; Special Population Dosing
Lithium salts		
Lithium carbonate (Eskalith)[a,b] (Eskalith CR) (Lithobid) Lithium citrate (Cibalith-S)[a,b]	300 mg twice daily	900–2400 mg/day in two to four divided doses, preferably with meals
		Renal impairment: lower doses required with frequent serum monitoring
		There is wide variation in the dosage needed to achieve therapeutic response
		Trough serum lithium concentration (ie, 0.6–1.2 mEq/L [mmol/L] for maintenance therapy and 0.8–1.2 mEq/L [mmol/L] for acute mood episodes taken 12 hours after the last dose)
Antiseizure medications		
Divalproex sodium (Depakote)[a] (Depakote ER) Valproic acid[a] (Depakene) Valproate sodium (Depacon)	250–500 mg twice daily A loading dose of divalproex (20–30 mg/kg/day) can be given	750–3000 mg/day (20–60 mg/kg/day) given once daily or in divided doses
		Titrate to clinical response
		Dose adjustment needed with hepatic impairment
Lamotrigine (Lamictal)[b]	25 mg daily	50–400 mg/day in divided doses. Dosage should be slowly increased (eg, 25 mg/day for 2 weeks, then 50 mg/day for weeks 3 and 4, and then 50-mg/day increments at weekly intervals up to 200 mg/day)
		Dose adjustment needed with hepatic impairment
Carbamazepine (Equetro)[a] (Tegretol) (Epitol) (Tegretol-XR) (Carbatrol)	200 mg twice daily	200–1800 mg/day in two to four divided doses
		Titrate to clinical response
		Dose adjustment needed with hepatic impairment
Oxcarbazepine (Trileptal)	300 mg twice daily	300–1200 mg/day in two divided doses
		Titrate based on clinical response
		Dose adjustment required with severe renal impairment

(Continued)

TABLE 68-4   Agents Used in the Treatment of Bipolar Disorder (*Continued*)

Drug (Brand Name)	Initial Dosing	Usual Dosing; Special Population Dosing
Second-generation antipsychotics		
Aripiprazole (Abilify)[a,b] (Abilify Maintena)[b]	10–15 mg daily	10–30 mg/day once daily
Asenapine (Saphris)[b]	5–10 mg twice daily sublingually	5–10 mg twice daily sublingually
Cariprazine (Vraylar)[a]	1.5 mg daily	3–6 mg daily
Lumateperone (Caplyta)[c]	42 mg daily	42 mg daily
Lurasidone (Latuda)[c]	20 mg daily	20–120 mg daily with food
Olanzapine (Zyprexa)[a,b] (Zyprexa Zydis)	2.5–5 mg twice daily	5–20 mg/day once daily or in divided doses
Olanzapine and fluoxetine (Symbyax)[c]	6 mg olanzapine and 25 mg fluoxetine daily	6–12 mg olanzapine and 25–50 mg fluoxetine daily
Quetiapine (Seroquel)[a,b]	50 mg twice daily	50–800 mg/day in divided doses or once daily when stabilized
Risperidone (Risperdal)[a] (Risperdal M-Tab) (Risperdal Consta)[b]	0.5–1 mg twice daily	0.5–6 mg/day once daily or in divided doses
Ziprasidone (Geodon)[a]	40–60 mg twice daily	40–160 mg/day in divided doses
Benzodiazepines		
Various	Dosage should be slowly adjusted up and down according to response and adverse effects	Use in combination with other medications (eg, antipsychotics, lithium, valproate) for the acute treatment of mania or mixed episodes Use as a short-term adjunctive sedative–hypnotic agent

[a]FDA-approved for acute mania.
[b]FDA-approved for maintenance.
[c]FDA-approved for acute bipolar depression.

Lithium

- **Lithium** is a first-line agent for acute mania, and maintenance treatment of bipolar I and II disorders. It is considered second line for acute bipolar II depression.
- It is rapidly absorbed, neither protein bound nor metabolized, and excreted unchanged in the urine and other body fluids.
- It may require 6–8 weeks to show antidepressant efficacy. It produces a prophylactic response in up to two-thirds of patients and reduces suicide risk.
- Abrupt discontinuation or noncompliance with lithium therapy can increase the risk of relapse.
- Initial GI and CNS adverse effects are often dose related and are worse at peak serum concentrations (1–2 hours postdose). Lowering the dose, taking doses with food, using extended-release products, and once-daily dosing at bedtime may help. Diarrhea can sometimes be improved by switching to a liquid formulation.
- A benign fine hand tremor occurs in many patients whereas a coarse hand tremor may be a sign of toxicity. The fine tremor may be treated by switching to a long-acting preparation, lowering the dose, or adding propranolol, 20–120 mg/day.
- Polydipsia with polyuria with or without nephrogenic diabetes insipidus (DI) can occur. About 20%–40% of patients develop nephrogenic DI soon after initiating lithium, and it persists in about 10%–25% of patients. It is typically reversible with lithium discontinuation. Nocturia is common and managed by changing to once-daily dosing at bedtime.
- Lithium reduces the kidneys' ability to concentrate urine and may cause a nephrogenic DI with low urine-specific gravity and low osmolality polyuria (urine volume >3 L/day). This may be treated with loop or thiazide diuretics. If a thiazide diuretic is used, lithium doses should be decreased by 50% and lithium and potassium levels monitored. Amiloride has weaker natriuretic effects and seems to have little effect on lithium clearance.
- Hypothyroidism can occur in lithium-treated patients (more common in females) and does not require discontinuation of lithium. Exogenous thyroid hormone (ie, levothyroxine) can be added to the regimen. If lithium is discontinued, the need for levothyroxine should be reassessed because hypothyroidism can be reversible.
- Lithium may cause cardiac effects including T-wave flattening or inversion (up to 30% of patients), atrioventricular block, and bradycardia. In patients with significant cardiac disease, an ECG and consultation with a cardiologist are recommended at baseline and periodically during therapy.
- Other late-appearing lithium adverse effects are benign reversible leukocytosis, acne, folliculitis, and weight gain.
- Lithium toxicity can occur with serum levels greater than 1.5 mEq/L (mmol/L), but older persons may have toxic symptoms at lower levels. Severe toxic symptoms (eg, vomiting, diarrhea, incontinence, incoordination, impaired cognition, arrhythmias, seizures, permanent neurologic impairment, and kidney damage) may occur with serum concentrations above 2 mEq/L (mmol/L).
  - ✓ Factors predisposing to lithium toxicity include sodium restriction, dehydration, vomiting, diarrhea, age greater than 50 years, heart failure, cirrhosis, medication interactions that decrease lithium clearance, heavy exercise, sauna baths, hot weather, and fever. Tell patients to maintain adequate sodium and fluid intake and to avoid excessive use of alcohol and caffeine-containing beverages.
  - ✓ If lithium toxicity is suspected, discontinue lithium and send the patient immediately to the emergency department.
  - ✓ Consider intermittent hemodialysis in these situations:
    - o In lithium-naive patients, when lithium serum concentrations are at least 4 mEq/L (mmol/L).
    - o In patients previously taking lithium, when lithium serum concentrations are 2.5 mEq/L (mmol/L) or greater and moderate-to-severe neurologic toxicity is present or as clinically indicated.
    - o Continue hemodialysis until serum lithium concentration is below 1 mEq/L (mmol/L) when drawn 8 hours after the last dialysis.

✓ Thiazide diuretics, nonsteroidal anti-inflammatory drugs, angiotensin-converting enzyme inhibitors, and salt-restricted diets can elevate lithium levels. Neurotoxicity can occur when lithium is combined with antipsychotics, methyldopa, metronidazole, phenytoin, and verapamil. Combining lithium with calcium channel blockers is not recommended because of reports of neurotoxicity. Acetaminophen or aspirin and loop diuretics are less likely to interfere with lithium clearance. Caffeine and theophylline can enhance renal elimination of lithium. Activated charcoal is not useful.

- Lithium is usually initiated with 600 mg/day for prophylaxis and 900–1200 mg/day for acute mania. Give immediate-release preparations two or three times daily and extended-release products once or twice daily. After patients are stabilized, many patients can switch to once-daily dosing.

- In general, lithium serum concentrations should be maintained between 0.6 and 1.0 mEq/L (mmol/L). Lithium levels are considered to be at steady state after approximately 5 days with samples drawn 12 hours postdose. Initially, check serum lithium concentrations once or twice weekly. After a desired serum concentration is achieved, check levels in 2 weeks, and when stable, check them every 3–6 months.

- Lithium clearance increases by 50%–100% during pregnancy. Monitor serum levels monthly during pregnancy and weekly the month before delivery. At delivery, reduce dose to prepregnancy levels and maintain hydration.

- A reasonable therapeutic trial in outpatients is at least 4–6 weeks with lithium serum concentrations of 0.6–1.2 mEq/L (mmol/L). Although serum concentrations less than 0.6 mEq/L (mmol/L) may be associated with higher relapse rates, some patients can do well at 0.4–0.7 mEq/L (mmol/L). Patients with acute mania can require serum concentrations of 1–1.2 mEq/L (mmol/L), and some need up to 1.5 mEq/L (mmol/L). For bipolar prophylaxis in older patients, serum concentrations of 0.4–0.6 mEq/L (mmol/L) are recommended.

Antiseizure Medications

- For more in-depth information on the adverse medication effects, pharmacokinetics, and interactions, refer to Chapter 54.

Valproate Sodium and Valproic Acid

- **Divalproex sodium** (sodium valproate) is as effective as lithium and **olanzapine** for mania, and it can be more effective than lithium for rapid cycling, mixed states, and bipolar disorder with substance use disorder. It reduces the frequency of (or prevents) recurrent mania, depressive, and mixed episodes.

- Lithium, carbamazepine, antipsychotics, or benzodiazepines can augment the antimania effects of valproate. Valproate can be added to lithium to achieve synergistic effects in patients who are treatment refractory and are rapid cyclers or have mixed features, and the combination is effective as maintenance therapy for bipolar I disorder. The potential for medication interactions necessitate blood level monitoring of both agents. SGAs can be added to valproate for breakthrough mania, but they can increase the risk of sedation and weight gain. Combining valproate with lamotrigine increases the risk of rashes, ataxia, tremor, sedation, and fatigue.

- The most frequent dose-related adverse effects of valproate are GI complaints, fine tremor, and sedation. Giving it with food, reducing the initial dose and making gradual increases, or switching to the extended-release formulation can help alleviate the GI complaints. Reducing the dose or adding a β-blocker may alleviate tremors. Giving the total dose at bedtime can minimize daytime sedation. Other adverse effects are ataxia, lethargy, alopecia, pruritus, prolonged bleeding, transient increases in liver enzymes, weight gain, and hyperammonemia. Thrombocytopenia can occur at higher doses; lowering the valproate dose may normalize platelet counts. Fatal necrotizing hepatitis is rare and idiosyncratic, occurring in children on multiple anticonvulsants. Life-threatening pancreatitis has been reported.

- For healthy inpatient adults with acute mania, the initial starting dose of valproate is typically 20 mg/kg/day given in divided doses over 12 hours. The daily dose is adjusted by 250–500 mg every 1–3 days based on response and tolerability. The maximum dose is 60 mg/kg/day (see **Table 68-4**).

✓ For outpatients with hypomania or euthymia, or for older patients, the initial dose is generally lower (5–10 mg/kg/day in divided doses) and gradually titrated to avoid adverse effects.

✓ After establishing the optimal dose, the dose can be given twice daily or at bedtime if tolerated. Extended-release divalproex can be given once daily, but bioavailability can be 15% lower than that of immediate-release products.

• Most clinicians seek a serum concentration range of 50–125 mcg/mL (347–866 μmol/L) measured 12 hours after the last dose. Patients with cyclothymia or bipolar II disorder respond at lower blood levels, while patients with more severe forms may require up to 150 mcg/mL (1040 μmol/L). Serum levels are most useful when assessing adherence or toxicity.

Carbamazepine

• Because of interactions, **carbamazepine** is usually reserved for use after treatment failure with lithium or divalproex sodium. Patients with a history of head trauma, anxiety, or substance use may respond to treatment with carbamazepine.

• It has acute antimania effects, but its long-term effectiveness is less clear. It may be less effective than lithium for maintenance therapy and bipolar depression. The combination of carbamazepine with lithium, valproate, and antipsychotics is often used for mania episodes in treatment-resistant patients.

• Carbamazepine adverse effects are summarized in Chapter 54.

• Carbamazepine induces the hepatic metabolism of antidepressants, ASMs, antipsychotics, and other medications. Individuals taking oral contraceptives who receive carbamazepine should be counseled to use alternative contraception.

• Certain medications that inhibit CYP3A4 (eg, cimetidine, diltiazem, erythromycin, fluoxetine, fluvoxamine, itraconazole, ketoconazole, nefazodone, and verapamil) added to carbamazepine therapy may cause carbamazepine toxicity. When carbamazepine is combined with valproate, reduce the carbamazepine dose, as its free levels can be increased. Do not combine clozapine and carbamazepine because of possible additive bone marrow suppression.

• For inpatients in an acute mania episode, doses can be started at 400–600 mg/day in divided doses with meals and increased by 200 mg/day every 2–4 days up to 1200–1600 mg/day. Outpatients should be started at lower doses and titrated upward more slowly to avoid adverse effects. Many patients tolerate once-daily dosing after stabilization.

• During the first month of therapy, serum concentrations may decrease because of autoinduction of cytochrome P450 3A4 enzymes, requiring a dose increase.

• Carbamazepine serum levels are usually obtained every 1 or 2 weeks during the first 2 months, then every 6–12 months during maintenance. Serum samples are drawn 10–12 hours postdose and at least 2–5 days after dosage initiation or change. Most clinicians attempt to maintain levels between 6–10 mcg/mL (25–42 μmol/L), but some patients may require 12–14 mcg/mL (51–59 μmol/L).

• Use of carbamazepine in patients of Asian ancestry requires genetic testing for human leukocyte antigen (HLA) allele, HLA-B 1502, to help detect a higher risk of Stevens–Johnson syndrome and toxic epidermal necrolysis.

Oxcarbazepine

• **Oxcarbazepine** is typically recommended as a third-line option for mania, and is not recommended for treatment of bipolar depression.

• Initial dosing is usually 150–300 mg twice daily, which can be increased by 300–600 mg every 3–6 days up to 1200 mg/day in divided doses (with or without food).

• Discontinue oxcarbazepine at the first sign of a skin reaction, as severe dermatologic reactions have been reported (eg, Stevens–Johnson syndrome). Other adverse effects may include impaired cognitive or psychomotor performance, somnolence, fatigue,

incoordination, and hyponatremia. Severe hyponatremia is more common with oxcarbazepine than with carbamazepine.
* Oxcarbazepine is a CYP 2C19 inhibitor and a 3A4/5 inducer. It induces the metabolism of oral contraceptives, necessitating the use of alternative contraception measures. Oxcarbazepine does not autoinduce its own metabolism.

Lamotrigine

* **Lamotrigine** has both antidepressant and mood-stabilizing effects. It may have augmenting properties when combined with lithium or valproate. It has a low rate of switching patients to mania. Although it is less effective for acute mania compared with lithium and valproate, it may be beneficial for the maintenance therapy of treatment-resistant bipolar I and II disorders. It seems most effective for prevention of bipolar depression.
* Common adverse effects include headache, nausea, dizziness, ataxia, diplopia, drowsiness, tremor, maculopapular rash, and pruritus. Although most rashes resolve with continued therapy, some progress to life-threatening Stevens–Johnson syndrome. Discontinue lamotrigine if the rash is diffuse, involves mucous membranes, and is accompanied by fever or sore throat. The incidence of rash is greatest with concomitant administration of valproate, rapid dose escalation of lamotrigine, and higher than recommended lamotrigine initial doses.
* In patients taking valproate, dose lamotrigine at about one-half the standard doses, and titrate upward more slowly than usual.
* For maintenance treatment of bipolar disorder, the usual dosage range of lamotrigine is 50–300 mg/day. The target dose is generally 200 mg/day (100 mg/day when combined with valproate and 400 mg/day when combined with carbamazepine). For patients not taking medications that affect lamotrigine's clearance, the dose is 25 mg/day for the first 2 weeks, then 50 mg/day for weeks 3 and 4, 100 mg/day for the next week, then 200 mg/day. Patients who stop dosing for more than a few days should restart the dose escalation schedule.

Antipsychotics

* First-generation (eg, **fluphenazine, haloperidol**) and second-generation (eg, **aripiprazole, asenapine, clozapine, lurasidone, quetiapine, risperidone, ziprasidone**) antipsychotics are effective as monotherapy or as add-on therapy for acute mania. Long-term antipsychotics can be needed for some patients, but the risks versus benefits must be weighed in view of long-term adverse effects (eg, obesity, type 2 diabetes, hyperlipidemia, hyperprolactinemia, and tardive dyskinesia).
* Both first- and second-generation antipsychotics are effective in patients with acute mania associated with agitation, aggression, and psychosis.
* Clinical trials support the use of quetiapine and lurasidone as monotherapy and adjunctive treatment for bipolar depression. Data also support the use of combined fluoxetine/olanzapine for bipolar depression.
* Oral aripiprazole, olanzapine, sublingal asenapine, and long-acting risperidone are effective monotherapy options for maintenance treatment in bipolar disorder. First-generation depot antipsychotics (eg, haloperidol decanoate, fluphenazine decanoate) can be useful for maintenance treatment in patients who are noncompliant or treatment-resistant.
* Controlled studies in acute mania suggest that lithium or valproate plus an antipsychotic is more effective than any of these agents alone.
* Clozapine monotherapy has acute and long-term mood-stabilizing effects in refractory bipolar disorder but requires regular white blood cell monitoring for agranulocytosis.
* Higher initial antipsychotic doses (eg, olanzapine 20 mg/day) may be required for acute mania. After mania is controlled (usually 7–28 days), the antipsychotic can be gradually tapered and discontinued, and the patient maintained on mood-stabilizer monotherapy.
* For more information on the adverse effects, pharmacokinetics, and medication interactions of specific antipsychotics, refer to Chapter 72.

Alternative Medications

- High-potency benzodiazepines (eg, **clonazepam and lorazepam**) are common alternatives (or adjuncts) to antipsychotics for acute mania, agitation, anxiety, panic, and insomnia, or in patients who cannot take mood stabilizers. IM lorazepam may be used for acute agitation. When no longer required, benzodiazepines should be gradually tapered and discontinued to avoid withdrawal symptoms. A relative contra-indication for long-term use is a history of a substance use disorder or unhealthy use.
- Adjunctive **antidepressants** may be no better than placebo for acute bipolar depression when combined with mood stabilizers, but this is controversial. The rate of mood switching from depression to mania with tricyclic antidepressants and venla-faxine is higher than the rate associated with the use of selective serotonin reuptake inhibitors. Before initiating an antidepressant, be sure the patient has a therapeutic dose or blood level of a primary mood stabilizer. Be cautious in using antidepressants in those with a history of mania after a depressive episode, and those with frequent cycling. Generally, the antidepressant should be withdrawn 2–6 months after remission.

Special Populations

- Contraception and pre-conception counseling should be a part of the patient education plan for patients diagnosed with bipolar disorder who are able to become pregnant.
- The occurrence of Epstein anomaly in infants exposed to lithium during the first trimester is estimated to be between 1 and 10.78:1000, and the risk of neural tube defects is 13.4:1000. When lithium is used during pregnancy, use the lowest effective dose to prevent relapse, and lessen the risk of "floppy" infant syndrome, hypothyroidism, and nontoxic goiter in the infant. Monitor closely and adjust dose as appropriate.
- Breastfeeding is usually discouraged for individuals taking lithium.
- When valproate, carbamazepine, and lamotrigine are taken during the first trimester, the risk of neural tube defects is ~4%, ~3%, and ~2%, respectively. Administration of folic acid can reduce the risk of neural tube defects.
- Individuals taking valproate may breastfeed, but the lactating individual and infant should have identical laboratory monitoring.
- First-generation antipsychotics seem to have little teratogenic risk when used during pregnancy. Data on the SGAs are more limited. Risk to benefit ratio must be considered before using antipsychotics during pregnancy.
- Approximately one-third to two-thirds of patients diagnosed with bipolar disorder experience their first episode as a child or adolescent; however, there are few controlled studies in this population. Little is known about the long-term efficacy and safety of specific agents or combination therapies in this population. Different medications have different FDA approvals for use.
- Up-to-date guidelines should be consulted for the treatment of children and adolescents with bipolar disorder.
- The elimination half-life of lithium and valproate increases with age. Older patients can have many medical comorbidities and increased sensitivity to adverse effects of mood stabilizers and antipsychotics.

EVALUATION OF THERAPEUTIC OUTCOMES

- Mood episodes: Document symptoms on a daily mood chart (document life stressors, type of episode, length of episode, and treatment outcome); monthly and yearly life charts are valuable for documenting patterns of mood cycles.
- See Table 68-5 for guidelines for laboratory monitoring of patients on mood stabilizers.
- Assess medication adherence; missing medication doses is a primary reason for non-response and recurrence of episodes.
- Ask patients about adverse medication effects, especially sedation and weight gain; manage them rapidly and vigorously to avoid nonadherence.

TABLE 68-5 Guidelines for Baseline and Routine Laboratory Tests and Monitoring for Mood Stabilizers

	Physical Examination and General Chemistry[a]	Hematologic Tests[b]	Metabolic Tests[c]	Liver Function Tests[d]	Renal Function Tests[e]	Thyroid Function Tests[f]	Serum Electrolytes[g]	Dermatologic[h]	Pharmacogenomic Testing
SGAs[i]	Baseline		Baseline and 6–12 months						
Carbamazepine[j]	Baseline	Baseline and 6–12 months		Baseline and 6–12 months	Baseline		Baseline and 6–12 months	Baseline and 6–12 months	Baseline
Lamotrigine[k]	Baseline							Baseline and 6–12 months	
Lithium[l]	Baseline	Baseline and 6–12 months	Baseline and 6–12 months		Baseline and 6–12 months	Baseline and 6–12 months	Baseline and 6–12 months	Baseline and 6–12 months	
Oxcarbazepine[m]	Baseline		Baseline and 6–12 months				Baseline and 6–12 months		Baseline
Valproate[n]	Baseline	Baseline and 6–12 months	Baseline and 6–12 months	Baseline and 6–12 months				Baseline and 6–12 months	

SGAs, second-generation antipsychotics.

[a]Screen for substance use and serum pregnancy.
[b]Complete blood cell count (CBC) with differential and platelets.
[c]Fasting glucose, serum lipids, and weight.
[d]Lactate dehydrogenase, aspartate aminotransferase, alanine aminotransferase, total bilirubin, and alkaline phosphatase.
[e]Serum creatinine, blood urea nitrogen, urinalysis, urine osmolality, and specific gravity.
[f]Triiodothyronine, total thyroxine, thyroxine uptake, and thyroid-stimulating hormone.
[g]Serum sodium.
[h]Rashes, hair thinning, and alopecia.

(Continued)

jSecond-generation antipsychotics: Monitor for increased appetite with weight gain (primarily in patients with initial low or normal body mass index); monitor closely if rapid or significant weight gain occurs during early therapy; cases of hyperlipidemia and diabetes reported.

kCarbamazepine: Manufacturer recommends CBC and platelets (and possibly reticulocyte counts and serum iron) at baseline, and that subsequent monitoring be individualized by the clinician (eg, CBC, platelet counts, and liver function tests every 2 weeks during the first 2 months of treatment, and then every 3 months if normal). Monitor more closely if patient exhibits hematologic or hepatic abnormalities or if the patient is receiving a myelotoxic medication; discontinue if platelets are <100,000/mm³ (<100 × 10⁹/L), if white blood cell (WBC) count is <3000/mm³ (<3 × 10⁹/L), or if there is evidence of bone marrow suppression or liver dysfunction. Serum electrolyte levels should be monitored in the elderly or those at risk for hyponatremia. Carbamazepine interferes with some pregnancy tests.

lLamotrigine: If renal or hepatic impairment, monitor closely and adjust dosage according to manufacturer's guidelines. Serious dermatologic reactions have occurred within 2–8 weeks of initiating treatment and are more likely to occur in patients receiving concomitant valproate, with rapid dosage escalation, or using doses exceeding the recommended titration schedule.

lLithium: Obtain baseline electrocardiogram for patients older than 40 years or if preexisting cardiac disease (benign, reversible T-wave depression can occur). Renal function tests should be obtained every 2–3 months during the first 6 months, and then every 6–12 months; if impaired renal function, monitor 24-hour urine volume and creatinine every 3 months; if urine volume >3 L/day, monitor urinalysis, osmolality, and specific gravity every 3 months. Thyroid function tests should be obtained once or twice during the first 6 months, and then every 6–12 months; monitor for signs and symptoms of hypothyroidism; if supplemental thyroid therapy is required, monitor thyroid function tests and adjust thyroid dose every 1–2 months until thyroid function indices are within normal range, and then monitor every 3–6 months.

mOxcarbazepine: Hyponatremia (serum sodium concentrations <125 mEq/L [mmol/L]) has been reported and occurs more frequently during the first 3 months of therapy; serum sodium concentrations should be monitored in patients receiving medications that lower serum sodium concentrations (eg, diuretics or medications that cause inappropriate antidiuretic hormone secretion) or in patients with symptoms of hyponatremia (eg, confusion, headache, lethargy, and malaise). Hypersensitivity reactions have occurred in approximately 25%–30% of patients with a history of carbamazepine hypersensitivity and require immediate discontinuation.

nValproate: Weight gain reported in patients with low or normal body mass index. Monitor platelets and liver function during first 3–6 months if evidence of increased bruising or bleeding. Monitor closely if patients exhibit hematologic or hepatic abnormalities or in patients receiving medications that affect coagulation, such as aspirin or warfarin; discontinue if platelets are <100,000/mm³/L (<100 × 10⁹/L) or if prolonged bleeding time. Pancreatitis, hyperammonemic encephalopathy, polycystic ovary syndrome, increased testosterone, and menstrual irregularities have been reported; not recommended during first trimester of pregnancy due to risk of neural tube defects.

- Be aware of suicidal ideation or attempts. Suicide completion rates with bipolar I disorder are 10%–15%; suicide attempts are primarily associated with depressive episodes, mixed episodes with severe depression, or presence of psychosis.
- Assess patients with partial treatment response or nonresponse for accurate diagnosis, concomitant medical or psychiatric conditions, medication adherence, and use of medications or substances that exacerbate mood symptoms.
- Involve patients and family members in treatment to monitor target symptom response and adverse medication effects and to enhance adherence and reduce stressors. Standardized rating scales may be useful in monitoring for response.

See Chapter 86, Bipolar Disorder, authored by Jordan C. Cooler and Shannon J. Drayton, for a more detailed discussion of this topic.

Depressive Disorder 69

- The essential feature of *major depressive disorder* (MDD) is a clinical course characterized by one or more major depressive episodes without a history of manic or hypomanic episodes.
- Refer to guidelines published by the American Psychiatric Association, the British Association of Psychopharmacology, and the Canadian Network for Mood and Anxiety Treatments as they have similarities in their recommendations.

PATHOPHYSIOLOGY

- *Monoamine hypothesis:* Decreased brain levels of the neurotransmitters norepinephrine (NE), serotonin (5-HT), and dopamine (DA) may cause depression.
- *Postsynaptic changes in receptor sensitivity:* Studies have demonstrated that desensitization or downregulation of NE or 5-HT_{1A} receptors may relate to onset of antidepressant effects.
- *Dysregulation hypothesis:* Failure of homeostatic neurotransmitter regulation, rather than absolute increases or decreases in their activities.
- *Inflammatory hypothesis:* Chronic stress and inflammation may alter glutamatergic and GABA transmission. Brain-derived neurotrophic factor (BDNF) is a primary mediator of neuronal changes as well as synaptogenesis whose expression is reduced due to stress and may be associated with depression.
- Neuroactive steroids are a growing area of research for depression.

CLINICAL PRESENTATION

- *Emotional symptoms:* Diminished ability to experience pleasure, loss of interest in usual activities, sadness, pessimism, crying, hopelessness, anxiety, feelings of worthlessness or guilt, and psychotic features (eg, auditory hallucinations and delusions). Recurrent thoughts of death, suicidal ideation without a specific plan, suicide attempt, or a plan for committing suicide.
- *Physical symptoms:* Weight gain or loss, fatigue, pain (especially headache), sleep disturbance, decreased or increased appetite, loss of sexual interest, and gastrointestinal (GI) and cardiovascular complaints (especially palpitations).
- *Cognitive symptoms:* Decreased ability to concentrate, poor memory for recent events, confusion, and indecisiveness.
- *Psychomotor disturbances:* Psychomotor retardation (slowed physical movements, thought processes, and speech) or psychomotor agitation.

DIAGNOSIS

- MDD is characterized by one or more major depressive episodes, as defined by the *Diagnostic and Statistical Manual of Mental Disorders,* 5th ed. Five or more of the above symptoms must have been present nearly every day during the same 2-week period and cause significant distress or impairment. Depressed mood or loss of interest or pleasure must be present in adults (or irritable mood in children and adolescents). Table 69-1 outlines a common acronym for MDD diagnostic criteria.
- The depressive episode must not be attributable to physiological effects of a substance or medical condition.
- There must not be a history of manic-like or hypomanic-like episodes unless they were induced by a substance or medical condition.
- Diagnosis requires a medication review, physical examination, mental status examination, a complete blood count with differential, thyroid function tests, and electrolyte determination.

TABLE 69-1	Diagnostic Criteria for Major Depressive Episode
S	Suicidal ideation with or without plan, suicide attempt; recurrent thoughts of death
I	Interest—loss of interest or pleasure in activities; anhedonia
G	Guilt—inappropriate or excessive in nature; feelings of worthlessness
E	Energy decreased
C	Concentration decreased; difficulty making decisions
A	Appetite changes; typically decreased; resulting in 5% change in weight from baseline
P	Psychomotor agitation or retardation
S	Sleep impairment; typically insomnia but may be hypersomnia

- At least five symptoms must be consistently present over a 2-week period.
- Symptoms must include depressed mood or anhedonia.
- Symptoms must cause substantial distress or impairment in functioning.
- Other medical conditions or substance use do not account for symptoms.

- Many chronic illnesses (eg, stroke, Parkinson disease, traumatic brain injury, hypothyroidism) and substance use disorders are associated with depression. Medications associated with depressive symptoms include many antihypertensives, oral contraceptives, isotretinoin, interferon-β_{1a}, and many others.
- Standardized rating scale should be used to diagnose depression and evaluate treatment.

TREATMENT

- <u>Goals of Treatment</u>: Resolution of current symptoms (ie, remission), prevention of further episodes of depression (ie, relapse or recurrence), and prevention of suicide.

NONPHARMACOLOGIC THERAPY

- Psychotherapy (eg, cognitive therapy, dialectical behavior therapy, or interpersonal psychotherapy) is recommended as primary treatment for mild to moderately severe major depressive episode. For severe depression, it may be used in combination with medications as its effect is considered additive. Psychotherapy alone is not recommended for acute treatment of severe and/or psychotic MDD.
- Electroconvulsive therapy (ECT) may be considered when a rapid response is needed, risks of other treatments outweigh potential benefits, there is history of a poor response to medications, and the patient prefers ECT. A rapid therapeutic response (10–14 days) has been reported.
- Repetitive transcranial magnetic stimulation has demonstrated efficacy and does not require anesthesia as does ECT.
- Recent data suggest the benefit of physical activity in patients with MDD, and the American Psychiatry Association has endorsed inclusion of exercise into MDD treatment plans.

PHARMACOLOGIC THERAPY

General Approach

- Figure 69-1 shows an algorithm for treatment of uncomplicated MDD. Table 69-2 guides adult dosing of antidepressants.
- Antidepressants are considered first line and are equal in efficacy when administered in comparable doses. They are often classified by chemical structure and/or presumed mechanism.
- The initial choice of antidepressant is often made empirically and influenced by the patient's or family member's history of response, concurrent medical

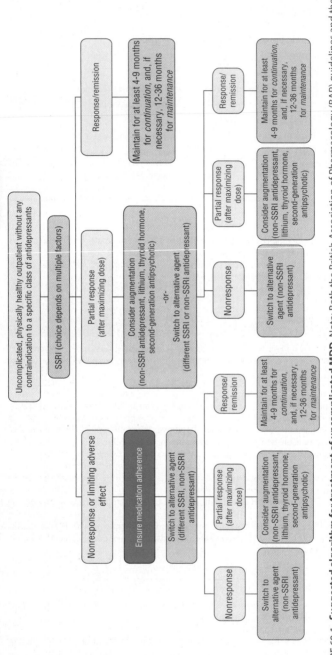

FIGURE 69-1. Suggested algorithm for treatment of uncomplicated MDD. Note: Both the British Association of Pharmacology (BAP) guidelines and the STAR*D trial suggest that switching and augmentation strategies are supported by stronger evidence compared to dose increases (among poor antidepressant responders). SSRI, selective serotonin reuptake inhibitor.

TABLE 69-2 Adult Dosing Guidance for Currently Available Antidepressant Medications

Medication (Brand Name)	Initial Dose (mg/day)	Usual Dosage Range (mg/day)	Comments (eg, Maximum Daily Dosage, Suggested Therapeutic Plasma Concentration)
Selective serotonin reuptake inhibitors (SSRIs)			
Citalopram (Celexa)	20	20–40	Doses >40 mg/day not recommended due to QT prolongation risk; maximum 20 mg/day for CYP2C19 poor metabolizers or coadministration with CYP2C19 inhibitors; 20 mg/day recommended for patients older than 60 years of age
Escitalopram (Lexapro)	5–10	10–20	Maximum 20 mg/day; dose may be increased to maximum daily dose after at least 1 week
Fluoxetine (Prozac)	10–20	20–60	Maximum 80 mg/day; dose may be increased in 20 mg increments
Fluvoxamine (Luvox)	25–50	50–300	Maximum 300 mg/day; daily doses >100 mg total dose should be divided twice daily, with the larger dose given at night Maximum 300 mg/day (ER formulation)
Paroxetine (Paxil)	10–20	20–50	Maximum 50 mg/day (IR formulation); titrate 10 mg/day increments weekly Maximum 62.5 mg/day (CR formulation); titrate 12.5 mg/day increments weekly
Sertraline (Zoloft)	25–50	50–200	Maximum 200 mg/day; titrate 25 mg/day increments weekly
Serotonin–norepinephrine reuptake inhibitors (SNRIs)			
Desvenlafaxine (Pristiq)	50	100	Doses up to 400 mg/day have been studied; however, tolerability decreases with doses >50 mg. Dose reductions or discontinuation may be required if sustained hypertension occurs
Duloxetine (Cymbalta)	30	30–90	Maximum 120 mg/day (given once or twice daily); doses exceeding 60 mg/day not shown to provide increased efficacy for the treatment of MDD
Venlafaxine (Effexor)	37.5–75	75–225	Maximum 375 mg/day (IR); maximum 225 mg/day (ER); may increase in increments up to 75 mg/day at a minimum of every 4 days. Dose reductions or discontinuation may be required if sustained hypertension occurs

(Continued)

TABLE 69-2	Adult Dosing Guidance for Currently Available Antidepressant Medications *(Continued)*		
Medication (Brand Name)	**Initial Dose (mg/day)**	**Usual Dosage Range (mg/day)**	**Comments (eg, Maximum Daily Dosage, Suggested Therapeutic Plasma Concentration)**
Levomilnacipran (Fetzima)	20	40–120	Initial dose (20 mg) for 2 days before dose increases is recommended at intervals of 2 or more days. Dose adjustment or discontinuation may be required if sustained elevated heart rate or hypertension occurs
Tricyclic antidepressants (TCAs)			
Amitriptyline (Elavil)	25	100–200	Maximum 300 mg/day for MDD; depending on the total dose, it may be given as a single daily dose at bedtime or in divided doses throughout the day; therapeutic serum level 100–250 ng/mL (mcg/L; 370–925 nmol/L); parent drug plus metabolite (nortriptyline)
Desipramine (Norpramin)	25	100–200	Maximum 300 mg/day; suggested therapeutic concentration range for combined imipramine + desipramine: 100–300 ng/mL (mcg/L; ~370–1100 nmol/L)
Doxepin (Sinequan)	25	100–200	Maximum 300 mg/day; may be given in a single daily dose at bedtime (if tolerated) or in divided doses throughout the day; a single dose should not exceed 150 mg
Imipramine (Tofranil)	25	100–200	Maximum 300 mg/day; may be given in a single daily dose at bedtime (if tolerated) or divided doses; suggested therapeutic concentration range for combined imipramine + desipramine: 100–300 ng/mL (mcg/L; ~370–1100 nmol/L)
Nortriptyline (Pamelor)	25	50–150	Maximum 150 mg/day; total daily may be given as a single daily dose (if tolerated) or 25 mg doses given three to four times daily; therapeutic serum level 50–150 ng/mL (mcg/L; 190–570 nmol/L)
Norepinephrine and dopamine reuptake inhibitor (NDRI)			
Bupropion (Wellbutrin)	150 (75 mg given twice daily)	150–450	Maximum 450 mg/day (IR, ER), 400 mg/day (SR); ER dosed once or twice daily; SR dosed once or twice daily; IR may be dosed up to three times daily. Adhering to labeled maximum daily and maximum single doses minimizes effect on seizure threshold
Mixed serotonergic effects (mixed 5-HT)			
Nefazodone (Serzone)	100	200–400	Maximum 600 mg/day; daily doses should be divided twice daily

Trazodone (Desyrel)	50	150–300	Maximum 600 mg/day
Vilazodone (Viibryd)	10	20–40	Target dose 20–40 mg/day unless coadministered with CYP3A4 inhibitor (dose not to exceed 20 mg/day). Dose titration: 10 mg/day for 7 days, 20 mg/day for 7 days, and then may increase to 40 mg/day. Dose must be taken with food to ensure adequate absorption

Serotonin and α₂-adrenergic antagonist

Vortioxetine (Brintellix)	10	20	Maximum 20 mg/day

Monoamine oxidase inhibitors (MAOIs)

Mirtazapine (Remeron)	15	15–45	Maximum 45 mg/day
Phenelzine (Nardil)	15	30–90	Maximum 90 mg/day; divided dosing; increase by 15 mg at 1- to 3-week intervals
Selegiline (transdermal) (Emsam)	6	6–12	Not to exceed 12 mg/24 hours; dose may be increased by 3 mg/day increments every 2 weeks; site of application should be rotated
Tranylcypromine (Parnate)	10	20–40	Maximum 60 mg/day; divided dosing; increase by 10 mg at 1- to 3-week intervals
Isocarboxazid (Marplan)	10–20	30–60	Maximum 60 mg/day; divided dosing

Second-generation antipsychotics (SGA) as augmentation (5-HT₂ₐ and D₂ modulators)

Aripiprazole (Abilify)	2	2–15	FDA-approved for augmentation; CANMAT Level 1 evidence, 1st line
Brexpiprazole (Rexulti)	1	1–3	FDA-approved for augmentation; CANMAT Level 1 evidence, 2nd line
Olanzapine (Zyprexa)	2.5	2.5–10	Not FDA-approved for augmentation; CANMAT Level 1 evidence, 2nd line
Olanzapine/fluoxetine (Symbyax)	3/25	6–12/25–50	FDA-approved for treatment-resistant depression
Quetiapine (Seroquel)	50	150–300	FDA-approved for augmentation; CANMAT Level 1 evidence, 1st line
Risperidone (Risperdal)	1	1–3	Not FDA-approved for augmentation; CANMAT Level 1 evidence, 1st line

(Continued)

783

TABLE 69-2 Adult Dosing Guidance for Currently Available Antidepressant Medications *(Continued)*

Medication (Brand Name)	Initial Dose (mg/day)	Usual Dosage Range (mg/day)	Comments (eg, Maximum Daily Dosage, Suggested Therapeutic Plasma Concentration)
Alternative augmentation agents (not FDA-approved for antidepressant augmentation)			
Buspirone (Buspar)	10	10–60	Divided dosing 2–3 times daily
			5-HT$_{1A}$ partial agonist
Lithium	300	600–1200	Dose based on therapeutic levels (target 0.6–1 mEq/L [mmol/L])
			Mechanism in depression not fully understood
Triiodothyronine (Cytomel)	0.025	0.025–0.05	Once daily dosing; monitor free T3 levels

CR, continuous release; ER, extended release; IR, immediate release; MDD, major depressive disorder; SR, sustained release; CANMAT, Canadian Network for Mood and Anxiety Treatments.

conditions, medications the patient is taking, presenting symptoms, potential for medication interactions, medication adverse effect profiles, patient preference, and medication cost.

- An individual's pharmacogenomics may be useful when choosing therapy as a way to better predict antidepressant adverse effects or response. Dosing recommendations to aid in the interpretation of results are available through the Clinical Pharmacogenomics Implementation Consortium (CPIC) as well as the FDA-approved package inserts.
- About 50%–60% of patients with varying types of depression improve with pharmacologic treatment.
- At least a 6-week trial of an antidepressant at maximum dosage is considered an adequate trial.
- The acute phase of treatment lasts 6–12 weeks, and the goal is remission (ie, absence of symptoms). The continuation phase (4–9 months after remission) seeks to eliminate residual symptoms or prevent relapse. The maintenance phase (12–36 months or more) seeks to prevent recurrence of a new episode of depression. Some guidelines recommend lifelong maintenance therapy for persons at greatest risk for recurrence (ie, younger than 40 years of age with two or more prior episodes or any age with three or more prior episodes).
- Give older patients one-half of the initial dose given to younger adults, and increase the dose more slowly. Older patients may require 6–12 weeks of treatment to achieve the desired antidepressant response.
- Early in treatment, all antidepressants can increase suicidal thinking and behavior in children, adolescents, and young adults less than 25 years of age. Suicide risk may also be elevated in the 30 days after discontinuation.
- Educate patients and their support systems about the delay in antidepressant response (typically 2–4 weeks) and the importance of adherence before starting therapy and throughout treatment.
- Occurrence of a withdrawal syndrome with some antidepressants may be reduced with a slow taper over weeks or months when the medication is being discontinued.
- **Table 69-3** shows antidepressant potency and relative selectivity for inhibition of various receptors. Specific adverse effects seen with select antidepressants are given in **Table 69-4**.
- The ability of any antidepressant to inhibit or induce the CYP450 enzymes can be a significant factor determining its capability to cause a pharmacokinetic interactions.

Selective Serotonin Reuptake Inhibitors

- The SSRIs inhibit the reuptake of 5-HT into the presynaptic neuron. They are generally chosen as first-line antidepressants because of their relative safety in overdose and improved tolerability compared with earlier agents (**Fig. 69-1**).
- Nonresponse to one SSRI does not predict nonresponse to an alternative SSRI.
- The SSRIs may have a nonlinear pattern of accumulation with chronic dosing. Hepatic impairment, renal impairment, and age can influence SSRI pharmacokinetics which are summarized in **Table 69-5**.
- Any antidepressant that enhances serotonergic activity can be associated with serotonin syndrome characterized by mental status changes, autonomic instability, and neuromuscular abnormalities. Combining an SSRI with another 5-HT augmenting agent is also a risk.
- The primary adverse effects for SSRIs are nausea, vomiting, diarrhea, headache, insomnia, fatigue, and sexual dysfunction and have a reduced incidence of sedative, anticholinergic, and cardiovascular adverse effects or weight gain.
- A few patients have anxiety symptoms early in treatment which may be reduced by starting with lower doses and slowly titrating up.
- **Citalopram** and **escitalopram** may to an increase in QT interval at doses above 40 mg/day.

TABLE 69-3	Relative Potencies of Norepinephrine and Serotonin Reuptake Blockade and Selected Receptor Antagonism Profile of Antidepressants				
	Reuptake		**Antagonism**		
	NE	5-HT	M1	H1	α1
Selective serotonin reuptake inhibitors (SSRIs)					
Citalopram	0	++++	0	+	0
Escitalopram	0	++++	0	0	0
Fluoxetine	+	++++	0	0	0
Fluvoxamine	0	++++	0	+	0
Paroxetine	++	++++	++	+	0
Sertraline	0	++++	0	0	+
Serotonin–norepinephrine reuptake inhibitors (SNRIs)					
Duloxetine	+++	++++	0	0	0
Levomilnacipran	++++	+++	+	0	0
Venlafaxine[a] and desvenlafaxine	+++	++++	0	0	0
Tricyclic antidepressants (TCAs)					
Amitriptyline	++	++++	++++	++++	+++
Desipramine	++++	++	+	++	++
Doxepin	++	++	+++	++++	+++
Imipramine	++	++++	+++	+++	+++
Nortriptyline	++++	++	++	+++	++
Mixed serotonergic (mixed 5-HT)					
Nefazodone	0	++	0	+++	+++
Trazodone	0	++	0	++	+++
Vilazodone	0	++++	0	+	0
Vortioxetine	0	++++	0	+	0
Norepinephrine and dopamine reuptake inhibitor (NDRI)					
Bupropion[b]	+	0	+	0	0
Serotonin and α₂-receptor antagonist					
Mirtazapine	0	0	0	+++	+

α1, antiadrenergic, hypotension; H1, antihistamine, sedation; M1, antimuscarinic/anticholinergic adverse effects.
[a]Venlafaxine: primarily 5-HT at lower doses, NE at higher doses, and DA at very high doses.
[b]Bupropion: also blocks dopamine reuptake.
++++, high; +++, moderate; ++, low; +, very low; 0, absent or not adequately studied.

- Potentially fatal reactions may occur when any SSRI and MAOI are coadministered. A 5-week washout after fluoxetine discontinuation is critical before starting an MAOI.
- If an SSRI is added to a regimen which includes interacting medications the SSRI starting dose should be low and slowly titrated.
- Table 69-6 compares second- and third-generation antidepressants for their effects on CYP450 enzymes. CYP2D6 and 3A4 are responsible for the metabolism of more than 80% of current medications. Consult the literature for detailed information concerning any real or potential psychotherapeutic interactions.

TABLE 69-4 Adverse Medication Reactions and Monitoring Parameters Associated with Select Antidepressants

Medication	Adverse Reaction	Monitoring	Comments
Antidepressants from each pharmacologic class			
Common to all antidepressants			
	Suicidality	Behavioral changes Mental status	(US black box warning) for all antidepressants; caregivers should be alerted to monitor for acute changes in behavior (especially early in treatment)
Selective serotonin reuptake inhibitors (SSRIs)			
Common to all SSRIs			
	Anxiety or nervousness	Assess severity and impact on patient functioning and quality of life	Most prominent on initial treatment; lower initial doses recommended in patients with prominent anxiety
	Hyponatremia	Serum sodium	More likely in older females; sodium may decrease within 72 hours of initiating antidepressant
	Nausea	Frequency and severity	May improve with slower dose titration
	Sleep changes (insomnia and somnolence)	Sleep patterns	Among SSRI class: fluoxetine may be more activating; fluvoxamine and paroxetine may be more sedating
	Sexual dysfunction	Assess severity and impact on patient functioning and quality of life	Spontaneous self-reporting may be low; clinician should assess symptoms; reversible on drug discontinuation
SSRI-specific			
Citalopram (possibly escitalopram)	QTc interval prolongation	Electrocardiogram; electrolytes (eg, potassium, magnesium)	Caution use in "at-risk" patients (eg, electrolyte disturbance; discontinue if QTc persistently >500 msec or increased >50 msec over baseline
Paroxetine	Anticholinergic effects	Symptoms: dry mouth, constipation, urinary retention, mental status	Avoid in older adults

(Continued)

TABLE 69-4	Adverse Medication Reactions and Monitoring Parameters Associated with Select Antidepressants *(Continued)*		
Medication	Adverse Reaction	Monitoring	Comments
Serotonin–norepinephrine reuptake inhibitors (SNRIs)			
Common to all SNRIs			
	Cardiovascular changes	Increases in blood pressure; heart rate	Possibly less likely with duloxetine; may need to lower/discontinue dose
	Insomnia	Sleep patterns	Possibly less likely with duloxetine
	Nausea	Frequency and severity	May improve with slower dose titration
	Sexual dysfunction	Assess severity and impact on patient functioning and quality of life	Spontaneous self-reporting may be low; clinicians should assess symptoms; reversible on drug discontinuation
	Sweating	Frequency and severity	May require change in therapy
SNRI-specific			
Desvenlafaxine	Dose-related hyperlipidemia	Lipid profile	Elevations in total cholesterol, low-density lipoproteins, and triglycerides
Duloxetine	Liver toxicity	Liver function tests	May be transient upon initiation or sustained
Mixed serotonergic effects (mixed 5-HT)			
Nefazodone	Liver toxicity	Liver function tests	Nefazodone black box warning in the United States for hepatotoxicity
Trazodone	Orthostatic hypotension	Blood pressure, pulse	May be more severe as compared with other antidepressants; rate-limiting adverse effect
	Priapism	Patient report of sexual adverse effects, especially painful erection	Patient should seek medical attention for prolonged erection (ie, >4 hours)
Vilazodone and vortioxetine	Nausea	Frequency and severity	Most common dose-limiting adverse effect
Serotonin and α₂-adrenergic antagonist			
Mirtazapine	Weight gain	Body weight	Frequently occurring and significant (> 7% over baseline) weight gain among adults; diet mediated
Norepinephrine and dopamine reuptake inhibitor (NDRI)			
Bupropion	Seizure activity	Electroencephalogram if indicated	See Table 69-2 for proper dosing, which can help decrease seizure risk; caution use in patients with eating disorders or alcohol use disorders

TABLE 69-5	Pharmacokinetic Properties of Antidepressants	
Generic Name	**Elimination Half-Life[a]**	**Plasma Protein Binding (%)**
Selective serotonin reuptake inhibitors (SSRIs)		
Citalopram	33 hours	80
Escitalopram	27–32 hours	56
Fluoxetine	4–6 days[b]	94
Fluvoxamine	15–26 hours	77
Paroxetine	24–31 hours	95
Sertraline	27 hours	99[c]
Serotonin–norepinephrine reuptake inhibitors (SNRIs)		
Desvenlafaxine	11 hours	30
Duloxetine	12 hours	90
Levomilnacipran	12 hours	22
Venlafaxine	5 hours	27–30
Norepinephrine/Dopamine reuptake inhibitor (NDRI)		
Bupropion	10–21 hours	82–88
Tricyclic antidepressants (TCAs)		
Amitriptyline	9–46 hours	90–97
Desipramine	11–46 hours	90–97
Doxepin	8–36 hours	68–82
Imipramine	6–34 hours	63–96
Nortriptyline	16–88 hours	87–95
Mixed serotonergic (mixed 5-HT)		
Nefazodone	2–4 hours	99
Trazodone	6–11 hours	92
Vilazodone	25 hours	>95
Vortioxetine	66 hours	98
Serotonin and α2-adrenergic antagonists		
Mirtazapine	20–40 hours	85

[a]Biologic half-life in slowest phase of elimination
[b]Four to 6 days with chronic dosing; norfluoxetine, 4–16 days.
[c]Increases 30%–40% when taken with food.

Serotonin–Norepinephrine Reuptake Inhibitors and Antidepressants with Mixed Serotonin Effects

- **Venlafaxine** may have a slight efficacy advantage compared to other antidepressants.
- Common adverse effects may be dose-related and include nausea, sexual dysfunction, activation, and hyperhidrosis.
- Venlafaxine may cause a dose-related increase in diastolic blood pressure, which may require dosage reduction or discontinuation if sustained hypertension occurs. Nausea and vomiting may be worse with venlafaxine and there may be higher adverse effect-related discontinuation rates with venlafaxine and duloxetine than with the SSRIs.
- The most common adverse effects of **duloxetine** are nausea, dry mouth, constipation, decreased appetite, insomnia, and increased sweating.
- **Mirtazapine** enhances central noradrenergic and serotonergic activity by antagonizing central presynaptic α_2-adrenergic autoreceptors and heteroreceptors. It also

TABLE 69-6	Second- and Third-Generation Antidepressants and Cytochrome (CYP) P450 Enzyme Inhibitory Potential			
	CYP Enzyme			
Medication	**1A2**	**2C**	**2D6**	**3A4**
Bupropion	0	0	+++	0
Citalopram	0	0	+	NA
Duloxetine	0	0	+++	0
Escitalopram	0	0	+	0
Fluoxetine	0	++	++++	++
Fluvoxamine	++++	++	0	+++
Mirtazapine	0	0	0	0
Nefazodone	0	0	0	++++
Paroxetine	0	0	++++	0
Sertraline	0	++	+	+
(des)-Venlafaxine	0	0	0/+	0
Vilazodone	0	0	0	0
Vortioxetine	0	0	0	0

++++, high; +++, moderate; ++, low; +, very low; 0, absent.

antagonizes 5-HT$_2$ and 5-HT$_3$ receptors and blocks histamine receptors. It may be an option for patients experiencing sexual dysfunction with other antidepressants. Mirtazapine's most common adverse effects are somnolence, and weight gain.

- **Levomilnacipran** is a single-isomer, extended-release form of milnacipran (FDA-approved to treat fibromyalgia). It inhibits NE reuptake more than 5-HT reuptake and may increase blood pressure and heart rate. Its place in therapy for MDD is unknown.
- **Trazodone** and **nefazodone** antagonize the 5-HT$_2$ receptor and inhibit the reuptake of 5-HT. They can also enhance 5-HT$_{1A}$ neurotransmission. Trazodone blocks α_1-adrenergic and histaminergic receptors increasing dizziness and sedation.
  - ✓ Trazodone cause minimal anticholinergic effects and sedation, dizziness, and cognitive slowing are the most frequent dose-limiting adverse effects. Common adverse effects with nefazodone are dizziness, orthostatic hypotension, and somnolence.
  - ✓ Priapism occurs rarely with trazodone (1 in 6000 male patients). Surgical intervention may be required, and impotence may result.
  - ✓ Nefazodone carries a black box warning for life-threatening liver failure. Do not initiate nefazodone in individuals with active liver disease or elevated serum transaminases.
- **Vilazodone** and **vortioxetine** are antidepressants with mixed serotonin effects that are a combination SSRI and 5-HT$_{1A}$ presynaptic receptor partial agonists. Vilazodone may be particularly useful for depressed patients with anxiety, and vortioxetine may be helpful for depressed patients with cognitive difficulties.
  - ✓ Vilazodone is associated with nausea, diarrhea, dizziness, insomnia, and decreased libido, especially in males.
  - ✓ Vortioxetine causes nausea and constipation and sexual dysfunction in males at the highest dose (20 mg/day).

Bupropion

- **Bupropion** inhibits both the NE and DA reuptake making it one of the most activating antidepressants.

✓ The occurrence of seizures with bupropion is dose related and may be increased by predisposing factors (eg, history of head trauma or central nervous system [CNS] tumor). At the ceiling dose (450 mg/day), the incidence of seizures is 0.4%.

✓ Other adverse effects are nausea, vomiting, tremor, insomnia, dry mouth, and skin reactions. It is contraindicated in patients with bulimia or anorexia nervosa, due to a higher risk for seizures. It causes less sexual dysfunction than SSRIs.

Tricyclic Antidepressants

- Tricyclic antidepressant (TCA) use has diminished given other equally effective therapies that are safer on overdose and better tolerated. They inhibit the reuptake of NE and 5-HT and have affinity for adrenergic, cholinergic, and histaminergic receptors.

- TCAs cause anticholinergic effects (eg, dry mouth, blurred vision, constipation, urinary retention, tachycardia, memory impairment, and delirium) and sedation. Additional adverse effects include weight gain, orthostatic hypotension, cardiac conduction delay, and sexual dysfunction.

- **Desipramine** carries an increased risk of death in patients with a family history of sudden cardiac death, cardiac dysrhythmias, or cardiac conduction disturbances.

- Abrupt withdrawal of TCAs (especially high doses) may result in cholinergic rebound (eg, dizziness, nausea, diarrhea, insomnia, and restlessness).

- TCA metabolism appears to be linear within the usual dosage range. Dose-related kinetics cannot be ruled out in older patients. Factors reported to influence TCA plasma concentrations include renal or hepatic dysfunction, genetics, age, cigarette smoking, and concurrent medications.

- In acutely depressed patients, there is a correlation between antidepressant effect and plasma concentrations for some TCAs (eg, **amitriptyline, nortriptyline, imipramine,** and **desipramine**). The best-established therapeutic range is for **nortriptyline**, and data suggest a therapeutic window (Table 69-2).

- Some indications for TCA plasma level monitoring include inadequate response or relapse; adverse effects; use of higher than standard doses; suspected non-adherence; pharmacokinetic interactions; older, pediatric, and adolescent patients; pregnant patients; pharmacogenomic indications; and cardiac disease. Obtain steady state plasma concentrations usually after a minimum of 1 week at constant dosage, during the elimination phase 12 hours after the last dose.

- TCAs may interact with other medications that modify hepatic cytochrome P450 (CYP450) enzyme activity or hepatic blood flow. TCAs also are involved in interactions through displacement from protein-binding sites.

- Increased plasma concentrations of TCAs and symptoms of toxicity may occur when CYP2D6 inhibitors are added.

Monoamine Oxidase Inhibitors

- **Isocarboxazide**, **phenelzine,** and **tranylcypromine** increase the concentrations of NE, 5-HT, and DA within the neuronal synapse through inhibition of monoamine oxidase (MAO). They are nonselective inhibitors of MAO-A and MAO-B. **Selegiline**, available as a transdermal patch for treatment of major depression, inhibits brain MAO-A and MAO-B but has reduced effects on MAO-A in the gut.

- Table 69-7 shows dietary and medication restrictions for patients taking phenelzine or tranylcypromine.

- The most common medication adverse effect is postural hypotension (more likely with phenelzine than tranylcypromine), which can be minimized by divided dosing.

- Phenelzine is mildly to moderately sedating, but tranylcypromine is often stimulating, and the last dose of the day is administered in the early afternoon. Sexual dysfunction in both genders is common. Phenelzine has been associated with hepatocellular damage and weight gain.

- The potentially fatal hypertensive crisis can occur when MAOIs are taken concurrently with foods high in tyramine, and with certain medications (see Table 69-7). Symptoms include occipital headache, stiff neck, nausea, vomiting, sweating, and

TABLE 69-7	Dietary and Medication Restrictions for Monoamine Oxidase Inhibitors[a]	
Foods to Avoid Completely	**Foods to Eat in Moderation**	
Aged cheeses (eg, cheddar, blue, Swiss, Camembert)	American cheese, Parmesan cheese	
	Canned, filtered beer	
Chicken liver	Havarti, brie	
Dry aged meats (eg, mortadella, salami, prosciutto)	Pepperoni	
Fava beans	Pizza (large commercial chains generally safe; avoid gourmet with aged cheeses and meats)	
Kim chee	White wine	
Red wine	**Foods Without Restrictions**	
Sauerkraut	Fresh dairy products (cottage cheese, cream cheese, fresh milk, ice cream, ricotta, sour cream, yogurt)	
Smoked or pickled fish (eg, lox, caviar, pickled herring)	Fresh meats (including fresh sausage)	
Soy sauce, fermented soy, miso	Processed meats (eg, lunch meat, hot dogs, ham)	
Tap beer	Spirits (eg, bourbon, gin, rum, vodka)	
Yeast extract	Yeast bread products	
Medications to Avoid Completely		
Antidepressants[a]	Dextromethorphan	Meperidine
Amphetamines	Dopamine	Methyldopa
Appetite suppressants	Ephedrine	Methylphenidate
Asthma inhalants	Epinephrine	Reserpine
Buspirone	Guanethidine	Sympathomimetics
Carbamazepine	Levodopa	Tryptophan
Decongestants	Local anesthetics[b]	

[a]Tricyclic antidepressants may be used with caution by experienced clinicians in treatment-refractory populations.
[b]Those containing sympathomimetic vasoconstrictors.

sharply elevated blood pressure. It can be treated with agents such as captopril. Education regarding dietary and medication restrictions is critical. Patients taking transdermal selegiline patch doses greater than 6 mg/24 hours must follow the dietary restrictions.

- Potentially fatal reactions may occur when any SSRI or TCA is coadministered with an MAOI. However, TCAs and MAOIs can be combined in refractory patients by experienced clinicians with careful monitoring.

Ketamine

- **Ketamine** modulates glutamate activity via extrasynaptic N-methyl-D-aspartate (NMDA) receptor antagonism resulting in increased BDNF activity and synaptogenesis.
- It has rapid antidepressant effects when used in intravenous doses of 0.5mg/kg for treatment of treatment-resistant depression (TRD).
- **Esketamine** is the single s-isomer of ketamine that has a higher affinity for the NMDA receptor than the r-isomer. Intranasal esketamine is FDA-approved and requires supervised, in-clinic self-administration (1–3 sprays in each nostril per session) followed by 2 hours of in-clinic observation. In trials, patients received doses twice weekly for 4 weeks and variable dosing thereafter.
- Medication adverse effects include transient psychotomimetic/dissociative effects and blood pressure elevation (10–20 mm Hg) with both agents. It has a mandatory Risk Evaluation and Mitigation Strategies (REMS).

Brexanolone

- **Brexanolone** (exogenous allopregnanolone) is thought to exert antidepressant effect by allosteric modulation of $GABA_A$ receptors, which may increase 5-HT and NE transmission and is FDA-approved for postpartum depression. Administration involves a 60-hour stepped dose, intravenous infusion which is very costly.
- Common adverse effects are headache, dizziness, and somnolence. It also has a REMS program with Elements to Ensure Safe Use (ETASU) due to the incidence of excessive sedation or loss of consciousness.

Alternative Pharmacotherapy

- **St. John's wort**, a herb containing hypericum, may be effective some with mild-to-moderate depression. It is associated with several medication interactions.
- **Omega-3 fatty acids**, **S-adenosyl-L-methionine** (SAMe), and **folate** are additional pharmacotherapies that could be considered. Evidence regarding their use is conflicting or still emerging. All of these agents should be used with caution.

SPECIAL POPULATIONS

Older Patients

- In older patients, depressed mood may be less prominent than other symptoms, such as loss of appetite, cognitive impairment, sleeplessness, fatigue, physical complaints, and loss of interest in usual activities.
- The SSRIs are often considered first-choice antidepressants for older patients. Bupropion, venlafaxine, and mirtazapine are also effective and well tolerated.
- Hyponatremia is more common in older patients.

Pediatric Patients

- Symptoms of depression in childhood include boredom, anxiety, failing adjustment, and sleep disturbance.
- Data supporting efficacy of antidepressants in children and adolescents are sparse. Fluoxetine and escitalopram are FDA-approved for patients below 18 years of age.
- All antidepressants carry a black box warning for use in this population regarding increased risk for suicidal ideation and behavior. The FDA recommends specific monitoring parameters.
- Several cases of sudden death have been reported in children and adolescents taking desipramine and baseline electrocardiogram (ECG) is recommended.

Pregnancy and Lactation

- Individuals who discontinued antidepressant therapy during pregnancy were five times more likely to have a relapse during their pregnancy than those who continued treatment.
- The absolute risk of antidepressant use in pregnancy is unknown.
- Risks reported with SSRIs use in pregnancy include low birth weight, respiratory distress, and congenital heart defects.
- The risks and benefits of drug therapy during pregnancy must be weighed, including concerns about untreated depression.
- There is a great deal of uncertainty regarding long-term antidepressant exposure in infants exposed through human milk due to the lack of data. More information can be found in Chapter 32.

Relative Resistance and Treatment-Resistant Depression

- One in three patients who did not achieve remission with an antidepressant may become symptom-free when an additional medication (eg, bupropion SR or buspirone) is added. One in four may achieve remission after switching to a different antidepressant (eg, venlafaxine XR or bupropion, or sertraline).
- The current antidepressant may also be augmented by addition of another agent (eg, lithium or triiodothyronine [T_3]), or another antidepressant can be added.

A second generation antipsychotic (eg, aripiprazole, quetiapine, brexpiprazole) can be used to augment antidepressant response. New medications such as ketamine and esketamine may be considered.

- The practice guideline of the American Psychiatric Association recommends that after 6–8 weeks of treatment, partial responders should consider changing the dose, augmenting the antidepressant, or adding psychotherapy or ECT. For patients with no response, options include changing to another antidepressant or the addition of psychotherapy or ECT. **Figure 69-1** is an algorithm for treatment of depression including refractory patients.

- Before changing treatment, evaluate the adequacy of the medication dosage and adherence, as most "treatment-resistant" depressed patients have received inadequate therapy.

- Issues to be addressed in assessing the patient who has not responded to treatment include asking: (1) Is the diagnosis correct?; (2) Does the patient have a psychotic depression?; (3) Is the dose and duration of treatment adequate?; (4) Do adverse medication reactions preclude adequate dosing?; (5) Is patient adherence appropriate?; (6) Was a stepwise approach to treatment used?; (7) Was treatment outcome adequately measured?; (8) Is there a coexisting or pre-existing medical or psychiatric disorder?; (9) Are there other factors interfering with treatment?; (10) May pharmacogenomics be impacting treatment?

EVALUATION OF THERAPEUTIC OUTCOMES

- Several monitoring parameters, in addition to plasma concentrations, are useful. Monitor regularly for adverse effects (**Table 69-4**), remission of target symptoms, and changes in social or occupational functioning. Assure regular monitoring for several months after discontinuation of antidepressants.

- Regularly monitor blood pressure of patients given serotonin–norepinephrine reuptake inhibitors.

- A pretreatment ECG is recommended before starting TCA therapy in children, adolescents, and patients over 40 years of age, and perform follow-up ECGs periodically.

- Monitor for suicidal ideation after initiation of any antidepressant, especially in the first few weeks of treatment and up to 30 days after treatment discontinuation.

- In addition to the clinical interview, use psychometric rating instruments to rapidly and reliably measure the nature and severity of depressive and associated symptoms.

See Chapter 88, Major Depressive Disorder, authored by Amy M. VandenBerg, for a more detailed discussion of this topic.

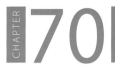

CHAPTER 70

Insomnia

- Approximately 70 million Americans suffer with a sleep-related problem, and as many as 60% of those experience a chronic disorder.

SLEEP PHYSIOLOGY

- Humans typically have four to six cycles of non-rapid eye movement (NREM) and rapid eye movement (REM) sleep each night, each cycle lasting 70–120 minutes. Usually, there is progression through the three stages of NREM sleep before the first REM period.
- Stage 1 of NREM is the stage between wakefulness and sleep. Stages 3 and 4 sleep are called *delta sleep* (ie, slow-wave sleep).
- In REM sleep, there is a low-amplitude, mixed-frequency electroencephalogram, increased electrical and metabolic activity, increased cerebral blood flow, muscle atonia, poikilothermia, vivid dreaming, and fluctuations in respiratory and cardiac rate.
- Older individuals have lighter more fragmented sleep with more arousals and gradual reduction in slow-wave sleep.
- REM sleep is turned on by cholinergic cells. Dopamine has an alerting effect. Neurochemicals involved in wakefulness include norepinephrine and acetylcholine in the cortex and histamine and neuropeptides (eg, substance P and corticotropin-releasing factor) in the hypothalamus.
- Polysomnography (PSG) measures multiple electrophysiologic parameters simultaneously during sleep (eg, electroencephalogram, electrooculogram of each eye, electrocardiogram, electromyogram, air thermistors, abdominal and thoracic strain belts, and oxygen saturation) to characterize sleep and diagnose sleep disorders.

CLINICAL PRESENTATION

- Insomnia is subjectively characterized as trouble initiating or maintaining sleep or waking up early with the inability to fall back asleep. The consequence of this disrupted sleep is daytime sleepiness.
- Transient (two or three nights) and short-term (less than 3 months) insomnia is common. Chronic insomnia (more than 3 months duration) occurs in 9%–12% of adults and in up to 20% of older individuals.

DIAGNOSIS

- A complete diagnostic examination should include routine laboratory tests, physical and mental status examinations, as well as ruling out any medication- or substance-related causes.
- Causes of insomnia include stress; jet lag or shift work; pain or other medical problems; mood or anxiety disorders; substance withdrawal; stimulants, steroids, or other medications.

TREATMENT

- Goals of Treatment: To correct the underlying sleep complaint, improve daytime functioning, and avoid adverse medication effects.

NONPHARMACOLOGIC THERAPY

- Behavioral and educational interventions that may help include short-term cognitive behavioral therapy, relaxation therapy, stimulus control therapy, cognitive therapy, sleep restriction, paradoxical intention, and sleep hygiene education (Table 70-1).

TABLE 70-1	Nonpharmacologic Recommendations for Managing Insomnia

Stimulus control procedures

1. Establish regular time to wake up and to go to sleep (including weekends).

2. Sleep only as much as necessary to feel rested.

3. Go to bed only when sleepy. Avoid long periods of wakefulness in bed. Use the bed only for sleep or intimacy; do not read or watch television in bed.

4. Avoid trying to force sleep; if you do not fall asleep within 20–30 minutes, leave the bed and perform a relaxing activity (eg, read, listen to music) until drowsy. Repeat this as often as necessary.

5. Avoid blue spectrum light from television, smart phones, tablets, and other mobile devices.

6. Avoid daytime naps.

7. Schedule worry time during the day. Do not take your troubles to bed.

Sleep hygiene recommendations

1. Exercise routinely (three to four times weekly) but not close to bedtime because this can increase wakefulness.

2. Create a comfortable sleep environment by avoiding temperature extremes, loud noises, and illuminated clocks in the bedroom.

3. Discontinue or reduce the use of alcohol, caffeine, and nicotine.

4. Avoid drinking large quantities of liquids in the evening to prevent nighttime trips to the restroom.

5. Do something relaxing and enjoyable before bedtime.

- Management includes identifying and correcting the cause of insomnia, educating about sleep hygiene, managing stress, monitoring for mood symptoms, and eliminating unnecessary pharmacotherapy.
- In patients aged 55 years and older, cognitive behavioral therapy may be more effective than pharmacologic therapy at improving certain measures of insomnia.
- Transient and short-term insomnia should be treated with good sleep hygiene and careful use of sedative–hypnotics if necessary. Chronic insomnia calls for careful assessment for a medical cause, nonpharmacologic treatment, and careful use of sedative–hypnotics if necessary (Fig. 70-1).

PHARMACOLOGIC THERAPY

Antidepressants

- Antihistamines (eg, **diphenhydramine, doxylamine**, and **pyrilamine**) are available without a prescription. Their anticholinergic adverse effects may be problematic, especially in older individuals.
- Antidepressants are good alternatives for patients who should not receive benzodiazepines, especially those with depression, pain, or a history of substance use disorder or unhealthy substance use.
  - ✓ **Amitriptyline, doxepin**, and **nortriptyline** are effective, but medication adverse effects include sedation, anticholinergic effects, adrenergic blockade effects, and cardiac conduction prolongation.
  - ✓ Low-dose doxepin is approved for sleep maintenance insomnia.
  - ✓ Mirtazapine may improve sleep, but may cause daytime sedation and weight gain.
  - ✓ **Trazodone**, 25–100 mg at bedtime, is often used for insomnia induced by selective serotonin reuptake inhibitors or bupropion and in patients prone to unhealthy substance use. Medication adverse effects include risk for serotonin syndrome

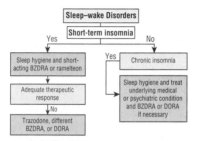

FIGURE 70-1. Algorithm for treatment of insomnia. BZDRA, benzodiazepine receptor agonist; DORA, dual orexin A and orexin B receptor antagonists.

(when used with other serotonergic drugs), oversedation, α-adrenergic blockade, dizziness, and rarely, priapism.

Miscellaneous Agents

- **Suvorexant** and **lemborexant** are dual orexin A and orexin B receptor antagonists (DORA). Instead of inducing sleepiness, they turn off wake signaling. Suvorexant doses of 10–20 mg or lemborexant doses of 5–10 mg at bedtime are indicated for difficulty initiating or maintaining sleep. Adverse effects include sedation and rarely narcolepsy-like symptoms. Use caution in patients with depression because they can worsen depression and trigger suicidal thinking in a dose-dependent manner.
- **Ramelteon** is a melatonin receptor agonist selective for the MT_1 and MT_2 receptors. The dose is 8 mg at bedtime. It is well tolerated, but adverse effects include headache, dizziness, and somnolence. It is not a controlled substance, and does not cause acute drowsiness similar to other insomnia agents. It is effective for patients with chronic obstructive pulmonary disease and sleep apnea.
- **Valerian**, an herbal product, is available without a prescription. The recommended dose is 300–600 mg. Data supporting its efficacy are lacking.

Benzodiazepine Receptor Agonists

- The benzodiazepine receptor agonists (BZDRAs) are the most commonly used drugs for insomnia. They include the newer nonbenzodiazepine γ-aminobutyric acid$_A$ (GABA$_A$) agonists and the traditional benzodiazepines, which also bind to GABA$_A$. The United States Food and Drug Administration (FDA) requires labeling regarding anaphylaxis, facial angioedema, complex sleep behaviors (eg, sleep driving, phone calls, and sleep eating).
- The pharmacokinetics and dosing of BZDRAs approved by the FDA for insomnia are summarized in Table 70-2. Other BZDRAs are often used off label for the treatment of insomnia.
- Benzodiazepines have sedative, anxiolytic, muscle relaxant, and anticonvulsant properties. They increase stage 2 sleep and decrease REM and delta sleep.
- Overdose fatalities are rare unless benzodiazepines are taken with other central nervous system (CNS) depressants.
- **Triazolam** is distributed quickly because of its high lipophilicity, and it has a short duration of effect. Erythromycin, nefazodone, fluvoxamine, and ketoconazole reduce the clearance of triazolam and increase plasma concentrations.
- The effects of **flurazepam** and **quazepam** are long because of active metabolites and therefore they should not be used as first-line agents.
  - ✓ Adverse effects include drowsiness, psychomotor incoordination, decreased concentration, cognitive deficits, and anterograde amnesia, which are minimized by using the lowest dose possible.
  - ✓ Tolerance to daytime CNS effects (eg, drowsiness, decreased concentration) may develop in some individuals.

TABLE 70-2	Pharmacokinetics of Benzodiazepine Receptor Agonists				
Generic Name (Brand Name)	t_{max} (hours)[a]	Half-Life[b] (hours)	Daily Dose Range (mg)	Metabolic Pathway	Clinically Significant Metabolites
Estazolam (ProSom)	2	12–15	1–2	Oxidation	–
Eszopiclone (Lunesta)	1–1.5	6	2–3	Oxidation	
				Demethylation	
Flurazepam (Dalmane)	1	8	15–30	Oxidation	Hydroxyethylflurazepam, flurazepam aldehyde
				N-dealkylation	N-desalkylflurazepam[c]
Quazepam (Doral)	2	39	7.5–15	Oxidation, N-dealkylation	2-Oxo-quazepam, N-desalkylflurazepam[c]
Temazepam (Restoril)	1.5	10–15	15–30	Conjugation	–
Triazolam (Halcion)	1	2	0.125–0.25	Oxidation	–
Zaleplon (Sonata)	1	1	5–10	Oxidation	–
Zolpidem (Ambien; Intermezzo)	1.6	2–2.6	1.75–10[d]	Oxidation	–

[a]Time to peak plasma concentration.
[b]Half-life of parent drug.
[c]N-desalkylflurazepam, mean half-life 47–100 hours.
[d]Oral and sublingual dosing 5–10 mg; sublingual tablets for middle-of-the night dosing 1.75–3.5 mg (1.75 mg for women, 3.5 mg for men).

✓ Rebound insomnia is minimized by using the lowest effective dose and tapering the dose upon discontinuation.

✓ Long elimination half-life benzodiazepines are associated with falls and hip fractures; thus, flurazepam and quazepam should be avoided in older individuals. **Lorazepam**, **oxazepam**, and **temazepam** are the three BZDRAs often suggested to be used for older patients as they are primarily broken down by conjugation. Not all of these agents are FDA approved for insomnia.

Nonbenzodiazepine GABA_A Agonists

- In general, the nonbenzodiazepine hypnotics do not have significant active metabolites, and they are associated with less physical withdrawal, tolerance, and rebound insomnia than the benzodiazepines.
- **Zolpidem** is comparable in effectiveness to benzodiazepine hypnotics, and it has little effect on sleep stages. Its duration is approximately 6–8 hours. Common adverse effects are drowsiness, amnesia, dizziness, headache, and gastrointestinal (GI) complaints. It appears to have minimal effects on next-day psychomotor performance. The usual dose is 5 mg in females, older persons, and those with liver impairment, and 5–10 mg in males. Sleep eating has been reported. It should be taken on an empty stomach.
- **Zaleplon** has a rapid onset, a half-life of ~1 hour, and no active metabolites. It decreases time to sleep onset, but does not reduce nighttime awakenings or increase the total sleep time. It does not appear to cause next-day psychomotor impairment.

The most common adverse effects are dizziness, headache, and somnolence. The recommended dose is 10 mg (5 mg in older patients).

- **Eszopiclone** has a rapid onset and duration of action of up to 6 hours. The most common adverse effects are somnolence, unpleasant taste, headache, and dry mouth. It may be taken nightly for up to 6 months.

EVALUATION OF THERAPEUTIC OUTCOMES

- Assess patients with short-term or chronic insomnia after 1 week of therapy for drug effectiveness, adverse events, and adherence to nonpharmacologic recommendations. Patients should maintain a daily recording of awakenings, medications taken, naps, and an index of sleep quality.

See Chapter 92, Sleep Disorders, authored by John M. Dopp, and Bradley G. Phillips, for a more detailed discussion of this topic.

Opioid Use Disorder

- *Opioid use disorder* (OUD) is a chronic lifelong disorder that consists of intoxication and withdrawal from opioids. Seventy percent of overdose deaths involve opioid substances including prescription opioids (ie, natural opioids, semisynthetic opioids, and methadone), as well as heroin and synthetic opioids (ie, illicitly manufactured fentanyl). Deaths from opioids have reached epidemic levels.

PATHOPHYSIOLOGY

- The true etiology behind OUD is unknown. In general, it is felt that there needs to be a triad of the right patient, with the right genetic risk factors, being exposed to opioids in order for it to occur.

CLINICAL PRESENTATION

- Signs and symptoms of opioid intoxication include euphoria, dysphoria, slurred speech, miosis, apathy, sedation, and attention impairment.
- Pinpoint pupils, decreased breathing, pulmonary edema, loss of consciousness, and death may occur with opioid intoxication.
- Signs and symptoms of withdrawal include lacrimation, mydriasis, piloerection, diaphoresis, diarrhea, yawning, muscle aches, and insomnia.
- Withdrawal symptoms begin within 8–24 hours for opioids with a short half-life (eg, heroin), and can last up to 7–10 days. For agents with a long half-life (eg, methadone), symptoms can begin about 24 hours following the last dose but takes up to 96 hours to peak with gradual reduction over 2 weeks or longer.
- Occurrence of delirium suggests withdrawal from another substance (eg, alcohol).
- Laboratory tests include a comprehensive metabolic panel to monitor serum electrolyte concentrations in the setting of significant vomiting or diarrhea; check liver function tests if using buprenorphine. Arterial blood gases, pulse oximetry, and capnography are useful to assess respiratory depression in opioid intoxication.
- **Heroin** can be snorted, smoked, and given IV. Complications of heroin use include overdoses, anaphylactic reactions to impurities, nephrotic syndrome, septicemia, endocarditis, and acquired immunodeficiency.
- **Hydrocodone** is the most widely misused pharmaceutical controlled substance in the United States.
- **Fentanyl** is a synthetic short-acting opioid which is 50–100 times more potent than morphine and approved for management of acute or chronic pain associated with advanced cancer. Most fentanyl-related morbidity and mortality have been linked to illicitly manufactured fentanyl and fentanyl analogs. It is often mixed with heroin or cocaine, with or without the user's knowledge. Several states have reported spikes in overdose deaths due to fentanyl and its analogs (eg, carfentanil).
- Opioids are commonly combined with stimulants (eg, cocaine [speedball]) or alcohol in individuals with unhealthy use.
- **Methadone** has caused an increased number of deaths in recent years. Converting to methadone from other opioid agonists can be tricky, and lethal when done improperly. Peak respiratory depressant effects occur later and last longer than peak analgesic effects.
- **Dextromethorphan** and **loperamide** are over-the-counter medications that cause central nervous system (CNS) depression and mild hallucinogenic effects in high doses and significant hallucinations and CNS depression in excessive doses. Loperamide is sometimes taken with medications or foods that enhance its ability to cross

the blood-brain barrier (ie, verapamil, methadone, cimetidine, or grapefruit juice) to obtain CNS effects.
- Loperamide at supratherapeutic doses can cause possible cardiac arrhythmias including QTc interval prolongation, torsades de pointes, ventricular dysrhythmias, syncope, and cardiac arrest.
- Acute overdoses of dextromethorphan can be treated with naloxone.

DIAGNOSIS

- The *Diagnostic and Statistical Manual of Mental Disorders*, 5th edition (*DSM-5*) defines OUD as "problematic pattern of substance use leading to clinically significant impairment or distress as manifested by at least two of eleven criteria occurring in the preceding 12-month period."
- These behaviors fall into the categories of: (1) impaired control, (2) social impairment, (3) risky use, and (4) pharmacological criteria, including tolerance and withdrawal.
- OUDs occur in a broad range of severity from mild (2–3 symptoms) to moderate (4–5 symptoms) to severe (6 or more symptoms).
- The Clinical Opiate Withdrawal Scale (COWS) or the Objective Opioid Withdrawal Scale (OOWS) are clinician-rated assessment tools used to trend the severity of opioid withdrawal symptoms and medication efficacy.

TREATMENT

- <u>Goals of Treatment</u>: Cessation of use of the medication or substance, termination of substance-seeking behaviors, and return to normal functioning. The goals of treatment of withdrawal include prevention of progression to life-threatening severity, thus enabling comfort and functionality conducive to participation in a treatment program. OUD is a chronic disorder, and providing long-term medication decreases the risk of an accidental overdose or relapse.

NONPHARMACOLOGIC THERAPY

- Many patients can achieve recovery with proper treatment, counseling programs, or 12-step programs such as Narcotics Anonymous. Participation in this should not be required for receiving medications and behavioral therapy should be introduced if and when the patient is ready.

PHARMACOLOGIC THERAPY

- **Naloxone** is a key strategy in reducing opioid-related deaths because it may revive unconscious patients with respiratory depression. Naloxone is a competitive mu-opioid receptor antagonist that can be used in the reversal of an opioid overdose, but it may precipitate physical withdrawal in dependent patients. Table 71-1 outlines the naloxone delivery options.
- Patients and their caregivers should be educated on the availability of naloxone and the proper use of this agent. The World Health Organization (WHO) recommends that anyone who might witness an overdose should have access to naloxone and proper training. Many states have simplified the process to obtain naloxone to prevent opioid-related overdoses.

Withdrawal

- A variety of treatment regimens are used for patients during the acute opioid withdrawal phase and are summarized in Tables 71-2 and 71-3.
- Avoid unnecessary pharmacologic detoxification if possible (eg, if symptoms are tolerable), and provide patient-specific supportive care measures, such as fluids, until the patient stabilizes.
- The three Food and Drugs Administration (FDA) approved medications used in OUD include **methadone, buprenorphine**, and **naltrexone**, all of which work by blocking the effects of the opioids and effectively treat OUD.

TABLE 71-1 Naloxone Delivery Options

	Intramuscular Injection	Auto-Injector (Evzio)	Nasal Spray (Narcan)	Intranasal Spray (Atomizer)
Description of what is provided to patient	Two single-use 0.4 mg/mL vials Two single-use 3 mL syringes, 23–25 gauge, 1–1.5 inch needles	One box of 2 mg/0.4 mL prefilled auto injectors that includes 2 devices and a trainer device	One box of two 4 mg/0.1 mL intranasal devices	2 mg/2 mL prefilled naloxone needleless syringe Two mucosal atomizer devices
Directions for use	Inject 1 mL intramuscularly in shoulder or thigh upon signs of opioid overdose. Call 911 immediately. May repeat once in 2–3 minutes if minimal or no response	Use one auto-injector on outer thigh by depressing and holding for 5 seconds. Voice automation will direct the patient. Call 911. May repeat × 1 in 2–3 minutes if minimal or no response	Use full contents of spray in one nostril upon signs of opioid overdose. Call 911. May repeat × 1 in 2–3 minutes using other nostril if minimal or no response	Spray one-half of contents of syringe into each nostril upon signs of opioid overdose. Call 911. May repeat × 1 in 2–3 minutes if minimal or no response

Pearls

- Naloxone does not cause severe effects or adverse medication effects if administered to patients who are currently not taking opioids
- Naloxone should be given if the patient is intoxicated by a combination of products since the naloxone will still work for the opioid but not for other products such as benzodiazepines or alcohol

Naloxone counseling topics

- Overdose recognition, response, prevention, and importance of seeking emergency medical care
- Proper device use and counseling of family members and caregivers about proper storage, shelf life, and checking expiration date
- Potential adverse medication effects associated with naloxone
- Availability of treatment programs

General opioid safety counseling

- Take medication only prescribed for you, only take prescribed doses
- Do not mix opioids with alcohol or sleeping pills
- Always store all medications in a locked and secure place and dispose of unused medications appropriately
- Do not use opioids/medications in seclusion
- Never buy opioids/medication from unknown source
- Do not restart opioid at same dose if there is a period of abstinence as overdose is possible due to lower tolerance

TABLE 71-2 Differences Between Medications Used to Treat OUD

	Methadone	Extended-Release Injectable Naltrexone (XR-NTX)	Buprenorphine
Pharmacology	Full opioid agonist at mu-opioid receptor with long half-life to allow for once-daily dosing	Antagonist at mu-opioid receptor (*note: does not provide analgesia*)	Partial agonist at mu-opioid receptor with long half-life (up to 36 hours via sublingual administration); blocks intoxicating effects of other opioids
Phase of treatment in OUD; effect	Medically supervised withdrawal, maintenance; reduces or eliminates withdrawal symptoms and cravings to use opioids, blocks or blunts the effects of opioids	Prevention of relapse following medically supervised withdrawal; reduces or eliminates cravings to use opioids and blunts or blocks the effects of opioids	Medically supervised withdrawal, maintenance; reduces or eliminates withdrawal symptoms and cravings and blocks or blunts the effects of opioids
Route of administration	Provided orally once daily: commonly given as liquid concentrate in OTPs but current guidelines also allow solid oral-dosage forms as well	IM extended-release (depot naltrexone) (*Note: oral not as effective and use is not common in the treatment of OUD*)	Sublingual, buccal tablet, buccal film Other routes of administration available after meeting specific criteria: subdermal implant, subcutaneous extended-release injection
Restrictions for prescribing	CII; patient must meet Federal Opioid-Treatment Program standards; can be used in hospital settings for OUD treatment	Not a controlled substance but requires a prescription. All naltrexone products can be prescribed by general practitioners and in OUD treatment	CIII; requires waiver to prescribe outside of OTPs; prescribers receive separate DEA number with a "X" upon meeting requirements; to confirm practitioner verification: https://www.samhsa.gov/bupe/lookup-form; laws on this are changing, and the X waiver may no longer apply

(*Continued*)

		Extended-Release Injectable	
TABLE 71-2	Differences Between Medications Used to Treat OUD (*Continued*)		
	Methadone	**Naltrexone (XR-NTX)**	**Buprenorphine**
Restrictions for prescribing (*continued*)			Implant: prescribers must be certified in Probuphine REMS program to insert/remove implants
			Subcutaneous: healthcare settings and pharmacies must be certified in the Sublocade REMS program and only dispense the medication directly to a provider for administration
Patients that are commonly considered for this type of therapy	Patients with OUD; physiologically dependent on opioids and meet federal OTP admission criteria	Patients with OUD; patients who are abstinent from short-acting opioids for 7–10 days and long-acting opioids 10–14 days	Patients with OUD; physiologically dependent on opioids
Major adverse effects	Constipation, vomiting, dizziness, sedation, QTc prolongation, respiratory depression (risk is highest during initiation of methadone or dose titration and concurrent use of benzodiazepines or alcohol)	Injection site pain and tenderness, risk of injection site induration, toothache, LFT elevation, insomnia, nasopharyngitis	Constipation, vomiting, dizziness, sedation, insomnia, blurred vision, respiratory depression (highest risk with concurrent use of CNS depressants including benzodiazepines); sublingual buprenorphine/naloxone sublingual and buccal film: oral hypoesthesia, oral mucosal erythema, glossodynia

CII, Schedule II prescription; CIII, Schedule III prescription; CNS, central nervous system; IM, intramuscular; LFT, liver function test; OTP, Opioid Treatment Program; OUD, opioid use disorder; REMS, Risk Evaluation and Mitigation Strategy.

TABLE 71-3 Extended-Release Products Approved by FDA for OUD

Medication (Brand Name)	Dose	Comments
Naltrexone tablets (Revia)	Following a 7–10 day opioid-free period for short-acting opioids or a 10–14 day opioid-free period for long-acting opioids: begin with dose of 25 mg daily with food. If no signs of withdrawal, increase dose to 50 mg po daily	Should be part of a comprehensive treatment plan that includes psychosocial support Reports of elevated LFTs have been reported; use with caution Use with caution in patients with renal impairment as naltrexone and active metabolite are renally excreted
Naltrexone XR injection (Vivitrol)	Following a 7–10 day opioid-free period for short-acting opioids or a 10–14 day opioid-free period for long-acting opioids: 380 mg IM in gluteal area alternating buttocks; every 4 weeks or once a month	Must be administered by a healthcare provider Must use manufacturer provided needle and assess body size of patient at each visit so proper needle size is used Monitor injection site closely for any signs of abnormal pain and contact healthcare provider immediately if this occurs Dose adjustment is required in mild or moderate hepatic impairment. No data available in severe hepatic impairment Use caution in patients with moderate-to-severe renal impairment; naltrexone and active metabolite are renally excreted
Buprenorphine (Probuphine)	Four implants are inserted subdermally in the inner side of the upper arm and should remain in place for 6 months	Patients must meet specific criteria for use: • Only indicated for patients who are opioid tolerant • Demonstrates clinical stability on trans-mucosal buprenorphine with Subutex or Suboxone 8 mg/day or less (or transmucosal equivalent) for ≥3 months without requiring supplemental dose adjustments Must be inserted or removed within a facility and by a certified provider who has completed the required live training It is recommended to not prescribe as-needed transmucosal buprenorphine products Not recommended with moderate-to-severe hepatic impairment Limited data in renal impairment, currently no dosage adjustments listed

(Continued)

Medication (Brand Name)	**Dose**	**Comments**
T ABLE 71-3		Extended-Release Products Approved by FDA for OUD *(Continued)*
Buprenorphine (Sublocade)	For patients who have achieved clinical stability on equivalent of 8–24 mg of a transmucosal buprenorphine product daily *Available in two extended-release solutions:* • *100 mg/0.5 mL* • *300 mg/1.5 mL* Directions: inject 300 mg subcutaneously once a month in abdominal area for 2 months, then decrease dose to 100 mg once monthly in abdominal area	Must be administered by a healthcare provider Steady state occurs after 4–6 months; Detectable buprenorphine levels could occur 12 months or longer after discontinuation; urine and plasma concentration correlations are not known Injections must occur at least 26 days apart following all manufacturer directions for preparation and injection Do not give the injection at the belt or waistband area where pressure will occur Counsel regarding small bump at the injection site that will decrease in size over the next several weeks. Do not rub or massage this area if needed, the most recently injected depot can be removed within the 14 days of injection under local anesthesia Doses can be adjusted back to 300 mg monthly for patients in whom benefits exceed risks Examine injection site each month for evidence of tampering Not recommended with moderate-to-severe hepatic impairment Limited data in renal impairment, currently no dosage adjustments listed

IM, intramuscularly; LFTs, liver function tests; mg, milligram; mL, milliliters.

Methadone

- **Methadone** is a mu-opioid agonist that suppresses withdrawal symptoms and controls cravings for maintenance therapy.
- Once-daily dosing can range from 10 to 30 mg, depending on the patient's use pattern. This dose should be reduced to 10–20 mg for those over the age of 60, or if medication interactions are identified.
- Dose adjustments of 5–10 mg should occur gradually, no sooner than every 4–7 days based on clinical response. Maintenance doses range between 60 and 120 mg/day.
  - ✓ Adverse medication effects include sedation and respiratory depression. Methadone has many cytochrome P450 interactions. Concomitant use of alcohol or benzodiazepines can lead to overdose and should be assessed. There is a risk of QT prolongation, which is increased when given with other medications that prolong the QT interval.
- The use of methadone for OUD treatment is only approved through the Opioid Treatment Program (OTP), controlled by the Drug Enforcement Agency (DEA) and Substance Abuse and Mental Health Services Administration (SAMHSA). Methadone for the treatment of OUD may be provided to patients during a hospital admission for treatment of other health conditions.

Buprenorphine

- **Buprenorphine** is a partial mu-receptor agonist available as buprenorphine alone or buprenorphine/naloxone formulations. Table 71-4 outlines the products used in the treatment of OUD. Due to its partial agonist activity, buprenorphine does provide some intrinsic pain control and has a ceiling effect for respiratory depression. Buprenorphine can be misused.
- Initiation in the emergency room for patients who present with opioid withdrawal symptoms is a treatment option, and federal guidelines state that buprenorphine should be offered to patients with OUD who are appropriate candidates.
- Buprenorphine is a Schedule III controlled substance with specific prescribing restrictions. Refer to the DEA webpage for the most up-to-date regulations regarding buprenorphine prescribing. Sedation or intoxication is the main adverse effect seen with use.
- It is recommended that treatment starts with a COWS score of 12 or higher for the first dose, based on buprenorphine Risk Evaluation and Mitigation Strategy (REMS).
- Medically supervised withdrawal with buprenorphine consists of an induction phase and a dose reduction phase followed by maintenance. SAMHSA has evidence-based recommendations for use of buprenorphine for OUD. The same buprenorphine preparation is commonly used for induction, stabilization, and maintenance for most patients.
- Induction helps patients switch from the misused opioid to buprenorphine. The goal is to find the minimum dose of buprenorphine at which the patient discontinues or markedly diminishes use of the misused opioid and experiences no withdrawal symptoms or craving, and minimal or no adverse effects. The initial induction doses should be administered as observed treatment.
- The stabilization phase starts when the patient is experiencing no withdrawal symptoms or uncontrollable cravings, and has minimal or no adverse effects.
- The maintenance phase may be indefinite and should focus on psychosocial issues that contribute to a patient's OUD.
- Patient education is important (Table 71-5).

Naltrexone

- **Naltrexone** is a mu-opioid antagonist available for OUD in both an oral tablet and an extended-release injectable formulation.
- After confirming patients have been opioid free for 7–10 days, the initial dose is 25 mg given once daily, which can be increased to 50 mg/daily. Extended-release injectable naltrexone (Vivitrol) is FDA-approved for use following opioid detoxification to help prevent relapse.
  - ✓ The main adverse effects include swelling, bruising, and pruritus at the injection site. Elevations in liver function tests may occur with oral use.

Alpha-2 Agonists

- **Clonidine** or **lofexidine** may be used to attenuate withdrawal symptoms such as anxiety, tachycardia, hypertension, chills, and piloerection.
  - ✓ Adverse effects include hypotension, dizziness, and sedation.

EVALUATION OF THERAPEUTIC OUTCOMES

- OUD is a chronic disorder that requires pharmacological treatment and psychosocial and educational support. Consistent monitoring for efficacy and appropriateness through treatment is critical.
- Monitoring for withdrawal reactions utilizing proper assessment scales (ie, COWS or OOWS) can aid in evaluating the patient appropriately.
- Medication safety has to be considered based on unique adverse effect profiles and medication interaction concerns for the selected treatment regimen.

TABLE 71-4	Oral Buprenorphine Products Used in Treatment of OUD				
	Buprenorphine SL Tablet	**Suboxone SL Tablet**	**Zubsolv SL Tablet**	**Suboxone SL or Buccal Film**	**Bunavail Buccal Film**
Strengths of products commercially available/Routes of administration	2 mg 8 mg	Buprenorphine/Naloxone 2 mg/0.5 mg 8 mg/2 mg	Buprenorphine/Naloxone 0.7 mg/0.18 mg 1.4 mg/0.36 mg 2.9 mg/0.71 mg 5.7 mg/1.4 mg 8.6 mg/2.1 mg 11.4 mg/2.9 mg	Buprenorphine/Naloxone 2 mg/0.5 mg 4 mg/1 mg 8 mg/2 mg 12 mg/3 mg	Buprenorphine/Naloxone 2.1 mg/0.3 mg 4.2 mg/0.7 mg 6.3 mg/1 mg
Recommended once-daily target maintenance dose and dosing ranges	<u>Target maintenance dose</u> 16 mg **Dosing range** 4–24 mg[a]	<u>Target maintenance dose</u> 16 mg/4 mg **Dosing range** 4 mg/1 mg to 24 mg/6 mg[b]	<u>Target maintenance dose</u> 11.4 mg/2.9 mg **Dosing range** 2.9 mg/0.71 mg to 17.2 mg/4.2 mg[b]	<u>Target maintenance dose</u> 16 mg/4 mg **Dosing range** 4 mg/1 mg to 24 mg/6 mg[a]	<u>Target maintenance dose</u> 8.4 mg/1.4 mg **Dosing range** 2.1 mg/0.3 mg to 12.6 mg/2.1 mg

SL, sublingual.

[a]Doses higher than 24 mg/6 mg have not been shown to offer any further benefit.

[b]Doses higher than 17.2 mg/4.2 mg have not been shown to offer any added benefit.

Note: Refer to individual product dosing information when switching formulations due to possible bioequivalence variability. Monitoring is recommended following a switch in products due to possible variation in response to different formulations.

| **TABLE 71-5** | Patient Education Points for Buprenorphine Treatment |

Prior to Starting Buprenorphine Therapy and Repeat Education at Induction:

- **Communication with prescriber:** Tell your doctors about all medications, including over-the counter, herbal, creams, injections, inhalants, and street medications, that you are currently taking. This is important so your doctor is aware of what is in your body and if there are any chances of a dangerous interaction. Additionally, tell all of your doctors you are taking buprenorphine. If you are being treated for pain, it is very important to tell your doctor you are taking buprenorphine.
- **Goals of therapy:** The goal of any your first week of treatment is to improve the symptoms of withdrawal without causing any oversedation (making you too tired or feeling over medicated). Notify your doctor/prescriber if you are feeling overly tired/sedated or euphoric within 1–4 hours of your dose. Dose adjustments might occur initially and it will take a little time for the buprenorphine to become stable in your system. The goals of therapy include finding the right dose to eliminate withdrawal, decrease or even eliminate cravings for opioids, and block the effects of other opioids without severe medication adverse effects.
- **Product use:**
- Buprenorphine products (tablets, sublingual film, and buccal film) are not equivalent. If you have to transition to a new buprenorphine product, a dose adjustment might be required.
- Take your dose at regular intervals and only as prescribed.
- If you miss a dose, take the dose as soon as possible. If it is almost time for the next dose, do not double your dose, take only the dose that is prescribed.
- Leave medication in packaging until you are ready to use.
- Do not swallow sublingual tablets or film. This can reduce the effect of buprenorphine and lead to withdrawal symptoms.
- Sublingual tablets

  - ✓ Place tablets under your tongue and allow the tablet to fully dissolve, which can take several minutes.

  - ✓ If your dose requires multiple tablets, all tablets can be placed under the tongue at one time. If this is uncomfortable, only place two tablets under the tongue at a time.
- Sublingual film

  - ✓ Drink water prior to placing the film to help the film dissolve easily.

  - ✓ Place film under the tongue, to the left or right of the center of the tongue, and allow to completely dissolve.

  - ✓ If you are prescribed two films at a time, place the second film on the opposite side of the tongue. Do not allow the films to touch.

  - ✓ If you are prescribed more than two films at a time, wait until previous films have dissolved and repeat the process.
- Buccal film

  - ✓ Wet the inside of your cheek with your tongue or rinse with water prior to placing film.

  - ✓ Hold the film by the edges with two fingers and place on inside of cheek until fully dissolved, which can take up to 30 minutes.

  - ✓ If you are prescribed two films, place the second film inside the opposite cheek.

  - ✓ Do not adjust the film placement or touch the film, do not chew or swallow the film.

  - ✓ Do not drink or eat until the film has completely dissolved.
- **Common adverse effects:** Some adverse effects can occur when taking buprenorphine. These do not happen all of the time and do not happen to everyone. If you are experiencing any of these adverse effects, please tell your doctor immediately. Do not stop taking buprenorphine without first speaking to your doctor. The most common adverse effects include headache, nausea, constipation, abdominal pain, insomnia, sweating, and a possible feeling of weakness or lack of energy.

(Continued)

TABLE 71-5 Patient Education Points for Buprenorphine Treatment *(Continued)*

· **Precautions and warnings**
· Using alcohol while taking buprenorphine is very dangerous and can lead to increased risk of overdose and possibly death.
· There is a risk of overdose and possibly death if taking buprenorphine with benzodiazepines or alcohol.
· Using tobacco products prior to using buprenorphine decreases the absorption of buprenorphine, thereby decreasing its effectiveness.
· Long-term buprenorphine maintenance is recommended in many cases. If you stop buprenorphine, there is a high risk of overdose if you return to opioid use.
· Buprenorphine is an opioid that can cause physical dependence. Do not stop taking buprenorphine without consulting your doctor. If you stop buprenorphine abruptly, you could experience withdrawal symptoms.
· All medications, including buprenorphine, should be stored in a secure area, preferably in a locked cabinet or safe. It is important to keep medication away from children.
· It is recommended that you do not drive, operate heavy machinery, or perform any dangerous activities until you are fully aware of how this medication affects you.
· If you feel you have taken too much buprenorphine, you will need emergency medical attention immediately. Some possible signs include dizziness, confusion, unsteady or faint, slowed reflexes, or breathing slower.
· Do not inject these products. Serious life-threatening infections could occur. Additionally, serious withdrawal reactions can also occur upon injecting many of these buprenorphine products.
· **Pregnancy:** It is very important to inform your doctors if you become pregnant or if you are planning to become pregnant.
· **Counseling options:** Recovery resources and counseling resources are available for you and your family. We can give you further information on this when you are ready.

Maintenance:

· **Adherence assessment:** If any discrepancies arise, initiate discussion to identify reasons for discrepancies
  · Complete pill/film count.
  · Review Prescription Drug Monitoring Program (PDMP).
  · Confirm current buprenorphine dose.
  · Review results of urine toxicology screen.
· **Treatment assessment and counseling**
  · Review treatment goals and assess progress.
  · Review and assess benefits and risks of continuing buprenorphine treatment.
  · Discuss participation in counseling or encourage counseling if not receiving counseling.

· Data from urine toxicology screens and profiles from the Prescription Drug Monitoring Program (PDMP) can provide critical information on the full clinical picture for each patient.
· Continual patient education must occur to ensure proper medication administration and safety as the therapy continues.

See Chapter 85, Substance Use Disorders I: Opioids, Cannabis, and Stimulants by Patrick Leffers, Brittany Johnson, and Patrick Aaronson for a more detailed discussion of the topic.

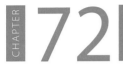
Schizophrenia

- *Schizophrenia* is a chronic illness characterized by positive symptoms (eg, delusions and hallucinations); negative symptoms (eg, anhedonia and social isolation); and cognitive dysfunction (eg, impaired working memory, and executive function) all leading to impaired psychosocial functioning.

PATHOPHYSIOLOGY

- Schizophrenia causation theories include genetics, obstetric complications with hypoxia, neurodevelopmental disorders, neurodegenerative theories, dopamine receptor defect, and regional brain abnormalities including hyper- or hypoactivity of dopaminergic processes in specific brain regions. Increased ventricular size and decreased gray matter have been reported.
- Alterations in glutamatergic neurotransmission resulting in increased neuronal pruning have also been implicated in schizophrenia pathogenesis. Genes controlling N-methyl-D-aspartate (NMDA) receptor activity are hypothesized to be part of this process.
- There is now a plethora of diverse findings pointing to immune dysfunction in schizophrenia, as well as abnormalities of autoantibodies and cytokine functioning.
- Positive symptoms may associate with dopamine receptor hyperactivity in the mesocaudate, whereas negative and cognitive symptoms relate to dopamine receptor hypofunction in the prefrontal cortex.

CLINICAL PRESENTATION

- Symptoms may include positive symptoms: hallucinations (especially hearing voices); delusions (fixed false beliefs); ideas of influence (actions controlled by external influences); disconnected thought processes (loose associations); illogical conversation; ambivalence (contradictory thoughts); negative symptoms: alogia (poverty of speech), avolition, flat affect, anhedonia, and social isolation; and cognitive dysfunction (eg, impaired attention, working memory, and executive function). These may be accompanied by uncooperativeness, hostility, and verbal or physical aggression; impaired self-care skills; and disturbed sleep and appetite.
- After the acute psychotic episode has resolved, there may be residual features (eg, anxiety, suspiciousness, lack of motivation, poor insight, impaired judgment, social withdrawal, difficulty in learning from experience, and poor self-care skills).
- Comorbid psychiatric and medical disorders (eg depression, anxiety disorders, substance use, and general medical disorders such as respiratory disorders, cardiovascular disorders, and metabolic disturbances) can also occur. Medication nonadherence is also common.

DIAGNOSIS

- The *Diagnostic and Statistical Manual of Mental Disorders*, 5th ed. (*DSM-5*), specifies the following diagnostic criteria:
  - ✓ Continuous symptoms persisting for ≥6 months with ≥1 month of active symptoms (Criterion A). May include prodromal or residual symptoms.
    - Criterion A: For ≥1 month, two of the following must be present for a significant time: delusions, hallucinations, disorganized speech, grossly disorganized or catatonic behavior, and negative symptoms. At least one symptom must be delusions, hallucinations, or disorganized speech.
    - Criterion B: Significantly impaired functioning.

- Before treatment, perform a mental status and neurologic examination, a physical examination (vitals including height and weight), complete family and social history, psychiatric diagnostic interview, and laboratory workup (complete blood count [CBC], electrolytes, hepatic function, renal function, electrocardiogram [ECG], fasting serum glucose, serum lipids, thyroid function, and urine toxicology screen).

TREATMENT

- <u>Goals of Treatment</u>: The goal is to alleviate target symptoms, avoid medication adverse effects, improve psychosocial functioning and productivity, achieve compliance with the prescribed regimen, and prevent relapse. Involve the patient in treatment planning.

NONPHARMACOLOGIC THERAPY

- Psychosocial rehabilitation programs to improve adaptive functioning are the mainstay of nonpharmacologic therapy for schizophrenia. Programs involving the family aimed at supportive employment and housing are considered "best practices" and decrease rehospitalization while improving functioning in the community.
- Clinical decision making should be a mutual process involving the patient and clinician.

PHARMACOLOGIC THERAPY

- Both first-generation antipsychotics (FGAs, also known as traditional) and second-generation antipsychotics (SGAs, also known as atypical) treat schizophrenia symptoms. Available antipsychotics and dosage ranges are shown in Table 72-1.
- Table 72-2 summarizes the long-acting injectable antipsychotics (LAIAs), including dosage range, conversion from oral to LAIA, and injection method/technique.
- The antipsychotic's mechanism of action is unknown. FGAs have high D_2 antagonism and low serotonin-2 receptor [5-HT_{2A}] antagonism. SGAs exhibit moderate-to-high D_2 antagonism and high 5-HT_{2A} antagonism, and **clozapine** shows low D_2 antagonism and high 5-HT_{2A} antagonism.
- Base antipsychotic selection on: (1) avoidance of certain adverse medication effects, (2) concurrent medical or psychiatric disorders, and (3) patient or family history of response. Figure 72-1 is an algorithm for schizophrenia management. Clozapine has superior efficacy for suicidal behavior.
- In first-episode schizophrenia, initiate dosing at the lower end of the range. Use of SGAs during the first acute episode results in greater treatment retention and relapse prevention compared to FGAs. **Aripiprazole, risperidone**, or **ziprasidone** may be preferred first line.
- Risperidone injection is more effective than oral risperidone in preventing relapse over a 1-year period for first episode schizophrenia. A long-acting antipsychotic should be considered during stages 1A, 1B, and 2 as they have consistently demonstrated an advantage in reduced hospitalizations and relapse prevention in patients with schizophrenia.
- In Stage 3, clozapine monotherapy is recommended.
- For Stage 4, minimal evidence exists for any treatment option for patients with adequate symptom improvement with clozapine. Use of antipsychotic combinations is controversial, as limited evidence supports increased efficacy, despite this practice being somewhat common.
- Predictors of response include prior response to the medication, absence of alcohol or substance use, acute onset and short duration of illness, later age of onset, affective symptoms, family history of affective illness, medication adherence, employment, and good premorbid adjustment. Negative symptoms are generally less responsive to antipsychotic therapy.
- An initial dysphoric response (eg, dislike of the medication or feeling worse, combined with anxiety or akathisia) portends a poor response, adverse effects, and nonadherence.

TABLE 72-1 Available Antipsychotics, Dosage Ranges, and Major Metabolic Pathways

Generic Name	Starting Dose (mg/day)	Usual Dosage Range (mg/day)	Comments	Major Metabolic Pathways
First-generation antipsychotics				
Chlorpromazine	50–150	300–1000	Most weight gain among FGAs	FMO3, CYP3A4
Fluphenazine	5	5–20		
Haloperidol	2–5	2–20	Higher dropout rate in first episode	**CYP2D6**, CYP1A2, CYP3A4
Loxapine	20	50–150		
Loxapine inhaled	10	10	Maximum 10 mg per 24 hours; Approved REMS program only	
Perphenazine	4–24	16–64		**CYP2D6**
Thioridazine	50–150	100–800	Significant QTc prolongation	
Thiothixene	4–10	4–50		
Trifluoperazine	2–5	5–40		
Second-generation antipsychotics				
Aripiprazole	5–15	15–30		**CYP2D6, CYP3A4**
Asenapine	5	10–20	Sublingual only, no food or drink for 10 minutes after administration	**CYP1A2, UGT1A4**, CYP2D6, CYP3A4
Brexpiprazole	1	2–4		**CYP2D6, CYP3A4**
Cariprazine	1.5	1.5–6	Due to long half-life, steady state is not reached for several weeks	**CYP3A4**, CYP2D6
Clozapine	25	100–800	REMS program, Check plasma level before exceeding 600 mg	**CYP1A2, CYPD6, CYP3A4**
Iloperidone	1–2	6–24	Care with dosing in CYP2D6 slow metabolizers	**CYP2D6, CYP3A4**
Lumateperone	42	42	Bioavailability increased by 9% with high-fat meal	**CYP3A4**, CYP1A2, CYP2C8, Aldoketoreductase 1C1, UGT1A1, UGT1A4, UGT 2B15
Lurasidone	20–40	40–120	Take with food, ≥350 calories (1460 J)	**CYP3A4**, CYP1A2

(Continued)

TABLE 72-1		Available Antipsychotics, Dosage Ranges, and Major Metabolic Pathways (*Continued*)		
Generic Name	**Starting Dose (mg/ day)**	**Usual Dosage Range (mg/day)**	**Comments**	**Major Metabolic Pathways**
Olanzapine	5–10	10–20	Avoid in first episode because of weight gain	CYP1A2, CYP3A4, FMO3
Paliperidone	3–6	3–12	Bioavailability increased when administered with food	Renal unchanged (59%) CYP3A4 and multiple pathways
Quetiapine	50	300–800		**CYP3A4,** CYP3A5
Quetiapine XR	300	400–800		**CYP3A4,** CYP3A5
Risperidone	1–2	2–8		**CYP2D6,** CYP3A4
Ziprasidone	40	80–160	Take with food, ≥500 calories (2100 J)	Aldehyde oxidase, CYP3A4, CYP1A2

CrCl, creatinine clearance; IM, intramuscular; LAIA, long-acting injectable; PO, oral; T_{ss}, time to steady state.

Note: In first-episode patients, starting dose and target dose should generally be 50% of the usual dose range. See LAIAs in text for dosing of these agents.

- The importance of developing a therapeutic alliance between the patient and the clinician cannot be overemphasized.
- Table 72-3 outlines the incidence for common antipsychotics adverse effects, which often follows their binding affinities.
- Anticholinergic effects occur most commonly with low-potency FGAs, clozapine, and olanzapine. These include impaired memory, dry mouth, constipation, tachycardia, blurred vision, inhibition of ejaculation, and urinary retention. Older patients are especially sensitive to these effects.
- Sedation can be reduced if most or the entire daily dose is taken at bedtime.
- Antipsychotics are highly lipophilic, bind highly to membranes and plasma proteins, have large volumes of distribution, and are largely metabolized by cytochrome P450 (CYP) pathways (Table 72-1). Pharmacogenetics may impact their pharmacokinetics.
- Most antipsychotics, except quetiapine and ziprasidone, have elimination half-lives ≥24 hours and can be dosed once daily.
- Antipsychotic pharmacokinetics can be significantly affected by concomitant enzyme inducers or inhibitors. Smoking induces hepatic enzymes and may increase antipsychotic clearance by as much as 50%. **Asenapine**, an inhibitor of CPY2D6, is the only antipsychotic that significantly affects the pharmacokinetics of other medications. Fluvoxamine, an inhibitor of CYP1A2, increases clozapine serum concentrations by two- to three-fold. Ketoconazole profoundly decreases lurasidone metabolism, and concomitant use is not recommended. Carbamazepine can decrease aripiprazole serum concentrations. Reduce the **iloperidone** dose by 50% when used with CYP2D6 inhibitors such as fluoxetine or paroxetine.

Initial Therapy

- The goals for the first 7 days of treatment are decreased agitation, hostility, anxiety, and aggression and normalization of sleep and eating.
- Titrate the antipsychotic dose over the first few days to an effective dose in the middle of the ranges shown in Table 72-1. The starting dose for first episode psychosis is half of that used for chronically ill patients. Rapid titration is not recommended.

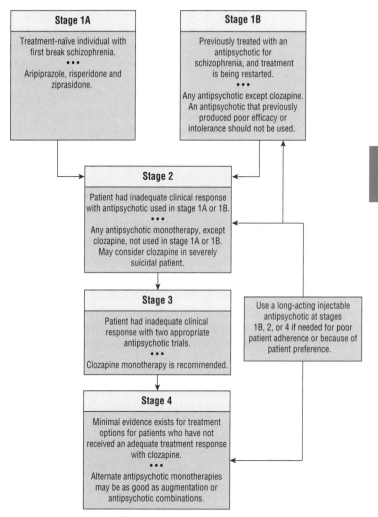

FIGURE 72-1. Suggested pharmacotherapy algorithm for treatment of schizophrenia. Schizophrenia should be treated in the context of an interprofessional model that addresses the psychosocial needs of the patient, necessary psychiatric pharmacotherapy, psychiatric co-occurring mental disorders, treatment adherence, and any medical problems the patient may have (See the text for a description of the algorithm stages).

TABLE 72-2	Summary of Available Long Acting Injectable Antipsychotics (LAIAs)				
Medication Name	**Fluphenazine Decanoate**	**Haloperidol Decanoate**	**Risperidone (Risperdal Consta)**	**Risperidone (PERSERIS)**	**Paliperidone Palmitate (Invega Sustenna) (1MPP)**
Dose Range (mg)	12.5–100	20–450	12.5–50	90–120	39–234
PO Overlap	None	4 weeks (none if loading); use PO dose patient was taking prior to injection	3 weeks after first injection: use PO dose patient was taking prior to injection	None	None
Recommended maximum dose	100 mg every 2–3 weeks	450 mg every 4 weeks	50 mg every 2 weeks	120 mg monthly	234 mg every 4 weeks
Initiation or Loading	Can Load	Can Load	None	None	Initiation required
Time to peak	8–24 hours	4–11 days	4–5 weeks	4–6 hours	13 days
T_{ss}	2–3 months	2–3 months	6–8 weeks	60 days	7–11 months
Half-life	14 ± 2[a] days	21 days	3–6 days	9–11 days	25–49 days
Injection Site Gluteal	Yes	Yes	Yes	Abdominal only	Yes after second dose
Deltoid	Yes	Yes	Yes		Yes
Injection Method/ Technique	Z-Track	Z-Track			Subcutaneous Injection
Notes			A starting dose of 12.5 mg is recommended in patients with hepatic or renal impairment	90 mg = 3 mg PO Risperidone 120 mg = 4 mg PO Risperidone	Avoid use in patients with moderate-to-severe renal impairment (CrCl <50 mL/min [0.83 mL/s])

1MPP, monthly paliperidone palitate; 3MPP, every three months paliperidone palmitate; 6MPP, every six months paliperidone palmitate; CrCl, creatinine clearance; IM, intramuscular; LAIA, long-acting injectable; PO, oral; T_{ss}, time to steady state.
[a]Based on multiple-dose data. Single-dose data indicate a β-half-life of 6–10 days.
[b]Additional dosing regimens include extended intervals up to 1064 mg every 8 weeks; loading protocol with Aristada Initio 675 mg + maintenance Aristada dose + PO 30 mg × 1 dose does not require PO overlap.

Paliperidone Palmitate (Invega Trinza) (3MPP)	Paliperidone Palmitate (Invega Hafyera) (6MPP)	Olanzapine Pamoate (Zyprexa Relprevv)	Aripiprazole Monohydrate (Abilify Maintena)	Aripiprazole (Lauroxil Aristada)
273–819	1092–1560	150–405	300–400	441–882[b]
None	None	None	2 weeks PO dose ranges from 10 to 20 mg/day	21 days PO overlap after first injection
819 mg every 3 months	1560 mg every 6 months	300 mg every 2 weeks or 405 mg every 4 weeks	400 mg monthly	882 mg monthly
None required, dose based on last Invega Sustenna dose: If 78 mg give 273 mg If 117 mg give 410 mg If 156 mg give 546 mg If 234 mg give 819 mg	None required, dose used depends on last Invega Sustenna or Trinza dose For Invega Sustenna: If 156 mg give 1092 mg If 234 mg give 1560 mg For Invega Trinza: If 546 mg give 1092 mg If 819 mg give 1560 mg	Initiation required	None	None required, dose based on PO dose: If 10 mg/day give 441 mg If 15 mg/day give 662 mg If 20 mg give 882 mg
30–33 days	29–32 days	<1 week	5–7 days	5–6 days
Continues steady state	Continues steady state	3 months	3–4 months	4 months
84–89 days (deltoid) 118–139 days (gluteal)	148–159 days	30 days	30–47 days	29–35 days
Yes	Yes	Yes	Yes	Yes
Yes	No	No	No	Yes, but only 441 mg dose
Requires at least a 4-month trial with 1MPP; not recommended in patients with moderate or severe renal impairment (CrCl <50 mL/min [0.83 mL/s])	Requires at least a 4-month trial with 1MPP or at least 1 cycle of 3MPP; not recommended in patients with moderate or severe renal impairment (CrCl <50 mL/min [0.83 mL/s])	Monitor for PDSS Subject to REMS	Maintenance dose reduced to 300 mg if patient experiences adverse events. Dose adjustment needed in CYP2D6 slow metabolizers Avoid use in patients taking CYP 3A4 inhibitors >14 days	May require 2-week PO trial to establish efficacy before initiating LAIA Avoid use of strong CYP2D6 and 3A4 inhibitors for 662 and 882 mg dose, no adjustment needed for 441 mg dose

TABLE 72-3 Relative Incidence of Adverse Medication Effects from Commonly Used Antipsychotics[a,b]

	Sedation	EPS	Anticholinergic	Orthostasis	Weight Gain	Prolactin
Aripiprazole	+	+[c]	+	+	+	±
Asenapine	++	+/++	+	+	++	+
Brexpiprazole	+	+	±	+	+	+
Cariprazine	±	+/++[c]	±	+	+	+
Chlorpromazine	+++	+++	+++	++++	++	++
Clozapine	++++	±	++++	++++	++++	±
Fluphenazine	+	++++	+	+	+	+++
Haloperidol	++	++++	+	+	+	+++
Iloperidone	+	±	+++	+++	+++	+
Lumateperone	+	±	+	+	+	++
Lurasidone	++	+/++[c]	+	++	+	+
Olanzapine	++	+	+++	++	++++	+
Paliperidone	+	++	+	++	++	++++
Perphenazine	+	++++	+	+	+	+++
Quetiapine	+++	+	+++	++	+++	+
Risperidone	++	++	+	++	++	++++
Thioridazine	++	+++	++++	++++	+	+++
Thiothixene	++	++++	+	+	+	+++
Ziprasidone	++	++	+	+	+	+

[a]Adverse effects shown are relative risk based on doses within the recommended therapeutic range.
[b]Individual patient risk varies depending on patient-specific factors.
[c]Primarily akathisia.

EPS, extrapyramidal side effects—include dystonias, pseudoparkinsonism, akathisia, and tardive dyskinesia.
Relative adverse effect risk: ±, negligible; +, low; ++, moderate; +++, moderately high; ++++, high.

If there is no improvement within 2 weeks at a therapeutic dose, then move to the next treatment stage (Fig. 72-1).

- In partial responders who are tolerating the antipsychotic well, titration above the usual dose range for 2–4 weeks with close monitoring is appropriate.
- Intramuscular (IM) antipsychotic administration (eg, aripiprazole 5.25–9.75 mg, ziprasidone 10–20 mg, olanzapine 2.5–10 mg, or haloperidol 2–5 mg) can be used for agitation. This approach does not improve the extent of response, time to remission, or length of hospitalization. IM **lorazepam**, 2 mg, as needed for agitation added to the maintenance antipsychotic is a rational alternative to an injectable antipsychotic. Combining IM lorazepam with olanzapine or clozapine is not recommended because of the risk of hypotension, central nervous system (CNS) depression, and respiratory depression.
- Inhaled **loxapine** powder, approved for acute agitation, can be administered only in a healthcare facility and through the FDA-approved Risk Evaluation and Mitigation Strategy (REMS). Use is limited to one 10-mg inhaled dose per 24 hours. Patients with any lung disease associated with bronchospasm (eg, asthma, chronic obstructive pulmonary disease) are excluded. It may offer no advantage over IM and oral products.

Stabilization Therapy

- During weeks 2 and 3, the goal is to improve socialization, self-care, and mood. Dose titration may continue every 1–2 weeks as long as the patient has no adverse effects.
- If the patient begins to show an adequate response at a particular dose, then continue that dosage as long as symptoms continue to improve. Improvement in formal thought disorder may require an additional 6–8 weeks.

Maintenance Therapy

- The goal of maintenance therapy is relapse prevention. Continue medication for at least 12 months after remission of the first psychotic episode. Many experts recommend treatment for at least 5 years, and lifetime pharmacotherapy at the lowest effective dose is necessary in most patients with schizophrenia.
- When switching from one antipsychotic to another, the first should be tapered and discontinued over at least 1–2 weeks while the second antipsychotic is initiated and tapered upward. Slow titration, especially FGAs and clozapine, can be done to avoid cholinergic rebound.

Management of Treatment-Resistant Schizophrenia

- Only clozapine has shown superiority over other antipsychotics, with improvement occurring slowly. About 60% of patients improve if used for up to 6 months.
- Clozapine is usually titrated more slowly than other antipsychotics to reduce orthostatic hypotension. If a 12.5-mg test dose does not produce hypotension, then 25 mg at bedtime is recommended. After 3 days, this is increased to 25 mg twice daily and then increased in 25–50 mg/day increments every 3 days until a dose of at least 300 mg/day is reached.
- A 12-hour postdose clozapine serum concentration of at least 350 ng/mL (1.07 μmol/L) is associated with efficacy. Monitor serum concentrations before exceeding 600 mg daily, in patients with unusual or severe adverse effects, those concomitantly taking potentially interacting medications, those with age or pathophysiologic changes suggesting altered kinetics, and in those suspected of medication nonadherence.
- Mood stabilizers (eg, **lithium, valproic acid**, and **carbamazepine**) may improve labile affect and agitation in patients with refectory schizophrenia. Selective serotonin reuptake inhibitors (SSRIs) may improve obsessive-compulsive symptoms that worsen or arise during clozapine treatment.
- Little data supports or refutes combining antipsychotcs, but this strategy is often employed. One of the medications should be discontinued if there is no improvement within 6–12 weeks.

TABLE 72-4	Agents Used to Treat Extrapyramidal Side Effects	
Generic Name	**Equivalent Dose (mg)**	**Daily Dosage Range (mg)**
Antimuscarinics		
Benztropine[a]	1	1–8[b]
Biperiden[a]	2	2–8
Trihexyphenidyl	2	2–15
Antihistaminic		
Diphenhydramine[a]	50	50–400
Dopamine agonist		
Amantadine	NA	100–400
Benzodiazepines		
Lorazepam[a]	NA	1–8
Diazepam	NA	2–20
Clonazepam	NA	2–8
β-Blockers		
Propranolol	NA	20–160

NA, not applicable.
[a]Injectable dosage form can be given intramuscularly for relief of acute dystonia.
[b]In treatment-refractory cases, dosage can be titrated to 12 mg/day with careful monitoring; nonlinear pharmacokinetics has been reported.

Extrapyramidal Side Effects

Dystonias

- Dystonias are prolonged tonic muscle contractions (occurring usually within 24–96 hours of dosage initiation or dosage increase); they may be life-threatening (eg, pharyngeal–laryngeal dystonias). Other dystonias are trismus, glossospasm, tongue protrusion, blepharospasm, oculogyric crisis, torticollis, and retrocollis. Risk factors include younger (male) patients and use of FGA, high-potency agents, and high dose.
- Treatment includes IM or IV anticholinergics (**Table 72-4**) or benzodiazepines. **Benztropine** 2 mg, or **diphenhydramine** 50 mg, may be given IM or IV, or **diazepam**, 5–10 mg by slow IV push, or **lorazepam**, 1–2 mg IM, may be given. Relief usually occurs within 15–20 minutes of IM injection or 5 minutes of IV administration.
- Prophylactic anticholinergic medications are reasonable when using high-potency FGAs (eg, haloperidol and fluphenazine) in young males or with a prior dystonia. Risk can be minimized by using lower initial doses or by using an SGA.

Akathisia

- Akathisia occurs in 20%–40% of patients treated with high-potency FGAs and consists of subjective complaints (feelings of inner restlessness) and/or objective symptoms (pacing, shifting, shuffling, or tapping feet).
- Reduction in dose is the best intervention when feasible. Switching to an SGA is an option, although akathisia may still occur. Iloperidone, quetiapine, and clozapine appear to have the lowest risk. Benzodiazepines should be avoided in patients with a history of substance use. **Propranolol** (up to 160 mg/day) is reported to be effective. Emerging literature suggests that agents with antagonist activity at the 5-HT$_2$ receptor (**cyproheptadine**, **mirtazapine**, and **trazodone**) may be protective against akathisia.

Parkinsonism

- There are four cardinal symptoms: (1) akinesia, bradykinesia, or decreased motor activity, including mask-like facial expression, micrographia; (2) tremor, primarily at rest; decreasing with movement; (3) cogwheel rigidity; limbs yield in jerky, ratchet-like fashion when moved passively by the examiner; (4) stooped, unstable posture and slow, shuffling, or festinating gait.

- Possible accessory symptoms include seborrhea, sialorrhea, hyperhidrosis, fatigue, weakness, dysphagia, and dysarthria.
- Risk factors include FGA use (especially in high dose), increasing age, and possibly female sex.
- Symptoms start 1–2 weeks after antipsychotic initiation or dose increase. Risk with SGAs is low except with risperidone in doses greater than 6 mg/day. Quetiapine, aripiprazole, brexpiprazole, iloperidone, asenapine, lumateperone, and clozapine are reasonable alternatives in a patient experiencing EPS with other SGAs.
- **Benztropine** has a half-life that allows once- to twice-daily dosing. Typical dosing is 1–2 mg twice daily up to a maximum of 8 mg daily. **Diphenhydramine** produces more sedation (**Table 72-4**). All of the anticholinergics have been misused for euphoriant effects. **Amantadine** is as effective as anticholinergics with less effect on memory.
- Attempt to taper and discontinue these agents 6 weeks to 3 months after symptoms resolve.

Tardive Dyskinesia

- Tardive dyskinesia (TD) is characterized by abnormal involuntary movements. The classic presentation is buccolingual-masticatory or orofacial movements interfering with chewing, wearing dentures, speech, respiration, or swallowing. Facial movements include frequent blinking, brow arching, grimacing, upward deviation of the eyes, and lip smacking. Restless choreiform and athetotic movements of the limbs occur in later stages. Movements may worsen with stress, decrease with sedation, and disappear with sleep.
- Screen at baseline using the Abnormal Involuntary Movement Scale (AIMS) and the Dyskinesia Identification System Condensed User Scale (DISCUS). Repeat monitoring every 6 months for those at high risk and every 12 months for all others.
- TD prevention includes: (1) use SGAs first-line; (2) biyearly TD screening; and (3) discontinue antipsychotics or switch to SGAs at the earliest symptoms of TD, if possible.
- Risk factors for TD include duration of antipsychotic therapy, higher dose, possibly cumulative dose, possibly female sex, increasing age, occurrence of acute extrapyramidal symptoms, poor antipsychotic response, diagnosis of organic mental disorder, diabetes mellitus, and mood disorders. With FGAs the prevalence of TD ranges from 20%–50%. With SGAs, the risk of TD is ~3.0% per year in younger adults compared to 7.7% per year for FGAs.
- **Deutetrabenazine** and **valbenazine** are vesicular monoamine transporter-2 (VMAT2) inhibitors approved for TD treatment in adults. Warnings associated with their use include suicidality, depression, and QT interval prolongation.

Other Antipsychotic Adverse Effects

Seizures

- The highest risk is with chlorpromazine or clozapine and they are more likely with treatment initiation, higher doses, and rapid dose increases.
- Dosage reduction should occur for an isolated seizure, and antiseizure medication is usually not recommended.
- If a change in antipsychotic therapy is required, aripiprazole, risperidone, thioridazine, haloperidol, pimozide, trifluoperazine, and fluphenazine may be considered.

Thermoregulation

- Poikilothermia, the body temperature adjusting to the ambient temperature, can be a serious antipsychotic adverse effect. Hyperpyrexia, leading to heat stroke, may be dangerous in hot weather or during exercise. Hypothermia is also a risk, especially in older individuals. These problems are more common with the use of low-potency FGAs and can occur with the more anticholinergic SGAs.

Neuroleptic Malignant Syndrome

- Neuroleptic malignant syndrome (NMS) occurs in <1% of patients with high potency FGAs having the greatest risk.
- Symptoms develop rapidly over 24–72 hours: body temperature exceeding 38°C [100.4°F]), altered level of consciousness, autonomic dysfunction (tachycardia, labile blood pressure, diaphoresis, and tachypnea), and rigidity.
- Myoglobinuria, leukocytosis, increases in creatine kinase (CK), aspartate aminotransferase (AST), alanine aminotransferase (ALT), and lactate dehydrogenase (LDH) are common.
- Discontinue antipsychotics and provide supportive care. **Dantrolene**, **bromocriptine**, or **amantadine** may be useful in severe cases as all have reports of reduced time to clinical improvement and reduction in mortality rates.
- Antipsychotic rechallenge with the lowest effective dose of an SGA or low-potency FGA may be considered after at least 2 weeks without antipsychotics. Monitor carefully and titrate the dose slowly.

Endocrine Effects

- Prolactin elevations are associated with galactorrhea, gynecomastia, decreased libido, and menstrual irregularities. They are common and are likely with FGAs, risperidone, and paliperidone. Possible management strategies include switching to an agent with lower risk (eg, aripiprazole, asenapine, iloperidone, lurasidone, brexpiprazole, lumateperone, and cariprazine). Dopamine agonists are not recommended due to potential psychosis exacerbation.
- Weight gain with antipsychotic therapy may be most likely with olanzapine, clozapine, risperidone, quetiapine, and iloperidone. Ziprasidone, aripiprazole, lumateperone, lurasidone, brexpiprizole, and cariprazine appear to cause minimal weight gain.
- Patients with schizophrenia have a high prevalence of type 2 diabetes, which antipsychotics can worsen. Olanzapine and clozapine have the highest risk of causing new-onset diabetes, followed by risperidone and quetiapine. The risk with aripiprazole and ziprasidone is likely less than with other SGAs. Asenapine, iloperidone, lurasidone, brexpiprazole, cariprazine, and lumateperone also appear to have a lower risk, but more data is needed.
- Genetic variation within the dopamine, serotonin, melanocortin-4, and alpha 2 receptors have been associated with antipsychotic weight gain. However, it is most likely polygenic and impacted by the environment.

Cardiovascular Effects

- Orthostatic hypotension (defined as >20 mm Hg drop in systolic blood pressure upon standing) is greatest with low-potency FGAs, clozapine, iloperidone, quetiapine, and combination antipsychotics. Older patients and those with diabetes and cardiovascular disease are predisposed. Dose reduction or changing to an antipsychotic with less α-adrenergic blockade may help, and tolerance may develop within 2–3 months.
- The low-potency piperidine phenothiazines (thioridazine), clozapine, iloperidone, and ziprasidone are the most likely to cause ECG changes, including increased heart rate, flattened T waves, ST-segment depression, and prolongation of QT and PR intervals. Thioridazine prolongs the QTc on average about 20 milliseconds longer than haloperidol, risperidone, olanzapine, or quetiapine. For thioridazine, the effect is dose related, and the medication's labeling carries a boxed warning for torsades de pointes and sudden death.
- Iloperidone pharmacogenomic metabolism may increase the risk of QTc prolongation in CYP2D6 poor metabolizers. High IV doses of haloperidol also can prolong the QTc, and it also carries a boxed warning.
- Medication discontinuation should occur with QTc prolongation consistently exceeding 500 milliseconds. Torsades rarely happens in the absence of additional risk factors (eg, age greater than 60, female sex, preexisting cardiac or cerebrovascular disease, hepatic impairment, hypokalemia, hypomagnesemia, additional medications

that prolong the QTc interval, metabolic inhibition by another medication, or preexisting QTc prolongation).

- In patients older than 50 years, pretreatment ECG and serum potassium and magnesium levels are recommended.
- Myocarditis is an infrequent and dose-independent adverse effect that is most likely to occur with clozapine but has been reported with quetiapine, and possibly with olanzapine. Recommended laboratory monitoring has been proposed with baseline and weekly monitoring of C-reactive protein (CRP) for the first 4 weeks, while troponin (I or T) and B-type natriuretic peptide monitoring has also been suggested. Cardiomyopathy, a potentially life-threatening adverse effect, can also be seen with clozapine, which typically presents later in the course of treatment than myocarditis, with an average time of onset of 14 months. Clozapine rechallenge after myocarditis is debated, and not recommended after cardiomyopathy.
- Those taking FGAs or SGAs have twice the risk of sudden cardiac death than nonusers. Antipsychotics are associated with a 1.53-fold increase in ventricular arrhythmia or sudden cardiac death.
- Compared to the general population, the risk of venous thromboembolism (VTE) is twofold higher in individuals with schizophrenia treated with an antipsychotic. Although the mechanism of this risk is unknown, increased sedative adverse effects, metabolic effects, antipsychotic effect on platelet aggregation, and hyperprolactinemia indirectly increasing venous stasis have been proposed.

Lipid Effects

- Some SGAs and phenothiazines cause serum triglycerides and cholesterol elevations. Olanzapine, clozapine, and quetiapine have the highest risk for dyslipidemia.
- Weight gain, diabetes, and lipid abnormalities during antipsychotic therapy are consistent with development of metabolic syndrome (consisting of raised triglycerides, ≥ 150 mg/dL [1.70 mmol/L]), low high-density lipoprotein cholesterol (≤ 40 mg/dL [1.03 mmol/L] for males, ≤ 50 mg/dL [1.29 mmol/L] for females), elevated fasting glucose (≥ 100 mg/dL [5.6 mmol/L]), blood pressure elevation ($\geq 130/85$ mm Hg), and weight gain (abdominal circumference >102 cm [40 in.] for males, >89 cm [35 in.] for females).

Psychiatric Effects

- Aripiprazole is associated with impulse control disorders such as pathological gambling, uncontrolled sexual urges, uncontrolled spending, binge or compulsive eating, and other intense urges.

Ophthalmologic Effects

- Exacerbation of narrow-angle glaucoma can occur with antipsychotics and/or anticholinergic use.
- Opaque deposits in the cornea and lens may occur with chronic phenothiazine treatment, especially chlorpromazine. Although visual acuity is not usually affected, periodic slit-lamp examinations are recommended with long-term phenothiazine use. Baseline and periodic slit-lamp examinations are also recommended for quetiapine-treated patients because of cataract development in animal studies.
- Thioridazine doses greater than 800 mg daily (the recommended maximum dose) can cause retinitis pigmentosa with permanent visual impairment or blindness.

Genitourinary System

- Urinary hesitancy and retention are common, especially with low-potency FGAs and clozapine, and males with benign prostatic hyperplasia.
- Urinary incontinence resulting from α-blockade, by the SGAs, is especially problematic with clozapine.
- Risperidone and paliperidone produce as much sexual dysfunction as FGAs, but other SGAs with weaker prolactin effects pose less risk. Priapism, an unprovoked painful erection that persists for longer than an hour, is increasingly reported with antipsychotic use.

Hematologic System

- Antipsychotics can cause transient leukopenia, that usually does not progress to clinical significance. Clozapine, chlorpromazine, and olanzapine have the highest risk for neutropenia.
- The risk of developing neutropenia or agranulocytosis with clozapine is approximately 3% and 0.8%, respectively. Increasing age and female sex increase risk. The greatest risk is between 1 and 6 months of initiating treatment. The baseline absolute neutrophil count (ANC) must be $\geq$ 1500/μL (1.5 $\times$ 10^9/L) to start clozapine. Weekly ANC monitoring for the first 6 months is FDA mandated. After this time, if it remains >1500/μL (1.5 $\times$ 10^9/L), ANC monitoring can be decreased to every 2 weeks for the next 6 months. Subsequently, if all ANCs remain >1500/μL (1.5 $\times$ 10^9/L) monitoring can be decreased to monthly. If at any time the ANC drops to <500/μL (0.5 $\times$ 10^9/L), discontinue clozapine and monitor the ANC daily until it is >1500/μL (1.5 $\times$ 10^9/L). Refer to the product labeling for more detailed information, including monitoring for mild and moderate leukopenia.
- Agranulocytosis also occurs in 0.01% of patients receiving FGAs, and it may occur more frequently with chlorpromazine and thioridazine. The onset is usually within the first 8 weeks of therapy and can manifest as sore throat, leukoplakia, erythema, and ulcerated pharynx. Patients with these symptoms and a ANC <500/μL (0.5 $\times$ 10^9/L), should discontinue the antipsychotic with close monitoring for secondary infection.

Dermatologic System

- Allergic reactions are rare and usually occur within 8 weeks of initiating therapy. They manifest as maculopapular, erythematous, or pruritic rashes.
- Contact dermatitis, on the skin or oral mucosa, may occur. Swallowing of the FGA oral concentrates quickly may decrease rashes on the oral mucosa.
- Ziprasidone carries a warning about a rare but fatal skin reaction called Drug Reaction with Eosinophilia and Systemic Symptoms (DRESS).
- Both FGAs and SGAs can cause photosensitivity with severe sunburns. Patients should use maximal blocking sunscreens, hats, protective clothing, and sunglasses when in the sun.
- Blue-gray or purplish discoloration of skin exposed to sunlight may occur with higher doses of low-potency phenothiazines (especially chlorpromazine) given long term. This may occur with concurrent corneal or lens pigmentation.

Use in Pregnancy and Lactation

- Haloperidol is the best-studied FGA with approximately 400 reported exposures. A small study found a twofold elevated risk of preterm birth in pregnant persons with schizophrenia taking FGAs as compared with those not taking antipsychotics. Risk of neonatal EPS is increased with in-utero exposure to FGAs, with effects in the infant lasting for 3–12 months after birth.
- All SGAs cross the blood–placental barrier to varying degrees. A meta-analysis found a greater risk of birth defects and preterm births with first-trimester exposure to SGA, but no specific abnormality was identified. Other larger studies also suggest that aripiprazole, olanzapine, quetiapine, risperidone, and ziprasidone collectively do not increase the risk of congenital malformations or cardiac malformation. Large, well-controlled studies are needed to clarify the safety of SGAs during pregnancy.
- For all of the FGAs, the overall relative infant doses (RID) obtained through human milk is thought to be less than 10%, which is a common threshold indicating safe use. Olanzapine and quetiapine have reported RIDs of <4%. Risperidone and aripiprazole have higher RIDs up to ~9%. Nursing while on clozapine is not recommended due to the risk of severe neutropenia and seizures in the infant.

EVALUATION OF THERAPEUTIC OUTCOMES

- Table 72-5 summarizes antipsychotic adverse effects, patient monitoring parameters, and frequency of monitoring parameters.
- The four-item Positive Symptom Rating Scale and the Brief Negative Symptom Assessment are brief enough to be useful in the outpatient setting to measure changes in symptomatology. Patient-rated self-assessments can also be useful, as they engage the patient in treatment and can open the door for patient education and addressing misconceptions. Clinicians should be assertive in attempting to achieve symptom remission.

TABLE 72-5	Antipsychotic Adverse Reaction and Monitoring Parameters		
Adverse Reaction	**Monitoring Parameter**	**Frequency**	**Comments**
Adverse Reaction Monitoring Parameters for All Antipsychotic Medications			
Akathisia	Ask about restlessness or anxiety. Observe patient for restlessness. Barnes Akathisia Scale can also be used	Every visit	
Anticholinergic adverse effects	Ask patient about constipation, blurry vision, urinary retention, or unusual dry mouth	Every visit	
Glucose intolerance	FBS or HbA1c	At baseline, after 3 months, and if normal, then annually	
Hyperlipidemia	Lipid profile	At baseline, after 3 months, and if normal, then annually	
Orthostatic hypotension	Ask patient about dizziness on standing. If present, check BP and HR in sitting and standing positions	Every visit	The degree of orthostatic change in BP to produce symptoms varies. In general, a BP change of 20 mm Hg or more is significant
Hyperprolactinemia	In females, ask about expression of milk from the breast and menstrual irregularities. In males, ask about breast enlargement or expression of milk from nipples. If symptoms present, check serum prolactin level	Every visit	In the absence of symptoms, there is no need to monitor serum prolactin

(Continued)

TABLE 72-5	Antipsychotic Adverse Reaction and Monitoring Parameters (Continued)		
Adverse Reaction	**Monitoring Parameter**	**Frequency**	**Comments**
Sedation	Ask patient about unusual sedation or sleepiness	Every visit	
Sexual dysfunction	Ask patient about decreased sexual desire, difficulty being aroused, or problems with orgasm	Every visit	Patients with schizophrenia have more sexual dysfunction than the normal population. Compare symptoms with medication-free state
Tardive dyskinesia	Standardized rating scale such as the AIMS or the DISCUS	At baseline, and then every 6 months for FGAs and every 12 months for SGAs	
Weight gain	Measure body weight, BMI, and waist circumference	At baseline, monthly for the first 6 months, and then quarterly	Waist circumference is the single best predictor of cardiac morbidity
Adverse Reaction Monitoring Parameters For Specific Antipsychotics			
Agranulocytosis	ANC	At baseline, weekly for 6 months, then every 2 weeks for 6 months, and then monthly	Clozapine only
Sialorrhea or excess drooling	Ask patient about problems with excess drooling, waking in the morning with a wet ring on their pillow. Visual observation of the patient for drooling	Every visit	Clozapine only

(Continued)

TABLE 72-5	Antipsychotic Adverse Reaction and Monitoring Parameters (*Continued*)		
Adverse Reaction	**Monitoring Parameter**	**Frequency**	**Comments**
Bronchospasm, respiratory distress, respiratory depression, respiratory arrest	Before administration, screen patients for a history of asthma, chronic obstructive pulmonary disease, or other lung disease associated with bronchospasm. Monitor patient every 15 minutes for a minimum of 1 hour after medication administration for signs and symptoms of bronchospasm (ie, vital signs and chest auscultation). Only one 10-mg dose can be given every 24 hours	Every dose administration	Inhaled loxapine only. Can only be administered in approved healthcare facilities registered in REMS program
Postinjection sedation/ delirium syndrome	Observe the patient for at least 3 hours after administration. Monitor for possible sedation, altered level of consciousness, coma, delirium, confusion, disorientation, agitation, anxiety, or other cognitive impairment	Every dose administration	Long-acting olanzapine pamoate monohydrate only. Can only be administered in approved healthcare facilities registered in REMS program

AIMS, abnormal involuntary movement scale; ANC, absolute neutrophil counts; BMI, body mass index; BP, blood pressure; DISCUS, dyskinesia identification system condensed user scale, FBS, fasting blood sugar; FGA, first-generation antipsychotic; HbA1c, Hemoglobin A1c; HR, heart rate; REMS, Risk Evaluation and Mitigation Strategy; SGA, second-generation antipsychotic.

See Chapter 87, Schizophrenia, authored by M. Lynn Crismon, Tawny L. Smith, and Peter F. Buckley, for a more detailed discussion of this topic.

Substance Use Disorders: Non-Opioid

- *Substance use disorder* (SUD) is a lifelong illness that consists of intoxication and withdrawal from the substance that may cause euphoria. Because this illness affects the brain and behavior, it results in the inability to limit or control the use of legal and illegal substances.

PATHOPHYSIOLOGY

- The true etiology behind SUD is unknown. In general, it is felt that there needs to be a triad of the right patient, with the right genetic risk factors, being exposed to the right medication or substance in order for a SUD to occur.

CENTRAL NERVOUS SYSTEM DEPRESSANTS: CLINICAL PRESENTATION

ALCOHOL

- Table 73-1 relates the effects of **alcohol** to the blood alcohol concentration (BAC).
- Alcohol withdrawal includes (1) a history of cessation or reduction in heavy and prolonged alcohol use and (2) the presence of two or more of the symptoms of alcohol withdrawal.
- There is 14 g of alcohol in 12 oz of beer, 5 oz of wine, or 1.5 oz (one shot) of 80-proof whiskey. This amount will increase the BAC by approximately 20–25 mg/dL (4.3–5.4 mmol/L) in a healthy 70-kg (154-lb) man. Deaths generally occur when BACs are greater than 400–500 mg/dL (87–109 mmol/L).
- Absorption of alcohol begins in the stomach within 5–10 minutes of ingestion. Peak concentrations are usually achieved 30–90 minutes after finishing the last drink.
- Alcohol is metabolized by alcohol dehydrogenase to acetaldehyde, which is metabolized to carbon dioxide and water by aldehyde dehydrogenase. Catalase and the microsomal alcohol oxidase system are also involved.
- Most clinical laboratories report BAC in milligrams per deciliter. In legal cases, results are reported in percentage (grams of alcohol per 100 mL of whole blood). Thus, a BAC of 150 mg/dL = 0.15% = 34 mmol/L.

BENZODIAZEPINES AND OTHER SEDATIVE HYPNOTICS

- Benzodiazepine intoxication is manifested as slurred speech, poor coordination, swaying, drowsiness, hypotension, nystagmus, and confusion.
- Likelihood and severity of withdrawal are a function of dose and duration of exposure. Gradual tapering of dosage is necessary to minimize withdrawal and rebound anxiety.
- Signs and symptoms of benzodiazepine withdrawal are similar to those of alcohol withdrawal (Table 73-1). Withdrawal from short-acting benzodiazepines (eg, **oxazepam, lorazepam**, and **alprazolam**) has an onset within 12–24 hours of the last dose. **Diazepam, chlordiazepoxide**, and **clorazepate** have elimination half-lives (or active metabolites with elimination half-lives) of 24 to more than 100 hours. Thus, withdrawal may be delayed for up to 7 days after their discontinuation.
- **Flunitrazepam** (Rohypnol) is often called a *date-rape drug*, it has been given to individuals (without their knowledge) to lower their inhibitions.
- **Zolpidem** is reported to have little liability for physical dependence, but tolerance and withdrawal have been reported.
- **Carisoprodol** is a muscle relaxant used for muscle spasms and back pain. **Meprobamate** is one of its metabolites. Symptoms of overdose and unhealthy use are similar to alcohol (Table 73-1).

TABLE 73-1	Specific Effects of Alcohol Related to Blood Alcohol Concentration	
BAC (%) (mmol/L)	Type of Impairment	Effect(s)
0.0–0.05 (0–12)	Mild	Mild speech/memory/attention/coordination/balance impairment, relaxation, sleepiness
0.06–0.15 (13–34)	Increased	Impaired speech/memory/attention/coordination/balance, risk of aggression, significantly impaired driving skills, increased risk of injury to self and others, moderate memory impairment
0.16–0.30 (35–65)	Severe	Impaired speech/memory/attention/coordination/reaction time, balance significantly impaired, driving skills dangerously impaired, judgment and decision making dangerously impaired, blackouts, vomiting, and signs of alcohol poisoning common, loss of consciousness
0.31–0.45 (66–98)	Life-threatening	Loss of consciousness, danger of life-threatening alcohol poisoning, significant risk of death

BAC, blood alcohol concentration.

DIAGNOSIS

- The *Diagnostic and Statistical Manual of Mental Disorders*, 5th ed. (*DSM-5*) defines SUD as "problematic pattern of substance use leading to clinically significant impairment or distress as manifested by at least two of eleven criteria occurring in the preceding 12-month period."
- The CAGE questionnaire or alcohol use disorders identification test (AUDIT) can be used to assess unhealthy alcohol and sedative hypnotic use. The USAUDIT has been adapted to the United States and may be more accurate to detect unhealthy use of alcohol.

TREATMENT

- Goals of Treatment: The cessation of use of the substance, termination of substance-seeking behaviors, and return to normal functioning. The goals of treatment for withdrawal include prevention of progression to life-threatening severity, thus enabling comfort and functionality conducive to participation in a treatment program.

NONPHARMACOLOGIC THERAPY

- Treatment of substance use disorders is primarily behavioral and a lifelong process. Most treatment programs embrace the Alcoholics Anonymous approach (ie, a 12-step model).
- Both psychosocial interventions and pharmacologic therapy can be beneficial to reduce the frequency of drinking.

PHARMACOLOGIC THERAPY

Alcohol

Intoxication

- In treating acute intoxications of central nervous system depressants, support of vital functions is critical.
- When toxicology screens are desired, blood or urine should be collected immediately upon arrival for treatment.

Withdrawal

- Treatment of withdrawal for alcohol is summarized in Table 73-2.
- Most clinicians agree that symptom-triggered treatment with benzodiazepines is the standard of care for alcohol detoxification where medication is given when the patient has symptoms and the Clinical Institute Withdrawal Assessment–Alcohol, Revised (CIWA-AR) score is ≥8. Various benzodiazepines may be used (Table 73-2) depending on patient-specific factors (ie, age and liver function). The patient should be reassessed hourly with continued doses given if the score is ≥8. The assessment timeframe can be extended to every 4–8 hours once the patient appears stable and their CIWA-AR score is <8.
- The front-loading method is recommended if the CIWA-AR scores is ≥19. This approach uses a long-acting benzodiazepine such as **diazepam** 10–20 mg or **chlordiazepoxide** 100 mg, repeated every 1–2 hours until the patient is sedated. The short-acting benzodiazepine lorazepam is also preferred because it can be administered IV, intramuscularly, or orally with predictable results (Table 73-2). Fluid, electrolyte, and vitamin deficiencies should also be addressed (Table 73-2).
- Alcohol withdrawal seizures do not require antiseizure medications unless they progress to status epilepticus or there is an underlying seizure disorder. An increase in the dosage and slowing of the tapering schedule of the benzodiazepine used for detoxification or a single injection of a benzodiazepine may be necessary to prevent further seizure activity. Otherwise treat seizures supportively.

Alcohol Use Disorder

- Table 73-3 shows dosing and monitoring of medication therapy for alcohol use disorder and unhealthy use. Duration of treatment is dependent on several, patient-specific factors, such as clinical response, tolerability, patient preference, history of relapses, and severity of the disorder.
- **Disulfiram** deters a patient from drinking by producing an aversive reaction if the patient drinks. It inhibits aldehyde dehydrogenase in the pathway for alcohol metabolism, allowing acetaldehyde to accumulate, resulting in flushing, vomiting, headache, palpitations, tachycardia, fever, and hypotension.
  - ✓ Severe reactions include respiratory depression, arrhythmias, MI, seizures, and death. Inhibition of the enzyme continues for as long as 2 weeks after stopping disulfiram.
  - ✓ Prior to starting disulfiram, obtain baseline liver function tests (LFTs), and repeat at 2 weeks, 3 months, and 6 months, then twice yearly. Wait at least 24 hours after the last drink before starting disulfiram, usually at a dose of 250 mg/day.
- **Naltrexone** reduces craving and the number of drinking days. Do not prescribe it to patients currently taking opioids because it can precipitate severe withdrawal syndrome. A depot formulation allows monthly administration in a usual dose of 380-mg intramuscularly.
  - ✓ Naltrexone is hepatotoxic and contraindicated in patients with hepatitis, liver failure, or serum aminotransferase levels greater than five times normal. LFTs should be done at baseline and 1–3 months after starting therapy, then annually. Use with caution in patients with moderate-to-severe renal impairment.
  - ✓ Adverse medication effects include nausea, headache, dizziness, nervousness, insomnia, and somnolence.
- **Acamprosate** is a glutamate modulator that reduces alcohol craving.
  - ✓ The most common acamprosate adverse effect is diarrhea.
  - ✓ Undergoes renal elimination.

Benzodiazepines and Other Sedative Hypnotics

Intoxication

- **Flumazenil** can be used for benzodiazepine overdoses and is contraindicated when cyclic antidepressant use is known or suspected due to seizure risk. Use may precipitate physical withdrawal.

TABLE 73-2 Dosing and Monitoring of Pharmacologic Agents Used in the Treatment of Alcohol Withdrawal

Agent/Route	Dosage Range Per Day (Unless Otherwise Noted)	Indication	Monitoring	Duration of Dosing	Level of Evidence for Efficacy
Multivitamin oral/IV	1 tablet	Malnutrition	Diet	At least until eating a balanced diet at caloric goal	B3
Thiamine oral/IV	100 mg	Deficiency	CBC, WBC, nystagmus	Empiric for 5 days. More if evidence of deficiency	B2
Crystalloid fluids IV (NS or D5-0.45 NS with 20 mEq [mmol] of KCl per liter)	50–100 mL/h	Dehydration	Weight, electrolytes urine output, nystagmus if dextrose	Until intake and outputs stabilize and oral intake is adequate	A3
Clonidine oral (Catapres)	0.05–0.3 mg Consider dose reduction in older individuals	Autonomic tone rebound and hyperactivity, hypertensive urgency	Shaking, tremor, sweating, blood pressure	3 days or less	B2
Clonidine transdermal (Catapres-TTS)	TTS-1 to TTS-3 Consider dose reduction in older individuals	Autonomic tone rebound and hyperactivity	Shaking, tremor, sweating, blood pressure	1 week or less. One patch only	B3
Haloperidol oral/IV (Haldol)	2.5–5 mg every 2–4 hours	Agitation unresponsive to benzodiazepines, hallucinations (tactile, visual, auditory, or otherwise), or delusions	Subjective response plus rating scale (CIWA-AR or equivalent), ECG	Individual doses as needed	B1
Antipsychotics, second generation Quetiapine oral (Seroquel)	25–200 mg; dosage adjustment is necessary in hepatic impairment	Agitation unresponsive to benzodiazepines, hallucinations, or delusions in patients intolerant of first-generation antipsychotics	Subjective response plus rating scale (CIWA-AR or equivalent)	Individual doses as needed in addition to scheduled antipsychotic	C3
Aripiprazole oral (Abilify)	5–15 mg				

(Continued)

TABLE 73-2 Dosing and Monitoring of Pharmacologic Agents Used in the Treatment of Alcohol Withdrawal *(Continued)*

Agent/Route	Dosage Range Per Day (Unless Otherwise Noted)	Indication	Monitoring	Duration of Dosing	Level of Evidence for Efficacy
Benzodiazepines					
Lorazepam oral/IV/IM (Ativan)	0.5–8 mg	Tremor, anxiety, diaphoresis, tachypnea, dysphoria, seizures	Subjective response plus rating scale (CIWA-AR or equivalent)	Individual doses as needed. Underdosing is more common than overdosing	A2
Chlordiazepoxide oral (Librium)	25–300 mg				
Diazepam oral/IV/IM (Valium)	5–40 mg				
Oxazepam oral (Serax) oral	15–30 mg				
Dexmedetomidine IV (Precedex)	0.2 mcg/kg/h, titrate based on response	Adjunct to BZD for autonomic hyperactivity, sympathetic symptom control	Tremor, blood pressure, heart rate	5 days or less	B2
Phenobarbital oral/IV (Luminal)	30–260 mg	Adjunct to BZD, promotes BZD binding to $GABA_A$ receptor	Sedation, respiratory depression, blood pressure	5 days or less	B2
Alcohol oral/IV		Prevent withdrawal	Subjective signs of withdrawal	Wide variation	C3

Quality of evidence: (1) evidence from more than one properly randomized controlled trial; (2) evidence from more than one well-designed clinical trial with randomization, from cohort or case-control analytic studies or multiple time series, or dramatic results from uncontrolled experiments; and (3) evidence from opinions of respected authorities, based on clinical experience, descriptive studies, or reports of expert communities.

CBC, complete blood count; CIWA-Ar, Clinical Institute Withdrawal Assessment for Alcohol, revised; D5, dextrose 5%; ECG, electrocardiogram; KCl, potassium chloride; NS, normal saline; WBC, white blood cell count.

Withdrawal

- For benzodiazepine withdrawal, use the same medication and dosages used for alcohol withdrawal (see Table 73-3).
- The onset of withdrawal from long-acting benzodiazepines may be up to 7 days after medication discontinuation. Initiate treatment at usual doses and maintain this dose for 5 days. Then taper over 5 days. Alprazolam use may require a more gradual taper of the benzodiazepine used for withdrawal.

EVALUATION OF THERAPEUTIC OUTCOMES

ALCOHOL

- Treating alcohol withdrawal takes precedence over the treatment of alcohol dependence.
- Close monitoring of withdrawal symptoms is essential to avoid progression to severe withdrawal.
- Patient counseling on medications' adverse effects used for alcohol use discomfort, followed by close monitoring and follow-up are necessary to assess therapeutic response and adherence.

TABLE 73-3	Dosing and Monitoring of Pharmacologic Agents Used in the Treatment of Alcohol Use Disorder		
	Dosage Range Per Day	**Indication**	**Monitoring**
Disulfiram (Antabuse)	125–500 mg; use with caution in patients with hepatic disease or insufficiency	Deterrence	Facial flushing, liver enzymes
Acamprosate (Campral)	999–1998 mg and higher (333 mg tablets) Dosage adjustment necessary in renal impairment	Craving	Patient-reported craving, renal function
Naltrexone (ReVia)	50–100 mg; dosage adjustment may be needed in renal and liver impairment	Craving	Patient-reported craving
Naltrexone (Vivitrol)	380-mg intramuscularly once every 4 weeks	Craving	Patient-reported craving, liver enzymes, injection site reactions
Antiseizure Medications (eg, topiramate [Topamax], carbamazepine [Tegretol], valproic acid [Depakote], gabapentin [Neurontin], oxcarbazepine [Trileptal])	Seizure disorder doses	Craving	Patient-reported craving, plasma medication levels
Antidepressants (eg, fluoxetine [Prozac], amitriptyline [Elavil], citalopram [Celexa], sertraline [Zoloft])	Depression doses	Craving, depression, anxiety	Patient-reported craving

BENZODIAZEPINES AND OTHER SEDATIVE HYPNOTICS

- Gradual taper of benzodiazepines should occur over 4–8 weeks and sometimes longer depending on the duration of use.
- Reduce the daily dose 10%–25% every 2 weeks to decrease the risk of severe withdrawal reactions and seizures.
- Minor abstinence symptoms (ie, anxiety, insomnia, irritability, sensitivity to light and sound, and muscle spasms) can remain for several weeks after the acute phase of withdrawal.

CENTRAL NERVOUS SYSTEM STIMULANTS: CLINICAL PRESENTATION

NICOTINE

- **Nicotine** is a ganglionic cholinergic-receptor agonist with dose-dependent pharmacologic effects, including stimulation and depression in the central and peripheral nervous systems; respiratory stimulation; skeletal muscle relaxation; catecholamine release by the adrenal medulla; peripheral vasoconstriction; and increased blood pressure, heart rate, cardiac output, and oxygen consumption. Low doses produce increased alertness and improved cognitive functioning. Higher doses stimulate the "reward" center in the brain. Cigarette smoking is the leading cause of preventable morbidity and mortality in the United States. It increases the risks of cardiovascular diseases, lung cancer, other cancers, and nonmalignant respiratory diseases.
- Abrupt cessation of nicotine results in withdrawal symptoms usually within 24 hours, including anxiety, cravings, difficulty concentrating, frustration, irritability, hostility, insomnia, and restlessness.

COCAINE

- **Cocaine** may be the most behaviorally reinforcing of all substances. Ten percent of people who begin to use the substance "recreationally" go on to heavy use. Pharmacologically it blocks reuptake of catecholamine neurotransmitters.
- Signs and symptoms of cocaine intoxication include agitation, euphoria, loquacity, sweating or chills, nausea, tachycardia, arrhythmias, respiratory depression, mydriasis, altered blood pressure, and seizures. Adverse effects seen with use include ulceration of nasal mucosa and nasal septal collapse.
- Withdrawal symptoms begin within hours of discontinuation and last up to several days. Signs and symptoms of withdrawal include fatigue, sleep disturbances, nightmares, depression, substance craving, changes in appetite, bradyarrhythmias, myocardial infarction (MI), and tremors.

  ✓ The hydrochloride salt of cocaine is inhaled or injected. The high from snorting lasts 15–30 minutes. Smoking cocaine base (crack or rock) is almost instantly absorbed and causes intense euphoria. The high from smoking lasts 5–10 minutes. Tolerance to the "high" develops quickly. The elimination half-life of cocaine is 1 hour.

  ✓ In the presence of alcohol, cocaine is metabolized to cocaethylene, a longer-acting compound than cocaine with a greater risk for causing death.

METHAMPHETAMINE

- **Methamphetamine** (known as speed, meth, and crank) can be taken orally, rectally, intranasally, by IV injection, and by smoking. Inhalation or IV injection results in an intense rush that lasts a few minutes. Methamphetamine has a longer duration of effect than cocaine. Ephedrine and pseudoephedrine can be extracted from cold and allergy tablets and converted to methamphetamine. In the United States, federal law requires that pseudoephedrine-containing products be kept behind a counter and that identification be shown at the time of purchase.
- Intoxication may present as increased wakefulness, increased physical activity, decreased appetite, dental caries, increased respiration, hyperthermia, euphoria,

irritability, insomnia, confusion, tremors, anxiety, paranoia, aggressiveness, convulsions, increased heart rate and blood pressure, stroke, and death.
- Individuals in withdrawal may exhibit depression, cognitive impairment, substance craving, dyssomnia, and fatigue, but they are usually not in acute distress. Duration of withdrawal ranges from 2 days to several months. Occurrence of delirium suggests withdrawal from another substance (eg, **alcohol**).

ECSTASY (MDMA)

3,4-methylenedioxymethamphetamine (MDMA; Ecstasy or Molly) is usually taken by mouth as a tablet, capsule, or powder, but it can also be smoked, snorted, or injected; if taken by mouth, effects last 4–6 hours.

- It stimulates the CNS, causes euphoria and relaxation, and produces a mild hallucinogenic effect. It can cause muscle tension, nausea, impaired memory, impaired attention and reasoning, impaired incidental learning, chills, sweating, panic, anxiety, depression, hallucinations, convulsions, and paranoid thinking. It increases heart rate and blood pressure and destroys serotonin (5-HT)–producing neurons in animals. It is considered to be neurotoxic in humans.

DIAGNOSIS

- See previous Diagnosis section. Several screening scales such as the Amphetamine Withdrawal Questionnaire, CAGE Questionnaire Modified for Smoking Behavior, and Drug Abuse Screening Test (DAST-10) can be used.

TREATMENT

- <u>Goals of Treatment</u>: The goals include cessation of substance use, termination of substance-seeking behaviors, and return to normal functioning.

NONPHARMACOLOGIC THERAPY

Nicotine Use Disorder

- The Agency for Healthcare Research and Quality (AHRQ) and the United States Preventive Services Task Force (USPSTF) have developed treatment guidelines that use the 5 As (**A**sk about tobacco use, **A**dvise the person to quit through clear individualized messages, **A**ssess the patient's willingness to quit, **A**ssist in quitting, and **A**rrange follow-up and support).
- The USPSTF statement emphasized counseling sessions and highlighted the goal of reaching at least four in-person sessions with total contact time between 90 to 300 minutes.
- Minimal contacts, lasting <3 minutes that include the 5As, are more successful in increasing cessation rates than interventions involving no contact.
- Motivational interviewing is a collaborative approach with moderate efficacy when used with other cessation approaches.
- Counseling alone can be effective but is further augmented by the addition of pharmacotherapy.

Cocaine, Methamphetamine, and MDMA Use

- Active monitoring and management of vital organ functions are required for a positive outcome.

PHARMACOLOGIC THERAPY

Nicotine Use Disorder

- First-line pharmacotherapies for smoking cessation include Nicotine Replacement Therapy (NRT), **bupropion sustained release**, and **varenicline**. Combinations of these should be considered if a single agent has failed. Second-line pharmacotherapies include **clonidine** and **nortriptyline** and should be considered if first-line therapy fails.

- The USPSTF concluded that the current evidence is insufficient to assess the balance of benefits and harms of pharmacotherapy interventions for tobacco cessation in pregnant persons.

Nicotine Replacement Therapy

- Dosing and monitoring of pharmacotherapy for smoking cessation are shown in Table 73-4. Nicotine replacement therapy increases quit rates by 50%–60%, and all products were tolerated with very limited reports of serious adverse events. Only the nasal inhaler and the nasal spray are prescription products, as all others are available without a prescription.

- The 2- and 4-mg gum and lozenge doses are recommended for those who experience time to first cigarette (TTFC) less than 30 minutes and greater than 30 minutes, respectively. The 4 mg gum may increase chance of smoking cessation in heavy users compared to the 2 mg dose. The gum should be chewed slowly until a peppery or minty taste emerges and then parked between the cheek and gums to facilitate nicotine absorption. Generally, the gum should be used for up to 12 weeks at no more than 24 pieces per day and no more than 20 lozenges should be used in 1 day for up to 12 weeks. Patients should be given specific dosing and usage instructions for both the gum and lozenges to improve efficacy.

- The patch has the highest adherence rate and may be combined with as needed gum, lozenge, or nasal spray use. The initial patch dosage should be worn from 4 to 6 weeks, and then the dose should be tapered to the next strength every 2 weeks. A new patch should be placed on a relatively hairless location each morning. Patients who experience sleep disruption should remove the 24-hour patch prior to bedtime or use the 16-hour patch.

- Nicotine nasal spray more than doubles long-term abstinence rates compared to placebo spray. Recommended duration of therapy is 3–6 months.

- Nicotine oral inhaler consists of a mouthpiece and plastic cartridge that is placed into the inhaler and delivers 4 mg of nicotine through vapor inhalation, of which ~2 mg is absorbed systemically. Patients should actively puff on the inhaler for 5 minutes, adjusting use based on effect, as the cartridge can be used for up to 20 minutes of active puffing. The initial dosing is 6–16 cartridges/day for up to 12 weeks. A taper should be initiated after 6 weeks.

- NRT products may cause nausea and light-headedness which may indicate nicotine overdose. Rotate the patch site to minimize skin irritation. Sleep disturbances are reported in 23% of patients using the patch. Eating or drinking anything except water should be avoided for 15 minutes before and during administration of the lozenge and gum. Long-term NRT may be needed in some patients.

- Electronic nicotine delivery systems (ENDS, or e-cigarettes) usage is highly controversial and continued research is needed to evaluate their efficacy and safety. A severe lung illness related to use of e-cigarettes and vaping and referred to "E-cigarette or Vaping use-Associated Lung Injury (EVALI) has been reported with most cases linked to tetrahydrocannabinol (THC) continuing products.

Bupropion and Varenicline

- Bupropion sustained release (SR) inhibits neuronal reuptake, and potentiates the effects of norepinephrine and dopamine. Its use is contraindicated in patients with current or past seizure disorder, current or prior diagnosis of bulimia or anorexia nervosa, and use of a monoamine oxidase inhibitor within the last 14 days. Concurrent use of medications that lower the seizure threshold is a concern.
  - ✓ Bupropion adverse effects may include neuropsychiatric symptoms (in adults and pediatric patients), including depression, anxiety, agitation, hostility, suicidal thoughts/behavior, and attempted suicide.

- **Varenicline** is a partial agonist that binds selectively to nicotinic acetylcholine receptors with a greater affinity than nicotine, producing a lesser response than nicotine. It

TABLE 73-4 First-Line Pharmacotherapy Treatment Options for Smoking Cessation

Medication	Dosing (For individuals 18 years or older. For those <18 years, discuss with a prescriber before use)	Duration	Comments/Monitoring Parameters
Nicotine Replacement Therapies (NRTs)			
Nicotine patch	Based on cigarettes smoked per day: **>10 cigs/day:** Step 1: 21 mg/day: Weeks 1–6 Step 2: 14 mg/day: Weeks 7–8 Step 3: 7 mg/day: Weeks 9–10 **<10 cigs/day:** Step 2: 14 mg/day: 6 Weeks Step 3: 7 mg/day: 2 Weeks	8–10 weeks	• Patch can be worn for up to 24 hours per day • If patient has sleep disturbances, remove patch at night and place one patch in morning (~16 hours per day) • If waking up with cravings, patch should be worn for 24 hours • Recommended to place patch on stop day. However, if patient smokes with patch on, there is no major risk • Place a new patch on each day, hold patch on for 10 seconds to help adherence • Rotate patches to avoid skin irritation • Do not cut patches, do not wear patches for greater than 24 hours, do not use more than one patch at a time
Nicotine gum	1st cigarette ≤30 minutes after waking: 4 mg 1st cigarette ≥30 minutes after waking: 2 mg Weeks 1–6: 1 piece of gum every 1–2 hours prn Weeks 7–9: 1 piece every 2–4 hours prn Weeks 10–12: 1 piece every 4–8 hours prn Then stop Do not exceed 24 pieces/day	12 weeks	• Continuous use can lead to adverse effects (pyrosis, nausea, hiccups) • 4-mg strength has shown to be more efficacious in heavy smokers over 6-week time period • If patient uses with a cigarette, there is no major risk • Counseling on proper use of gum: • Do not eat or drink 15 minutes before or during use of gum • Chew each piece slowly • Park between cheek and gum after a peppery sensation becomes apparent • Repeat process until peppery sensation does not reoccur (approximately 30 minutes) • Use alternate sides of mouth when using chew and park method • Use at least 9 pieces of gum per day for first 6 weeks to improve cessation

(Continued)

TABLE 73-4 First-Line Pharmacotherapy Treatment Options for Smoking Cessation (*Continued*)

Medication	Dosing (For individuals 18 years or older. For those <18 years, discuss with a prescriber before use)	Duration	Comments/Monitoring Parameters
Lozenge available as Nicorette lozenge or Nicorette mini lozenge	1st cigarette ≤30 minutes after waking: 4 mg 1st cigarette ≥30 minutes after waking: 2 mg Weeks 1–6: 1 lozenge by mouth every 1–2 hours prn Weeks 7–9: 1 lozenge by mouth every 2–4 hours prn Weeks 10–12: 1 lozenge by mouth every 4–8 hours prn Then stop Do not exceed 5 lozenges in 6 hours or 20 lozenges/day	12 weeks	Counseling points • Do not eat or drink anything 15 minutes prior to or during lozenge use • Allow the lozenge to dissolve slowly, approximately 20–30 minutes • Nicotine release could create a tingling or warm sensation • Do not chew or swallow the lozenge • Periodically rotate the lozenge to different areas of the mouth • Use at least 9 lozenges per day for first 6 weeks to improve cessation.
Nicotine oral inhaler + cartridge plus mouthpiece (Nicotrol®)	10-mg nicotine/cartridge; supplies 80 puffs 1. Stop smoking completely before use. 2. Initial dose: 1 cartridge every 1–2 hours 3. Begin gradual reduction of device after 3 months of use 4. Gradual dose taper over 6–12 weeks	6 months	• Patients should stop smoking prior to starting this product • Most successful patients in trials; use ranged from 6–16 cartridges per day, 20 minutes continuous puffing • Recommended duration of treatment: 3 months with subsequent weaning with gradual reduction over 6–12 weeks • Treatment longer than 6 months has not been studied • Precautions: patients with asthma, chronic pulmonary disease, history of recent myocardial infarction, serious arrhythmias, or worsening angina • Counseling: • Insert cartridge into mouthpiece and inhale medication quickly by puffing on mouthpiece for continuously for 20 minutes or four 5 minute sessions • Deep inhalation is not necessary when using this product • Change cartridge when nicotine taste is no longer detected • Dosing is individualized; initially it is recommended to use at least 6 cartridges per day for 3–6 weeks. Do not exceed 16 cartridges per day.

Nicotine metered nasal spray (Nicotrol NS)	Availed in 10 mg/mL bottle 1 spray (0.5-mg nicotine/spray) into each nostril 1–2 times each hour when craving cigarette Max dose: 10 sprays per hour (max of 80 sprays per day)	3–6 months	• Two sprays is considered **1 dose** • Treatment duration is 3 months; safety beyond 6 months has not been studied • Counseling: • Breathe normally while administering spray, do not sniff or inhale deeply while administering spray • Wait at least 2–3 minutes before blowing nose after using product • For best results, use at least 16 sprays per day which has been found as the minimum effective dose • Pregnancy Category D

Non-Nicotine Replacement Options

Bupropion (Zyban)	150 mg by mouth daily × 3 days, then 150 mg by mouth twice daily (dosing interval should be > 8 hours)	3–6 months	• Do not exceed 300 mg/day • Recommend initiating therapy 1–2 weeks prior to set "quit" day • Tapering is not needed with discontinuing agent • Black box warning for neuropsychiatric warning and suicide warnings removed in 2016; downgraded to warning • Pregnancy category: C, excreted into breastmilk • Monitor patients with renal/hepatic impairment • Counseling points: • May cause dry mouth • May cause insomnia, avoid bedtime dosing • May help with post-cessation weight gain • Recommended dosing interval: more than 8 hours when taking twice daily

(Continued)

TABLE 73-4 First-Line Pharmacotherapy Treatment Options for Smoking Cessation (Continued)

Medication	Dosing (For individuals 18 years or older. For those <18 years, discuss with a prescriber before use)	Duration	Comments/Monitoring Parameters
Varenicline (Chantix)	Start with dose titration: Days 1–3: 0.5 mg by mouth once daily Days 3–7: 0.5 mg by mouth twice daily Week 2 until end of treatment: 1 mg by mouth twice daily	12 weeks; an additional 12 week course may be used in select patients	• Take with food and a full glass of water • Quit day can be flexible with 4 options: • Start varenicline 1 week after quit day • Start varenicline and establish quit day between days 8 and 35 • Start varenicline and gradually reduce smoking with goal of cessation by week 12 of therapy • If patient has difficulty with cessation, taper smoking by 50% each month with a goal of smoking abstinence in 12 weeks, continue varenicline for another 12 weeks for a full 24 week therapy • Maintenance up to 6 months therapy is approved • Renal impairment dosing for CrCl ≤30 mL/min (0.5 mL/sec) • No dosing adjustment needed in hepatic impairment • Neuropsychiatric adverse events: black box warning removed in December 2016, warning remains • Counseling Points: • Varenicline works in two ways by relieving symptoms of nicotine withdrawal and blocking rewards of smoking • Most common adverse medication effects: nausea, sleep problems, constipation, gas, vomiting • Consider dose reduction if experiencing insomnia

is also FDA-approved for 6 months of maintenance therapy. It may result in a higher rate of cessation than bupropion and single forms of NRT.

✓ Varenicline adverse effect may include suicidal thoughts and erratic and aggressive behavior. Screen patients for psychiatric illness or behavior change after starting varenicline. It may also be associated with a small increased risk of cardiovascular events.

• Combining either bupropion or varenicline with NRT may be more effective than monotherapy for either agent but may result in higher medication adverse effects.

Other Therapies

• **Clonidine** is an effective smoking-cessation treatment in doses varying from 0.15 to 0.75 mg/day orally and from 0.1 to 0.2 mg/day transdermally.

✓ Clonidine adverse effects include dry mouth, dizziness, hypotension, sedation, and constipation. Monitor blood pressure. Abrupt discontinuation may result in nervousness, agitation, headache, tremor, and elevation in blood pressure.

• **Nortriptyline** is initiated 10–28 days before the quit date. The dose is initiated at 25 mg/day, gradually increasing to 75–100 mg/day. In trials, treatment duration was commonly 12 weeks.

✓ Adverse effects include sedation, dry mouth, blurred vision, urinary retention, tremor, and light-headedness.

Cocaine, Methamphetamine, and MDMA

• No pharmacologic therapies are available for these agents. When toxicology screens are desired, blood or urine should be collected immediately upon arrival for treatment.

• Treat pharmacologically only if the patient is agitated or psychotic. Injectable lorazepam 2–4 mg IM every 30 minutes to 6 hours can be used for agitation. Low-dose antipsychotics can be used short term for psychosis. Treat seizures supportively, but IV lorazepam or diazepam can be used for status epilepticus.

EVALUATION OF THERAPEUTIC OUTCOMES

NICOTINE USE DISORDER

• Tobacco cessation is a process that could take an extended period of time with extensive education and continual monitoring being vital to this process.

• The most effective treatment strategy for smoking cessation is a combination of behavioral and pharmacological treatment and frequent monitoring of both early on in the process is recommended.

• Patient counseling is vital to ensure maximum efficacy. Frequent reassessment should occur to evaluate breakthrough cravings, withdrawal symptoms, and relapses. Patients should be asked to immediately report any adverse effects to ensure adherence and prevent relapse.

COCAINE, METHAMPHETAMINE, AND MDMA USE

• When considering therapeutic outcomes, each treatment must be evaluated to determine efficacy and safety. Ongoing psychosocial and educational support is important to maximize outcomes.

OTHER SUBTANCES: CLINICAL PRESENTATION

CANNABIS

• **Cannabis** (known as reefer, pot, grass, and weed) is a commonly used substance. Federally this substance continues to be illegal, although many states have passed laws allowing use. The active compounds within marijuana include the principal psychoactive component Δ^9-**tetrahydrocannabinol** (THC) and **cannabidiol** (CBD), which does not have psychoactive effects. Cannabis is most commonly smoked, but it can be orally ingested. After inhalation, the pharmacologic effects can be seen in about 10 minutes. Both THC and CBD are poorly bioavailable; therefore, peak concentrations occur in about 2 hours after ingestion. The single use terminal half-life of 24 hours is significantly elongated with chronic use due to accumulation and redistribution from fatty tissues. In chronic users, THC is detectable on toxicologic screening for up to 4–5 weeks after cessation of use.

- A growing number of synthetically derived cannabinoids (spice, K2, dream, red X dawn, and others) are often misused for their psychoactive effects. The product is inert dry plant material sprayed with these compounds.
- Initial effects of cannabis include increased heart rate, dilated bronchial passages, and bloodshot eyes. Subsequent effects include euphoria, dry mouth, hunger, tremor, sleepiness, anxiety, fear, distrust, panic, incoordination, poor recall, amotivation, and toxic psychosis. Other physiologic effects include sedation, difficulty in performing complex tasks, and disinhibition. Endocrine effects include amenorrhea, decreased testosterone production, and inhibition of spermatogenesis. Recent findings suggest a neurotoxic effect on the adolescent brain.
- Cannabis use impairs driving performance, and is associated with increased risk of motor vehicle crashes.
- After abrupt discontinuation, heavy users may have a withdrawal syndrome characterized by irritability, anger, aggression, anxiety, depressed mood, restlessness, sleep difficulty, decreased appetite, or weight loss.
- Cannabinoid hyperemesis syndrome (CHS) is a syndrome of cyclical vomiting in habitual users that abates after discontinuation of cannabis.
- The toxic symptoms of synthetic cannabinoids are similar to the effects of cannibus plus sympathomimetic effects, including agitation, anxiety, tachycardia, hypertension, nausea and vomiting, muscle spasms, seizures, tremors, paranoid behavior, nonresponsiveness, diaphoresis, hallucinations, and suicidal thoughts and behaviors.

LYSERGIC ACID DIETHYLAMIDE

- **Lysergic acid diethylamide (LSD)** can cause either agonist or antagonist effects on 5-HT activity. It is sold as tablets, capsules, a liquid, and on squares of decorated paper. Research is currently ongoing to determine if LSD is effective therapeutically for depression.
- Signs and symptoms of LSD intoxication include mydriasis, tachycardia, diaphoresis, palpitations, blurred vision, tremor, incoordination, dizziness, weakness, and drowsiness; psychiatric signs and symptoms include perceptual intensification, depersonalization, derealization, illusions, psychosis, synesthesia, and flashbacks. It produces tolerance but is not addictive. There is no withdrawal syndrome.

SYNTHETIC CATHINONES (BATH SALTS)

- **Catha edulis (Khat)** is a shrub native to the horn of Africa that when chewed produces stimulating effects. The psychoactive properties of this plant are due to several alkaloids including cathine and cathinone (thus the name cathinones). The pharmacology of the various cathinones and related substances is not well studied. **Bath salts** (schedule I controlled substances) are synthetic, sympathomimetic, designer substances that can cause intoxication, dependence, and death. **Flakka** is a potent cathinone that has become popular.
- In addition to the stimulant effects of bath salts adverse effects include tachycardia, hypertension, diabetic ketoacidosis, paranoid psychosis, hyperthermia, agitation, headache, hyponatremia, and suicide.

INHALED ORGANIC SOLVENTS

- Inhaled **organic solvents** include gasoline, glue, aerosols, amyl nitrite, butyl nitrite, typewriter correction fluid, lighter fluid, cleaning fluids, paint products, nail polish remover, waxes, and varnishes. Chemicals in these products include nitrous oxide, toluene, benzene, methanol, methylene chloride, acetone, methylethyl ketone, methylbutyl ketone, trichloroethylene, and trichloroethane.

- Physiologic effects include CNS depression, headache, nausea, anxiety, hallucinations, and delusions. With chronic use, the substances are toxic to virtually all organ systems. Death may occur from arrhythmias or suffocation.

DIAGNOSIS

- See previous Diagnosis section. Cannabis use disorder (CUD) is often associated with multiple failed attempts at halting cannabis use.

TREATMENT

- <u>Goals of Treatment</u>: The goals include cessation of use of the substance, termination of substance-seeking behaviors, and return to normal functioning.

NONPHARMACOLOGIC THERAPY

- Treatment for all most often centers on psychosocial interventions and supportive care.
- For cannabis use, nonpharmacologic therapy includes cognitive behavioral therapy (CBT), motivational enhancement therapy (MET), or a combination, which is synergistic. Hot bathing may be effective for CHS.

PHARMACOLOGIC THERAPY

- See Pharmacologic Therapy for Cocaine, Methamphetamine, and MDMA above.
- **Dronabinol, nabilone, nabiximiol, gabapentin**, N-Acetylcysteine **(NAC)** have been used to abate cannabis withdrawal symptoms with some success, but additional research is needed.
- **Antiemetics, haloperidol** and topical **capsaicin** may help for CHS symptoms.

EVALUATION OF THERAPEUTIC OUTCOMES

- When considering therapeutic outcomes, each treatment must be evaluated to determine efficacy and safety. Ongoing psychosocial and educational support is important to maximize outcomes.

See Chapter 86, Substance Use Disorders I: Alcohol, Nicotine, and Caffeine, authored by Lori Dupress and Robin Moorman Li, and Chapter 85, Substance Use Disorders I: Opioids, Cannabis, and Stimulants by Patrick Leffers, Brittany Johnson, and Patrick Aaronson for a more detailed discussion of the topic.

74

Acid–Base Disorders

- *Acid–base disorders* are caused by disturbances in hydrogen ion (H^+) homeostasis, which is ordinarily maintained by extracellular buffering, renal regulation of hydrogen ion and bicarbonate excretion, and ventilatory regulation of carbon dioxide (CO_2) elimination.

GENERAL PRINCIPLES

- Buffering refers to the ability of a solution to resist change in pH after the addition of a strong acid or base. The body's most abundant extracellular buffer system is the carbonic acid/bicarbonate (H_2CO_3/HCO_3^-) system.
- Most of the body's acid production is in the form of CO_2 and is produced from catabolism of carbohydrates, proteins, and lipids.
- There are four primary types of acid–base disturbances, which can occur independently or together as a compensatory response.
- Metabolic acid–base disorders are caused by changes in plasma bicarbonate concentration (HCO_3^-). Metabolic acidosis is characterized by decreased HCO_3^-, and metabolic alkalosis is characterized by increased HCO_3^-.
- Respiratory acid–base disorders are caused by altered alveolar ventilation, producing changes in the partial pressure of carbon dioxide from arterial blood ($PaCO_2$). Respiratory acidosis is characterized by increased $PaCO_2$, whereas respiratory alkalosis is characterized by decreased $PaCO_2$.

DIAGNOSIS

- Blood gases (Table 74-1), serum electrolytes, medical history, and clinical condition are the primary tools for determining the cause of acid–base disorders and for designing therapy.
- Arterial blood gases (ABGs) are measured to determine oxygenation and acid–base status (Fig. 74-1). Low pH values (<7.35) indicate acidemia, whereas high values (>7.45) indicate alkalemia. The $PaCO_2$ value helps determine whether there is a primary respiratory abnormality, whereas the HCO_3^- concentration helps determine whether there is a primary metabolic abnormality. Steps in acid–base diagnosis and interpretation based on observed compensatory responses are described in Tables 74-2 and 74-3, respectively.

Metabolic Acidosis

PATHOPHYSIOLOGY

- Metabolic acidosis is characterized by a decrease in pH as a result of a primary decrease in serum HCO_3^- concentration, which can result from the buffering of an exogenous acid (consumption of HCO_3^-), accumulation of an organic acid because of a metabolic disturbance (eg, lactic acid and ketoacids), loss of bicarbonate-rich body fluids (eg, diarrhea, biliary drainage, or pancreatic fistula), or progressive accumulation of endogenous acids secondary to impaired kidney function (eg, phosphates and sulfates). Rapid administration of non–alkali-containing IV fluids can cause dilutional acidosis.

TABLE 74-1	Normal Blood Gas Values	
	Arterial Blood	**Mixed Venous Blood**
pH	7.40 (7.35–7.45)	7.38 (7.33–7.43)
PO_2	80–100 mm Hg (10.6–13.3 kPa)	35–40 mm Hg (4.7–5.3 kPa)
SaO_2	95% (0.95)	70–75% (0.70–0.75)
PCO_2	35–45 mm Hg (4.7–6.0 kPa)	45–51 mm Hg (6.0–6.8 kPa)
HCO_3^-	22–26 mEq/L (mmol/L)	24–28 mEq/L (mmol/L)

HCO_3^-, bicarbonate; PCO_2, partial pressure of carbon dioxide; PO_2, partial pressure of oxygen; SaO_2, saturation of arterial oxygen.

TABLE 74-2	Steps in Acid–Base Diagnosis

1. Obtain ABG and electrolyte panel simultaneously.
2. Compare $[HCO_3^-]$ on ABG and electrolyte panel to verify accuracy.
3. Calculate SAG (corrected for albumin when appropriate).
4. Is acidemia (pH <7.35) or alkalemia (pH >7.45) present?
5. Is the primary abnormality respiratory (alteration in $PaCO_2$) or metabolic (alteration in HCO_3^-)?
6. Estimate compensatory response (Table 71-7).
7. Compare change in $[Cl^-]$ with change in $[Na^+]$.
8. Compare the relative change of HCO_3^- and SAG to rule out mixed disorder(s).

ABG, arterial blood gases; $[Cl^-]$, chloride ion concentration; $[HCO_3^-]$, bicarbonate concentration; $[Na^+]$, sodium ion concentration; PCO_2, partial pressure of carbon dioxide from arterial blood; SAG, serum anion gap.

- Serum anion gap (SAG) can be used to determine whether an organic or mineral acidosis is present. SAG is calculated as follows:

$$SAG = [Na^+] - [Cl^-] - [HCO_3^-]$$

The normal SAG is approximately 10 mEq/L (mmol/L), with a range of 8–12 mEq/L (mmol/L). SAG is a relative rather than an absolute indication of the cause of metabolic acidosis.

CLINICAL PRESENTATION

- Acute, mild metabolic acidosis is relatively asymptomatic; the patient may complain of loss of appetite, nausea, and vomiting. Chronic acidemia causes bone demineralization with the development of growth failure and short stature in children and osteomalacia and osteopenia in adults.
- Acute severe metabolic acidemia (pH <7.2) involves the cardiovascular, respiratory, and central nervous systems (CNS). Hyperventilation is often the first sign of metabolic acidosis. Respiratory compensation may occur as Kussmaul respirations (ie, deep, rapid respirations characteristic of diabetic ketoacidosis).
- The compensatory response for metabolic acidosis is to increase CO_2 excretion by increasing the respiratory rate.

TREATMENT

- The primary treatment is to correct the underlying disorder. Additional treatment depends on the severity and onset of acidosis.

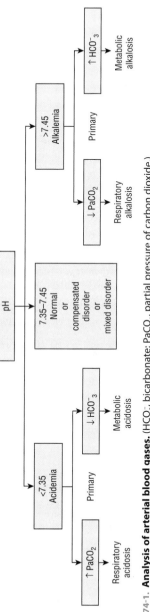

FIGURE 74-1. **Analysis of arterial blood gases.** (HCO_3^-, bicarbonate; $PaCO_2$, partial pressure of carbon dioxide.)

TABLE 74-3	Guidelines for Interpretation of Acid–Base Disorders Based on Compensatory Responses
Acidosis	**Compensation**
Metabolic	$PaCO_2$ (in mm Hg) should decrease by 1.25 times the fall in plasma $[HCO_3^-]$ (in mEq/L or mmol/L)
Acute respiratory	Plasma $[HCO_3^-]$ should increase by 0.1 times the increase in $PaCO_2$ (in mm Hg)
Chronic respiratory	Plasma $[HCO_3^-]$ should increase by 0.4 times the increase in $PaCO_2$ (in mm Hg)
Alkalosis	**Compensation**
Metabolic	$PaCO_2$ (in mm Hg) should increase by 0.6 times the rise in plasma $[HCO_3^-]$ (in mEq/L or mmol/L)
Acute respiratory	Plasma $[HCO_3^-]$ should decrease by 0.2 times the decrease in $PaCO_2$ (in mm Hg), but usually not to <18 mEq/L (mmol/L)
Chronic respiratory	Plasma $[HCO_3^-]$ should fall by 0.4 times the decrease in $PaCO_2$ (in mm Hg), but usually not to <14 mEq/L (mmol/L)

$[HCO_3^-]$, bicarbonate; $PaCO_2$, partial pressure of carbon dioxide from arterial blood; multiply values expressed in kPa by 7.519 to convert to mm Hg.

- Manage asymptomatic patients with mild to moderate acidemia (HCO_3^- 12–20 mEq/L [mmol/L]; pH 7.2–7.4) with gradual correction of the acidemia over days to weeks using oral **sodium bicarbonate** or other alkali preparations (Table 74-4).
- The dose of bicarbonate can be calculated as follows:

$$LD\ (mEq\ or\ mmol/L) = (V_D \times BW) \times (desired\ [HCO_3^-] - current\ [HCO_3^-])$$

where V_D is the volume of distribution of bicarbonate (0.5 L/kg) and BW is body weight in kg.

- Intravenous alkali therapy can be used to treat patients with acute severe metabolic acidosis due to hyperchloremic acidosis, but its role is controversial in patients with lactic acidosis. Therapeutic options include **sodium bicarbonate** and historically, tromethamine, which is no longer available in the United States. If IV sodium bicarbonate is used, the goals are to increase, not normalize, pH (to approximately 7.2) and plasma bicarbonate (to 8–10 mEq/L [mmol/L]). While sodium bicarbonate administration provides fluid and electrolyte replacement and increases arterial pH, it does not improve cardiac function, organ perfusion, or intracellular pH.

Metabolic Alkalosis

PATHOPHYSIOLOGY

- Metabolic alkalosis is *initiated* by increased pH and HCO_3^-, which can result from reduced renal bicarbonate excretion, excessive losses of hydrogen ions from the kidneys or stomach, or from a gain secondary to the ingestion or administration of bicarbonate-rich fluids.
- Metabolic alkalosis is *maintained* by abnormal renal function that prevents the kidneys from excreting excess bicarbonate.

CLINICAL PRESENTATION

- No unique signs or symptoms are associated with mild to moderate metabolic alkalosis. Some patients complain of symptoms related to the underlying disorder (eg, muscle weakness with hypokalemia or postural dizziness with volume depletion) or have a history of vomiting, gastric drainage, or diuretic use.

TABLE 74-4 Therapeutic Alternatives for Oral Alkali Replacement

Product	Milliequivalents of Alkali	Dosage Form(s)
Sodium citrate/citric acid	1 mL contains 1 mEq sodium and is equivalent to 1 mEq bicarbonate	Solution, sodium citrate 500 mg, citric acid 334 mg per 5 mL
Sodium bicarbonate	3.9 mEq bicarbonate per tablet (325 mg)	Tablet, 325 mg
	7.8 mEq bicarbonate per tablet (650 mg)	Tablet, 650 mg
	60 mEq bicarbonate per teaspoon (5 g per teaspoon)	Baking soda powder
Potassium citrate	Each tablet contains 5, 10, or 15 mEq potassium and delivers approximately 5, 10, or 15 mEq bicarbonate	Tablet extended-release, 5 mEq
		Tablet extended-release, 10 mEq
		Tablet extended-release, 15 mEq
Potassium bicarbonate/ potassium citrate	Each tablet contains 10, 20, or 25 mEq potassium and delivers approximately 10, 20, or 25 mEq bicarbonate	Tablet effervescent, 10 mEq
		Tablet effervescent, 20 mEq
		Tablet effervescent, 25 mEq
Potassium citrate/citric acid	Each packet contains 30 mEq potassium and delivers approximately 30 mEq bicarbonate	Powder for solution, potassium citrate monohydrate 3300 mg, citric acid monohydrate 1002 mg per packet
	Each mL contains 2 mEq potassium and delivers approximately 2 mEq bicarbonate	Solution, potassium citrate monohydrate 1100 mg, citric acid monohydrate 334 mg per 5 mL
Sodium citrate/potassium citrate/citric acid	1 mL contains 1 mEq potassium and 1 mEq sodium ion, and delivers approximately 2 mEq bicarbonate	Solution, citric acid 334 mg, sodium citrate 500 mg, and potassium citrate 550 mg per 5 mL

- Severe alkalemia (pH >7.55) can be associated with cardiac arrhythmias, hyperventilation, hypoxemia, and neuromuscular irritability.
- The compensatory response to metabolic alkalosis is respiratory, manifested as hypoventilation which increases $PaCO_2$.

TREATMENT

- Treatment is aimed at correcting the factor(s) responsible for maintaining the alkalosis and depends on whether the disorder is sodium chloride responsive or resistant (Fig. 74-2).
- Sodium chloride–responsive disorders usually result from volume depletion and chloride loss, which can accompany severe vomiting, prolonged nasogastric suction, and diuretic therapy. Initially, therapy is directed at expanding intravascular volume and replenishing chloride stores.
- Management of sodium chloride-resistant disorders usually consists of treatment of the underlying cause of the mineralocorticoid excess.

Respiratory Alkalosis

PATHOPHYSIOLOGY

- Respiratory alkalosis is characterized by a decrease in $PaCO_2$ that leads to an increase in pH.
- $PaCO_2$ decreases when ventilatory CO_2 excretion exceeds metabolic CO_2 production, usually because of hyperventilation.
- Causes include increases in neurochemical stimulation via central or peripheral mechanisms, or physical increases in ventilation via voluntary or artificial means (eg, mechanical ventilation).

CLINICAL PRESENTATION

- Although usually asymptomatic, respiratory alkalosis can cause adverse neuromuscular, cardiovascular, and GI effects.
- Light-headedness, confusion, decreased intellectual functioning, syncope, and seizures can be caused by decreased cerebral blood flow.
- Nausea and vomiting can occur, probably due to cerebral hypoxia.
- Cardiac arrhythmias can occur in severe respiratory alkalosis.
- Serum electrolytes can be altered; serum chloride is usually increased; serum potassium, phosphorus, and ionized calcium are usually decreased.
- The initial compensatory response is to chemically buffer excess bicarbonate by releasing hydrogen ions from intracellular proteins, phosphates, and hemoglobin. If prolonged (>6 hours), proximal tubular bicarbonate reabsorption is inhibited, and the serum bicarbonate concentration decreases.

TREATMENT

- Treatment is often unnecessary because most patients have few symptoms and only mild pH alterations (ie, pH not exceeding 7.50).
- Direct measures to correct the underlying cause (eg, treatment of pain, hypovolemia, fever, infection, or salicylate overdose) can be effective. A rebreathing device (eg, paper bag) can help control hyperventilation in patients with anxiety/hyperventilation syndrome.
- Correct respiratory alkalosis associated with mechanical ventilation by decreasing the number of mechanical breaths per minute, using a capnograph and spirometer to adjust ventilator settings more precisely, or increasing dead space in the ventilator circuit.

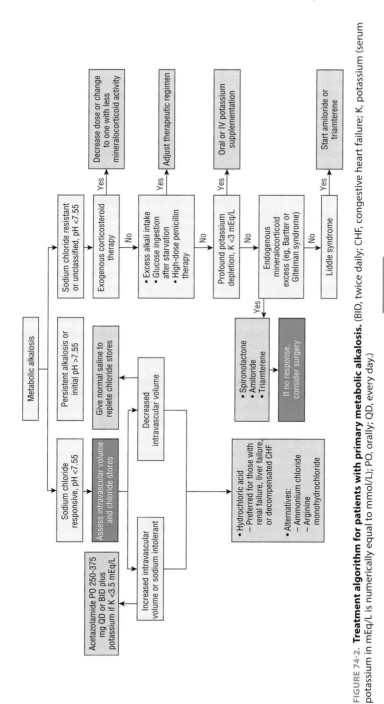

FIGURE 74-2. **Treatment algorithm for patients with primary metabolic alkalosis.** (BID, twice daily; CHF, congestive heart failure; K, potassium (serum potassium in mEq/L is numerically equal to mmol/L); PO, orally; QD, every day.)

Respiratory Acidosis

PATHOPHYSIOLOGY

- Respiratory acidosis is characterized by an increase in $PaCO_2$ and a decrease in pH.
- Respiratory acidosis results from conditions that centrally inhibit the respiratory center, diseases that interfere with pulmonary perfusion or neuromuscular function, and intrinsic airway or parenchymal pulmonary disease. Acute respiratory acidosis with hypoxemia, hypercarbia, and acidosis is life-threatening.

CLINICAL PRESENTATION

- Neurologic symptoms include altered mental status, abnormal behavior, seizures, stupor, and coma. Hypercapnia can mimic a stroke or CNS tumor by producing headache, papilledema, focal paresis, and abnormal reflexes. CNS symptoms are caused by increased cerebral blood flow and are variable, depending in part on the acuity of onset.
- Initial compensatory response to acute respiratory acidosis is chemical buffering. Metabolic compensation occurs when respiratory acidosis is prolonged beyond 12–24 hours. In response to hypercapnia and acidemia, proximal tubular bicarbonate reabsorption, ammoniagenesis, and distal tubular hydrogen secretion are enhanced, resulting in an increase in the serum bicarbonate concentration that raises the pH toward normal.

TREATMENT

- Provide adequate ventilation if CO_2 excretion is acutely and severely impaired ($PaCO_2$ >80 mm Hg [>10.6 kPa]) or if life-threatening hypoxia is present (arterial oxygen tension [PaO_2] <40 mm Hg [<5.3 kPa]). Ventilation can include maintaining a patent airway (eg, emergency tracheostomy, bronchoscopy, or intubation), clearing excessive secretions, administering oxygen, and providing mechanical ventilation.
- Treat underlying cause aggressively (eg, administration of bronchodilators for bronchospasm; narcotic or benzodiazepine antagonists to reverse effect of these agents on the respiratory center). Bicarbonate administration is rarely necessary and is potentially harmful.
- Chronic respiratory acidosis (eg, chronic obstructive pulmonary disease [COPD]) is treated essentially the same as acute respiratory acidosis with a few important exceptions. Oxygen therapy should be initiated carefully and only if the PaO_2 is less than 50 mm Hg (6.7 kPa) because the drive to breathe depends on hypoxemia rather than hypercarbia.
- For information on chronic respiratory acidosis, see Chapter 79.

Mixed Acid–Base Disorders

PATHOPHYSIOLOGY

- Failure of compensation is responsible for mixed respiratory and metabolic acidosis, or mixed respiratory and metabolic alkalosis. In contrast, excess compensation is responsible for metabolic acidosis and respiratory alkalosis, or metabolic alkalosis and respiratory acidosis (see Table 74-3).
- Respiratory and metabolic acidosis can develop in patients with cardiorespiratory arrest, with chronic lung disease who are in shock, and with metabolic acidosis who develop respiratory failure.
- The most common mixed acid–base disorder is respiratory and metabolic alkalosis, which occurs in critically ill surgical patients with respiratory alkalosis caused by mechanical ventilation, hypoxia, sepsis, hypotension, neurologic damage, pain, or

medications; and with metabolic alkalosis caused by vomiting or nasogastric suctioning and massive blood transfusions.

- Mixed metabolic acidosis and respiratory alkalosis occur in patients with advanced liver disease, salicylate intoxication, and pulmonary–renal syndromes.
- Mixed metabolic alkalosis and respiratory acidosis can occur in patients with COPD and chronic respiratory acidosis who are treated with salt restriction, diuretics, and possibly glucocorticoids.

TREATMENT

- Treat mixed respiratory and metabolic acidosis by initiating oxygen delivery to improve hypercarbia and hypoxia. Mechanical ventilation can be needed to reduce $PaCO_2$. During initial therapy, give appropriate amounts of alkali to reverse the metabolic acidosis.
- Correct the metabolic component of mixed respiratory and metabolic alkalosis by administering **sodium and potassium chloride solutions**. Readjust the ventilator or treat the underlying disorder causing hyperventilation to treat the respiratory component.
- Treatment of mixed metabolic acidosis and respiratory alkalosis should be directed at the underlying cause.
- In metabolic alkalosis and respiratory acidosis, pH does not usually deviate significantly from normal, but treatment can be required to maintain PaO_2 and $PaCO_2$ at acceptable levels. Aim treatment at decreasing plasma bicarbonate with sodium and potassium chloride therapy, allowing renal excretion of retained bicarbonate from diuretic-induced metabolic alkalosis.

EVALUATION OF THERAPEUTIC OUTCOMES

- Monitor patients closely because acid–base disorders can be serious and even life-threatening.
- ABGs are the primary tools for the evaluation of therapeutic outcome.

See Chapter 71, Acid–Base Disorders, authored by Anne M. Tucker and Tami N. Johnson, for a more detailed discussion of this topic.

Acute Kidney Injury

- *Acute kidney injury* (AKI) is a clinical syndrome generally defined by an abrupt reduction in kidney function as evidenced by changes in serum creatinine (SCr), blood urea nitrogen (BUN), and urine output.
- RIFLE (Risk, Injury, Failure, Loss of Kidney Function, and End-Stage Renal Disease), AKIN (Acute Kidney Injury Network), and the Kidney Disease: Improving Global Outcomes (KDIGO) clinical practice guidelines are three criteria-based classification systems developed to define and stage AKI in different patient populations (Table 75-1).
- KDIGO criteria are most commonly used; these criteria have been validated across different patient populations, and their staging correlates closely with hospital mortality, cost, and length of stay. SCr and urine output are the main diagnostic criteria.
- AKI becomes acute kidney disease (AKD) if kidney function is impaired beyond 7 days, and can ultimately transition into chronic kidney disease (CKD) if the duration exceeds 90 days.

PATHOPHYSIOLOGY

- AKI can be categorized as prerenal (resulting from decreased renal perfusion in the setting of undamaged parenchymal tissue), intrinsic (resulting from structural damage to the kidney, most commonly the tubule from an ischemic or toxic insult), and postrenal (caused by obstruction of urine flow downstream from the kidney) (Fig. 75-1).
- The risk of AKI increases substantially with decreasing glomerular filtration rate (GFR) and presence of albuminuria and underlying CKD.

CLINICAL PRESENTATION

- Patient presentation varies widely and depends on the underlying cause. Early recognition and cause identification are critical, as they directly affect the outcome of AKI. Time of injury onset can be difficult to determine in outpatients who present with nonspecific or seemingly unrelated symptoms. AKI in hospitalized patients may be detected earlier due to frequent laboratory studies and patient assessment.
- Symptoms in the outpatient setting include acute change in urinary habits, edema, electrolyte disturbances, sudden weight gain, or severe abdominal or flank pain. Signs include edema, colored or foamy urine, and, in volume-depleted patients, postural hypotension, decreased jugular venous pressure (JVP), and dry mucous membranes. Fluid overload is often reflected by elevated JVP, pitting edema, ascites, and pulmonary crackles.

DIAGNOSIS

- Thorough medical and medication histories, physical examination, assessment of laboratory values, and, if needed, imaging studies are important in the diagnosis of AKI.
- SCr cannot be used alone to diagnose AKI because it is insensitive to rapid changes in GFR. SCr lag behind the GFR's decline by 1–2 days, leading to a significant overestimation of GFR in the early stages of AKI and a potential delay in diagnosis of the syndrome. The use of BUN in AKI is very limited because urea production and renal clearance are heavily influenced by extrarenal factors such as critical illness, volume status, protein intake, and medications.
- Urine output measured over a specified period of time allows for short-term assessment of renal function, but its utility is limited to cases in which it is significantly decreased.
- In addition to BUN and SCr, selected blood and urine tests, and urinary sediment are used to differentiate the cause of AKI and guide patient management (Tables 75-2 and 75-3).

TABLE 75-1	RIFLE, AKIN, and KDIGO Classification Schemes for AKI[a]	
RIFLE Category	**SCr and GFR[b] Criteria**	**Urine Output Criteria**
Risk	SCr increase to 1.5-fold or GFR decrease >25% from baseline	<0.5 mL/kg/h for ≥6 hour
Injury	SCr increase to 2-fold or GFR decrease >50% from baseline	<0.5 mL/kg/h for ≥12 hour
Failure	SCr increase to 3-fold or GFR decrease >75% from baseline, or SCr ≥4 mg/dL (354 μmol/L) with an acute increase of at least 0.5 mg/dL (44 μmol/L)	Anuria for ≥12 hour
Loss	Complete loss of function (RRT) for >4 weeks	
ESKD	RRT >3 months	
AKIN Criteria	**SCr Criteria**	**Urine Output Criteria**
Stage 1	SCr increase ≥0.3 mg/dL (27 μmol/L) or 1.5- to 2-fold from baseline	<0.5 mL/kg/h for ≥6 hour
Stage 2	SCr increase >2- to 3-fold from baseline	<0.5 mL/kg/h for ≥12 hour
Stage 3	SCr increase >3-fold from baseline, or SCr ≥4 mg/dL (354 μmol/L) with an acute increase of at least 0.5 mg/dL (44 μmol/L), or need for RRT	<0.3 mL/kg/h for ≥24 hour or anuria for ≥12 hour
KDIGO Criteria	**SCr Criteria**	**Urine Output Criteria**
Stage 1	SCr increase ≥0.3 mg/dL (27 μmol/L) or 1.5–1.9 times from baseline	<0.5 mL/kg/h for 6–12 hour
Stage 2	SCr increase 2–2.9 times from baseline	<0.5 mL/kg/h for ≥12 hour
Stage 3	SCr increase three times from baseline, or SCr ≥4 mg/dL (354 μmol/L), or need for RRT, or eGFR[c] <35 mL/min/1.73 m^2 (0.34 mL/sec/m^2) in patients <18 years	Anuria for ≥12 hour

AKI, acute kidney injury; AKIN, Acute Kidney Injury Network; ESKD, end-stage kidney disease; eGFR, estimated glomerular filtration rate; hr, hours; KDIGO, Kidney Disease: Improving Global Outcomes; RIFLE, Risk, Injury, Failure, Loss of Kidney Function, and End-Stage Kidney Disease; RRT, renal replacement therapy; SCr, serum creatinine.
[a]For all staging systems, the criterion that leads to worst possible diagnosis should be used.
[b]GFR calculated using the Modification of Diet in Renal Disease (MDRD) equation.
[c]GFR calculated using the Schwartz formula.

- Simultaneous measurement of urine and serum electrolytes and calculation of the fractional excretion of sodium (FE$_{Na}$) can help determine the etiology of AKI (see Table 75-2).
- The FE$_{Na}$ is one of the better diagnostic parameters to differentiate the cause of AKI and is calculated as:

$$FE_{Na} = (U_{Na} \times SCr \times 100)/(U_{Cr} \times S_{Na})$$

where U$_{Na}$ = urine sodium, SCr = serum creatinine, U$_{Cr}$ = urine creatinine, and S$_{Na}$ = serum sodium.
- A number of new serum and urinary biomarkers have been investigated to detect and predict the clinical outcomes of AKI, including tissue inhibitor of metalloproteinases 2 (TIMP-2) and insulin-like growth factor binding protein 7 (IGFBP7). Other biomarkers of kidney damage include neutrophil gelatinase–associated lipocalin (NGAL), kidney injury molecule 1 (KIM-1), interleukin 18 (IL-18), liver-type fatty acid binding protein (L-FABP), and N-acetyl-beta-D-glucosaminidase (NAG). They

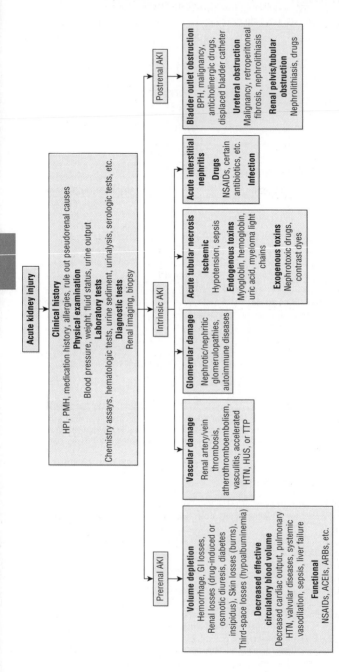

FIGURE 75-1. Classification of acute kidney injury (AKI) based on etiology. ACEIs, angiotensin–converting enzyme inhibitors; ARBs, angiotensin receptor blockers; BPH, benign prostatic hyperplasia; GI, gastrointestinal; HPI, history of present illness; HTN, hypertension; HUS, hemolytic uremic syndrome; NSAIDs, nonsteroidal anti-inflammatory drugs; PMH, past medical history; TTP, thrombotic thrombocytopenic purpura.

TABLE 75-2	Diagnostic Parameters for Differentiating Causes of AKI[a]		
Laboratory Test	**Prerenal AKI**	**Intrinsic AKI**	**Postrenal AKI**
Urine sediment	Hyaline casts, may be normal	Granular casts, cellular debris	Cellular debris
Urinary RBC	None	2–4+	Variable
Urinary WBC	None	2–4+	1+
Urine Na (mEq/L or mmol/L)	<20	>40	>40
FE_{Na} (%)	<1	>2	Variable
Urine specific gravity	>1.018	<1.012	Variable

AKI, acute kidney injury; FE_{Na}, fractional excretion of sodium; Na, sodium; RBC, red blood cell; SCr, serum creatinine; WBC, white blood cell.

[a]Common laboratory tests are used to classify the cause of AKI. Functional AKI, which is not included in this table, would have laboratory values similar to those seen in prerenal AKI. The laboratory results listed under intrinsic AKI are those seen in acute tubular necrosis, the most common cause of intrinsic AKI.

TABLE 75-3	Urinary Findings as a Guide to the Etiology of AKI	
Type of Urinary Evaluation	**Presence of**	**Suggestive of**
Urinalysis	Leukocyte esterases	Pyelonephritis
	Nitrites	Pyelonephritis
	Protein	
	Mild (<0.5 g/day)	Tubular damage
	Moderate (0.5–3 g/day)	Glomerulonephritis, pyelonephritis, tubular damage
	Large (>3 g/day)	Glomerulonephritis, nephrotic syndrome
	Hemoglobin	Glomerulonephritis, pyelonephritis, renal infarction, renal tumors, kidney stones
	Myoglobin	Rhabdomyolysis-associated tubular necrosis
	Urobilinogen	Hemolysis-associated tubular necrosis
Urine sediment	Microorganisms	Pyelonephritis
Cells	Red blood cells	Glomerulonephritis, urinary tract infection, renal infarction, papillary necrosis, renal tumors, kidney stones
	White blood cells	Pyelonephritis, interstitial nephritis
	Eosinophils	Drug-induced interstitial nephritis, renal transplant rejection
	Epithelial cells	Tubular necrosis
Casts	Granular casts	Tubular necrosis
	Hyaline casts	Prerenal azotemia
	White blood cell casts	Pyelonephritis, interstitial nephritis
	Red blood cell casts	Glomerulonephritis, renal infarct, lupus nephritis, vasculitis
Crystals	Urate	Postrenal obstruction
	Calcium phosphate	Postrenal obstruction

have been used for risk assessment, early detection, classification, and prognosis of AKI in addition to and not as a replacement for clinical assessment and standardized tests for kidney function.

- Two new terms "functional change" and "kidney damage" have been proposed in recognition of subclinical kidney injury. Functional change refers to changes in glomerular and tubular function and includes markers such as SCr, eGFR, and cystatin C. Kidney damage describes the presence of tubular and/or glomerular injury and includes markers such as TIMP-2 and IGFBP7.

PREVENTION

- Goals of Prevention: The goals are to screen and identify patients at risk; monitor high-risk patients until the risk subsides; and implement prevention strategies when appropriate.
- The choice of preventive strategy depends on the patient's risk factors for AKI such as comorbidities, planned procedures, and medications, to name a few.

NONPHARMACOLOGIC AND PHARMACOLOGIC STRATEGIES FOR PREVENTION OF AKI

- Electronic alerts within electronic health records have been used for early detection of AKI and increased surveillance of patients on nephrotoxic medications. In general, alerts lead to greater implementation of the intervention, lower loss of kidney function, and decreased exposure to nephrotoxins.
- Intravenous fluids are routinely used in the prevention of AKI, particularly with hemodynamic instability secondary to intravascular volume depletion and for prevention of contrast-induced acute kidney injury (CI-AKI). KDIGO guidelines recommend isotonic crystalloids over colloids for intravascular volume expansion. Balanced solutions may offer some benefit compared to normal saline solutions.
- Both hyper- and hypoglycemia are associated with adverse patient outcomes. Hyperglycemia can occur secondary to stress, inflammation, or medications (eg, steroids) while hypoglycemia develops secondary to decreased clearance of insulin, interruptions in nutrition support prior to procedures, or tight insulin protocols. Guidelines from the American Diabetes Association and Surviving Sepsis Campaign recommend a glycemic target range of 140–180 mg/dL (7.8–10 mmol/L) and less than 180 mg/dL (10 mmol/L), respectively, in critically ill patients.

TREATMENT OF ACUTE KIDNEY INJURY

- Goals of Treatment: Short-term goals include minimizing the degree of insult to the kidney, reducing extrarenal complications, and expediting recovery of renal function. Restoration of renal function to pre-AKI baseline is the ultimate goal.

GENERAL APPROACH TO TREATMENT

- There is no cure for AKI. Management of AKI focuses on supportive care and managing resultant complications, which includes hemodynamic instability, fluid overload, electrolyte imbalances, and acid-base abnormalities.
- Prerenal AKI should be managed with hemodynamic support and volume replacement, intrinsic AKI management relies on managing the cause and providing supportive care, and postrenal AKI therapy should focus on removing the cause of the obstruction.

PHARMACOLOGIC AND NONPHARMACOLOGIC STRATEGIES FOR TREATMENT OF AKI

- Fluid therapy is used to maintain or restore intravascular volume to assure adequate renal perfusion. Use IV fluids judiciously to prevent volume depletion and/or fluid overload which adversely affect kidney function and increase morbidity and mortality.

- Loop diuretics (eg, **furosemide**) are frequently prescribed to manage fluid overload in patients with established kidney injury and often as a precursor to renal replacement therapy (RRT). Loop diuretics increase urine output but may not improve patient outcomes (ie, mortality, need for RRT). Therefore, the KDIGO guidelines recommend limiting their use to the management of fluid overload and avoiding their use for the purpose of treatment of AKI. Diuretic resistance is a relatively common problem in patients with AKI; see Table 75-4 for strategies to counteract diuretic resistance.

- Hyperkalemia is the most common and serious electrolyte disorder in AKI; frequent monitoring is essential. Hyperphosphatemia and hypocalcemia are also common and unlike potassium, not efficiently removed by dialysis. Metabolic acidosis can occur; determining and correcting the underlying cause of the acid–base imbalance is imperative.

- Nutritional management of critically ill patients with AKI is complex due to multiple mechanisms for metabolic derangements. Loss of the normal physiologic and metabolic functions of the kidney and the hypercatabolic response to stress and injury impact the metabolism of nutrients.

- In severe AKI, RRT, such as hemodialysis, is used to treat fluid overload, electrolyte disturbances (eg, hyperkalemia), acid–base imbalances, uremic complications, oliguria or anuria, and pulmonary edema from fluid overload. See Table 75-5 for indications for RRT in AKI. Intermittent and continuous (CRRT) options have different advantages (and disadvantages); the choice usually depends on physician preference and resources available. No difference in mortality or dialysis dependence has been shown; however, CRRT is generally preferred in hemodynamically unstable patients.

- Intermittent hemodialysis (IHD) is the most frequently used RRT and has the advantage of widespread availability and the convenience of lasting only 3–4 hours. Disadvantages include difficult venous dialysis access in hypotensive patients and hypotension due to rapid removal of large amounts of fluid.

TABLE 75-4	Common Causes of Diuretic Resistance in Patients with AKI
Causes of Diuretic Resistance	**Potential Therapeutic Solutions**
Excessive sodium intake (sources may be dietary, IV fluids, and drugs)	Remove sodium from nutritional sources and medications
Inadequate diuretic dose or inappropriate regimen	Increase dose, increase frequency, use continuous infusion, or add thiazide
Reduced oral bioavailability (usually furosemide)	Use parenteral therapy, switch to oral torsemide or bumetanide
Nephrotic syndrome (loop diuretic protein binding in tubule lumen)	Increase dose, add thiazide
Reduced renal blood flow	
Drugs (NSAIDs, ACEIs, vasodilators)	Discontinue these drugs if possible
Intravascular depletion	Intravascular volume expansion
Increased sodium resorption	
Distal nephron hypertrophy	Add thiazide, sodium restriction
Postdiuretic sodium retention	Dietary sodium restriction, use continuous infusion
Heart failure	Assess effective circulatory volume, increase dose, increase frequency, use continuous infusion
Cirrhosis	Assess effective circulatory volume, consider paracentesis
Acute tubular necrosis	Increase diuretic dose, diuretic combination therapy

ACEIs, angiotensin-converting enzyme inhibitors; NSAIDs, nonsteroidal anti-inflammatory drugs.

TABLE 75-5	Common Indications for Renal Replacement Therapy
Indication for RRT	**Clinical Setting**
A: acid–base abnormalities	Metabolic acidosis (especially if pH <7.2)
E: electrolyte imbalance	Severe hyperkalemia and/or hypermagnesemia
I: intoxications	Salicylates, lithium, methanol, ethylene glycol, theophylline, phenobarbital
O: fluid overload	Fluid overload (especially pulmonary edema unresponsive to diuretics)
U: uremia	Uremia or associated complications (neuropathy, encephalopathy, pericarditis)

- Several CRRT variants have been developed including continuous venovenous hemo-filtration (CVVH), continuous venovenous hemodialysis (CVVHD), and continuous venovenous hemodiafiltration (CVVHDF) which differ in fluid clearance and solute removal. CRRT gradually removes solute over 24 hours a day which is tolerated better in critically ill patients. Disadvantages include limited availability of equipment, need for intensive nursing care, and the need to individualize IV replacement, dialysate fluids, and medication therapy adjustments.
- Circuit clotting and filter patency limit CRRT performance requiring anticoagulation. The KDIGO Work Group recommends regional citrate as the preferred anticoagulant. The approach to anticoagulation is patient specific; if the patient requires systemic anticoagulation for an underlying comorbidity (eg, atrial fibrillation, artificial heart valve) no additional anticoagulation for RRT is needed.

Medication Dosing Considerations in AKI

- Medication therapy optimization in AKI is a challenge. Variables include residual drug clearance, fluid accumulation, comorbidities, and use of RRTs. In general, medication elimination may be more robust in AKI compared to chronic kidney disease (CKD), suggesting some caution with utilizing CKD data for dosing decisions.
- Pharmacotherapy decisions should take into consideration the four distinct phases of AKI: initiation, extension, maintenance, and recovery phase. This requires frequent monitoring and adjustment of medication dosing to optimize therapy as kidney function stabilizes.
- Volume of distribution for water soluble drugs is significantly increased due to edema. Use of dosing guidelines for chronic kidney disease (CKD) does not reflect the clearance and volume of distribution in critically ill AKI patients. In addition to volume overload, reductions in cardiac output or liver function can alter the pharmacokinetic profile of most medications. Patients with AKI may have a higher residual nonrenal clearance than those with CKD with similar creatinine clearances, possibly resulting in more robust elimination leading to lower than expected, possibly subtherapeutic, serum concentrations.
- Physicochemical and pharmacokinetic characteristics that can alter medication clearance during RRT include molecular weight (inversely related to clearance), protein binding, volume of distribution, and degree of renal clearance or fraction eliminated by the kidneys. Medication-dosing requirements for patients with AKI or CKD who are receiving CRRT are complex.
- Individualization of pharmacotherapy for a patient receiving RRT is dependent on the patient's residual kidney function, the clearance of the medication by CRRT, as well as the properties of the medication (ie, molecular weight, V_D, protein binding, and sieving coefficient).

TABLE 75-6	Key Monitoring Parameters for Patients with Established AKI
Parameter	**Frequency**
Fluid ins and outs	Hourly/Every shift
Patient weight	Daily
Hemodynamics (blood pressure, heart rate, mean arterial pressure, etc.)	Hourly/Every shift
Blood chemistries	
Sodium, potassium, chloride, bicarbonate, calcium, phosphate, magnesium	Daily
Blood urea nitrogen/serum creatinine	Daily
Drugs and their dosing regimens	Daily
Nutritional regimen	Daily
Blood glucose	Daily (minimum)
Therapeutic drug monitoring of renally cleared drugs (eg, vancomycin aminoglycosides)	Highly variable, about three times weekly
Times of administered doses	Daily
Doses relative to administration of renal replacement therapy	Daily (unless unanticipated changes occur)
Urinalysis	
Calculate measured creatinine clearance	Every time measured urine collection performed
Calculate fractional excretion of sodium	Every time measured urine collection performed
Plans for renal replacement therapy	Daily

EVALUATION OF THERAPEUTIC OUTCOMES

- Vigilant monitoring of patient status is essential, especially in those who are critically ill (**Table 75-6**).
- Perform therapeutic drug monitoring for drugs that have a narrow therapeutic index if results can be obtained in a timely manner.

See Chapter 61, Acute Kidney Injury, authored by Jenana Maker, Lauren Roller, and William Dager, for a more detailed discussion of this topic.

- *Chronic kidney disease* (CKD) is defined as abnormalities in kidney structure or function, present for 3 months or longer.
- CKD is staged based on cause, glomerular filtration rate (GFR), and albuminuria based on the Kidney Disease: Improving Global Outcomes (KDIGO) guidelines for evaluation and management of CKD.
- Prognosis of CKD depends on cause of kidney disease, GFR at time of diagnosis, degree of albuminuria measured by albumin-to-creatinine ratio (ACR), and presence of other comorbid conditions. Please refer to *Pharmacotherapy: A Pathophysiologic Approach*, 12th ed., Chapter 62, Figure 62-1: KDIGO GFR and albuminuria categories and prognosis of CKD by category.

PATHOPHYSIOLOGY

- Clinical and sociodemographic risk factors for susceptibility to and initiation of CKD are useful for identifying individuals at risk of developing CKD. Clinical factors include, but are not limited to, diabetes, hypertension, obesity, smoking, autoimmune diseases, systemic infections, reduction in kidney mass, and low birth weight. Sociodemographic factors include older age, ethnic minority status, low income or education, and exposure to certain chemical and environmental conditions.
- KDIGO recommends that prognosis be considered to help guide testing and treatment decisions. Validated estimating equations such as the kidney failure risk equation (KFRE) provide an accurate 2- and 5-year risk of progression to kidney failure for individuals with stage 3–5 CKD.
- Progression risk factors are associated with further decline in kidney function. Persistence of the underlying initiation factors (eg, diabetes mellitus, hypertension) is the most important predictor of progressive CKD.
- Most progressive nephropathies share a final common pathway to irreversible renal parenchymal damage and end stage renal disease (ESRD) (**Fig. 76-1**). Key elements of the pathway to ESRD include loss of nephron mass, glomerular capillary hypertension, and albuminuria.

CLINICAL PRESENTATION

- Progression of CKD from category 1 to 5 occurs over decades in the majority of people who are asymptomatic until they reach CKD 4 or 5. Signs and symptoms seen with stages 4–5 include fatigue, weakness, shortness of breath, mental confusion, nausea, vomiting, bleeding, anorexia, itching, cold intolerance, peripheral neuropathies, edema, weight gain, changes in urine output, and "foaming" of urine.

TREATMENT OF CKD

GENERAL APPROACH

- Goals of Treatment: The goal is to delay or prevent the progression of CKD.
- Consult KDIGO consensus guidelines for management of CKD; these guidelines are based on evidence and expert recommendations.
- General nonpharmacologic recommendations for all CKD patients include exercise 30 minutes five times/week, weight loss if BMI >25 kg/m^2, smoking cessation, limit alcohol intake, and follow a low-sodium diet if hypertensive.

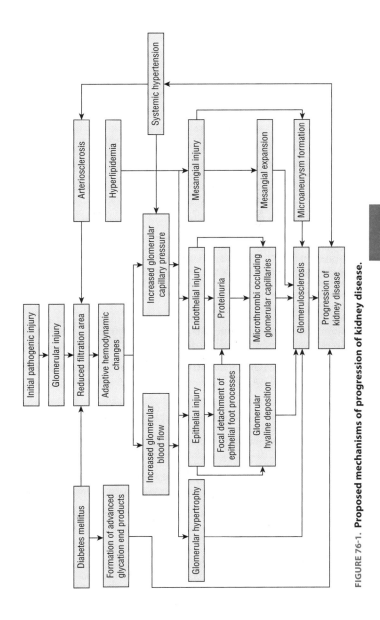

FIGURE 76-1. **Proposed mechanisms of progression of kidney disease.**

- General pharmacologic recommendations for all CKD patients include to adjust medication doses for kidney function, avoid herbal medicines, discuss over-the-counter medicines with pharmacist or other provider before self-medicating, discontinue potentially nephrotoxic/renally excreted drugs if estimated GFR (eGFR) <60 mL/min/1.73 m^2, adhere to vaccine recommendations, take aspirin as secondary prevention if indicated, and avoid oral phosphate-containing bowel preparations if GFR <60 mL/min/1.73 m^2.

PHARMACOLOGIC THERAPY

- Pharmacologic therapies to slow CKD progression include drugs with demonstrated benefits to reduce albuminuria and to manage the causal factors for CKD, primarily hypertension and diabetes.

Albuminuria

- First-line therapy should include an **angiotensin-converting enzyme inhibitor (ACEI)** or an **angiotensin II receptor blocker (ARB)** if the patient's urine albumin excretion is in category A2 or greater (ACR >30 mg/g [>3.4 mg/mmol]). The antiproteinuric effect of ACEIs and ARBs is a class effect. Initiate therapy with the lowest recommended dose and increase dose until albuminuria is reduced by 30%–50% or side effects such as when a greater than 30% increase in serum creatinine (SCr) or elevation in serum potassium occurs or the maximum dose is achieved (Fig. 76-2).
- Sodium glucose transport-2 inhibitors (SGLT2i) slow progression of Type 2 diabetic and nondiabetic proteinuric CKD by reducing glucose and sodium reabsorption in the proximal tubule of the kidney, resulting in decreased glomerular hyperfiltration and reduced glomerular hypertension. SGLT2i significantly slow progression of kidney disease, reduce the need for dialysis or transplantation, and decrease mortality. Continue SGLT2i until dialysis or kidney transplantation. See Chapter 19 for more information on SGLT2i.
- Finererone is a novel, selective, nonsteroidal mineralcorticoid receptor antagonist (MRA) studied in patients with CKD due to Type 2 diabetes. It is an option in patients who cannot tolerate SGLT2i; it has not been studied in combination with SGLT2i plus ACEI/ARB.
- **Nondihydropyridine calcium channel blockers** are third-line antiproteinuric drugs when an ACEI/ARB and SGLT2 inhibitor is contraindicated or not tolerated.

Hypertension

- Figure 76-2 provides an algorithm for recommended blood pressure goals based on the degree of albuminuria present and the choice of antihypertensive agent.
- For more information on hypertension, see Chapter 10.

Diabetes

- Screen patients with diabetes annually for CKD starting at the time of diagnosis of type 2 diabetes and 5 years after diagnosis of type 1 diabetes by ordering serum creatinine, eGFR, and a urine ACR.
- Management of diabetes in patients with CKD includes reduction of proteinuria and achievement of target blood pressure and HbA1C.
- For more information on diabetes, see Chapter 19.

MANAGEMENT OF SECONDARY COMPLICATIONS

- Base management of complications of CKD on the KDIGO consensus guidelines which are based on evidence, when available, and expert recommendations.
- Use an interdisciplinary team approach that includes individuals trained to address the complex secondary complications of CKD to emphasize patient-centered care.

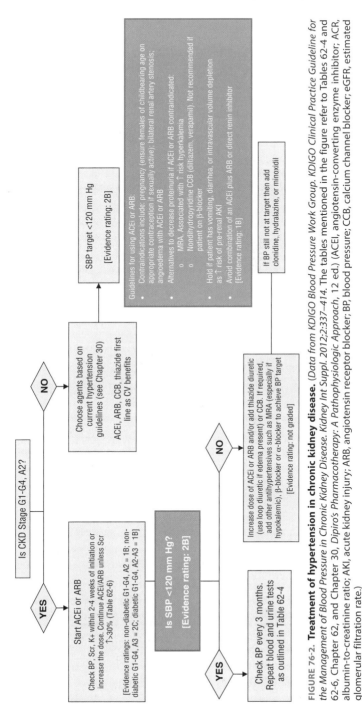

FIGURE 76-2. Treatment of hypertension in chronic kidney disease. *(Data from KDIGO Blood Pressure Work Group. KDIGO Clinical Practice Guideline for the Management of Blood Pressure in Chronic Kidney Disease. Kidney Int Suppl. 2012;2:337–414. The tables mentioned in the figure refer to Tables 62-4 and 62-6, Chapter 62, and Chapter 30, Dipiro's Pharmacotherapy: A Pathophysiologic Approach, 12 ed.) (ACEI, angiotensin-converting enzyme inhibitor; ACR, albumin-to-creatinine ratio; AKI, acute kidney injury; ARB, angiotensin receptor blocker; BP, blood pressure; CCB, calcium channel blocker; eGFR, estimated glomerular filtration rate.)*

Anemia of CKD

- The primary cause of anemia of CKD is a relative deficiency in production of erythropoietin in the kidney; other causes include decreased gastrointestinal (GI) absorption of iron, inflammation, frequent blood testing, blood loss from hemodialysis (HD) for patients with ESRD, and increased iron demands from erythropoiesis stimulating agent (ESA) therapy. Additional factors are decreased red cell life span, the effects of accumulation of uremic toxins and inflammatory cytokines, and vitamin B_{12} and folate deficiencies.
- Desired outcomes of anemia management are to safely achieve target hemoglobin (Hb) levels that increase oxygen-carrying capacity to decrease signs and symptoms of anemia and reduce the need for blood transfusions.
- Guide initiation of iron or ESA therapy by the patient's Hb, transferrin saturation (TSat), and ferritin (Table 76-1). The risk of mortality and cardiovascular events is higher in CKD patients treated to higher Hb target values with an ESA. The target range for Hb in the CKD population is a topic of much debate. The current labeling for all ESAs warns that dosing ESAs to target Hb levels greater than 11 g/dL (110 g/L; 6.83 mmol/L) for CKD patients increases the risk for death, serious CV reactions, and stroke.
- Oral or intravenous (IV) **iron** supplementation is recommended in non-HD patients (eg, CKD category 3 or higher and peritoneal dialysis [PD] patients), and IV supplementation in ESRD. Supplementation with oral products (see Table 33-1) is more convenient but patients are likely to require IV iron supplementation to correct absolute iron deficiency, especially if they are receiving an ESA. Adverse effects of oral iron are primarily GI in nature and include constipation, nausea, and abdominal cramping which may negatively influence adherence.

TABLE 76-1	KDIGO Recommendations for Initiation of ESAs and Iron in Adults with Anemia of CKD	
	ND-CKD	**ESRD**
ESA initiation	If Hb <10 g/dL (100 g/L; 6.21 mmol/L). Consider rate of fall of Hb, prior response to iron, risk of needing a transfusion, risk of ESA therapy, and presence of anemia symptoms before initiating an ESA. [2C]	Use ESAs to avoid drop in Hb to <9 g/dL (90 g/L; 5.59 mmol/L) by starting an ESA when Hb is between 9 and 10 g/dL (90 and 100 g/L; 5.59 and 6.21 mmol/L). [2B]
	Do not initiate if Hb ≥10 g/dL (100 g/L; 6.21 mmol/L). [2D]	
Hb level	Do not use ESAs to *intentionally* increase Hb above 13 g/dL (130 g/L, 8.07 mmol/L). [1A]	Do not use ESAs to *intentionally* increase Hb above 13 g/dL (130 g/L, 8.07 mmol/L). [1A]
	Do not use ESAs to maintain Hb above 11.5 g/dL (115 g/L; 7.14 mmol/L). [2C]	Do not use ESAs to maintain Hb above 11.5 g/dL (115 g/L; 7.14 mmol/L). [2C]
Iron initiation[a]	If TSat is ≤30% (0.30) and ferritin is ≤500 ng/mL (mcg/L; 1120 pmol/L). [2C]	If TSat is ≤30% (0.30) and ferritin is ≤500 ng/mL (mcg/L; 1120 pmol/L). [2C]

CKD, chronic kidney disease; ESA, erythropoiesis-stimulating agent; ESRD, end-stage renal disease; Hb, hemoglobin; ND-CKD, nondialysis CKD patients; QOL, quality of life; TSat, transferrin saturation.
[a]If TSat and serum ferritin are below suggested levels, consider iron supplementation if goal is to increase Hb and/or decrease ESA dose. *Note:* Serum ferritin is an acute-phase reactant—use clinical judgment when above 500 ng/mL (mcg/L; 1120 pmol/L).
The strength of recommendation is indicated as Level 1, Level 2, or Not Graded. The quality of the supporting evidence is shown as A, B, C, or D.

- Soluble **ferric pyrophosphate citrate** is an iron compound added to the dialysate used for HD allowing for continuous iron administration during the procedure. Ferric pyrophosphate binds directly to transferrin, bypassing the reticuloendothelial system and resulting in increased Hb concentrations and reduction in ESA dose and IV iron requirements.
- IV iron preparations have different pharmacokinetic profiles determined by the size of the iron-containing core and the composition of the surrounding carbohydrate shell. Such differences affect the rate of dissociation of iron from the complex, the rate of distribution, and the maximum tolerated dose and rate of infusion (Table 76-2).
- Adverse effects of IV iron include allergic reactions, hypotension, dizziness, dyspnea, headaches, lower back pain, arthralgia, syncope, and arthritis. Some of these reactions can be minimized by decreasing the dose or rate of infusion. Non-dextran IV iron formulations have a better safety record than iron dextran. An analysis of anaphylaxis risk in patients newly exposed to IV iron products (including **dextran**, **gluconate**, **sucrose**, or **ferumoxytol**) reported the highest risk with iron dextran and the lowest risk with iron sucrose. Fatal and serious hypersensitivity reactions including anaphylaxis have occurred with ferumoxytol.
- Long-term IV iron administration introduces a risk of iron overload leading to hepatic, pancreatic, and cardiac dysfunction. Maintain target serum ferritin and TSat values to minimize risk.
- All available ESAs may be administered either IV or subcutaneously (SubQ) (Table 76-3). The biosimilar **epoetin alfa-epbx** is available in the United States with the same indications as the biological drug, **epoetin alfa**. SubQ administration of epoetin results in a prolonged absorption phase leading to an extended half-life allowing target Hb to be maintained at doses 15%–30% lower than IV doses.
- The prolonged half-lives of **darbepoetin alfa** and **methoxy PEG-epoetin beta** allow for less frequent dosing.
- Causes of ESA resistance include iron deficiency, acute illness, inflammation, infection, chronic bleeding, aluminum toxicity, malnutrition, hyperparathyroidism, cancer, and chemotherapy.
- ESAs are well tolerated. Hypertension is the most common adverse event and may be associated with the rate of rise in Hb.
- Figure 76-3 provides an approach to management of anemia in patients with CKD. For more information on anemia, see Chapter 33.

Mineral and Bone Disorder

- Desired outcomes for management of disorders of mineral and bone metabolism (CKD-MBD) are to "normalize" the biochemical parameters and prevent bone manifestations, cardiovascular and extravascular calcification, and associated morbidity and mortality.
- The KDIGO-recommended targets for calcium, phosphorus, and parathyroid hormone (PTH) and the frequency of monitoring based on CKD category are given in Table 76-4.
- Guidelines emphasize avoiding hypercalcemia based on evidence linking higher calcium levels with mortality and nonfatal cardiovascular events. The phosphorus recommendation is to maintain levels "toward the normal" based on evidence linking both high- and low-phosphate concentrations with increased mortality.
- Calcium-phosphorus homeostasis is mediated through a complex interplay of hormones and their effects on bone, the GI tract, kidneys, and the parathyroid gland. As kidney function declines, phosphate elimination decreases resulting in hyperphosphatemia and a decrease in serum calcium concentration. Hypocalcemia stimulates secretion of PTH. Serum calcium balance can be maintained only at the expense of increased bone resorption, leading to alterations in structural integrity of bone and other consequences.

Treatment

- Dietary phosphorus restriction, dialysis, and parathyroidectomy are nonpharmacologic approaches to management of hyperphosphatemia and CKD-MBD.

TABLE 76-2	Intravenous Iron Agents			
Iron Compounds	Brand Names	Molecular Weight (Daltons)	FDA-Approved Indications	FDA-Approved Dosing[a,b]
Ferric carboxymaltose	Injectafer	150,000	Adult patients with intolerance to oral iron or who have had an unsatisfactory response to oral iron and adult patients with CKD not on dialysis	Give 2 doses separated by at least 7 days of 750 mg per dose (if body weight is ≥50 kg) or 15 mg/kg per dose (if body weight is <50 kg) not to exceed 1500 mg per course; give either IV push (100 mg/min) or diluted in not more than 250 mL of 0.9 NaCl as an infusion over at least 15 minutes
Ferric derisomaltose	Monoferric	155,000	Treatment of iron deficiency anemia in adults with ND-CKD or who have intolerance to oral iron or unsatisfactory response to oral iron	If weight ≥50 kg: 1000 mg as a single dose If weight <50 kg administer 20 mg/kg actual body weight as a single dose
Ferric pyrophosphate citrate	Triferic AVNU	1313	Iron replacement to maintain Hb in adult patients with ESKD on hemodialysis	6.75 mg iron over 3–4 hours at each HD session via pre-dialyzer infusion line, post-dialyzer infusion line, or a separate connection to the venous blood line
	Triferic			Add the appropriate ampule or powder packet* to the bicarbonate concentrate solution to achieve a final concentration of ferric pyrophosphate citrate of 110 µg/L *Add one 5 mL ampule to 2.5 gallons (9.5 L) of bicarbonate concentrate or one 50 mL ampule to 25 gallons (95 L) of bicarbonate or one packet of powder to each 25 gallons ampule (95 L)
Ferumoxytol	Feraheme	750,000	Adult patients with iron-deficiency anemia associated with chronic kidney disease	510 mg (17 mL) as a single dose, followed by a second 510-mg dose 3–8 days after the initial dose; dilute in 50–200 mL of 0.9% NaCl or 5% dextrose and administer as an IV infusion over 15 minutes
Iron dextran	INFeD	96,000	Patients with iron deficiency in whom oral iron is unsatisfactory or impossible	100 mg over 2 minutes (25-mg test dose required) Note: Equation provided by manufacturer to calculate dose based on desired Hb

Iron sucrose	Venofer	43,000	Adult and pediatric ESKD patients on HD age 2 years and older	Adult: 100 mg over 2–5 minutes or 100 mg in maximum of 100 mL of 0.9% NaCl over 15 minutes per consecutive HD session
				Pediatric: 0.5 mg/kg not to exceed 100 mg per dose over 5 minutes or diluted in 25 mL of 0.9% NaCl administered over 5–60 minutes (give dose every 2 weeks for 12 weeks)
			Adult and pediatric ND-CKD patients age 2 years and older	Adult: 200 mg over 2–5 minutes on five different occasions within 14-day period; there is limited experience with administration of 500 mg diluted in a maximum of 250 mL of 0.9% NaCl over 3.5–4 hours on days 1 and 14
				Pediatric: see pediatric dosing for CKD 5HD (give dose every 4 weeks for 12 weeks)
			Adult and pediatric ESKD patients on PD, age 2 years and older	Adult: give 3 divided doses within 28 days as 2 infusions of 300 mg over 1.5 hours 14 days apart followed by one 400 mg infusion over 2.5 hours 14 days later; dilute in a maximum of 250 mL of 0.9% NaCl
				Pediatric: see pediatric dosing for CKD 5HD (give dose every 4 weeks for 12 weeks)
Sodium ferric gluconate	Ferrlecit	350,000	Adult and pediatric ESKD patients on HD age 6 years and older receiving ESA therapy	Adult: 125 mg over 10 minutes or 125 mg in 100 mL of 0.9% NaCl over 60 minutes
				Pediatric: 1.5 mg/kg in 25 mL of 0.9% NaCl over 60 minutes; maximum dose 125 mg per dose

CKD, chronic kidney disease; ESA, erythropoiesis stimulating agent; ESKD, end-stage kidney disease; Hb, hemoglobin; HD, hemodialysis; IV, intravenous; ND-CKD, non-dialysis CKD patients.

[a]Monitor for 30 minutes following an infusion; KDIGO guidelines recommend monitoring for 60 minutes (1B recommendation for iron dextran, 2C recommendation for non-dextran products).

[b]With the exception of ferric carboxymaltose, ferric derisomaltose, and ferumoxytol, small doses (eg, 25–150 mg/wk) are generally used for maintenance regimens. Larger doses (eg, 1 g) should be administered in divided doses. The IV form of ferric pyrophosphate citrate (Triferic AVNU) is administered in smaller increments (6.75 mg).

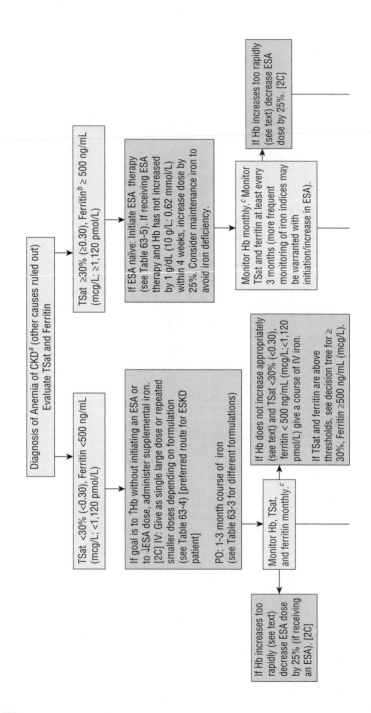

Diagnosis of Anemia of CKD[a] (other causes ruled out)
Evaluate TSat and Ferritin

TSat <30% (<0.30), Ferritin <500 ng/mL (mcg/L; <1,120 pmol/L)

If goal is to ↑Hb without initiating an ESA or to ↓ESA dose, administer supplemental iron. [2C] IV: Give as single large dose or repeated smaller doses depending on formulation (see Table 63-4) [preferred route for ESKD patient]

PO: 1-3 month course of iron (see Table 63-3 for different formulations)

Monitor Hb, TSat, and ferritin monthly.[c]

If Hb increases too rapidly (see text) decrease ESA dose by 25% (if receiving an ESA). [2C]

If Hb does not increase appropriately (see text) and TSat <30% (<0.30), ferritin < 500 ng/mL (mcg/L;<1,120 pmol/L) give a course of IV iron.

If TSat and ferritin are above thresholds, see decision tree for ≥ 30%, Ferritin ≥500 ng/mL (mcg/L).

TSat ≥30% (≥0.30), Ferritin[b] ≥ 500 ng/mL (mcg/L; ≥1,120 pmol/L)

If ESA naïve: Initiate ESA therapy (see Table 63-5). If receiving ESA therapy and Hb has not increased by 1 g/dL (10 g/L; 0.62 mmol/L) within 4 weeks, increase dose by 25%. Consider maintenance iron to avoid iron deficiency.

Monitor Hb monthly.[c] Monitor TSat and ferritin at least every 3 months (more frequent monitoring of iron indices may be warranted with initiation/increase in ESA).

If Hb increases too rapidly (see text) decrease ESA dose by 25%. [2C]

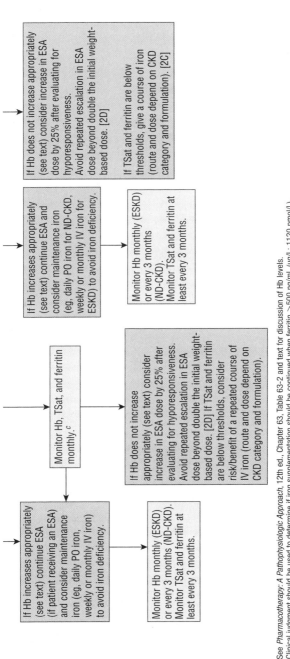

Monitor Hb, TSat, and ferritin monthly.[c]

If Hb increases appropriately (see text) continue ESA (if patient receiving an ESA) and consider maintenance iron (eg, daily PO iron, weekly or monthly IV iron) to avoid iron deficiency.

Monitor Hb monthly (ESKD) or every 3 months (ND-CKD). Monitor TSat and ferritin at least every 3 months.

If Hb does not increase appropriately (see text) consider increase in ESA dose by 25% after evaluating for hyporesponsiveness. Avoid repeated escalation in ESA dose beyond double the initial weight-based dose. [2D] If TSat and ferritin are below thresholds, consider risk/benefit of a repeated course of IV iron (route and dose depend on CKD category and formulation).

If Hb increases appropriately (see text) continue ESA and consider maintenance iron (eg, daily PO iron for ND-CKD, weekly or monthly IV iron for ESKD) to avoid iron deficiency.

Monitor Hb monthly (ESKD) or every 3 months (ND-CKD). Monitor TSat and ferritin at least every 3 months.

If Hb does not increase appropriately (see text) consider increase in ESA dose by 25% after evaluating for hyporesponsiveness. Avoid repeated escalation in ESA dose beyond double the initial weight-based dose. [2D]

If TSat and ferritin are below thresholds, give a course of iron (route and dose depend on CKD category and formulation). [2C]

[a]See *Pharmacotherapy: A Pathophysiologic Approach,* 12th ed., Chapter 63, Table 63-2 and text for discussion of Hb levels.

[b]Clinical judgment should be used to determine if iron supplementation should be continued when ferritin >500 ng/mL (μg/L; 1120 pmol/L).

[c]Weekly monitoring of Hb may be warranted. Wait at least 1 week after an IV dose of iron to measure TSat and ferritin. The tables mentioned in the figure refer to Tables 63-3 and 63-4, Chapter 63, *Dipiro's Pharmacotherapy: A Pathophysiologic Approach,* 12 ed.

FIGURE 76-3. Algorithm for management of anemia of CKD in adults. (CKD, chronic kidney disease; ESKD, end-stage kidney disease; ESA, erythropoiesis-stimulating agent; Hb, hemoglobin; ND-CKD, nondialysis CKD patients; TSat, transferrin saturation. Evidence grading in brackets.)

TABLE 76-3 ESAs in CKD

Drug Name	Brand Name(s)	Starting Dose	Route of Administration	Half-Life (Hours)
Epoetin alfa	Epogen, Procrit	Adults: 50–100 units/kg three times per week	IV or SubQ	8.5 (IV)
				24 (SubQ)
		Pediatrics: 50 units/kg three times per week		
Epoetin alfa-epbx	Retacrit	See epoetin alfa information		
Darbepoetin alfa	Aranesp	Adults:	IV or SubQ	25 (IV)
		ND-CKD: 0.45 mcg/kg once every 4 weeks		48 (SubQ)
		ESKD: 0.45 mcg/kg once per week or 0.75 mcg/kg every 2 weeks		
		Pediatrics:		
		0.45 mcg/kg once weekly; may give 0.75 mcg/kg once every 2 weeks in ND-CKD patients		
Methoxy PEG-epoetin beta	Mircera	All adult CKD patients: 0.6 mcg/kg every 2 weeks; once Hb stabilizes, double the dose and administer monthly (eg, if administering 0.6 mcg/kg every 2 weeks, give 1.2 mcg/kg every month)	IV or SubQ	134 (IV)
				139 (SubQ)

CKD, chronic kidney disease; ESKD, end-stage kidney disease; ND-CKD, nondialysis CKD patients; PEG, polyethylene glycol; SubQ, subcutaneous.

Phosphate-Binding Agents

- Oral calcium compounds bind phosphate thereby decreasing phosphorus absorption from the gut and are first-line agents for controlling both serum phosphorus and calcium concentrations (Table 76-5). **Calcium carbonate** and **calcium acetate** are the primary preparations used. **Sevelamer** is a nonabsorbable, nonelemental hydrogel that effectively lowers phosphorus and also lowers LDL and increases HDL.
- **Lanthanum carbonate** controls phosphorus and maintains PTH in the target range with less risk of hypercalcemia than calcium-containing binders. **Ferric citrate** and **sucroferric oxyhydroxide** are iron-based phosphate-binding agents.
- Adverse effects of all phosphate binders are generally limited to GI effects, including constipation, diarrhea, nausea, vomiting, and abdominal pain. Risk of hypercalcemia may necessitate restriction of calcium-containing binder use and/or reduction in dietary intake. Aluminum and magnesium binders are not recommended for regular use in CKD. The potential for iron overload should be considered with ferric citrate.

Vitamin D Therapy

- **Calcitriol**, 1,25-dihydroxyvitamin D_3, and vitamin D analogs directly inhibit or suppress PTH synthesis and also stimulate absorption of serum calcium by intestinal cells, which decreases PTH secretion by the parathyroid glands.
- Serum calcium and phosphorus should be within the normal range before initiation and during continued vitamin D therapy. Adjust vitamin D dose every 2–4 weeks based on PTH concentrations and trends in calcium and phosphorus (Table 76-6).

TABLE 76-4 KDIGO Monitoring and Goals for Calcium, Phosphorus, and Parathyroid Hormone

	Chronic Kidney Disease Stage			
Parameter	G3	G4	G5	ESKD
Corrected calcium[a]				
Monitoring frequency[b]	Every 6–12 months	Every 3–6 months	Every 1–3 months	Every 1–3 months
Goal	Avoid hypercalcemia	Avoid hypercalcemia	Avoid hypercalcemia	Avoid hypercalcemia
Phosphorus				
Monitoring frequency[b]	Every 6–12 months	Every 3–6 months	Every 1–3 months	Every 1–3 months
Goal	Toward the normal range	Toward the normal range	Toward the normal range	Toward the normal range
Intact PTH				
Monitoring frequency[b]	Based on baseline level and CKD progression	Every 6–12 months	Every 3–6 months	Every 3–6 months
Goal	Avoid progressively rising levels or levels persistently above the upper limit of normal	Avoid progressively rising levels or levels persistently above the upper limit of normal	Avoid progressively rising levels or levels persistently above the upper limit of normal	2–9 times the upper normal limit

ESKD, end-stage kidney disease.
[a]Corrected for albumin.
[b]Not graded.

TABLE 76-5	Phosphate-Binding Agents for Treatment of Hyperphosphatemia in Chronic Kidney Disease Patients				
Category	Drug	Brand Name	Compound Content	Starting Doses	Dose Titration[a]	Comments[b]
Calcium-based binders	Calcium acetate (25% elemental calcium)	PhosLo	25% Elemental calcium (169 mg elemental calcium per 667 mg capsule)	1334 mg three times a day with meals	Increase or decrease by 667 mg meal (169 mg elemental calcium)	Comparable efficacy to calcium carbonate with lower dose of elemental calcium Approximately 45 mg phosphorus bound per 1 g calcium acetate Evaluate for drug interactions with calcium
		Phoslyra	667 mg calcium acetate per 5 mL			
	Calcium carbonate[c]	Tums, Os-Cal, Caltrate	40% Elemental calcium	0.5–1 g (elemental calcium) three times a day with meals	Increase or decrease by 500 mg/ meal (200 mg elemental calcium)	Dissolution characteristics and phosphate binding may vary from product to product Approximately 39 mg phosphorus bound per 1 g calcium carbonate Evaluate for drug interactions with calcium
Iron-based binders	Ferric citrate	Auryxia	210 mg elemental iron per tablet (= 1 g ferric citrate)	420 mg ferric iron three times daily with meals	Increase or decrease dose by 1 or 2 tablets per meal	May increase serum iron, ferritin, and TSat May cause discolored (dark) stools Evaluate for drug interactions with iron
	Sucroferric oxyhydroxide	Velphoro	500 mg elemental iron per chewable tablet (= 2.5 g sucroferric oxyhydroxide)	500 mg three times daily with meals	Increase or decrease by 500 mg/day	May cause discolored (dark) stools Evaluate for drug interactions with iron

Class	Drug	Brand	Available formulations	Dose	Titration	Comments
Resin binders	Sevelamer carbonate	Renvela	800 mg tablet; 0.8 and 2.4 g powder for oral suspension	800–1600 mg three times a day with meals (once-daily dosing also effective)	Increase or decrease by 800 mg/meal	Also lowers low-density lipoprotein cholesterol; Consider in patients at risk for extraskeletal calcification; Risk of metabolic acidosis with sevelamer hydrochloride (less risk with carbonate formulation); May interact with cipro and mycophenolate mofetil
	Sevelamer hydrochloride	Renagel	400 and 800 mg caplets	800–1600 mg three times a day with meals	Increase or decrease by 800 mg/meal	
Other elemental binders	Lanthanum carbonate	Fosrenol	500, 750, and 1000 mg chewable tablets; 750 and 1000 mg oral powder	1500 mg daily in divided doses with meals	Increase or decrease by 750 mg/day	Potential for accumulation of lanthanum due to GI absorption (long-term consequences unknown); Evaluate for drug interactions (eg, cationic antacids, quinolone antibiotics)
	Aluminum hydroxide (NOT PREFERRED)	AlternaGel	Content varies (range 100–600 mg/unit)	300–600 mg three times a day with meals	Not for long-term use requiring titration	Not a first-line agent; risk of aluminum toxicity; do not use concurrently with citrate-containing products; Reserve for short-term use (4 weeks) in patients with hyperphosphatemia not responding to other binders; Evaluate for drug interactions

TSat, transferrin saturation.

aBased on phosphorus levels, titrate every 2–3 weeks until phosphorus goal is reached.

bGI side effects are possible with all agents (eg, nausea, vomiting, abdominal pain, diarrhea, or constipation).

cMultiple preparations available that are not listed.

TABLE 76-6 Vitamin D Agents

Nutritional vitamin D

Generic Name	Brand Name	Form of Vitamin D	Dosage Forms	Initial Dose	Dosage Range	Frequency of Dosing or Dose Titration[a]
Ergocalciferol	Drisdol	D_2	po	Varies based on 25(OH)D levels	400–50,000 international units	Daily (doses of 400–2000 international units)
Cholecalciferol[b]	Generic	D_3	po			Weekly or monthly for higher doses (50,000 international units)
Calcifediol	Rayaldee	D_3	po	30 mcg daily	30–60 mcg	Increase after 3 months if PTH above desired range

Vitamin D and analogs

Generic Name	Brand Name	Form of Vitamin D	Dosage Forms	Initial Dose[c,d]	Dosage Range	Dose Titration[a]
Calcitriol	Rocaltrol	D_3	po	0.25 mcg daily	0.25–5 mcg	Increase by 0.25 mcg/day at 4–8 week intervals
	Calcijex		IV	1–2 mcg three times per week	0.5–5 mcg	Increase by 0.5–1 mcg at 2–4 week intervals
Doxercalciferol[e]	Hectorol	D_2	po	ND-CKD: 1 mcg daily	5–20 mcg	Increase by 0.5 mcg at 2-week intervals for daily dosing or by 2.5 mcg at 8-week intervals for three times per week dosing
				ESKD: 10 mcg three times per week		
			IV	ESKD: 4 mcg three times per week	2–8 mcg	Increase by 1–2 mcg at 8-week intervals

| Paricalcitol | Zemplar | D_2 | po | ND-CKD: 1 mcg daily or 2 mcg three times per week if PTH ≤500 pg/mL (ng/L; 54 pmol/L); 2 mcg daily or 4 mcg three times per week if PTH >500 pg/mL (ng/L; 54 pmol/L) | 1–4 mcg | Increase by 1 mcg (for daily dosing) or 2 mcg (for three times per week dosing) at 2–4 week intervals |
| | | | IV | ESKD: 0.04–1 mcg three times per week | 2.5–15 mcg | Increase by 2–4 mcg at 2–4 week intervals |

ESKD, end-stage kidney disease; IV, intravenous; ND-CKD, nondialysis chronic kidney disease; PTH, parathyroid hormone.

[a]Based on PTH, calcium, and phosphorus levels. Decreases in dose are necessary if PTH is oversuppressed and/or if calcium and phosphorus are elevated.

[b]Multiple preparations are available that are not listed.

[c]Dose ratios are as follows: 1:1 for IV paricalcitol to oral doxercalciferol, 1.5:1 for IV paricalcitol to IV doxercalciferol, and 1:1 for IV to oral calcitriol.

[d]Daily oral dosing most common for nonhemodialysis CKD patients, IV or PO dosing three times per week more often used in the hemodialysis population.

[e]Prodrug that requires activation by the liver.

- KDIGO does not advocate for routine use of calcitriol and vitamin D analogs in the nondialysis CKD population and suggests that they be reserved for patients with CKD stages 4–5.
- The newer vitamin D analogs **paricalcitol** and **doxercalciferol** may be associated with less hypercalcemia and hyperphosphatemia. Observational studies show all-cause and cardiovascular survival benefit with these agents.

Calcimimetics

- **Cinacalcet** and **etelcalcetide** reduce PTH secretion by increasing the sensitivity of the calcium-sensing receptor. The most common adverse events include nausea and vomiting.
- Since these agents lower serum calcium they should not be started if the serum calcium is less than the lower limit of normal. Start cinacalcet at 30 mg daily, which can be titrated to the desired PTH and calcium concentrations every 2–4 weeks to a maximum of 180 mg daily. Initiate etelcalcetide at 5 mg IV three times per week at the end of hemodialysis.
- Measure calcium and phosphorus 1 week after initiating therapy and measure PTH within 1–4 weeks or per protocol of the dialysis center.

CARDIOVACULAR COMPLICATIONS OF CKD

CARDIOVASCULAR DISEASE

- CKD patients are at increased risk of CVD, independent of the etiology of their kidney disease and this is associated with much higher mortality rates. Traditional risk factors include diabetes, dyslipidemia, hypertension, smoking, and obesity. Nontraditional risk factors include proteinuria, anemia, inflammation, and abnormal calcium and phosphate metabolism, resulting in vascular calcification oxidative stress.
- CKD patients benefit from treatment of traditional and nontraditional risk factors. Aspirin is recommended for secondary prevention in all patients based on decreased mortality in observational studies. Non-dialysis CKD patients have multiple options to delay CKD progression including sodium-glucose co-transporter type 2 inhibitors, glucagon-like-peptide-1 receptor agonists, and mineralocorticoid receptor antagonists.

HYPERLIPIDEMIA

- CKD with or without nephrotic syndrome is frequently accompanied by abnormalities in lipoprotein metabolism.
- KDIGO Lipid Guidelines recommend:
  1. Complete a fasting lipid profile in all adults with newly identified CKD.
  2. **Statin** treatment in adults ages 18–49 years with CKD but not treated with chronic dialysis or kidney transplantation, who have one or more of the following: known coronary disease; diabetes mellitus; prior ischemic stroke; estimated 10-year incidence of coronary death or nonfatal MI greater than 10%.
  3. Statin or statin/**ezetimibe** combination in adults >50 years with eGFR <60 mL/min/1.73 m² but not treated with chronic dialysis or kidney transplantation.
  4. Do not initiate statins or statin/ezetimibe combination therapy in adults with dialysis-dependent CKD. Continue these agents if patient is already taking them at the time of dialysis initiation.

See Chapter 62, Chronic Kidney Disease, authored by Lori D. Wazny, and Chapter 63, Chronic Kidney Disease: Management of Secondary Complications, authored by Joanna Q. Hudson, for a more detailed discussion of this topic.

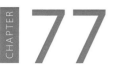
- *Fluid and electrolyte homeostasis* is maintained by feedback mechanisms, hormones, and many organ systems, and is necessary for the body's normal physiologic functions. Disorders of sodium and water, calcium, phosphorus, potassium, and magnesium homeostasis are addressed separately in this chapter.

DISORDERS OF SODIUM AND WATER HOMEOSTASIS

- Total body water (TBW) ranges from 45% to 80% of body weight depending on sex, age, gestational age, and disease states and is distributed primarily into two compartments: intracellularly (ICF; two-thirds [67%] of TBW), and one-third (33%) is contained in the extracellular space.
- *Effective osmoles* are solutes that cannot freely cross cell membranes, such as sodium and potassium. Addition of an isotonic solution to the extracellular fluid (ECF) does not change ICF volume because there is no change in effective ECF osmolality. Adding a hypertonic solution to the ECF decreases ICF volume, whereas adding a hypotonic solution increases it. Table 77-1 summarizes the composition of commonly used IV solutions and their expected distribution into the ECF and ICF compartments.
- Hypernatremia and hyponatremia can be associated with conditions of high, low, or normal ECF sodium and volume. Both conditions are most commonly the result of abnormalities of water metabolism. It's important to understand the difference between *dehydration* (loss of TBW producing hypertonicity) and *hypovolemia* (volume depletion due to a symptomatic deficit in ECF volume).

HYPONATREMIA (SERUM SODIUM <135 mEq/L [mmol/L])

Pathophysiology

- Results from an excess of extracellular water relative to sodium because of impaired water excretion.
- Causes of nonosmotic release of arginine vasopressin (AVP), commonly known as *antidiuretic hormone*, include hypovolemia and decreased effective circulating volume as seen in patients with chronic heart failure (HF), nephrotic syndrome, cirrhosis, and syndrome of inappropriate antidiuretic hormone (SIADH).
- Hyponatremia is classified as isotonic, hypertonic, or hypotonic depending on serum osmolity (Fig. 77-1).
- Hypotonic hyponatremia, the most common form of hyponatremia, can be further classified as hypovolemic, euvolemic, or hypervolemic.
- Hypovolemic hypotonic hyponatremia is associated with a loss of ECF volume and sodium, with the loss of more sodium than water. It is seen with fluid losses caused by diarrhea, excessive sweating, and diuretics.
- Euvolemic hyponatremia is associated with a normal or slightly decreased ECF sodium content and increased TBW and ECF volume. It is most commonly caused by SIADH which is seen with certain cancers, CNS disorders, and lung disease in addition to medications.
- Hypervolemic hyponatremia is associated with an increase in ECF volume in conditions with impaired renal sodium and water excretion, such as cirrhosis, HF, and kidney failure.

Clinical Presentation

- Most patients with hyponatremia are asymptomatic.
- Presence and severity of symptoms are related to the magnitude and rapidity of onset of hyponatremia. Hyponatremia that is severe or develops rapidly is associated with symptoms that progress from nausea and malaise to headache and lethargy and, eventually, to seizures, coma, and death.

TABLE 77-1 Composition of Common IV Solutions

Solution	Dextrose g/dL (kcal/L)	Na+ (mEq/L or mmol/L)	K+ (mEq/L or mmol/L)	Cl- (mEq/L or mmol/L)	Other (mEq/L)	Osmolality (mOsm/kg or mmol/kg)	Tonicity	Distribution		
								% ECF	% ICF	Free water (mL/L)
Dextrose 5% in water	5 (170)	0	0	0	---	253	Hypotonic	33	67	1000 mL
0.2% NaCl[a]	0	34	0	34	---	68	Hypotonic	50	50	750 mL
0.45% NaCl[b]	0	77	0	77	---	154	Hypotonic	67	33	500 mL
0.9% NaCl[c]	0	154	0	154	---	308	Isotonic	100	0	0 mL
Lactated Ringer's[d]	0	130	4	105	Lactate 28 Ca 4.8	273	Isotonic	97	3	0 mL
Plasma-Lyte A[e] Plasma-Lyte 148[e]	0.44 (21)	140	5	98	Acetate 27 Mg 3 Gluc 23	294	Isotonic	100	0	0 mL
Normosol-R[f] Normosol-R pH 7.4	0	140	5	98	Acetate 27 Mg 3 Gluc 23	294	Isotonic	100	0	0 mL
3% NaCl[g]	0	513	0	513	---	1026	Hypertonic	100	0	−2331 mL

Ca, calcium; Cl−, chloride; ECF, extracellular fluid; ICF, intracellular fluid; IV, intravenous; K+, potassium; Mg, magnesium; NA, not applicable; Na+, sodium; NaCl, sodium chloride; For conversion of kcal/L to kJ/L multiply by 4.184).

[a]Also referred to as quarter normal saline.
[b]Also referred to as half normal saline.
[c]Also referred to as normal saline.
[d]Also referred to as LR; also available commercially as Dextrose 5% LR.
[e]Plasma-Lyte A pH 7.4; Plasma-Lyte 148 pH 5.5.
[f]Normosol-R available with pH 6.6 and Normosol-R pH 7.4.
[g]Hypertonic solution; results in osmotic removal of water from the ICF.

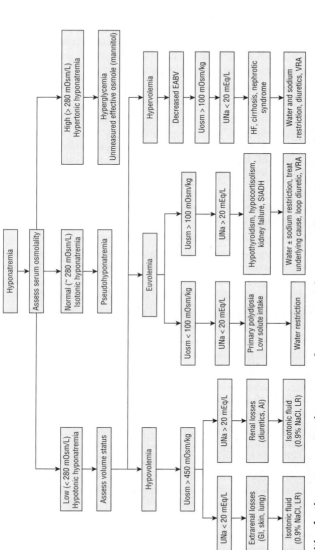

FIGURE 77-1. **Algorithm for the assessment and treatment of nonemergent hyponatremia.** AI, adrenal insufficiency; EABV, effective arterial blood volume; GI, gastrointestinal; HF, heart failure; LR, lactated Ringers; NaCl, sodium chloride; SIADH, syndrome of inappropriate antidiuretic hormone; UNa, urine sodium concentration [values in mEq/L are numerically equivalent to mmol/L]; Uosm, urine osmolality [values in mOsm/kg are numerically equivalent to mmol/kg]; VRA, vasopressin receptor antagonist.

- Patients with hypovolemic hyponatremia present with neurologic symptoms and also symptoms of hypovolemia, including decreased skin turgor, orthostatic hypotension, tachycardia, and dry mucous membranes.

Treatment

- <u>Goals of Treatment</u>: Resolve underlying cause of the sodium and ECF volume imbalance and safely correct the sodium and water derangements. Too rapid correction of serum sodium concentration can lead to an acute decrease in brain cell volume, contributing to the development of osmotic demyelination syndrome (ODS).

Acute or Severely Symptomatic Hypotonic Hyponatremia

- Symptomatic patients, regardless of fluid status, should initially be treated with 3% NaCl (513 mEq/L [mmol/L]) until symptoms resolve. Resolution of severe symptoms may require only a 5% increase in serum sodium; some clinicians suggest an initial target serum sodium of ~120 mEq/L (mmol/L).
- Treat SIADH with 3% saline plus, if the urine osmolality exceeds 300 mOsm/kg (mmol/kg), a loop diuretic (**furosemide**, 20–40 mg IV every 6 hours or **bumetanide**, 0.5–1 mg IV every 2–3 hours for several doses). Consider a continuous infusion if intermittent doses are not sufficient to manage edema.
- Treat hypovolemic hypotonic hyponatremia with 0.9% NaCl.
- Treat hypervolemic hypotonic hyponatremia with 3% NaCl and prompt initiation of fluid restriction. Loop diuretic therapy or **arginine vasopressin receptor antagonist (VRA)** is often required to facilitate urinary excretion of free water.

Nonemergent Hypotonic Hyponatremia

- Treatment of SIADH involves water restriction and correction of the underlying cause; discontinue medications that could be a contributing factor. Restrict water intake to approximately 1000–1200 mL/day. Treat patients unable to restrict water sufficiently with NaCl tablets and a loop diuretic or **demeclocycline** (300 mg orally two to four times daily; onset of action in 3–6 days).
- VRAs or "vaptans" (eg, **conivaptan** [available IV only] and **tolvaptan** [15 mg orally daily]) are therapeutic options for both euvolemic and hypervolemic hypotonic hyponatremia but are contraindicated in hypovolemic hyponatremia, in patients with HF, cirrhosis, and SIADH. The vaptans have dramatic effects on water excretion; fluid restriction should be avoided for the first 24–48 hours of starting VRA therapy when active sodium correction is occurring. Tolvaptan labeling currently includes a warning to avoid use for more than 30 days in patients with chronic liver disease. Consult product labeling for drug interactions, adverse drug reactions, and contraindications.
- Treatment of asymptomatic hypervolemic hypotonic hyponatremia involves correction of the underlying cause and restriction of water intake to less than 1000–1500 mL/day. Dietary intake of sodium chloride should be restricted to 1000–2000 mg/day.

HYPERNATREMIA (SERUM SODIUM >145 mEq/L [mmol/L])

Pathophysiology and Clinical Presentation

- Hypernatremia results from insensible water loss (evaporative water loss through skin and lungs), from hypotonic GI losses, or when patients are exposed to high temperatures. Diabetes insipidus (DI) causes a water diuresis. Hypernatremia may also result from hypertonic NaCl administration or from excess sodium intake from IV and enteral fluids and medications.
- Increase in serum sodium concentration and osmolality causes acute water movement from the ICF to the ECF. Symptoms are primarily caused by decreased brain cell volume and can include weakness, lethargy, restlessness, irritability, twitching, and confusion. Symptoms of a more rapidly developing hypernatremia include seizures, coma, and death.

Treatment

- <u>Goals of Treatment</u>: Correct serum sodium concentration at a rate that restores and maintains brain cell volume.

- Begin treatment of hypovolemic hypernatremia with 0.9% NaCl. After hemodynamic stability is restored and intravascular volume is replaced, replace free-water deficit with 5% dextrose or 0.45% NaCl or another hypotonic fluid.
- The correction rate should be approximately 1 mEq/L (1 mmol/L) per hour for hypernatremia that developed in less than 48 hours and 0.5 mEq/L (0.5 mmol/L) per hour for hypernatremia that developed more slowly.
- Treat central DI with intranasal **desmopressin**, beginning with 5–10 mcg once or twice daily, titrated to a maximum dose of 40 mcg given every 8 hours. Oral tablets are available; poor bioavailability contributes to unpredictable response when transitioning between dosage forms.
- Treat nephrogenic DI by decreasing ECF volume with a thiazide diuretic and dietary sodium restriction (2000 mg/day), which can decrease urine volume by as much as 50%. Other treatment options include drugs with antidiuretic properties (Table 77-2).
- Treat sodium overload with loop diuretics (furosemide, 20–40 mg IV every 6 hours) and 5% dextrose at an appropriate rate.

EDEMA

Pathophysiology and Clinical Presentation

- Edema, defined as a clinically detectable increase in interstitial fluid volume, develops when excess sodium is retained either as a primary defect in renal sodium excretion or as a response to a decrease in the effective circulating volume despite an already expanded or normal ECF volume.
- Edema is usually due to heart, kidney, or liver failure, or a combination of these conditions.
- Edema is initially detected in the feet or pretibial area in ambulatory patients and in the presacral area in bed-bound individuals, and is described as "pitting" when a depression caused by briefly exerting pressure over a bony prominence does not rapidly refill.

Treatment

- Diuretics are the primary pharmacologic therapy for edema when severe or when treatment of the underlying disease and sodium and water restriction are insufficient. Loop diuretics are the most potent, followed by thiazide diuretics and then potassium-sparing diuretics.

TABLE 77-2 Medications Used in Central and Nephrogenic DI

Drug	Indication	Dose
Desmopressin acetate	Central and nephrogenic	IN: 5–20 mcg q12–24h
		IV/SQ: Initial, 0.25–1 mcg q12–24h
		PO: Initial: 0.05–0.2 **mg** qhs; Usual: 0.1–0.8 **mg** in 2–3 doses, max 1.2 mg daily
		SL: 60 mcg TID; usual, 120–720 mcg daily in 2–3 doses
Chlorpropamide	Central	125–250 mg orally daily
Carbamazepine	Central	100–300 mg orally twice daily
Hydrochlorothiazide	Central and nephrogenic	25 mg orally q12–24 h
Amiloride	Nephrogenic	5–10 mg orally daily
		Pediatrics: 0.2 mg/kg/day in 3 doses or 20 mg/1.73 m^2/day
Indomethacin	Central and nephrogenic	50 mg orally q8–12 h

DI, diabetes insipidus; IN, intranasal; IV, intravenous; PO, oral; SL, sublingual; SQ, subcutaneous.

DISORDERS OF CALCIUM HOMEOSTASIS

- ECF calcium is moderately bound to plasma proteins (40% to 50%), primarily albumin. Ionized or free calcium is the physiologically active form that is homeostatically regulated.
- Each 1 g/dL (10 g/L) drop in serum albumin concentration less than 4 g/dL (40 g/L) decreases total serum calcium concentration by 0.8 mg/dL (0.20 mmol/L).

HYPERCALCEMIA (TOTAL SERUM CALCIUM >10.2 mg/dL [>2.55 mmol/L])

Pathophysiology and Clinical Presentation

- Cancer and hyperparathyroidism are the most common causes of hypercalcemia. Primary mechanisms include increased bone resorption, increased GI absorption, and increased tubular reabsorption by the kidneys.
- Clinical presentation depends on the degree of hypercalcemia and rate of onset. Mild-to-moderate hypercalcemia (serum calcium concentration <13 mg/dL [<3.25 mmol/L] or ionized calcium concentration <6 mg/dL [<1.50 mmol/L]) can be asymptomatic.
- Hypercalcemia of malignancy develops quickly and is associated with anorexia, nausea and vomiting, constipation, polyuria, polydipsia, and nocturia. Hypercalcemic crisis is characterized by acute elevation of serum calcium to greater than 15 mg/dL (>3.75 mmol/L), acute kidney injury, and obtundation. Untreated hypercalcemic crisis can progress to oliguric acute kidney injury, coma, and life-threatening ventricular arrhythmias.
- Complications of chronic hypercalcemia (ie, hyperparathyroidism) include metastatic calcification, hypercalciuria, and chronic kidney disease secondary to interstitial nephrocalcinosis.
- Electrocardiographic (ECG) changes include shortening of the QT interval and coving of the ST-T wave.

Treatment

- Treatment approach depends on the degree of hypercalcemia, acuity of onset, and presence of symptoms requiring emergent treatment (Fig. 77-2).
- Management of asymptomatic, mild-to-moderate hypercalcemia begins with attention to the underlying condition and correction of fluid and electrolyte abnormalities.
- Hypercalcemic crisis and acute symptomatic hypercalcemia are medical emergencies requiring immediate treatment. Rehydration with normal saline followed by loop diuretics (eg, furosemide, bumetanide) can be used in patients with normal to moderately impaired renal function. Normalization of total calcium may be seen within 24–48 hours.
- Initiate treatment with **calcitonin** in patients in whom saline hydration is contraindicated (Table 77-3). Onset of action is seen within 1–2 hours; however, the degree and extent of calcium reduction is often unpredictable.
- **Bisphosphonates** (eg, **pamidronate** and **zoledronic acid**) are indicated for hypercalcemia of malignancy. Total serum calcium decline begins within 2 days and nadirs in 7 days. Duration of normocalcemia varies but usually does not exceed 2–3 weeks, depending on treatment response of underlying malignancy.
- **Denosumab** is a monoclonal antibody approved for treatment of hypercalcemia of malignancy in patient's refractory to bisphosphonate therapy; corrected serum calcium remains above 12.5 mg/dL (3.13 mmol/L) more than 7 days of therapy.
- **Prednisone** or an equivalent agent is usually effective by reducing GI calcium absorption when hypercalcemia results from multiple myeloma, leukemia, lymphoma, sarcoidosis, and hypervitaminoses A and D. Onset of action is relatively slow.
- **Cinacalcet** administered at a starting dose of 30 mg orally twice daily is used for treatment of hypercalcemia secondary to parathyroid carcinoma.

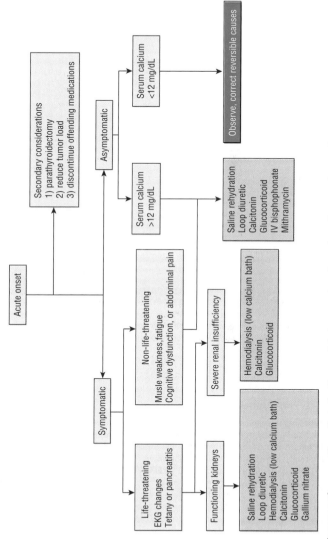

FIGURE 77-2. Pharmacotherapeutic options for the acutely hypercalcemic patient. Serum calcium of 12 mg/dL is equivalent to 3 mmol/L.

TABLE 77-3 Medication Dosing Table for Hypercalcemia

Drug/Brand Name	Starting Dosage	Time Frame to Initial Response	Monitoring and Special Population Considerations
0.9% saline ± electrolytes	200–300 mL/h	24–48 hours	Electrolyte abnormalities, fluid overload, CI in advanced kidney disease, congestive heart failure
Loop diuretics Furosemide/Lasix® Bumetandide/Bumex® Torsemide/Demadex®	40–80 mg IV q1–4h of furosemide or equivalent	N/A	Electrolyte abnormalities (potassium and magnesium), CI in patients with allergy to sulfas (use ethacrynic acid)
Calcitonin/Miacalcin®	4 units/kg q12h SC/IM	1–2 hours	Facial flushing, nausea/vomiting, allergic reaction, CI in patients with allergy to calcitonin
Pamidronate/Aredia®	30–90 mg IV over 2–24 hours	2 days	Fever, fatigue, skeletal pain, CI in kidney disease
Zoledronate/Reclast®	4 mg IV over 15 minutes	1–2 days	Fever, fatigue, skeletal pain, CI in kidney disease
Corticosteroids	40–60 mg oral prednisone equivalents daily	3–5 days	Diabetes mellitus, osteoporosis, infection, CI in patients with serious infections, hypersensitivity

CI, contraindicated; SC, subcutaneous.

HYPOCALCEMIA (TOTAL SERUM CALCIUM <8.6 mg/dL [<2.15 mmol/L])

Pathophysiology

- Hypocalcemia results from altered effects of parathyroid hormone and vitamin D on the bone, gut, and kidney. Primary causes are postoperative hypoparathyroidism and vitamin D deficiency.
- Hypomagnesemia can be associated with severe symptomatic hypocalcemia that is unresponsive to calcium replacement therapy. Calcium normalization is dependent on magnesium replacement.

Clinical Presentation

- Clinical manifestations are variable and depend on the onset of hypocalcemia. Tetany is the hallmark sign of acute hypocalcemia, which manifests as paresthesias around the mouth and in the extremities; muscle spasms and cramps; carpopedal spasms; and, rarely, laryngospasm and bronchospasm.
- Cardiovascular manifestations result in ECG changes characterized by a prolonged QT interval and symptoms of decreased myocardial contractility often associated with HF. Acute and chronic hypocalcemia can result in a reversible syndrome characterized by acute myocardial failure or refractory HF. Other cardiovascular manifestations include arrhythmias, bradycardia, and hypotension that are unresponsive to fluid and vasopressor administration.

Treatment

- Acute, symptomatic hypocalcemia requires IV administration of soluble calcium salts (Fig. 77-3). Initially, 100–300 mg of elemental calcium (eg, 1 g **calcium chloride**, 2–3 g **calcium gluconate**) should be given IV over 10–30 minutes (≤60 mg of elemental calcium per minute).

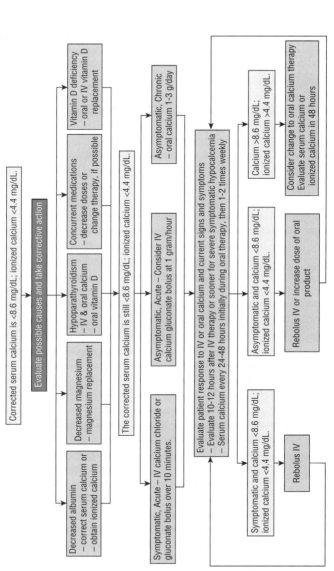

FIGURE 77-3. Hypocalcemia diagnostic and treatment algorithm. Serum calcium of 8.6 mg/dL is equivalent to 2.15 mmol/L. Ionized calcium of 4.4 mg/dL is equivalent to 1.1 mmol/L.

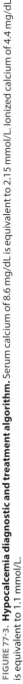

- The initial bolus dose is effective for only 1–2 hours; therefore, repeat doses should be given hourly as needed until severe, symptomatic patients are stabilized.
- Calcium gluconate is preferred over calcium chloride for peripheral administration because the latter is more irritating to veins.
- After acute hypocalcemia is corrected, the underlying cause and other electrolyte problems should be corrected. Magnesium supplementation is indicated for hypomagnesemia.
- Oral calcium supplementation (eg, 1–3 g/day of elemental calcium initially, then 2–8 g/day in divided doses) is indicated for chronic hypocalcemia due to hypoparathyroidism and vitamin D deficiency. If serum calcium does not normalize, add a vitamin D preparation.

DISORDERS OF PHOSPHORUS HOMEOSTASIS

HYPERPHOSPHATEMIA (SERUM PHOSPHORUS >4.5 mg/dL [>1.45 mmol/L])

Pathophysiology

- Most commonly caused by decreased phosphorus excretion, secondary to decreased glomerular filtration rate (GFR) seen in chronic kidney disease or acute kidney injury.
- Intracellular phosphate release can occur with rhabdomyolysis, hemolysis, and tumor lysis syndrome, a complication of chemotherapy associated with massive cell lysis with highest incidence in patients with acute leukemias and Burkitt's lymphoma.

Clinical Presentation

- Acute symptoms include nausea, vomiting, diarrhea, lethargy, obstruction of the urinary tract, and, rarely, seizures. Calcium phosphate crystals are likely to form when the product of the serum calcium and phosphate concentrations exceeds 50–60 mg^2/dL^2 (4–4.8 mmol^2/L^2) which precipitate into soft tissues, and cause nephrolithiasis or obstructive uropathy in the kidneys.
- The major effects of long-term hypophosphatemia are related to the development of hypocalcemia.
- For more information on hyperphosphatemia and renal failure, see Chapter 76.

Treatment

- The most effective way to treat nonemergent hyperphosphatemia is to decrease phosphate absorption from the GI tract with phosphate binders (see Chapter 76, **Table 76-5**) and decreasing the dietary content of phosphate.
- Severe symptomatic hyperphosphatemia manifesting as hypocalcemia and tetany is treated by the IV administration of calcium salts.

HYPOPHOSPHATEMIA (SERUM PHOSPHORUS <2.7 mg/dL [<0.87 mmol/L])

Pathophysiology

- Hypophosphatemia results from decreased GI absorption, reduced tubular reabsorption, or extracellular to intracellular redistribution.
- Hypophosphatemia is associated with alcohol use disorder, parenteral nutrition with inadequate phosphate supplementation, chronic ingestion of antacids, diabetic ketoacidosis, and prolonged hyperventilation.

Clinical Presentation

- Severe hypophosphatemia (serum phosphorus <1.5 mg/dL [<0.5 mmol/L]) has diverse clinical manifestations that affect many organ systems, including the following:
  - ✓ Neurologic manifestations: Progressive syndrome of irritability, apprehension, weakness, numbness, paresthesias, dysarthria, confusion, obtundation, seizures, and coma.
  - ✓ Skeletal muscle dysfunction: Myalgia, bone pain, weakness, and potentially fatal rhabdomyolysis.

✓ Respiratory muscle weakness and diaphragmatic contractile dysfunction resulting in acute respiratory failure.

✓ Congestive cardiomyopathy, arrhythmias, hemolysis, and increased risk of infection can also occur.

• Chronic hypophosphatemia can cause osteopenia and osteomalacia because of enhanced osteoclastic resorption of bone and limited crystallization constituents (phosphate), respectively.

Treatment

• Treat severe (<1.5 mg/dL; <0.5 mmol/L) or symptomatic hypophosphatemia with IV phosphorus replacement at a dose of 0.32–0.64 mmol/kg with normal kidney function. In critically ill trauma patients, doses up to 1 mmol/kg have been used.

• Asymptomatic patients or those who exhibit mild-to-moderate hypophosphatemia (1.5–2.7 mg/dL [0.5–0.9 mmol/L]) can be treated with oral phosphorus supplementation in doses of 1–2 g (32–64 mmol) daily in divided doses, with the goal of correcting serum phosphorus concentration in 7–10 days (Table 77-4).

• Monitor patients with frequent serum phosphorus and calcium determinations, especially if phosphorus is given IV or if renal dysfunction is present.

DISORDERS OF POTASSIUM HOMEOSTASIS

HYPOKALEMIA (SERUM POTASSIUM <3.5 mEq/L [mmol/L])

Pathophysiology

• Results from a total-body potassium deficit or shifting of serum potassium into the intracellular compartment.

• Many medications can cause hypokalemia (Table 77-5), and it is most commonly seen with use of loop and thiazide diuretics. Other causes of hypokalemia include diarrhea, vomiting, and hypomagnesemia.

Clinical Presentation

• Signs and symptoms are nonspecific and variable and depend on the degree of hypokalemia and rapidity of onset. Mild hypokalemia is often asymptomatic.

• Moderate hypokalemia is associated with muscle weakness, cramping, malaise, and myalgias.

• Cardiovascular manifestations include cardiac arrhythmias (eg, heart block, atrial flutter, paroxysmal atrial tachycardia, ventricular fibrillation, and digitalis-induced

TABLE 77-4	Oral Phosphorus Replacement Therapy with Phosphate, Potassium, and Sodium Content per Packet or Tablet		
Product	**Phosphate Content**	**Potassium Content**	**Sodium Content**
Packet			
Phos-NaK	250 mg (8 mmol)	280 mg (7.1 mEq)	160 mg (6.9 mEq)
Tablet			
Av-Phos 250 Neutral	250 mg (8 mmol)	45 mg (1.1 mEq)	298 mg (13 mEq)
K-Phos Neutral	250 mg (8 mmol)	45 mg (1.1 mEq)	298 mg (13 mEq)
K-Phos No. 2	250 mg (8 mmol)	88 mg (2.3 mEq)	134 mg (5.8 mEq)
Phospha 250 Neutral	250 mg (8 mmol)	45 mg (1.1 mEq)	298 mg (13 mEq)
Phospho-Trin 250 Neutral	250 mg (8 mmol)	45 mg (1.1 mEq)	298 mg (13 mEq)
Virt-Phos 250 Neutral	250 mg (8 mmol)	45 mg (1.1 mEq)	298 mg (13 mEq)

Phosphorus 31 mg = 1 mmol; potassium 39 mg = 1 mEq = 1 mmol; sodium 23 mg = 1 mEq = 1 mmol.

TABLE 77-5	Mechanism of Medication-Induced Hypokalemia	
Transcellular Shift	**Enhanced Renal Excretion**	**Enhanced Fecal Elimination**
β₂-Receptor agonists	Diuretics	Laxatives
Epinephrine	Acetazolamide	Sodium polystyrene sulfonate
Albuterol	Thiazides	Sorbitol
Terbutaline	Indapamide	Patiromer
Fomoterol	Metolazone	Sodium zirconium cyclosilicate
Salmeterol	Furosemide	
Isoproterenol	Torsemide	
Ephedrine	Bumetanide	
Pseudoephedrine	Ethacrynic acid	
Theophylline	High-dose penicillins	
Levothyroxine	Nafcillin	
Decongestants	Ampicillin	
Caffeine	Penicillin	
Insulin overdose	Mineralocorticoids	
Verapamil overdose	Miscellaneous	
Barium overdose	Aminoglycosides	
	Amphotericin B	
	Cisplatin	

arrhythmias). In severe hypokalemia (serum concentration <2.5 mEq/L; mmol/L), ECG changes include ST-segment depression or flattening, T-wave inversion, and U-wave elevation.

Treatment

- In general, every 1 mEq/L (mmol/L) decrease in potassium below 3.5 mEq/L (mmol/L) corresponds with a total body deficit of 100–400 mEq (mmol). To correct mild deficits, patients receiving chronic loop or thiazide diuretics generally need 40–100 mEq (mmol) of potassium.
- Whenever possible, potassium supplementation should be administered by mouth. Of the available salts, potassium chloride is most commonly used because it is the most effective for common causes of potassium depletion, use of diuretics, and with diarrhea.
- Limit IV administration to severe hypokalemia, patients exhibiting signs and symptoms such as ECG changes or muscle spasms, or inability to tolerate oral therapy. IV supplementation is more dangerous than oral therapy due to the potential for hyperkalemia, phlebitis, and pain at the infusion site. Potassium should be administered in saline because dextrose can stimulate insulin secretion and worsen intracellular shifting of potassium. Generally, 10–20 mEq (mmol) of potassium is diluted in 100 mL of 0.9% NaCl and administered through a peripheral vein over 1 hour. ECG monitoring should be performed to detect cardiac changes.

HYPERKALEMIA (SERUM POTASSIUM >5 MEQ/L [MMOL/L])

Pathophysiology

- Hyperkalemia develops when potassium intake exceeds excretion or when the transcellular distribution of potassium is disturbed.
- Primary causes of true hyperkalemia include increased potassium intake, decreased potassium excretion, tubular unresponsiveness to aldosterone, and redistribution of potassium to the extracellular space.

Clinical Presentation

- Hyperkalemia is frequently asymptomatic; patients might complain of heart palpitations or skipped heartbeats.
- The earliest ECG change (serum potassium 5.5–6 mEq/L; mmol/L) is peaked T waves. The sequence of changes with further increases in serum potassium concentration is widening of the PR interval, loss of the P wave, widening of the QRS complex, and merging of the QRS complex with the T wave resulting in a sine-wave pattern.

Treatment

- Treatment depends on the desired rapidity and degree of lowering and the patient's clinical condition (Fig. 77-4, Table 77-6).
- Calcium administration rapidly reverses ECG manifestations and arrhythmias, but it does not lower serum potassium concentrations. Calcium is short acting and therefore must be repeated if signs or symptoms recur.
- Rapid correction of hyperkalemia requires administration of drugs that shift potassium intracellularly (eg, insulin and dextrose, sodium bicarbonate, or albuterol).

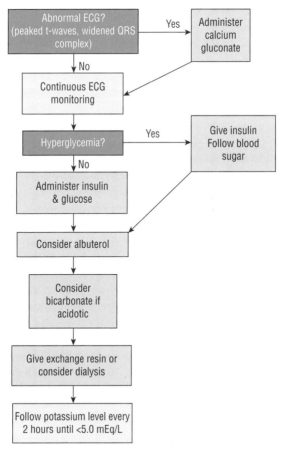

FIGURE 77-4. **Treatment approach for hyperkalemia.** Serum potassium of 5.0 mEq/L is equivalent to 5.0 mmol/L.

TABLE 77-6 Therapeutic Alternatives for the Management of Hyperkalemia

Medication	Dose	Route of Administration	Onset/Duration of Action	Acuity	Mechanism of Action	Expected Result
Calcium gluconate or chloride	1 g	IV over 5–10 minutes	1–2 minutes/ 10–30 minutes	Acute	Raises cardiac threshold potential	Reverses electrocardiographic effects
Furosemide	20–40 mg	IV	5–15 minutes/ 4–6 hours	Acute	Inhibits renal Na⁺ reabsorption	Increased urinary K⁺ loss
Regular insulin	5–10 units	IV or SC	30 minutes/2–6 hours	Acute	Stimulates intracellular K⁺ uptake	Intracellular K⁺ redistribution
Dextrose 10%	1000 mL (100 g)	IV over 1–2 hours	30 minutes/2–6 hours	Acute	Stimulates insulin release	Intracellular K⁺ redistribution
Dextrose 50%	50 mL (25 g)	IV over 5 minutes	30 minutes/2–6 hours	Acute	Stimulates insulin release	Intracellular K⁺ redistribution
Sodium bicarbonate	50–100 mEq (50–100 mmol)	IV over 2–5 minutes	30 minutes/2–6 hours	Acute	Raises serum pH	Intracellular K⁺ redistribution
Albuterol	10–20 mg	Nebulized over 10 minutes	30 minutes/1–2 hours	Acute	Stimulates intracellular K⁺ uptake	Intracellular K⁺ redistribution
Hemodialysis	4 hours	N/A	Immediate/variable	Acute	Removal from serum	Increased K⁺ elimination
Sodium polystyrene sulfonate	15–60 g	Oral or rectal	1 hour/variable	Nonacute	Resin exchanges Na⁺ for K⁺	Increased K⁺ elimination
Patiromer	8.4–25.2 g	Oral	Hours/variable	Nonacute	Resin exchanges Ca⁺⁺ for K⁺	Increased K⁺ elimination
Sodium zirconium cyclosilicate	5–15 g	Oral	1 hour/variable	Nonacute	Resin exchanges Na⁺ for K⁺	Increased K⁺ elimination

- **Sodium polystyrene sulfonate** is a cation-exchange resin suitable for asymptomatic patients with mild-to-moderate hyperkalemia. Each gram of resin exchanges 1 mEq (1 mmol) of sodium for 1 mEq (1 mmol) of potassium. The sorbitol component promotes excretion of exchanged potassium by inducing diarrhea. The oral route is better tolerated and more effective than the rectal route.

DISORDERS OF MAGNESIUM HOMEOSTASIS

HYPOMAGNESEMIA (SERUM MAGNESIUM
<1.4 mEq/L [<1.7 mg/dL; <0.70 mmol/L])

Pathophysiology

- Hypomagnesemia is usually associated with disorders of the intestinal tract or kidneys. Medications (eg, aminoglycosides, amphotericin B, cyclosporine, diuretics, digitalis, and cisplatin) or conditions that interfere with intestinal absorption or increase renal excretion of magnesium can cause hypomagnesemia.
- Commonly associated with alcoholism.

Clinical Presentation

- Although typically asymptomatic, the dominant organ systems involved are the neuromuscular and cardiovascular systems. Symptoms include heart palpitations, tetany, twitching, and generalized convulsions.
- Ventricular arrhythmias are the most important and potentially life-threatening cardiovascular effect.
- ECG changes include widened QRS complexes and peaked T waves in mild deficiency. Prolonged PR intervals, progressive widening of the QRS complexes, and flattening of T waves occur in moderate-to-severe deficiency.
- Many electrolyte disturbances occur with hypomagnesemia, including hypokalemia and hypocalcemia.

Treatment

- The severity of magnesium depletion and the presence of symptoms dictate the route of magnesium supplementation. Intramuscular magnesium is painful and is reserved for patients with severe hypomagnesemia and limited venous access. IV bolus injection is associated with flushing, sweating, and a sensation of warmth.
- The optimal oral magnesium regimen is unknown; 8–12 g of magnesium sulfate in divided doses over 24 hours followed by 4–6 g/day for 3–5 days is one widely accepted regimen when the serum magnesium concentration is greater than 1 mEq/L (1.2 mg/dL [0.5 mmol/L]). Sustained-release products are preferred due to improved patient compliance and less GI side effects (eg, diarrhea).
- Administer IV magnesium if serum concentrations are less than 1 mEq/L (<1.2 mg/dL [<0.5 mmol/L]) or if signs and symptoms are present regardless of serum concentration. Infuse 4–6 g of magnesium over 12–24 hours and repeat as needed to maintain serum concentrations above 1 mEq/L (1.2 mg/dL [0.5 mmol/L]). Continue until signs and symptoms resolve. Reduce magnesium dose by 25%–50% with renal insufficiency.

HYPERMAGNESEMIA (SERUM MAGNESIUM
>2 mEq/L [>2.4 mg/dL; >1 mmol/L])

Pathophysiology

- Magnesium concentrations steadily increase as the GFR decreases below 30 mL/min/1.73 m^2 and is generally associated with advanced CKD.
- Other causes include magnesium-containing antacids in patients with renal insufficiency, enteral or parenteral nutrition in patients with multiorgan system failure, magnesium for treatment of eclampsia, lithium therapy, hypothyroidism, and Addison disease.

Clinical Presentation

- Symptoms are rare when the serum magnesium concentration is less than 4 mEq/L (<4.9 mg/dL [<2 mmol/L]).
- The sequence of neuromuscular signs as serum magnesium increases from 5 to 12 mEq/L (6.1–14.7 mg/dL [2.5–6 mmol/L]) is sedation, hypotonia, hyporeflexia, somnolence, coma, muscular paralysis, and, ultimately, respiratory depression.
- The sequence of cardiovascular signs as serum magnesium increases from 3 to 15 mEq/L (3.7–18.4 mg/dL [1.5–7.5 mmol/L]) is hypotension, cutaneous vasodilation, QT-interval prolongation, bradycardia, primary heart block, nodal rhythms, bundle branch block, QRS- and then PR-interval prolongation, complete heart block, and asystole.

Treatment

- IV calcium (100–200 mg of elemental calcium; eg, calcium gluconate 2 g IV) is indicated to antagonize the neuromuscular and cardiovascular effects of magnesium. Doses should be repeated as often as hourly in life-threatening situations.
- Forced diuresis with 0.45% NaCl and loop diuretics (eg, furosemide, 40 mg IV) can promote magnesium elimination in patients with normal renal function or stage 1, 2, or 3 CKD. In dialysis patients, change to a magnesium-free dialysate.

EVALUATION OF THERAPEUTIC OUTCOMES

- The primary end point for monitoring treatment of fluid and electrolyte disorders is the correction of the abnormal serum electrolyte. In general, monitoring is initially performed at frequent intervals and, as homeostasis is restored, subsequently performed at less frequent intervals.
- Monitor all electrolytes as individual electrolyte abnormalities typically coexist with another abnormality (eg, hypomagnesemia with hypokalemia and hypocalcemia, or hyperphosphatemia with hypocalcemia).
- Monitor patients for resolution of clinical manifestations of electrolyte disturbances and for treatment-related complications.

See Chapter 68, Disorders of Sodium and Water Homeostasis, authored by Katherine H. Chessman and Jason S. Haney; Chapter 69, Disorders of Calcium and Phosphorus Homeostasis, authored by Angela L. Bingham; and Chapter 70, Disorders of Potassium and Magnesium Homeostasis, authored by Rachel W. Flurie, for a more detailed discussion of this topic.

CHAPTER

78 | Allergic Rhinitis

- *Allergic rhinitis* involves inflammation of nasal mucous membranes in sensitized individuals when inhaled allergenic particles contact mucous membranes and elicit a response mediated by immunoglobulin E (IgE). There are two types: seasonal and persistent (formerly called "perennial") allergic rhinitis.

PATHOPHYSIOLOGY

- Airborne allergens enter the nose during inhalation and are processed by lymphocytes, which produce antigen-specific IgE, sensitizing genetically predisposed hosts to those agents. On nasal reexposure, IgE bound to mast cells interacts with airborne allergens, triggering release of inflammatory mediators.
- An immediate reaction occurs within seconds to minutes, resulting in rapid release of preformed and newly generated mediators from the arachidonic acid cascade. Mediators of immediate hypersensitivity include histamine, leukotrienes, prostaglandin, tryptase, and kinins. These mediators cause vasodilation, increased vascular permeability, and production of nasal secretions. Histamine produces rhinorrhea, itching, sneezing, and nasal obstruction.
- A late-phase reaction may occur 4–8 hours after initial allergen exposure due to cytokine release from mast cells and thymus-derived helper lymphocytes. This inflammatory response causes persistent chronic symptoms, including nasal congestion.

CLINICAL PRESENTATION

- Seasonal (hay fever) allergic rhinitis occurs in response to specific allergens (eg, pollen from trees, grasses, and weeds) present at predictable times of the year (spring and/or fall) and typically causes more acute symptoms.
- Persistent allergic rhinitis occurs year-round in response to nonseasonal allergens (eg, dust mites, animal dander, molds) and typically results in less variable, chronic symptoms.
- Many patients have a combination of both types, with symptoms year-round and seasonal exacerbations.
- Symptoms include clear rhinorrhea, sneezing, nasal congestion, postnasal drip, allergic conjunctivitis, and pruritic eyes, ears, or nose.
- In children, physical examination may reveal dark circles under the eyes (allergic shiners), a transverse nasal crease caused by repeated rubbing of the nose, adenoidal breathing, edematous nasal turbinates coated with clear secretions, tearing, and periorbital swelling.
- Patients may complain of loss of smell or taste, with sinusitis or polyps the underlying cause in many cases. Postnasal drip with cough or hoarseness can be bothersome.
- Untreated rhinitis symptoms may lead to disturbed sleep, malaise, fatigue, and poor work or school performance.
- Allergic rhinitis is associated with other conditions, including asthma, chronic rhinosinusitis, otitis media, nasal polyposis, respiratory infections, and dental malocclusions.
- Complications include recurrent and chronic sinusitis and epistaxis.

DIAGNOSIS

- Medical history includes careful description of symptoms, environmental factors and exposures, results of previous therapy, use of medications, previous nasal injury or surgery, and family history.
- Allergy testing can help determine whether rhinitis is caused by immune response to allergens. Immediate-type hypersensitivity skin tests are commonly used. Percutaneous testing is safer and more generally accepted than intradermal testing, which is usually reserved for patients requiring confirmation. The radioallergosorbent test (RAST) can detect IgE antibodies in the blood that are highly specific for a given antigen, but it may be slightly less sensitive than percutaneous tests.

TREATMENT

- <u>Goals of Treatment</u>: Minimize or prevent symptoms, prevent long-term complications, avoid or minimize medication side effects, provide economical therapy, and maintain normal lifestyle.
- **Figure 78-1** depicts a treatment algorithm for allergic rhinitis.

NONPHARMACOLOGIC THERAPY

- Avoiding offending allergens is important but difficult to accomplish, especially for perennial allergens. Mold growth can be reduced by keeping household humidity below 50% and removing obvious growth with bleach or disinfectant.

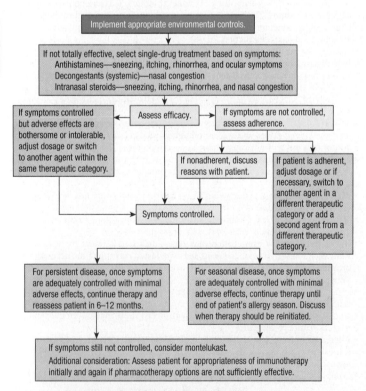

FIGURE 78-1. Treatment algorithm for allergic rhinitis.

- Patients sensitive to animals benefit most by removing pets from the home, if feasible. Reducing exposure to dust mites by washing bedding on a hot cycle, replacing carpets with hard flooring, and using vacuum cleaners with HEPA filters has not been shown to provide a clinical benefit. Only encasing bedding in impermeable covers has some clinical benefit in children but not adults.
- Steps to prevent poor air quality in homes include avoiding wall-to-wall carpeting, using moisture control to prevent mold accumulation, and controlling sources of pollution such as cigarette smoke.
- Patients with seasonal allergic rhinitis should keep windows closed and minimize time spent outdoors during pollen seasons. Filter masks can be worn while gardening or mowing the lawn.
- Nasal saline irrigations may improve nasal symptoms and reduce medicine consumption. Adhesive nasal strips can facilitate breathing and reduce nasal obstruction.

PHARMACOLOGIC THERAPY

Antihistamines

- Histamine H_1-receptor antagonists bind to H_1 receptors without activating them, preventing histamine binding and action. They are effective in preventing the histamine response but not in reversing its effects after they have occurred. Antihistamines antagonize increased capillary permeability, wheal-and-flare formation, and itching.
- *Oral antihistamines* are divided into two categories: (1) nonselective (first-generation or sedating antihistamines) and (2) peripherally selective (second-generation or nonsedating antihistamines). However, individual agents should be judged on their specific sedating effects because variation exists among agents within these categories (Table 78-1).
- Antihistamines help control symptoms of sneezing, rhinorrhea, itching, and conjunctivitis. Symptom relief is caused in part by an anticholinergic drying effect that reduces nasal, salivary, and lacrimal gland hypersecretion.
- Antihistamines are only fully effective when taken 1–2 hours before anticipated exposure to the offending allergen. For seasonal allergic rhinitis, start treatment before the expected allergy season begins. Guidelines recommend that nonsedating agents be tried first, but tolerance to sedation from first-generation agents can develop after 4 days of treatment. If nonsedating agents are ineffective or too expensive, first-generation agents may be used. For persistent allergic rhinitis, use an intranasal corticosteroid as an alternative to or in combination with systemic antihistamines.
- Drowsiness is the most frequent antihistamine side effect, and it can interfere with driving ability or adequate functioning. Sedative effects can be beneficial in patients who have difficulty sleeping because of rhinitis symptoms.
- Adverse anticholinergic such as dry mouth, difficulty in voiding urine, constipation, and cardiovascular effects may occur (Table 78-1). Antihistamines should be used with caution in patients predisposed to urinary retention and in those with increased intraocular pressure, hyperthyroidism, and cardiovascular disease.
- Other side effects include loss of appetite, nausea, vomiting, and epigastric distress. Taking medication with meals or a full glass of water may prevent gastrointestinal (GI) side effects.
- Table 78-2 lists recommended doses of oral agents.
- *Intranasal antihistamines*: **Azelastine** is a prescription-only intranasal antihistamine that relieves sneezing, rhinorrhea, and nasal pruritus of seasonal allergic rhinitis. The 0.1% product can be used in children for seasonal allergies, whereas the 0.15% product is labeled only for adults with either type of allergic rhinitis. However, guidelines favor use of intranasal antihistamines for seasonal but not persistent allergic rhinitis. Caution patients about the potential for drowsiness because systemic availability is ~40%. Patients may also experience drying effects, headache, and diminished effectiveness over time. **Olopatadine** is another intranasal antihistamine; it may cause less drowsiness because it is a selective H_1-receptor antagonist.

897

	Relative Sedative Effects	Relative Anticholinergic Effects
TABLE 78-1 Relative Adverse-Effect Profiles of Antihistamines		
Medications		
Alkylamine class, nonselective		
Brompheniramine maleate	Low	Moderate
Chlorpheniramine maleate	Low	Moderate
Dexchlorpheniramine maleate	Low	Moderate
Ethanolamine class, nonselective		
Carbinoxamine maleate	High	High
Clemastine fumarate	Moderate	High
Diphenhydramine hydrochloride	High	High
Phenothiazine class, nonselective		
Promethazine hydrochloride	High	High
Piperidine class, nonselective		
Cyproheptadine hydrochloride	Low	Moderate
Phthalazinone class, peripherally selective		
Azelastine (nasal only)	Low to none	Low to none
Bepotastine (ophthalmic only)	Low to none	Low to none
Piperazine class, peripherally selective		
Cetirizine	Low to moderate	Low to none
Levocetirizine	Low to moderate	Low to none
Piperidine class, peripherally selective		
Desloratadine	Low to none	Low to none
Fexofenadine	Low to none	Low to none
Loratadine	Low to none	Low to none
Olopatadine (nasal only)	Low to none	Low to none

- *Ophthalmic antihistamines*: **Levocabastine**, **olopatadine**, and **bepotastine** are ophthalmic antihistamines that can be used for conjunctivitis associated with allergic rhinitis. Systemic antihistamines are also usually effective for allergic conjunctivitis. Ophthalmic agents are a useful addition to nasal corticosteroids for ocular symptoms.

Decongestants

- Topical and systemic decongestants are sympathomimetic agents that act on adrenergic receptors in nasal mucosa to produce vasoconstriction, shrink swollen mucosa, and improve ventilation. They should only be used when nasal congestion is present. Decongestants work well in combination with antihistamines when nasal congestion is present.
- Topical decongestants are applied directly to swollen nasal mucosa via drops or sprays (Table 78-3). They result in little or no systemic absorption.
- Treatment should not exceed 3–5 days to avoid rhinitis medicamentosa (rebound vasodilation with congestion). Patients with this condition use more spray more often with less response. Abrupt cessation is an effective treatment, but rebound congestion may last for several days or weeks. Nasal corticosteroids have been used successfully but take several days to work. Weaning off the topical decongestant can be accomplished by decreasing dosing frequency or concentration over several weeks. Combining the weaning process with nasal corticosteroids may be helpful.

TABLE 78-2	Medication Dosing for Allergic Rhinitis		
Drugs	**Brand Names**	**Dosage for Adolescents[a] and Adults**	**Recommended Pediatric Doses**
Antihistamines			
Oral			
<u>Nonselective</u>			
Chlorpheniramine maleate	Various	Plain: 4 mg every 6 hours Extended release: 12 mg every 12 hours	6–11 years: 2 mg every 4–6 hours 2–5 years: 1 mg every 4–6 hours
Clemastine fumarate	Tavist	1.34 mg (1 mg base) twice daily, up to 2.68 mg 3 times daily; max. 8.04 mg/day (6 mg base/day)	6–11 years: syrup 0.67 mg (0.5 mg base) twice daily; max. 4.02 mg/day (3 mg base/day)
Diphenhydramine HCl	Benadryl, others	25–50 mg every 4–6 hours (max. 300 mg/day)	6–11 years: 12.5–25 mg every 4–6 hours; max. 150 mg/day
<u>**Peripherally selective**</u>			
Cetirizine	Zyrtec	5–10 mg once daily	6–11 years: 5–10 mg once daily6 mo. to 5 years: 2.5 mg once daily
Fexofenadine	Allegra	60 mg every 12 hours or 180 mg once daily	2–11 years: 30 mg once daily
Levocetirizine	Xyzal	5 mg once daily (in the evening)	6–11 years: 2.5 mg once daily (in the evening) 6 months–5 years: 1.25 mg once daily (in the evening)
Loratadine	Alavert, Claritin	10 mg once daily	6–12 years: 10 mg once daily or 5 mg twice daily 2–5 years: 5 mg once daily
Nasal			
Azelastine	Astelin, Astepro	1–2 sprays per nostril once or twice daily	2–11 years: 1 spray per nostril twice daily
Olopatadine	Patanase	Two sprays per nostril twice daily	6–11: 1 spray per nostril twice daily
Ophthalmic			
Bepotastine	Bepreve	1 drop into the affected eye(s) twice daily	2–11 years: 1 drop into the affected eye(s) twice daily
Levocabastine	Livostin	1 drop into the affected eye(s) 4 times daily	(Safety and efficacy not established)
Olopatadine	Patanol	1 drop into the affected eye(s) twice daily at intervals of 6–8 hours	3–11 years: 1 drop into the affected eye(s) twice daily at intervals of 6–8 hours

(Continued)

TABLE 78-2	Medication Dosing for Allergic Rhinitis (*Continued*)		
Drugs	**Brand Names**	**Dosage for Adolescents[a] and Adults**	**Recommended Pediatric Doses**
Decongestants			
Oral			
Pseudoephedrine	Various	60 mg every 4–6 hours	6–11 years: 30 mg every 4–6 hours
		Sustained release: 120 mg every 12 hours	2–5 years: 15 mg every 4–6 hours
		Controlled release: 240 mg once daily	
Phenylephrine	Various	0–20 mg every 4 hours	6–11 years: 5 mg every 4 hours
			2–5 years: 2.5 mg every 4 hours
Nasal			
Oxymetazoline	Various	2–3 sprays twice daily	6–11 years: 2–3 sprays twice daily
Phenylephrine	Various	2–3 sprays every 4 hours (0.25%–1%)	6–11 years: 2–3 sprays every 4 hours (0.25%)
			2–5 years: 2–3 sprays every 4 hours (0.125%)
Nasal corticosteroids			
Beclomethasone	Beconase AQ	1–2 sprays in each nostril twice daily	6–11 years: 1 spray in each nostril twice daily
	Qnasl	2 sprays in each nostril once daily	4–11 years: 1 spray in each nostril once daily
Budesonide	Rhinocort Aqua	1 spray in each nostril once daily	6–11 years: 1 spray in each nostril once daily
Flunisolide	Various	Two sprays in each nostril twice daily	6–14 years: 2 sprays in each nostril twice daily
Fluticasone	Flonase	1–2 sprays in each nostril daily once daily	2–11 years: 1 spray in each nostril once daily
Mometasone	Veramyst, Nasonex, Nasacort	2 sprays in each nostril once daily	2–11 years: 1 spray in each nostril once daily
Triamcinolone	Nasacort AQ	2 sprays in each nostril once daily	2–11 years: 1 spray in each nostril once daily
Other nasal medications			
Cromolyn	Nasalcrom	1 spray in each nostril 3–4 times daily	2–11 years: 1 spray in each nostril 3–4 times daily
Ipratropium	Atrovent	2 sprays in each nostril 4 times daily	5–11 years: 2 sprays in each nostril 4 times daily

(*Continued*)

	Brand Names	**Dosage for Adolescents[a] and Adults**	**Recommended Pediatric Doses**
TABLE 78-2	Medication Dosing for Allergic Rhinitis (*Continued*)		
Drugs			
Leukotriene-receptor antagonist			
Montelukast	Singulair	10 mg orally once daily	6–14 years: 5 mg chewable tablet once daily
			2–5 years: 4 mg chewable tablet or oral granules once daily
			6–23 months: 4 mg oral granules once daily

[a]Adolescent age is ≥ 12 years except for flunisolide and montelukast (≥ 15 years).

- Other adverse effects of topical decongestants are burning, stinging, sneezing, and dryness of the nasal mucosa.
- These products should be used only when absolutely necessary (eg, at bedtime) and in doses that are as small and infrequent as possible. Duration of therapy should be limited to 3 days or less.
- **Pseudoephedrine** (Table 78-2) is an oral decongestant that has a slower onset of action than topical agents but may last longer and cause less local irritation. Rhinitis medicamentosa does not occur with oral decongestants. Doses up to 180 mg produce no measurable change in blood pressure or heart rate. However, higher doses (210–240 mg) may raise both blood pressure and heart rate. Systemic decongestants should be avoided in hypertensive patients unless absolutely necessary. Severe hypertensive reactions can occur when pseudoephedrine is given with monoamine oxidase inhibitors. Pseudoephedrine can cause mild CNS stimulation, even at therapeutic doses. Because of misuse as a component in the illegal manufacture of methamphetamine, pseudoephedrine is restricted to behind-the-counter sale with a limit on monthly purchases.
- **Phenylephrine** has replaced pseudoephedrine in many nonprescription antihistamine–decongestant combination products because of legal restrictions on pseudoephedrine sales.
- Combination oral products containing a decongestant and antihistamine are rational because of different mechanisms of action. However, antihistamines must be taken on a regular schedule, but decongestants should only be used when needed. Consumers should read product labels carefully to avoid therapeutic duplication and use combination products only for short courses.

TABLE 78-3	Duration of Action of Topical Decongestants
Medications	**Durations of Action (hours)**
Short acting	
Phenylephrine hydrochloride	Up to 4
Intermediate acting	
Naphazoline hydrochloride	2–6
Tetrahydrozoline hydrochloride	
Long acting	
Oxymetazoline hydrochloride	Up to 12
Xylometazoline hydrochloride	

Nasal Corticosteroids

- Intranasal corticosteroids reduce inflammation by reducing mediator release, suppressing neutrophil chemotaxis, reducing intracellular edema, causing mild vasoconstriction, and inhibiting mast cell–mediated, late-phase reactions.
- They relieve sneezing, rhinorrhea, itching, and nasal congestion (Table 78-2). Blocked nasal passages should be cleared with a decongestant or saline irrigation before administration to ensure adequate penetration of the spray. Advise patients to avoid sneezing or blowing their nose for at least 10 minutes after administration. Some patients improve within a few days, but peak response may require 2–3 weeks. The dosage may be reduced once a response is achieved.
- These agents are an excellent choice for persistent rhinitis and can also be excellent for seasonal rhinitis, especially if begun before exposure and the onset of symptoms. Recent guidelines suggest that nasal corticosteroids should be recommended as initial therapy for allergic rhinitis.
- Side effects are minimal and include sneezing, stinging, headache, epistaxis, and rare infections with *Candida albicans*.

Cromolyn Sodium

- **Cromolyn sodium**, a mast cell stabilizer, is available as a nonprescription nasal spray for symptomatic prevention and treatment of allergic rhinitis. It prevents antigen-triggered mast cell degranulation and release of mediators, including histamine. The most common side effect is local irritation (sneezing and nasal stinging).
- Nasal passages should be cleared before administration, and inhaling gently through the nose during administration enhances distribution to the entire nasal lining. Dosing must be repeated at 6-hour intervals to maintain the effect (Table 78-2).
- For seasonal rhinitis, treatment should be initiated just before the start of the offending allergen's season and continue throughout the season.
- In persistent rhinitis, improvement may not be seen for 2–4 weeks; antihistamines or decongestants may be needed during this initial phase of therapy.

Ipratropium Bromide

- **Ipratropium bromide** nasal spray is an anticholinergic agent that exhibits antisecretory properties when applied locally. It provides symptomatic relief of rhinorrhea associated with allergic and other forms of chronic rhinitis.
- It is not included in current treatment guidelines for allergic rhinitis and should be reserved for patients who fail or cannot tolerate other therapies. The optimal dose should be determined based on the specific patient's symptoms and response.
- Adverse effects are mild and include headache, epistaxis, and nasal dryness.

Montelukast

- **Montelukast** is a leukotriene-receptor antagonist approved for treatment of persistent allergic rhinitis in children as young as 6 months and for seasonal allergic rhinitis in children as young as 2 years (Table 78-2).
- Montelukast is a third-line choice after antihistamines and nasal corticosteroids. Monotherapy is no more effective than peripherally selective antihistamines and is less effective than intranasal corticosteroids; however, the combination of montelukast and an antihistamine is more effective than an antihistamine alone. Montelukast monotherapy has been recommended for children with mild persistent asthma and coexisting allergic rhinitis.

Immunotherapy

- Immunotherapy is the process of administering doses of antigens responsible for eliciting allergic symptoms into a patient with the intent of inducing tolerance to the allergen when natural exposure occurs. Until recently, immunotherapy was only available for subcutaneous injection; sublingual dosage forms are now available for a limited number of allergens.

- Beneficial effects of immunotherapy may result from induction of IgG-blocking antibodies, reduction in specific IgE (long-term), reduced recruitment of effector cells, altered T-cell cytokine balance, T-cell anergy, and alteration of regulatory T-cell activity.
- Good candidates for immunotherapy include patients with a strong history of severe symptoms unsuccessfully controlled by avoidance and pharmacotherapy and patients unable to tolerate adverse effects of drug therapy. Poor candidates include patients with medical conditions that compromise the ability to tolerate an anaphylactic-type reaction, patients with impaired immune systems, and patients with a history of nonadherence.
- For subcutaneous immunotherapy, very dilute solutions are given initially once or twice weekly. The concentration is increased until the maximum tolerated dose or highest planned dose is achieved. This maintenance dose is continued in slowly increasing intervals over several years, depending on clinical response. Better results are obtained with year-round rather than seasonal injections.
- Sublingual immunotherapy is available for ragweed, certain grasses, and house dust mite allergen. Ragweed and grass allergens are started 12 weeks before the allergen season and continued throughout the season. Because house dust mites cause persistent allergic rhinitis, this treatment is given year-round. The first dose is administered in the physician's office to allow observation of the patient for 30 minutes for hypersensitivity reactions. The patient places the tablet under the tongue where it dissolves; patients should not swallow for at least 1 minute. After the first dose is administered without incident, patients can take sublingual immunotherapy at home, but an auto-injectable epinephrine must be prescribed and available for immediate use.
- Adverse reactions with subcutaneous immunotherapy include mild induration and swelling at the injection site. More severe reactions (generalized urticaria, bronchospasm, laryngospasm, vascular collapse, and death from anaphylaxis) occur rarely. Severe reactions are treated with epinephrine, antihistamines, and systemic corticosteroids. The most common reactions with sublingual immunotherapy are pruritus of the mouth, ears, and tongue; throat irritation; and mouth edema. Sublingual immunotherapy is only approved for persons age 18 year and older.

EVALUATION OF THERAPEUTIC OUTCOMES

- Monitor patients regularly for reduction in severity of identified target symptoms and presence of side effects.
- Ask patients about their satisfaction with the management of their allergic rhinitis. Management should result in minimal disruption to their normal lifestyle.
- The Medical Outcomes Study 36-Item Short Form Health Survey and the Rhinoconjunctivitis Quality of Life Questionnaire measure symptom improvement and parameters such as sleep quality, nonallergic symptoms (eg, fatigue and poor concentration), emotions, and participation in a variety of activities.

See Chapter e14, Allergic Rhinitis, authored by J. Russell May, for a more detailed discussion of this topic.

Asthma

- *Asthma* is defined by the Global Initiative for Asthma (GINA) as a heterogeneous disease usually characterized by chronic airway inflammation. It is defined by a history of respiratory symptoms such as wheezing, shortness of breath, chest tightness, and cough that vary over time and in intensity, together with variable expiratory airflow limitation.

PATHOPHYSIOLOGY

- Numerous inflammatory cells and mediators cause chronic airway inflammation that leads to expiratory airway limitation. Airway narrowing results from smooth muscle contraction, with remodeling due to structural changes and airway plugging by mucous hypersecretion that leads to wheezing, shortness of breath, chest tightness, and cough.

- Bronchial hyperresponsiveness (BHR) is a heightened response to a stimulus (eg, cat dander) that enhances susceptibility to airway narrowing.

- Allergen inhalation in allergic patients causes an early-phase allergic reaction (within minutes) with activation of cells bearing allergen-specific immunoglobulin E (IgE). After rapid activation, airway mast cells and macrophages release proinflammatory mediators such as histamine and eicosanoids that induce contraction of airway smooth muscle, mucus secretion, edema, and exudation of plasma in the airways. Plasma protein leakage induces a thickened, engorged, edematous airway wall and narrowing of lumen with reduced mucus clearance.

- A late-phase inflammatory reaction occurs 6–9 hours after allergen provocation and involves recruitment and activation of eosinophils, T lymphocytes, basophils, neutrophils, and macrophages.

- Bronchial epithelial cells release cytokines such as eicosanoids, peptidases, matrix proteins, periostin, cytokines, chemokines, and nitric oxide (NO). Epithelial shedding may heighten BHR and enhance airway sensitivity to provocative stimuli.

- Eosinophils migrate to airways and release inflammatory mediators such as leukotrienes and granule proteins that injure airway tissue.

- T-lymphocyte activation leads to release of cytokines from type 2 T-helper (TH_2) cells that mediate allergic inflammation (interleukin [IL]-4, IL-5, and IL-13). Conversely, type 1 T-helper (TH_1) cells produce IL-2 and interferon-γ which are essential for cellular defense mechanisms. Allergic asthmatic inflammation may result from imbalance between TH_1 and TH_2 cells.

- Mast cell degranulation results in release of mediators such as histamine; eosinophil and neutrophil chemotactic factors; leukotrienes C_4, D_4, and E_4; prostaglandins; and platelet-activating factor (PAF). Histamine can induce smooth muscle constriction and bronchospasm and may contribute to mucosal edema and mucus secretion.

- Alveolar macrophages release inflammatory mediators, including proinflammatory and anti-inflammatory cytokines, reactive oxygen species, and eicosanoids. Production of neutrophil chemotactic factor and eosinophil chemotactic factor furthers the inflammatory process. Neutrophils also release mediators (PAFs, prostaglandins, thromboxanes, and leukotrienes) that contribute to BHR and airway inflammation. Leukotrienes C_4, D_4, and E_4 are released during inflammatory processes in the lung and produce bronchospasm, mucus secretion, microvascular permeability, and airway edema.

- The airway smooth muscle is innervated by parasympathetic, sympathetic, and nonadrenergic inhibitory nerves. Normal resting tone of airway smooth muscle is maintained by vagal efferent activity, and bronchoconstriction can be mediated by vagal stimulation in small bronchi. Airway smooth muscle contains noninnervated β_2-adrenergic receptors that produce bronchodilation. The nonadrenergic, noncholinergic (NANC) nervous system in the trachea and bronchi may amplify inflammation by releasing nitric oxide.

CLINICAL PRESENTATION

CHRONIC ASTHMA

- Symptoms include episodes of shortness of breath, chest tightness, coughing (particularly at night), wheezing, or a whistling sound when breathing. These often occur with exercise but may occur spontaneously or in association with known allergens.
- Signs include expiratory wheezing (rhonchi) on auscultation; dry, hacking cough; and atopy (eg, allergic rhinitis or atopic dermatitis).
- Asthma can vary from chronic daily symptoms to only intermittent symptoms. Intervals between symptoms may be days, weeks, months, or years.
- Severity is determined by lung function, symptoms, nighttime awakenings, and interference with normal activity prior to therapy. Patients can present with mild intermittent symptoms that require no medications or only occasional short-acting inhaled β_2-agonists (SABAs) to severe chronic symptoms despite multiple medications.

ACUTE SEVERE ASTHMA

- Uncontrolled asthma can progress to an acute state in which inflammation, airway edema, mucus accumulation, and severe bronchospasm result in profound airway narrowing that is poorly responsive to bronchodilator therapy.
- Patients may be anxious in acute distress and complain of severe dyspnea, shortness of breath, chest tightness, or burning. They may be able to say only a few words with each breath. Symptoms are unresponsive to usual measures (ie, SABAs).
- Signs include expiratory and inspiratory wheezing on auscultation; dry, hacking cough; tachypnea; tachycardia; pallor or cyanosis; and hyperinflated chest with intercostal and supraclavicular retractions. Breath sounds may be diminished with severe obstruction.

DIAGNOSIS

CHRONIC ASTHMA

- Diagnosis is made primarily by history of recurrent episodes of coughing, wheezing, chest tightness, or shortness of breath and confirmatory spirometry.
- Patients may have family history of allergy or asthma or symptoms of allergic rhinitis or atopic dermatitis. History of exercise or cold air precipitating dyspnea or increased symptoms during specific allergen seasons suggests asthma. Patient may have excessive variability in twice-daily peak expiratory flows (PEF) over 2 weeks.
- Spirometry demonstrates obstruction (forced expiratory volume in 1 second [FEV_1]/forced vital capacity [FVC] <80%) with reversibility after inhaled β_2-agonist administration (at least 12% and 200 mL increase in FEV_1). If baseline spirometry is normal, challenge testing with exercise, methacholine, or mannitol can be used to elicit BHR.

ACUTE SEVERE ASTHMA

- PEF and FEV1 are <40% of normal predicted values. Pulse oximetry reveals decreased arterial oxygen and O_2 saturations.
- Arterial blood gases may reveal metabolic acidosis and low partial pressure of oxygen (Pao_2).
- Obtain the history and physical examination while initial therapy is provided, assessing for onset and causes of the exacerbation; severity of symptoms and if associated with anaphylaxis; medication use, adherence, and response to current therapy; and risk factors for asthma-related death (history of near-fatal asthma requiring intubation and mechanical ventilation, hospitalization or emergency care in the past year, recent use of oral corticosteroids, no current use of inhaled corticosteroids [ICS],

overuse of SABA therapy [more than 1 canister/month], history of psychiatric disease or psychosocial problems, poor medication adherence, lack of a written asthma action plan, and food allergy). During the physical exam, assess vital signs and identify any complicating factors (eg, pneumonia, anaphylaxis) and comorbid conditions that could be causing acute shortness of breath such as inhaled foreign body, heart failure, pulmonary infection, and pulmonary embolism.

- Measure lung function testing by PEF or FEV_1 before treatment if possible, 1 hour after start of treatment, and then periodically until response is achieved or no further improvement is evident. Monitor oxygen saturation closely, preferably by pulse oximetry.

- Arterial blood gases are typically reserved for patients who are poorly responsive to initial treatment or deteriorating.

- Obtain a complete blood count if there are signs of infection (fever and purulent sputum).

TREATMENT

- <u>Goals of Treatment</u>: The GINA long-term goals for asthma management include (1) to achieve good control of symptoms and maintain normal activity levels, and (2) to minimize future risk of exacerbations, fixed airflow limitation, and side effects. For acute severe asthma, the primary goal is to prevent death by recognizing the signs of deterioration and providing rapid treatment.

NONPHARMACOLOGIC THERAPY

- Patient education is mandatory to improve medication adherence, self-management skills, and use of healthcare services.

- Short-term (approximately 2 weeks) home PEF monitoring can be used to assess treatment response. Longer-term PEF monitoring is generally recommended only for patients with a history of sudden severe asthma exacerbations, difficult to control severe asthma, or poor symptom perception.

- Avoidance of known allergenic triggers can improve symptoms, reduce medication use, and decrease BHR. Environmental triggers (eg, animals) should be avoided in sensitive patients, and smokers should be encouraged to quit.

- In acute asthma exacerbations, initiate oxygen therapy to achieve an arterial oxygen saturation of 93%–95% in adolescents and adults and 94%–98% in school-aged children and pregnant women or those with cardiac disease.

- Correct dehydration if present; urine specific gravity may help guide therapy in children when assessment of hydration status is difficult.

PHARMACOTHERAPY

General Approach

- Table 79-1 summarizes GINA recommendations for initial controller treatment in adults and adolescents with persistent asthma. A stepped-care approach is used to manage persistent asthma for all ages. If newly diagnosed, the initial step is based upon levels of impairment and risk, which determine asthma severity. All patients with persistent asthma (mild, moderate, or severe) should be started on inhaled corticosteroid therapy. Therapy is escalated as needed by increasing the ICS dose or adding a second and then a third inhaled controller medication, typically a long-acting β_2 adrenergic receptor agonist (LABA) (preferred) or a long-acting muscarinic agonist (LAMA). All patients should have quick-relief reliever therapy available for acute symptoms. Assess disease control 2–6 weeks after the start of therapy and adjust therapy accordingly. Follow-up every 2–3 months thereafter as appropriate.

- Figure 79-1 describes the stepwise approach for managing asthma in ages 12 years and older.

TABLE 79-1 GINA Recommendations for Initial Controller Treatment in Adults and Adolescents

Symptom Presentation	Preferred Treatment (Evidence Level)
Symptoms or need for SABA less than 2×/mo; no waking due to asthma in last month; and no risk factors for exacerbations, including in prior year	No controller (D)
Infrequent symptoms, but patient has one or more risk factors for exacerbation (eg, low lung function, use of OCS in prior year, intensive care treatment for asthma ever)	Low-dose ICS (D)
Symptoms or need for SABA between 2×/mo and 2×/week, or patient wakes due to asthma more than once/mo	Low-dose ICS (D)
Symptoms or need for SABA >2×/week	Low-dose ICS[a] (A)
Troublesome symptoms most days or waking ≥1 ×/week, esp. if any risk factors exist	Medium/high-dose ICS or low-dose ICS/LABA[b] (A)
Symptoms consistent with severely uncontrolled asthma, or with an acute exacerbation	OCS short course AND start of high-dose ICS or moderate-dose ICS/LABA[b] (D)

[a]Less effective options are LTRA or theophylline.
[b]Not recommended for initial controller treatment in children ages 6–11 years.
(A), (B), (C), (D) = grade of evidence with A as the highest grade and D as the lowest grade.

- Step-down of therapy is warranted if symptoms have been well controlled and lung function has been stable for 3 months or longer. While engaging the patient in this effort, monitor symptoms and PEF and schedule follow-up. Stepping down ICS doses by 25%–50% at 3-month intervals is feasible and safe for most patients.
- Personalized asthma management emphasizes three components: (1) ASSESS symptom control and risk factors, (2) ADJUST therapy and treat modifiable risk factors, and (3) REVIEW RESPONSE and optimize control about every 3 months.
- The primary therapy of acute exacerbations includes inhaled SABAs and (depending on severity) systemic corticosteroids, inhaled ipratropium, intravenous (IV) magnesium sulfate, and oxygen. Treatments are typically administered concurrently to facilitate rapid improvement. Measure initial response 1 hour after the first three inhaled bronchodilator treatments.
- Figure 79-2 outlines strategies for self-management of worsening asthma in adolescents and adults with a written asthma action plan.
- Figure 79-3 is an algorithm for management of acute asthma exacerbations in acute care facilities (eg, emergency departments).

β_2-Agonists

- SABAs (eg, **albuterol**) are the most effective bronchodilators and the treatment of first choice for managing acute severe asthma. A SABA is also indicated for as-needed treatment of intermittent episodes of bronchospasm (eg, exercise-induced bronchospasm). Aerosol administration enhances bronchoselectivity and provides more rapid response and greater protection against provocations (eg, exercise, allergen challenges) than systemic administration. In adults, administration as either continuous nebulization or intermittent administration (every 20 minutes for 3 doses) administration over 1-hour results in equivalent improvement. There is no role for IV β_2 agonists in severe asthma.

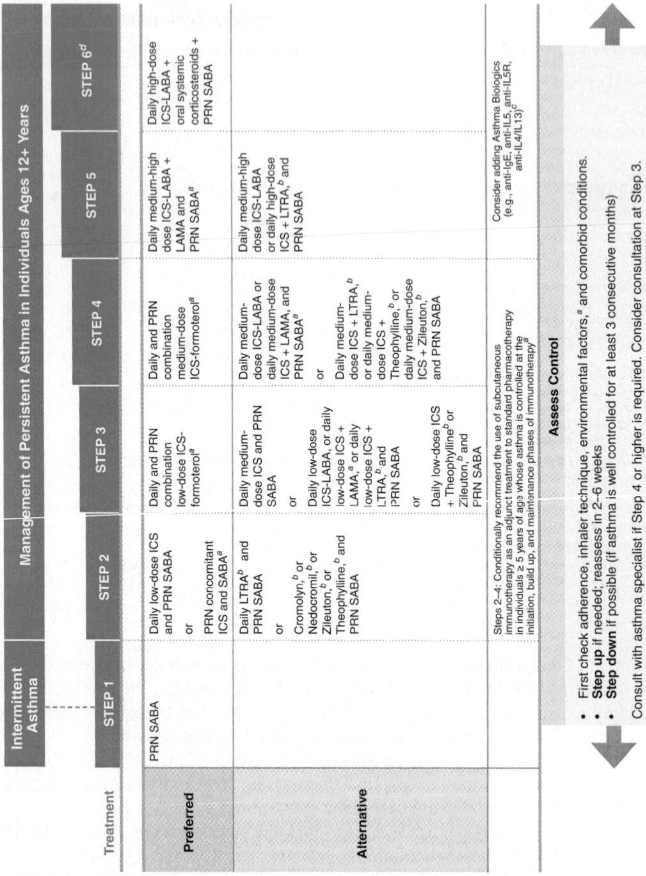

FIGURE 79-1. Stepwise approach for management of asthma in ages 12 years and older. ICS, inhaled corticosteroids; LABA, long-acting β2-agonist; LAMA, long-acting muscarinic antagonist; LTRA, leukotriene receptor antagonist; SABA, inhaled short-acting β2-agonist. [a]Updated based on the 2020 guidelines. [b]Cromolyn, nedocromil, LTRAs including zileuton and montelukast, and theophylline were not considered for this update and/or have limited availability for use in the United States, and/or have an increased risk of adverse consequences and need for monitoring that makes their use less desirable. The FDA issued a Boxed Warning for montelukast in March 2020. [c]The AHRQ systematic reviews that informed this report did not include studies that examined the role of asthma biologics (eg, anti-IgE, anti-IL5, anti-IL5R, anti-IL4/IL13). Thus this report does not contain specific recommendations for the use of biologics in asthma in Steps 5 and 6. [d]Data on the use of LAMA therapy in individuals with severe persistent asthma (Step 6) were not included in the AHRQ systematic review and thus no recommendation is made.

- Nonprescription inhaled **epinephrine** as Primatene Mist metered-dose inhaler is less effective than prescription SABAs and is only to be used for temporary relief of mild symptoms of intermittent asthma in patients ≥12 years old; patients should see a physician immediately if improvement is not seen within 20 minutes, symptoms

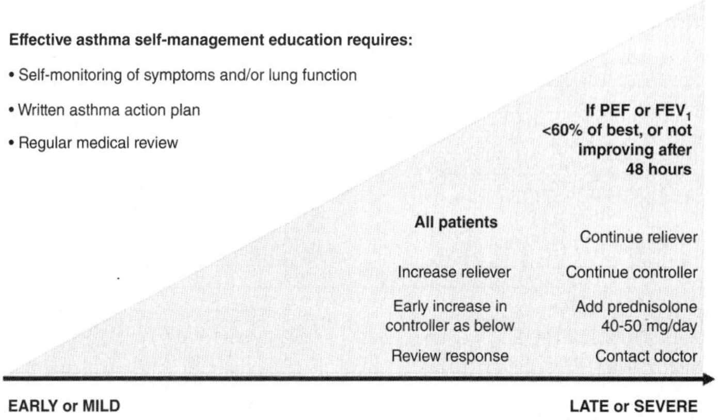

Effective asthma self-management education requires:

- Self-monitoring of symptoms and/or lung function
- Written asthma action plan
- Regular medical review

	All patients	**If PEF or FEV$_1$ <60% of best, or not improving after 48 hours**
		Continue reliever
	Increase reliever	Continue controller
	Early increase in controller as below	Add prednisolone 40-50 mg/day
	Review response	Contact doctor

EARLY or MILD → **LATE or SEVERE**

Medication	Short-term change (1-2 weeks) for worsening asthma	Evidence Level
Increase usual reliever:		
Low dose ICS/formoterol[a]	Increase frequency of reliever use (maximum formoterol total 72 mcg/day	A
Short-acting beta2-agonist (SABA)	Increase frequency of SABA use For pMDI, add spacer	A A
Increase usual controller:		
Maintenance and reliever ICS/formoterol[a]	Continue maintenance ICS/formoterol and increase reliever ICS/formoterol as needed[a] (maximum formoterol total 72 mcg/day)	A
Maintenance ICS with SABA as reliever	At least double ICS; consider increasing ICS to high dose (maximum 2000 mcg/day BDP equivalent)	B
Maintenance ICS/formoterol with SABA as reliever	Quadruple maintenance ICS/formoterol (maximum formoterol 72 mcg/day)	B
Maintenance ICS/other LABA with SABA as reliever	Step up to higher dose formulation of ICS/other LABA, or consider adding a separate ICS inhaler (to maximum total 2000 mcg/day BDP equivalent)	D
Add oral corticosteroids (OCS) and contact doctor		
OCS (prednisone or prednisolone)	Add OCS for severe exacerbations (eg, PEF or FEV$_1$ <60% personal best or predicted), or patient not responding to treatment over 48 hours. Once started, morning dosing is preferable.	A
	Adults: prednisolone 40-50 mg/day (maximum 50 mg) usually for 5-7 days. *Children 6-11 years*: 1-2 mg/kg/day (maximum 40 mg) usually for 3-5 days	D
	Tapering is not needed if OCS are prescribed for <2 weeks	B

FIGURE 79-2. Self-management of worsening asthma in adults and adolescents with a written asthma action plan.

become worse, or require more than 8 inhalations in a 24-hour period, or there are more than two episodes in a week.

- Two long-acting β_2-agonists (LABAs), **formoterol** (Foradil) and **salmeterol** (Serevent), provide bronchodilation for 12 hours or longer and are dosed twice daily. When combined with an ICS, formoterol may be dosed on a daily and as-needed basis (thus, more frequently than twice daily).

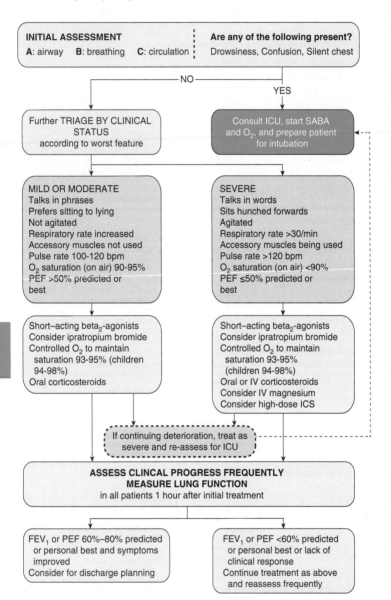

FIGURE 79-3. Management of asthma exacerbations in an acute care facility, for example, the emergency department. To obtain O2 saturation in SI units (fraction) multiply the results expressed as a percentage by 0.01.

- Three ultra-LABAs (**indacaterol** [Arcapta Neohaler], **olodaterol** [Striverdi Respimat], and **vilanterol**) have a 24-hour bronchodilator duration of effect. Only vilanterol in combination with fluticasone furoate (with and without umeclidinium) is available for once-daily dosing for asthma in adults ≥18 years old in the United States. Products containing indacaterol and olodaterol are only indicated for COPD but are being evaluated for asthma.
- Table 79-2 contains dosing guidelines for acute severe asthma exacerbations.

TABLE 79-2	**Drug Doses for Treatment of Acute Severe Exacerbations of Asthma**		
	Dosages		
Medications	**≥12 Years Old**	**<12 Years Old**	**Comments**
Inhaled β-agonists			
Albuterol nebulizer solution (5 mg/mL, 0.63 mg/3 mL, 1.25 mg/3 mL, 2.5 mg/3 mL)	2.5–5 mg every 20 minutes for three doses, and then 2.5–10 mg every 1–4 hours as needed, or 10–15 mg/h continuously	0.15 mg/kg (minimum dose 2.5 mg) every 20 minutes for three doses, and then 0.15–0.3 mg/kg up to 10 mg every 1–4 hours as needed, or 0.5 mg/kg/h by continuous nebulization	Only selective β$_2$-agonists are recommended. For optimal delivery, dilute aerosols to minimum of 4 mL at gas flow of 6–8 L/min. Use face mask if <4 years of age
Albuterol MDI (90 mcg/puff)	4–8 puffs every 30 minutes up to 4 hours, and then every 1–4 hours as needed	4–8 puffs every 20 minutes for three doses, and then every 1–4 hours as needed	In patients in severe distress, nebulization is preferred; use VHC-type spacer with face mask if <4 years old
Levalbuterol nebulizer solution (0.31 mg/3 mL, 0.63 mg/3 mL, 2.5 mg/1 mL, 1.25 mg/3 mL)	Give one-half the milligram dose of albuterol above	Give one-half the milligram dose of albuterol above	The single isomer of albuterol is twice as potent on a milligram basis Not recommended
Levalbuterol MDI (45 mcg/puff)	See albuterol MDI dose	See albuterol MDI dose above	See albuterol MDI dose; one-half as potent as albuterol on a microgram basis Not recommended
Anticholinergics			
Ipratropium bromide nebulizer solution (0.25 mg/mL)	500 mcg every 30 minutes for three doses, and then every 2–4 hours as needed	250 mcg every 20 minutes for three doses, and then 250 mcg every 2–4 hours	May mix in same nebulizer with albuterol; only add to β$_2$-agonist therapy

(Continued)

| TABLE 79-2 | Drug Doses for Treatment of Acute Severe Exacerbations of Asthma (Continued) |

| | Dosages | | |
Medications	**≥12 Years Old**	**<12 Years Old**	**Comments**
Ipratropium bromide MDI (18 mcg/puff)	8 puffs every 20 minutes as needed for up to 3 hours	4–8 puffs as needed every 2–4 hours	Not to be continued once hospitalized
Corticosteroids			
Prednisone, methylprednisolone, prednisolone	50 mg in one or two divided doses (prednisone equivalent)	1 mg/kg (maximum 40 mg/day) in two divided doses (prednisone equivalent)	For outpatient "burst" use 1–2 mg/kg/day, maximum 60 mg, for 3–5 days in children and 40–60 mg/day in one or two divided doses for 5–7 days in adults

Note: No advantage has been found for very-high-dose corticosteroids in acute severe asthma, nor is there any advantage for IV administration over oral therapy. The usual regimen is to continue the oral corticosteroid for the duration of hospitalization. The final duration of therapy following a hospitalization or emergency department visit may be from 3 to 10 days. If patients are then started on an ICS, there is no need to taper the systemic corticosteroid dose. An ICS can be started at any time during the exacerbation.

Corticosteroids

- ICS are the preferred long-term control therapy for persistent asthma because of potency and consistent effectiveness; they are the only therapy shown to reduce risk of dying from asthma. See Table 79-3 for comparative ICS doses; all agents are approved for once- or twice-daily dosing.
- Response to ICS is delayed; symptoms improve in most patients within the first 1–2 weeks and reach maximum improvement in 4–8 weeks. Maximum improvement in FEV_1 and PEF rates may require 3–6 weeks.

| TABLE 79-3 | Inhaled Corticosteroids and Comparative Daily Dosages in Adults and Adolescents (12 Years and Older) |

| | Comparative Daily Dosages (mcg) of Inhaled Corticosteroids | | |
	Low Dose	**Medium Dose**	**High Dose**
Beclomethasone dipropionate DPI[a]	80–240	>240–480	>480
Budesonide DPI	180–540	>540-1080	>1080
Budesonide Nebules	unknown	unknown	unknown
Ciclesonide HFA[b] MDI[c]	160–320	320–640	>640
Flunisolide HFA MDI	320	320–640	>640
Fluticasone furoate DPI		100	200
Fluticasone propionate HFA MDI	888–264	264–440	>440
Fluticasone propionate DPI	100–300	300–500	>500
Mometasone furoate DPI	110–220	>220–440	>440

[a]Dry powder inhaler.
[b]Hydrofluoroalkane
[c]Metered-dose inhaler.

- Systemic toxicity of ICS is minimal with low-to-moderate doses, but risk of systemic effects increases with high doses (eg, growth suppression in children, osteoporosis, cataracts, dermal thinning, easy bruising, adrenal insufficiency). Local adverse effects include dose-dependent oropharyngeal candidiasis and dysphonia, which can be reduced by using a spacer device.
- Systemic corticosteroids (Table 79-4) are indicated in all patients with acute severe asthma not responding completely to initial inhaled β_2-agonist administration (every 20 minutes for 3 doses) and should be administered within 1 hour of presentation to reduce the risk of hospitalization. IV therapy offers no advantage over oral administration except in patients unable to take oral medications. Adults are treated effectively with 5–7 days of oral prednisone (or equivalent), but children may require only 3–5 days. Dexamethasone for 1–2 days is an option for children and has the benefit of less vomiting. Continue full doses until the PEF reaches 70% of predicted normal or personal best. Tapering the dose after discharge is unnecessary if patients are prescribed an ICS for outpatient therapy.
- Adverse effects of systemic corticosteroids can occur even after a short course (<14 days). The ideal strategy is to use systemic corticosteroids in a short "burst" and then maintain the patient on appropriate long-term control therapy with ICS.

Anticholinergics

- Anticholinergics reverse cholinergic-mediated bronchoconstriction and are effective bronchodilators in asthma.
- Ipratropium bromide is useful as adjunctive therapy in acute severe asthma not completely responsive to SABA alone. Patients with persistent asthma who are intolerant to short-acting β_2-agonists may be prescribed ipratropium for rescue inhaler use.
- Time to reach maximum bronchodilation from aerosolized ipratropium is longer than from aerosolized SABAs (30–60 minutes vs. 5–10 minutes). However, some bronchodilation is seen within 30 seconds, and 50% of maximum response occurs within 3 minutes. Ipratropium bromide has a duration of action of 4–8 hours; tiotropium bromide has a duration of 24 hours.
- I
- **Tiotropium bromide** (Spiriva) and **umeclidinium bromide** are long-acting inhaled anticholinergics with a duration of 24 hours. Tiotropium may be considered as an add-on therapy in patients whose asthma is not well controlled with a medium to high dose of ICS and LABA combination therapy. Umeclidinium bromide is available as a combination inhaler with fluticasone and vilanterol (Anoro Ellipta) but is not FDA approved for relief of acute bronchospasm or for treatment of asthma.

Leukotriene Modifiers

- **Zafirlukast** (Accolate) and **montelukast** (Singulair) are oral leukotriene receptor antagonists (LTRA) that reduce the proinflammatory and bronchoconstriction effects of leukotriene D$_4$. However, they are less effective than low-dose ICS, and they are less effective than LABAs when added to ICS for moderate persistent asthma. They are not used to treat acute exacerbations and must be taken on a regular basis,

TABLE 79-4	Comparison of Systemic Corticosteroids			
Systemic	Anti-Inflammatory Potency	Mineralocorticoid Potency	Duration of Biologic Activity (Hours)	Elimination Half-Life (Hours)
Hydrocortisone	1	1	8–12	1.5–2
Prednisone	4	0.8	12–36	2.5–3.5
Methylprednisolone	5	0.5	12–36	3.3
Dexamethasone	25	0	36–72	3.4–4

even during symptom-free periods. The adult zafirlukast dose is 20 mg twice daily, taken at least 1 hour before or 2 hours after meals; the dose for children ages 5–11 years is 10 mg twice daily. The adult montelukast dose is 10 mg once daily, taken in the evening without regard to food; the dose for children ages 6–14 years is one 5 mg chewable tablet daily in the evening.

- Use of montelukast and zafirlukast has fallen out of favor due to increased observance of unusual adverse effects and modest therapeutic efficacy. An idiosyncratic syndrome similar to the Churg–Strauss syndrome, with marked circulating eosinophilia, heart failure, and associated eosinophilic vasculitis, has been reported rarely. Because of reports of adverse neuropsychiatric events especially within a few weeks of starting therapy, monitor patients for signs of irritability, aggressiveness, and sleep disturbances; suicidality has also been reported rarely. There have been reports of fatal hepatic failure associated with zafirlukast.

- **Zileuton** (Zyflo) is a 5-lipoxygenase inhibitor; its use is limited due to potential for elevated hepatic enzymes, especially in the first 3 months of therapy, and inhibition of metabolism of drugs metabolized by CYP3A4 (eg, theophylline, warfarin). The dose of zileuton tablets is 600 mg four times daily with meals and at bedtime. The dose of zileuton extended-release tablets is two 600 mg tablets twice daily, within 1 hour after the morning and evening meals (total daily dose 2400 mg).

Biologic Agents

- These agents target the IgE pathway (relevant to allergic asthma) or IL-4, IL-13, and IL-5 pathways (relevant to the Th2 pathway and eosinophilic disorders) and are indicated for patients with moderate or severe asthma (depending upon the drug) along with other biomarkers or clinical indicators associated with treatment response. They are typically reserved for patients with moderate to severe persistent asthma who have poor symptom control despite treatment with high-dose ICS-LABA with relevant allergic (or eosinophilic) biomarkers or need maintenance oral corticosteroids.

- **Omalizumab** (Xolair) is an anti-IgE antibody approved for treatment of allergic asthma not well controlled by oral or ICS. Dosage is determined by baseline total serum IgE (international units/mL [kIU/L]) and body weight (kg). Doses range from 150 to 375 mg subcutaneously (SC) at either 2- or 4-week intervals. Omalizumab is recommended for treating patients >6 years of age with moderate-to-severe asthma not adequately controlled by ICS, ICS/LABA, and in some cases, oral corticosteroids. Elevated levels of the fraction of exhaled nitric oxide (FeNO) at ≥24 ppb and eosinophil levels >260 eosinophils/mcg/L while taking high-dose ICS are predictive of an exacerbation reduction response. Patients taking omalizumab reported local injection site reactions (similar to all subcutaneous biologics) and rates of anaphylaxis at 0.1%, which resulted in a Boxed Warning. Treatment must be administered in a clinical setting to observe for anaphylaxis after each dose.

- **Mepolizumab** (Nucala) and **reslizumab** (Cinqair) are monoclonal antibodies directed against IL-5 to block activation of the IL-5 receptor on eosinophils. **Benralizumab** (Fasenra) binds to the alpha subunit of the IL-5 receptor of eosinophils and prevents binding of IL-5, thus mitigating downstream eosinophilic inflammation. Mepolizumab and benralizumab are approved for patients ≥12 years old with severe asthma and are administered SC; reslizumab is approved for severe asthma in patients ≥18 years old and is administered IV. Mepolizumab and reslizumab are dosed every 4 weeks; benralizumab is dosed every 4 weeks for 3 months then every 8 weeks. Doses are to be administered in a healthcare setting by professionals who are prepared to manage anaphylaxis. Each of these drugs is indicated for patients with an "eosinophilic phenotype" (which has not been formally defined). However, a reduction in exacerbation rate of ~50% is observed when patients have a certain minimum peripheral blood eosinophil count that varies by drug.

- **Dupilumab** (Dupixent) targets the IL-4α receptor, thus blocking signaling of IL4 and IL-13, which are cytokines that promote IgE synthesis and inflammatory cell recruitment. Dupilumab is approved for patients with moderate-to-severe asthma age ≥ 12 years old with an eosinophilic phenotype and is administered SC every 2 weeks. Unlike mepolizumab, reslizumab, and benralizumab, FeNO levels >25 ppb in addition to blood eosinophil levels ≥ 150 cells/μL (0.15×10^9/L) is predictive of a response in reducing the asthma exacerbation rate by $\sim 50\%$.

Magnesium Sulfate

- Magnesium sulfate is a moderately potent bronchodilator, producing relaxation of smooth muscle by blocking calcium ion influx into smooth muscles; it may also have anti-inflammatory effects.

- For patients with severe asthma exacerbations, a single 2 g IV infusion may reduce hospital admissions in adults who have an FEV_1 <25%–30% predicted upon arrival in the emergency department, children and adults who have persistent hypoxemia after standard treatment, and children whose FEV_1 remains <60% predicted after 1 hour of standard treatment. Adverse effects include hypotension, facial flushing, sweating, depressed deep tendon reflexes, hypothermia, and CNS and respiratory depression.

Methylxanthines

- Methylxanthines are rarely used today because of the high risk of severe life-threatening toxicity, numerous drug interactions, and decreased efficacy compared with ICS, LABAs, and biologics. **Theophylline** is a moderately potent bronchodilator with mild anti-inflammatory properties and is available for oral and IV administration. It is not recommended in the GINA guidelines for acute exacerbations or persistent asthma. Theophylline dosing requires monitoring of serum concentrations for both efficacy and toxicity, including seizures and death. In addition, theophylline is eliminated primarily by metabolism via the hepatic CYP P450 microsomal enzymes (primarily CYP1A2 and CYP3A4), and drug interactions affecting metabolism significantly affect blood concentrations.

EVALUATION OF THERAPEUTIC OUTCOMES

- Focus the initial encounters on the patient's concerns, expectations, and goals of treatment. Basic education should include discussion of asthma as a chronic lung disease, the types of medications, and how they are to be used. Teach inhaler technique, advise the patient about when to seek medical advice, and provide written action plans. Both peak flow-based and symptom-based self-monitoring can be effective, if taught and followed correctly.

- At the first follow-up visit, reinforce the educational messages from the first visit and review the patient's current medications, adherence, and any difficulties related to therapy.

- The two key components of effective asthma control are "symptom control" and "future risk of adverse outcomes." Assess symptom control by frequency of daytime and nighttime asthma symptoms, reliever medication use, and activity limitations; poor symptom control is also an indicator of future risk for exacerbations.

- Future risk of adverse outcomes includes assessment of risks for future exacerbations, fixed airflow limitation (and thus diminished response to therapy), and medication adverse effects. To assess the risk for future exacerbations, measure lung function before the start of treatment and then 2 months later when maximum response to controller medications is likely attained.

- During ongoing care, measure spirometry yearly but reserve long-term PEF monitoring for patients with severe asthma.

- Validated questionnaires can be administered regularly, such as the Asthma Control Test, Asthma Therapy Assessment Questionnaire, and Asthma Control Questionnaire.

- Ask patients about exercise tolerance because perceived good exercise tolerance may be biased by a sedentary lifestyle adapted to the frequency of bothersome symptoms.

- All patients on inhaled drugs should have their inhalation technique evaluated monthly initially and then every 3–6 months.
- After initiation of anti-inflammatory therapy or increase in dosage, most patients should experience decreased symptoms within 1–2 weeks and achieve maximum improvement within 4–8 weeks. Improvement in baseline FEV_1 or PEF should follow a similar time course, but decrease in BHR as measured by morning PEF, PEF variability, and exercise tolerance may take longer and improve over 1–3 months.

See Chapter 44, Asthma, authored by Kathryn V. Blake and Jean Y. Moon, for a more detailed discussion of this topic.

Chronic Obstructive Pulmonary Disease

- Chronic obstructive pulmonary disease (COPD) is characterized by progressive airflow limitation that is not fully reversible. Two principal conditions (referred to as phenotypes) include:
  - ✓ *Chronic bronchitis*: Chronic or recurrent excess mucus secretion with cough that occurs on most days for at least 3 months of the year for at least 2 consecutive years.
  - ✓ *Emphysema*: Abnormal, permanent enlargement of the airspaces distal to the terminal bronchioles, accompanied by destruction of their walls, without fibrosis.

PATHOPHYSIOLOGY

- The most common cause of COPD is exposure to tobacco smoke. Inhalation of noxious particles and gases activates neutrophils, macrophages, and $CD8^+$ lymphocytes, which release chemical mediators, including tumor necrosis factor-α, interleukin-8, and leukotriene B_4. Inflammatory cells and mediators lead to widespread destructive changes in airways, pulmonary vasculature, and lung parenchyma, resulting in chronic airflow limitation.

- Oxidative stress and imbalance between aggressive and protective defense systems in the lungs (proteases and antiproteases) may also occur. Oxidants generated by cigarette smoke react with and damage proteins and lipids, contributing to cell and tissue damage. Oxidants also promote inflammation and exacerbate protease–antiprotease imbalance by inhibiting antiprotease activity.

- The protective antiprotease α_1-antitrypsin (AAT) inhibits protease enzymes, including neutrophil elastase. AAT deficiency increases risk for premature emphysema.

- Inflammatory exudate in airways leads to increased number and size of goblet cells and mucus glands. Mucus secretion increases and ciliary motility is impaired. There is thickening of the smooth muscle and connective tissue in airways. Chronic inflammation leads to scarring, fibrosis, and airflow obstruction.

- Arterial blood gas (ABG) abnormalities result from impaired gas transfer due to parenchymal damage and loss of alveolar-capillary networks. Significant ABG changes are usually not present until airflow limitation is very severe. In such patients, *hypoxemia* (low arterial oxygen tension—Pao_2 45–60 mm Hg [6.0–8.0 kPa]) and *hypercapnia* (elevated arterial carbon dioxide tension—$Paco_2$ 50–60 mm Hg [6.7–8.0 kPa]) can become chronic problems. Hypoxemia is initially associated with exertion but develops at rest as the disease progresses. Hypoxemia results from hypoventilation (V) of lung tissue relative to perfusion (Q) of the area. This low V/Q ratio progresses over several years, resulting in a consistent decline in Pao_2. As gas exchange worsens with disease progression, patients may exhibit chronic hypercapnia and are referred to as CO_2 retainers. In such patients, central respiratory response to chronically increased $Paco_2$ is blunted. Serum pH is usually near normal because the kidneys compensate by retaining bicarbonate. If acute respiratory distress develops (eg, as with pneumonia or COPD exacerbation with respiratory failure) $Paco_2$ may rise sharply, resulting in worsening respiratory acidosis.

- Chronic hypoxemia and changes in pulmonary vasculature lead to increases in pulmonary pressures, especially during exercise. Sustained elevated pulmonary pressures can lead to right-sided heart failure (cor pulmonale) characterized by right ventricle hypertrophy in response to increased pulmonary vascular resistance.

- Chronic airflow obstruction leads to air trapping, resulting in thoracic hyperinflation and flattening of diaphragmatic muscles, making them less efficient muscles of ventilation and predisposing patients to muscle fatigue, especially during exacerbations. Patients with thoracic hyperinflation have increased functional residual capacity (FRC), which is the amount of air left in the lungs after exhalation. Increased FRC limits the amount of air the patient can inhale to fill the lungs and shortens the inhalation time, which may increase complaints of dyspnea.

- Loss of skeletal muscle mass and decline in overall health status can lead to ischemic cardiovascular events, cachexia, weight loss, osteoporosis, anemia, and muscle wasting.

CLINICAL PRESENTATION

- Initial symptoms include chronic cough and sputum production; patients may experience cough for several years before dyspnea develops. Dyspnea is worse with exercise and progressive over time, with decreased exercise tolerance or decline in physical activity. Chest tightness or wheezing may be present.
- Physical examination may be normal in milder stages. When airflow limitation progresses, patients may have shallow breathing, increased resting respiratory rate, "barrel chest" due to lung hyperinflation, pursed lips during expiration, use of accessory respiratory muscles, and cyanosis of mucosal membranes.

DIAGNOSIS

- Diagnosis is based on patient symptoms, history of exposure to risk factors such as tobacco smoke and occupational substances, and confirmation by pulmonary function testing, such as spirometry.
- Spirometry assesses lung volumes and capacities. Forced vital capacity (FVC) is the total volume of air exhaled after maximal inhalation, and FEV_1 is the total volume of air exhaled in 1 second. Postbronchodilator spirometry results should be used to assess lung function in patients with COPD. FEV_1 is measured 10–15 minutes after inhalation of a short-acting β_2-agonist or 30–45 minutes after a short-acting anticholinergic or a combination of the two agents. Airflow limitation is confirmed by a postbronchodilator FEV_1/FVC <70% (0.70).
- The Global Initiative for Chronic Obstructive Lung Disease (GOLD) guidelines suggest a four-grade classification of airflow limitation based on the FEV_1/FVC <70% (0.70), measured FEV_1 compared to predicted FEV_1 (%), and presence of symptoms: (1) mild, (2) moderate, (3), severe, or (4) very severe.
- Recommended patient assessment questionnaires to assess dyspnea and other measures of health status include the COPD Assessment Test (CAT), modified Medical Research Council (mMRC) Dyspnea Questionnaire, and the COPD Control Questionnaire (CCQ).

TREATMENT

- Goals of Treatment: Prevent or slow disease progression, relieve symptoms, improve exercise tolerance, improve overall health status, prevent and treat exacerbations, prevent and treat complications, and reduce morbidity and mortality.

NONPHARMACOLOGIC THERAPY

- Educate patients about their disease, treatment plans, and strategies to slow progression and prevent complications.
- Smoking cessation is the most important intervention to prevent development and progression of COPD. Reducing exposure to occupational dust and fumes as well as other environmental toxins is also important.
- Pulmonary rehabilitation programs include exercise training, breathing exercises, optimal medical treatment, psychosocial support, and health education.
- Administer the influenza vaccine annually during each influenza season. Vaccination against pneumococcal infection is recommended for all adults with COPD. Patients who have not previously received a pneumococcal conjugate vaccine (PCV) should receive either PCV20 or PCV15 followed by a pneumococcal polysaccharide vaccine (PPSV23) at least one year later. Patients who have previously received PPSV23 should be given either PCV15 or PCV20 at least one year later.

- All individuals over the age of 5 years should receive a viral vector or mRNA vaccine to prevent severe illness and death associated with coronavirus infection and disease (COVID-19).
- Once patients are stabilized as outpatients and pharmacotherapy is optimized, institute long-term oxygen therapy if either of the following conditions is documented twice in a 3-week period: (1) resting Pao_2 <55 mm Hg (7.3 kPa) or Sao_2 <88% (0.88) with or without hypercapnia, or (2) resting Pao_2 55–60 mm Hg (7.3–8.0 kPa) or Sao_2 <88% (0.88) with evidence of right-sided heart failure, polycythemia, or pulmonary hypertension. Oxygen can be delivered by nasal cannula at 1–2 L/min, providing 24%–28% (0.24–0.28) fraction of inspired oxygen (Fio_2) with a goal to raise Pao_2 above 60 mm Hg (8.0 kPa).

PHARMACOLOGIC THERAPY

- No COPD medication has been conclusively shown to slow lung function decline or prolong survival. The GOLD guidelines recommend that a combined "ABCD" classification system based on symptom severity and risk of future exacerbations be used as a stepwise approach to pharmacotherapy rather than FEV_1 measurements (Table 80-1). Symptom assessment should be measured at baseline and then during routine visits using CAT or mMRC. Defined cut points for patients exhibiting "more symptoms" and "less symptoms" have been established for CAT and mMRC. Frequency of exacerbations is assessed by reviewing exacerbation history for the past 12 months. Patients are assigned to an ABCD category based on these two assessments. Patients with at least two exacerbations in the last 12 months, or one exacerbation requiring hospitalization, are considered high risk for future exacerbations (category C or D). Guidelines recommend that initial and escalation therapy (Table 80-2) be based on ABCD category classification.
- Bronchodilators are the mainstay of drug therapy; classes include short- and long-acting β_2-agonists, short- and long-acting muscarinic antagonists (anticholinergics), and methylxanthines. Short-acting inhaled bronchodilators relieve symptoms (eg, dyspnea) and increase exercise tolerance. Long-acting inhaled bronchodilators relieve symptoms, reduce exacerbation frequency, and improve quality of life and health status. Bronchodilators do not significantly improve measurements of expiratory airflow such as FEV_1.

TABLE 80-1	Recommended Initial Pharmacotherapy for Stable COPD
Patient Category	**Initial Therapy**
A (less symptoms, less exacerbation risk)	Offer either short- or long-acting bronchodilator, depending on symptoms
B (more symptoms, less exacerbation risk)	Start LAMA or LABA for symptom control
C (less symptoms, more exacerbation risk)	Start long-acting bronchodilator for exacerbation prevention; LAMA is preferred over LABA for initial therapy
D (more symptoms, more exacerbation risk)	Start long-acting bronchodilator for exacerbation prevention; LAMA is preferred over LABA for initial monotherapy
	May start dual LAMA/LABA for severe breathlessness
	If blood eosinophils ≥300/μL (0.3 × 10⁹/L), start ICS/LABA as initial dual therapy

CAT, COPD Assessment Test; FEV_1, forced expiratory volume in 1 second; ICS, inhaled corticosteroid; LABA, long-acting β-agonist; LAMA, long-acting muscarinic antagonist; mMRC, modified Medical Research Council questionnaire; SABA, short-acting β-agonist; SAMA, short-acting muscarinic antagonist.

TABLE 80-2	Recommended Escalation Pharmacotherapy for Stable COPD

Target Symptom	Current Therapy	Escalation Therapy
Dyspnea	LABA or LAMA monotherapy	Add additional long-acting bronchodilator if persistent symptoms on monotherapy (LAMA + LABA) If dual bronchodilators do not improve symptoms, change device or active ingredient and/or step back to monotherapy If patient becomes high risk for future exacerbations, choose escalation therapy based on the target symptom of "Exacerbations"
Dyspnea	LABA + ICS	Add additional long-acting bronchodilator if persistent symptoms on dual therapy (LAMA + LABA + ICS) If pneumonia, inappropriate indication, or lack of response to ICS, consider deescalation back to LABA + LAMA only
Exacerbations	LABA or LAMA monotherapy	Add long-acting bronchodilator if persistent exacerbations on monotherapy (LABA + LAMA) If current therapy is LABA and blood eosinophils ≥ 300, consider adding ICS to LABA (LABA + ICS) If current therapy is LABA and blood eosinophils ≥ 100 AND ≥ 2 moderate exacerbations/1 hospitalization, consider adding ICS to LABA (LABA + ICS)
Exacerbations	LABA + ICS	Add long-acting bronchodilator if persistent exacerbations on dual therapy (LAMA + LABA + ICS) If pneumonia, inappropriate indication or lack of response to ICS, consider deescalation back to LABA + LAMA only
Exacerbations	LABA + LAMA + ICS	If FEV1 <50% and presence of chronic bronchitis, consider adding roflumilast If a former or never smoker, consider adding azithromycin daily or three times a week for 12 months If pneumonia, inappropriate indication, or lack of response to ICS, consider deescalation and withdrawal of ICS

Short-Acting Bronchodilators

- Either a short- or long-acting bronchodilator is recommended initially for patients with occasional symptoms (Table 80-1, category A). Short-acting bronchodilators are also recommended for all patients (categories A–D) as rescue or as-needed therapy to manage symptoms. Choices among short-acting bronchodilators include short-acting β_2-agonists (SABAs) or short-acting muscarinic antagonists (SAMAs). Both drug classes have a relatively rapid onset of action, relieve symptoms to a similar degree, and improve exercise tolerance and lung function. Short-acting bronchodilators do not reduce the frequency or severity of COPD exacerbations. If a patient does not achieve adequate symptom control with one agent, combining a SABA with a SAMA is reasonable.

- **Short-acting β_2-agonists (SABAs)** stimulate adenyl cyclase to increase formation of cyclic adenosine monophosphate (cAMP), which mediates relaxation of bronchial smooth muscle. They may also improve mucociliary clearance. SABAs have a rapid onset of effect; they cause only a small improvement in FEV_1 acutely but may still improve symptoms and exercise tolerance. The SABA choices include **albuterol** and **levalbuterol** (Table 80-3). Albuterol is most frequently used and is a racemic mixture of

(R)-albuterol (responsible for bronchodilation) and (S)-albuterol (which has no thera-peutic effect). Levalbuterol is a single-isomer formulation of (R)-albuterol that offers no clear efficacy or safety advantages over albuterol, and it is more expensive. Inhalation is the preferred route for SABAs, and administration via metered-dose or dry powder inhalers (MDIs, DPIs) is at least as effective as nebulization therapy and is more conve-nient and less costly. Inhaled SABAs are generally well tolerated; they can cause sinus tachycardia and rhythm disturbances rarely in predisposed patients. Skeletal muscle tremors can occur initially but generally subside as tolerance develops. Older patients may be more sensitive and experience palpitations, tremors, and "jittery" feelings.

- **Short-acting muscarinic antagonists (SAMAs)** produce bronchodilation by inhibit-ing muscarinic receptor subtypes M_1, M_2, and M_3 in bronchial smooth muscle and mucus glands. This blocks acetylcholine, reducing cyclic guanosine monophosphate (cGMP), which normally acts to constrict bronchial smooth muscle, and decreasing

TABLE 80-3 Select Medications Used for Treatment of COPD[a]

Generic (Brand) Name	Dosage Form	Dosage Frequency[b]
Short-acting β_2-agonists		
Albuterol sulfate (Proventil HFA, Ventolin HFA, Proair HFA)	MDI	Every 4–6 hours PRN
Albuterol sulfate (Proair RespiClick)	DPI	Every 4–6 hours PRN
Levalbuterol hydrochloride (Xopenex, generic)	NEB solution	Every 6–8 hours PRN
Levalbuterol tartrate (Xopenex HFA)	MDI	Every 4–6 hours PRN
Short-acting muscarinic antagonists (SAMAs)		
Ipratropium bromide (Atrovent HFA)	MDI	4 times/day PRN
Ipratropium bromide (generic)	NEB solution	3–4 times/day PRN
Long-acting β_2-agonists (LABAs)		
Arformoterol tartrate (Brovana)	NEB solution	Every 12 hours
Formoterol fumarate (Perforomist)	NEB solution	Every 12 hours
Indacaterol maleate (Arcapta Neohaler)	DPI	Once daily
Olodaterol hydrochloride (Striverdi Respimat)	SMI	Once daily
Salmeterol xinafoate (Serevent Diskus)	DPI	Twice daily
Long-acting muscarinic antagonists (LAMAs)		
Aclidinium bromide (Tudorza Pressair)	DPI	Twice daily
Tiotropium bromide (Spiriva Respimat)	SMI	Once daily
Tiotropium bromide (Spiriva Handihaler)	DPI	Once daily
Glycopyrrolate (Lonhala Magnair)	NEB solution	Twice daily
Glycopyrrolate (Seebri Neohaler)	DPI	Twice daily
Umeclidinium bromide (Incruse Ellipta)	DPI	Once daily
Inhaled corticosteroids		
Beclomethasone dipropionate (Qvar 40, 80)	MDI	Twice daily
Budesonide (Pulmicort Flexhaler)	DPI	Twice daily
Flunisolide (Aerospan HFA)	MDI	Twice daily
Fluticasone propionate (Flovent HFA)	MDI	Twice daily
Mometasone furoate (Asmanex Twisthaler)	DPI	Twice daily

(Continued)

TABLE 80-3 Select Medications Used for Treatment of COPD[a] (*Continued*)		
Generic (Brand) Name	**Dosage Form**	**Dosage Frequency[b]**
Combination inhalers		
SABA/SAMA: albuterol sulfate + ipratropium bromide (Duoneb, generic)	NEB solution	4–6 times/day PRN
SABA/SAMA: albuterol sulfate + ipratropium bromide (Combivent Respimat)	SMI	4–6 times/day PRN
LAMA/LABA: umeclidinium bromide + vilanterol trifenatate (Anoro Ellipta)	DPI	Once daily
LAMA/LABA: tiotropium bromide + olodaterol hydrochloride (Stiolto Respimat)	SMI	Once daily
LAMA/LABA: glycopyrrolate + indacaterol maleate (Utibron Neohaler)	DPI	Twice daily
LAMA/LABA: glycopyrrolate + formoterol fumarate (Bevespi Aerosphere)	MDI	Twice daily
ICS/LABA: budesonide + formoterol fumarate dehydrate (Symbicort)	MDI	Twice daily
ICS/LABA: fluticasone furoate + vilanterol trifenatate (Breo Ellipta)	DPI	Once daily
ICS/LABA: fluticasone propionate + salmeterol xinafoate (Advair Diskus, Airduo RespiClick)	DPI	Twice daily
ICS/LABA: fluticasone propionate + salmeterol xinafoate (Advair HFA)	MDI	Twice daily
ICS/LABA: mometasone furoate + formoterol fumarate (Dulera)	MDI	Twice daily
ICS/LAMA/LABA: fluticasone furoate + umeclidinium bromide + vilanterol trifenatate (Trelegy Ellipta)	DPI	Once daily
Oral medications		
Roflumilast (Daliresp)	Oral tablets	Once daily
Theophylline (Theo-24, generic)	Oral tablets, capsules	Once or twice daily (extended release)

DPI, dry power inhaler; ICS, inhaled corticosteroid; inh, inhalations; LABA, long-acting β_2-agonist; LAMA, long-acting muscarinic antagonist; MDI, metered-dose inhaler; NEB, nebulized; PRN, as needed; SABA, short-acting β_2-agonist; SAMA, short-acting muscarinic antagonist; SMI, soft mist inhaler.
[a]Not all medications are FDA-approved for treatment of COPD.
[b]Consult official product labeling or the medical literature for dosages used for COPD treatment.

mucus secretion. **Ipratropium bromide** is the most commonly prescribed SAMA in the United States (Table 80-3). Improvements in pulmonary function are similar to inhaled SABAs, although ipratropium has a slower onset of action (15–20 minutes vs. 5 minutes for albuterol) and more prolonged effect. Because of its slower onset, ipratropium may be less suitable for as-needed use but is often prescribed in this manner. In contrast to albuterol, patients may experience additional symptom improvement with a larger number of inhalations (eg, 6 puffs every 6 hours, maximum 24 puffs/day), whereas no additional improvement occurs with more frequent use than every 6 hours. The most frequent patient complaints are dry mouth, nausea, and occasionally metallic taste. Because it is poorly absorbed systemically, anticholinergic side effects are uncommon (eg, blurred vision, constipation, urinary retention, nausea, and tachycardia). Inhaled anticholinergics may rarely precipitate narrow-angle glaucoma symptoms.

Long-Acting Bronchodilators

- Long-acting bronchodilators are recommended for patients with persistent symptoms or in whom short-acting therapies do not provide adequate relief (Table 80-1, category B). Long-acting agents are also recommended for patients at high risk for exacerbation (categories C and D). Therapy can be administered as an inhaled long-acting β₂-agonist (LABA) or muscarinic antagonist (LAMA). Compared with short-acting agents, long-acting bronchodilators are more convenient for patients with persistent symptoms and are superior in improving lung function, relieving symptoms, reducing exacerbation frequency and need for hospitalization, and improving quality of life. LABAs and LAMAs are equally effective in managing symptoms, but LAMAs are more effective for preventing exacerbations and should be considered first-line monotherapy for patients at high risk for exacerbation. Treatment selection should consider individual patient response, tolerability, adherence, and economic factors.
- The available LABAs differ primarily by dosing frequency and device type (Table 80-3). **Arformoterol**, **formoterol**, **indacaterol**, and **olodaterol** have an onset of action similar to albuterol (<5 minutes), whereas **salmeterol** has a slower onset (15–20 minutes); however, none of these agents are recommended for acute relief of COPD symptoms. **Vilanterol** is available in the United States only in combination with an inhaled corticosteroid (fluticasone) or LAMA (umeclidinium). There is no dose titration for any of these agents; the starting dose is the effective and recommended dose for all patients.
- The available LAMAs differ in dosing frequency and device type (Table 80-3). They are more selective than ipratropium at blocking muscarinic receptors and dissociate slowly from M₃ receptors, resulting in prolonged bronchodilation. **Aclidinium**, **glycopyrrolate**, and **umeclidinium** have a faster onset of action (5–15 minutes) than **tiotropium** (80 minutes); however, none of these agents are recommended for acute relief of symptoms. There is no dose titration for any of these agents; the starting dose is the effective and recommended dose for all patients.

Combination Muscarinic Antagonists and β₂-Agonists

- Combination bronchodilator regimens are often used as symptoms worsen over time. Combining bronchodilators with different mechanisms of action allows use of the lowest possible effective doses and reduces potential adverse effects from individual agents. Short-acting bronchodilators may be combined for patients experiencing persistent symptoms, although step-up to long-acting bronchodilator monotherapy is usually preferred (Table 80-1).
- Guidelines recommend combining long-acting bronchodilators (LAMA/LABA) for patients who have persistent symptoms or recurrent exacerbations on bronchodilator monotherapy. The combination provides significant improvement in lung function, symptoms, and quality-of-life measures compared with LABA or LAMA monotherapy. In addition, dual long-acting bronchodilator therapy decreases the frequency of moderate-to-severe exacerbations compared to either LAMA or LABA monotherapy.

Methylxanthines

- **Theophylline** and **aminophylline** may produce bronchodilation by several mechanisms, including inhibition of phosphodiesterase, thereby increasing cAMP levels.
- Chronic theophylline use in COPD may improve lung function and gas exchange. Subjectively, theophylline reduces dyspnea, increases exercise tolerance, and improves respiratory drive.
- Methylxanthines have a limited role in COPD therapy because of the availability of LABAs and LAMAs as well as significant methylxanthine drug interactions and interpatient variability in dosage requirements. Theophylline may be considered in patients intolerant of or unable to use inhaled bronchodilators.
- Sustained-release theophylline preparations are most appropriate for long-term COPD management; they improve adherence and achieve more consistent serum concentrations than rapid-release products. Caution should be used in switching

from one sustained-release preparation to another because of variability in sustained-release characteristics.

- Initiate theophylline therapy with 200 mg twice daily and titrate upward every 3–5 days to the target dose; most patients require 400–900 mg daily. Make dose adjustments based on trough serum concentrations. A therapeutic range of 8–15 mcg/mL (44–83 μmol/L) is targeted to minimize risk of toxicity. Once a dose is established, monitor concentrations once or twice a year unless the disease worsens, medications that interfere with theophylline metabolism are added, or toxicity is suspected.

- Common theophylline side effects include dyspepsia, nausea, vomiting, diarrhea, headache, dizziness, and tachycardia. Arrhythmias and seizures may occur, especially at toxic concentrations.

- Factors that decrease theophylline clearance and lead to reduced dosage requirements include advanced age, bacterial or viral pneumonia, heart failure, liver dysfunction, hypoxemia from acute decompensation, and drugs such as cimetidine, macrolides, and fluoroquinolone antibiotics.

- Factors that may enhance theophylline clearance and result in need for higher doses include tobacco and marijuana smoking, hyperthyroidism, and drugs such as phenytoin, phenobarbital, and rifampin.

Corticosteroids

- Anti-inflammatory mechanisms of corticosteroids in COPD include reducing capillary permeability to decrease mucus, inhibiting release of proteolytic enzymes from leukocytes, and inhibiting prostaglandins.

- Inhaled corticosteroid (ICS) therapy is recommended for initial treatment in patients at high risk of exacerbation and with eosinophils >300 cells/μL (Table 80-1, categories C and D). For escalation therapy, ICS may be considered for patients who have recurrent exacerbations despite optimal therapy with inhaled bronchodilators.

- The clinical benefits of ICS therapy (including decreased exacerbation frequency and improved lung function and health status) have been observed with combination therapy, primarily as an addition to LABA monotherapy. Given lack of supporting evidence, ICS monotherapy is not recommended for patients with COPD.

- For patients with recurrent exacerbations despite optimal long-acting bronchodilator monotherapy, combination therapy with dual long-acting bronchodilators (LAMA/LABA) is preferred over combination therapy with ICS/LABA (Table 80-1). Dual therapy with ICS/LABA may be considered instead of LAMA/LABA for patients with blood eosinophil counts ≥300 cells/μL (0.3×10^9/L).

- For patients with persistent symptoms and recurrent exacerbations on dual inhaled therapy, triple therapy with LAMA/LABA/ICS is recommended as initial escalation therapy (Table 80-1). Given the risk of adverse ICS effects, some clinicians avoid triple inhalation therapy for patients with persistent exacerbations and lower blood eosinophil counts (<100 cells/μL [0.1×10^9/L]) in favor of oral alternatives such as roflumilast or azithromycin.

- Short-term systemic corticosteroids may also be considered for acute exacerbations. Chronic systemic corticosteroids should be avoided in COPD because of questionable benefits and high risk of toxicity.

- The moderate-to-high ICS doses used in clinical trials of COPD have been associated with an increased risk of pneumonia and mycobacterial pulmonary infections. Other adverse effects include hoarseness, sore throat, oral candidiasis, and skin bruising. Severe side effects such as adrenal suppression, osteoporosis, and cataract formation occur less frequently than with systemic corticosteroids, but clinicians should monitor patients receiving high-dose chronic inhaled therapy. Treat patients with the lowest effective ICS dose to minimize risk of fracture.

Roflumilast

- **Roflumilast** is a phosphodiesterase 4 (PDE4) inhibitor that relaxes airway smooth muscle and decreases activity of inflammatory cells and mediators such as TNF-α and IL-8. Roflumilast is recommended for patients with recurrent exacerbations despite treatment with triple inhalation therapy (LAMA/LABA/ICS; Table 80-1). It may also be considered as escalation therapy for patients with recurrent exacerbations on dual long-acting bronchodilators (LAMA/LABA) who are not candidates for ICS, such as those with low blood eosinophil count (<100 cells/μL [0.1×10^9/L]) or who are at higher risk of adverse effects associated with ICS. Because theophylline and roflumilast have similar mechanisms of action, they should not be used together.

- Major adverse effects include diarrhea, nausea, decreased appetite, weight loss, headache, and neuropsychiatric effects such as suicidal thoughts, insomnia, anxiety, and new or worsened depression. Although most symptoms usually resolve over time, a low starting dose (250 mcg orally once daily) is recommended for the first 4 weeks before increasing to the maintenance dose (500 mcg once daily). Caution is advised in patients with a history of depression or suicidality.

- Roflumilast is metabolized by CYP3A4 and 1A2; coadministration with strong CYP P450 inducers is not recommended due to potential for subtherapeutic plasma concentrations. Use caution when administering roflumilast with strong CYP P450 inhibitors due to potential for adverse effects.

Azithromycin

- Chronic **azithromycin** has been associated with lower rates of COPD exacerbation but also with colonization with macrolide resistant bacteria and hearing deficits. In addition, the azithromycin product labeling includes a precaution about QT prolongation after a retrospective study reported increased cardiac events with short courses of azithromycin.

- Based on limited evidence supporting long-term treatment (beyond 1 year), current guidelines recommend to consider adding chronic azithromycin only for patients with recurrent exacerbations despite optimal therapy and who are not active smokers (Table 80-1). Clinicians may consider azithromycin for individual patients at high risk for exacerbations but must carefully weigh the risks and benefits of therapy.

α1-Antitrypsin Replacement Therapy

- For patients with inherited AAT deficiency-associated emphysema, treatment focuses on reduction of risk factors such as smoking, symptomatic treatment with bronchodilators, and augmentation therapy with replacement AAT.

- Several proprietary **alpha$_1$-proteinase inhibitors** are available: Glassia, Prolastin-C, Aralast, Aralast-NP, and Zemaira. Augmentation therapy is intended to maintain serum concentrations above the protective threshold of 10 μmol/L throughout the dosing interval. The recommended dosing regimen is 60 mg/kg IV given once weekly, usually at a rate of 0.08 mL/kg/min (consult individual product labeling), adjusted to patient tolerance. Augmentation therapy can cost over $50,000 annually.

COPD EXACERBATIONS

- A COPD exacerbation is defined as a change in the patient's baseline symptoms (dyspnea, cough, or sputum production) beyond day-to-day variability sufficient to warrant a change in management.

- The primary physiologic change is often a worsening of ABG values due to poor gas exchange and increased muscle fatigue. With severe exacerbations, profound hypoxemia and hypercapnia can be accompanied by respiratory acidosis and respiratory failure.

- Although criteria used to define acute exacerbations vary, most rely on a change in one or more of the following clinical findings: worsening dyspnea, increased sputum volume, or increased sputum purulence (Table 80-4).

- Additional symptoms may include chest tightness, increased need for bronchodilators, malaise, fatigue, and decreased exercise tolerance. Physical exam may reveal fever, wheezing, and decreased breath sounds. Obtain a sputum sample for Gram stain and culture and a chest x-ray to evaluate for new infiltrates.

TABLE 80-4	Staging Acute Exacerbations of COPD
Mild (type 1)	One cardinal symptom[a] plus at least one of the following: upper respiratory tract infection within 5 days, fever without other explanation, increased wheezing, increased cough, increase in respiratory or heart rate >20% above baseline
Moderate (type 2)	Two cardinal symptoms
Severe (type 3)	Three cardinal symptoms

[a]Cardinal symptoms include worsening of dyspnea, increase in sputum volume, and increase in sputum purulence.

- The diagnosis of acute respiratory failure is made based on an acute change in ABGs: an acute drop in Pao_2 of 10–15 mm Hg (1.3–2.0 kPa) or any acute increase in $Paco_2$ that decreases the serum pH to 7.3 or less. Additional indications of respiratory failure include restlessness, confusion, tachycardia, diaphoresis, cyanosis, hypotension, irregular breathing, miosis, and unconsciousness.
- Goals of Treatment: (1) Minimize the negative consequences of the acute exacerbation (ie, reduce symptoms, prevent hospitalization, shorten hospital stay, prevent acute respiratory failure or death) and (2) prevent future exacerbations.

NONPHARMACOLOGIC THERAPY

- Provide oxygen therapy for patients with significant hypoxemia (eg, oxygen saturation <90% [0.90]). Use caution because many COPD patients rely on mild hypoxemia to trigger their drive to breathe. Overly aggressive oxygen administration to patients with chronic hypercapnia may result in respiratory depression and respiratory failure. Adjust oxygen to achieve Pao_2 >60 mm Hg (8.0 kPa) or oxygen saturation (Sao_2) >90% (0.90). Obtain ABG after oxygen initiation to monitor CO_2 retention resulting from hypoventilation.
- Noninvasive positive-pressure ventilation (NPPV) provides ventilatory support with oxygen and pressurized airflow using a face or nasal mask without endotracheal intubation. NPPV is not appropriate for patients with altered mental status, severe acidosis, respiratory arrest, or cardiovascular instability. Intubation and mechanical ventilation may be needed in patients failing NPPV or who are poor candidates for NPPV.

PHARMACOLOGIC THERAPY

Bronchodilators

- Dose and frequency of bronchodilators are increased during acute exacerbations to provide symptomatic relief. SABAs are preferred because of rapid onset of action. Muscarinic antagonists may be added if symptoms persist despite increased doses of β_2-agonists. LABAs or LAMAs should not be used for quick relief of symptoms or on an as-needed basis.
- Bronchodilators may be administered via MDI, DPI, or nebulization with equal efficacy. Nebulization may be considered for patients with severe dyspnea who are unable to hold their breath after actuation of an MDI.
- Theophylline should generally be avoided due to lack of evidence documenting benefit and the concern for adverse effects.

Corticosteroids

- Treatment with systemic corticosteroids in acute exacerbations improves oxygenation and recovery time, shortens hospitalization, and reduces risk of relapse.
- Although the optimal corticosteroid dose and duration are unknown, prednisone 40 mg orally daily (or equivalent) for 5 days is effective for most patients. Longer courses have been associated with increased risk of pneumonia, hospitalization, and all--cause mortality, and shorter courses (5–7 days) are preferred to avoid adverse effects.

Antimicrobial Therapy

- In order to limit unnecessary use, antibiotics should be initiated in any of these clinical situations: (1) patients presenting with three cardinal symptoms of acute exacerbation, (2) patients presenting with two cardinal symptoms as long as one is increased sputum purulence, and (3) patients requiring mechanical ventilation regardless of symptoms. Utility of sputum Gram stain and culture is questionable because some patients have chronic bacterial colonization of the bronchial tree between exacerbations. Use of C-reactive protein (CRP) as a biomarker to guide antimicrobial therapy decisions may be reasonable.
- Selection of empiric antimicrobial therapy should be based on the most likely organisms: *Haemophilus influenzae, Moraxella catarrhalis, Streptococcus pneumoniae,* and *Haemophilus parainfluenzae.* Drug-resistant pneumococci, β-lactamase–producing *H. influenzae* and *M. catarrhalis,* and enteric gram-negative organisms, including *Pseudomonas aeruginosa,* may be present in complicated acute exacerbations.
- Table 80-5 summarizes the most common organisms based on patient presentation and recommended antimicrobial therapy. Continue antimicrobial therapy for at least 5–7 days. If the patient deteriorates or does not improve as anticipated, hospitalization may be necessary, and more aggressive attempts should be made to identify potential pathogens responsible for the exacerbation.

TABLE 80-5	Recommended Antimicrobial Therapy for Acute Exacerbations of COPD	
Patient Characteristics	**Likely Pathogens**	**Recommended Therapy**
Uncomplicated exacerbations (<4 exacerbations per year, no comorbid illness)	*S. pneumoniae* *H. influenzae* *M. catarrhalis* *H. parainfluenzae* Resistance uncommon	Macrolide (azithromycin, clarithromycin) Second- or third-generation cephalosporin Doxycycline Therapies not recommended[a]: TMP/SMX, amoxicillin, first-generation cephalosporins, erythromycin
Complicated exacerbations (Age ≥65 and >4 exacerbations per year, presence of comorbid illness)	As above plus drug-resistant pneumococci, β-lactamase–producing *H. influenzae* and *M. catarrhalis*	Amoxicillin/clavulanate Fluoroquinolone with enhanced pneumococcal activity (levofloxacin, gemifloxacin, moxifloxacin)
Presence of risk factors for colonization and infection with multidrug resistant pathogens: ✓ Need for chronic corticosteroid therapy ✓ Recent hospitalization (90 days) ✓ Recent antibiotic therapy (90 days) ✓ Resident of long-term care facility	Some enteric gram-negatives As above plus *P. aeruginosa*	Fluoroquinolone with enhanced pneumococcal and *P. aeruginosa* activity (levofloxacin) IV therapy if required: β-lactamase–resistant penicillin with antipseudomonal activity, third- or fourth-generation cephalosporin with antipseudomonal activity

TMP-SMX, trimethoprim-sulfamethoxazole.
[a]TMP/SMX should not be used due to increasing pneumococcal resistance; amoxicillin and first-generation cephalosporins are not recommended due to β-lactamase susceptibility; and erythromycin is not recommended due to insufficient activity against *H. influenzae.*

EVALUATION OF THERAPEUTIC OUTCOMES

- In chronic stable COPD, assess pulmonary function tests annually and with any treatment additions or discontinuations. Other outcome measures are symptom scores, quality-of-life assessments, exacerbation rates, emergency department visits, and hospitalizations.
- In acute exacerbations of COPD, assess white blood cell count, vital signs, chest x-ray, and changes in frequency of dyspnea, sputum volume, and sputum purulence at the onset and throughout treatment of the exacerbation. In more severe exacerbations, ABG and Sao_2 should also be monitored.
- Evaluate patient medication adherence, side effects, and potential drug interactions at every encounter.

See Chapter 45, Chronic Obstructive Pulmonary Disease, authored by Sharya V. Bourdet and Dennis M. Williams, for a more detailed discussion of this topic.

CHAPTER

81 | Benign Prostatic Hyperplasia

- *Benign prostatic hyperplasia* (BPH), is a non-cancerous condition in which an enlarged prostate compresses the urethra, blocking the outflow of urine. It is characterized by three stages: BPH, benign prostatic enlargement (BPE), and benign prostatic obstruction (BPO).

PATHOPHYSIOLOGY

- Three types of prostate gland tissue are epithelial or glandular, stromal or smooth muscle, and capsule. Both stromal tissue and capsule are embedded with α_1-adrenergic receptors.
- The precise pathophysiologic mechanisms that cause BPH are not clear. Both intraprostatic dihydrotestosterone (DHT) and type II 5α-reductase are believed to be involved.
- BPH commonly results from both static (gradual enlargement of the prostate) and dynamic (agents or situations that increase α-adrenergic tone and constrict the gland's smooth muscle) factors. Examples of drugs that can exacerbate symptoms include testosterone, α-adrenergic agonists (eg, decongestants), and those with significant anticholinergic effects (eg, antihistamines, phenothiazines, tricyclic antidepressants, antispasmodics, and antiparkinsonian agents).

CLINICAL PRESENTATION

- Patients present with a variety of signs and symptoms categorized as obstructive or irritative. Symptoms vary over time.
- Obstructive signs and symptoms result when dynamic and/or static factors reduce bladder emptying. Patients experience urinary hesitancy, urine dribbles out of the penis, and the bladder feels full even after voiding.
- Irritative signs and symptoms are common and result from long-standing obstruction at the bladder neck. Patients experience urinary frequency, urgency, and nocturia.
- Obstructive and irritative voiding symptoms are referred to as lower urinary tract symptoms (LUTS) which are not limited to BPH but may also be caused by neurogenic bladder or urinary tract infections.
- BPH progression may produce complications including urinary retention, chronic kidney disease, gross hematuria, urinary incontinence, recurrent urinary tract infection, bladder diverticula, and bladder stones.

DIAGNOSIS

- Includes careful medical history, physical examination, objective measures of bladder emptying (eg, peak and average urinary flow rate and postvoid residual [PVR] urine volume), and laboratory tests (eg, urinalysis and prostate-specific antigen [PSA]).
- On digital rectal examination, the prostate is usually but not always enlarged (>20 g), soft, smooth, and symmetric.

TREATMENT

- <u>Goals of Treatment</u>: The goals are to control symptoms, prevent progression of complications, and delay need for surgical intervention.

- Management options include watchful waiting, pharmacologic therapy, and surgical intervention. The choice depends on severity of signs and symptoms (Table 81-1).
- Watchful waiting is appropriate for patients with mild disease (Fig. 81-1). Patients are reassessed at 6–12 month intervals and educated about behavior modification, such as fluid restriction before bedtime, minimizing caffeine and alcohol intake, frequent emptying of the bladder, and avoiding drugs that exacerbate voiding symptoms.

PHARMACOLOGIC THERAPY

- Pharmacologic therapy is appropriate for patients with moderate BPH symptoms and as an interim measure for patients with severe BPH.
- Pharmacologic therapy interferes with the stimulatory effect of testosterone on prostate gland enlargement (reduces the static factor), relaxes prostatic smooth muscle (reduces the dynamic factor), or relaxes bladder detrusor muscle (Table 81-2).
- Initiate therapy with an α_1-adrenergic antagonist for faster onset of symptom relief. Select a 5α-reductase inhibitor in patients with a prostate gland of more than 40 g who cannot tolerate the cardiovascular adverse effects of α_1-adrenergic antagonists. Consider combination therapy for symptomatic patients with a prostate gland of more than 40 g and PSA of 1.4 ng/mL (1.4 mcg/L) or more.
- Consider monotherapy with a phosphodiesterase inhibitor (PI) or use in combination with an α-adrenergic antagonist when erectile dysfunction and BPH are present.
- Combination therapy may reduce bothersome symptoms but may also result in an increased risk of adverse effects and drug interactions, higher cost of treatment, lower rates of adherence, and modest improvement in objective measures of BPH improvement.

α-Adrenergic Antagonists

- α-Adrenergic antagonists relax smooth muscle in the prostate and bladder neck, increasing urinary flow rates by 2–3 mL/sec in 60%–70% of patients and reducing PVR urine volumes. These agents do not decrease prostate volume or PSA levels. Second- and third-generation α_1-adrenergic antagonists are considered equally effective for treatment of BPH.
- **Prazosin, terazosin, doxazosin**, and **alfuzosin** are second-generation nonselective α_1-adrenergic antagonists. They antagonize peripheral vascular α_1-adrenergic receptors in addition to those in the prostate resulting in adverse effects such as first-dose syncope, orthostatic hypotension, and dizziness. Dose titration is recommended for immediate-release formulations of doxazosin and terazosin to minimize these adverse effects. Current practice guidelines do not recommend prazosin due to multiple doses/day and significant cardiovascular adverse effects. Alfuzosin is less likely to cause cardiovascular adverse effects than other second-generation agents and is considered functionally and clinically uroselective.

TABLE 81-1	Categories of BPH Disease Severity Based on Symptoms and Signs	
Disease Severity	**AUA Symptom Score**	**Typical Symptoms and Signs**
Mild	≤7	Asymptomatic
		Peak urinary flow rate <10 mL/sec
		PVR urine volume >25–50 mL
Moderate	8–19	All of the above signs plus obstructive voiding symptoms and irritative voiding symptoms (signs of detrusor instability)
Severe	≥20	All of the above plus one or more complications of BPH

AUA, American Urological Association; BPH, benign prostatic hyperplasia; PVR, postvoid residual volume.

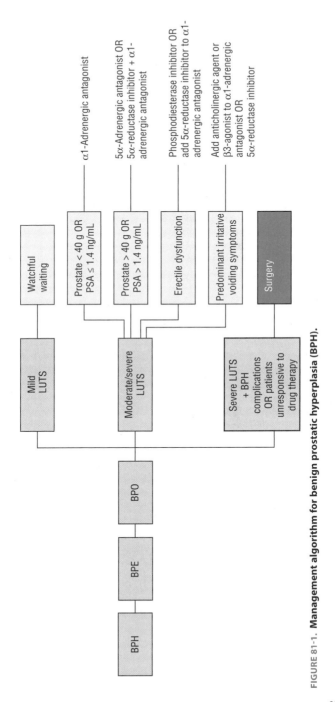

FIGURE 81-1. Management algorithm for benign prostatic hyperplasia (BPH).

TABLE 81-2 Dosing of Drugs Used in Treatment of Benign Prostatic Hyperplasia

Drug	Brand Name	Initial Dose	Usual Dose	Special Population Dose
α-Adrenergic Antagonists				
Prazosin	Minipress	0.5 mg twice a day orally	1–5 mg twice a day orally	To up-titrate the dose, double the dose every 2 weeks.
Terazosin	Hytrin	1 mg at bedtime orally	10–20 mg daily orally	Take extra care if the patient is taking other drugs that lower blood pressure. No dosage adjustment is required for patients with renal or hepatic impairment.
Doxazosin	Cardura Cardura XL	1 mg daily orally 4 mg daily orally	8 mg daily orally 4–8 mg daily	When switching from the immediate- to the extended-release formulation, start with 4 mg of the extended-release formulation no matter what maintenance dose of immediate-release doxazosin the patient is taking. No dosage adjustment is required for patients with renal or hepatic impairment.
Alfuzosin	Uroxatral	10 mg daily orally	10 mg daily orally (no dose titration)	This is an extended-release formulation, and it should not be chewed or crushed. The drug should be taken after meals and used cautiously in patients with creatinine clearance less than 30 mL/min (0.5 mL/sec). No dosage adjustment is required for patients with mild hepatic impairment. It is contraindicated in patients with moderate-to-severe hepatic impairment.
Tamsulosin	Flomax	0.4 mg daily orally	0.4–0.8 mg daily orally	This is an extended-release formulation, and it should not be chewed or crushed. The drug should be taken after meals. No dosage adjustment is needed in patients with renal or liver impairment.
Silodosin	Rapaflo	8 mg daily orally	8 mg daily orally (no dose titration)	This drug is contraindicated when creatinine clearance is less than 30 mL/min (0.5 mL/sec). If creatinine clearance is 30–50 mL/min (0.5–0.83 mL/sec), use 4 mg daily orally, preferably after the same meal each day. No dosage adjustment is required for patients with mild-to-moderate hepatic impairment. Should not be given to patients on potent CYP 3A4 inhibitors or with severe hepatic impairment.

5α-Reductase Inhibitors

Finasteride	Proscar	5 mg daily orally	No dosage adjustment in patients with renal impairment. Use cautiously in patients with hepatic impairment.
Dutasteride	Avodart	0.5 mg daily orally	No dosage adjustment in patients with renal impairment. Use cautiously in patients with hepatic impairment.
Dutasteride + tamsulosin	Jalyn	1 tablet (equivalent to 0.5-mg dutasteride + 0.4-mg tamsulosin) daily orally	1 tablet daily orally	No dosage adjustment needed in patients with renal or moderate hepatic impairment.

Phosphodiesterase Inhibitor

Tadalafil	Cialis	5 mg daily orally	5 mg daily orally	If creatinine clearance is 30–50 mL/min (0.5–0.83 mL/sec), use 2.5 mg daily orally. Do not use if creatinine clearance is less than 30 mL/min (0.5 mL/sec). Use cautiously in patients with mild-moderate hepatic impairment. Avoid in patients with severe hepatic impairment.

Anticholinergic Agents

Darifenacin	Enablex	7.5 mg daily orally	7.5–15 mg daily orally	This is an extended-release formulation and it should not be chewed or crushed. To up-titrate the dose, double the dose after 2 weeks. If the patient is taking a potent CYP3A4 inhibitor (eg, ketoconazole, itraconazole, ritonavir, nelfinavir, and clarithromycin), do not exceed 7.5 mg daily orally. No dosage adjustment is needed for patients with renal impairment. Use a maximum dose of 7.5 mg daily for patients with moderate hepatic impairment. Do not use in patients with severe hepatic impairment.
Fesoterodine	Toviaz	4 mg daily orally	4–8 mg daily orally	This is an extended-release formulation, and it should not be chewed or crushed. If the patient is taking a potent CYP3A4 inhibitor (eg, ketoconazole, itraconazole, ritonavir, nelfinavir, and clarithromycin), do not exceed 4 mg daily orally. If the creatinine clearance is less than 30 mL/min (0.5 mL/sec), do not exceed 4 mg daily orally. Use is not recommended in patients with severe hepatic impairment.

(Continued)

TABLE 81-2 Dosing of Drugs Used in Treatment of Benign Prostatic Hyperplasia (Continued)

Drug	Brand Name	Initial Dose	Usual Dose	Special Population Dose
Oxybutynin	Ditropan	5 mg two to three times a day orally	5–10 mg two to three times a day orally	Increase daily dose at 5-mg increments at weekly intervals. No specific dosing modifications available for patients with renal or hepatic impairment; use cautiously in these patients.
	Ditropan XL	5 mg daily orally	5–30 mg daily orally	This is an extended-release formulation, and it should not be crushed or chewed. Increase daily dose at 5-mg increments at weekly intervals. No specific dosing modifications available for patients with renal impairment; use cautiously in these patients.
	Oxytrol TDS	1 patch (3.9-mg oxybutynin) twice weekly	1 patch (3.9 mg) twice weekly	This is a transdermal patch. Apply to abdomen, hip, or buttock. Rotate application site. Do not expose patch to sunlight. No specific dosing modifications available for patients with renal or hepatic impairment; use cautiously in these patients.
	Gelnique 10% gel	1-g gel (100-mg oxybutynin) daily	1-g gel (100-mg oxybutynin) daily	This is available as premeasured dose packets. Apply to abdomen, thighs, upper arms, or shoulders. Wash hands after application. Do not bathe, shower, or swim for 1 hour after application. Cover application site with clothing until medication dries on skin. Rotate application site daily. No specific dosing modifications available for patients with renal or hepatic impairment; use cautiously in these patients.
Solifenacin	VESIcare	5 mg daily orally	5–10 mg daily orally	If the creatinine clearance is less than 30 mL/min (0.5 mL/sec) or the patient has moderate hepatic impairment, do not exceed 5 mg daily orally. Do not use if the patient has severe hepatic impairment. If the patient is taking a potent CYP3A4 inhibitor (eg, ketoconazole, itraconazole, ritonavir, nelfinavir, and clarithromycin), do not exceed 5 mg daily orally
Tolterodine	Detrol	2 mg twice daily orally	1–2 mg twice daily orally	If the patient has significant renal impairment or severe hepatic impairment, limit dose to 1 mg twice a day.
	Detrol LA	4 mg daily orally	2–4 mg daily orally	This is an extended-release formulation, and it should not be chewed or crushed. If the creatinine clearance is 10–30 mL/min (0.17–0.5 mL/sec) or the patient has mild-moderate hepatic impairment, do not exceed 2 mg daily orally. If the creatinine clearance is less than 10 mL/min (0.17 mL/sec), do not use Detrol LA. If the patient has severe hepatic impairment, use of the extended-release formulation is not recommended.

Trospium	Sanctura	20 mg twice daily orally	20 mg twice daily orally	Avoid alcohol ingestion for 2 hours after a dose. Use cautiously in patients with moderate-severe hepatic impairment. In patients older than 75 years, use the immediate-release formulation and start with 20 mg daily orally. If the creatinine clearance is less than 30 mL/min (0.5 mL/sec), use 20-mg immediate-release formulation
	Sanctura XR	60 mg daily orally	60 mg daily orally	This is an extended-release formulation, and it should not be chewed or crushed. This is not recommended in patients with creatinine clearance less than 30 mL/min (0.5 mL/sec). This should be used cautiously in patients with severe hepatic impairment.

β₃-Adrenergic Agonist

Mirabegron	Myrbetriq	25 mg daily orally	25–50 mg daily orally	This is an extended-release formulation. Do not chew, crush, or divide tablet. In patients with a creatinine clearance of 15-29 mL/min (0.25–0.48 mL/sec) or those with moderate hepatic impairment, the maximum daily dose should be 25 mg daily. This drug is not recommended in patients with creatinine clearance less than 15 mL/min (0.25 mL/sec) or those with severe hepatic impairment.
Vibegron	Gemtesa	75 mg daily orally	75 mg daily orally (no dose titration)	This tablet may be crushed and administered in applesauce or put into a glass of water for ease of administration. No dosage adjustment for patients with a creatinine clearance of 15 mL/min (0.25 mL/sec) or more. Do not use in patients with creatinine clearance less than 15 mL/min (0.25 mL/sec). No dosage adjustment for patients with mild-to-moderate hepatic impairment. Do not use in patients with severe hepatic impairment.

- **Tamsulosin** and **silodosin**, third-generation α_1-adrenergic antagonists, are selective for prostatic α_{1A}-receptors. Therefore, they do not cause peripheral vascular smooth muscle relaxation and associated hypotension. Dose titration is minimal and the onset of peak action is seen within a week.
- Potential drug interactions include decreased metabolism of α_1-adrenergic antagonists with CYP 3A4 inhibitors (eg, cimetidine and diltiazem) and increased catabolism of α_1-adrenergic antagonists with concurrent use of CYP 3A4 stimulators (eg, carbamazepine and phenytoin).

5α-Reductase Inhibitors

- 5α-Reductase inhibitors interfere with the stimulatory effect of testosterone. These agents slow disease progression and decrease the risk of complications.
- Compared with α_1-adrenergic antagonists, disadvantages of 5α-reductase inhibitors include 6–12 months of use to maximally shrink the prostate, less likelihood of inducing objective urinary symptom improvement, and more sexual dysfunction. They are considered second-line therapy in sexually active males.
- **Dutasteride** inhibits types I and II 5α-reductase, whereas **finasteride** inhibits only type II.
- 5α-Reductase inhibitors may be preferred in patients with uncontrolled arrhythmias, poorly controlled angina, requirement for multiple antihypertensives, or intolerance to the hypotensive effects of α_1-adrenergic antagonists.
- Measure PSA at baseline and again after 6 months of therapy. If PSA does not decrease by 50% after 6 months of therapy in an adherent patient, evaluate the patient for prostate cancer.
- 5α-Reductase inhibitors are in FDA pregnancy category X and are therefore contraindicated in pregnant women. Women who are pregnant or seeking to become pregnant should not handle the tablets or have contact with semen from men taking 5α-reductase inhibitors.

Phosphodiesterase Inhibitors

- Increase in cyclic GMP by PIs relaxes smooth muscle in the prostate, urethra, pelvic blood vessels, and bladder neck.
- **Tadalafil** 5 mg daily improves voiding symptoms but does not increase urinary flow rate or reduce PVR urine volume. Combination therapy with α-adrenergic antagonist results in significant improvement in LUTS, increased urinary flow rates, and decreased PVR volume.

Anticholinergic Agents

- Addition of **oxybutynin** and **tolterodine** to α-adrenergic antagonists relieves irritative voiding symptoms including urinary frequency, urgency, and nocturia. Start with lowest effective dose to determine tolerance of CNS adverse effects and dry mouth. Measure PVR urine volume before initiating treatment (should be less than 150 mL).
- Consider transdermal (eg, oxybutynin) or extended-release formulations (eg, tolterodine) or uroselective agents (eg, **darifenacin** or **solifenacin**) if systemic anticholinergic adverse effects are poorly tolerated.
- **Trospium** or **fesoterodine** have a lower propensity to cross the blood-brain barrier making them an option for older adults at risk of sedation and confusion.

B$_3$-Adrenergic Agonist

- **Mirabegron** and **vibegron** are β_3-adrenergic agonists that relax the detrusor muscle reducing irritative voiding systems, increase urinary bladder capacity and the interval between voidings. They do not cause anticholinergic adverse effects and are alternatives to anticholinergic agents in patients with LUTS.

SURGICAL INTERVENTION

- Prostatectomy, performed transurethrally or suprapubically, is the gold standard for treatment of patients with moderate-to-severe symptoms, who are not responsive to or cannot tolerate adverse effects of drug therapy, who are noncompliant with drug therapy, or who prefer surgical intervention. Surgical intervention is always indicated for patients with complications of BPH, including acute urinary retention not responsive to drug treatment, chronic urinary retention associated with decreased renal function or overflow urinary incontinence, urolithiasis, recurrent urinary tract infection, or recurrent hematuria.
- Retrograde ejaculation complicates up to 75% of transurethral prostatectomy procedures. Other complications seen in 2%–15% of patients are bleeding, urinary incontinence, and erectile dysfunction.

PHYTOTHERAPY

- Although widely used in Europe for BPH, phytotherapy with products such as saw palmetto berry (*Serenoa repens*), stinging nettle (*Urtica dioica*), and African plum (*Pygeum africanum*) are not recommended. Studies are inconclusive, and these agents are not regulated by the FDA.

EVALUATION OF THERAPEUTIC OUTCOMES

- The primary therapeutic outcome of BPH therapy is restoring adequate urinary flow with minimal treatment-related adverse effects. Assess efficacy 6–12 weeks after starting treatment.
- Outcome depends on the patient's perception of effectiveness and acceptability of therapy. The American Urological Association Symptom Score is a validated standardized instrument that can be used to assess patient quality of life.
- Objective measures of bladder emptying (eg, urinary flow rate and PVR urine volume) are useful measures in patients considering surgery.
- Monitor laboratory tests (eg, blood urea nitrogen, creatinine, and PSA) and urinalysis regularly. An annual digital rectal examination and PSA are recommended if life expectancy is at least 10 years.

See Chapter 104, Benign Prostatic Hyperplasia, authored by Mary Lee and Roohollah Sharifi, for a more detailed discussion of this topic.

Erectile Dysfunction

- *Erectile dysfunction* (ED) is the persistent (minimum of 3 months) or recurrent failure to achieve or maintain a penile erection suitable for sexual intercourse. Patients often refer to it as impotence.

PATHOPHYSIOLOGY

- ED can result from any single abnormality or combination of abnormalities of the four systems necessary for a normal penile erection. Vascular, neurologic, or hormonal etiologies of ED are referred to as *organic ED*. Patients who do not respond to psychogenic stimuli and have no organic cause for dysfunction have *psychogenic ED*.
- The penis has two corpora cavernosa and one corpus spongiosum, which contain interconnected sinuses that fill with blood to produce an erection that is sustained by occlusion of venous outflow from the corpora.
- Acetylcholine works with other neurotransmitters (ie, cyclic guanylate monophosphate [cGMP], cyclic adenosine monophosphate [cAMP], or vasoactive intestinal polypeptide) to produce penile arterial vasodilation and ultimately an erection.
- Organic ED is associated with diseases that compromise vascular flow to the corpora cavernosum (eg, peripheral vascular disease, arteriosclerosis, and essential hypertension), impair nerve conduction to the brain (eg, Parkinson's disease, epilepsy, spinal cord injury, and stroke), or impair peripheral nerve conduction (eg, diabetes mellitus). Secondary ED is associated with hypogonadism.
- Psychogenic ED is associated with malaise, reactive depression or performance anxiety, sedation, Alzheimer disease, hypothyroidism, and mental disorders. Patients with psychogenic ED generally have a higher response rate to interventions than those with organic ED.
- Social habits (eg, cigarette smoking and excessive ethanol intake) and medications (Table 82-1) can also cause ED.

CLINICAL PRESENTATION

- Signs and symptoms of ED can be difficult to detect. The patient's partner is often the first to report ED to the healthcare provider.
- Nonadherence to drugs thought to cause ED can be a sign of ED.

DIAGNOSIS

- Key diagnostic assessments include description of ED severity, medical, psychological, and surgical histories, review of concurrent medications, physical examination, assessment of cardiac reserve, and laboratory tests (ie, serum blood glucose, lipid profile, and testosterone level).
- Assess the severity of ED with a standardized questionnaire, such as the International Index of Erectile Function (IIEF).

TREATMENT

- <u>Goals of Treatment</u>: The goal is to improve the quantity and quality of penile erections suitable for intercourse.
- The Third Princeton Consensus Conference recommendations (2012) are a widely accepted multidisciplinary approach to managing erectile dysfunction. The first step in the management of ED is to identify and, if possible, reverse underlying causes. Psychotherapy can be used as monotherapy for psychogenic ED or as an adjunct to specific treatments.
- Treatment options include vacuum erection devices (VEDs), medications (Table 82-2), and surgery. Although no option is ideal, the least invasive options are chosen first (Fig. 82-1).

TABLE 82-1 Medication Classes That Can Cause Erectile Dysfunction

Drug Class	Proposed Mechanism by Which Drug Causes Erectile Dysfunction	Special Notes
Anticholinergic agents (antihistamines, antiparkinsonian agents, tricyclic antidepressants, phenothiazines)	Anticholinergic activity	• Second-generation nonsedating antihistamines (eg, loratadine, fexofenadine, or cetirizine) are associated with less erectile dysfunction than first-generation agents. • Selective serotonin reuptake inhibitor (SSRI) and multiple receptor reuptake inhibitor antidepressants cause less erectile dysfunction than tricyclic antidepressants. Of the SSRIs, paroxetine, sertraline, fluvoxamine, and fluoxetine cause erectile dysfunction more commonly than venlafaxine, nefazodone, trazodone, bupropion, duloxetine, mirtazapine, escitalopram, or vilazodone. • Phenothiazines with less anticholinergic effect (eg, chlorpromazine) can be substituted in some patients if erectile dysfunction is a problem.
Dopamine antagonists (eg, metoclopramide, phenothiazines)	Inhibit prolactin inhibitory factor, thereby increasing prolactin levels	• Increased prolactin levels inhibit testicular testosterone production; decreased libido results.
Estrogens or drugs with antiandrogenic effects (eg, luteinizing hormone-releasing hormone superagonists, digoxin, spironolactone, ketoconazole, cimetidine)	Suppress testosterone-mediated stimulation of libido	• In the face of decreased libido, a secondary erectile dysfunction develops because of diminished sexual drive.
CNS depressants (eg, barbiturates, narcotics, benzodiazepines, short-term use of large doses of alcohol, anticonvulsants)	Suppress perception of psychogenic stimuli	

(Continued)

TABLE 82-1 Medication Classes That Can Cause Erectile Dysfunction (Continued)

Drug Class	Proposed Mechanism by Which Drug Causes Erectile Dysfunction	Special Notes
Agents that decrease penile blood flow (eg, diuretics, peripheral β-adrenergic antagonists, or central sympatholytics [methyldopa, clonidine, guanethidine])	Reduce arteriolar flow to corpora	• Any diuretic that produces a significant decrease in intravascular volume can decrease penile arteriolar flow. • Spironolactone has estrogenic effects, and has a high potential to decrease libido and cause erectile dysfunction when used in large doses. • First-generation β-blockers (eg, propranolol) or second-generation agents (eg, atenolol or metoprolol) are associated with more erectile dysfunction than newer generation agents (eg, nebivolol), which possess vasodilatory actions through blockade of alpha adrenoreceptors and release of nitric oxide. • Safer antihypertensives include angiotensin-converting enzyme inhibitors, postsynaptic alpha$_1$-adrenergic antagonists (terazosin, doxazosin), calcium channel blockers, and angiotensin II receptor antagonists.
Miscellaneous • Finasteride, dutasteride	Erectile dysfunction from 5-alpha reductase inhibitors is thought to result from inhibition of androgen-mediated nitric oxide production by vascular endothelial cells.	• Sexual dysfunction has been reported to persist even after the 5-alpha reductase inhibitor is discontinued.
Lithium carbonate	Unknown mechanism	
Gemfibrozil	Unknown mechanism	
Interferon	Unknown mechanism	
Clofibrate	Unknown mechanism	
Monoamine oxidase inhibitors (eg, phenelzine, isocarboxazid, tranylcypromine)	Unknown mechanism	
Opiates	Unknown mechanism	

CNS, central nervous system.

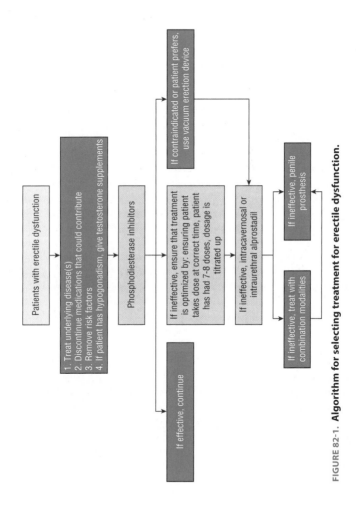

FIGURE 82-1. Algorithm for selecting treatment for erectile dysfunction.

TABLE 82-2 Dosing Regimens for Selected Drug Treatments for Erectile Dysfunction

Drug	Brand Name[a]	Initial Dose	Usual Range	Special Population Dose	Other
Phosphodiesterase Inhibitor					
Sildenafil	Viagra	50 mg orally 1 hour before intercourse	25–100 mg 1 hour before intercourse. Limit to one dose per day	In patients aged 65 years and older, start with 25-mg dose. In patients with creatinine clearance less than 30 mL/min (0.5 mL/sec) or severe hepatic impairment, limit starting dose to 25 mg. In patients with mild-to-moderate hepatic impairment or those taking strong CYP3A4 inhibitors (eg, itraconazole, ketoconazole, or erythromycin), consider starting with 25 mg. In patients taking protease inhibitors, limit starting dose to 25 mg.	Generic formulations are available. Titrate dose so that erection lasts no more than 1 hour. High-fat foods decrease the rate of absorption by 1 hour. Avoid taking dose with grapefruit juice. Contraindicated with nitrates by any route of administration.
Vardenafil	Levitra[b]	5–10 mg orally 1 hour before intercourse	5–20 mg 1 hour before intercourse. Limit to one dose per day	In patients aged 65 years and older, start with 5-mg Levitra. No dosage adjustment is required in patients with decreased creatinine clearance or mild hepatic impairment. In patients with moderate hepatic impairment, start with 5-mg Levitra. Use not recommended in patients with severe hepatic impairment. In patients taking strong P450 CYP3A4 inhibitors (eg, atazanavir, erythromycin, clarithromycin, ketoconazole, itraconazole), limit starting dose to 2.5 mg in a 24-hour period. In patients on ritonavir, limit dose to 2.5 mg every 72 hours. Not recommended in patients with congenital prolonged QT interval or in patients taking Type 1A or Type 3 antiarrhythmics.	Generic formulations are available. Titrate dose so that erection lasts no more than 1 hour. High-fat foods decrease the rate of absorption by 1 hour. Avoid taking the dose with grapefruit juice. Contraindicated with nitrates by any route of administration.

Staxyn[c]	10-mg tablet to dissolve on the tongue 1 hour before intercourse	10-mg tablet to dissolve on the tongue 1 hour before intercourse. Limit to one dose per day	Dose of Staxyn requires no adjustment in patients aged 65 years or older, patients with creatinine clearance less than 30 mL/min (0.5 mL/sec), or those with mild hepatic impairment. Do not use in patients with moderate or severe hepatic impairment or those taking moderately or highly potent P450 CYP3A4 inhibitors. Do not initiate Staxyn in patients taking *alpha*-adrenergic antagonists.	Generic formulations are available. Staxyn should be taken without any liquid or food. The tablet should be placed on the tongue where it will dissolve. No up-titration of dose is recommended. Do not substitute Staxyn for Levitra, or vice versa.
Tadalafil	Cialis	5–10 mg orally at least 30 minutes before intercourse OR 2.5–5 mg orally once daily	10–20 mg at least 30 minutes before intercourse. Limit to one dose per day 2.5–5 mg once daily. Limit to one dose per day	Dose of tadalafil requires no dosage adjustment in patients aged 65 years or older. In patients with creatinine clearance of 30–50 mL/min (0.5–0.83 mL/sec), limit starting dose to 10 mg every 48 hours; if less than 30 mL/min (0.5 mL/sec), limit starting dose to 5 mg every 72 hours. In patients with mild-to-moderate hepatic impairment, limit starting dose to 10 mg every 24 hours. Do not use in patients with severe hepatic impairment. In patients taking potent P450 CYP3A4 inhibitors, limit starting dose to 10 mg every 72 hours (if using it on demand) or 2.5 mg daily (if using a continuous daily regimen).	Generic formulations are available. Titrate dose so that erection lasts no more than 1 hour. Food does not affect rate or extent of drug absorption. Avoid taking dose with grapefruit juice. Contraindicated with nitrates by any route of administration. When taken with large amounts of ethanol, tadalafil may cause orthostatic hypotension.

(*Continued*)

943

TABLE 82-2	Dosing Regimens for Selected Drug Treatments for Erectile Dysfunction (*Continued*)			
Drug	Brand Name[a]	Initial Dose	Usual Range	Special Population Dose	Other
Avanafil	Stendra	100 mg orally 15 minutes before intercourse	50–200 mg orally 15 minutes before intercourse. Limit to one dose per day	Dosage adjustment needed in patients aged 65 years or older. In patients with creatinine clearance of 30–89 mL/min (0.5–1.49 mL/sec) or those with mild-to-moderate hepatic impairment, no dosage adjustment is needed. Not recommended if creatinine clearance is less than 30 mL/min (0.5 mL/sec), if the patient has severe hepatic disease, or if the patient is taking potent P450 CYP3A4 inhibitors. If the patient is taking moderate P450 CYP3A4 inhibitors (eg, erythromycin, fluconazole), the maximum recommended dose is 50 mg every 24 hours.	Titrate dose so that erection lasts no more than 1 hour. May be taken with or without food. Avoid taking dose with grapefruit juice. Contraindicated with nitrates by any route of administration. When taken with large amounts of ethanol, avanafil may cause orthostatic hypotension.
Prostaglandin E₁					
Alprostadil intracavernosal injection	Caverject, Edex	2.5 mcg intracavernosally 5–10 minutes before intercourse	10–40 mcg 5–10 minutes before intercourse. Maximum recommended dose is 60 mcg. Limit to not more than one injection per day and not more than three injections per week with a 24-hour interval between doses. Give each dose over 5–10 seconds	In older adults, use the lowest effective dose. No specific dosage adjustment provided in labeling for patients with hepatic or renal impairment.	Titrate dose to achieve an erection that lasts 1 hour. Patient will require training on aseptic intracavernosal injection technique. Avoid intracavernosal injections in patients with sickle cell anemia, multiple myeloma, leukemia, severe coagulopathy, schizophrenia, poor manual dexterity, severe venous incompetence, severe cardiovascular disease, or Peyronie's disease.

Alprostadil intraurethral pellet	Muse	125–250 mcg intraurethrally 5–10 minutes before intercourse	250–1,000 mcg just before intercourse. Limit to not more than two doses per day	In older adults, use the lowest effective dose. No specific dosage adjustment provided in labeling for patients with hepatic or renal impairment.	Patient will require training on proper intraurethral administration techniques. Use applicator provided to administer medications to avoid urethral injury.

Testosterone Supplements[d]

Methyltestosterone	Methitest	10 mg once daily	10–50 mg once daily	No dosage adjustment provided in labeling for patients with renal or hepatic impairment or older adults.	Not recommended for use due to extensive first-pass hepatic catabolism and because it is associated with hepatotoxicity. May cause fluid retention in patients with renal or hepatic disease.
Testosterone cypionate intramuscular injection	Depo-Testosterone	100–200 mg every 2–4 weeks	200–400 mg every 2–4 weeks (up to 6 weeks)	No dosage adjustment provided in labeling for patients with renal or hepatic impairment or older adults.	During the dosing interval, supraphysiologic serum concentrations of testosterone are produced during a portion of the dosing interval. This has been linked to mood swings and infertility.
Testosterone enanthate intramuscular injection		100–200 mg every 2–4 weeks	200–400 mg every 2–4 weeks (up to 6 weeks)	No dosage adjustment provided in labeling for patients with renal or hepatic impairment or older adults.	During the dosing interval, supraphysiologic serum concentrations of testosterone are produced during a portion of the dosing interval. This has been linked to mood swings and infertility.

(Continued)

TABLE 82-2	Dosing Regimens for Selected Drug Treatments for Erectile Dysfunction (*Continued*)				
Drug	Brand Name[a]	Initial Dose	Usual Range	Special Population Dose	Other
Testosterone undecanoate intramuscular injection	Aveed	750 mg as a single dose	750 mg as a single dose on Day 0, Week 4, and then 750 mg every 10 weeks	No dosage adjustment: provided in labeling for patients with renal or hepatic impairment or older adults. Contraindicated in patients with serious hepatic or renal disease.	Only available in facilities certified through a Risk Evaluation and Mitigation Strategy Program. Administer by deep intramuscular injection into gluteal muscle. Avoid intravascular injection, which can lead to pulmonary oil embolism.
Testosterone transdermal patch	Androderm	4 mg as a single dose at bedtime	2–6 mg as a single dose at bedtime. Titrate dose 2 weeks after initiating a dose. Multiple patches may be needed to achieve dose needed.	No dosage adjustment is provided in labeling for patients with renal or hepatic impairment or older adults.	When administered at bedtime, serum concentrations of testosterone in the usual circadian pattern are produced. Apply to those body sites recommended in the package labeling: upper arm, back, abdomen, and thigh. Rotate application sites every 7 days. May have to apply multiple patches at one time to achieve appropriate serum testosterone level. Avoid swimming, showering, or washing administration site for 3 hours after patch application.

| Testosterone gel | AndroGel 1% (25 mg/2.5 g) Testim 1% (25 mg/2.5 g) | 5–10 g of gel (equivalent to 50–100 mg testosterone, respectively) as a single dose in the morning | 5–10 g of gel (equivalent to 50–100 mg testosterone, respectively) as a single dose in the morning. Titrate dose at 14-day intervals | No dosage adjustment provided in labeling for patients with renal or hepatic impairment or older adults. | Cover application site to avoid inadvertent transfer to others. Avoid swimming, showering, or washing administration site for 2 hours after gel application. Apply to those sites recommended in the product labeling. For Androgel, apply to shoulders, upper arms, or abdomen. For Testim, apply to shoulders or upper arms only. Children and women should avoid contact with unclothed or unwashed application sites. Patients should wash hands with soap and water after administration of transdermal testosterone product. For patients who have difficulty measuring the appropriate dose using tubes of gel, it is also available in premeasured dose packets or from a pump dispenser. REMS assessments must be submitted to the FDA. |
| | AndroGel 1.62% (20.25 mg/1.25 g) | 2 pumps (equivalent to 40.5-mg testosterone) as a single dose in the morning | 2–4 pumps (equivalent to 40.5–81 mg) as a single dose in the morning. Titrate dose 14–28 days after starting treatment | No dosage adjustment provided in labeling for patients with renal or hepatic impairment or older adults. | Apply to shoulders and upper arms. Avoid swimming, showering, or washing administration site for 2 hours after application. Same precautions as listed above for 1% gel. REMS assessments must be submitted to the FDA. |

(*Continued*)

TABLE 82-2 Dosing Regimens for Selected Drug Treatments for Erectile Dysfunction (*Continued*)

Drug	Brand Name[a]	Initial Dose	Usual Range	Special Population Dose	Other
Testosterone transdermal spray	Fortesta 2% (10 mg/actuation)	4 sprays (equivalent to 40-mg testosterone) every morning	4–7 sprays (equivalent to 40–70 mg testosterone) every morning. Titrate dose up at 14- to 35-day intervals	No dosage adjustment: provided in labeling for patients with renal or hepatic impairment or older adults.	Must prime pump by pushing on pump three times. Apply to front or inner thighs only. Cover application site to avoid inadvertent transfer to others. Avoid swimming, showering, or washing administration site for 2 hours after spray application. Children and women should avoid contact with unclothed or unwashed application sites. Patients should wash hands with soap and water after administration of transdermal testosterone product. REMS assessments must be submitted to the FDA.
Testosterone transdermal solution	Axiron (30 mg/actuation)	One pump spray (equivalent to 30-mg testosterone) to left or right axilla daily	1–4 pump sprays (equivalent to 30–120 mg testosterone, respectively) to axilla daily. If dose is more than one pump spray, divide total dose between axillae. Titrate dose at 14- to 35-day intervals	No dosage adjustment provided in labeling for patients with renal or hepatic impairment or older adults.	Limit application to axilla. Apply antiperspirant or deodorant before Axiron. If applying multiple spray doses to an axilla, apply one spray, let dry, then apply second dose. Avoid swimming, showering, or washing administration site for 2 hours after application. REMS assessments must be submitted to the FDA.

				Dosage Adjustment	Administration
Testosterone intranasal gel	Natesto (5.5 mg/actuation)	2 pump actuations in nostrils (equivalent to 1 pump actuation per nostril, total dose of 11 mg) three times a day	2 pump actuations in nostrils (equivalent to 1 pump actuation per nostril, total dose of 11 mg) three times a day. If serum testosterone level is not corrected with this dose, it is recommended to switch to an alternative testosterone supplement	No dosage adjustment provided in labeling for patients with renal or hepatic impairment or older adults.	Administer each dose 6 to 8 hours apart. Prime pump by inverting and depressing pump 10 times. Blow nose before application. After administration, press on nostrils and lightly massage. Do not blow nose or sniff for 1 hour after administration. Do not administer with any other intranasal product, except decongestants. Discontinue if patient has rhinitis. If patient develops severe rhinitis, temporarily switch to an alternative testosterone replacement product until rhinitis resolves. Avoid use in patients with chronic nasal conditions, sinusitis, or after nasal or sinus surgery.
Testosterone subcutaneous implant pellet	Testopel 75 mg/pellet	150–450 mg (equivalent to 2–6 pellets) as a single dose every 3–6 months	150–450 mg as a single dose every 3–6 months	No dosage adjustment recommended for renal or hepatic impairment or older adults.	Trained health professional is required to administer the dose. Use sterile implanter kit. Administration of the dose requires a forearm incision and local anesthesia to subcutaneously implant dose. Clinical onset is delayed for 3–4 months after initial dose. Generic formulations are available in higher strengths: 100 or 200 mg per pellet.

aCommon brand names are included in this table. Medications may be available with other brand names or as generic formulation.
bLevitra brand was discontinued in April 2021. Vardenafil is available as generic formulation.
cStaxyn brand was discontinued in April 2021. Vardenafil is available as generic formulation.
dThis listing includes only those testosterone supplements approved for treating hypogonadism associated with aging. Testosterone enanthate autoinjector and oral testosterone undecanoate are not included for this reason.

NONPHARMACOLOGIC TREATMENT

Vacuum Erection Device

- First-line therapy for older patients in stable relationships. Onset of action is slow (ie, 3–20 minutes). An erection can be sustained through use of constriction bands or tension rings.
- Consider VEDs as second-line therapy after failure of oral or injectable drugs. Response rate improves with addition of **alprostadil** or a phosphodiesterase inhibitor (PI).
- VEDs are contraindicated in patients with sickle cell disease or a history of prolonged erections. Use cautiously in patients taking warfarin as the likelihood of penile bruising is increased.

Surgery

- Surgical insertion of a penile prosthesis, the most invasive treatment for ED, is reserved for patients who do not respond to or who are not candidates for less invasive medical treatments or devices.

PHARMACOLOGIC TREATMENTS

Phosphodiesterase Type 5 Inhibitors

- Phosphodiesterase decreases catabolism of cGMP, a vasodilatory neurotransmitter in the corporal tissue.
- PIs used for ED exhibit variable selectivity for isoenzyme type 5 in genital tissue. Inhibition of this isoenzyme in nongenital tissues (eg, peripheral vascular tissue, tracheal smooth muscle, and platelets) can produce adverse effects.
- Available agents (**avanafil, sildenafil, tadalafil,** and **vardenafil**) have different pharmacokinetic and pharmacodynamics profiles (Table 82-3). They are considered equally effective and comparable in safety despite no comparative clinical trial data.
- PIs are first-line therapy for younger patients. Effectiveness appears to be dose related; nonresponse rate is 30%–40%. Patient education is critical for clinical success.
- Hepatic metabolism of all four PIs can be inhibited by enzyme inhibitors of CYP 3A4. Use a lower starting dose to minimize dose-related adverse effects.
- Avoid exceeding prescribed doses due to increased frequency of adverse effects and inconsistent erectile responses.
- In usual doses, the most common adverse effects include headache, facial flushing, dyspepsia, nasal congestion, and dizziness that are all dose related.
- Sildenafil and vardenafil decrease systolic/diastolic blood pressure by 8–10/5–8 mm Hg for 1–4 hours after a dose. Although most patients are asymptomatic, multiple antihypertensives, nitrates, and baseline hypotension increase the risk of developing adverse effects. Avanafil and tadalafil are associated with similar decreases in blood pressure. Use PI with caution in patients with cardiovascular disease because of the inherent cardiac risk associated with vigorous sexual activity.
- Guidelines are available for stratifying patients on the basis of their cardiovascular risk (Table 82-4).
- Sildenafil, vardenafil, and avanafil cause increased sensitivity to light, blurred vision, or transient loss of blue–green color discrimination in 2%–3% of patients. Use cautiously in patients at risk for retinitis pigmentosa; evaluate patients with sudden vision loss before continuing treatment.
- Nonarteritic anterior ischemic optic neuropathy (NAION) is a sudden, unilateral, painless blindness, which may be irreversible. Isolated cases of NAION have been associated with PI use, although a cause–effect relationship has not been established.
- PIs are contraindicated in patients taking nitrates. Use cautiously in patients taking α-adrenergic antagonists.

TABLE 82-3 Pharmacodynamics and Pharmacokinetics of Phosphodiesterase Inhibitors

	Sildenafil (Viagra)	Vardenafil (Levitra/Staxyn)	Tadalafil (Cialis)	Avanafil (Stendra)
Inhibits PDE-5	Yes	Yes	Yes	Yes
Inhibits PDE-1	Yes	Yes	Minimally	Minimally
Inhibits PDE-6	Yes	Yes	No	Mildly
Inhibits PDE-11	No	No	Yes	No
Time to peak plasma level (hours)	0.5–1	0.7–0.9/1.5	2	0.5–0.8
Oral bioavailability (%)	40	15/21–44	36	15
Fatty meal decreases rate and/or extent of oral absorption?	Yes	Yes/No[a]	No	Yes - rate
Mean plasma half-life (hours)	3.7	4.4–4.8/4–6	18	5
Active metabolite	Yes	Yes/Yes	No	Yes
Is CYP 3A4 principally responsible for metabolism?	Yes	Yes/Yes	Yes	Yes
Other CYP enzymes responsible for metabolism	CYP 2C9, CYP 2C19, CYP 2D6, CYP 1A2	CYP 3A5, CYP 2C9	None	CYP 2C9
Percentage of dose excreted in feces	80	91–95/91–95	61	62
Percentage of dose excreted in urine	13	2–6/2–6	36	21
Clinical onset (minutes)	60	30/60	60	25–40
Duration (hours)	2–4, up to 12	4–5/4–6	24–36	6+

[a]When Staxyn is taken with water, the area under the curve decreases by 29%.

TABLE 82-4	Recommendations of the Third Princeton Consensus Conference for Cardiovascular Risk Stratification of Patients Being Considered for Phosphodiesterase Inhibitor Therapy	
Risk Category	**Description of Patient's Condition**	**Management Approach**
Low risk	Has asymptomatic cardiovascular disease with <3 risk factors for cardiovascular disease	Patient can be started on phosphodiesterase inhibitor
	Has well-controlled hypertension	
	Has mild CHF (NYHA class I or II)	
	Has mild valvular heart disease	
	Has had a myocardial infarction >8 weeks ago	
Intermediate risk	Has ≥3 risk factors for cardiovascular disease	Patient should undergo complete cardiovascular workup and treadmill stress test to determine tolerance to increased myocardial energy consumption associated with increased sexual activity. Then, reclassify in low- or high-risk category
	Has mild or moderate, stable angina	
	Had a recent myocardial infarction or stroke within the past 2–8 weeks	
	Has moderate CHF (NYHA class III)	
	History of stroke, transient ischemic attack, or peripheral artery disease	
High risk	Has unstable or refractory angina, despite treatment	Phosphodiesterase inhibitor is contraindicated; sexual intercourse should be deferred
	Has uncontrolled hypertension	
	Has severe congestive heart failure (NYHA class IV)	
	Has had a recent myocardial infarction or stroke within past 2 weeks	
	Has moderate or severe valvular heart disease	
	Has high-risk cardiac arrhythmias	
	Has obstructive hypertrophic cardiomyopathy	

NYHA, New York Heart Association.

Reprinted with permission from Nehra A, Jackson G, Miner M, et al. The Princeton III Consensus Recommendations for the Management of Erectile Dysfunction and Cardiovascular Disease. Mayo Clin Proc. 2012;87(8):766–778.

Testosterone-Replacement Regimens

- **Testosterone**-replacement regimens restore serum testosterone levels to the normal range (300–1100 ng/dL; 10.4–38.2 nmol/L). These regimens are indicated for symptomatic patients with hypogonadism as confirmed by low serum testosterone concentrations.
- Testosterone-replacement regimens correct secondary ED by improving libido. Libido, mood, and quality of life may improve in 3–4 weeks, erectile function may improve in 6 months, but other symptoms of hypogonadism (eg, bone density) may take longer to resolve.
- Oral, buccal, intranasal, parenteral, and transdermal products are available (see Table 82-2). Injectable regimens are preferred because they are effective, inexpensive, and do not have the bioavailability problems or adverse hepatotoxic effects of oral

regimens. Continue treatment for 3–6 months before an increase in dosage is considered. Testosterone patches, gels, and sprays are more expensive than other forms and should be reserved for patients who refuse injections.

- Testosterone replacement can cause sodium retention which can result in weight gain or exacerbate hypertension, congestive heart failure, and edema; gynecomastia; serum lipoprotein changes; and erythrocytosis.

- Oral testosterone-replacement regimens are usually avoided as they cause hepatotoxicity which ranges from mildly elevated hepatic transaminases to serious liver diseases including peliosis hepatitis, hepatocellular and intrahepatic cholestasis, and benign or malignant tumors.

- Topical testosterone patches may cause contact dermatitis that responds to topical corticosteroids.

Alprostadil

- **Alprostadil**, or prostaglandin E_1, stimulates adenyl cyclase to increase production of cAMP, a neurotransmitter that ultimately enhances blood flow to and blood filling of the corpora.

- Alprostadil is approved as monotherapy for the management of ED. It is generally prescribed after failure of VEDs and PIs and for patients who cannot use these therapies. The intracavernosal route is more effective than the intraurethral route.

- *Intracavernosal* alprostadil is effective in 70%–90% of patients, but 30%–50% discontinue therapy during first 6–12 months. Perceived ineffectiveness, inconvenience of administration, unnatural, nonspontaneous erection, needle phobia, loss of interest, and cost of therapy are reasons given for discontinuation.

- *Intracavernosal* alprostadil is used successfully in combination with VEDs or vasoactive agents (eg, papaverine and phentolamine) that act by different mechanisms.

- *Intracavernosal* alprostadil acts rapidly, with an onset of 5–15 minutes. Duration of action is dose related and, within the usual dosage range, lasts less than 1 hour. To avoid adverse effects, the maximum number of injections is one daily and three weekly, with at least 24 hours between doses.

- Usual dose is 10–20 mcg up to a maximum of 60 mcg. The manufacturer recommends slow dose titration, but in clinical practice, most patients start with 10 mcg and titrate quickly.

- Local adverse effects (eg, hematoma and bruising) occur during the first year of therapy. Other adverse effects include cavernosal plaques or fibrosis at the injection site (2%–12% of patients), penile pain (10%–44%), and priapism (1%–15%). Penile pain is usually mild and self-limiting, but priapism (ie, painful, drug-induced erection lasting >1 hour) necessitates immediate medical attention.

- Use cautiously in patients at risk of priapism (eg, sickle cell disease, leukemia, or multiple myeloma) and bleeding complications secondary to injections.

- Instill *intraurethral* alprostadil, 125–1000 mcg 5–10 minutes before intercourse after emptying the bladder. No more than two doses daily are recommended.

- *Intraurethral* administration is associated with mild pain in 24%–32% of patients. Prolonged painful erections are rare.

- Female partners may experience vaginal burning, itching, or pain, which is probably related to transfer of alprostadil during intercourse.

Unapproved Agents

- A variety of commercially available and investigational agents have been used for management of ED. Examples include **yohimbine** (6–15 mg orally three times daily), **papaverine** (7.5–60 mg [single-agent therapy] or 0.5–20 mg [combination therapy] intracavernosal injection), and **phentolamine** (0.5–1 mg in combination with 30-mg papaverine; dose administered ranges from 0.1 to 1 mL of the mixture as an intracavernosal injection).

EVALUATION OF THERAPEUTIC OUTCOMES

- The primary therapeutic outcomes for ED are improving the quantity and quality of penile erections suitable for intercourse and avoiding adverse drug reactions and interactions.
- Assess the patient at baseline and after a treatment trial period of several weeks.
- Identify patients with unrealistic expectations and counsel accordingly to avoid adverse effects due to excessive use of erectogenic agents.

See Chapter 103, Erectile Dysfunction, authored by Mary Lee and Roohollah Sharifi, for a more detailed discussion of this topic.

83 Urinary Incontinence

- *Urinary incontinence* (UI) is defined as involuntary loss of urine.

PATHOPHYSIOLOGY

- The urethral sphincter, a combination of smooth and striated muscles within and external to the urethra, maintains adequate resistance to the flow of urine from the bladder until voluntary voiding is initiated.
- Volitional and involuntary bladder contractions are mediated by activation of post-synaptic muscarinic receptors by acetylcholine. Bladder smooth muscle cholinergic receptors are mainly of the M_2 variety; however, M_3 receptors are responsible for both emptying contractions of normal micturition and involuntary bladder contractions, which can result in UI. Therefore, most pharmacologic antimuscarinic therapy is anti-M_3 based, resulting in detrusor smooth muscle relaxation and reduction in bladder overactivity.
- Stimulation of β_3-adrenergic receptors in the detrusor muscle results in smooth muscle relaxation. β_3-agonists attenuate bladder contractility, which is useful for treatment of overactive bladder (OAB) and urgency incontinence.
- UI occurs as a result of overactivity or underactivity of the urethra, bladder, or both.
- Urethral underactivity, known as *stress UI* (SUI), occurs during activities such as exercise, running, lifting, coughing, and sneezing. The urethral sphincter no longer resists the flow of urine from the bladder during periods of physical activity.
- Bladder overactivity, known as *urgency UI* (UUI), is a symptom syndrome characterized by urinary urgency, usually accompanied by increased daytime frequency and/or nocturia, with urinary incontinence (OAB-wet) or without (OAB-dry), in the absence of urinary tract infection or other detectable diseases. The detrusor muscle is overactive and contracts inappropriately during urinary storage.
- Urethral overactivity and/or bladder underactivity is known as overflow incontinence or chronic urinary retention. The bladder is filled to capacity but is unable to empty, causing urine to leak from a distended bladder past a normal outlet and sphincter. Common causes of urethral overactivity include benign prostatic hyperplasia (see Chapter 80); prostate cancer (see Chapter 64); and, in women, cystocele formation or surgical overcorrection after SUI surgery.
- Mixed incontinence includes the combination of bladder overactivity and urethral underactivity.
- Functional incontinence is not caused by bladder- or urethra-specific factors but rather occurs in patients with conditions such as dementia or cognitive or mobility deficits.
- Many medications may precipitate or aggravate voiding dysfunction and UI (Table 83-1).

CLINICAL PRESENTATION

- Signs and symptoms of UI depend on the underlying pathophysiology (Table 83-2). Patients with SUI generally complain of urine leakage with physical activity, whereas those with UUI complain of frequency, urgency, high-volume incontinence, and nocturia and nocturnal incontinence.
- Urethral overactivity and/or bladder underactivity is a rare but important cause of UI. Patients complain of lower abdominal fullness, hesitancy, straining to void, decreased force of stream, interrupted stream, and sense of incomplete bladder emptying. Patients can also have urinary frequency, urgency, and abdominal pain.

TABLE 83-1	Medications That Influence Lower Urinary Tract Function
Medications	**Effect**
Diuretics, acetylcholinesterase inhibitors	Polyuria resulting in urinary frequency, urgency
α-Receptor antagonists	Urethral muscle relaxation and stress urinary incontinence
α-Receptor agonists	Urethral muscle contraction (increased urethral closure forces) resulting in urinary retention (more common in men)
Calcium channel blockers	Urinary retention due to reduced bladder contractility
Narcotic analgesics	Urinary retention due to reduced bladder contractility
Sedative hypnotics	Functional incontinence caused by delirium, immobility
Antipsychotic agents	Anticholinergic effects resulting in reduced bladder contractility and urinary retention
Anticholinergics	Urinary retention due to reduced bladder contractility
Antidepressants, tricyclic	Anticholinergic effects resulting in reduced bladder contractility (urinary retention), and α-antagonist effects resulting in reduced urethral smooth muscle contraction (stress incontinence)
Alcohol	Polyuria resulting in urinary frequency, urgency
ACEIs	Cough as a result of ACEIs may aggravate stress urinary incontinence

ACEIs, angiotensin-converting enzyme inhibitors.

DIAGNOSIS

- A complete medical history, physical examination (ie, abdominal examination to exclude distended bladder, pelvic examination in women looking for evidence of prolapse or hormonal deficiency, and genital and prostate examination in men), and brief neurologic assessment of the perineum and lower extremities are recommended.
- For SUI, the preferred diagnostic test is observation of urethral meatus while the patient coughs or strains.

TABLE 83-2	Differentiating Bladder Overactivity-Related UI (Urgency Urinary Incontinence) from Urethral Underactivity-Related UI (Stress Urinary Incontinence)	
Symptoms	**Bladder Overactivity (UUI)**	**Urethral Underactivity (SUI)**
Urgency (strong, sudden desire to void)	Yes	Not common
Frequency with urgency	Yes	Rarely
Leaking during physical activity (eg, coughing, sneezing, lifting)	No	Yes
Amount of urinary leakage with each episode of incontinence	Large if present	Usually small
Ability to reach the toilet in time following an urge to void	No or just barely	Yes
Nocturnal incontinence (presence of wet pads or undergarments in bed)	Yes	Rare
Nocturia (waking to pass urine at night)	Usually	Seldom

- For UUI, the preferred diagnostic tests are urodynamic studies. Perform urinalysis and urine culture to rule out urinary tract infection.
- For urethral overactivity and/or bladder underactivity, perform digital rectal examination or transrectal ultrasound to rule out prostate enlargement. Perform renal function tests to rule out renal failure.

TREATMENT

- <u>Goals of Treatment</u>: Restoration of continence, reduction in the number of UI episodes, and prevention of complications while minimizing adverse treatment consequences and cost. Improvement in the patient's quality of life, lesser care burden, and reduced risk of nursing home placement are also important.

NONPHARMACOLOGIC TREATMENT

- Nonpharmacologic, nonsurgical treatment options include behavioral interventions, external neuromodulation, anti-incontinence devices, and supportive interventions. Behavioral interventions (eg, lifestyle modifications, voiding schedule regimens, and pelvic floor muscle rehabilitation) are generally first-line treatment for SUI, UUI, and mixed UI.
- Surgery rarely plays a role in initial management of UI but can be required for secondary complications (eg, skin breakdown or infection). The decision to surgically treat symptomatic UI requires that lifestyle compromise warrant an elective operation and that nonsurgical therapy be proven undesirable or ineffective.

PHARMACOLOGIC TREATMENT

Bladder Overactivity: Urgency Urinary Incontinence

- The pharmacotherapy of first choice for UUI includes antimuscarinic agents and β_3-adrenergic agonists drugs, which antagonize muscarinic cholinergic receptors (Table 83-3).

Oxybutynin

- **Oxybutynin immediate-release** (IR) is the oldest and least expensive treatment for UUI.
- Many patients discontinue oxybutynin IR because of adverse effects due to nonurinary antimuscarinic effects (eg, dry mouth, constipation, vision impairment, confusion, cognitive impairment, and tachycardia), α-adrenergic inhibition (eg, orthostatic hypotension), and histamine H_1 inhibition (eg, sedation and weight gain).
- **Oxybutynin extended-release** (XL) is better tolerated than oxybutynin IR. Maximum benefits may take up to 4 weeks after dose initiation or escalation.
- **Oxybutynin transdermal system** (TDS) has similar efficacy but is better tolerated than oxybutynin IR presumably because this route avoids first-pass metabolism in the liver, which generates the metabolite thought to cause adverse events, especially dry mouth.
- **Oxybutynin gel** causes significantly less dry mouth than oxybutynin IR, but patients must be monitored for anticholinergic affects during long-term therapy, particularly frail patients.

Tolterodine

- **Tolterodine**, a competitive muscarinic receptor antagonist, is as effective as oxybutynin IR in efficacy outcomes with lower drug discontinuation rates.
- Tolterodine undergoes hepatic metabolism involving cytochrome (CYP) 2D6 and 3A4 isoenzymes. Therefore, elimination may be impaired by CYP 3A4 inhibitors, including **fluoxetine, sertraline, fluvoxamine**, macrolide antibiotics, azole antifungals, and grapefruit juice.

TABLE 83-3 Dosing of Medications Approved for OAB or UUI

Drug	Brand Name	Initial Dose	Usual Range	Special Population Dose	Comments
Anticholinergics/Antimuscarinics					
Oxybutynin IR	Ditropan	2.5 mg twice daily	2.5–5 mg two to four times daily		Titrate in increments of 2.5 mg/day every 1–2 months; available in oral solution
Oxybutynin XL	Ditropan XL	5–10 mg once daily	5–30 mg once daily		Adjust dose in 5-mg increments at weekly interval; swallow whole
Oxybutynin TDS	Oxytrol, Oxytrol for Women (OTC)		3.9 mg/day apply one patch twice weekly		Apply every 3–4 days; rotate application site
Oxybutynin gel 10%	Gelnique		One sachet (100 mg) topically daily		Apply to clean and dry, intact skin on abdomen, thighs, or upper arms/shoulders; contains alcohol
Oxybutynin gel 3%	Gelnique 3%		Three pumps (84 mg) topically daily		Same as above
Tolterodine IR	Detrol		1–2 mg twice daily	1 mg twice daily if patient is taking CYP3A4 inhibitors, or with renal/hepatic impairment	Avoid in patients with creatinine clearance less than 10 mL/min (0.17 mL/s) or severe hepatic impairment
Tolterodine LA	Detrol LA		2–4 mg once daily	2 mg once daily in those who are taking CYP3A4 inhibitors (ketoconazole, itraconazole, clarithromycin, or ritonavir), those with hepatic impairment (Child-Pugh class A or B) or severe renal impairment (creatinine clearance 10–30 mL/min [0.17–0.50 mL/s])	Swallow whole; avoid in patients with creatinine clearance ≤10 mL/min (0.17 mL/s) or severe hepatic impairment

	Brand			
Trospium chloride IR	Sanctura		20 mg twice daily	20 mg once daily in patient age ≥75 years or creatinine clearance ≤30 mL/min (0.5 mL/s)	Take 1 hour before meals or on empty stomach; patient age ≥75 years should take at bedtime
Trospium chloride ER	Sanctura XR		60 mg once daily	Avoid in patient age ≥75 years or creatinine clearance ≤30 mL/min (0.5 mL/s)	Take 1 hour before meals or on empty stomach; swallow whole
Solifenacin	VESIcare	5 mg daily	5–10 mg once daily Pediatric: use suspension dose based on body weight	5 mg daily if patient is taking CYP3A4 inhibitors or with creatinine clearance ≤30 mL/min (0.5 mL/s) or moderate hepatic impairment; avoid in severe hepatic impairment	Swallow whole
Darifenacin ER	Enablex	7.5 mg once daily	7.5–15 mg once daily	7.5 mg daily if patient is taking potent CYP3A4 inhibitors or with moderate hepatic impairment; avoid in severe hepatic impairment	Titrate dose after at least 2 weeks; swallow whole
Fesoterodine ER	Toviaz	4 mg once daily	4–8 mg once daily	4 mg daily if patient is taking potent CYP3A4 inhibitors or with creatinine clearance ≤30 mL/min (0.5 mL/s); avoid in severe hepatic impairment	Prodrug (metabolized to 5-hydroxymethyl tolterodine); swallow whole

β₃-Adrenergic Agonist

	Brand			
Mirabegron ER	Myrbetriq	25 mg once daily	25–50 once daily	25 mg once daily if creatinine clearance 15–29 mL/min (0.25–0.49 mL/s) or moderate hepatic impairment; avoid in patients with ESRD or severe hepatic impairment	Swallow whole
Vibegron	Gemtase	75 mg once daily		Avoid in patients with end-stage kidney disease with or without hemodialysis, or severe hepatic impairment	Swallow whole. Tablets may be crushed and mixed with apple sauce

CYP, cytochrome P450 enzyme; ER, extended-release; ESRD, end-stage renal disease; IR, immediate release; LA, long acting; OAB, overactive bladder; OTC, over-the-counter; TDS, transdermal system; UUI, urge urinary incontinence; XL, extended release.

- Tolterodine's most common adverse effects include dry mouth, dyspepsia, headache, constipation, and dry eyes. The maximum benefit of tolterodine is not realized for up to 8 weeks after therapy initiation or dose escalation.
- **Tolterodine long acting** (LA) offers once-daily dosing and may also take up to 8 weeks after therapy initiation or dose escalation to see maximum benefit.
- **Fesoterodine fumarate** is a prodrug for tolterodine and is considered an alternative first-line therapy for UI in patients with urinary frequency, urgency, or urge incontinence.

Other Pharmacologic Therapies for Urgency Urinary Incontinence

- **Trospium chloride IR**, a quaternary ammonium anticholinergic, was shown to be noninferior to oxybutynin IR but was associated with less dry mouth. It causes the expected anticholinergic adverse effects with increased frequency in patients age 75 years or older. An extended-release product is also available.
- **Solifenacin succinate** and **darifenacin** are second-generation antimuscarinic agents. Both have been shown to improve urinary symptoms and quality-of-life. Drug interactions are possible if CYP 3A4 inhibitors or inducers are given with solifenacin succinate or CYP 2D6 or 3A4 inhibitors with darifenacin.
- **Mirabegron** is a β_3-adrenergic agonist alternative to anticholinergic/antimuscarinic drugs for managing UUI. It has modest efficacy as compared with placebo. Hypertension, nasopharyngitis, urinary tract infection, and headache are the most common adverse effects. It is a moderate inhibitor of CYP2D6. **Vibegron** is a second β_3-adrenergic agonist approved for the treatment of OAB with symptoms of UUI, urgency, and urinary frequency.
- Use of other agents, including tricyclic antidepressants, **propantheline, flavoxate, hyoscyamine**, and **dicyclomine hydrochloride**, is not recommended as these agents lack better efficacy and have the potential for serious adverse effects.
- A systematic review of 94 randomized controlled trials with antimuscarinic drugs for UUI showed similar, small benefits for all drugs studied. Selection of initial drug therapy depends on side-effect profile, comorbidities, concurrent drug therapy, and patient preference in drug delivery methods (Table 83-4).

TABLE 83-4	Adverse Event Incidence Rates (%) with Approved Drugs for Bladder Overactivity[a]			
Drug	**Dry Mouth**	**Constipation**	**Dizziness**	**Vision Disturbance**
Oxybutynin IR	71	15	17	10
Oxybutynin XL	61	13	6	14
Oxybutynin TDS	7	3	NR	3
Oxybutynin gel	10	1	3	3
Tolterodine	35	7	5	3
Tolterodine LA	23	6	2	4
Trospium chloride IR	20	10	NR	1
Trospium chloride XR	11	9	NR	2
Solifenacin	20	9	2	5
Darifenacin ER	24	18	2	2
Fesoterodine ER	27	5	NR	3
Mirabegron ER	3	3	3	NR
Vibegron	<1	2	<1	<1

IR, immediate release; LA, long acting; NR, not reported; TDS, transdermal system; XL, extended release; XR/ER, extended release.
[a]All values constitute mean data, predominantly using product information from the manufacturers.

- **Botulinum toxin A** temporarily paralyzes smooth or striated muscle. It is indicated for the treatment of detrusor overactivity associated with neurologic conditions and OAB; it is considered third-line treatment. Multiple intravesical injections are administered directly into the bladder muscle without general anesthesia; therapeutic and adverse effects are seen 3–7 days after injection and subside after 6–8 months. Increased bladder capacity, increased bladder compliance, and improved quality of life have been reported in patients with refractory OAB. Adverse effects of botulinum toxin A include dysuria, hematuria, urinary tract infection, and urinary retention (up to 20%).

Urethral Underactivity: Stress Urinary Incontinence

- Treatment of SUI is aimed at improving urethral closure by stimulating α-adrenergic receptors in smooth muscle of the bladder neck and proximal urethra, enhancing supportive structures underlying the urethral epithelium, or enhancing serotonin and norepinephrine effects in the micturition reflex pathways.

Estrogens

- Historically, local and systemic **estrogens** have been the mainstays of pharmacologic management of SUI.
- A meta-analysis of 34 trials evaluating the use of local or systemic estrogen therapy on UI in postmenopausal women found that systemic administration of estrogen alone or in combination with progesterone resulted in UI worsening. There was some evidence that vaginal estrogen may improve UI, and reduce urgency and frequency.
- A meta-analysis of 17 trials of local estrogen compared to placebo or no treatment found beneficial effects on UI and OAB symptoms and some urodynamic parameters.
- Based on the results of these analyses, only topical estrogen products should be used for treatment of UI or OAB in postmenopausal women.

α-Adrenergic Receptor Agonists

- Many open trials support the use of a variety of α-adrenergic receptor agonists in SUI. Combining an α-adrenergic receptor agonist with an estrogen yields somewhat superior clinical and urodynamic responses compared with monotherapy.
- Contraindications to these agents include hypertension, tachyarrhythmias, coronary artery disease, myocardial infarction, cor pulmonale, hyperthyroidism, renal failure, and narrow-angle glaucoma.

Duloxetine

- **Duloxetine**, a dual inhibitor of serotonin and norepinephrine reuptake indicated for depression and painful diabetic neuropathy, is approved in many countries for the treatment of SUI, but not in the United States. Duloxetine is thought to facilitate the bladder-to-sympathetic reflex pathway, increasing urethral and external urethral sphincter muscle tone during the storage phase.
- Six placebo-controlled studies showed that duloxetine reduces incontinent episode frequency and the number of daily micturitions, increases micturition interval, and improves quality-of-life scores. These benefits were statistically significant but clinically modest.
- Monitor patients taking concurrent CYP 2D6 and 1A2 substrates or inhibitors closely.
- The adverse event profile might make adherence problematic. Adverse events include nausea, headache, insomnia, dizziness, constipation, and dry mouth.

Overflow Incontinence

- Overflow incontinence secondary to benign or malignant prostatic hyperplasia may be amenable to pharmacotherapy (see Chapters 65 and 81).

EVALUATION OF THERAPEUTIC OUTCOMES

- Total elimination of UI signs and symptoms may not be possible. Therefore, realistic goals should be established for therapy.
- In the long-term management of UI, the clinical symptoms of most distress to the individual patient need to be monitored.
- Survey instruments used in UI research along with quantitating the use of ancillary supplies (eg, pads) can be used in clinical monitoring.
- Therapies for UI frequently have nuisance adverse effects, which need to be carefully elicited. Adverse effects can necessitate drug dosage adjustments, use of alternative strategies (eg, chewing sugarless gum, sucking on hard sugarless candy, or use of saliva substitutes for xerostomia), or even drug discontinuation.

See Chapter 105, Urinary Incontinence, authored by Eric S. Rovner, Kristine Talley, and Sum Lam, for a more detailed discussion of this topic.

Pediatric Pharmacotherapy, Nutrition, and Neonatal Critical Care

TABLE A1-1	Opioid Administration for Acute and Severe Pain in Pediatrics
Intermittent IV or PO bolus administration (not as needed)	In 2018, the FDA announced limiting use of prescription opioid cough and cold medications containing codeine or hydrocodone in children <18 years old. Weak opioids (eg, codeine, hydrocodone, and oxycodone) often are combined with acetaminophen or an NSAID for moderate pain. With dose escalation of combination oral products, be aware that the dose does not exceed recommended daily amounts for acetaminophen or ibuprofen. One percent to 7% of the general population and up to 28% of some ethnic groups have a genetic variation in the enzyme cytochrome P450 2D6 that causes codeine to be converted to morphine faster and more completely. In 2012, the FDA issued a Drug Safety Communication stating that codeine use in certain children after tonsillectomy or adenoidectomy for obstructive sleep apnea syndrome led to deaths and life-threatening respiratory depression. Consider alternative analgesics for children undergoing tonsillectomy or adenoidectomy. If codeine or codeine-containing products are prescribed, then use the lowest effective dose for the shortest period of time on an as-needed basis. IV administration of codeine has been associated with allergic reactions related to histamine release. Parenteral administration of codeine is not recommended. Intermittent opioid administration is associated with wide fluctuation between peak and trough concentrations, so the patient may alternate between peak blood concentrations associated with untoward effects and trough concentrations associated with inadequate pain relief when being treated for severe pain. Oxycodone and morphine are available in a sustained-release formulation for use with chronic pain (not acute pain). The tablet must be swallowed whole and cannot be administered to patients through gastric tubes.
IV continuous infusion	Loading dose is administered to rapidly achieve a therapeutic blood concentration and pain relief (ie, morphine loading dose of 0.05–0.15 mg/kg in children; 0.1 mg/kg infused over 90 minutes in neonates). Loading dose is followed by a maintenance continuous infusion. Doses that are considered safe in children can cause respiratory depression and seizures in neonates because of decreased clearance, immature blood–brain barrier at birth that is more permeable to morphine, and an increased unbound fraction of morphine that increases CNS effects of the drug.

(Continued)

TABLE A1-1	Opioid Administration for Acute and Severe Pain in Pediatrics (*Continued*)
PCA	Gives patient some control over his or her pain therapy. PCA allows the patient to self-administer small opioid doses. The PCA-Plus (Abbott, Chicago, IL) pump allows the patient to receive a continuous infusion together with a set number of self-administered doses per hour. PCA helps to eliminate wide peak and trough fluctuations so that blood concentrations remain in a therapeutic range. Children as young as 5 or 6 years of age can master the use of PCA.
Epidural and intrathecal analgesia	Effective in the management of severe postoperative, chronic, or cancer pain. Spinal opioids can be administered by a single bolus injection into the epidural or subarachnoid space or by continuous infusion via an indwelling catheter. Dosage requirement by these routes is significantly less than that required with IV administration. Morphine, hydromorphone, fentanyl, and sufentanil are effective when administered intrathecally. Bupivacaine is the most commonly used local anesthetic in continuous epidural infusions. Fentanyl, morphine, or hydromorphone usually is combined with bupivacaine for epidural infusions.
Transdermal administration	Fentanyl and buprenorphine are available as a transdermal formulation. Multiple patches of an agent may be applied for patients who require higher doses. Disadvantage of transdermal administration is the requirement for an alternative short-acting opioid for breakthrough pain.
Transmucosal administration	Fentanyl lozenge is absorbed transmucosally. It is useful for providing analgesia during painful procedures. Advantages include rapid onset of action (within 15 minutes), short duration of action (60–90 minutes), and painless administration because no injection is needed. Common side effects are vomiting and mild-to-moderate oxygen desaturation. Doses of 10–15 mcg/kg provide blood concentrations equivalent to 3–5 mcg/kg IV.

FDA, Food and Drug Administration; IM, intramuscular; NSAID, nonsteroidal anti-inflammatory drug; PCA, patient-controlled analgesia; PO, by mouth.

TABLE A1-2	Frequency and Volume of Feedings in Infants	
Age	Feedings Per Day	Volume Per Feeding, mL (ounces)
Birth–1 week	6–10	30–90 (1–3)
1 week–1 month	7–8	60–120 (2–4)
1–3 months	5–7	120–180 (3–6)
3–6 months	4–5	180–210 (6–7)
6–9 months	3–4	210–240 (7–8)
9–12 months	3	210–240 (7–8)

TABLE A1-3 Composition of Human Milk Fortifiers[a] (Select Products and Nutrients)

Nutrient	Similac HMF[b,c] Powder (Per Packet)	Enfamil HMF Powder (Per Packet)[b]	Similac HMF Hydrolyzed Protein Concentrated Liquid[b,c] (Per 5 mL)	Enfamil HMF Acidified Liquid[b,c] (Per 5 mL)
Calories, kcal	3.5	3.5	7	7.5
Protein, g	0.25	0.275	0.35	0.55
Fat, g	0.09	0.25	0.27	0.575
Sodium, mg	3.75	4	5	6.75
Potassium, mg	15.75	7.25	21	11.25
Calcium, mg	29.25	22.5	35	29
Magnesium, mg	1.75	0.25	2.2	0.46
Phosphorus, mg	16.75	12.5	20	15.75
Selenium, mcg	0.125	-	0.2	-
Iron, mg	0.08	0.36	0.11	0.44
Zinc, mg	0.25	0.18	0.3	0.24
Vitamin A, IU	155	237.5	197	290
Vitamin C, mg	6.25	3	7.7	3.8
Vitamin D, IU	30	37.5	35	47
Vitamin E, IU	0.8	1.15	1	1.4
Vitamin K, mcg	2	1.1	2.4	1.425

HMF, human milk fortifier.
[a]Mix 1 packet (powder) or 5 mL (liquid) in 25 mL to make 24 kcal/oz (3.4 kJ/mL) concentration.
[b]Also contains linoleic acid, thiamin, riboflavin, pyridoxine, cyanocobalamin, niacin, folic acid, pantothenic acid, biotin, manganese, and copper.
[c]Also contains iodine, choline, and inositol.
Data from Abbott Nutrition, www.abbottnutrition.com; Mead Johnson Nutrition, www.meadjohnson.com.

TABLE A1-4	Formulas for Premature Infants[a]						
Formula	Energy (kcal/dL) (kcal/oz)	Protein (g/dL)	Fat (g/dL)	Vitamin D (IU/mL)	Calcium (mg/dL)	Phosphorus (mg/dL)	Iron (mg/dL)
Mature human milk	65–70 (19.5–21)	1.03	3.5	Variable (based on mother's intake)	20–25	12–14	0.3–0.9
Premature infant formulas							
Similac Special Care 20	67.6 (20)	2.03	3.67	101.4	121.7	67.6	1.22
Similac Special Care 24	81.2 (24)	2.43	4.41	101.4	146.1	81.2	1.46
Similac Special Care 24 High Protein	81.2 (24)	2.68	4.41	121.7	146.1	81.2	1.46
Similac Special Care 30	101.4 (30)	3.04	6.71	182.6	152.2	101.4	1.83
Enfamil Premature 20	67.6 (20)	2.2	3.4	200	112	61	1.22
Enfamil Premature 24	81.2 (24)	2.7	4.1	240	134	73	1.46
Enfamil Premature 24 HP	81.2 (24)	2.9	4.1	240	134	73	1.46
Enfamil Premature 30	101.4 (30)	3.3	5.1	300	167	91	1.83
Postdischarge formulas							
Similac Neosure	74 (22)	2.1	4.1 MCT 25%	52	78	46	1.3
Enfamil EnfaCare/Enfamil NeuroPro EnfaCare	74 (22)	2.1	4 MCT 20%	53	90	50	1.3

[a]For results expressed in SI units: For energy expressed in kcal/dL multiply by 41.84 to convert to kJ/L; for energy expressed in kcal/oz multiply by 0.1415 to convert to kJ/mL; for fat or protein expressed in g/dL multiply by 10 to convert to g/L; for vitamin D expressed in IU/mL multiply by 1000 to convert to IU/L; and for calcium, phosphorus, or iron expressed in mg/dL multiply by 10 to convert to mg/L.

MCT, medium-chain triglycerides.

Data from Abbott Nutrition, www.abbottnutrition.com; Mead Johnson Nutrition, www.meadjohnson.com.

TABLE A1-5 World Health Organization (WHO) Guidelines for Oral Rehydration in Children

Recommended Volume of ORT to Correct Dehydration

Weight (kg)[a]	Age[a]	ORS, mL in the First 4 Hours[b]
<5	<4 months	200–400
5–7.9	4–11 months	200–400
8–9.9	12–23 months	600–800
10–15.9	2–4 years	800–1200
16–29.9	5–14 years	1200–2200
≥30	≥15 years	2200–4000

Recommended Volume after Stooling to Prevent Dehydration

Age (y)	Recommended Volume (mL)	Maximum Daily Volume (mL)
<2	50–100	500
2–9	100–200	1000
≥10	At least 100–200, but as much as desired	2000

[a]Use age only if weight is not available.
[b]Volume for the first 4 hours can also be calculated by multiplying the weight (kg) by 75.

TABLE A1-6 Oral/Enteral Hydration Solutions (Examples Only)

Product	Sodium (mEq/L)	Potassium (mEq/L)	Chloride (mEq/L)	Base (mEq/L)	CHO (g/L)	Osm (mOsm/L)	Other
Recommended Concentration	60–90	15–25	50–80	8–12	Equal to sodium; <111 mmol/L	200–310	
Rehydration solutions—replace fluid deficits							
WHO (UNICEF), original[a]	90	19.2	21	30	13.5	333	
WHO (UNICEF), modified	75	20	65	10	13.5	245	
Bana—Adult	68.6	10.3			2		
Ceralyte 70 (packets)	70	20	60	30	40 (rice)	<260	
Ceralyte 90 (packets)	90	20	80	30	40 (rice)	<275	
Drip Drop Solution	60	20	8	80	16	<200	
Pedialyte Advanced Care+[b]	60	20					Zinc
Maintenance solutions—prevent fluid deficits							
Pedialyte®, Pedialyte® Freezer Pops, Pedialyte Advanced Care[b]	45	20	35	30	25	388	Zinc
Ceralyte 50 (packets)	50	20	40	30	40 (rice)	<260	
Enfamil® Enfalyte®	50	20	40	30	20	251	
Clear liquids and sports drinks (for comparison only—not rehydration or maintenance solutions)							
Juice	2	30	–	0	69	730	
Soda	3	–	–	13	70	700	
Gatorade (G2)[c]	20	3.2	17	30	21	305	
Gatorade Prime[c]	40.5	7.6	17	30	195	305	

[a]Gold standard for rehydration solutions.
[b]Contains prebiotics.
[c]Other forms available; sugar-free Gatorade available; caution with sugar substitutes.
Data from Manufacturers' websites; World Health Organization, apps.who.int/medicinedocs/en/d/Js4950e/2.4.html.

TABLE A1-7 Antimicrobial Dosage Regimens for Neonates

Medication	Chronologic Age ≤ 28 days				Chronologic Age > 28 days
	Dosage expressed in mg/kg/dose				
	Weight ≤ 2,000 g		Weight > 2,000 g		All Weights
	PNA 0-7 days[a]	PNA 8-28 days[a]	PNA 0-7 days[a]	PNA 8-28 days[a]	PNA 29-60 days[a]
Antibiotics					
Ampicillin	50 Q 12 h	75 Q 12 h	50 Q 8 h	50 Q 8 h	50 Q 6 h
Ampicillin *(GBS meningitis)*	100 Q 8 h	75 Q 6 h	100 Q 8 h	75 Q 6 h	75 Q 6 h
Cefazolin	25 Q 12 h	25 Q 12 h	25 Q 8 h	25 Q 8 h	25 Q 8 h
Cefepime	30 Q 12 h	30 Q 12 h	50 Q 12 h	50 Q 12 h	50 Q 8 h
Cefotaxime	50 Q 12 h	50 Q 8 h	50 Q 12 h	37.5 Q 6 h	50 Q 6 h
Ceftazidime	50 Q 12 h	50 Q 8 h	50 Q 12 h	50 Q 8 h	50 Q 8 h
Clindamycin	5 Q 8 h	5 Q 8 h	7 Q 8 h	9 Q 8 h	10 Q 8 h
Meropenem[b]	20 Q 12 h	20 Q 8 h	20 Q 8 h	30 Q 8 h[c]	30 Q 8 h
Metronidazole	7.5 Q 12 h	7.5 Q 12 h	7.5 Q 8 h	10 Q 8 h	10 Q 8 h
Nafcillin/Oxacillin	25 Q 12 h	25 Q 8 h	25 Q 8 h	25 Q 6 h	37.5 Q 6 h
Penicillin G *(GBS meningitis)*	150,000 Units Q 8 h	125,000 Units Q 6 h	150,000 Units Q 8 h	125,000 Units Q 6 h	125,000 Units Q 6 h
Penicillin G *(Congenital syphilis)*	50,000 Units Q 12 h	50,000 Units Q 8 h	50,000 Units Q 12 h	50,000 Units Q 8 h	50,000 Units Q 6 h
Piperacillin/ Tazobactam	100 Q 8 h	80 Q 6 h[d]	80 Q 6 h	80 Q 6 h	80 Q 6 h
Vancomycin	15 Q 12–18 h	15 Q 8–12 h	15 Q 8–12 h	15 Q 6–8 h	15 Q 6–8 h
Antiviral					
Acyclovir	20 Q 12 h	20 Q 8 h	20 Q 8 h	20 Q 8 h	20 Q 8 h
Antifungals					
Amphotericin B Deoxycholate	1 Q 24 h	1 Q 24 h	1 Q 24 h	1 Q 24 h	1 Q 24 h
Liposomal/ Lipid Complex Amphotericin B	5 Q 24 h	5 Q 24 h	5 Q 24 h	5 Q 24 h	5 Q 24 h
Fluconazole[e]	12 Q 24 h	12 Q 24 h	12 Q 24 h	12 Q 24 h	12 Q 24 h

[a]PNA (postnatal age).
[b]Higher dosage may be required for meningitis.
[c]Adjust dosage after 14 days of age instead of 7 days of age.
[d]When postmenstrual age reaches 30 weeks.
[e]Load with 25 mg/kg/dose followed maintenance dose 24 hours later; adjust for renal dosing if serum creatinine ≥ 1.3 mg/dL (115 μmol/L).

TABLE A1-8	Medications Used for Patient Ductus Arteriosus (PDA) Closure	
Medication	**Dosing Regimen**	**Monitoring Parameters**
Indomethacin	**Intravenous, intermittent:** PNA <48 hours: 0.1 mg/kg/dose Q 12–24 h × 3 doses PNA 2–7 days: 0.2 mg/kg/dose Q 12–24 h × 3 doses PNA >7 days: 0.25 mg/kg/dose Q 12–24 h × 3 doses	Urine output (hold dose if <0.6 mL/kg/h), serum creatinine (hold dose if >1.6 mg/dL [141 μmol/L]), platelets, signs of bleeding Blood pressure, murmur, respiratory status, echocardiogram
Ibuprofen	**Intravenous, intermittent:** "Standard-dose": 10 mg/kg/dose × 1 dose followed by 5 mg/kg/dose Q 24 h × 2 doses "High-dose": 20 mg/kg/dose × 1 dose followed by 10 mg/kg/dose Q 24 h × 2 doses High-dose regimen found to have higher closure rates compared to standard-dose without more frequent adverse medication reactions	Urine output (hold dose if <0.6 mL/kg/h), serum creatinine, platelets, signs of bleeding Blood pressure, murmur, respiratory status, echocardiogram
Acetaminophen	**Intravenous, intermittent:** 15 mg/kg/dose Q 6 h × 3–7 days	Liver function tests Blood pressure, murmur, respiratory status, echocardiogram

PNA, postnatal age.

TABLE A1-9	Neonatal Dosing Recommendations for Commonly Used Analgesics and Sedatives		
Medication	**Uses**	**Dosing Regimen**	**Comments**
Sucrose 24% solution	Analgesia; mild procedural pain	<1 kg: 0.1 mL/dose 1–2 kg: 0.1–0.2 mL/dose >2 kg: 0.1–0.5 mL/dose	Administer 1–2 minutes prior to procedure May be applied to pacifier or directly to tongue Do not exceed 3 doses per procedure
Acetaminophen	Analgesia; mild-to-moderate postoperative or prolonged pain Analgesia; moderate-to-severe postoperative pain when used in combination with an opioid	**Oral:** GA 28–32 weeks: 10–12 mg/kg/dose Q 6–8 h; max. dose 40 mg/kg/day GA 33–37 weeks: 10–15 mg/kg/dose Q 6 h; max. dose 60 mg/kg/day Term, ≥10 days: 10–15 mg/kg/dose Q 4–6 h; max. dose 75 mg/kg/day	Not effective for acute procedural pain

(Continued)

TABLE A1-9	Neonatal Dosing Recommendations for Commonly Used Analgesics and Sedatives (*Continued*)		
Medication	**Uses**	**Dosing Regimen**	**Comments**
		Intravenous:	
		PMA 28–32 weeks: 10 mg/kg/dose Q 12 h; max. dose 22.5 mg/kg/day	
		PMA 33–36 weeks: 10 mg/kg/dose Q 8 h; max. dose 40 mg/kg/day	
		PMA ≥37 weeks: 10 mg/kg/dose Q 6 h; max. dose 40 mg/kg/day	
Morphine	Analgesia; moderate-to-severe prolonged or postoperative pain	**Intravenous, intermittent:** 0.05–0.1 mg/kg/dose Q 4–6 h	Preterm neonates may be more susceptible to hypotension, respiratory depression, apnea
		Intravenous, continuous: 0.01–0.03 mg/kg/h	Titrate to effect
			Practitioners should be aware of potential adverse effects on neurodevelopment
Fentanyl	Analgesia; moderate-to-severe acute procedural pain, prolonged, or postoperative pain	**Intravenous, intermittent:** 0.5–3 mcg/kg/dose Q 2–4 h	Administer bolus over 3–5 minutes; more rapid rates may cause chest wall rigidity
		Intravenous, continuous: 0.5–3 mcg/kg/h	Titrate to effect
Midazolam	Sedation; procedural or prolonged	**Intravenous, intermittent:** 0.05–0.1 mg/kg/dose	Myoclonus may occur especially in preterm neonates
		Intravenous, continuous:	Titrate to effect
		GA 24–26 weeks: 0.02–0.03 mg/kg/h	Practitioners should be aware of potential adverse effects on neurodevelopment
		GA 27–29 weeks: 0.03–0.04 mg/kg/h	
		GA ≥30 weeks: 0.03–0.06 mg/kg/h	
Dexmedetomidine	Sedation, analgesia; prolonged	**Intravenous, continuous:** 0.1–0.3 mcg/kg/h	Limited neonatal data

GA, gestational age; PMA, postmenstrual age.

(*See the following chapters for more detailed discussions of these topics:*

- e/Chapter 20, Pediatrics: General Topics in Pediatric Pharmacotherapy, authored by Milap C. Nahata and Carol Taketomo

- e/Chapter 21, Pediatrics: Oral nutrition and Rehydration of Infants and Children, authored by Katherine H. Chessman

- e/Chapter 22, Pediatrics: Neonatal Critical Care, authored by Kirsten H. Ohler and Jennifer T. Pham)

Geriatric Assessment and Pharmacotherapy

TABLE A2-1	Physiologic Changes with Aging
Organ System	**Manifestation**
Body composition	↓ Total body water
	↓ Lean body mass
	↑ Body fat
	↔ or ↓ Serum albumin
	↑ α_1-Acid glycoprotein (↔ or ↑ by several disease states)
Cardiovascular	↓ Cardiovascular response to stress
	↓ Baroreceptor activity leading to decreased exercise tolerance
	↓ Cardiac output
	↑ Systemic vascular resistance with loss of arterial elasticity and dysfunction of systems maintaining vascular tone
	↑ Systolic blood pressure and increased risk of arrhythmias
	↓ Compliance of the left ventricle, increasing the risk of positional hypotension
Neurological	↓ Size of the hippocampus and frontal and temporal lobes
	↓ Number of receptors of all types and ↑ sensitivity of remaining receptors
	↓ Short-term memory, coding and retrieval, and executive function
	Altered sleep patterns
	↑ Blood–brain barrier permeability
Endocrine	↓ Estrogen, testosterone, thyroid hormone
	Altered insulin signaling
	Decreased basal metabolic rate
Gastrointestinal	↓ Gastric motility
	↓ Vitamin absorption by active transport mechanisms
	↓ Splanchnic blood flow
	↓ Bowel surface area
Genitourinary	Atrophy of the vagina with decreased estrogen
	Prostatic hypertrophy with androgenic hormonal changes
	Detrusor hyperactivity may predispose to incontinence
Hepatic	↓ Hepatic mass
	↓ Hepatic blood flow
	↓ Phase I (oxidation, reduction, hydrolysis) metabolism
Immune	↓ Antibody production in response to antigen
	↑ Autoimmunity
Oral	Altered dentition
	↓ Ability to taste salt, bitter, sweet, and sour
Pulmonary	↓ Respiratory muscle strength
	↓ Chest wall compliance
	↓ Arterial oxygenation and impaired carbon dioxide elimination
	↓ Lung tissue elasticity

(Continued)

TABLE A2-1	Physiologic Changes with Aging (*Continued*)
Organ System	**Manifestation**
Renal	↓ Glomerular filtration rate
	↓ Renal blood flow
	↓ Number of functioning nephrons
	↓ Tubular secretory function
	↓ Renal mass
Sensory	Presbyopia (diminished ability to focus on near objects)
	↓ Night vision
	Presbycusis (high-pitch, high-frequency hearing loss)
	↓ Sensation of smell and taste
Musculoskeletal	↓ Skeletal bone mass (osteopenia)
	↓ Muscle mass
	Joint stiffening due to reduced water content in tendons, ligaments, and cartilage
	Altered gait and posture
Skin/Hair	Thinning of stratum corneum
	↓ Melanocytes
	↓ Depth and extent of the subcutaneous fat layer
	Atrophy of sweat glands
	Thinning and graying of hair

Data from Drenth-van Maanen AC, Wilting I, Jansen PAF. Prescribing medicines to older people: How to consider the impact of ageing on human organ and body functions. Br J Clin Pharmacol. 2020 Oct;86(10):1921–1930. Clinical implications of the aging process. In: Kane RL, Ouslander JG, Resnick B, Malone ML, eds. Essentials of Clinical Geriatrics. 8th ed. McGraw Hill; 2017.

TABLE A2-2	Age-Related Changes in Drug Pharmacokinetics
Pharmacokinetic Phase	**Pharmacokinetic Parameters**
Gastrointestinal absorption	Unchanged passive diffusion and no change in bioavailability for most drugs
	↓ Active transport and ↓ bioavailability for some drugs
	↓ First-pass metabolism, ↑ bioavailability for some drugs, and ↓ bioavailability for some prodrugs
Distribution	↓ Volume of distribution and ↑ plasma concentration of water-soluble drugs
	↑ Volume of distribution and ↑ terminal disposition half-life ($t_{1/2}$) for lipid-soluble drugs
Hepatic metabolism	↓ Clearance and ↑ $t_{1/2}$ for some drugs with poor hepatic extraction (capacity-limited metabolism). Phase I metabolism may be affected more than Phase II
	↓ Clearance and ↑ ($t_{1/2}$ for drugs with high hepatic extraction ratios (flow-limited metabolism)
Renal excretion	↓ Clearance and ↑ $t_{1/2}$ for renally eliminated drugs and active metabolites

Data from Maher D, Ailabouni N, Mangoni AA, Wiese MD, Reeve E. Alterations in drug disposition in older adults: a focus on geriatric syndromes. Expert Opin Drug Metab Toxicol. 2021 Jan;17(1):41–52. Thürmann PA. Pharmacodynamics and pharmacokinetics in older adults. Curr Opin Anaesthesiol. 2020 Feb;33(1):109–113.

TABLE A2-3	Comparison of American Geriatrics Society Beers Criteria and STOPP Criteria
Criteria	**Organization**
Beers	Criteria are organized into five tables:
	1. PIMs for all older adults, organized according to organ system and therapeutic category
	2. PIMs for some older adults due to drug–disease or drug–syndrome interactions that might exacerbate disease/syndromes (eg, syncope, delirium, dementia, history of falls or fractures, history of gastrointestinal ulcers, urinary incontinence, benign prostatic hyperplasia, heart failure)
	3. PIMs to be used with caution (eg, aspirin for primary prevention, dabigatran/rivaroxaban—gastrointestinal bleeding in people >75 years)
	4. Potentially clinically important drug–drug interactions that should be avoided (eg, opioids, lithium, phenytoin, warfarin, avoid total of ≥3 CNS active drugs to reduce falls risk)
	5. Medications that should be avoided or have dosage reduced with varying levels of kidney function
STOPP	1. Organized according to physiological system (11 sections) and includes drugs to avoid, drug–drug, dosing considerations for reduced renal function, and drug–disease interactions
	2. A section focused on general concepts that are not medication specific and include drug prescribed without evidence-based clinical indication, drug prescribed without recommended duration, and therapeutic duplication

PIM, potentially inappropriate medication.
Data from O'Mahony D, O'Sullivan D, Byrne S, O'Connor MN, Ryan C, Gallagher P. STOPP/START criteria for potentially inappropriate prescribing in older people: Version 2. Age Ageing. 2015;44:213–218; 2019 American Geriatrics Society Beers Criteria Update Expert Panel. American Geriatrics Society 2019 updated Beers Criteria for potentially inappropriate medication use in older adults. J Am Geriatr Soc. 2019. doi:10.1111/jgs.15767.

TABLE A2-4	Medication Appropriateness Index

Questions to ask about each individual medication

1. Is there an indication for the medication?

2. Is the medication effective for the condition?

3. Is the dosage correct?

4. Are the directions correct?

5. Are the directions practical?

6. Are there clinically significant drug–drug interactions?

7. Are there clinically significant drug–disease interactions?

8. Is there unnecessary duplication with other medication(s)?

9. Is the duration of therapy acceptable?

10. Is this medication the least expensive alternative compared with others of equal utility?

Reprinted from Hanlon JT, Schmader KE, Samsa GP, et al. A method for assessing drug therapy appropriateness. J Clin Epidemiol. 1992;45:1045–1051.

TABLE A2-5	Examples of Clinically Important Drug–Disease Interactions Determined by Expert Panel Consensus

Disease	Drug or Drug Class
Heart failure	NSAIDs, COX-2 inhibitors, thiazolidinediones, dronedarone
Heart failure with reduced ejection fraction	Nondihydropyridine calcium channel blockers
Syncope	Acetylcholinesterase inhibitors, peripheral nonselective α_1-blockers, tertiary tricyclic antidepressants, antipsychotics
Delirium	Anticholinergics, antipsychotics, benzodiazepines, corticosteroids, H_2-receptor antagonists, zolpidem and zoleplon ("z-hypnotics")
Cognitive impairment	Anticholinergics, antipsychotics, benzodiazepines, nonbenzodiazepine hypnotics, z-hypnotics
History of falls	Antiepileptics, antipsychotics, benzodiazepines, antidepressants, z-hypnotics, opioids
Parkinson disease	Antipsychotics (except quetiapine, clozapine, pimavanserin), metoclopramide, prochlorperazine, promethazine
Peptic ulcer disease	Aspirin in doses of 325 mg/day or more, NSAIDs
Chronic kidney disease stage IV and higher	NSAIDs
Urinary incontinence in women	Peripheral α_1-blockers

COX-2, cyclooxygenase 2; NSAIDs, nonsteroidal anti-inflammatory drugs.
Data from 2019 American Geriatrics Society Beers Criteria Update Expert Panel. American Geriatrics Society 2019 updated Beers Criteria for potentially inappropriate medication use in older adults. J Am Geriatr Soc. 2019. doi:10.1111/jgs.15767.

TABLE A2-6	Atypical Disease Presentation in Older Adults

Disease	Presentation
Acute myocardial infarction	Only ~50% present with chest pain. In general, older adults present with weakness, confusion, syncope, and abdominal pain; however, electrocardiographic findings are similar to those in younger patients.
Congestive heart failure	Instead of dyspnea, older patients may present with hypoxic symptoms, lethargy, restlessness, and confusion.
Gastrointestinal bleed	Although the mortality rate is ~10%, presenting symptoms are nonspecific, ranging from altered mental status to syncope with hemodynamic collapse. Abdominal pain often is absent.
Upper respiratory infection	Older patients typically present with lethargy, confusion, anorexia, and decompensation of a preexisting medical condition. Fever, chills, and productive cough may or may not be present.
Urinary tract infection	Dysuria, fever, and flank pain may be absent. More commonly, older adults present with incontinence, confusion, abdominal pain, nausea or vomiting, and azotemia.

(See the following chapters for more detailed discussions of these topics:

- *e/Chapter 23, Geriatrics: Physiology of Aging, authored by Krista L. Donohoe, Elvin T. Price, Tracey L. Gendron, and Patricia W. Slattum*

- *e/Chapter 24: Geriatrics: Medication Use in Older Adults, authored by Emily R. Hajjar, Lauren R. Hersh, and Shelly L. Gray*

- *e/Chapter 25: Geriatrics: Assessing Health and Delivering HealthCare to Older Adults, authored by Leigh Ann Mike, Zachary A. Marcum, and Shelly L. Gray)*

Critical Care: Patient Assessment and Pharmacotherapy

TABLE A3-1	Pharmacokinetic Changes in Critical Illness		
Pharmacokinetic Parameter	Changes in the Critically Ill	Etiologies	Example Drugs Affected
Absorption	↓ Absorption	Perfusion abnormalities	Enteral, intramuscular, or subcutaneous drugs
		Decreased GI motility	*Itraconazole (capsules need an acidic medium for absorption), phenytoin (significant drug–nutrient interactions), subcutaneous enoxaparin (incompletely absorbed in the setting of vasopressors and edema)*
		Altered gastric pH	
		Bowel wall edema	
		Drug–nutrient interactions	
Distribution	↑ V_d	Large-volume resuscitation	Hydrophilic drugs
		Capillary leak syndrome	*Aminoglycosides, beta-lactams, daptomycin, hydromorphone, morphine, vancomycin*
		Ascites	
		Mechanical ventilation	
		Hypoalbuminemia	Albumin-bound drugs
			Amiodarone, ceftriaxone, midazolam, morphine, phenytoin, propofol, valproic acid, warfarin
		Extracorporeal circuits with expansive surface area (ECMO)	Lipophilic drugs
			Diazepam, fentanyl, fluoroquinolones, macrolides, midazolam, propofol
	↓ V_d	Decreased α1-acid glycoprotein	Drugs bound to α1-acid glycoprotein
			Azithromycin, carvedilol, fentanyl, lidocaine, olanzapine, phenobarbital
Metabolism	↑ Metabolism	Hepatic enzyme induction	Flow-dependent drugs (hepatic extraction ratio >0.7)
		Augmented hepatic blood flow	*Propofol, midazolam, morphine, metoprolol*
	↓ Metabolism	Hepatic enzyme inhibition	Flow-independent drugs (hepatic extraction ratio <0.3)
		Decreased hepatic blood flow	*Warfarin, diazepam, phenytoin*

(Continued)

TABLE A3-1	Pharmacokinetic Changes in Critical Illness (*Continued*)		
Pharmacokinetic Parameter	**Changes in the Critically Ill**	**Etiologies**	**Example Drugs Affected**
Excretion	↑ Clearance	Augmented renal clearance	Renally eliminated medications
			Beta-lactam antibiotics, vancomycin, enoxaparin, gabapentin, levetiracetam
		Extracorporeal removal	
	↓ Clearance	Acute kidney injury	Nephrotoxic medications
			Aminoglycosides, NSAIDs, antivirals, contrast

ECMO, extracorporeal membrane oxygenation; GI, gastrointestinal; NSAIDs, nonsteroidal anti-inflammatory drugs; V_d, volume of distribution.

TABLE A3-2	Management of Pain, Agitation, and Delirium (PAD)

Assess for presence of PAD

Pain	≥4 times per nursing shift and as needed with NRS, BPS, CPOT
Agitation/Sedation	≥4 times per nursing shift and as needed with RASS and SAS
Delirium	Once per nursing shift and as needed with CAM-ICU and ICDSC

Identify and correct inciting factors when possible

Establish patient-specific treatment goals

Nonpharmacologic management

Pain	Massage therapy, relaxation techniques, cold packs, manipulative medicine
Agitation	Manage pain and discomfort; provide reassurance, support, and empathetic explanations for procedures, diagnostic tests, and diagnoses; avoid excessive noise, immobility, constipation, and physical restraints
Delirium	Correct modifiable risk factors; promote diurnal sleep patterns and orientation to person, place, and circumstance; encourage family visitation; provide cognitive stimulation and mobility efforts; and limit sedation

Pharmacologic management

Pain	Opioids and nonopioids for non-neuropathic pain, gabapentinoids for neuropathic pain, multimodal options for both
Agitation	Analgosedation, propofol, or dexmedetomidine for most patients. Reserve benzodiazepines for specific indications
Delirium	Dexmedetomidine for agitated delirium that interferes with weaning from mechanical ventilation. The role of antipsychotics is uncertain

Assess response to therapy; if not adequate, consider alternative approach

Determine plan for withdrawal of pharmacotherapy and transition of care

BPS, Behavioral Pain Scale; CAM-ICU, Confusion Assessment Method for the ICU; CPOT, Critical Care Pain Observational Tool; ICDSC, Intensive Care Delirium Screening Checklist; NRS, Numeric Rating Scale; RASS, Richmond Agitation Scale; SAS, Sedation Agitation Scale.

TABLE A3-3 Common ICU Medications Associated with Agitation and Delirium

Category	Medication or Class	Agitation	Delirium	With Use	With Withdrawal
Antibiotic	Cefepime	X	X	X	
	Macrolides	X		X	
	Fluoroquinolones	X	X	X	
	Voriconazole		X	X	
Anticholinergic	Diphenhydramine		X	X	
Anticonvulsant	Gabapentin	X			X
	Levetiracetam	X		X	
	Pregabalin	X			X
Antidepressant	Amitriptyline	X	X		X
	Selective serotonin reuptake inhibitors	X	X	X	X
	Serotonin norepinephrine reuptake inhibitors	X	X	X	X
Gabaminergic	Benzodiazepines	X	X	X	X
Miscellaneous	Corticosteroids	X	X	X	
	Digoxin	X	X	X	
	Ketamine	X	X	X	X
	Psychoactive medications	X	X	X	X

TABLE A3-4   Selected Pharmacotherapy Recommendations from the 2018 PADIS Guidelines

Recommendation	Recommendation Grade[a]
Pain	
Use multimodal approach to decrease opioid exposure	Conditional
Use enteral gabapentin, pregabalin, or carbamazepine with opioids for neuropathic pain	Strong
Use enteral gabapentin, pregabalin, or carbamazepine with opioids for pain <u>after cardiovascular surgery</u>	Conditional
Use opioid at the lowest effective dose or NSAID as an opioid alternative for procedural pain along with nonpharmacologic interventions	Conditional
Use an assessment-driven, protocol-based stepwise approach for pain management	Conditional
Use thoracic epidural anesthesia/analgesia for pain associated with abdominal aortic aneurysm surgery	Strong
Agitation/Sedation	
Use an assessment-driven, protocol-based, stepwise approach for sedation management	Conditional
Titrate sedatives to light (vs. deep) sedation	Conditional
Propofol or dexmedetomidine are preferred over benzodiazepines for sedation	Conditional
Delirium	
Do not use haloperidol or atypical antipsychotics to prevent delirium	Conditional
Do not routinely use haloperidol or atypical antipsychotics to treat delirium	Conditional
Use dexmedetomidine for delirium in ventilated patients where agitation is precluding weaning or extubation	Conditional

[a]Strong recommendation that applies to almost all patients is based on moderate- to high-quality data where the benefits clearly outweigh the burdens; conditional recommendation that applies to most patients but with significant exceptions based on context using data that are conflicting, low quality, insufficient, or involve limited patient populations where there may be a close balance between benefits and burdens.

Data from Devlin JW, Skrobik Y, Gelinas C, et al. Clinical practice guidelines for the prevention and management of pain, agitation/sedation, delirium, immobility, and sleep disruption in adult patients in the intensive care unit. *Crit Care Med*. 2018;46:e825–e873.

TABLE A3-5 Common ICU Analgesics and Sedatives Administered as Infusions

Drug	MOA	Dosing Range[a]	PK/PD Properties	ADR and Special Populations	Comments
Analgesics					
Fentanyl	μ agonist	25–200 mcg/h LD = 50–100 mcg	1–2 min onset; 2–4 h half-life; CYP3A metabolism; no active metabolites	Serotonin syndrome; caution with SSRI and SNRI	Rapid onset and offset Useful in kidney disease Less hypotension vs. morphine Interaction with CYP3A metabolized drugs (midazolam)
Hydromorphone	μ agonist	0.5–4 mg/h LD = 0.5–2 mg	5–10 min onset; 2–3 h half-life; glucuronidation; neurotoxic metabolite	Rare neurotoxicity due to metabolite accumulation in kidney disease	Slower onset than fentanyl, but longer duration No CYP interactions and no serotonin syndrome
Morphine	μ agonist	2–30 mg/h LD = 2–5 mg	5–10 min onset; 3–4 h half-life; demethylation and glucuronidation; active metabolites	Hypotension Accumulation of active metabolites in kidney disease	Venodilation from histamine release
Remifentanil	μ agonist	0.5–15 mcg/kg/h LD = 1.5 mcg/kg	1–3 min onset; 3–4 min half-life; esterase metabolism; no active metabolites	Allows frequent evaluations of neurologic function	Drug clearance unaffected by organ dysfunction Use IBW to dose obese patients Costly
Ketamine	NMDA receptor antagonist	0.05–0.4 mg/kg/h	1 min onset; 2–3 h half-life; demethylation; active metabolite	Possible hypertension Psychological disturbances	Does not interfere with respiratory function Useful for opioid-tolerant patients

Sedatives

Dexmedetomidine	Central α_2 agonist	0.2–1.4 mcg/kg/h	5–10 min onset; 3 h half-life; CYP2A6 metabolism and glucuronidation; no active metabolites	Bradycardia and hypotension	Does not interfere with respiratory function Allows "cooperative sedation" Opioid-sparing properties Less delirium than midazolam
Midazolam	GABA agonist	1–5 mg/h LD = 1–5 mg	2–3 min onset; 3–11 h half-life; CYP3A metabolism; active metabolites	Delirium Context-sensitive half-life	Less hypotension than propofol or dexmedetomidine Allows deep sedation and amnesia CYP3A interactions
Propofol	GABA agonist	5–50 mcg/kg/min	1–2 min onset; 3–12 h half-life; CYP2B6 and CYP3A metabolism; no active metabolites	Hypotension PRIS Hypertriglyceridemia Pancreatitis	Allows easy goal titration and neurologic evaluations Can provide deep sedation with amnesia No analgesia Interacts with midazolam

ADR, adverse drug reaction; cooperative sedation, ability to participate in care and follow commands; CYP, cytochrome P450; GABA, γ-aminobutyric acid; h, hour; IBW, ideal body weight; LD, loading dose; min, minute; MOA, mechanism of action; NMDA, N-methyl-**d**-aspartate; PK/PD, pharmacokinetic/pharmacodynamic; PRIS, propofol-related infusion syndrome; SNRI, serotonin norepinephrine reuptake inhibitor; SSRI, selective serotonin reuptake inhibitor.

aTypical dosing range for adult ICU patients; analgesic dosing requirements for pain relief may exceed these recommendations as will sedative dosing requirements to produce deep sedation.

(See the following chapters for more detailed discussions of these topics:

- *e/Chapter 26, Critical Care: Considerations in Medication Drug Selection, Dosing, Monitoring, and Safety, authored by Erin F. Barreto and Amy L. Dzierba*

- *e/Chapter 27, Critical Care: Pain, Agitation, and Delirium, authored by Caitlin S. Brown and Gilles L. Fraser)*

Drug Allergy

| TABLE A4-1 | Classification of Allergic Drug Reactions | | | |

Type	Descriptor	Characteristics	Typical Onset	Clinical Manifestations
I	Immediate (IgE mediated)	Allergen binds to IgE on basophils or mast cells, resulting in release of inflammatory mediators	Within 1 hour (may be within 1–6 hours)	Anaphylaxis, angioedema, hives, itching, wheezing, hypotension
II	Delayed; cytotoxic	Cell destruction occurs because of cell-associated antigen that initiates cytolysis by antigen-specific antibody (IgG) and complement. Most often involves blood elements	Typically >72 hours to weeks	Hemolytic anemia, thrombocytopenia
III	Delayed; immune complex	Antigen–antibody (IgG or IgM) complexes form and deposit on blood vessel walls and activate complement, which results in a serum sickness-like syndrome or vasculitis	>72 hours to weeks	Serum sickness, fever, rash, lymphadenopathy, joint pain
IV	Delayed; T cell–mediated	Antigens cause activation of T lymphocytes, which release cytokines and recruit effector cells	>72 hours	
	IVa	Th1 cells, interferon-γ, monocytes, and eosinophils respond to the antigen	1–21 days	Tuberculin reaction, contact dermatitis
	IVb	Th2 cells, interleukin-4, and interleukin-5 respond to the antigen	1–6 weeks	Maculopapular rashes with eosinophilia
	IVc	Cytotoxic T cells, perforin, granzyme B, FasL respond to the antigen	4–28 days	Bullous exanthems; fixed drug eruptions
	IVd	T cells and interleukin-8 respond to the antigen	>72 hours	Acute generalized exanthematous pustulosis

TABLE A4-2	Treatment of Anaphylaxis

1. Remove the inciting allergen, if possible.

2. Assess airway, breathing, circulation, and orientation. Support the airway.

3. Cardiopulmonary resuscitation: Start chest compressions (100/min) if cardiovascular arrest occurs at any time.

4. Administer epinephrine 1:1000 (adults: 0.3–0.5 mg; children: 0.01 mg/kg) IM in the lateral aspect of the thigh.

5. Place the patient in a recumbent position.

6. Administer oxygen 8–10 L/min through facemask or up to 100% oxygen as needed; monitor by pulse oximetry, if available.

7. Repeat IM epinephrine every 5–15 minutes for up to 3 injections if the patient is not responding.

8. Establish IV line for venous access. Keep line open with 0.9% saline solution. For hypotension or failure to respond to epinephrine, administer 1–2 L at a rate of 5–10 mL/kg in the first 5–10 minutes. Children should receive up to 30 mL/kg in the first hour.

9. Consider nebulized albuterol 2.5–5 mg in 3 mL of saline for lower airway obstruction; repeat as necessary.

10. In cases of refractory bronchospasm or hypotension not responding to epinephrine because a β-adrenergic blocker is complicating management, glucagon 1–5 mg IV (20–30 mcg/kg; maximum, 1 mg in children) should be given IV over 5 minutes.

11. Give norepinephrine or epinephrine by continuous IV infusion for patients with inadequate response to IM epinephrine and IV saline. For epinephrine, add 1 mg (1 mL of 1:1000) of epinephrine to 1000 mL of 0.9% saline solution; start infusion at 2 mcg/min and increase up to 10 mcg/min based on blood pressure, heart rate, and cardiac function.

12. Consider intraosseous access for either adults or children if attempts at IV access are unsuccessful.

13. Consider diphenhydramine (adults 25–50 mg; children 1 mg/kg, up to 50 mg) IM or by slow IV infusion.

14. Consider ranitidine 50 mg in adults and 12.5–50 mg (1 mg/kg) in children. The dose may be diluted in 5% dextrose in water to a volume of 20 mL and injected over 5 minutes.

15. Consider methylprednisolone 1–2 mg/kg/dose up to 125 mg (or an equivalent steroid) to reduce the risk of recurring or protracted anaphylaxis. Prednisone 20 mg orally can be given in mild cases. These doses can be repeated every 6 hours as required.

IM, intramuscular; IV, intravenous.
Adapted from Shaker MS, Wallace DV, Golden DB, et al. Anaphylaxis: A 2020 practice parameter update, systematic review, and grading of recommendations, assessment, development and evaluation (GRADE) analysis. J Allergy Clin Immunol. 2020;145:1082-1123.

TABLE A4-3 Procedure for Performing Penicillin Skin Testing

Step 1: Prick Test

This will be performed first on the patient, before proceeding to intradermal testing.

a. Clean the volar surface of either forearm with an alcohol swab.

b. Using an ink pen, draw 3 vertical lines approximately 1 in (2.5 cm) apart on the designated testing site of the arm.

c. Draw up 0.1 mL of the 4 solutions (Pre-pen, diluted Penicillin G, histamine positive control, and saline negative control) in 4 separate allergy syringes.

d. Apply a small drop of each solution to the separate premarked sites on the testing arm.

e. The histamine test site should be the most distal site from the elbow, followed up the arm by saline, Pre-Pen, and Pen G.

f. Puncture the epidermis using a twisting motion with a sterile 22–28 gauge needle at each drop site. Do not draw blood. Very little pressure is required.

g. Read the test in 15–20 minutes: (document test results below)

1. Test is <u>negative:</u> change in diameter of the wheal is **less than** 3 mm than that observed with the negative control. <u>Proceed to intradermal test.</u>

2. Test is <u>positive:</u> change in diameter of the wheal is **greater than** 3 mm than that observed with the negative control. As soon as a positive response is observed, the solution should be wiped off the skin. <u>Do not proceed to intradermal test.</u>

3. The positive control (histamine skin test) should be positive to ensure the results are not falsely negative.

4. The negative control (saline skin test) should be negative. If a wheal >2–3 mm develops after 20 minutes, repeat prick skin test. Upon retesting, if control still creates a wheal >2–3 mm after 20 minutes, discontinue test and notify the ID Physician and/or the ID Stewardship Pharmacist.

Step 2: Intradermal Test

Only conduct this test if the patient produced a negative result with the prick test in step 1.

a. Select 5 sites on the volar surface on the forearm. These sites should be on the opposite arm from the prick test if possible.

b. Using a 26–30 gauge, short bevel needle, intradermally inject 0.02 mL of Pre-Pen solution **twice** (separate at least 2 cm apart). Mark the margins of the initial blebs with an ink pen.

c. Using separate needles and syringes, intradermally inject diluted Pen G (0.02 mL = 200 units of penicillin) **twice** (separate at least 2 cm apart) and 0.02 mL of saline (separate at least 5 cm apart from other sites).

d. Read in 20 minutes: (document test results below)

1. Test is <u>negative:</u> there is no increase in the original bleb and no greater reaction than the negative control site.

2. Test is <u>positive:</u> bleb or wheal increases >2 mm from its original size or is >2 mm larger than the negative control. <u>Patient is NOT to receive penicillin.</u>

Step 3: (Optional) Oral Penicillin Challenge

a. If deemed necessary by ordering physician

1. Oral penicillin (eg, amoxicillin 250 mg) challenge or graded challenge of target drug in a monitored setting for 30–45 minutes.

Data from Jones BM, Bland CM. Penicillin skin testing as an antimicrobial stewardship initiative. Am J Health Syst Pharm. 2017;74:232–237.

TABLE A4-4	Characteristics of Drug Tolerance Protocols			
Underlying Mechanism	Initial Dose	Duration of Protocol	Potential Outcome of Process	Example
Immunologic IgE (desensitization)	Micrograms	Hours	Desensitization; render mast cells less responsive to degranulation	Anaphylaxis to β-lactam antibiotics; taxanes
Immunologic non-IgE	Milligrams	Hours to days (eg, 6 hours–10 days)	Not known	Delayed cutaneous reactions to trimethoprim–sulfamethoxazole
Pharmacologic	Milligrams	Hours to days (eg, 2 hours–5 days)	Cautious induction of a reaction followed by a shift in a metabolic process	NSAID-exacerbated respiratory disease
Undefined	Micrograms to milligrams	Prolonged; days to weeks	Not known	Isolated cutaneous reactions to allopurinol

Data from Solensky R, Khan DA. Drug allergy: An updated practice parameter. Ann Allergy Clin Immunol. 2010;105:259–273.

TABLE A4-5　Induction of Drug Tolerance Protocol for IV Cephalosporin[a]

Preparation of Solutions

	Volume of Diluents (eg, 0.9% NSS)	Total to be Injected in Each Bottle	Final Concentration (mg/mL)
Solution 1	250 mL	10 mg	0.04
Solution 2	250 mL	100 mg	0.4
Solution 3	250 mL	1000 mg	4

Induction of Drug Tolerance Protocol

Step	Solution	Rate (mL/h)	Time (min)	Administered Dose (mg)	Cumulative Dose (mg)
1	1	2	15	0.02	0.02
2	1	5	15	0.05	0.07
3	1	10	15	0.1	0.17
4	1	20	15	0.2	0.37
5	2	5	15	0.5	0.87
6	2	10	15	1	1.87
7	2	20	15	2	3.87
8	2	40	15	4	7.87
9	3	10	15	10	17.87
10	3	20	15	20	37.87
11	3	40	15	40	77.87
12	3	75	184.4	922.13	1000

NSS, normal saline solution.
[a]Full dose equals 1000 mg. Total time was 349.4 minutes.
Data from Solensky R, Khan DA. Drug allergy: An updated practice parameter. Ann Allergy Clin Immunol. 2010;105:259–273.

(See e/Chapter 108, Drug Allergy, authored by Mary L. Staicu, Christopher M. Bland, and Bruce M. Jones, for a more detailed discussion of this topic.)

Drug-Induced Hematologic Disorders

TABLE A5-1	Drugs Associated with Aplastic Anemia

Observational study evidence
Carbamazepine
Furosemide
Gold salts
Mebendazole
Methimazole
Nonsteroidal anti-inflammatory drugs
Oxyphenbutazone
Penicillamine
Phenobarbital
Phenothiazines
Phenytoin
Propylthiouracil
Sulfonamides
Thiazides

Case report evidence (*probable* or *definite* causality rating)
Acetazolamide
Aspirin
Captopril
Chloramphenicol
Chloroquine
Chlorothiazide
Chlorpromazine
Dapsone
Felbamate
Interferon alfa
Lisinopril
Lithium
Nizatidine
Pentoxifylline
Quinidine
Sulindac
Ticlopidine

MedWatch postmarketing reports 2009–2020
Adalimumab
Aliskiren
Amlodipine
Carvedilol
Dantrolene
Etanercept
Infliximab
Oxcarbazepine
Pembrolizumab
Posaconazole
Valsartan

TABLE A5-2	Drugs Associated with Agranulocytosis		
Observational Study Evidence	**Case Report Evidence (*Probable* or *Definite* Causality Rating)**		**MedWatch Postmarketing Reports 2009–2020**
β-Lactam antibiotics	Acetaminophen	Levodopa	Amlodipine
Carbamazepine	Acetazolamide	Meprobamate	
Carbimazole	Ampicillin	Methazolamide	
	Aripiprazole		
Clomipramine	Captopril	Methyldopa	Bocepravir
Digoxin	Carbenicillin	Metronidazole	Clozapine
	Cefepime		
Dipyridamole	Cefotaxime	Nafcillin	Defarasirox
Ganciclovir	Cefuroxime	NSAIDs	Fluoxetine
		Ostreotide	
Glyburide	Chloramphenicol	Olanzapine	Haloperidol
Gold salts	Chlorpromazine	Oxacillin	Hydrochlorothiazide
Imipenem–cilastatin	Chlorpropamide	Penicillamine	Iacosamide
			Ibrutinib
Indomethacin	Chlorpheniramine	Penicillin G	Leflunomide
Macrolide antibiotics	Clindamycin	Pentazocine	Levitiracetam
			Linezolid
Methimazole	Clozapine	Phenytoin	Memantine
			Metformin
Mirtazapine	Colchicine	Primidone	Molindone
Phenobarbital	Doxepin	Procainamide	Olanzapine
			Oseltamivir
Phenothiazines	Dapsone	Propylthiouracil	Oxcarbazepine
Prednisone	Desipramine	Pyrimethamine	Paliperidone
Propranolol	Ethacrynic acid	Quinidine	Pantoprazole
Spironolactone	Ethosuximide	Quinine	Pimozide
Sulfonamides	Flucytosine	Rifampin	Propafenone
Sulfonylureas	Gentamicin	Streptomycin	Quetiapine
Ticlopidine	Griseofulvin	Terbinafine	Rifabutin
Valproic acid	Hydralazine	Ticarcillin	Risperidone
		Tocainide	
Zidovudine	Hydroxychloroquine	Tolbutamide	Sulfasalazide
		Valganciclovir	
	Imipenem–cilastatin	Vancomycin	Thiothixene
	Imipramine		Trandolapril
			Ustekinumab
	Lamotrigine		Ziprasidone

NSAID, nonsteroidal anti-inflammatory drug.

TABLE A5-3	Drugs Associated with Hemolytic Anemia

Observational study evidence
Phenobarbital
Phenytoin
Ribavirin

Case report evidence (*probable* or *definite* causality rating)
Acetaminophen
Angiotensin-converting enzyme inhibitors
β-Lactam antibiotics
Cephalosporins
Ciprofloxacin
Clavulanate
Dabigatran
Dimethyl fumarate
Efavirenz
Erythromycin
Etoricoxib
Hydrochlorothiazide
Indinavir
Interferon alfa
Iomeprol
Ketoconazole
Lansoprazole
Levodopa
Levofloxacin
Methyldopa
Minocycline
NSAIDs
Omeprazole
p-Aminosalicylic acid
Phenazopyridine
Probenecid
Procainamide
Quinidine
Rifabutin
Rifampin
Streptomycin
Sulbactam
Sulfonamides
Sulfonylureas
Tacrolimus
Tazobactam
Teicoplanin
Tolbutamide
Tolmetin
Triamterene

MedWatch postmarketing reports 2009–2020
Amlodipine
Bevacizumab
Chlorpropamide
Deferasirox
Fludarabine
Pegademase
Pioglitazone
Rosiglitazone

NSAID, nonsteroidal anti-inflammatory drug.

TABLE A5-4 Drugs Associated with Metabolic Hemolytic Anemia

Observational study evidence

Dapsone

Rasburicase

Case report evidence (*probable* or *definite* causality rating)

Ascorbic acid

Metformin

Methylene blue

Nalidixic acid

Nitrofurantoin

Phenazopyridine

Primaquine

Sulfacetamide

Sulfamethoxazole

Sulfanilamide

TABLE A5-5 Drugs Associated with Megaloblastic Anemia

Case report evidence (*probable* or *definite* causality rating)

Azathioprine

Chloramphenicol

Colchicine

Cotrimoxazole

Cyclophosphamide

Cytarabine

5-Fluorodeoxyuridine

5-Fluorouracil

Hydroxyurea

6-Mercaptopurine

Methotrexate

Oral contraceptives

p-Aminosalicylate

Phenobarbital

Phenytoin

Primidone

Pyrimethamine

Sulfasalazine

Tetracycline

Vinblastine

MedWatch Postmarketing reports 2009-2020

Adalimumab

Aripiprazole

Carbamazepine

Esomeprazole

Metformin

Risperidone

Rivaroxaban

Telaprevir

TABLE A5-6 Drugs Associated with Thrombocytopenia

Observational study evidence

Carbamazepine
Oxaliplatin
Phenobarbital
Phenytoin
Valproic acid

Case report evidence (*probable* or *definite* causality rating)

Abciximab
Acetaminophen
Acyclovir
Albendazole
Aminoglutethimide
Aminosalicylic acid
Amiodarone
Amphotericin B
Ampicillin
Aspirin
Atorvastatin
Bevacizumab
Bisoprolol
Capecitabine
Captopril
Chlorothiazide
Chlorpromazine
Chlorpropamide
Cimetidine
Ciprofloxacin
Clarithromycin
Clopidogrel
Dabigatran
Danazol
Deferoxamine
Diazepam
Diazoxide
Diclofenac
Diethylstilbestrol
Digoxin

Ethambutol
Enzalutamide
Felbamate
Fenofibrate
Fluconazole
Fondaparinux
Gabapentin
Gold salts
Haloperidol
Heparin
Hydrochlorothiazide
Ibuprofen
Inamrinone
Indinavir
Indomethacin
Interferon alfa-2b
Isoniazid
Isotretinoin
Itraconazole
Levamisole
Levetiracetam
Levofloxacin
Linezolid
Lithium
Low-molecular-weight heparins
Lurasidone
Measles, mumps, and rubella vaccine
Meclofenamate
Mesalamine
Methyldopa
Minoxidil
Morphine
Moxifloxacin
Nalidixic acid
Naphazoline
Naproxen
Nitroglycerin
Octreotide

Olmesartan
Oseltamivir
Oxacillin
p-Aminosalicylic acid
Pantoprazole
Penicillamine
Pentamidine
Pentoxifylline
Piperacillin
Primidone
Procainamide
Pyrazinamide
Quinidine
Quinine
Ranitidine
Recombinant hepatitis B vaccine
Red Bush Tea (Rooibos)
Rifampin
Rivaroxaban
Sevoflurane
Simvastatin
Sirolimus
Sulfasalazine
Sulfonamides
Sulindac
Tacrolimus
Tamoxifen
Tolmetin
Trastuzumab
Trimethoprim
Vancomycin

Medwatch postmarketing reports 2009–2020

Acarbose
Adalimumab
Ado-trastuzumab
Alfuzosin
Aliskirin

(Continued)

TABLE A5-6	Drugs Associated with Thrombocytopenia (*Continued*)	
Amlodipine	Eptifibatide	Pamidronate
Benazepril	Ethionamid	Pemetrexed
Bocepravir	Filgrastim	Pioglitazone
Bortezomib	Fondaparinux	Pomalidomide
Chlorambucil	Glimepiride	Propylthiouracil
Cladribine	Heparin	Quinine
Cotrimoxazole	Hydrochlorothiazide	Raltegravir
Dalteparin	Indomethacin	Rosiglitazone
Dantrolene	Iloprost	Rosuvastatin
Deferasirox	Interferon beta 1a	Spironolactone
Didanosine	Leflunomide	Sunitinib
Drotecogin alfa	Losartan	Telmisartan
Efalizumab	Montelukast	Torsemide
Eltrombopag	Obinutuzumab	Trepostinil
Enoxaparin	Octreotide	Ursodiol
Epirubicin	Oxcarbazepine	
Epoprostenol	Palivizumab	

(See e/Chapter 125, Drug-Induced Hematologic Disorders, authored by Elisa M. Greene and Tracy M. Hagemann, for a more detailed discussion of this topic.)

TABLE A6-1	Roussel Uclaf Causality Assessment Method (RUCAM)				
Criteria	**Result**	**Score**	**Result**	**Score**
Timing (days) from…				
…start of therapy	5–90	+2	<5 or >90	+1
… or cessation of therapy (except slowly metabolized drugs)			≥30	+1
Result of unintentional rechallenge of drug/herb alone	Alk Phos > 2XN	+3	Alk Phos ≤ Normal	−2
Result of unintentional rechallenge drugs/herbs given	Alk Phos > 2XN	+1	Alk Phos ≤ Normal	0
Previous reports of this drug and this reaction in…	Product labeling	+2	Published literature	+1
Concurrent hepatotoxic drug/herb?	No	0		
If yes, Is hepatoxic drug/herb timing…	Consistent	−2	Inconsistent	0
Concurrent drug/herb more likely?	Positive Rechallenge	−3	Validated Test	−3
Risk Factor: Drinks/day Alcohol > 2 (female) > 3 (male)	Yes	+1	No	0
Risk Factor: Pregnant?	Yes	+1	No	0
Risk Factor: Age > 55 years old	Yes	+1	No	0
Alternatives to Rule Out				
Group I Alternative: Hepatitis A Virus via + Anti-HAV-IgM				
Group I Alternative: Hepatitis B Virus via + Anti-HBV-IgM or + HBV-DNA				
Group I Alternative: Hepatitis C Virus via + Anti-HCV-IgM or + HCV-RNA				
Group I Alternative: Hepatitis E Virus via + Anti-HEV-IgM, + Anti-HEV-IgG or + HEV-RNA				
Group I Alternative: Other positive test for other liver diseases or disorders, such as Hepatobiliary Sonography, Color Doppler Sonography, Endosonography, Liver CT Scan, Liver MRI				
Group I Alternative: Diagnosis of Alcoholism with elevated AST of ALT > 2				
Group I Alternative: Recent hypotensive history (particularly with underlying heart disease)				
Group II Alternatives: Autoimmune Hepatitis, Chronic Viral Hepatitis, Biliary or Sclerosing Cholangitis				
Group II Alternatives: Complications of Sepsis, Metastatic Malignancy, Genetic Liver Diseases				
Group II Alternatives: Positive Test for Infection Cytomegaly, Epstein-Bar, Herpes Simplex, Varicella-Zoster Viruses				
All Alternatives Ruled Out	Groups I and II	+2	Group I only	+1
Some Alternatives Ruled Out	5–6 of Group I	0	<5 of Group I	−2
An Alternative Cause is…	Highly Likely	−3	Somewhat Likely	0

Total Score ≤0 means the drug or herb is not a likely cause; ≤2 means it is unlikely to be the cause; ≤5 means the drug or herb possibly may have caused this reaction; ≤8 means the drug or herb is a probable cause of the reactions, and >8 means the drug or herb is highly probable to be the cause. (2 × N = Two Times the Normal Upper Limit)

TABLE A6-2 Relative Patterns of Hepatic Enzyme Elevation versus Type of Hepatic Lesion

Enzyme	Abbreviations	Necrotic	Cholestatic	Chronic
Alkaline phosphatase	Alk Phos, AP	↑	↑↑↑	↑
5'-Nucleotidase	5-NC, 5NC	↑	↑↑↑	↑
γ-Glutamyltransferase	GGT, GGTP	↑	↑↑↑	↑↑
Aspartate aminotransferase	AST, SGOT	↑↑↑	↑	↑↑
Alanine aminotransferase	ALT, SGPT	↑↑↑	↑	↑↑
Lactate dehydrogenase	LDH	↑↑↑	↑	↑

(See e/Chapter 56, Drug-Induced Liver Injury, authored by William Kirchain and Rondall E. Allen, for a more detailed discussion of this topic.)

TABLE A7-1 Summary of Drug-Induced Pulmonary Disease—Presentation, Diagnosis, Causative Agents, and Management

Disease	Presentation	Key Diagnostic Components	Causative Agents	Management
Reactions involving the interstitium				
Interstitial pneumonitis and fibrosis	Can be acute or chronic Dyspnea, cough, Clubbing, crackles	History of drug exposure Bilateral localized or diffuse opacities and reduced lung volumes on CXR "Honeycombing" on chest CT Elevated ESR with amiodarone Restrictive/normal PFTs	Amiodarone, bleomycin, gemcitabine, carmustine, cyclophosphamide, taxanes, EGFR inhibitors, dasatinib, mTORi, busulfan, sulfasalazine, methotrexate, leflunomide, phenytoin, nitrofurantoin, daptomycin	Drug discontinuation, dose reduction or interruption Corticosteroids Supplemental oxygen
Organizing pneumonia	Nonproductive cough, shortness of breath, bilateral crackles Less commonly, fever	History of drug exposure Bilateral patchy infiltrates on CXR Rarely, eosinophilia present	Amiodarone, bleomycin, minocycline, nitrofurantoin, gold, sulfasalazine, interferon alpha, carbamazepine, L-tryptophan, cocaine	Drug discontinuation Corticosteroids Supplemental oxygen
Eosinophilic pneumonia	Can be acute or chronic Dry cough, dyspnea, chest pain, fever	History of drug exposure Bilateral reticular ground-glass opacities on chest CT Acute: elevated peripheral neutrophils with high BAL eosinophils Chronic: elevated peripheral eosinophils, elevated IgE, CRP, ESR	Daptomycin, mesalamine, sulfasalazine, minocycline	Drug discontinuation Corticosteroids Omalizumab Supplemental oxygen Acute: mechanical ventilation common

Hypersensitivity pneumonitis	Usually, immediate Urticaria, angioedema, rhinitis, conjunctivitis, dyspnea, and bronchospasm	History of drug exposure Based on presentation	NSAIDS (dose-dependent), methotrexate, nitrofurantoin	Drug discontinuation Corticosteroids Antihistamines Supplemental oxygen
Noncardiac pulmonary edema	Dyspnea, chest discomfort, tachypnea, hypoxemia	History of drug exposure Interstitial and alveolar infiltrates Laboratory values and PFTs not helpful	Cytarabine, gemcitabine, immune globulins, interleukin, muronomab-CD3, pentostatin, tretinoin, tricyclic antidepressants, methotrexate, mitomycin aspirin (dose-dependent), methadone, morphine, oxytocin, protamine, heroin, cocaine, cytarabine, infliximab GM-CSF, vinca alkaloids, amiodarone, nitrofurantoin, talc	Drug discontinuation Diuretics Supplemental oxygen Mechanical ventilation Uncertain role corticosteroids
Diffuse alveolar damage	Typically acute, can be subacute Hemoptysis, cough, dyspnea, acute respiratory failure	History of drug exposure New or unexplained infiltrates on CXR Dropping hematocrit Hemorrhagic BAL	Chemotherapy, all-trans-retinoic acid, propylthiouracil, penicillin, sulfasalazine, hydralazine, leukotriene antagonists, mitomycin, amiodarone, nitrofurantoin, crack cocaine, thrombolytics, anticoagulants, antiplatelet agents, dextran 70	Drug discontinuation Reversal of coagulation Corticosteroids for chemotherapy-induced Supplemental oxygen

(Continued)

TABLE A7-1 Summary of Drug-Induced Pulmonary Disease—Presentation, Diagnosis, Causative Agents, and Management (*Continued*)

Disease	Presentation	Key Diagnostic Components	Causative Agents	Management
Reactions involving the pleura				
Nonlupus-related pleural effusion	Pleuritic chest pain, pleural effusions	History of drug exposure Pleural fluid eosinophilia (nonspecific) Elevated peripheral eosinophils	Sclerotherapy agents (most common), amiodarone, minoxidil, methysergide, bromocriptine, bleomycin, mitomycin, procarbazine, methotrexate, cyclophosphamide, dasatinib	Drug discontinuation Corticosteroids Supplemental oxygen
Lupus-related pleural effusion	Pleuritic chest pain, pleural effusions	History of drug exposure Similar to idiopathic lupus Pleural fluid: exudative, ANA higher than serum values, lupus erythematosus cells may be present	Procainamide (most common), hydralazine, chlorpromazine, isoniazid, D-penicillamine, methyldopa, quinidine	Drug discontinuation Supplemental oxygen
Reactions without direct toxic effect to the lung tissue				
Bronchospasm	Wheezing	History of drug exposure Based on presentation	Acetaminophen, aspirin, NSAIDs, beta-blockers, iodinated radiocontrast dye	Drug discontinuation Corticosteroids Supplemental oxygen
Cough	Can occur within hours to months Persistent dry cough, "tickle" in throat	History of drug exposure Based on presentation	ACE-inhibitors, calcium channel blockers, fentanyl, latanoprost ophthalmic	Drug discontinuation
Pulmonary arterial hypertension	Dyspnea	History of drug exposure mPAP ≥25 mm Hg at rest during RHC	Anorectic agents, amphetamines, dasatinib, selective serotonin inhibitors (risk to newborn if mother taking)	Drug discontinuation Pulmonary vasodilators

Thromboembolic disorders	Dyspnea	History of drug exposure; Pulmonary embolism on chest CT	Bleomycin, cyclophosphamide, alkylating/alkylating-like agents, mitomycin, high-dose combined oral contraception, immune checkpoint inhibitors	Drug discontinuation; Anticoagulation; Thrombolysis; Supplemental oxygen
Apnea	Hypoventilation	History of drug exposure; Based on presentation	Opioids, neuromuscular blockers	Dose reduction or discontinuation of drug; Naloxone (for opioids)
Chest wall rigidity	Decreased compliance of chest wall, respiratory muscles, or laryngeal structures	History of drug exposure; Based on presentation	Synthetic opioids (fentanyl, remifentanil, methadone), also morphine	Dose reduction or discontinuation of drug

ANA, antinuclear antibodies; BAL, bronchoalveolar lavage; CRP, c-reactive protein; CT, computerized tomography scan; CXR, chest X-ray; EGFR, epidermal growth factor receptor; ESR, erythrocyte sedimentation rate; GM-CSF, granulocyte-macrophage colony-stimulating factor; mPAP, mean pulmonary arterial pressure; mTORi, mechanistic target of rapamycin inhibitors; NSAIDS, nonsteroidal anti-inflammatory drugs; PFTs, pulmonary function tests; RHC, right heart catheterization.

TABLE A7-2	Diagnostic Criteria for the Presence of Drug-Induced Pulmonary Diseases (DIPD)

History

    Known or suspected exposure to a drug known to cause DILD

Current

    Clinical and histopathological findings correlate with previous reports of DILD

    Other causes of clinical and histopathological findings can be ruled out

Future

    Clinical manifestations improve after withdrawal of the drug

    Clinical manifestations recur after rechallenge

(See e/Chapter 48, Drug-Induced Pulmonary Diseases, authored by Margaret A. Miklich and Mojdeh Heavner, for a more detailed discussion of this topic.)

Drug-Induced Kidney Disease

TABLE A8-1	Drug-Induced Kidney Structural–Functional Alterations

Tubular epithelial cell damage

Acute tubular injury/necrosis	Osmotic nephropathy
Aminoglycoside antibiotics	Mannitol
Radiographic contrast media	Dextran
Chimeric antigen receptor T-cells	IV immunoglobulin (sucrose)
Cisplatin, carboplatin	Hydroxyethyl starch
Ifosfamide	SGLT-2 inhibitors
Amphotericin B	
Cyclosporine, tacrolimus	
Adefovir, cidofovir, tenofovir	
Pentamidine	
Foscarnet	
Zoledronate	

Hemodynamically mediated kidney injury

Angiotensin-converting enzyme inhibitors	NSAIDs
Angiotensin II receptor blockers	Cyclosporine, tacrolimus
SGLT-2 inhibitors	OKT3
Chimeric antigen receptor T-cells	High-dose interleukin-2

Obstructive nephropathy

Crystal nephropathy	Nephrolithiasis
Acyclovir	Sulfonamides
Sulfonamides	Triamterene
Indinavir, atazanavir	Indinavir, atazanavir
Foscarnet	Nephrocalcinosis
Methotrexate	Oral sodium phosphate solution
Ascorbic acid, ethylene glycol, orlistat	
Ciprofloxacin	

Glomerular disease

Minimal change disease	Focal segmental glomerulosclerosis
NSAIDs, COX-2 inhibitors	Pamidronate
Lithium	Interferon-α and β
Pamidronate	Lithium
Interferon-α and β	Sirolimus
Membranous disease	Anabolic steroids
NSAIDs	Tyrosine kinase inhibitors
Penicillamine	
Captopril	

(Continued)

TABLE A8-1	Drug-Induced Kidney Structural–Functional Alterations (*Continued*)

Tubulointerstitial disease

Acute allergic interstitial nephritis	Chronic interstitial nephritis
β-Lactams	Cyclosporine
Ciprofloxacin	Lithium
NSAIDs, cyclooxygenase-2 inhibitors	Aristolochic acid
Proton pump inhibitors	Combination analgesics
Loop diuretics	Papillary necrosis
Immune checkpoint inhibitors	NSAIDs, combined phenacetin, aspirin, and caffeine analgesics

Renal vasculitis, thrombotic microangiopathy, thrombosis, and cholesterol emboli

Vasculitis and thrombosis	Methamphetamines
Hydralazine	Cyclosporine, tacrolimus
Propylthiouracil	Adalimumab
Allopurinol	Bevacizumab
Penicillamine	Cholesterol emboli
Gemcitabine	Warfarin
Mitomycin C	Thrombolytic agents

TABLE A8-2	Potential Risk Factors for Aminoglycoside Nephrotoxicity

(A) Related to aminoglycoside dosing

Large total cumulative dose

Prolonged therapy

Trough concentration exceeding 2 mg/L[a]

Recent previous aminoglycoside therapy

(B) Related to synergistic nephrotoxicity. Aminoglycosides in combination with

Cyclosporine

Amphotericin B

Vancomycin

Diuretics

Iodinated radiographic contrast agents

Cisplatin

NSAIDs

(Continued)

| TABLE A8-2 | Potential Risk Factors for Aminoglycoside Nephrotoxicity (*Continued*) |

(C) Related to predisposing conditions in the patient

Preexisting kidney disease

Diabetes

Increased age

Poor nutrition

Shock

Gram-negative bacteremia

Liver disease

Hypoalbuminemia

Obstructive jaundice

Dehydration

Hypotension

Potassium or magnesium deficiencies

[a]The equivalent concentration in SI molar units is 4.3 μmol/L for tobramycin and 4.2 μmol/L for gentamicin.

| TABLE A8-3 | Recommended Interventions for Prevention of Contrast Nephrotoxicity |

Intervention	Recommendation	Recommendation Grade[a]
Contrast	Minimize contrast volume/dose	A-1
	Use noniodinated contrast studies	A-2
	Use low- or iso-osmolar contrast agents	A-2
Medications	Avoid concurrent use of potentially nephrotoxic drugs (eg, NSAIDs, aminoglycosides)	A-2
Isotonic sodium chloride (0.9%)	Initiate infusion 3–12 hours prior to contrast exposure and continue 6–24 hours postexposure	A-1
	Infuse at 1–1.5 mL/kg/h adjusting postexposure as needed to maintain a urine flow rate of 150 mL/h	
	Alternatively, in urgent cases, initiate infusion at 3 mL/kg/h, beginning 1 hour prior to contrast exposure, then continue at 1 mL/kg/h for 6 hours postexposure	

[a]*Strength of recommendations*: A, B, and C are good, moderate, and poor evidence to support recommendation, respectively. *Quality of evidence*: (1) evidence from more than one properly randomized, controlled trial; (2) evidence from more than one well-designed clinical trial with randomization, from cohort or case-controlled analytic studies or multiple time series, or dramatic results from uncontrolled experiments; and (3) evidence from opinions of respected authorities, based on clinical experience, descriptive studies, or reports of expert communities.

TABLE A8-4	Drugs Associated with Allergic Interstitial Nephritis

Antimicrobials

Acyclovir	Indinavir
Aminoglycosides	Rifampin
Amphotericin B	Sulfonamides
β-Lactams	Tetracyclines
Erythromycin	Trimethoprim–sulfamethoxazole
Ethambutol	Vancomycin

Diuretics

Acetazolamide	Loop diuretics
Amiloride	Triamterene
Chlorthalidone	Thiazide diuretics

Neuropsychiatric drugs

Carbamazepine	Phenytoin
Lithium	Valproic acid
Phenobarbital	

Nonsteroidal anti-inflammatory drugs

Aspirin	Ketoprofen
Indomethacin	Phenylbutazone
Naproxen	Diclofenac
Ibuprofen	Cyclooxygenase-2 inhibitors
Diflunisal	
Piroxicam	

Miscellaneous

Acetaminophen	Immune checkpoint inhibitors
Allopurinol	Lansoprazole
Interferon-α	Methyldopa
Aspirin	Omeprazole
Azathioprine	p-Aminosalicylic acid
Captopril	Phenylpropanolamine
Cimetidine	Propylthiouracil
Clofibrate	Radiographic contrast media
Cyclosporine	Ranitidine
Glyburide	Sulfinpyrazone
Gold	Warfarin sodium

(See Chapter 65, Drug-Induced Kidney Disease, authored by Thomas D. Nolin and Mark A. Perazella, for a more detailed discussion of this topic.)

TABLE A9-1	Common Drug-Induced Ophthalmic Disorders, Causative Agents, and Treatment Recommendations	
Reactions	**Causative Agents**	**Treatment Recommendations**
Cataracts	Alkylating agents (busulfan)	Surgical removal of cataract
	Antiestrogens (tamoxifen)	
	Corticosteroids	
	Statins	
Dry eye	Alpha-1 antagonists (alfuzosin, tamsulosin, terazosin)	Nonpharmacologic therapy: (1) warm compresses, (2) increase fluid intake, (3) use humidifier
	Alpha-2 agonists (apraclonidine, brimonidine)	
	Anticholinergics (atropine, homatropine, hyoscine, ipratropium, tolterodine)	
	Anticonvulsants (valproic acid)	
	Antihistamines (cetirizine, chlorpheniramine, diphenhydramine, doxylamine)	Increase tear volume: (1) consider artificial tears or other topical lubricants, (2) punctal occlusion
	Antimalarials (chloroquine, hydroxychloroquine)	
	Antineoplastics (busulfan, cyclophosphamide)	
	Antipsychotics (thioridazine)	Decrease inflammation: (1) 0.05% cyclosporine ophthalmic drugs, (2) LFA-1 antagonist ophthalmic drops, (3) short-term ophthalmic glucocorticoids
	Anxiolytics (lorazepam)	
	Beta-agonists (acebutolol)	
	Beta-blockers (atenolol, propranolol)	
	Benzalkonium chloride	
	Bisphosphonates	
	Cannabinoids (dronabinol)	
	Systemic decongestants (pseudoephedrine)	Medication changes: (1) discontinue medication, (2) use preservative-free ophthalmic drops
	Diuretics (furosemide, indapamide, metolazone)	
	Oral contraceptives	
	Retinoids (isotretinoin)	
	Topical decongestants (naphazoline)	
	Tricyclic antidepressants (amitriptyline)	

(Continued)

TABLE A9-1	Common Drug-Induced Ophthalmic Disorders, Causative Agents, and Treatment Recommendations (*Continued*)	
Reactions	**Causative Agents**	**Treatment Recommendations**
Floppy iris syndrome	Alpha-1 antagonists Benzodiazepines Chlorpromazine Donepezil Duloxetine Finasteride Quetiapine	Preoperative screening for previous and/or current use of causative agents Consider cataract surgery before initiation of alpha-1 antagonist therapy Intracameral alpha-adrenergic agonists (epinephrine, phenylephrine) Intraoperative devices: (1) iris retractors, (2) OVDs, (3) pupil expanders
Optic neuropathy	Amiodarone Ethambutol Linezolid PDE-5 inhibitors (avanafil, sildenafil, tadalafil, vardenafil)	Discontinuation of causative drug as medically appropriate Regular ophthalmic examinations
Retinopathy	Aminoquinolines (hydroxychloroquine, chloroquine) Antiestrogens (tamoxifen) Phenothiazines (chlorpromazine, thioridazine) Retinoids (isotretinoin)	Monitor via regular ophthalmic examinations, patient-reported signs and symptoms Vision loss is irreversible

LFA-1, lymphocyte function-associated antigen 1; OVDs, ophthalmic viscosurgical devices; PDE-5, phosphodiesterase 5.

(See Chapter e116, Drug-Induced Ophthalmic Disorders, authored by Rena Gosser, for a more detailed discussion of this topic.)

Index

Note: Page numbers followed by *"f"* and *"t"* denote figures and tables, respectively.

.